Specialized Aspects of ECG

Peter W. Macfarlane · Adriaan van Oosterom · Michiel Janse · Paul Kligfield ·
John Camm · Olle Pahlm (Eds.)

Specialized Aspects of ECG

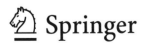 Springer

Editors
Peter W. Macfarlane
University of Glasgow
Glasgow
UK

Adriaan van Oosterom
Radboud University Nijmegen
Nijmegen
The Netherlands

Olle Pahlm
Lund University
Lund
Sweden

Paul Kligfield
Weill Cornell Medical College
New York, NY
USA

Michiel Janse
University of Amsterdam
Amsterdam
The Netherlands

John Camm
St. George's, University of London
London
UK

ISBN 978-0-85729-879-9
DOI 10.1007/978-0-85729-880-5

Library of Congress Control Number: 2011943336

First published in 2010 as part of Comprehensive Electrocardiology, 2nd Edition (ISBN 978-1-84882-045-6)

Printed on acid-free paper

Springer is part of Springer Science+Business Media (www.springer.com)

Editors-in-Chief

Peter W. Macfarlane
University of Glasgow
Glasgow
UK

Adriaan van Oosterom
Radboud University Nijmegen
Nijmegen
The Netherlands

Olle Pahlm
Lund University
Lund
Sweden

Paul Kligfield
Weill Cornell Medical College
New York, NY
USA

Michiel Janse
University of Amsterdam
Amsterdam
The Netherlands

John Camm
St. George's, University of London
London
UK

Preface

The first edition of *Comprehensive Electrocardiology* was published in 1989, when e-mail was still in its infancy (!!), and it was never envisaged at that time that a new edition would be prepared. It is probably fair to say that the majority of physicians would have regarded electrocardiography in particular as having reached its maximum usefulness with little additional information to be obtained therefrom. The intervening 20 years have shown how untrue this was.

An update to the book is long overdue. Sadly, some of our former contributors have died since the first edition was published and it is with regret that I note the passing of Philippe Coumel, Rudolph van Dam, Karel den Dulk, Ramesh Gulrajani, Kenici Harumi, John Milliken, Jos Willems and Christoph Zywietz. Where relevant, their contributions continue to be acknowledged but in some cases, chapters have been completely rewritten by new contributors. On the other hand, eight completely new chapters have been added and the appendices restructured.

The publisher felt it would be opportune to produce separate paperback versions of each of the four volumes of the second edition of *Comprehensive Electrocardiology* – hence this book entitled. *Specialized Aspects of Electrocardiography*.

In some ways, it is inconceivable what has taken place in the field of electrocardiology since the first edition. New ECG patterns have been recognised and linked with sudden death, new prognostic indices have been developed and evaluated, the ECG has assumed a pivotal role in the treatment of an acute coronary syndrome and among many other things, automated ECG interpretation is now commonplace. Significant advances have been made in the field of mathematical modeling and a solution to the inverse problem is now applied in routine clinical use. Electrophysiological studies have taken giant steps over the past 20 years and biventricular pacing is a relatively recent innovation. Electrocardiology has certainly not stood still in the last 20 years. Of course there have been parallel advances in imaging techniques but the ECG still retains a unique position in the armamentarium of the physician, let alone the cardiologist.

For this edition, my previous co editor, Professor T.D. Veitch Lawrie, decided to step aside and I wish to congratulate him on reaching his 91st birthday in September 2011. However, I am pleased that other very eminent individuals agreed to assist with the editing of the book, namely Adriaan van Oosterom, Olle Pahlm, Paul Kligfield, Michiel Janse and John Camm. In the nature of things, some of these co editors undertook much more work than others. For this book, I particularly have to acknowledge the support of Olle Pahlm. Without his support, this revised version of the material in the first edition would not have been possible.

Locally, I am very much indebted to my secretary Pamela Armstrong for a huge contribution in checking and subediting every chapter which went out from my office to the publisher. This was a Herculean task carried out with great aplomb. I would also like to thank Ms. Julie Kennedy for her contribution to a variety of tasks associated with preparing selected chapters, including enhancements to the English presentation on occasions.

I also wish to thank the publishers Springer for their considerable support throughout. Grant Weston initially commissioned the book and I am grateful to him for his confidence in supporting the preparation of a new edition. Jennifer Carlson and her team in New York also assisted significantly. I am also indebted to Mr. R. Samuel Devanand and his team at SPi Global, in India, for production of the paperback edition.

I again must thank my long suffering wife Irene who has had to fight to gain access to our home PC every night over these past few years!

Comprehensive Electrocardiology aims to bring together truly comprehensive information about the field and *Basic Electrocardiology* provides a strong theoretical foundation to the principles of electrocardiography. A book can never be completely up to date given the speed of publication of research findings over the internet these days but hopefully this publication will continue to be of significant use to readers for many years to come. *Basic Electrocardiology*, together with the other three paperback versions of the other volumes of *Comprehensive Electrocardiology*, contains much information that should be of use both to the practising clinician and the experienced researcher.

Now that this huge effort has been completed and the book is available electronically, it should be much easier to produce the next edition…!!

Peter Macfarlane
Glasgow
Autumn

Table of Contents

List of Contributors

K. Martijn Akkerhuis
Erasmus University Medical Centre
Rotterdam
The Netherlands

David K. Detweiler
University of Pennsylvania
Philadelphia, PA
USA

Gordon E. Dower
Loma Linda University Medical Centre
Loma Linda, CA
USA

Thomas Fåhraeus
University Hospital
Lund
Sweden

Johan Herlitz
Sahlgrenska University Hospital
Gothenburg
Sweden

Gerard Van Herpen
Erasmus University Medical Centre
Rotterdam
The Netherlands

V. Hombach
University Hospital of Ulm
Ulm
Germany

Per Johansson
Sahlgrenska University Hospital
Gothenburg
Sweden

Raija Jurkko
Helsinki University Central Hospital
Helsinki
Finland

Petri Korhonen
Helsinki University Central Hospital
Helsinki
Finland

Jan A. Kors
Erasmus University Medical Centre
Rotterdam
The Netherlands

Peter W. Macfarlane
University of Glasgow
Glasgow
UK

Markku Mäkijärvi
Helsinki University Central Hospital
Helsinki
Finland

Olle Pahlm
Lund University
Lund
Sweden

Pentti M. Rautaharju
Wake Forest University School of Medicine
Winston-Salem, NC
USA

Pentti Siltanen
Helsinki University Central Hospital
Helsinki
Finland

Maarten L. Simoons
Erasmus University Medical Centre
Rotterdam
The Netherlands

Michael B. Simson
Hospital of the University of Pennsylvania
Philadelphia, PA
USA

Leif Sörnmo
Lund University
Lund
Sweden

Maciej Sosnowski
Medical University of Silesia
Katowski
Poland

Leif Svensson
Stockholm Prehospital Center
Stockholm
Sweden

Elin Trägårdh-Johansson
Lund University
Lund
Sweden

Heikki Väänänen
Aalto University School of Science and Technology
Espoo
Finland

1 Ambulatory Electrocardiogram Monitoring

V. Hombach

P. W. Macfarlane et al. (eds.), *Specialized Aspects of ECG*, DOI 10.1007/978-0-85729-880-5_1,
© Springer-Verlag London Limited 2012

Abbreviations

AAD = Antiarrhythmic Drug
AECG = Ambulatory ECG
AF = Atrial Fibrillation
AFl = Atrial Flutter
AMI = Acute Myocardial Infarction
APB = Atrial Premature Beat
ARVCM = Arrhythmogenic Right Ventricular Cardiomyopathy
BRS = Baroreflex Sensitivity
CAD = Coronary Artery Disease
CHD = Coronary Heart Disease
CHF = Congestive Heart Failure
DCM = Dilatative Cardiomyopathy
EPS = Electrophysiological Study
HCM = Hypertrophic Cardiomyopathy
HOCM = Hypertrophic Obstructive Cardiomyopathy
HRV = Heart-Rate Variability
HRT = Heart-Rate Turbulence
ICD = Implantable Cardiac Defibrillator
LVEF = Left Ventricular Ejection Fraction
LVF = Left Ventricular Function
LVH = Left Ventricular Hypertrophy
MB = Megabyte
MI = Myocardial Infarction
NPV = Negative Predictive Value
PPV = Positive Predictive Value
PVC = Premature Ventricular Contraction (VPB)
PWD = P-Wave Duration
QTD = QT Dispersion
QTI = QT Interval
QTV = QT (Interval) Variability
SA-ECG = Signal-Averaged ECG
SCD = Sudden Cardiac Death
SI = Silent (Myocardial) Ischemia
SH = Systemic Hypertension
TO = Turbulence Onset
TS = Turbulence Slope
VEA = Ventricular Ectopic Activity
VF = Ventricular Fibrillation
VLP = Ventricular Late Potential
VPB = Ventricular Premature Beat
VT = Ventricular Tachycardia
nsVT = nonsustained Ventricular Tachycardia
sVT = sustained Ventricular Tachycardia

1.1   Introduction

Ambulatory electrocardiography (AECG) is a diagnostic procedure, which involves recording the electrical activity of the heart using a technique first described by Holter [1–5]. The method is therefore also known as Holter electrocardiography or Holter (ECG) monitoring. The technique has been most commonly employed for the detection of arrhythmias and transient ST-T changes. However, due to increased use of multichannel, digitized, and telemetered signals, this traditional use has been expanded to the analysis of heart-rate variability (HRV), heart-rate turbulence (HRT), QT-dispersion (QTD) and variability (QTV), and signal averaging of long-term ECGs for retrieval of P-wave duration (PWD) and ventricular late potentials (VLP). Current AECG equipment consists of a recorder and an analysis system and provides the basis for the detection and analysis of the above-mentioned parameters. A complete set of recommendations for equipment standards was proposed in 1985 [6], and more recently the official ACC/AHA guidelines on technical aspects and clinical applications of AECG have been published [7].

1.2 Holter Monitoring Hardware and Software

1.2.1 Electrodes and Electrode Preparations

By convention, bipolar leads (see ❯ Chap. 11 of *Basic Electrocardiology: Cardiac Electrophysiology, ECG Systems and Mathematical Modeling*) are normally used to record a potential difference between two sites on the thorax. The electrodes most commonly employed are disposable electrodes that are pregelled and self-adhesive. They usually have a true silver/silver chloride sensing element mounted on a self-adhesive tape or foam material, which is nonirritating and hypoallergenic to skin (❯ Fig. 1.1). It is the electrode adhesiveness and extent of skin irritation that generally affect the quality of the ambulatory electrocardiographic signal by producing baseline wander, a low signal-to-noise ratio, and a short duration of adequate performance. The coupling of the skin and electrode (the skin–electrode interface) acts as an additional circuit with a resistance and capacitance between the heart and the recorder (❯ Fig. 1.2).

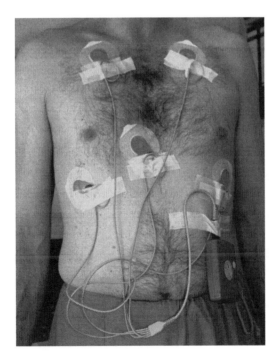

◘ Fig. 1.1

Electrode arrangement for three-channel AECG recording. Five pregelled disposable electrodes are used to record a CM₅ lead and a bipolar transthoracic lead. The fifth electrode is an indifferent electrode. The choice of these two bipolar leads provides high-amplitude ECG signals and the possibility of detecting the majority of changes in repolarization

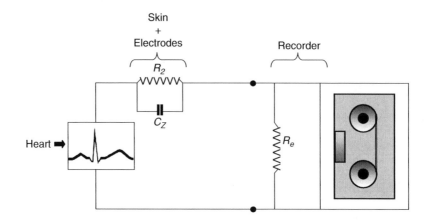

◻ Fig. 1.2
A model of the electrical circuit utilized in AECG recording. The coupling between skin and electrodes consists of a resistance and capacitance in parallel, which is responsible for diminishing the amplitude of the ECG signal if its impedance is high

The total impedance of this circuit depends mainly on the preparation of the skin. The surface-skin oil and dirt should be removed prior to recording by cleaning the skin with gauze moistened with ether, making the skin slightly erythematous. If necessary, the skin over the electrode area should be shaved, gently abraded with emery tape, and thoroughly cleansed with an alcohol swab. One electrode can then be placed on each of the prepared skin-surface sites (❷ Fig. 1.1), taking care to place the gelled pad firmly in contact with the abraded skin surface. The adequacy of the skin preparation for obtaining an optimum electrocardiographic signal can be checked by measuring the electrical impedance between the positive and negative poles of each bipolar lead. The measured resistance between electrodes should be ⩽5 kΩ, preferably ⩽2 kΩ. The impedance increases when the frequency of the signal decreases.

1.2.2   Selection of Lead Positions

Most AECG recorders utilize five or seven electrodes attached to the chest, which record two or three bipolar leads onto two or three channels [7–9], although systems employing multiple unipolar leads are now commercially available allowing a 12-lead ECG to be recorded. The first two channels may be used for arrhythmia and ischemia in the inferior myocardial wall. The lead positions recommended by the American Heart Association [6] are illustrated in ❷ Fig. 1.1, which provides an example of a three-bipolar lead/three-channel lead positioning. The practical advantages of multichannel Holter recording are increased reliability of the recorded ECG, improved recognition of ectopic cardiac beats, and enhanced detection of myocardial ischemia.

1.2.2.1   Leads for Recording Arrhythmias

A variety of bipolar lead configurations are used, the most common being a modified V_5 (CM$_5$), a modified V_3 (CM$_3$) or V_2 (CM$_2$), and a modified inferior lead (aVR, reverse Nehb I, Nehb D). No study has yet established the superiority of one lead over another; indeed, the choice of leads will differ according to the aim of the individual examination. A bipolar lead with positive electrode in the V_1 or V_2 position usually identifies atrial activity most clearly, showing the characteristic QRS patterns of right and left bundle branch block which help to distinguish supraventricular ectopic beats with aberrant conduction from ventricular ectopic beats. A bipolar lead with positive electrode in the V_5 position and the negative electrode in one of several other positions, such as the manubrium (lead CM$_5$), is the most sensitive single lead for the detection of ischemic ST-segment depression and provides a high-voltage ECG signal. However, with each of these two leads, some problems can occur in the presence of myocardial ischemia. One problem is that ST-segment depression might exist in only one lead (usually V_5), while the second (V_1 or V_2) remains quite normal, as shown in ❷ Fig. 1.3. If, during the period of ischemia, the first lead becomes unsuitable due to artifacts, some false-positive diagnoses may be made. For example, in ❷ Fig. 1.3, the run of ventricular tachycardia (VT) might have been interpreted as not being a result of myocardial ischemia, so, for example, an antiarrhythmic drug (AAD) would have been prescribed instead of an antianginal drug. A second problem is that leads V_1 and V_5 may fail to record ST-segment elevation owing to spasm of the right coronary artery or circumflex coronary artery. In such a situation, an inferior lead is useful, and the most convenient one is probably a bipolar anteroposterior lead. In ❷ Fig. 1.4, lead V_5 shows ST-segment depression (mirror image), while the anteroposterior lead shows ST-segment elevation owing to spasm of the right coronary artery as was demonstrated by coronary angiography. Thus, where coronary artery disease (CAD) is concerned, a combination of a bipolar V_5-type lead and an anteroposterior or inferior lead is probably the best. With standard 12-lead ECG, a simultaneous recording of leads III or aVF or Nehb J together with V_3 can detect almost all cases of ST-segment elevation. With 3-lead Holter monitoring, a combination of two bipolar precordial leads together with an inferior lead is recommended for ST-segment elevation monitoring. In the absence of suspected CAD, the recording of V_1- or V_2-type (CM$_2$) and V_5-type (CM$_5$) leads (see ❷ Chap. 11) provides the best chance of obtaining an ECG tracing with sufficient details to make an accurate diagnosis of any cardiac arrhythmia.

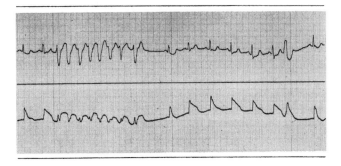

◨ **Fig. 1.3**

Sinus rhythm with a run of VT in a patient with variant angina. The two-channel recording confirms the diagnosis showing the characteristic marked ST elevation in the lower CM$_5$ lead. In the top channel (like V$_1$), only minor changes in repolarization occur. If the second lead had not been recorded, the variant angina would not have been detected and the VT would be considered as nonischemic in origin

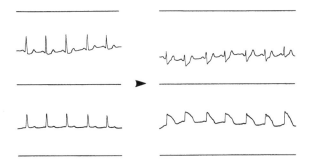

◨ **Fig. 1.4**

A two-channel recording in variant angina. The *left*-hand panel shows the baseline recordings while the *right*-hand panel shows the acute changes in the same patient. Note the characteristic marked ST elevation in the lower right CM$_5$ lead, whereas the mirror image in the other lead (like aVF) on its own might have led to a diagnosis of myocardial ischemia, but not of the variant form in the presence of chest pain

1.2.2.2 Leads for Recording ST-Segment Depression (Myocardial Ischemia)

For the detection of ischemic ST-segment depression, specially adapted 3-lead Holter recordings are recommended. In a study of Lanza et al. [8] of simultaneous recordings of a 3-lead AECG and a conventional 12-lead ECG recording during an exercise test, CM_5 was the single lead with the highest sensitivity (89%) in detecting myocardial ischemia. The addition of CM_3 to CM_5 increased the sensitivity to 94%, particularly for improved detection of isolated inferior myocardial ischemia, and the combination of all 3 AECG leads had a sensitivity of 96% with only 2% more than the best combination of 2 AECG leads (CM_5 plus an inferior lead). Osterhues et al. [9] could detect myocardial ischemia in 23 out of 54 patients (43%) with single vessel disease using standard CM_2 and CM_5 Holter leads (total number of ischemic episodes = 372). When adding a bipolar Nehb D-like lead, the detection rate could be increased to 30 out of 54 patients (55%, total number of ischemic episodes = 1,048), and the Nehb D-like lead was most sensitive for the detection of inferior ischemia in patients with right CAD. Alternatively, the use of an inverse Nehb J lead, in which the positive electrode is placed on the left posterior axillary line, may enhance the sensitivity to detect ischemia, as well [10]. Thus, routine identification of ischemic ST-segment deviation may only require two leads, most favorably the combination of CM_5 with an inferior lead (aVF, inverse Nehb J, Nehb D) [11].

1.2.3 Electrode Leads and Cable

Electrode lead wires are individually insulated and have a silver contact (❷ Fig. 1.1). The recorder cable is a shielded cable connected to the Holter recorder and is generally specific for each manufacturer's equipment. The electrode wires and the cable can both malfunction and be sources of artifacts.

1.2.4 Esophageal and Intracardiac Leads

One of the major problems in AECG with conventional electrode placements is the accurate detection of atrial depolarization. On account of various artifacts, P waves cannot always be recognized on a two- or three-channel recording, even during sinus rhythm. Moreover, during ectopic beats or tachycardia, the recognition of the P wave is often problematic. Therefore, the performance of ambulatory monitoring for the accurate diagnosis of arrhythmias remains doubtful compared to the more definitive results of an electrophysiological study (EPS). Several groups have attempted to record atrial activity during AECG using an esophageal bipolar lead [12, 13]. When the patient swallows the capsule, which contains a bipolar electrode, it is positioned so as to obtain an ECG signal with sufficient amplitude after the capsule has dissolved. The electrode wire should be fixed to the patient's cheek. However, difficulties experienced to date indicate that this technique cannot be easily used for the following reasons:

1. Difficulty is encountered in swallowing the capsule on account of its size (30 mm length).
2. The positioning of the electrode for recording an appropriate atrial ECG signal without significant ventricular depolarization is time consuming.

Nevertheless, the approach has been proved to be of considerable diagnostic value [13].

Some centers have preferred to use endoatrial leads to record atrial activity using a floating-catheter electrode. This technique permits a better atrial ECG signal to be obtained than does an esophageal lead. However, this procedure converts the AECG monitoring to an invasive examination [14]. The risk of local and general complications exists even if it appears relatively low. Thus, the use of intracardiac atrial leads remains confined to a few cases where an earlier attempt at recording the arrhythmia was unsuccessful and did not provide an exact diagnosis in patients in whom it is essential to determine the mechanism of the arrhythmia. In this case, AECG monitoring competes with an EPS because the benefits of the noninvasive technique disappear.

In practice, the interest of this technique remains confined to some cases where the knowledge of the exact mode of initiation of a tachycardia is useful for the management of the patient or in other patients in whom electrophysiological studies have been unable to provoke the arrhythmia.

1.2.5   Holter Recorders

Modern conventional AECG recorders are small, light-weight devices (110–320 g) that record two or three bipolar leads. They use a quartz digital clock and a separate recording track to keep time. The recorders are generally powered by a 9-V disposable alkaline battery (only rarely a rechargeable nickel–cadmium battery) and a calibration signal automatically inserted when the device is energized. In addition, a patient-activated event marker is conveniently placed on the device surface for the patient to note an event or indicate the presence of symptoms. The conventional format of the "first-generation" Holter recorders has been magnetic cassette-tape for directly recording the varying DC signals via the recording head onto the magnetic tape. Frequency-modulated (FM) systems are also available, although they are somewhat more prone to the generation of artifact. The tape-transport mechanism is driven by a hysteresis-synchronous motor assembly at speeds that are usually in the range of 1–2 mm/s; the speed is kept constant by an optical speed sensor on the flywheel and a crystal-controlled phase-locked loop.

1.2.5.1   Tape Recorders

Typically, such a unit records the ECG signal for between 24 and 48 h on a cassette or small magnetic tape, providing a permanent record of all electrical activity throughout the recording period and a playback as well as interrogation of the entire recording period (so-called "full disclosure"). ❷ Figure 1.5a shows the first Holter recorder developed by Avionics based on reel-to-reel magnetic-tape recording. This technology is adequate to detect abnormalities of conduction or rhythm, but it may be limited for recording low-frequency signals such as the ST segment. In some amplitude-modulated (AM) systems, an inadequate low-frequency response or a marked phase shift from the higher-frequency QRS signal may cause an artifactual distortion of the ST segment, which may be incorrectly interpreted as ischemic. It is usually claimed that only the FM type of recording system provides the necessary low-frequency response (down to 0.05 Hz) and less phase shift for accurate ST recording and reproduction, but this has to be counterbalanced against the higher costs, more baseline noise, and less clear display of such systems. This fact has been commented upon by Bragg-Remschell et al. [15]. More recent AM systems have been designed with improved low-frequency recording and playback characteristics and shown to record accurately ST-segment deviations [16, 17] and even T-wave alternans [18].

Caution should, therefore, be exercised with the older types of recorders in case ST-segment "depression" is a technical rather than a physiological phenomenon. One former development (Oxford Medical) has been the incorporation of a microprocessor inside the Holter recording unit itself so that signal analysis and classification can be carried out in real time. The ECG is also recorded on tape continuously because most cardiologists wish to have the acquired signal available for visual confirmation and assessment of any arrhythmia or ST-segment shift. Lastly, but not least, it should be noted

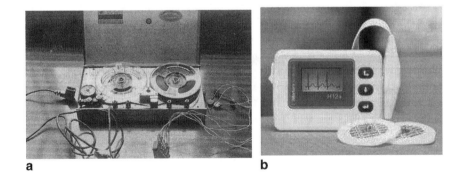
a   b

❏ Fig. 1.5
(a) Avionics 660 magnetic-tape recording system (one of the earliest systems used). **(b)** Mortara 12-lead Holter recorder (modern, solid-state recorder)

that regardless of whether AM or FM recording techniques are used, the tape itself may stretch and consequently distort the electrical signal.

1.2.5.2　Solid-State Recorders

Owing to the rapidly evolving technologies, nowadays direct recordings of the ECG signal in a digital format using solid-state recording devices are available ("second-generation" Holter recorders, ❷ Fig. 1.5b). Such direct digital recording avoids all of the biases introduced by the mechanical features of tape-recording devices and problems of analog recording formats that require analog-to-digital conversion before quantitative analysis. Digital ECG signals can be recorded up to 1,000 samples/s, which allow for the extremely accurate reproduction of the ECG signal necessary for highly sophisticated analysis methods like signal averaging or T-wave alternans measurements. Solid-state ECG recordings can be analyzed immediately and rapidly, and some recorders are equipped with microprocessors that can provide "on-line analysis" of the QRS complex and the ST segment and T waves as they are acquired. Also, the patient can be given feedback immediately in case of the detection of specific abnormalities, for example, ST-segment deviations. In addition, the solid-state format provides for ready electronic data transfer to a central analyzing unit. Limitations of this technology are the limited storage capacity of digital data, reliance on a computer algorithm in case of online analysis for identification of specific abnormalities, and the expense of the devices.

A full 24-h recording includes approximately 100,000 QRS-T complexes and requires about 20 megabytes (MB) of storage per channel. Therefore, compression of data is necessary, and at least two methods have been proposed, the "lossy" compression with very high compression ratios and the "loss-less" compression technique combined with an enhanced storage capacity. The problem with "lossy" compression is that the user is entirely dependent on the reliability of the microprocessor to distinguish important physiological abnormalities from artifact or wandering baseline, since, because of the lack of "full disclosure," confirmations of the decisions of the microcomputer cannot be made from the primary data, which are not recorded in their entirety and cannot be retrieved without error. Moreover, the accuracy of online interpretations may also be different for arrhythmia versus ischemia analyses [19]. However, it is essential for a physician using Holter monitoring that representative ECG tracings from all ischemic or arrhythmic episodes be confirmed by an experienced physician or technician, and thus, the lack of full disclosure may limit the reliability of the "lossy" compression method. The "loss-less" compression method in combination with enhanced storage capacity compresses ECG data by a factor of 3–5 by reducing the sampling rate from 256 to 64 or 16 Hz, respectively. Later, when the data are recalled, playback computer techniques recreate these abbreviated waveforms, whose sampling is often "weighted" about the R wave, to reproduce stored "full-disclosure" continuous electrocardiographic data. Some manufacturers have adopted the solid-state storage to their regular electrocardiographic instruments, whereby the recorder stores two channels of ECGs over 24 or 48 h on the recorder device, which subsequently is interfaced to the manufacturer's standard ECG cart or a data printer to provide 24 hourly continuous "full disclosure" printouts of all data recorded for visual interpretation.

Modern solid-state recorder devices provide special features such as an LCD display to control the quality of the ECG immediately after placement of the electrodes either by direct display (e.g., MT-101 from Schiller™, Lifecard from Delmar/Reynolds™, CardioMem from Getemed™), or by transfer via infrared to a Palm™ microcomputer (Medilog AR4 or AR12 from Oxford Instruments™). Some devices have a special loudspeaker incorporated for patient interaction, and most recorders provide pacemaker detection. Some provide recording of thoracic or respiratory activity as well (e.g., CardioMem from Getemed™, Medilog AR4 or AR12 from Oxford Instruments™). After the transfer of the full 24- or 48-h digital data, most analysis systems allow not only the analysis and presentation of normal and abnormal QRS complexes including bradycardias or tachycardias, but also the analysis of ST-segment deviations, HRV, QT duration and variability, and pacemaker function. Data transfer is usually completed within 2 min.

1.2.5.3　Storage Media

The storage media available are flash memory card or portable hard drive. Flash cards are about the size of a credit card, and have the capacity to store 20–40 MB of data (❷ Fig. 1.14). After completion of the recording, the flash cards are removed from the recording device and are inserted directly into the analysis unit or into a separate device by which the data can be transmitted electronically to another analyzing unit where the data can be played back and analyzed. Miniature hard drives can store more than 100 MB of data, and unlike flash cards, are not removed from the recorder, but the data are downloaded to another storage device or may be electronically transferred to a remote analysis unit.

1.2.5.4 Event Recorders

In contrast to the conventional 24-h Holter monitoring, both sampling and trans-telephonic devices record noncontinuous AECG data of an intermittent nature. There are two types of intermittent patient-worn recording devices (so-called event recorders), one that records and stores only a brief period of ECG activity, either by predefined criteria analyzed by the microcomputer (e.g., tachycardia, arrhythmia, bradycardia) or when activated by the patient in response to symptoms, and the other that records the ECG in a continuous manner but stores only brief periods of ECG recording (e.g., 5–300 s) in a memory when activated by the patient using the event marker at the time of a symptom (the so-called loop recorder). These event recorders can be used for prolonged periods of time, for example, many weeks, to identify infrequently occurring symptoms or arrhythmias that would not have been retrieved from a conventional 24-h AECG monitoring. A patient-activated event recorder needs rapid placement of electrodes, such as paddles connected to the recorder or a wrist bracelet, to record the ECG at the time of symptoms, whereas loop recorders use continuously worn electrodes. The recorded signal can be saved in memory and transferred at a later time to a central analysis unit or be transmitted to a receiving station by online transfer. Event recorders have the advantage of small size and light weight, their use is easy and they can be programmed to record many short episodes during an extended period of time (30 days to several weeks), and moreover, 1-, 2-, 3-, and mathematically reconstructed 12-lead formats are available.

A special type of event recorder is the implantable loop recorder (ILR), which may be used for identifying infrequent and transient symptoms of patients by long-term intermittent recordings. This device, of about the size of a pack of chewing gum is inserted under the skin at about the second rib on the left front of the chest and is activated by passing a special magnet over the device. It is capable of recording and storing up to 42 min of a single ECG channel, which can be partitioned for 1–7 episodes, with up to 20 min of preactivation ECG saved for subsequent downloading to a programming unit for analysis. The device can be configured to store patient-activated episodes, automatically activated recordings via, for example, low and high heart-rate limits, or a combination of both [20].

1.3 Artifacts in AECG Recording

An inherent problem with ambulatory monitoring is the almost inevitable occurrence of artifacts specific to this type of recording, resulting from a failure of one or more of the components of the system [4, 21–23]. Acknowledging these artifacts is of major importance because their misinterpretation can lead to erroneous clinical diagnoses and inappropriate therapeutic interventions. In addition, it is important to determine the cause of the artifact so that any fault in the equipment can be corrected. The major causes of artifact in Holter recordings are discussed in the following subsections. These essentially apply to recorders employing cassette tapes, as little experience has yet been gained with the newer solid-state technology (though problems with battery, electrodes, or cables are likely to be common to old and new systems).

1.3.1 Battery Failure

The most common artifact encountered during tape-based Holter monitoring is certainly the "pseudotachycardia" owing to the failure of the battery toward the end of the recording, as can be seen in ❷ Fig. 1.6, where a tachycardia characterized by a narrowing and lower voltage of the QRS complex occurs abruptly. The rhythm may be regular or irregular, simulating a paroxysmal supraventricular tachycardia (SVT). The replacement of the disposable or rechargeable batteries and, if necessary, the cassette or magnetic tape, could correct these artifacts. As a general rule, a new battery should be used with each recording, particularly in research studies where failure to record on a specific date can invalidate the whole study.

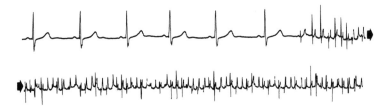

□ Fig. 1.6

An illustration of one form of artifact encountered during AECG, where failure of the batteries toward the end of the recording has produced a "pseudotachycardia," with a decrease of P, QRS, and T-wave durations in particular making the diagnosis straightforward

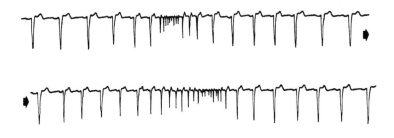

□ Fig. 1.7

Cyclic slackening of the magnetic tape on account of mechanical difficulty within the recorder

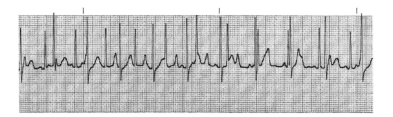

□ Fig. 1.8

An illustration of artifact resulting from the use of magnetic tape, which has not been erased properly before being used a second time, resulting in the superposition of two ECG tracings

1.3.2 Failure of the Magnetic-Tape Recording

Less frequently, a recording problem can occur intermittently, especially if some mechanical difficulty is present at each rotation of the cassette or magnetic tape. The characteristics of the artifact are the same as in battery failure, but they occur at periodic intervals (❷ Fig. 1.7). The use of a cassette or tape, which has not been properly erased, during a subsequent recording, can lead to the superposition of two ECGs and make the interpretation of the new ECG signals impossible, as shown in ❷ Fig. 1.8. Therefore, as a rule, new cassette tapes should be used for each new patient AECG study in order to avoid these tape problems.

1.3.3 Failure of Electrodes, Lead Wires, or Patient Cable

Any dysfunction of electrodes, lead wires, or patient cable contributes to artifacts. Permanent failure, such as a break in the cable or loss of electrode contact, is easily identified, as a permanent defect occurs in one of the two recording

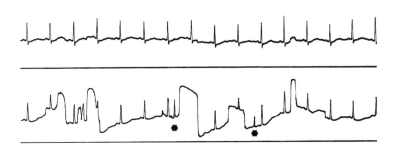

■ Fig. 1.9
An example of the value of using two-channel recording during AECG. The lower channel shows artifact caused by intermittent failure of the ECG cable, with temporary loss of the ECG tracing and marked baseline shift producing "pseudo-QRS" waves marked by asterisks

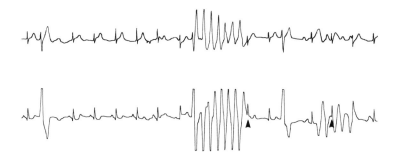

■ Fig. 1.10
"Pseudo-VT" is produced by shaking the ECG cable during Holter recording. This artifact can be identified by the presence of normal QRS complexes, as marked by arrows within the runs of pseudo-VT

leads. An intermittent failure, however, is more difficult to interpret. The use of at least two simultaneous leads in modern Holter recorders has considerably improved the detection of these artifacts. In a majority of cases, they occur only (or principally) in one lead as in ❷ Fig. 1.9. The intermittent loss of electrical contact in one of the two leads induces abrupt movements of the baseline without any recording of the ECG at that particular instant. However, in the other lead the normal ECG appearance easily permits the recognition of artifact. It should be noted that many analyzers, while displaying two channels, essentially analyze only one of the leads.

In some cases, the artifact can be present simultaneously in the two leads, particularly in the case of displacement of the patient's cable. In ❷ Fig. 1.10, the diagnosis of artifact is particularly difficult, because the presence of genuine VPBs can lead to an erroneous diagnosis of VT. Fortunately, two indices point to the diagnosis of artifact:

1. The second episode of pseudo-VT is not present in the upper tracing as it is in the lower tracing; and
2. The normal QRS rhythm can be observed within the artifact and coincides with the normal rhythm before and after the event.

As seen in the two preceding examples, the use of a second lead in the Holter recorder provides the most obvious means of identifying an artifact. In the absence of any displacement of the baseline, it is the only way to obtain an accurate diagnosis. In ❷ Fig. 1.11, for example, during a very short loss of electrical contact, only one PQRST complex disappears. In lead I, this is evidenced by a small undulation of the baseline. The presence of a normal QRS complex in lead II makes it possible

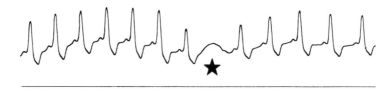

◘ Fig. 1.11

Transient loss of electrical contact in a lead wire or an electrode in the top channel producing the absence of one QRS complex (marked by a *star*). Its presence on the simultaneously recorded second channel permits its detection

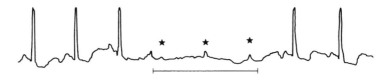

◘ Fig. 1.12

An example of an artifact during AECG recording producing pseudoatrioventricular block on account of a sudden decrease of QRS voltage owing to an increase of skin-electrode coupling impedance. The residual QRS complexes identified by *stars* may be wrongly identified as blocked P waves. The bar indicates the duration of the artifact

to exclude the diagnosis of a transient sinoatrial (SA) block. ❥ Figure 1.12 provides an example of pseudo-atrioventricular (AV) block due to a sudden decrease of QRS voltage.

1.4   Equipment for Analysis

1.4.1   Analog Holter Tape Recording

All methods of analysis require some form of playback system [4, 24–26] including those, which undertake real-time analysis of the AECG. All playback systems contain at least a magnetic-tape replay unit, while some older systems have an audio speaker and an ECG writer, which can provide samples. In addition, an oscilloscope or screen, an arrhythmia detector, a microprocessor-based analyzer (nowadays often a personal computer), an automatic ST-segment analysis system, and a fiber-optic or laser printer might form a part of such a system. Most current playback systems use generic computer hardware platforms and proprietary software protocols for data analysis and report generation. Signals recorded in analog format by magnetic tape are digitized at either a rate of 128 or 256 samples/s for subsequent analysis. The clock track on the tape can compensate for tape speed variations by a phase lock loop circuit. The resolution is usually at least eight bits and the sampling rate 128/s. The signal amplitude can be adjusted by the physician or technician based on the calibration signal recorded automatically at the beginning of each recording. Tape playback and scanning options include rapid playback with either superimposition of up to 1,000 times with or without audio-speaker control or page-type displays. Facsimile, modem, network, and internet integration allow for rapid distribution of AECG data and analyses throughout a hospital or larger health-care system.

The magnetic-tape unit, if required for playback, is a motor-driven assembly, which operates normally at 60 or 120 times the original recording speed, although more recently developed systems can function at 480 times the original recording speed. The magnetic heads detect and reproduce the original ECG signal for onward transmission to the

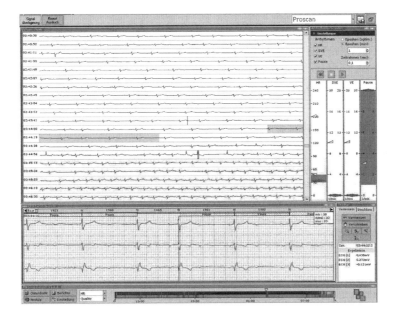

■ Fig. 1.13

Full disclosure of long sequences of a single ECG lead for quick paging up or down (*top*) and an arrhythmia-scanning mode (*right*) for rapid detection of phases of arrhythmias, three-channel real time ECG (*bottom*) (Oxford MedilogDarwin system)

remainder of the system. In FM systems, it is necessary for the replay unit to demodulate the signal in order to retrieve the original waveforms. In most modern tape-recording systems, the analog signal from the tape is digitized for quick and convenient quantitative data analysis.

In every Holter system, an oscilloscope or flat panel screen is an essential part to control and guide the whole analysis procedure. Practically, all Holter analysis systems have the option of presenting data in a superimposed fashion at 30, 60, 120, 240, or 480 times the original recording speed, which when coupled with an audio speaker constitutes the AVSEP (audiovisual superimposition electrocardiographic pattern) display. In the majority of instruments, the use of a storage oscilloscope makes it possible to "freeze" the display of a real-time ECG for a period of 2–3 s up to 180 s if desired. Either one or both recorded leads may be displayed in this way. By using a technique for "jogging," it is possible to jump forward or backward for a variable time in order to inspect quickly a series of "frozen" ECG displays (❯ Fig. 1.13). More recent systems sometimes use a graphics screen attached to a personal computer rather than a custom-engineered display (see ❯ Sect. 1.4.2).

In some older analog Holter systems, an audio speaker is incorporated that produces an audible sound, which is dependent on the detection of the R wave of the QRS complex. The tone can rise to a more shrill note in the presence of a fast heart rate or when an ectopic beat creates an isolated short R–R interval. On the contrary, with slow heart rates or longer R–R intervals, a low-pitched sound occurs. In some of the less-expensive units where there is no display, it is claimed that the ECG can be analyzed purely by listening to the audio signal produced by the replay unit.

The conventional form of a laser printer-ECG writer is incorporated into all Holter analysis systems and provides for up to three channels of ECG data to be written on standard (graphic) paper with an accompanying time printed on the edge track. It is evident that the production of specific examples of ECG abnormalities form a necessary part of the AECG report, providing essential material to enable the physician to interpret the 24-h recording. Moreover, graphic and tabulated AECG data, as well as a total 24-h ECG printout are provided by modern laser printers. Thus, this type of printout has supplanted the older fiber-optic printout system, which was able to print all or part of the ECG in a real-time format produced at high speed with a time reference frame. As previously mentioned, the display of the whole 24-h ECG on paper has become known as "full disclosure." This technique is very useful for giving information on the quality of the recording and for studying rare events, particularly when the major part of the Holter recording is normal. As can be seen in ❯ Fig. 1.13, a second degree AV block is easily detected on a compressed ECG tracing. However, this technique requires that the technician or physician who must examine the complete 24-h ECG tracing spends some considerable time in doing so. The most recent AECG analyzing units provide abnormal sequences such as pauses, arrhythmias, etc. automatically for direct technician or physician review. Usually, one lead is printed, but if necessary the two leads could be printed separately. For time reasons, the use of full AECG disclosure is normally confined to quality control, verification of rare events, evaluation of AAD efficacy, and similar specialized functions and is not recommended for widespread routine use. The most modern solid-state Holter analyzing units provide abnormal episodes within the full disclosure ECG (e.g., pauses, arrhythmias, etc.) automatically, line-by-line for direct and quick control by the technician or physician.

1.4.2   Solid-State Holter Recording

The newer solid-state Holter systems consist of the digital recording (solid-state) device, the electronic interface to transfer the data from flashcard or hard drive to the personal computer, the flat panel screen, the alpha-numeric keyboard, the personal computer with the proprietary software protocols for data analysis and report generation, and a laser printer (❯ Fig. 1.14). Some solid-state recorders are equipped with a microprocessor that provides "on-line analysis" of the QRS complex, the ST segment, as well as the T wave as they are acquired. Thus, a quick analysis and overview on the whole set of AECG data is immediately available at the technician's or physician's convenience, which facilitates and speeds up the interactive final analysis of the full 24h AECG. Details of the analysis workflow are given below.

1.5   Methods of Analysis

The approach to the analysis of 24-h ECG recordings varies from one manufacturer to another, and there are many systems commercially available worldwide. However, the different methods can be broken down into two very broad categories. Using discriminators, the hardware essentially differentiates between a normal (or dominant) QRS waveform and all others. The critical thresholds used to achieve the discrimination may (optionally) be adjusted by a technician. These are likely to be based on QRS width, amplitude or area, or some combination or derivative of these parameters. Various criteria based on the R–R interval, or the number of abnormal beats detected consecutively, can be set up to facilitate the detection and printout of arrhythmias. Using the method of a classifier, in microprocessor-based equipment the software automatically groups QRS complexes into a number of different categories ("templates"). This may be done in the recorder itself or in the laboratory-based analyzer. Thereafter, an operator may (optionally) adjust the classifications. Analysis of rhythm is then based on a study of the beat classifications, R–R intervals, and similar criteria. There are intermediate solutions where, for example, the second approach is used in the recorder to collect samples of arrhythmias

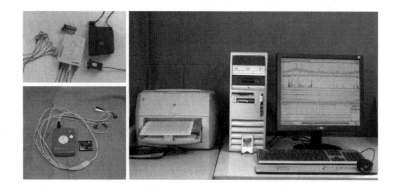

⬛ Fig. 1.14

Modern type of solid-state recorder systems: digital AECG recorder of Medset (*top left*), digital AECG recorder (*bottom left*), and complete analysis system of OxfordDarwin (*right*) with personal computer, keyboard, flatpanel screen, and laser printer

only, although details of heart rate over 24 h may also be stored. With some types of analyzers in either of the above categories, it is possible for the operator to view several minutes of an ECG on the screen in order to check visually for abnormalities or assess the quality of the recording.

1.5.1 Analog Tape Recordings

The first approach, that is, the use of the discriminator type, has the advantage that it can be used with a minimum of intervention by the operator and is thus suited to routine and automatic analysis of a large number of Holter recordings. On the other hand, experience shows that operator intervention can be valuable. The aim of using the discriminator approach in older Holter systems is not to provide an exact number of abnormal complexes (as is the case in the second approach), but to indicate their relative global frequency and, above all, to detect any arrhythmias. The principle of the technique is to use only a single pass of the tape (taking 12 or 24 min for 60 or 120 times real speed, respectively) in order to obtain data (e.g., trend plots) without intervention of the operator, or with minimal intervention such as an adjustment of the QRS width threshold, prior to the commencement of analysis, or to print any arrhythmias detected. This type of semiautomatic beat classification cannot provide the exact number of abnormal events because inevitably artifacts will be incorporated into QRS counts or because some normal QRS complexes will be considered abnormal or vice versa. However, if the original analog ECG signal is sufficiently high in amplitude without major artifacts, the QRS count is generally satisfactory with only a small percentage error. It is then possible to use such a system in order to obtain relatively quickly a large variety of presentations of the data contained on the recording.

1.5.2 Digital Solid-State Recordings

The most recent generation of automatic analyzers either undertakes the QRS analysis in real time using a microprocessor built into the recorder, or after replay using a similar technique whereby 64 or 128 different types of QRS complexes can be stored within the microprocessor memory. Each new QRS complex is compared with the different types already stored, and if it compares satisfactorily to one of these, the total count for that particular pattern is increased by one. If not, a new QRS morphology is then stored. At the end of the analysis, the various QRS morphologies can be displayed together with a count of beats in each group (❯ Fig. 1.15a, b). In some systems, it is possible for the operator to decide that a certain group of complexes consists of artifacts and have them deleted from the analysis. Alternatively, if there are only subtle differences between different groups, they can be merged and finally a categorization of normal or abnormal premature ventricular complexes (PVCs), premature supraventricular complexes (PSVCs), and so on can be added to each group so that the various counts can be accurately produced. This approach is now the standard technique of practically all modern AECG monitoring systems. Real-time analysis using the above technique has the advantage that at the end of the recording, the results can be instantly printed out via the appropriate replay and print-out unit.

1.5.3 Arrhythmia Analysis

1.5.3.1 From Tape Recorders

By using the main criteria, the R–R interval, and the QRS width, it is possible to develop algorithms that are able to detect automatically many types of arrhythmias in Holter analog tape recordings [27–29]. Each beat is classified as normal, ventricular ectopic, supraventricular ectopic, paced, other, or unknown, and a template for each type of abnormality is created. Enlarged premature beats (premature ventricular contractions (PVCs) or atrial premature beats (APBs) with aberrant intraventricular conduction) and narrow premature beats (supraventricular premature beats or PVCs narrower than sinus beats) are the easiest arrhythmias to detect. The ease of detection of such abnormalities, as well as of couplets does not differ greatly compared to that of isolated extrasystoles. However, all these phenomena can be detected more confidently with the assistance of an experienced technician to run the analyzer. All users of Holter monitoring know that the first generation of PVC counters could be grossly inaccurate in analyzing the ECG tracings in the presence of artifact.

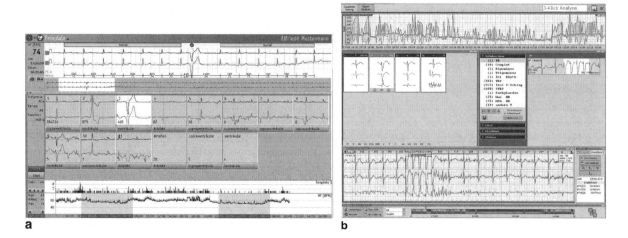

■ **Fig. 1.15**

(a) Overview on the analysis forms of the computer program (Medset system) showing real time three-channel ECG (*top*), templates of QRS complexes (*center*), and summary of arrhythmias and heart-rate trend (*bottom*). **(b)** Overview on the analysis forms of the computer program (Oxford MedilogDarwin system) including heart-rate trend curve (*top*), QRS complex templates (*left*), types of available templates (*center*), selected single lead strips (*right*), and three-channel real-time ECG (*bottom*)

In this context, the superiority of human intervention compared to the use of an automatic detector is evident. However, automatic detectors can be used for other purposes with more complex algorithms. An example is the recognition of atrial fibrillation (AF) as opposed to sinus arrhythmia on the basis of studying only the irregularity of the R–R interval distribution. Another example of the utility of the automatic analysis of arrhythmias is the detection of ventricular pauses caused by SA or AV block. Visually, this search is very difficult and the automated approach provides higher sensitivity at the slight expense of a larger number of false-positive reports.

The interactive technique, which requires an operator, uses variable criteria for the recognition of arrhythmias, principally for ventricular or supraventricular extrasystoles. The simplest method is to use the classical criteria of recognition, but with the possibility of modifying the thresholds of prematurity and QRS width according to the characteristics of the particular ECG under study. However, more sophisticated detectors have appeared recently using different criteria in order to obtain an improved separation between "normal" and "abnormal" QRS; that is to say, different QRS patterns. These criteria can include the slope of the first component of the QRS complex, its derivative, the QRS area, or the morphological pattern calculated from the analog signal or from a digitized ECG. These criteria can be utilized separately or together in order to define the similarity between each QRS complex and the basic "normal QRS," which is usually learned by the machine with some prompting by the operator at the onset of the recording. With this operator-based approach to setting up criteria, which can be adjusted – if necessary – during the tape analysis, the separation between supraventricular and ventricular complexes is usually achieved satisfactorily. ❷ Table 1.1 summarizes some important causes of false positive and false negative findings in the analysis of arrhythmias from AECG.

1.5.3.2   From Solid-State Recorders

In solid-state digital AECG systems, the total number of QRS complexes is analyzed and classified in different templates, which can be interactively controlled and categorized into normal or abnormal premature ventricular complexes (PVCs) or PSVCs. Together with the R–R intervals, every type of bradyarrhythmia, tachyarrhythmia, supraventricular, or ventricular premature complexes can be quantified by the computer protocol. A comparative real-time ECG printout provides interactive control of the classification result of the computer (❷ Figs. 1.15 and ❷ 1.16). In addition, most solid-state

Table 1.1

Some technical causes of false-positive and false-negative findings in arrhythmia detection and classification from the ambulatory electrocardiogram (AECG)

1. Battery failure with "pseudotachycardia"
2. Recorder malfunction with variable tape drive or inaccurate storage
3. Incomplete degaussing or erasure of data from previously used tapes or memory storage
4. Noise interference or lead-electrode baseline drift or artifact
5. Low-voltage recording
6. Physiologic variations in QRS form and voltage
7. Inadequate computer QRS detection and classification algorithms
8. Incorrect time stamping of AECG tracings
9. Inadequate or incorrect technician interpretation during analysis

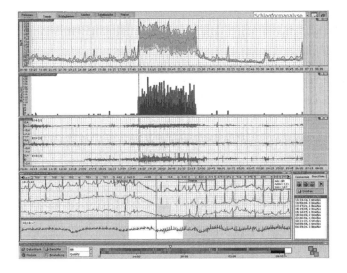

Fig. 1.16

Trend analysis of heart rate (*top*), counts of ventricular ectopic beats (*second top row*), ST-segment trends (*third row*), and three-channel real-time ECG and single lead "full disclosure" ECG (*bottom*) (Oxford MedilogDarwin system)

systems provide a separate channel for pacemaker spike analysis, and software for analyzing HRV either in the time or frequency domain or both.

After replay and digitizing the analog ECG signals from Holter magnetic tapes or – in case of solid-state ambulatory Holter systems – following transfer of the digital AECG data from the recorder to the computer via an interface, subsequent analysis of all ECG data is relatively easy, quick, and convenient if an appropriate software program is available. With most solid-state systems, a primary computer-based automatic analysis is performed and these data are presented on the screen as simultaneous multiple trend curves of heart rate (maximum, minimum, mean), PSVCs, PVCs, ST-segment deviation, and QRS complex templates together with a strip of two or three channels of the original ECG (❍ Figs. 1.15b and ❍ 1.17). Using the cursor at each time of the heart-rate trend or arrhythmia strip, a control and reclassification of QRS templates, arrhythmia classification, or ST-segment analysis can be made instantaneously. Moreover, further trend curves of pacemaker activity, HRV trends and instantaneous values at a given period of the 24 h recording, and respiratory activity may be displayed. Some modern systems also provide a 12-lead ECG, which is either recalculated mathematically from the 3-lead orthogonal X–Y–Z data using a transformation or an actual 12-lead ECG where the limb electrodes are placed on the chest (see ❍ Chap. 11 of *Basic Electrocardiology: Cardiac Electrophysiology, ECG*

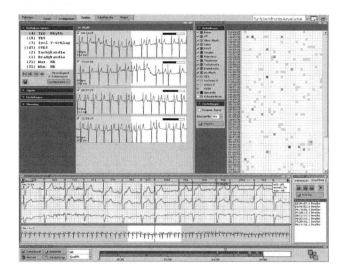

◘ Fig. 1.17
Arrhythmia overview including counts of single arrhythmic events (*left*), single lead arrhythmic episodes extracted from the overview on left side, survey on QRS templates over the full 24-h period with 30 s segments (*right*), and three-channel real-time ECG (*bottom*) (Oxford MedilogDarwin system)

Systems and Mathematical Modeling). Alternatively, a full disclosure ECG may be presented first page by page and by quick paging up or down and reading all ECG sequences. Abnormal episodes such as bradycardias, pauses, PVCs, or tachycardias can easily be identified, marked by the mouse, presented in real-time, and finally confirmed or corrected if necessary.

1.5.4   ST-Segment Analysis for Myocardial Ischemia

1.5.4.1   Technical Aspects – Analysis of Ischemic Episodes

With respect to ST-segment analysis for detecting myocardial ischemia, some important technical, electrocardiographic, and clinical aspects have to be considered, for which the following recommendations have been given [7]. The QRS-T morphology must be carefully scrutinized to ensure that it is suitable for interpretation. Cardiac rhythm should be sinus rhythm, the baseline ST segment should have ⩽0.1 mV deviation, and the ST segment ideally should be gently upsloping with an upright T wave. A flat ST segment associated with an inverted T wave may still be interpretable. However, downsloping or scooped ST-segment morphology should be avoided. The height of the R wave of the monitored lead should be ⩾1.0 mV. The lead selected for ischemia monitoring should not have a Q wave ⩾ 0.04 s or marked baseline ST-segment distortion. Patients with left-ventricular hypertrophy in the 12-lead ECG, left bundle branch block, nonspecific intraventricular conduction delay ⩾100 ms, or pre-excitation are not suitable for monitoring myocardial ischemia in the AECG. Medication with digitalis or some antidepressant drugs may distort the ST segment and preclude accurate interpretation of ST-segment deviations. ST-segment deviation is tracked by the use of a cursor within the PR segment to define the isoelectric reference point, and another cursor at the J-point and/or 60–80 ms beyond the J point to identify the presence of ST-segment depression. Myocardial ischemia is diagnosed by a sequence of flat or downsloping ST-segment depression of ⩾0.1 mV, with a gradual onset and offset that lasts for a minimum period of 1 min. Each episode of transient ischemia must be separated by a minimum duration of at least 1 min, during which the ST segment returns to baseline (the so-called 1 × 1 × 1 rule [30, 31]). Many investigators prefer a duration of at least 5 min between episodes, and the ACC/AHA Task Force also recommends a 5-min interval between episodes because the end of one episode and the onset of the next will take longer than 1 min to be physiologically distinct. Episodes of ST-segment deviation are characterized by identification of an onset and offset time, magnitude of deviation, and heart rate before and during the episode.

■ Table 1.2

Some causes of false-positive and false-negative findings in detection and interpretation of myocardial ischemia from the ambulatory electrocardiogram (AECG)

1.	Inadequate lead system employed
2.	Incorrect or lack of lead calibration
3.	Inadequate recording fidelity
4.	Recording signal processing that compresses or filters the data, altering the ST-segment characteristics
5.	Height of R wave <1.0 mV and Q wave ⩾0.04 s
6.	Downsloping or scooped ST-segment morphology
7.	Positional changes on the ST-segment
8.	Hyperventilation
9.	Vasoregulatory or Valsalva-induced ST segment changes
10.	Sudden excessive exercise-induced ST segment changes
11.	Preexcitation (WPW-syndrome)
12.	Intraventricular conduction disorders (LBBB, RBBB)
13.	Undiagnosed or unappreciated left ventricular hypertrophy
14.	ST segment changes secondary to tachyarrhythmias
15.	False ST segment changes from atrial fibrillation or atrial flutter
16.	ST segment changes secondary to electrolyte disturbance or drugs

Representative ECG strips at the time of ST-segment deviation in real time should be provided in the report format. Trend curves and/or a summary table of all ischemic episodes may be displayed in the final report. Alternatively, a miniaturized full-disclosure display can be printed out for all or part of the 24-h recording [7]. ❷ Table 1.2 summarizes some important causes of false positive and false negative findings regarding ST-segment analysis from the AECG.

One special problem is ST-segment elevation in variant angina, where the role of Holter monitoring is of considerable importance. During the playback analysis, the ST segment can be studied in two ways, either by visual examination or by automatic measurement, which can provide a trend of the ST amplitude. Some systems continuously monitor the ST amplitude, which is automatically compared to the baseline, defined by the onset of the accompanying QRS complex. In this case, the point of measurement can usually be placed by the operator at an appropriate distance from the J point in order to eliminate the detection of "physiological" ascent of the ST-segment depression. Other systems measure ST-segment depression automatically during the 24-h recording. This approach is subject to error in relating the ST measurement point to a fixed QRS trigger, which may vary with different QRS morphologies, that is, from patient to patient.

1.5.4.2 Beat-to-Beat Analysis

The most recent technical developments are fully automatic algorithms for beat-to-beat ST-segment amplitude measurements. Rather than identifying discrete sequential short episodes of ST-segment deviation, this approach utilizes frequency distributions of the ST-segment amplitude measurements for each 24-h recording (typically of 50,000–100,000 beats) in order to yield a better global perspective of ST-segment shifts that have occurred during the whole recording period [32, 33]. Following QRS detection and elimination of abnormal complexes, beat-by-beat isoelectric baseline estimation by cubic splines, and noise determination, the initial (R-ST1) and end point (R-ST2) of the regression line of the ST-slope is determined by the computer algorithm using the empiric formula for timing of the two points: $R\text{-}ST1 = 40 + K1\sqrt{RR}$ and $R\text{-}ST2 = 40 + K2\sqrt{RR}$. For a heart rate of 60 bpm, K1 was set to 70 ms and K2 to 110 ms, and the whole range of K1 and K2 was evaluated over a spectrum of heart rates up to R − R intervals of 1,600 ms. From the frequency distribution (histogram) of the average displacement of the ST-segment (AVD) time series over 24 h, several parameters indicative of transient myocardial ischemia were extracted. As expected, transient and ischemic episodes lasting only several minutes were shown to be skewed to the left and to be asymmetrically spread around an average deviation of

1

less than 0 mm, whereas nonischemic frequency distribution was narrow and symmetric with an average deviation close to 0 mm. Using several parameters like percentiles, spread measures, skewness, and clustering, the authors were able to distinguish between a normal cohort of 63 individuals and 37 patients with CAD by a cut-off point of 0.45 for the estimated probability of ischemia in ambulatory monitoring [32]. In a second study, the influence of the autonomic nervous system (ANS) on ST-segment variability was tested [33], using the same technique of computerized ST-segment analysis including a demodulator algorithm to compensate for respiratory baseline shifts. Nine healthy volunteers underwent the following experimental protocol: control period (breathing room air at 10 cycles/min = 0.17 Hz for 5 min), fast respiration period (breathing room air at 15 cycles/min = 0.25 Hz for another 5 min), metabolic period (breathing 100% oxygen at 10 cycles/min for about 8 min), and neurogenic period (after 10 min breathing pure air, administration of atropine iv. with breathing room air at 10 cycles/min for other 10 min). Analysis of power spectral densities of the AVD signal during the four different periods of the experimental protocol showed no effect of 100% oxygen inhalation, only a small effect of mechanical respiratory activity, but a significant decrease of both total variability and relative power with atropine intervention. The results were similar for HRV, and the conclusion of this study was that the ANS plays a significant role in the regulation of AVD time series. This is a new important physiological finding and should encourage further systematic studies by using the ST segment not only as a simple detector of myocardial ischemia, but rather as a target and component of comprehensive cardiovascular equilibrium [33].

1.5.5   Analysis of HRV

Twenty-four-hour Holter AECG recordings represent a near ideal source for both short- and long-term assessment of HRV. Analysis of HRV itself refers to beat-to-beat oscillations of the R – R interval, which in the absence of physical activity, postural changes, or emotional stimuli represents the balance between cardiac sympathetic and parasympathetic (vagal) efferent activity and in particular the autonomically mediated alterations of the sinus node discharge rate (R – R tachogram, ❷ Fig. 1.18). In general, two methods of HRV analysis have been described, namely, time domain and spectral analysis [34, 35]. The term "time domain" reflects the fact that the majority of methods used provide measures in units of time (e.g., milliseconds) and time domain parameters involve computing indexes that are not directly related to specific cycle lengths. This method offers a simple means of defining patients with decreased variability in the mean and standard deviations of the R – R intervals. In general, two methods of time domain analysis – statistical and geometric – are in use [34].

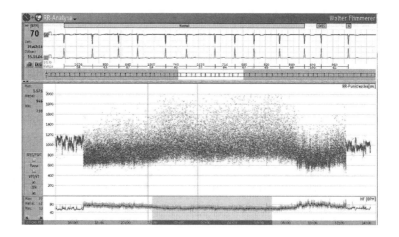

◨ Fig. 1.18

Trend of heart-rate tachogram (*center*) during sinus rhythm (*extreme left and extreme right*) and AF (*left* and *right center*) as a rough overview on HRV. Real time two-channel ECG (*top*) and heart-rate trend (*bottom*) are also included (Medset system)

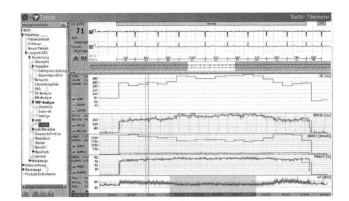

◙ Fig. 1.19

Trend curves of different time domain parameters of HRV (SDNN, rMSSD, SDNN50, and pNN50) and heart rate (*center* and *bottom*) together with a two-channel real-time ECG (*top*), same patient as in ❷ Fig. 1.18 (Medset system)

1.5.5.1 Statistical Methods for HRV Analysis

Among the statistical methods, time domain parameters analyzed include the mean R – R interval, the mean coupling interval between all normal beats, SDANN = standard deviation of the averaged normal sinus R – R intervals for all 5-min segments of the entire 24-h recording, SDNN = standard deviation of all normal sinus R – R intervals, SDNN index = mean of the standard deviations of all normal R – R intervals for all 5-min segments of the entire recording, NN50 = count of the number of pairs of adjacent R – R intervals differing by more than 50 ms in the entire recording, pNN50 = the percentage of adjacent R – R intervals that varied by more than 50 ms, and the rMSSD = root mean square of the difference between the coupling intervals of adjacent R – R intervals. Solid state recorders provide hour-to-hour trend analyses of different time-domain parameters (❷ Fig. 1.19). rMSSD, NN50, and pNN50 correlate highly and are markers of high-frequency variations (vagal influence) in heart rate [34]. Of all parameters, rMSSD seems the most statistically stable (in standard clinical populations, the distribution of rMSSD data is more normal than that of pNN50 or NN50 values) and should be preferred, particularly since it correlates highly with others.

1.5.5.2 Geometric Measures for HRV Analysis

The main practical limitation of statistical methods is the time-consuming and extensive offline-manual editing of the ECG signals in order to ensure good quality R – R interval series. The use of filters to exclude outliers of R – R intervals, for example, perhaps those differing by more than 20% of the preceding R – R interval, is sometimes unsuccessful and may provide substantially inaccurate results. Therefore, a solution to eliminate incorrect R – R intervals is geometric measures, that is, the conversion of R – R interval data into a geometric pattern, such as the sample-density histogram of R – R interval duration, the sample-density histogram of the differences between successive R – R intervals (there exists little experience with this method), and the duration of each R – R interval against the immediately preceding R – R interval (so called Lorenz plots or Poincaré maps) (❷ Fig. 1.20). Since the incorrect R – R intervals are usually substantially shorter (due to premature ectopic beats) or longer (due to sinus or compensatory pauses) than the population of correct R – R intervals, these incorrect R – R intervals fall outside the major peak of the distribution histogram and can easily be suppressed. Of the three geometric methods, the triangular index is the most important and most frequently used measure of HRV. It is calculated by dividing the total number of all R – R intervals by the height of the histogram of all R – R intervals measured on a discrete scale with bins of 7.8 ms, when using a sampling frequency of 128 Hz. A modification of the triangular index is the triangular interpolation of the R – R interval histogram (TINN), which is less dependent on the sampling frequency. This method interpolates the R – R interval histogram by a triangle, which has its base on the horizontal axis and its peak at the maximum point of the histogram, whereby the computation of the method identifies a triangle for which the square

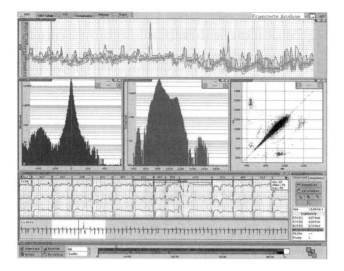

⬤ Fig. 1.20

HRV histogram: Trend curve of heart rate (*top row*), histogram of the R–R interval differences (*center left*), R–R interval histogram (*center*), scatterplot with plotting the duration of each R–R interval against the immediately preceding R–R interval (so called Lorenz plots, *center right*), and three-channel real-time ECG (*bottom*) (Oxford MedilogDarwin system)

difference between the histogram and the triangle is the minimum among all possible triangles. The length of the base of such a triangle is used as the measure of HRV. Both the HRV triangular index and TINN, measured over 24 h, express overall HRV and are more influenced by lower than by higher frequencies [34].

Because many studies in the past have used different HRV parameters leading to a lack of standardization and given that many measures correlate closely, the ESC/NASPE Task Force developed guidelines [36] to standardize nomenclature and methods of measurement. They recommended four time-domain HRV parameters:

1. SDNN (as an estimate of the overall HRV)
2. HRV triangular index (as an estimate of overall HRV)
3. SDANN (as an estimate of long-term components of HRV), and
4. RMSSD (as an estimate of short-term components of HRV)

1.5.5.3   Frequency-Domain Analysis of HRV

The basic assumption underlying the technique of frequency-domain analysis is that every periodic signal such as systolic arterial pressure or heart rate (R − R intervals) may be decomposed into a series of oscillatory components with different frequency and amplitude. When considering short-term recordings (5–10 min), spectral analysis of HRV is characterized by three components:

1. A high-frequency (HF) band in the range of 0.15–0.40 Hz, which can be considered as a measure of the physiological respiratory sinus arrhythmia;
2. A low-frequency (LF) band in the range of 0.04–0.15 Hz that corresponds to the LF rhythmicity of systolic arterial pressure frequently observed in conditions of sympathetic activation; and
3. A very low-frequency (VLF) band in the range of 0.0033–0.04 Hz that often shows a progressive decrease of power instead of a discrete spectral peak [37].

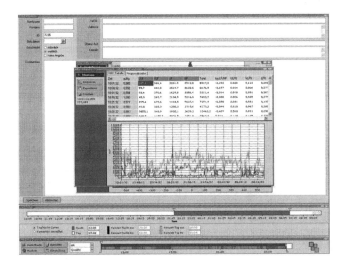

◘ Fig. 1.21

Trend curves of frequency-domain parameters of HRV (*bottom*) and numeric printout for the various parameters ULF, VLF, LF, and HF for every 5 min interval (*top*) (Oxford MedilogDarwin system)

◘ Table 1.3

Correlation of the different time and frequency components of heart rate variability (HRV)

Spectral component	Time-domain correlates	Normal measures for 24 hours
HF	rMSSD	<15 h
	pNN50	<0.75%
LF	SDNN index	<30 ms
VLF	SDNN index	<30 ms
ULF	SDNN	<50 ms
	SDANN	<40 ms
	HRV index	...
TP	SDNN	<50 ms
	HRV index	...

Abbreviations: *VLF* very-low frequency, *ULF* ultra-low frequency, *TP* total power, *SDNN index* mean of standard deviation of R-Rs, *HRV index* integral of the total number of normal R-Rs divided by the maximum of the density distribution

In practical terms, parasympathetic tone is primarily reflected in the HF component, the LF component is influenced by both sympathetic and parasympathetic nervous systems, and the LF/HF ratio is considered a measure of sympathovagal balance, reflecting sympathetic modulations [37]. The spectral profile of long-term recordings is completely different from that of short-term recordings, because most of the energy (up to 90% of total power) is distributed within the ultra-low-frequency (ULF) range ($\leqslant 0.003$ Hz) and the VLF range, whereas power of LF and HF accounts for only 10% of total power. Therefore, an alternative approach to the analysis of long-term recordings is to divide the entire 24-h period into a series of around 250 consecutive 5-min periods that are analyzed as short-term recordings [36, 37] (◉ Fig. 1.21). In general, it should be stressed that the two analytical techniques of time and frequency-domain HRV are complementary in that they are different mathematical analyses of the same phenomenon, which explains why certain time and frequency-domain variables correlate strongly with each other, as shown in ◉ Table 1.3.

1.5.5.4   Pitfalls and Limitations of HRV Analysis

Some technical aspects and pitfalls of HRV analysis have to be borne in mind. HRV increases with increased periods of observations, and it is important to distinguish ranges on the basis of duration of recordings. In practice, long-term 24-h and short-term 5-min recordings are used. Frequency-domain methods are preferable for short-term, and time-domain methods are mainly used for 24-h recordings (e.g., using SDNN, SDANN, and HRV triangular index), but also for short-term recordings (e.g., using rMSSD). The recording period should last at least ten times the duration of the wavelength of the lowest frequency under investigation (for HF components at least 1 min, for LF components 2 min). Most systems contain and use computer-digitized data with a sampling rate of 128 Hz, which is suboptimal for some experimental short-term recordings, but useful for long-term recordings in adults. In such cases, template matching or interpolation algorithms should be used to optimize the temporal accuracy of R-wave peak identification. If an analog recorder is used, the digitization rate is not relevant, but magnetic tape data may introduce errors related to noise, motion-related artifacts with missing R waves or spuriously detected beats, or other errors in R-wave timing such as might be related to magnetic tape stretch. In addition, arrhythmias may introduce difficulties in the analysis of HRV, for example, persistent AF renders HRV analysis impossible. If more than 20% of the detected beats are ectopic, because the interval before and after each ectopic beat is usually eliminated from the analysis, numerical estimates of HRV will not be accurate. Two methods exist for handling abnormal heartbeats, namely interpolation of occasional abnormal beats [38] and limiting analysis to segments that are free of abnormal beats, respectively.

1.5.6   Analysis of Heart-Rate Turbulence (HRT)

1.5.6.1   Pathophysiological Background

The new parameter of heart-rate-turbulence (HRT) was initially described by Schmidt et al. in 1999 [39]. The concept depends on the influence of single ventricular ectopic beats on the post-extrasystolic oscillations of baroreflex activity. Heart rate is controlled by vagal nerve activity with its direct effect on sinus node depolarization rate and AV-nodal conduction, the latency time is very short (450–700 ms) and thus, the heart responds in a beat-to-beat manner to any changes in vagal nerve activity [40, 41]. Following a single VPB, an instant drop of systolic and diastolic blood pressure ensues with a compensatory pause both in normals and in patients with compromised cardiac function that unloads carotid and aortic baroreceptors with a subsequent decrease of tonic vagal nerve activity [40]. In healthy normals, the drop of blood pressure is prolonged for the first 2–4 post-VPBs together with a transient loss of vagal activity, which seems to be responsible for the acceleration of heart rate. There then follows a steady increase of blood pressure with subsequent baroreceptor loading and an increase of vagal activity leading to a final deceleration phase of cardiac rhythm. In patients with depressed LV function, there is a sudden increase of systolic and diastolic blood pressure in the first post-VPB beat due to post-extrasystolic potentiation that compensates for the drop of blood pressure and activates the baroreceptors. The ensuing increased vagal nerve activity limits the initiation of early acceleration phase and prevents late deceleration phase of cardiac rhythm, that is, HRT cannot be observed [40]. HRT is therefore considered as a parameter of baroreflex sensitivity (BRS) that can be measured much more easily than the classic and complicated baroreflex testing approach.

1.5.6.2   Parameters of Heart-Rate Turbulence

HRT can be quantified by two parameters: turbulence onset (TO) and turbulence slope (TS). TO quantifies the brief phase of early acceleration (usually lasting for 2–4 sinus cycles) and is defined as the difference between the mean duration of the first two sinus beats following a VPB and the mean duration of the last two sinus beats preceding the VPB, divided by the mean duration of the last two sinus beats preceding the VPB. TO is expressed as a percentage. TS describes the speed of the late heart-rate deceleration phase and is defined as the maximum positive slope of a regression line assessed over any sequence of five subsequent R – R intervals within the first 20 sinus rhythm intervals after a VPB. TS is expressed in ms/R – R interval. In patients at low risk for mortality, VPB triggers an early acceleration of heart rate followed by a late deceleration phase, whereas in high-risk patients, HRT is blunted. For prognostic use of HRT, it is important to have appropriate cut-off values. TO and TS cut-off values were calculated by the group of Schmidt et al. [39, 42] with the use of a "training sample" composed of 100 patients with AMI. The log-rank test statistics for all possible cut-off points revealed optimal dichotomies of 0% for TO and 2.5 ms/R – R interval for TS.

1.5.6.3 Pitfalls and Limitations

It is important to note that Holter AECG data are very useful for evaluation of HRT, in case single VPBs are present in the entire recording, because different interesting time periods can be analyzed separately and, for example, diurnal variations of HRT in relation to clinical events can be detected. Some limitations of this method have to be mentioned. HRT analysis is limited to patients with dominant sinus rhythm. It cannot be used in patients with atrial flutter (AFl) or fibrillation, nor in those with second degree AV block or complete sinoatrial block. It cannot be used in patients with permanently firing cardiac pacemakers, while it is clear that the presence of VPBs in short- or long-term AECG recordings is essential for estimating HRT.

1.5.7 Analysis of QT Interval Variability (QTV)

1.5.7.1 Pathophysiological Background

QT interval (QTI) measurements, particularly in AECG recordings are of special interest, since prolonged ventricular repolarization with abnormal T-wave configuration and increased dispersion of QT-interval duration has been associated with increased risk of life-threatening ventricular arrhythmias both in congenital and in acquired conditions. In normal individuals, the QTI is modulated by multiple factors such as heart rate, circadian rhythm, and autonomic nervous-system activity. Acquired QT prolongation can be induced by myocardial ischemia, cardiac failure, electrolyte imbalances, diabetic neuropathy, and certain cardiac or non-cardiac drugs, while congenital QT prolongation and variability is caused by the abnormal function of cardiac ion channels following specific gene mutations. The main problems that limit the routine measurement of QTI are the absence of unequivocal criteria for determining T-wave offset, particularly in the presence of superimposed U waves, the absence of a general consensus on the best formula for adjusting the QTI to heart rate, and the diffusion of appropriate age- and gender-related normal values for corrected QTIs [43].

1.5.7.2 Technical Aspects

In 12-lead as well as in 3-lead Holter ECG recordings, the end of the T wave for assessing QTI may be determined either by the tangent method (drawing a tangent to the steepest point of downslope of T wave with T-wave offset being at the crossing of the tangent with the isoelectric line) [44], or visually by the return of the T wave to the TP baseline. In the case of U waves interrupting the T wave, the QT offset is measured at the nadir of the curve between T and U waves [45]. Finally, for AECG recordings analyzed by a computer-based technique, T-wave end may be automatically defined on a beat-to-beat basis by calculating the first derivative of the ECG signal and comparing it in the vicinity of expected T end with a threshold value [46].

The dynamic assessment of QTI during AECG monitoring requires computerized automatic measurements, with some technical problems due to low sampling rates, isoelectric baseline shifts, low signal-to-noise ratio, and difficult determination of the T-wave end at faster heart rates [43]. A low-noise ECG can be generated by averaging procedures that require the alignment of several consecutive beats over a given time interval with respect to R-wave peak (generally estimated by parabolic interpolation), and the averaged templates are then analyzed by specific algorithms that automatically detect QRS-T-wave features [47]. Averaging methods provide robust QTI measurements, but they lose the instantaneous variations in QT duration in the function of cycle length changes. Beat-to-beat analysis can explore instantaneous fluctuations of QT duration as a function of cycle length. However, this approach often requires the removal of large proportions of non-physiological data due to baseline noise. Therefore, beat-to-beat QTI measurements are best applied in short-term high-quality ECG recordings obtained under controlled conditions.

For evaluating long-term QTI dynamicity, two methods have been proposed, namely, the evaluation of the circadian excursion of the rate-corrected QTI (QTc), and the long-term evaluation of the QT/R−R relation, based on either beat-to-beat or averaging procedures. These two methods are increasingly implemented on modern commercial Holter systems and thus, are now available for routine clinical application.

1.5.8   Analysis of QT Dispersion (QTD)

1.5.8.1   Pathophysiological Background

The concept of measuring inter-lead variations of the QTI as a noninvasive parameter of QTD is based on observations made early in the 1950s, when Lepeschkin and Surawicz [44] reported QTI differences of 40 ms between leads I, II, and III, and of observations of Han and Moe, who demonstrated that nonuniform (asynchronous) recovery of excitability in the myocardium is an important factor for triggering ventricular tachyarrhythmias. They found meaningful differences in refractory periods even in adjacent (atrial and ventricular) myocardial fibers, for example, for ventricular refractory periods of 43 ms at a cycle length of 700 ms [48]. More recently, Antzelevich et al. showed important differences in refractory periods of myocardial slices due to the significantly longer depolarization and repolarization processes of the M cells in the midventricular myocardial wall compared to cells in the epicardial and endocardial layers [49]. QTD measured as the difference between the longest and shortest QTI within a 128-lead body surface mapping ECG, or a conventional 12-lead or a 3-lead Holter ECG is considered as a parameter of dispersion of ventricular repolarization and might be a prognostic marker of the propensity of a patient to life-threatening ventricular tachyarrhythmias.

1.5.8.2   Technical Aspects

Evaluation of repolarization duration in surface ECGs does not necessarily require a multi-lead system, as demonstrated by Sylvén et al. [50], who showed that the average QT duration computed from Frank's orthogonal leads highly correlates ($r = .885$, $p < .001$) with average QT duration obtained from 120-lead body-surface mapping. Zareba et al. [51] could show that in comparison to 12-lead ECGs, dispersion parameters calculated from 3 orthogonal-like leads (I, aVF, V_2) were equally effective in identifying patients who had arrhythmic cardiac death during follow-up. Thus, X, Y, and Z bipolar leads may be used for 24-h Holter AECG recordings to assess QTD at various time segments of the entire recording period.

1.5.8.3   Pitfalls and Limitations

There are several serious arguments against equating QTD with dispersion of ventricular repolarization that have been summarized by Rautaharju (2002) [52]. These arguments are as follows:

1. Measured QTD is determined primarily by dipolar components and does not represent dispersion of ventricular repolarization (the range of QTD in leads generated from strictly dipolar components is of the same order of magnitude as in the original 12-leads)
2. Inter-lead differences of QT duration are largely determined by T-wave "loop morphology" and by the projection of the terminal T-wave vector on individual leads (longest QT occurs in leads with the T-wave vector along the lead axis and shortest when near $90°$ angle)
3. Abnormal T-wave morphology has a strong influence on QTD (abnormal strictly dipolar morphological patterns can cause large inter-lead QT differences, which represent variability in amplitude/time domain rather than any physiologically meaningful intervals related to repolarization)

4. Overall technical variability of QTD measurement in the short- and long-range is too large to establish feasible thresholds and to separate normal from abnormal QTD (current consensus is that QTD values $\geqslant$100 ms are considered abnormal, but such large variations are commonly occurring with grossly abnormal T-wave morphology)

5. Variations in T-wave amplitude, lead vector strength, and noise level cause additional QTD variation (most T_{offset} detection algorithms use fixed thresholds so that T-wave amplitude variations via projection of strictly dipolar components may cause large QTD variations)

6. The presence of non-dipolar components in body surface ECG during repolarization has not been demonstrated as yet (the presence of non-dipolar components is necessary for detection of the end of localized ventricular repolarization and localized dispersion from QT measurements).

Regarding the many positive as well as negative studies on the prognostic value of QTD measurements and these problematic technical and physiological arguments, it is rather unclear at present whether QTD measurements either from 12-lead or from 3-lead Holter AECG recordings should be further used for stratifying patients with structural heart disease prone to sudden cardiac death (SCD) from ventricular tachyarrhythmias [51–53].

1.5.9 Signal Averaging of the AECG

1.5.9.1 Pathophysiological Background and Parameters of VLP

The technique of signal averaging was developed in order to retrieve small electrical signals at the microvolt level that arise from areas of slow and inhomogeneous conduction in diseased ventricular myocardium. In the early 1980s, advanced techniques were introduced for refinement of filtering of the signals (bi-directional filtering), the selection of bipolar orthogonal X, Y, and Z leads, and their combination into a vector magnitude for maximal sensitivity. In addition, computer algorithms were developed to identify QRS offset and provide numerical values for signals in the terminal part of the QRS complex [54]. A task force of the ESC, AHA, and ACC [55] published standards for acquisition and analysis of VLP and provided clinical indications for a signal-averaged ECG (SA-ECG). Three common parameters for detecting the presence of VLP have been accepted, and suggested cut-off values were given for two conditions, namely, when noise levels <1 μV with 25 Hz high pass filtering or <0.7 μV with 40 Hz high pass filtering are obtained:

1. fQRS = filtered QRS duration; fQRS >114 ms is regarded as abnormal
2. LAS40 = duration of the low-amplitude fQRS signal <40 μV immediately prior to QRS offset; LAS40 >38 ms is regarded as abnormal, and
3. RMS40 = the root mean square voltage of the terminal 40 ms of the fQRS; RMS40 < 20 μV is regarded as abnormal.

1.5.9.2 Pitfalls and Limitations

From a theoretical point of view, signal averaging from Holter tapes may have some technical limitations such as those due to speed stability of the recording and playback processes, a possible increase of background noise due to the patient's activities or inadequate electrode contact, and a restricted frequency bandwidth of the tape recorder. Most of these shortcomings can now be avoided with modern solid-state digital recorders, which provide a wide frequency bandwidth for retrieving microvolt potentials and also have an appropriately high sampling rate (between 1,000 and 4,000 samples/s), thus enhancing the quality of SA-ECGs and allowing frequency analysis methods without the current frequency restrictions. Despite some technical differences between ambulatory and real-time signal averaging, both methodologies have examined orthogonal XYZ leads, but AECG signal averaging has shown that bipolar leads V1, V5, and aVF also correlate closely with orthogonal leads XYZ. In addition, despite appreciable differences between real time and AECG signal-averaging technologies for bandwidth sampling rate and bit resolution, clinical studies have found close correlation and percent agreement between the two methodologies [56, 57]. Finally, the ability to record and analyze signal-averaged high-resolution ECGs from Holter tapes or solid-state recorders offers clear advantages: easy handling of the recordings, the option of several different recording periods during 24-h of registration, and the chance to assess arrhythmias, ST-segment changes, HRV, heart-rate turbulence, QTV, and late potentials from one data source and to correlate the results with each other.

1.5.10 Reports

There exists no established standard for an adequate AECG report. Most modern Holter recording systems provide composite trend curves for various parameters such as heart rate, arrhythmias, ST-segment deviations, and/or pacemaker activity, histograms of HRV or pacemaker stimulation, tabular summaries of various data, and ECG strips of relevant events either detected from the recordings or patient activated. Real-time ECG strips should provide samples of the ECG at times during which the patient has complained of symptoms, and present a variety of real-time ECG data including samples of each arrhythmia and any ST-segment changes. In many cases, the use of automated computer-based results together with a laser scanning printout of the ECG is useful, particularly for summarizing the data from a lengthy period of recording.

Twenty-four-hour heart-rate trend curves show a mean trend together with the maximum and minimum heart-rate trends calculated over brief time intervals. The difference between these two curves represents the HRV (❷ Fig. 1.20). This visual representation is often useful in understanding the causes of events over a relatively long period of time and for comparison with other events, for example, supraventricular or ventricular arrhythmias or ST-segment depression. Combined with the enumeration of the QRS complexes, it provides some indices, which indicate the variation of the dominant heart rate (usually sinus rate) according to the influence of autonomic tone. In general terms, the difference between day time and night time heart-rate curves is a good index of the importance of sympathetic tone. Moreover, depending on the different special features of Holter systems, many manufacturers provide histograms of QT/R – R relation, HRV, pacemaker stimulatory activity (❷ Figs. 1.22 and ❷ 1.23), or respiratory behavior of the patient.

Diagrams of premature beats are mainly used for displaying counts of PVCs. They express the variation of the number of abnormal events as a function of time and hence give an indication of the 24-h variation. The coupling interval of

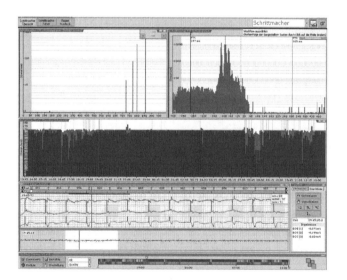

❏ Fig. 1.22

Pacemaker analysis: histogram of the intervals of successive pacemaker pulses (*top left*), histogram of the intervals of pacemaker pulses relative to the corresponding R waves (*top right*), trend diagram of pacemaker-induced ventricular stimulation in bpm over the whole monitoring period in a patient with predominant pacemaker activity (*second row*), and three-channel real-time ECG (*bottom*) (Oxford MedilogDarwin system)

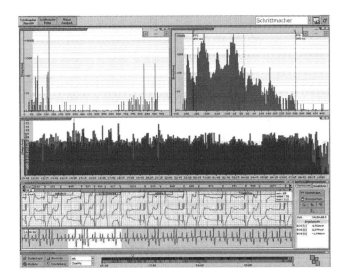

◘ Fig. 1.23

Pacemaker analysis: histogram of the intervals of successive pacemaker pulses (*top left*), histogram of the intervals of pacemaker pulses relative to the corresponding R waves (*top right*), trend diagram of pacemaker-induced ventricular stimulation in bpm over the whole monitoring period in a patient with intermittent pacemaker activity (*second row*), and three-channel real-time ECG (*bottom*) (Oxford MedilogDarwin system)

the premature beats can also be determined and displayed on a separate diagram. The comparison between the heart-rate trends and the PVC diagram is useful in presenting the relationship between heart rate and PVCs with their daily variations (❷ Fig. 1.17).

R – R interval or pacemaker stimulation histograms (❷ Figs. 1.22 and ❷ 1.23) are used by almost all manufacturers with some variations. A histogram of the R – R intervals presents all the QRS complexes arranged as a function of the preceding R – R interval. These R – R-interval histograms can be generated at fixed intervals during the 24 h of real time and superimposed to illustrate their progressive variation or the sudden appearance of an arrhythmia. Another type of graphic reporting is that of Lorenz or Poincaré plots, which summarize the data of HRV over a full AECG recording period. Recently, a novel application of these Lorenz plots has been developed for summarizing the full 24-h ECG data of AF (❷ Fig. 1.24) together with hill-like trend curves (❷ Fig. 1.25).

An essential part of a Holter AECG report is the presentation of a tabular summary of all relevant parameters on an hourly basis, for example, total number of QRS complexes, supraventricular and ventricular ectopic beats, couplets, triplets, or tachycardias, abnormal pauses of cardiac rhythm, HRV criteria both in the time and frequency domain, and pacemaker stimulation as well as pacemaker failures. In addition, full 24-h ECG disclosure – if desired – should be provided, as well as a variety of real-time ECG strips including samples of each arrhythmia or pauses of cardiac rhythm, any ST-segment changes and pacemaker dysfunction.

1.6   Incidence of Arrhythmias in Apparently Healthy Individuals

Before interpreting an AECG recording, the physician should be well acquainted with the findings in the apparently normal population. Some general points can be made from the literature [4, 26, 58–65] concerning the usual and unusual findings in apparently healthy persons.

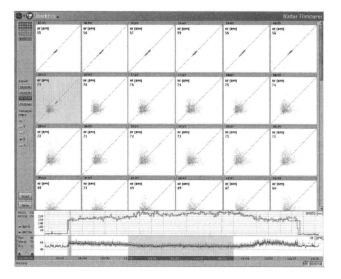

■ Fig. 1.24

Lorenz plots in a patient with sinus rhythm (*top row*) and AF for 20 min intervals each (*middle row*) and trend of HRV time domain parameters together with heart-rate trend (*bottom*) (Medset system)

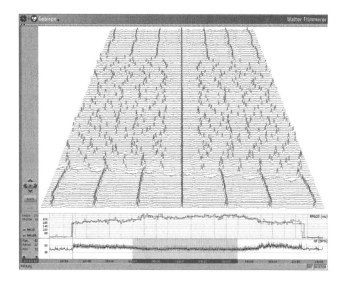

■ Fig. 1.25

Hill-like plot of consecutive ECG complexes in a patient with sinus rhythm (*upper* and *lower segments*) and AF and trend of HRV time domain parameters together with heart-rate trend (*bottom*, Medset system)

1.6.1 Maximal and Minimal Heart Rate

In general, the sinus rate tends to diminish with age as judged by AECG monitoring [58]. This is particularly obvious for the maximum heart rate during daytime. In elderly persons, the heart rate does not usually exceed 130 bpm. On the other hand, in a young population, it is not uncommon for the sinus rate to exceed 180 bpm during waking hours. According to the literature, the mean heart rates for 24-h AECG monitoring are 76.3 ± 11.8 bpm, between 10 a.m. and

6 p.m. they are 79.2 ± 11.0 bpm, and between 1 a.m. and 5 a.m. 66.1 ± 10.8 bpm. Women have a significantly higher mean heart rate than men (5–10 bpm higher [59]). The usual definition of sinus bradycardia (less than 60 bpm) is inappropriate for 24-h Holter ECG reports, because in all "normal" populations, a sinus rate between 40 and 60 bpm is commonly registered during sleep. The minimal sinus rate usually occurs at the end of sleep, that is, between 5 am and 6 am in persons with a normal diurnal cycle. Diurnal and nocturnal variations of sinus rate can easily be appreciated by ambulatory monitoring.

1.6.2 Sinoatrial Pauses

In association with sinus arrhythmia and bradycardia, sinus pauses ranging from 1.2 to 2 s are commonly encountered in 24-h ECG. However, pauses greater than 2 s have been seen in less than 1% of the normal population, usually during sleep and in young subjects. These pauses are probably caused in part by an enhanced vagal tone. Such findings are common in athletes. Therefore, only sinus pauses in excess of 2 s can be considered as abnormal, and therefore require further attention in adult or elderly subjects.

1.6.3 AV Block

First-degree and second-degree AV block are occasionally noted during ambulatory monitoring in healthy individuals. These blocks most commonly occur during sleep and are accompanied by sinus bradyarrhythmia. Second-degree AV block is always of the Mobitz type I, even if in some cases it occurs abruptly, thus making the increase of PR-interval duration less obvious. These episodes, which occur during sleep in young subjects, are always asymptomatic. In some rare cases, more significant conduction disturbances can be recorded, as in the example of ❷ Fig. 1.26. The ECGs are from a 37-year-old man submitted to ambulatory monitoring because of atypical chest pain. The symptoms were subsequently found to be unrelated to CAD, which was confirmed by coronary angiography and vasospastic provocative tests. During sleep, two episodes of second-degree AV block occurred with two or three P waves blocked in succession. Another recording performed one week later revealed the same phenomenon. This patient remained free of syncope or dizziness after a 4-year follow-up. ❷ Table 1.4 summarizes the arrhythmias that should be considered "normal for age" according to the literature.

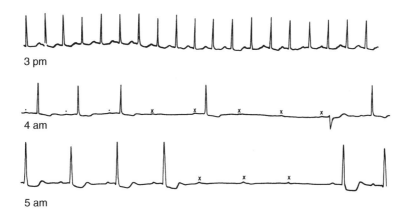

❏ Fig. 1.26

Paroxysmal AV block (blocked P waves are marked with crosses) occurring during the night in a young athletic man with no detectable heart disease. After four years of clinical follow up, this subject remained asymptomatic

⬛ Table 1.4

Normal findings of heart rate and arrhythmias on 24-hour ambulatory ECG monitoring according to age

Arrhythmias	Age ⩽ 25 years	Age 25–65 years	Age > 65 years
Sinus pauses	⩽2,500 ms	⩽2,000 ms	⩽2,000 ms
AV block	some occurring at night	none (except in case of regular physical training)	none
APCs	<10 h^{-1}	<10 h^{-1}	<100 h^{-1}
Atrial tachycardia (3 or more APCs)	none	none < 50 years some > 50 years	some
PVCs	<10 h^{-1}	<10 h^{-1}	<100 h^{-1}
Ventricular tachycardia (3 or more PVCs)	none	single <10 QRS	single <10 QRS

1.6.4 Atrial Arrhythmias

Atrial premature contractions (APCs) detected by AECG are reported to occur in 23–100% of normal persons studied [60–65]. The incidence of APCs increases significantly with age, being nearly absent in children (if it is distinguished from physiological sinus arrhythmia), but almost constantly present in healthy individuals of 65 years and more. Moreover, in these normal elderly patients, it is common to find frequent APCs (>1 min^{-1}) and/or episodes of paroxysmal atrial tachycardia (PAT). The incidence of PAT varies greatly from one report to another, but an awareness of the high incidence of PAT is of major importance for the interpretation of 24-h recordings in older patients complaining of symptoms. The discovery of a short isolated PAT in an 80-year-old subject does not imply any relationship with the symptom if it was not simultaneously felt during the recording.

1.6.5 Ventricular Arrhythmias

The occurrence of premature ventricular contractions (PVCs) in normal populations as detected by Holter recordings has been reported to range from 17% to 100% of individuals studied [60–65]. Depending on the variable length of ambulatory examination in these studies, one may conclude that the incidence of PVCs is approximately 50% in normal persons examined for 24 h and increases to approximately 75% in those studied for 48 h. Where various age groups have been studied, there is a clear relationship between age and the incidence of PVCs. Normally, healthy individuals have less than 100 PVCs per day without any runs of VT. In some healthy aged persons, however, numerous, perhaps multifocal, PVCs can occur and, more rarely, short runs of VT. In particular, accelerated idioventricular rhythm may occur during sleep.

According to these data, it is possible to consider as unusual the prevalence of frequent (>1 min^{-1}) or complex PVCs in individuals less than 65 years old. Such a prevalence and frequency of PVCs is not, of course, necessarily pathologic, but does require further examination to determine whether or not there is an underlying heart disease.

1.7 ST-Segment Changes in Apparently Healthy Persons

There are not many reports of ST-segment changes on 24-h ECGs in apparently healthy persons. However, three important studies have been published [66–68] involving 50, 120, and 182 volunteers, respectively.

In the first [66], ST-segment depression was defined as at least 0.1 mV horizontal or downsloping shift of the ST segment persisting 80 ms after the J point of the QRS complex. It occurred in 10–30% of the normal population in these studies, with multiple episodes in the majority of these during a single 24-h ECG recording. These changes usually took place at the same time as daily exercise, with a cardiac rate of over 100 beats per minute. Isolated T-wave inversion was even more frequent.

The frequency of ST-segment elevation (>0.1 mV) at the J point in these healthy subjects is a matter of some debate, being absent in the study of Armstrong et al. [66] but present in 23% of the volunteers of Quyyumi et al. [67]. In this study, ST-segment elevation occurred preferentially in young men, with a simultaneous low heart rate. At the same time, T waves became upright and peaked. The mean duration was usually very long (several hours). The difference between the two studies is probably caused by a difference in the criteria of positivity, while the pattern of ST changes is different from that observed in spontaneous angina. In these latter patients, ST elevation includes the T wave, with an aspect of the monophasic action potential, and the R wave increases. These modifications are progressive and persist for a few minutes only. Some studies have emphasized the fact that ST-T changes are more frequently encountered in female volunteers than in male volunteers; for example, 18% versus 1% in the Bjerregaard study [68].

Many ST-T abnormalities may be caused by positional change of the subject during the course of 24 h, and every effort should be made to assess whether ST-T change is indeed a genuine phenomenon. It should also be noted that most analyzers available at the present time do not detect major T-wave changes including a complete reversal of T-wave polarity. This is a significant shortcoming of all systems, although the operator could in fact position the ST marker at a point in the early part of the T wave if a search for T-wave changes is particularly desired. According to the literature, ST-segment elevation $\leqslant 0.3$ mV at night with T-wave increase upward or downward in individuals at ages below 40 years are considered normal, as is the case for ST-segment depression $\leqslant 0.2$ mV during tachycardia with upward or downward sloping ST segment accompanied by all types of T-wave changes as well.

Despite its shortcomings, 24-h ECG examination represents a useful diagnostic procedure in patients with spontaneous chest pain. In subjects with exercise-related symptoms, an exercise test provides more precise data with a higher specificity.

1.8 Clinical Relevance of AECG Recording

1.8.1 Evaluation of Patient's Symptoms

Patients often complain of symptoms, which are transient but suggest a cardiac origin. Holter ECG is an essential examination in such cases. This noninvasive technique is able to provide an accurate diagnosis, especially if the symptom coincides with any ECG abnormality detected during the recording. The most widely accepted use of AECG is the determination of patient's transient symptoms to cardiac arrhythmias. Some symptoms such as palpitation, syncope, near syncope, or dizziness are commonly caused by transient arrhythmias, whereas other transient symptoms such as shortness of breath, chest discomfort, diaphoresis, weakness, or transient ischemic cerebral attacks are less commonly related to cardiac arrhythmias. In principle, four possible outcomes may be expected with AECG monitoring: (1) typical symptoms may occur with the simultaneous documentation of a cardiac arrhythmia, (2) symptoms may occur at periods with no cardiac arrhythmias seen in the AECG, (3) during cardiac arrhythmias the patient may remain asymptomatic, and (4) the patient may remain symptomatic during AECG recording, and no arrhythmias are documented. With regard to situations (1) and (2), such findings are useful for further management of the patient in that either the symptoms can be related to arrhythmias or arrhythmias are not the cause of symptoms. The finding in the third situation is equivocal and in the fourth situation not helpful for further clarification of the patient's complaints.

1.8.1.1 Palpitations

Many patients complain of a variety of symptoms grouped under the term palpitations [4, 69–71]. If these symptoms are frequent, for example, every day, 24-h Holter ambulatory monitoring is the optimum way for their evaluation. In many cases, an abnormality can be seen at the time of the symptoms, signifying that they are related to a cardiac arrhythmia. Sometimes, a sinus tachycardia represents the electrocardiographic basis for palpitations. In contrast, it is well known that patients may have quite severe cardiac arrhythmias without being aware of them. This is particularly true for isolated PVCs, for frequent PVCs, and for short runs of VT. In any event, if palpitations are perceived during the recording, an accurate evaluation is easily provided by replaying the cassette tape or computer digitized ECG storage at the corresponding time. The problem is quite different in the absence of palpitations during ambulatory monitoring. In this case, the finding of one normal 24-h recording does not permit any conclusion to be drawn and the surveillance should be continued if symptoms have previously occurred with a reasonable frequency.

More difficult is the problem of the relevance of some arrhythmias recorded during ambulatory monitoring without simultaneous palpitations. Their significance depends on the incidence of the type of arrhythmia in the normal population. The occurrence of PVCs, even with some salvos, in an adult or aged patient, particularly if the patient suffers from coronary heart disease (CHD), is of little relevance; it is of limited importance to conclude that palpitations are caused by paroxysmal VT. Similarly, the discovery of short runs of atrial tachycardia in an elderly patient is irrelevant. However, if the arrhythmia observed is unusual according to the characteristics of the patient, it is probable that it may be the cause of the palpitations. This situation is variable according to the circumstances and the patient's activities. Nevertheless, the certainty of the diagnosis can only be assessed by an ECG recorded simultaneously with the symptom. For all these reasons, AECG monitoring is the preferred diagnostic method of examining such patients and is equally or more sensitive than other reported diagnostic techniques. The major exception is in relation to paroxysmal reciprocating junctional tachycardia where the attacks are very rare. The AECG recording is always normal between the attacks.

1.8.1.2   Dizziness or Syncope

Transient disturbances of consciousness producing dizziness or syncope are most commonly caused by a critical circulatory decrease in cerebral blood flow. Sinoatrial pauses or paroxysmal AV block may cause these symptoms, but modifications of heart rate alone may also cause disturbances of cerebral blood flow, mainly through tachycardia [4, 69–71]. It is now clear that healthy persons may tolerate a heart rate as low as 30 bpm and be asymptomatic, but ventricular rates higher than 150 bpm, particularly in elderly subjects or when underlying heart disease is present, often lead to a decrease in cerebral blood flow by causing inadequate ventricular diastolic filling and fall in cardiac output.

In several studies, a continuous ECG recording taken until symptoms have occurred shows that dizziness or loss of consciousness are, in the majority of cases, caused by a paroxysmal tachycardia (of atrial or ventricular origin) and not, as might be expected, by paroxysmal SA or AV blocks. Important inter-individual variations in the tolerance of arrhythmias are now well known. A normal young subject can tolerate an ectopic tachycardia with a heart rate in excess of 200 bpm or ventricular pauses of more than 3 s without producing symptoms of cerebral ischemia, whereas an older patient may faint after a few seconds of atrial tachycardia at 150 bpm. The state of the cerebral vessels, the presence or absence of cardiac disease, the body position and the duration of tachycardia or bradycardia are important considerations, and the occurrence or absence of symptoms depends on a combination of these factors.

Overall, the diagnostic yield of AECG monitoring for syncope or near syncope is relatively low. Seven to thirty-nine percent of patients with symptoms during AECG were reported to have no arrhythmia, and 1–26% to have arrhythmias. In patients without symptoms during AECG, 17–80% had no arrhythmia and 10–41% had episodes of arrhythmias [7]. In the study of Bass et al. [72], the value of three consecutive 24-h monitoring periods was evaluated. A major abnormality within the first 24-h recording was seen in 15% of patients, the additive yield was 11% on the second, and 4.2% in the third sequential recording. In this study, age, male sex, history of heart disease, and initial rhythm other than sinus were identified as factors that identified a useful recording [72].

1.8.1.3   Previous Ischemic Strokes

With the development of 24-h Holter recordings, previous ischemic cerebrovascular attacks become an important indication for this examination [73–76]. In most cases of this type of disease, the exact cause of the stroke remains unclear. Thus, the 24-h Holter examination is performed to search for a cardiac arrhythmia that might cause cerebral embolism.

Those arrhythmias able to induce a systemic embolism are almost always paroxysmal atrial arrhythmias and, in a few cases, VT, in the presence of left ventricular thrombus owing to previous myocardial infarction or cardiomyopathy. When an underlying cardiac disease is present, the diagnosis of systemic embolism is easier, but if clinical examination is completely normal, a 24-h AECG recording remains the best way of detecting a paroxysmal arrhythmia. However, the systematic use of this technique in all ischemic strokes is disappointing, since only a small proportion of patients with significant paroxysmal atrial arrhythmias may be identified. The great majority of these patients with previous stroke are over 60 years old and the relevance of these arrhythmias is unclear. As previously described, a significant proportion of "normal" elderly subjects can exhibit some short runs of atrial tachycardia. Therefore, the occurrence of such a disorder in a patient at risk of ischemic strokes does not prove by itself that the arrhythmia is the actual cause of the stroke. Only a sustained atrial tachycardia (lasting more than 10 min) should be considered as relevant in these elderly patients. As a result, the practical consequences (that is, the decision to begin anti-arrhythmic and/or anticoagulant therapy) are rarely directly related to the result of the 24-h AECG recording. In view of the economic and human costs of this technique, it is not recommended that it be performed systematically in all cases of stroke. It is preferable to reserve it for the younger patients (in which case an atrial arrhythmia is definitely relevant) or for cardiac patients, in whom there is the likelihood of a sustained arrhythmia.

1.8.1.4   Chest Pain

Transient unpredictable chest pain is a frequent symptom and may present a diagnostic problem for the clinician. Although exercise stress testing should be the first line of investigation, occasionally AECG may be a more practical and useful diagnostic test, particularly if the chest pain is unpredictable with respect to time of onset or cannot be provoked by exercise. Two- or three-channel AECG recording permits examination of anterior, inferior, and lateral myocardial leads for the detection of ischemic ST-segment changes during episodes of chest pain with or without cardiac arrhythmias [77–82].

Twenty-four-hour Holter ECG has emerged as a primary method of examination in patients with suspected variant angina in whom pain usually occurs unpredictably [78, 79]. The diagnostic value of this technique is demonstrated in the example of ❷ Fig. 1.273. In this case, considerable ST-segment elevation occurs during an episode of atypical chest pain, and there can be little doubt about the existence of variant angina probably caused by coronary artery spasm. The absence of ST-segment changes, however, appears to be of lesser value in reassuring the patient and the clinician that ischemic heart disease is absent because of the possibility of false-negative responses owing to inadequate lead positioning, short-lived ST-T changes, which are not detected during visual analysis of the replayed tape, as well as other factors. Finally, it should be stressed that only considerable deviation of the ST segment should be regarded as significant because of the frequency of minor abnormalities in normal persons during continuous ambulatory recordings.

1.8.2   Appraisal of the Mechanism of Arrhythmias

One of the major advantages of AECG is the facility to clarify the circumstances preceding the onset of arrhythmias. This technique enables the clinician to appreciate the many important characteristics concerning the mechanism of the arrhythmias, in particular the role of the autonomic nervous system (ANS) in more general terms, he/she can deduce the rhythmological explanation of the paroxysmal arrhythmia in question.

1.8.2.1   Sinoatrial Disorders

The main use of 24-h Holter ECG in this particular group of disorders [4, 83] is to indicate whether SA dysfunction is dependent on the daily cycle or on the sinus rate. This appears to be of importance in differentiating between "physiological" vagotonic SA pauses occurring in a young athletic subject during sleep or at rest and "pathological" SA block

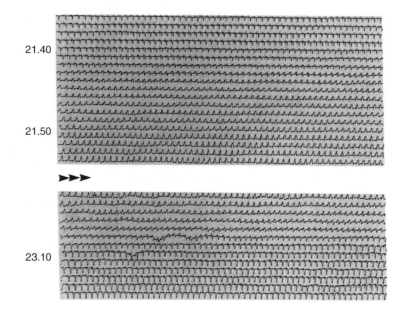

■ Fig. 1.27

An example of an ECG recorded during an episode of variant angina. The ECG is produced as a fiber-optic printout where one line represents 1 min. The time of recording is indicated on the *left*. Note the alteration between deep negative T waves on the one hand (as at 21.40) and marked ST elevation on the other (as at 21.50)

occurring at any time of the day or night. Moreover, in some cases, Holter monitoring is able to indicate that SA dysfunction occurs specifically when the sinus rate increases. This is a strong argument for concluding that a phase III SA block exists, and not merely a transient interruption of sinus automaticity. In this type of conduction disorder, the abnormalities are usually detected during the first 24-h Holter recording. A completely normal AECG recording constitutes a strong argument for the elimination of SA block from the differential diagnosis.

1.8.2.2 AV Block and Intraventricular Disorders

AECG monitoring is sometimes able to determine the mechanism of AV or intraventricular conduction disorders. This technique may be able to distinguish between proximal and distal AV block (between Mobitz type I and II) and between physiological and pathological blocks. In general terms, if a nodal AV block exists, it is usually present on numerous occasions during a 24-h recording, while it is easy to differentiate the physiological nodal AV block occurring abruptly during sleep in a young athletic subject from the permanent pathological block (of varying degrees) in an elderly patient. It is much rarer to capture a distal AV block during a single 24-h examination. However, in this case it is sometimes possible to discern a peculiar mechanism such as modifications of sinus rate or occurrence of long or short R–R cycles. A typical pattern of paroxysmal AV block caused by sinus tachycardia (phase III block) is shown in ❷ Fig. 1.28. This kind of tachycardia-dependent AV block is characteristic of a distal localization (intra-Hisian or infra-Hisian).

In these examples, all the usual characteristics of the conduction disorder are detected by AECG monitoring and an EPS becomes unnecessary. In the same way, the mechanism of some intermittent intraventricular conduction disturbances can be elicited by 24-h monitoring (phase III or phase IV blocks, succession of long and short R–R cycles). The discovery of an intermittent bundle branch block may be important clinically. A paroxysmal AV block seems less probable in the presence of an isolated intermittent bundle branch block than in the presence of a permanent bundle branch block.

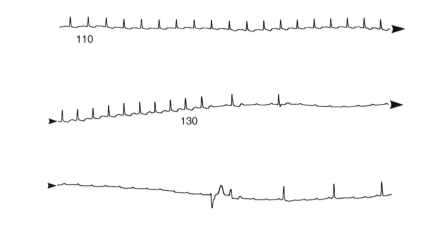

◘ Fig. 1.28
Paroxysmal AV block occurring during sinus tachycardia (phase III block) at 130 bpm (heart rate indicated on figure in bpm). A subsequent EPS showed intra-His bundle AV block reproduced by rapid atrial pacing

1.8.2.3 Paroxysmal Atrial Arrhythmias

In a large number of patients, the reason for the occurrence of a paroxysmal atrial arrhythmia [84, 85] remains unclear, particularly when no morphologic changes of the atria can be found. AECG monitoring is often useful in such cases since on many occasions it demonstrates the importance of the ANS in the genesis of the arrhythmia. Two opposite forms of paroxysmal arrhythmias can then be described, namely, vagally induced arrhythmias and adrenergically induced arrhythmias. With respect to the former, the atrial arrhythmia is preceded by a progressive decrease of sinus rate either during night or at rest, as demonstrated by heart-rate trend curves (e.g., ❷ Fig. 1.29). Usually, this heart-rate threshold is not unduly low (50–60 bpm). Middle-aged patients may experience palpitations, and sometimes peripheral embolisms. The atrial arrhythmia remains in paroxysmal form for a long period, commonly more than 10 years. It becomes progressively more frequent, occurring either daily or several times a day, and appears resistant to conventional therapy. Beta blockers, digitalis, and verapamil usually aggravate the arrhythmia and class I drugs are also unsatisfactory. Only amiodarone may be helpful when taken alone in the initial stages of the disease and in the later stages when combined with a class I drug. In some instances, sinus bradycardia preceding the onset of the atrial arrhythmia occurs abruptly during a few R–R cycles, suggesting a sudden increase in vagal tone as shown in ❷ Fig. 1.30. In these cases, it is sometimes possible to find a gastrointestinal reason for this enhanced vagal tone. Treating this condition may suppress the arrhythmia simultaneously. In some cases, which are resistant to all combinations of drugs, rapid atrial pacing may improve the clinical situation.

The opposite form, the paroxysmal adrenergic atrial arrhythmia, appears less frequent in contrast to the high frequency of palpitations experienced during exercise, emotion, or other high-hyperadrenergic states, which are mainly caused by isolated sinus tachycardia without rhythm disturbances. This type of arrhythmia is preceded by a progressive increase of sinus rate during daytime, which is not necessarily related to physical exercise (❷ Fig. 1.31). Except for some patients with an unsuspected hyperthyroidism, any organic cardiac disease may be present. Beta blockers are able to control the arrhythmia for some weeks or months, after which an escape phenomenon occurs, which requires additional class I drug therapy. Amiodarone or propafenone may be useful due to their noncompetitive inhibitive effect on the beta adrenoreceptors. The distinction between these two opposite forms of atrial paroxysmal arrhythmia often appears to be somewhat theoretical, because many patients cannot be easily classified into one or other type. On many occasions, however, ambulatory monitoring is of great value in these patients to provide a guideline for therapy.

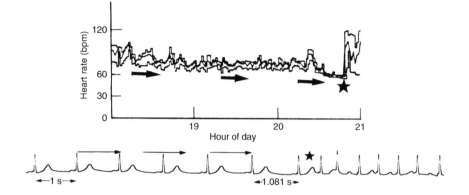

◻ Fig. 1.29

An example of a vagally induced atrial arrhythmia. A progressive sinus bradycardia with changes in atrial depolarization precedes the onset of AF. The change in rhythm marked by the *star* is also detected on the rate-trend curves

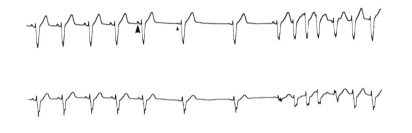

◻ Fig. 1.30

Another example of a vagally induced atrial arrhythmia. The onset of AF is preceded by a sudden sinus bradycardia

1.8.2.4   Paroxysmal Junctional Reciprocating Tachycardias

Usually, Holter monitoring is unprofitable in paroxysmal junctional reciprocating tachycardias because of the rarity of the attacks and the normality of the ECG recording between attacks. However, in some patients with frequent episodes of this type of tachycardia, ambulatory monitoring is able to demonstrate the mechanism that triggers its onset. When combined with the data from an EPS detailing the reentry circuit, the knowledge of the triggering mechanism often constitutes a guideline for therapy, for patients incapacitated by their arrhythmia. The most frequent initiation mode of the reciprocating tachycardia appears to be premature atrial contractions (PACs). It is interesting that in some patients, PACs are able to trigger the arrhythmia only if they occur during sinus tachycardia, reflecting an increase in sympathetic tone. This predisposing role of the adrenergic system is well known. Clinicians use isoprenaline during electrophysiological studies to induce the tachycardia more easily by atrial premature stimulation; this is because of the facilitation of conduction through normal and/or accessory pathways. In some of these patients, beta-blocking drugs should be added to previous antiarrhythmic therapy in order to obtain a satisfactory result.

Less frequently, the triggering mechanism of the tachycardia is PVCs, and in some patients with numerous PVCs it is remarkable that the tachycardia occurs only with a couplet and never with isolated PVCs. In a similar manner, during electrophysiological studies, a single ventricular extrastimulus is frequently unable to induce the tachycardia, which occurs with two or more extrastimuli. The practical consequence in this case is that there is a good chance of success for class I or III AADs being able to suppress the repetitive phenomena of PVCs. The three other mechanisms of triggering, specific for accessory pathways, require individual recognition and treatment. Induction of reciprocating tachycardias by sinus tachycardia (owing to a phase III block in concealed anterograde conduction through the accessory pathway) should be treated by beta-blocking agents or by amiodarone. The reverse situation, that is, induction by junctional escape beats (preventing concealed or patent anterograde conduction through a Kent bundle) or sinus bradycardia (with a phase

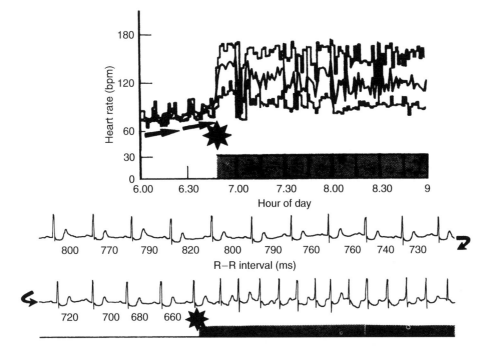

◘ Fig. 1.31

An example of an adrenergic atrial arrhythmia. Paroxysmal AF is preceded by a progressive sinus tachycardia. The change in rhythm labeled by the asterisk can also be seen on the heart-rate trend curves

IV block in the Kent bundle) usually requires pacemaker implantation or catheter ablation. The most recent and highly effective mode of therapy is catheter ablation of the accessory pathway based on a detailed mapping procedure using multiple intracardiac catheter electrodes.

1.8.2.5 Ventricular Arrhythmias

AECG monitoring is normally less useful than electrophysiological studies in elucidating an electrophysiological mechanism of ventricular arrhythmias [86–88]. The EPS is superior in providing criteria that suggest reentry, for example. In contrast, 24-h Holter monitoring is the examination of choice in the case of parasystolic beats, providing most useful data for the study of these rhythm disturbances [89]. In general, recording the onset of VT often reveals important information on the intrinsic mechanisms of the arrhythmia. Some examples illustrating these findings and their practical consequences are now discussed.

❷ Figure 1.32 shows a run of VT initiated by a compensatory pause following a single PVC with a morphological pattern different to those of the VT. This is a good demonstration of two different conditions necessary for the initiation of VT; that is, an isolated PVC as the trigger mechanism and a ventricular pause creating local conditions favorable to the sustaining mechanism of VT (focal or intraventricular reentry). In this situation, two therapeutic regimes can be proposed: suppression of the trigger mechanism or depression of the sustaining mechanism. ❷ Figure 1.33 is another example of a possible duality of the mechanisms involved in the genesis of a VT: an intraventricular reentry (as confirmed subsequently by EPS) triggered by APBs. In this case also, antiarrhythmic therapy may suppress the clinical VT in two different ways. The role of sympathetic tone, often important in the genesis of VT, is easily demonstrated by AECG monitoring, showing the relationship between VT and sinus tachycardia, which reflects an enhanced sympathetic activity. In the case presented in ❷ Fig. 1.34, paroxysmal VT occurs and persists during a period of sinus tachycardia owing to psychological stress, and disappears only when sinus tachycardia ceases. In the same manner, in some cases of sudden death,

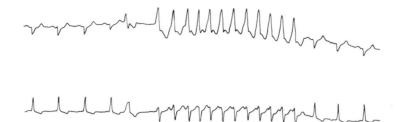

■ **Fig. 1.32**

A two-channel Holter ECG showing a run of VT initiated by a PVC of different morphological patterns followed by a compensatory pause. This spontaneous mode of initiation is unusual in patients with reentrant VT, which is easily induced by electrophysiological means

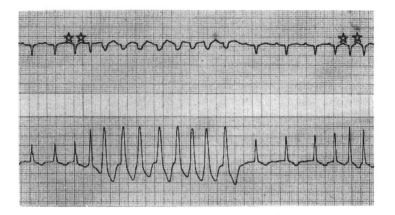

■ **Fig. 1.33**

An example of bitachycardia (coexistence of atrial and VT) in a patient with cardiomyopathy. A run of VT is initiated by a couplet of APCs indicated by the first pair of stars. Two simultaneously recorded leads are shown. In this case, the VT could be triggered by extra stimulation and was probably caused by a reentrant mechanism

sinus tachycardia indicating an increased sympathetic tone seems to play an important role in the triggering mechanism of the fatal arrhythmia.

The understanding of the mechanism of sudden death in cardiac patients is probably the best recent example. As demonstrated by some important series [90–92], the role of myocardial ischemia is practically confined to asystoles, and the vast majority of sudden deaths caused by a ventricular tachyarrhythmia are not directly caused by ischemia. Iatrogenic (drug-induced) "torsades de pointes" may be responsible for sudden death in noncoronary patients. Ventricular fibrillation (VF) is the usual mode of sudden death in coronary patients without preceding ischemia. VF usually follows a sustained VT, which accelerates before its transformation into VF. The electrophysiological phenomena leading to VT/VF are a shortening of the coupling interval of PVCs, a long R–R cycle (postextrasystolic pause) in half of the cases, an atrial arrhythmia or, more generally, an increase of heart rate reflecting an increase of sympathetic tone. This latter represents the main determinant of VT/VF.

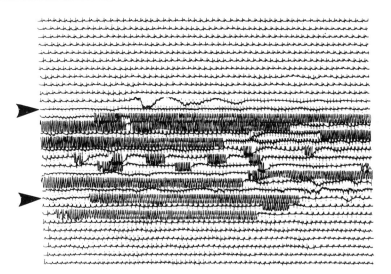

○ Fig. 1.34
A fiber-optic printout showing clearly the catecholergic mechanism of a ventricular arrhythmia. The salvos of VT are preceded by a marked acceleration of the sinus rhythm (indicated by *arrows*) and disappear when the sinus rate decreases

1.8.3   Monitoring for Myocardial Ischemia

1.8.3.1   General Considerations

In contrast to previous technical problems and limitations, with recent advancements of recorders with digital ECG and high-sampling rates, it is generally accepted that AECG monitoring provides accurate and clinically meaningful information about myocardial ischemia in patients with CAD [4, 91, 92]. After careful hook-up and testing for nonspecific ST-segment alterations due to hypoventilation or positional changes (testing in supine, prone, lateral, and sitting positions), the patients are asked to keep an accurate and complete diary of symptoms associated with specific events or activities, time of occurrence and disappearance of symptoms, and all other activities before the start of the recording. Upon return of the patient, a thorough review and confirmation of the diary entries has to be performed.

AECG provides a unique insight into the presence and severity of myocardial ischemia in patients with CAD. Unlike stress testing, AECG evaluates patients in their usual environment, allowing for assessment of ischemic jeopardy when the patient is exposed to the emotional or physical stress of daily life. Such insights concerning ischemia are fundamentally different from assessing ischemia in a supervised hospital or laboratory setting, where exercise stress testing is usually performed. The correlations between indices of ischemia during AECG monitoring and stress testing are quite weak [92]. An assessment of ischemic jeopardy by one technique is not a surrogate for ischemic jeopardy by the other technique [91, 93]. Most studies using AECG for ischemia assessment have been performed in patients with CAD, and there is a paucity of data regarding the role of AECG monitoring in asymptomatic individuals without known CAD or peripheral vascular disease. Thus, there is presently no evidence that AECG monitoring provides reliable information concerning ischemia in asymptomatic subjects without known CAD [93].

In addition to providing long-term monitoring for myocardial ischemia in an outpatient setting, AECG monitoring is also useful for detection of myocardial ischemia in preoperative risk stratification for patients who cannot exercise because of peripheral vascular disease, physical disability, or advanced lung disease. Moreover, it can be helpful for evaluation of patients with anginal episodes due to suspected variant angina, in whom an exercise test was negative. Finally, 24–48-h

AECG monitoring can provide information about the circadian pattern of myocardial ischemia and the pathophysiological mechanisms responsible for the ischemic episodes. It is particularly useful for detecting the extent of painless episodes of myocardial ischemia (so-called silent ischemia) that would otherwise remain undiagnosed, for example, by an exercise test.

1.8.3.2   Silent Myocardial Ischemia (SI)

The syndrome of painless myocardial ischemia was first described by Gettes in 1974 [94]. Since then, this syndrome, which is now usually referred to as SI, has attracted much attention, particularly its relation to sudden death [95–97]. The pathophysiology of painless (silent) ischemia in patients with stable CAD is not completely understood. Myocardial ischemia may occur either from episodic increase in myocardial oxygen demand, most conveniently identified by heart rate and blood pressure increase, or from an episodic decrease in myocardial oxygen supply related to either transient coronary artery vasoconstriction, transient platelet aggregation, or both. The actual identification of the presence of coronary vasoconstriction is deduced from heart-rate thresholds at which ischemia occurs: if heart-rate thresholds for ischemia vary in a given patient with stable CAD and ischemia occurs at lower heart-rate thresholds, it is likely that intermittent vasoconstriction is responsible, and when vasoconstriction is relieved, or vasodilation occurs, ischemia develops at higher heart-rate thresholds. If heart rate increases by $\geqslant 5$ bpm prior to an ischemic episode, this may suggest an increase of myocardial oxygen demand as the cause of ischemia, whereas the absence of heart-rate increase favors a decrease of oxygen supply as the ischemia-producing mechanism [98]. The fact that ischemia can be seen on AECG during normal daily activities at heart-rate thresholds 10–20% lower than heart-rate thresholds for ischemia during an exercise test suggests that episodes of ischemia during normal activities may at least in part be related to intermittent coronary vasoconstriction [92, 99]. Understanding the pathophysiology of ischemia in patients with stable CAD is made more complicated by the fact that many routine daily activities both increase myocardial oxygen demand and provoke coronary vasoconstriction such as mental or physical stress, exposure to cold, or cigarette smoking. In addition, elevated serum cholesterol or estrogen deprivation may create or exacerbate endothelial dysfunction that is responsible for coronary vasoconstriction. These pathophysiological considerations are important, since pharmacological treatment is often quite different with regard to the culprit mechanism of ischemia, and these different treatment options may also have important implications for prognosis.

From the literature, it is quite clear that the vast majority of episodes of transient ST-segment deviation during AECG monitoring occur in the absence of symptoms. Episodes of asymptomatic ischemia occur in 20–50% of patients with all types of CAD, that is, stable angina, unstable angina, and AMI, and the asymptomatic episodes may outnumber the symptomatic episodes by more than 20-fold. Explanations for the fact that some episodes are painful and some produce no symptoms include the following:

1. Episodes of silent ischemia may be less "severe" than symptomatic episodes, so the anginal threshold is not reached [100].
2. Disorders of the peripheral autonomic nerves, for example, diabetic neuropathy, may blunt the nociceptive signal of ischemia [101].
3. Increased beta-endorphin levels may decrease the central perception of myocardial pain [102, 103].
4. Abnormal central processing of afferent messages from the heart may occur due to non-myocardial factors and emotional or personality characteristics (so-called "gate theory": the cerebral cortex itself modulates the nociceptive signal that it receives) [104].

Cohn [96] has divided patients with SI into three groups:

1. Asymptomatic individuals who may suddenly die from CHD
2. Asymptomatic survivors of AMI; and
3. Anginal patients who have painless, as well as painful episodes

While detection of groups 1 and 2 relies on exercise testing, Holter monitoring is the most valuable method for detecting group 3. The clinical presentation of these 3 patient groups, as well as their prognosis, may be quite different. However, myocardial ischemia by itself represents an independent risk factor for patients with all types of CAD, that is, stable angina pectoris as well as unstable coronary syndromes (NSTEMI, STEMI).

1.8.3.3 Prevalence and Prognostic Significance of Myocardial Ischemia

In patients with stable CAD and angina pectoris, the prevalence of myocardial ischemia in AECG monitoring ranges between 20% and 45%, and in patients with unstable angina or with a previous myocardial infarction, it is between 30% and 40% [7]. Between 60% and 80% of ischemic episodes detected by AECG monitoring are reported to be asymptomatic. As to the prognostic significance in AECG monitoring, silent as well as symptomatic myocardial ischemia identifies patients at a significantly higher risk of future cardiac events and cardiac death [105–116]. ❷ Table 1.5 shows the results of these studies: at a mean follow-up between 10 and 37 months, the event rate for death, cardiac death, myocardial infarction, unstable angina, or revascularization ranged from 3% to 42% in patients without ischemic episodes, compared to event rates from 23% to 56% in patients with documented episodes of myocardial ischemia. These differences were statistically significant for all studies cited. Moreover, some studies have shown that ischemia detected by AECG monitoring can provide prognostic information additional to that obtained from established parameters during exercise testing [93, 106, 111, 115].

In the past, AECG monitoring has also been used to define the risk of perioperative events in patients without clinical evidence of CAD undergoing surgery for peripheral vascular disease. These patients were reported to have evidence of myocardial ischemia in 10–40% of cases, and the perioperative event rates were between 1% and 16% in those with a negative test as compared to those with event rates of 4–15% with a positive test [7]. From a clinical point of view, it should be emphasized that an exercise test alone, eventually combined with an echo or other imaging study, should suffice for preoperative evaluation. Only in patients who cannot undertake an exercise test, AECG monitoring for ischemia can be used for further evaluation.

AECG monitoring has also been used for evaluation of anti-ischemic therapy in patients with CAD. In this respect, it should be stressed that due to the significant day-to-day variability of ischemic ST-segment alterations, prolonged monitoring periods of at least 48 h should be performed. A number of studies have shown that 48-h AECG recording performed at baseline and after initiation of antianginal therapy can provide reliable information about the anti-ischemic efficacy and the prognosis of the patients. Some randomized clinical trials have demonstrated that suppression of myocardial ischemia as evaluated by AECG monitoring may improve the outcome in patients with CAD (❷ Table 1.6): the event rates in patients on antianginal drugs versus placebo, or for 100% responders versus non-100% responders, were significantly lower in patients with successful antianginal or anti-ischemic therapy [117–121]. Since data on this important application of AECG monitoring are relatively sparse, further large-scale prospective randomized clinical trials are needed to confirm these results, and to evaluate the definite role of AECG monitoring in the anti-anginal or anti-ischemic management of patients with CAD.

1.8.3.4 Limitations of Holter Monitoring for Myocardial Ischemia

When assessing patients with suspected myocardial ischemia, it is important to mention again that ST-segment changes and other repolarization abnormalities can occur for reasons other than myocardial ischemia, for example, LV hypertrophy, LV dysfunction, hyperventilation, systemic hypertension (SH), postural changes, conduction abnormalities, preexcitation, tachyarrhythmias, fluctuations of sympathetic tone, AADs, digitalis, psychotropic drugs, and electrolyte abnormalities. Moreover, the importance of proper electrode placement to retrieve myocardial ischemia from all parts of ventricular myocardium by using at least one anterior and one inferior lead has already been emphasized. A further potential limitation is the marked day-to-day variability in the frequency, degree and duration of ST-segment alterations, and ischemic episodes that makes the assessment of the effects of therapeutic interventions on ischemic indices very difficult. This problem may be overcome by prolonging the AECG recording period to 48 or 72 h and assessing similar physical and emotional activities of the patients during the serial monitoring sessions. Finally, in some patients, changes in T-wave polarity and morphology can be observed during Holter monitoring, but there are presently no data to suggest that such changes are specific for myocardial ischemia [7].

● Table 1.5

Observational studies on the incidence and prognostic significance of daily life ischemia (modified according to Cohn 1998)

Authors, year	No. patients	Incidence of AECG ischemia (%)	End points	Mean follow-up (months)	Event rates (%) With AECG ischemia	Event rates (%) Without ischemia	P-value	Comments
Rocco (1988)	86	57	Death, MI, UA, revasc.	12.5	40	3	0.003	Patients monitored once off Rx
Tzivoni (1988)	118	33	Cardiac death, MI, UA, revasc.	28	51	20	<0.001	All patients with previous MI
Hedblad (1989)	394	25	Cardiac death & nonfatal MI	43	15	3	<0.001	
Deedwania and Carbajal (1990)	107	43	Cardiac death	23	24	8	0.02	Monitored on Rx
Raby (1990)	176	18	Cardiac death, nonfatal MI	20	38	7	<0.0001	Patients with peripheral vascular disease
Yeung (1991)	138	59	Death, MI, revasc.	37	56	42	0.02	Monitored off Rx
Deedwania and Carbajal (1991)	86	45	Cardiac death	24	23	4	<0.008	Monitored on Rx which controlled symptoms
Quyyumi (1993)	116	39	MI, UA, revasc.	29	13	15	NS	Very low-risk patients
Moss (1993)	936	5	Cardiac death, nonfatal MI, or UA	23	27	24	NS	Very low-risk patients
deMarchena (1994)	50	32	Cardiac death, MI, UA, revasc.	10	56	21	<0.02	All patients monitored on Rx which controlled symptoms
Madjlessi-Simon (1996)	331	27	Death, MI, revasc., or worsening angina	21	33	17	0.004	All patients initially treated with a beta-blocker

Abbreviations: *AECG* ambulatory ECG, *MI* myocardial infarction, *UA* unstable angina, *revasc.* revascularization, *Rx* anti-anginal medication

□ Table 1.6

Clinical trials regarding the effect of anti-ischemic therapies on the prognostic significance of daily life ischemia (modified according to Cohn 1998)

Authors, year	No. patients	End points	Follow-up	Event rate by treatment group	P
Pepine (1994)	306	Death, MI, UA, worsening angina, or revascularization	1 year	25% placebo 11% atenolol	0.001
Rogers (1995)	558	Death, MI, revascularization, hospital admission	1 year	32% angina-guided medical strategy 31% ischemia-guided medical strategy 18% revascularization strategy	0.003
Dargie (1996)	682	Cardiac death, non-fatal MI, and UA Revascularization, worsening angina	2 years	13% atenolol 11% nifedipine 8% combination 8% atenolol 9% nifedipine SR 3% combination	n.s. n.s.
von Armin (1996)	520	Death, MI, UA, or revascularization	1 year	32% for non-100% responders 18% for 100% responders 33% for nifedipine 22% for bisoprolol	0.008 0.03

Abbreviations: *MI* myocardial infarction, *UA* unstable angina

1.8.4   Assessment of Risk in Patients with Cardiac Disease

When trying to stratify survivors of AMI or patients with congestive heart failure (CHF) with respect to their risk of dying from an arrhythmic death, specific noninvasive risk-stratification methods like detecting the type and frequency of ventricular arrhythmias, signal-averaged ECG, HRV, heart-rate turbulence, QTV, QTD, and, last but not least, assessment of LV function (ejection fraction) are mainly used. From an epidemiologic as well as therapeutic interventional point of view, a risk-stratifying test should provide a high positive predictive accuracy (PPA) combined with a reasonably high sensitivity, so that as few patients as possible are unnecessarily exposed to treatment. Moreover, the current tests used should not only predict total mortality, but also specific causes of death, particularly death from life-threatening ventricular arrhythmias. Another practical prerequisite for using different tests is that they should be available not only in specialized referral centers, but also to physicians in all hospitals that take care of cardiac patients. The performance of each of the tests should be properly standardized.

1.8.4.1   Post Myocardial Infarction

Prevalence of Ventricular Arrhythmias

Due to the widespread use of thrombolytic agents, and more recently due to routine acute mechanical recanalization (PCI) of occluded coronary arteries as well as the routine use of aspirin, beta blockers, and ACE inhibitors, inhospital mortality of patients with AMI has substantially decreased from 16% to 20% in the late 1970s to 6–10% in the early 1990s, while the 1-year risk of developing a malignant arrhythmia in AMI survivors after hospital discharge is 5% or less [7]. Arrhythmogenic death accounts for approximately 40–50% of total mortality in the first year after AMI, and thereafter, the risk of dying from a malignant arrhythmia decreases significantly in the next 12–24 months to below approximately 10%. It should be mentioned that mortality rates reported from controlled randomized trials are lower than those derived from more unselected consecutive series of patients due to strict adherence to exclusion criteria resulting in exclusion of higher risk patients such as older patients, those with recurrent MIs, MI after coronary bypass grafting, or ineligibility for thrombolysis or PCI.

Prognostic Significance of LV Function

For more than 20 years, depressed LV function assessed either by ejection fraction (EF) or by clinical signs of CHF represents the principal method of determining the risk of postinfarction patients. Numerous studies both in the pre- and post-thrombolysis, as well as the PCI era have demonstrated that depressed left ventricular ejection fraction (LVEF) < 35–40% is the most powerful predictor of total mortality in the first year after MI, while in patients with LVEF < 15–20% the vast majority of deaths are due to pump failure [7]. In a literature survey, Bailey et al. [121] have shown from 20 studies involving a total of 7,294 patients that sensitivity and PPA of impaired LV function was between 45% and 87% and between 9% and 33%, respectively, with a relative risk of 1.9–16.2 and an odds ratio of 2.0–21.6. It is quite clear that since the MADIT I and II trials in patients with an LVEF < 15–30% no further risk stratification is necessary and that these patients should receive an implantable cardiac defibrillator (ICD) [122]. In the remaining patients, at least in those with an LVEF $\geqslant$ 35–40%, further tests for risk stratification have to be performed.

Prognostic Significance of Ventricular Arrhythmias

Since the 1970s, premature ventricular contractions (PVCs) are considered as the "traditional" risk markers after AMI [123]. ❥ Table 1.7 with results from 20 studies in more than 11,000 patients [124–142] shows that sensitivity and positive predictive value (PPV) of PVCs was between 16% and 82% and between 7% and 52%, respectively, with a relative risk of 1.9–16.2 and an odds ratio of 2.0–21.6. In general, frequent PVCs (e.g., $\geqslant$10/h) and high-grade ventricular ectopy (e.g., repetitive PVCs, multiform PVCs, and non-sustained or sustained ventricular tachycardia (sVT)) have been associated with a higher mortality, but once the patients have at least 6 PVCs per hour, the risk of an arrhythmic event does not increase with more frequent PVCs [123]. The prognostic role of nonsustained VTs (nonsustained ventricular tachycardia [nsVT]) has received special interest. In contrast to previous findings, the GISSI investigators demonstrated that nsVT after AMI failed to predict arrhythmic death [123]. Similar results were reported by Hohnloser et al. [142], who could demonstrate that the prevalence of nsVT at the time of hospital discharge early after the index infarct was very low (95 of 325 consecutive infarct survivors) in a general postinfarction population of patients treated according to current therapeutic guidelines. During a mean follow-up of 30 months, the presence of nsVT was not an independent predictor of either arrhythmic or nonarrhythmic cardiac death. On multivariate stepwise regression analysis for the primary study endpoint of cardiac mortality and arrhythmic events, only the status of the infarct-related artery, HRV, and LV ejection fraction were found to be independent predictors.

In the MADIT I Trial, nsVTs were also used as a risk marker for inclusion of the patients into the study. In long-term survivors of MI with reduced LV function, it was shown that ICD implantation reduced the mortality rates by about 50% in MI survivors with reduced LVEF ($\leqslant$35%) and at least one symptomatic episode of nsVT, and in whom ventricular fibrillation or sustained VT was reproducibly induced during EPS and not suppressed by intravenous administration of procainamide [122]. At present, it is more or less accepted that in the thrombolysis or mechanical recanalization era (PCI in AMI patients), nsVT on its own is not a useful risk stratifier in patients after MI, but rather PVCs in general with a PPV between 5% and 15% should be combined with other risk markers such as impaired LV function, signal-averaged ECG (SAECG), parameters of HRV or of HRT to improve their prognostic impact.

Prognostic Significance of VLP

In the 1980s, the signal-averaged ECG (SAECG) was used to look for VLPs in patients after MI. VLPs were regarded as a sign of slow conduction in the peri-infarct zone that may facilitate the initiation of malignant ventricular tachyarrhythmias. Since then, numerous studies have been published on the prognostic significance of VLPs in survivors of MI before hospital discharge. In summary, the survey of Bailey et al. [121] on 22 studies in a total of 9,883 patients found that sensitivity and PPA of VLPs in the SAECG was between 35% and 83% and between 8% and 35%, respectively, with a relative risk of 1.8–31.5 and an odds ratio of 1.9–41.3. In this study, the SAECG was proposed as the first-step risk stratifier together with depressed LV function (see below). In a recent study on 1,800 consecutive survivors of MI in sinus rhythm and under 76 years, Bauer et al. [151] reported that the presence of VLPs before hospital discharge was not associated with the primary endpoint (SCD and serious arrhythmic events) in univariable and multivariable analysis after a follow-up period of median 34 months. In contrast, low LVEF ($\leqslant$30%) (hazard ratio 9.6, 95% CI 4.1–22.4), HRT turbulence category 1 (either TO or TS abnormal) (hazard ratio 5.1, 95% CI 1.9–14.4), and HRT category 2 (TO and TS abnormal) (hazard

■ Table 1.7

Yield of ventricular arrhythmias within the AECG for predicting arrhythmic events after acute myocardial infarction (AMI)

Author (year)	No. of Patients	Criteria	End points	Sensitivity, %	Specificity, %	PPV, %	NPV, %
Ruberman (1981)	1739	Complex VPBs (multiform, R on T, nsVT)	total death, SCD	54	76	15	95
Olson (1984)	115	≥10 PVCs/h or multiform or pair or VT	cardiac death	25	79	12	90
Mukharji (1984)	533	≥10 PVCs/h	sudden death	10	93	8	95
Kostis (1987)	1640	≥10 PVCs	sudden death	25	88	6	96
		≥10 PVCs/h or PVC pair or VT		43	75	8	96
		≥10 PVCs/h or (PVC pair or VT) or multiform		67	61	8	97
		≥10 PVCs/h and (PVC pair or VT) and multiform		16	94	11	96
Gomes (1989)	110	high grade VEA (couplets and nsVT)	arrhythmic event	81	57	25	94
Verzoni (1989)	208	PVCs-Lown grade 3-5	arrhythmic event	67	71	7	99
de Cock (1991)	99	≥10 PVCs/h	death or MI	44	83	52	78
		VT		26	100	100	75
		SVT		41	97	86	80
Farrell (1991)	416	PVCs >10/h	arrhythmic event	54	82	16	82
		Repetitive PVCs		54	81	15	97
Richards (1991)	358	PVCs-Lown 3-5	arrhythmic event	82	40	6	98
		PVCs-Lown 3-5	cardiac death	75	76	16	98
Steinberg (1992)	182	high grade VEA	sustained VT, SCD	44	73	14	93
Bigger (1992)	715	high rate of PVCs (≥ 3 per h)	all cause mortality, cardiac death, SCD	48	75	24	89
Kuchar (1993)	206	high grade VEA (couplets and nsVT)	symptomatic VT, SCD	73	68	15	97
McClements (1993)	301	≥10 PVCs/h or repetitive	arrhythmic event	38	74	6	96
Pedretti (1993)	305	≥2 runs nsVT	arrhythmic event	42	91	25	96
Hohnloser (1994)	173	PVCs-Lown 4	arrhythmic event	22	78	5	95
Hermosillo (1995)	200	complex ventricular arrhythmias	sVT, SCD	38	92	36	92
El-Sherif (1995)	1158	≥10 PVCs/h or VT	arrhythmic event	61	69	8	98
La Rovere (1998)	1170	complex ventricular arrhythmias	cardiac death	32	84	7	97
Hohnloser (1999)	325	nonsustained VT (nsVT)	cardiac death, sVT, resuscitated VF	16	85	8	92
Mäkikallio (2005)	2130	nonsustained VT, nsVT	sudden cardiac death	21	92	4.5	98

Abbreviations: NPV negative predictive value, VT ventricular tachycardia, SVT supraventricular tachycardia, nsVT nonsustained ventricular tachycardia, VEA ventricular ectopic activity, PVC premature ventricular complexes, SCD sudden cardiac death, sVT sustained Ventricular Tachycardia

ratio 7.5, 95% CI 2.4–23.9) were significant predictors of the primary endpoint in both univariable and multivariable analysis.

Prognostic Significance of HRV

The sympatho–vagal balance and its regulatory activity on the circulatory system is disturbed in survivors of myocardial infarction, as can be determined from a decrease of HRV and BRS, as well as from a blunted heart-rate turbulence (HRT). The specific mechanism of decreased vagal modulation remains unknown. Pragmatically, HRV, BRS, and HRT decrease early after MI with a nadir of 2–3 weeks and then increase back to normal levels by 6–12 months. Decreased HRV and BRS as well as blunted HRT are independent predictors of increased mortality rates, including sudden death, in patients after MI (❯ Table 1.8) [131, 134, 136, 142–149]. The optimal time-domain parameters of HRV for analysis of risk are SDNN and HRV triangular index, and high-risk patients have either an SDANN < 70 ms, an HRV triangular index < 15, a BRS < 3 ms/mm Hg, or HRT parameters TO $\geqslant$ 0% and TS $\leqslant$ 2.5 ms/R – R. Overall, the PPV of HRV parameters, BRS and HRT criteria using the cut-off points mentioned is relatively low in the range of 8–13% at a sensitivity level of 40% [141].

Prognostic Significance of Heart-Rate Turbulence

Heart-rate turbulence (HRT) has also been shown to be of prognostic significance in survivors of MI [150, 151]. In the validation study of the PILP-cohort and the EMIAT placebo arm cohort, a strong and significant association of TO and TS with total mortality was observed [153]. Two recent studies on large cohorts of postinfarction patients (1,800 and 3,130 consecutive patients, respectively) have substantiated the prognostic power of HRT. In the first study [152], both TO and TS were predictive of death or SCD with hazard ratios of 5.3 and 7.5 in multivariable analysis, and in the second study [152], reduced post-ectopic TS (hazard ratio for SCD 5.9) and nsVT (hazard ratio 2.3) were also significant predictors. However, the general problem is that using these predictors alone PPV is too low (between 6% and 13%), and the PPV can be increased by a combination of several parameters (HRV plus VLPs plus HRT plus LVEF) at the cost of constantly lowering the sensitivity down to 10% [7].

Stepwise Risk Stratification

To overcome these practical problems, Bailey et al. [121] proposed a clinically applicable risk stratification procedure in three steps, based on the total number of 25,543 patients collected with a weighted overall estimated two-year major adverse event (MAE) incidence of 7.9%, which was used as a prior probability. Furthermore, to explore the implications of combining tests, the analysis was simplified by using only the composite weighted mean values for sensitivity and specificity. The *first step* was the combination of LVEF and SAECG. If the two tests were both negative or both positive (as would be true for 64.2% of the patients), further testing would not be done, as the two-year probability of a MAE would be as low as 2.2% in the former, and high enough (38.7%) in the latter situation to warrant consideration of ICD implantation. The *second step* would be the performance of a 24-h AECG in the 35.8% of patients who had only a low LVEF or a positive SAECG, resulting in an intermediate two-year risk of 10.6% for a MAE. If severe ventricular arrhythmia (SVA) and abnormal HRV were both present or absent (25% of patient population), no further testing would be needed, because in the former case the posterior probability is still below the original prior probability, despite having either a low LVEF or an abnormal SAECG, and in the latter situation, the posterior probability would again be high enough to warrant consideration of ICD implantation. The *third step* would refer to the remaining 10.8% of the original patients, who would have an intermediate two-year risk of 17.5%. They would undergo an EPS, and 2.6% of the original group would have a positive EPS, again with a two-year risk of 45.1%, which is high enough to justify consideration of ICD implantation. At the end of applying all three stages of risk stratification, there remains a small proportion (8.2%) of unstratified patients with essentially the same risk of 8.9% as the original prior probability of 7.9% [121]. It should be noted that with the exception of assessing LVEF (by echocardiography, left ventricular angiography or cardiac magnetic resonance imaging [MRI]), all other parameters of step one and two can be derived from one 24-h AECG recording using modern solid-state digital recorder devices, so that only two investigational tools are necessary to reach step three, if applicable, according to the results of the different test parameters described.

◘ Table 1.8

Yield of heart rate variability (HRV) for predicting arrhythmic events after acute myocardial infarction (AMI)

Author (Reference)	No. of Patients	Criteria	End points	Sensitivity, %	Specificity, %	PPV, %	NPV, %
Kleiger (1987)	808	SDNN <50 ms*	all-cause death	34	88	34	88
Farrell (1991)	416	HRV triangular index <20† Mean R-R interval <750 ms	nonfatal VF	92 67	77 72	17 13	77 97
Odemuyiwa (1991)	385	HRV triangular index ≤30†	nonfatal VF	75	76		
Bigger (1992)	715	ULF VLF ULF+VLF	all-cause death	28 30 20	93 92 96	41 39 48	
Pedretti (1993)	294	HRV triangular index ≤29†	nonfatal VF	89	68	15	99
Zuanetti (1996)	567	SDNN, RMSSD, "NN50+"	total and CV mortality	42	87	24	93
Copie (1996)	551	24-h mean heart rate	cardiac death sudden death	46	88	16	97
Lanza (1998)	239	SDNN index, SDANN, VLF	sudden death	32	92	25	94
La Rovere (1998)	1,170 1,182	SDNN <70 ms* BRS <3.0 ms/mm Hg	nonfatal VF and cardiac death nonfatal VF and cardiac death	39 35	85 86	10 10	97 97
Hohnloser (1999)	325	SDNN <70ms	primary: cardiac death, sVT, resuscitated VF Secondary: arrhythmic event	60	82	22	96
Katz (1999)	185	Difference <10 bpm between shortest and longest RR-interval on 6 deep respirations in 1 minute	cardiovascular mortality	90	68	46	99
Malik (2000)	451	SDNN ≤50ms, HRV index ≤20	all cause mortality	50	73	18	92

Abbreviations: *NNP* negative predictive value, *PPV* positive predictive value, *VF* ventricular fibrillation, *CV* cardiovascular

1.8.4.2   Chronic Heart Failure

Prognostic Significance of Ventricular Arrhythmias

The majority of patients with CHF suffer from advanced structural heart disease, either ischemic or idiopathic dilated cardiomyopathy (IDCM), with progressive symptoms. Death results mostly from VT or fibrillation, bradyarrhythmia or asystole, progressive pump failure, recurrent ischemia or infarction, electromechanical dissociation, stroke, pulmonary emboli, or renal complications. Ventricular arrhythmias are extremely common in patients with CHF [153]. Ambient ventricular ectopic beats can be detected in ⩾90% of these patients, frequent VPCs in 70–95% of DCM and heart failure, while many of these patients have complex and multiform PVCs and episodes of nsVT. In the Captopril–Digoxin Multicenter study of 295 patients with mild to moderate heart failure and reduced LVEF < 40%, the frequency of VPBs was significantly higher in older patients, in those with LVEF < 20%, or IDCM. In such high-risk group patients, 50% also had episodes of nsVT compared to 30% with nsVT in the overall study. By multivariate analysis, only nsVT frequency was an independent predictor of risk of sudden death. Patients with frequent occurrences of nsVT (>2/day) had an almost threefold increase in total mortality [154]. In the V-HeFT II study on 715 patients, ventricular couplets were seen in 98% of patients and 28% had one or more episodes of nsVT. The presence of nsVT and ventricular couplets identified a group of patients with increased mortality [155]. In the GESICA-Trial [156], 34% of 516 patients showed nsVT. These episodes of nsVT were more frequent in patients with advanced heart failure, higher heart rate, lower systolic blood pressure, increased creatinine, or with Chagas disease. During a three year follow-up, the presence of nsVT was associated with an increased risk of total mortality (relative risk 1.69, p < .0002) and an increased rate of SCD (relative risk 2.77, p < .001). It can be concluded from these three large studies that in patients with advanced heart failure, the presence of nsVT identifies a subgroup with an increased risk of overall cardiac mortality and SCD. However, despite identifying this population with an increased relative risk of an adverse event, AECG monitoring for analysis of ventricular arrhythmias is either not sensitive enough or reveals a PPV that is too low for patient management purposes.

Prognostic Significance of HRV

The prognostic significance of HRV in patients with CHF was unclear in the past. In one of the first studies in 40 patients with CHF, compared with normals and those with a history of nsVT and normal cardiac function, there was no significant difference in the HRV parameters despite a significantly lowered HRV in heart failure patients [157]. In a prospective study of 71 patients with IDCM and CHF, Hoffman et al. [158] studied HRV by time- and frequency-domain methods. After a follow-up period of 15 ± 5 months, no significant difference of time or frequency-domain indices of HRV among patients with arrhythmic events compared with those without major arrhythmic events was found. In a further study of 159 patients with IDCM and CHF, 30 patients died during follow-up. There was a significant correlation between LVEF, increased SDNN, and pNN50 with an increased risk of cardiac death. However, the risk of SCD correlated only with LVEF in contrast to an increased low-frequency power (LFP) and impairment of pNN50 that strongly correlated with an increased risk of death from progressive pump failure. Further, two studies showed that HRV was reduced in patients with CHF and there was a strong correlation between HRV and LV function and peak oxygen consumption [159, 160].

More recently, several studies on larger patient populations have been published that showed a positive prognostic power of HRV in patients with CHF (❱ Table 1.9). Ponikowski et al. [161] studied 102 consecutive patients with CHF from ischemic or dilated cardiomyopathy, using AECG monitoring to assess all parameters of HRV both in the time and frequency domain. During follow-up of 584 ± 405 days, 19 patients died. In multivariate analysis, HRV parameters SDNN, SDANN, and LF were found to predict survival independently of NYHA functional class, EF, peak oxygen consumption, and the presence of VT within the AECG. The Kaplan–Meier survival curves revealed SDNN <100 ms to be a useful risk factor. Szabo et al. [162] investigated 159 patients with CHF due to ischemic or dilated cardiomyopathy, in whom both time and frequency-domain parameters were measured at entry to predict the endpoint of cardiac mortality. During a follow-up of 23 months (range 1–67), 30 of 159 patients died of cardiac causes. Both pNN50 < 2.0% and SDNN < 108 ms predicted cardiac death with a RR of 2.1 and 1.5 respectively, whereas pNN50 and LF power >14 ms^2 predicted death from pump failure with a RR of 5.4 and 6.8, respectively. Boveda et al. [163] reported on 190 patients with CHF and found the time-domain parameter SDNN < 67 ms to be significantly predictive for total death (RR 2.5, CI 1.5– 4.2). In the VA trial,

□ Table 1.9

Prognostic significance of heart rate variability (HRV) for predicting cardiovascular and total mortality in patients with congestive heart failure (CHF)

Author (Reference)	No. of patients	Criteria	End points	Adjusted RR (95% CI)
Szabo (1997)	159	pNN50 <2.00% SDNN <108 ms	cardiac mortality	2.1 (1.4–3.3) 1.5 (1.0–2.4)
		pNN50 <2.00% LFP >14 ms^2	death from pump failure	5.4 (1.7–17.5) 6.8 (2.2–20.9)
Boveda (2001)	190	SDNN <67 ms	total death	2.5 (1.5–4.2)
Bilchick (2002)	127	SDNN <65.3 ms (lowest quartile)	total death	3.7
			sudden death	2.4
La Rovere (2003)	242	LF ≤11 ms^2 (8 min controlled breathing)	sudden death	3.0 (1.2–7.6)
		≥ 83 VPB/hour	sudden death	3.7 (1.5–9.0)
Aronson (2004)	199	SDNN (lower tertile) SDANN Total power ULF	total mortality	2.2 (1.05–4.3) 2.1 (1.05–4.2) 2.2 (1.08–4.2) 2.6 (1.3–5.3)
Adamson (2004)	397	SDAAM <50 ms (5′) (from implanted resynchronisation devices)	total death	3.2
			cardiovascular death	4.4
Guzzetti (2005)	330	VLF night ≤509 ms^2	progressive pump failure	2.3 (1.4–3.8)
		LF night ≤20 ms^2	sudden death	2.7 (1.3–5.6)
		HF night ≤60 ms^2	sudden death	2.2 (1.0–4.6)

Abbreviations: *RR* relative risk, *CI* confidence interval, *nsVT* nonsustained ventricular tachycardia; *VT* ventricular tachycardia, *VPB* ventricular premature beat

Bilchik et al. [164] reported on 179 patients with CHF, in whom the lowest quartile of patients were compared with the remaining, using SDNN as the sole HRV parameter. Among 127 patients meeting the inclusion criteria, SDNN < 65.3 ms (the lowest quartile) was the sole independent factor predictive of survival in a multivariate model (p = .0001). A Cox proportional-hazards model revealed that each increase of 10 ms in SDNN conferred a 20% decrease in risk of mortality (p = .0001). Furthermore, patients with SDNN < 65.3 ms had a significantly increased risk of sudden death (p = .016). Thus, in this study, HRV was the only independent predictor of overall mortality and was significantly associated with sudden death. Aronson et al. [165] measured time and frequency HRV parameters from 24-h Holter recordings in 199 patients with NYHA class III or IV hospitalized for decompensated CHF, and during a mean follow-up after discharge of 312 ± 150 days, 40 patients (21.1%) died. Kaplan–Meier analysis indicated that patients with decreased values of SDNN over a 24-h period, SDANN, total power, and ULF power in the lower tertile were at higher risk of death. In a multivariate Cox regression model, the same indexes in the lower tertile were independent predictors of mortality (RR from 2.2 to 2.6). The conclusion was that the severity of autonomic dysfunction during hospital admission for CHF decompensation, as reflected by measures of overall HRV, can predict survival after hospital discharge.

La-Rovere et al. [166] developed a multivariate survival model for the identification of sudden (presumably arrhythmic) death from data of 202 consecutive patients with moderate to severe CHF. Both time- and frequency-domain HRV parameters obtained from 8-min ECG recordings at baseline and during controlled breathing were challenged against clinical and functional parameters. This model was then validated in 242 consecutive patients referred for CHF as the validation sample. Sudden death was independently predicted by a model that included LFP of HRV during controlled breathing ≤13 ms^2 and left ventricular end-diastolic diameter ≥ 77 mm (RR 3.7, 95% CI 1.5–9.3 and RR 2.6, 95% CI 1.1–6.3, respectively). LF ≤ 11 ms^2 during controlled breathing and ≥83 VPCs per hour on Holter monitoring were both independent predictors of sudden death (RR 3.0, 95% CI 1.2–7.6, and RR 3.7, 95% CI 1.5–9.0, respectively). The conclusion was that reduced short-term LFP during controlled breathing is a powerful and independent predictor of sudden death in patients with CHF. Similar results from the same group were reported by Guzzetti et al. [167], who studied 330 consecutive CHF patients. Using time, frequency, and fractal analyses, the risk of pump failure and of sudden death could be differentiated as follows: depressed power of night time HRV ($\leqslant$509 ms^2), VLP (<0.04 Hz), high-pulmonary wedge pressure ($\geqslant$18 mm Hg), and low left-ventricular EF ($\leqslant$24%) were independently related to pump failure, while reduction of LFP ($\leqslant$20 ms^2) and increased left ventricular end systolic diameter ($\geqslant$61 mm) were linked to sudden (arrhythmic) mortality. The dilemma, however, remains that there is no evidence that reducing the frequency of repetitive ventricular arrhythmias or increasing the HRV with medications can significantly reduce the incidence of total death or sudden death in patients with severe CHF.

From a technical point of view, it is interesting to note that HRV parameters may also be retrieved from the memory of implanted devices, as has been shown by Adamson et al. [168]. In 397 patients, continuous HRV was measured as the standard deviation of 5-min median atrial–atrial intervals (SDAAM) sensed by the biventricular pacing device. SDAAM < 50 ms, when averaged over 4 weeks, was associated with increased mortality risk (hazard ratio 3.2, p = .02), and SDAAM was persistently lower over the entire follow-up period in patients who required hospitalization or died. Automated detection of decreases in SDAAM was 70% sensitive in detecting cardiovascular hospitalizations, with 2.4 false-positives per patient-year follow-up.

Prognostic Significance of Heart-Rate Turbulence

Koyama et al. [169] measured heart-rate turbulence (HRT) in 50 patients with CHF, 34 with IDCM, and 16 with MI and compared this with 21 patients without obvious heart disease as a control group. HRT slope and HRT onset were measured by the original definition using digitized Holter ECG recordings, and cardiac pump function was assessed by echocardiography. The value of the HRT slope was significantly lower in CHF than in controls (3.7 ± 1.7 vs 16.4 ± 5.3, p < .01). The value of HRT onset in patients with CHF was significantly higher than in control patients (−1.1 ± 1.9 vs −3.6 ± 1.7, p < .05). The HRT slope and onset in CHF patients with VT were nearly identical to those without VT. It was concluded from this study that HRT slope appears to be a powerful prognostic marker that shows significant differences between CHF subgroups when divided by clinical events such as death or hospitalization from CHF. Kawasaki et al. [170] investigated 104 hypertrophic cardiomyopathy (HCM) patients, 44 MI patients, and 56 normal controls using HRT onset and slope. The latter parameters were abnormal in MI patients, but not in HCM patients as compared with normal control subjects. During a follow-up period of 27 ± 10 months, 7 HCM patients and 10 MI patients either died from cardiac death or were hospitalized for CHF. In MI patients, HRT onset was higher and the HRT slope was lower in patients with cardiac events than in patients without, whereas in HCM patients, the HRT onset or slope was similar between patients with and without cardiac events. It was concluded that, unlike MI patients, the HRT variables in selected HCM patients were not abnormal and failed to predict the clinical prognosis.

In the study of Grimm et al. [171] involving a cohort of 242 patients with IDCM, HRT analysis was performed in a blinded fashion. During 41 ± 23 months of follow-up, 54 patients (22%) died or underwent heart transplantation. On Cox univariate regression analysis, abnormal HRT onset, HRT slope, HRT onset combined with HRT slope, LV ejection, LV size, and NYHA functional class III showed a significant association with total mortality or the need for heart transplantation. On multivariable analysis, abnormal HRT onset identified patients without transplant-free survival, as did LV size and NYHA class III heart failure. Major arrhythmic events were observed in 42 patients (17%) during follow-up. On univariate analysis, abnormal HRT onset with HRT slope, male sex, NYHA class III, LV ejection fraction, and LV size were associated with a higher incidence of major arrhythmic events. On a multivariate analysis, only LV ejection fraction remained a significant arrhythmia risk predictor. It was concluded that in IDCM patients, HRT onset is a significant predictor of transplant-free survival, as well as LV size and NYHA class. For arrhythmia risk stratification, however, only LV ejection fraction remains a significant risk predictor. Again, the main problem is that, when using HRT parameters alone, their PPV is too low though sensitivity is reasonably high. In conclusion, at present there is not sufficient evidence to support routine use of AECG for HRT parameter analysis for therapeutic or prognostic purposes in patients with CHF.

1.8.4.3   Hypertrophic Cardiomyopathy (HCM)

The prevalence of ventricular arrhythmias detected from AECG monitoring is relatively high in patients with HCM [172–176]. It is widely accepted that the presence and severity of ventricular arrhythmias in HCM are related to severe impairment of left ventricular function (LVF). Moreover, SCD and syncope are common among patients with HCM. There are studies showing that there is some association between ventricular arrhythmias and adverse events. However, they differ on the nature of this association [173–176]. Studies on HRV in patients with HCM are sparse and the results equivocal, for example, Counihan et al. [177] found no association between HRV indexes and adverse events in HCM. Reduced HRV on ambulatory monitor recordings appears to be less useful in risk stratification in patients with HCM, as compared to those after acute MI, and thus is not widely used in this patient population. The features that most reliably identify the 10–20% of HCM patients at high risk of sudden death include prior cardiac arrest or sVT, multiple and repetitive episodes of nsVT, young age < 30 years at diagnosis (especially in those with extreme left ventricular hypertrophy (LVH) and wall thickness ⩾30 mm on echocardiography), a family history of HCM with sudden death, an abnormal blood pressure response to exercise especially in patients younger than 50 years, and genetic abnormalities associated with increased prevalence of sudden death [178]. In conclusion, the specific role of AECG monitoring to retrieve risk factors for prognostic reasons, such as ventricular (tachy-) arrhythmias, reduced HRV, or blunted HRT, remains unclear in the day-to-day treatment of HCM patients.

1.8.4.4   Valvular Heart Disease

The frequency of PVCs and the grade of arrhythmia (repetitive forms) are significantly correlated with LVF, but neither is related to the severity of valvular lesions (estimated valvular surface area or hemodynamically measured regurgitation). The occurrence of salvos of VT during an AECG recording in a patient with valvular disease (e.g., aortic stenosis or mitral regurgitation) is related in particular to a low LVEF and to an increased risk of sudden death [179]. Thus, the existence and severity of ventricular arrhythmias in valvular heart disease has an important prognostic value indicating poor myocardial performance, whatever the importance of the valvular lesion is.

A close relationship is now generally accepted between mitral valve prolapse and an increased frequency of ventricular arrhythmias during AECG monitoring compared to a normal population [180–183]. However, the prognostic significance of these findings remains unclear. Ventricular arrhythmias are unrelated to the severity of valvular disease. The prevalence of SVTs has been reported to be 5–10%. However, it includes usually only short runs of atrial beats and non-sustained tachycardias.

In conclusion, at present, the presence of mitral valve prolapse, chronic mitral regurgitation, aortic stenosis or regurgitation, or an aortic valve prosthesis without symptoms does not establish the need for AECG monitoring for analyzing the spectrum of ventricular arrhythmias, nor the parameters of HRV or HRT [7].

1.8.4.5   Systemic Hypertension (SH)

In most patients with SH, LVH is present. This is associated with an increased incidence of complex ventricular arrhythmias (VEA) and an increased risk of MI and sudden death [184, 185]. Because patients with SH and LVH with complex or frequent VEA have only a marginally significant risk of dying after adjusting for age, sex, and other clinical factors [186], AECG monitoring is of uncertain value in the management of asymptomatic patients with LVH. With respect to HRV, a few studies have shown an increase of low-frequency components of HRV in hypertensive patients compared to normals, with blunting of circadian patterns and reduced parasympathetic activity in hypertensives. In the Framingham Study, the predictive power of HRV parameters for the incidence of hypertension was tested and after adjustment for factors associated with hypertension, multiple regression analysis revealed that low-frequency components were associated with incident hypertension [187]. In the ARIC study of 2,061 normotensives, 64 participants developed hypertension during a 3-year follow-up, and a statistically significant inverse association between baseline HF band and the risk of incident hypertension was observed [188]. In a further study on dipper and non-dipper essential hypertensive individuals, both the LF and HF band were significantly lower in non-dipper hypertensives than in dipper hypertensive subjects throughout the day. In dipper hypertensives, the LF band showed a nocturnal decrease and the HF band an increase, whereas these diurnal changes in LF and HF bands were significantly blunted in non-dipper subjects [189]. These data show that hypertensives, and particularly non-dipper hypertensives, are characterized by decreased physiological circadian fluctuations of the ANS. However, because of paucity of relevant clinical data, the true role of HRV in the diagnosis and treatment of patients with essential hypertension remains unclear. In conclusion, there is not sufficient evidence to support routine use of AECG for arrhythmia or HRV parameter analysis for therapeutic or prognostic purposes in patients with essential hypertension and LVH.

1.8.4.6 Miscellaneous

Diabetes is associated among other things with diffuse degeneration of sympathetic and parasympathetic small nerve fibers, and more than 50% of patients with symptomatic diabetic neuropathy will die within 5 years [190]. High-frequency components of HRV may detect small changes in autonomic function in diabetic patients [191, 192] and distinguish diabetic subjects with neuropathy from those without neuropathy [193]. The clinical utility of HRV analysis as a reliable test for cardiac parasympathetic function is limited in diabetics due to the fact that a large number of diabetic subjects have reduced HRV and that there is no evidence that early identification of subclinical neuropathy will lead to improved patient outcomes. Therefore, routine HRV testing in diabetic subjects is not indicated at this time [7].

Patients with chronic renal failure who are on chronic hemodialysis bear an increased risk of CAD and of dying from a cardiovascular event. They show an increase in ventricular ectopy during dialysis. Hemodialysis patients with known CAD or peripheral vascular disease display the highest risk of having an abnormal AECG recording [194]. Though patients with higher grade VEA have a decreased survival compared to those without this type of VEA, it is unclear at present, whether AECG monitoring should be routinely performed in these patients [7].

Regarding pre- and postoperative evaluation, no association has been found between preoperative VEA and postoperative events when AECG monitoring was used before surgery in high-risk patients without myocardial ischemia and depressed LV function, who underwent non-cardiac surgery [195]. In addition, no association has been found between the occurrence of complex VEA after coronary artery bypass surgery and death after controlling for other clinical factors [195]. Therefore, at present there is no general recommendation for the routine use of AECG monitoring for risk stratification in preoperative and postoperative patients [7].

1.8.5 Evaluation of Therapeutic Interventions

1.8.5.1 Pacemaker and ICD Function

Once a pacemaker or ICD is implanted, an AECG is useful in assessing postoperative device function and in guiding appropriate programming of enhanced features such as rate responsiveness and automatic mode switching. Sometimes, the AECG can be a useful adjunct to continuous telemetric observation or pacemaker/ICD-based monitoring in assessing device function, though the present generation of pacemaker/ICD has limited monitoring capacity that is not capable of entirely supplanting conventional AECG. Tabular data derived from complexes classified by the pacemaker algorithm according to whether or not they are preceded by atrial sensed or paced beats can be obtained from the pacemaker memory, which summarizes the number or percentage of atrial and ventricular events that were either sensed or paced, including a separate quantification of sensed ventricular events preceding atrial activity. Current pacemaker devices do not generally provide electrogram confirmation of the counts, so the accuracy provided by the devices depends on accurate sensing and pacing functions. These tabular data can be used to broadly determine the frequency of VPBs, but the resolution of the data does not allow for minute-to-minute counts or detailed characterization of repetitive ventricular ectopy (rate, duration, or morphology of VT). Therefore, there is an important role for AECG monitoring in evaluating patients' symptoms, despite pacemaker implantation, or in detecting details of pacemaker failure.

Syncope, dizziness, and palpitations may persist or sometimes reappear in up to 30% of patients after pacemaker implantation, and persistent symptoms are frequently due to various types of arrhythmia. Thus, indications for AECG

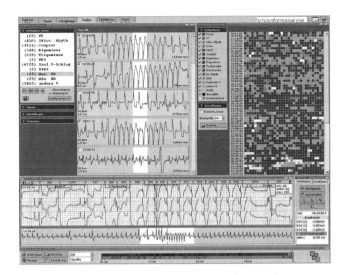

◘ Fig. 1.35
Arrhythmia overview in a patient with pacemaker-mediated tachycardia including counts of single arrhythmic events (*left*), single lead arrhythmic episodes extracted from the overview on left side, survey on QRS templates over the full 24-h period with 30 s segments (*right*), and three-channel real-time ECG and single lead "full disclosure" ECG (*bottom*) (Oxford MedilogDarwin system)

monitoring in patients with an implanted pacemaker include evaluation of frequent symptoms of palpitation, dizziness, syncope, or near syncope despite or due to pacemaker stimulation, for example, due to failure to sense, oversensing, failure to capture, or pacemaker pauses (myopotential inhibition) as well as due to pacemaker mediated tachycardia (endless loop tachycardia) (❷ Fig. 1.35). Moreover, AECG monitoring may assist in the programming of simple (lower rate interval, AV interval, ventricular and postventricular refractory period, and upper rate response of DDD pacemakers) and of enhanced features like rate responsiveness and automatic mode switching. Evaluation of suspected component failure by AECG monitoring is particularly important in cases where device interrogation is not definitive in establishing a conclusive diagnosis. Pacemaker syndrome is another important symptomatic situation that needs AECG recording to exclude the presence of pacemaker malfunction and to detect the appropriateness of atrio-ventricular synchrony. Pacemaker syndrome as first described in patients with VVI pacemakers may also occur in dual-chamber pacing systems when the programmed AV delay does not allow enough time for the atria to contract against open atrio-ventricular valves. This phenomenon may be observed in the following conditions: (1) programmed prolonged AV delay, (2) DDI or DDDIR pacing modes, (3) pacemaker-mediated tachycardia, (4) sinus bradycardia below the lower limit in the VDD pacing mode, (5) pace mode switching from DDD(R) to VVI(R), and (6) rate smoothing or fallback during DDD pacing. In some cases, it may be difficult to differentiate severe pacemaker syndrome from vasovagal syncope, and in these patients head-up tilt-testing may help to clarify the situation. Finally, the efficacy of AADs to suppress concomitant intermittent tachycardias, for example, paroxysmal AF or frequent VPBs that interfere significantly with pacemaker function, can also be assessed by AECG monitoring.

Patients following ICD implantation for the management of ventricular tachyarrhythmias often have ICD shock therapy during follow-up. AECG monitoring can be a useful alternative or adjunct to continuous telemetric monitoring or interrogation of ICD memory in establishing the appropriateness of such therapy. Moreover, the rate of SVTs (sinus tachycardia or AF with high ventricular rates) that eventually interfere with the cut-off parameters of the ICD device, with the consequence of the delivery of inappropriate shocks, may be evaluated and the efficacy of adjunctive pharmacological therapy in suppressing spontaneous arrhythmias in an attempt to minimize the frequency of device activation can be assessed by the AECG, as well.

1.8.5.2 Antiarrhythmic Drugs (AADs)

AECG monitoring has been widely used in the past to assess the effects of antiarrhythmic therapy, because it is a non-invasive technique that provides quantitative ECG data and permits correlation of symptoms with ECG phenomena. However, there are important limitations of AECG as a therapeutic guide such as the significant day-to-day variability in the type and frequency of arrhythmias in many patients, a lack of correlation between arrhythmia suppression after an intervention and subsequent outcome, uncertain guidelines for the degree of suppression required to demonstrate an effect, either clinical or statistical, and an absence of quantifiable spontaneous asymptomatic arrhythmias between episodes in many patients with a documented history of life-threatening ventricular tachyarrhythmias [7, 197].

AECG monitoring with quantitative analysis has not been widely used to guide the therapy of supraventricular arrhythmias because of the limited day-to-day occurrence of these arrhythmias and the uncertain significance of asymptomatic non-sustained atrial ectopy. But for evaluating the effects of AADs in patients with supraventricular arrhythmias, particularly AF, intermittent monitoring to confirm the presence of an arrhythmic episode during symptoms and to document arrhythmia-free intervals has become more or less a standard approach. Moreover, the AECG may also be used to monitor the effects of AV nodal blocking agents on heart rate in patients with atrial arrhythmias (beta blockers, digitalis, calcium channel blockers), particularly in AF. Since short-term reproducibility of the frequency and type of arrhythmia, especially in ventricular arrhythmias, between repeat AECG recordings is rather poor, a large reduction between 60% and 90% in arrhythmia frequency is required to ensure that the change is due to an antiarrhythmic effect of any intervention [7].

The best way of assessing the efficacy of a drug is probably to select a group of patients with the same arrhythmia and to measure the spontaneous variability between a control and a placebo period. If the variability is small with a good correlation between the two periods, a drug trial appears possible. It is then feasible to compare the respective efficacy of two drugs in the same group of patients. The appropriate statistical method (such as that developed by Sami et al. [198, 199]) uses a one-tailed 95% confidence interval calculated between baseline and placebo PVC measurements. The appreciation of the antiarrhythmic effect is based on the comparison with the relation between drug and control (❯ Fig. 1.36). If a drug shifts a PVC value under the 95% confidence interval line, its effectiveness can most likely be assumed in that patient. If a drug A shifts more patients under the 95% confidence interval line than drug B, A is probably more effective than B in this selected arrhythmia. This method is largely used to compare a new drug with an established treatment chosen as reference. An important limitation is the necessity to observe several periods without treatment (control, placebo, follow-up). Patients with severe symptomatic arrhythmias cannot be included in these studies. Open studies are indicated in such patients.

The data from the CAST trial, in which a higher mortality rate during follow-up was observed in those patients who had suppression of spontaneous VPBs after a titration phase and then received chronic encainide or flecainide therapy as opposed to placebo, led to a revision of the former concept that suppression of PVCs by AADs would improve the prognosis of patients with structural heart disease. Indeed, the trial showed that antiarrhythmic therapy with encainide or flecainide may be harmful to patients. More or less similar inconsistent results have been obtained with the empiric use of amiodarone, since some studies such as the BASEL, CASCADE, or GESICA trials showed a benefit in patients with preserved or depressed LV function [200–203], while others like EMIAT or CAMIAT revealed no significant change in mortality rate [204–206]. In one trial, amiodarone produced a significant reduction in arrhythmia frequency but had no effect on mortality rate [206].

In contrast to supraventricular tachy(arrhythmias), placebo-controlled trials of antiarrhythmic interventions in patients with sustained life-threatening ventricular tachyarrhythmias are problematic. Although in the study of Lampert et al. [207] improvements in arrhythmia-free survival in CHD patients who met certain criteria for drug response during serial AECG were reported, it is not possible to estimate the effects of the "healthy responder" phenomenon [208] on these observations, which means that patients who responded to the AECG-guided drug therapy had a different (more favorable) prognosis than those who did not. With respect to the method of choice for monitoring the outcome of an antiarrhythmic intervention, AECG as well as EP testing may be used. The ESVEM study [209], which used both tests in a randomized fashion on patients with an entry criterion of inducibility of sVT on two occasions and ⩾10 VPBs/h showed that there was no significant difference in predicting long-term success in either group, once a drug was determined to be effective (EPS: suppressing inducible VT, AECG: suppression of VPBs). However, AECG monitoring had the advantage in that it identified an AAD predicted to be effective more often than EPS in these patients. For practical reasons, despite

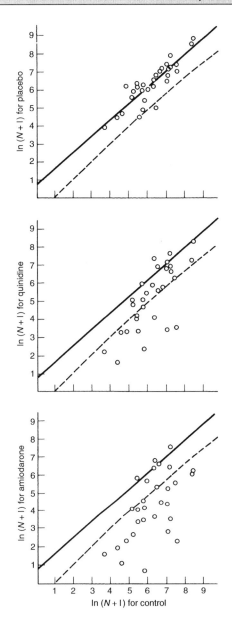

◘ Fig. 1.36

Results from a crossover comparative trial of quinidine (1 g day^{-1}) and amiodarone (400 mg day^{-1}) in 30 patients with frequent PVCs using the statistical methodology of Sami et al. [198, 199]. Each diagram shows a correlation line with a one-tailed 95% confidence interval indicated by the *dashed line*. In the top diagram, the control and placebo periods are compared with respect to the incidence of PVCs while similar comparisons are shown in the middle diagram for control versus quinidine and in the lower diagram for amiodarone versus control. The symbol *N* represents PVC frequency per hour. The effectiveness of the AAD therapy can be judged by the number of points beneath the 95% confidence interval line. In other words, the incidence of PVCs in patients on these drugs is lower than in control or placebo periods. It can also be seen that the antiarrhythmic efficacy is higher in patients with amiodarone than in those with quinidine

the many criticisms of the ESVEM trial, it may be concluded that AECG monitoring may be used to assess AAD efficacy in patients with frequent VPBs, but not in those with spontaneous sustained VTs.

The same holds true for assessing the phenomenon of proarrhythmia, which is defined as the aggravation of an arrhythmia, particularly of VEA, for example, either the increase of the number or complexity of VEA or the new incidence of a given ventricular arrhythmia, as well as sinus node dysfunction, or new or worsened AV conduction abnormalities. Proarrhythmia may occur early or late during the course of therapy, and an increase of arrhythmia needed to differentiate proarrhythmia from day-to-day variability may be estimated statistically on the basis of baseline arrhythmia frequency [198, 199, 210, 211]. A particular type of proarrhythmia is the induction of torsades de pointes that may be induced by drugs that prolong the QTI (e.g., class III AADs, tricyclic antidepressants, antihistamines, antibiotics, etc.). In such cases, AECG monitoring may be useful for the evaluation of new markers of this type of proarrhythmia, such as alternating QTIs or T waves, or altered QT-interval adaptation to changes in heart rate.

1.8.5.3   Antianginal Drugs

Most antianginal drugs are commonly assessed by counting the frequency of anginal attacks, and the number of nitroglycerin tablets consumed. This kind of investigation relies entirely on subjective symptom appreciation. Changes in lifestyle, environmental conditions, or daily activity may deeply affect the results. ST-segment monitoring provides an objective technique, as does stress testing, which is now routinely performed to evaluate these therapies. Thus, physicians should use repetitive stress tests or continuous AECG monitoring in cases of exercise angina. Twenty-four-hour ECGs are more efficient for characterizing the pharmacological properties of the drug, such as delay and duration of effect. In the case of spontaneous (Prinzmetal's) angina, ambulatory monitoring is the optimum technique allowing an accurate evaluation of the drugs, which are used in this condition (calcium antagonists) [212]. The development of AECG has also revealed that all patients with spontaneous angina exhibit painless episodes of ST-segment elevation in addition to experiencing painful attacks. When an antianginal treatment such as a calcium antagonist is not completely effective, only painless episodes persist. Repeated 24-h ECGs are then necessary to assess the efficacy of treatment and the need for an increase in dosage or a change to another drug. Thus, suspected Prinzmetal's angina is obviously a good indication for ambulatory monitoring, which is useful both as a diagnostic procedure and for evaluation of therapy.

1.9   Pediatric Patients

Similar to adult patients, the purposes of AECG monitoring in pediatric patients include the evaluation of symptoms, risk assessment in patients with cardiovascular disease, with or without symptoms of an arrhythmia, and the evaluation of cardiac rhythm after an intervention like drug therapy or device implantation [7]. Selection of the method of monitoring, for example, continuous versus patient activated recording, is predicated on the frequency and symptoms of the arrhythmia. AECG monitoring may be useful for evaluation of symptoms in patients with known cardiovascular disease and for medical therapy and intervention. In children with asymptomatic congenital heart block, a yearly Holter monitor is recommended. The escape rate at resting conditions is used as one criterion for the need of pacemaker implantation. In general, a resting heart rate greater than 60 bpm in children under 2 years, greater than 50 bpm in children 2–10 years, and greater than 40 bpm in children over 10 years of age is considered to be an adequate escape rhythm. In addition, the mean heart rate, the slowest heart rate, and the longest pause on AECG monitoring can also be used as supportive data, and the presence of ventricular ectopy (as single escape beats) is another indication for pacemaker implantation.

1.9.1   Evaluation of Symptoms

AECG in pediatric patients may be used for the evaluation of symptoms including palpitations, dizziness, syncope or near syncope, and chest pain and their relation to an underlying arrhythmia. Because of the paroxysmal nature of palpitations, an event recorder is usually recommended to detect the cause of these symptoms. In 10–15% of young individuals, an arrhythmia, in most cases SVT, has been reported to correlate with symptoms [213–218], (❷ Table 1.10), whereas ventricular ectopy or bradycardia was demonstrated in only other 2–5%. Interestingly, in about 50% of palpitations, sinus

◻ Table 1.10

Yield of Holter monitoring for evaluation of palpitation in pediatric patients with no structural heart disease

Author (year)	No. of patients	Method	Mean no. of days of monitoring	Symptoms during monitoring, n(%) Arrhythmia	No arrhythmia	No symptoms during monitoring, no arrhythmia, n (%)
Dick (1979)	6	TTM		2 (33)	4 (67)	0
Porter (1980)	25	TTM	1	3 (12)	9 (36)	13 (52)
Fyfe (1984)	41	HM	75	9 (22) (8 SVT)	12 (29)	20 (49)
Goldstein (1990)	48	TTM	14–90	10 (21) (7SVT)	15 (31)	23 (48)
Houyel (1992)[+]	201	TTM	85	24 (12) (23 SVT)	112 (56)	65 (32)
Karpawich (1993)	37	TTM	30	10 (27)	27 (73)	0
	45	HM	1	0	9 (20)	36 (80)
Total	403			58 (14)	188 (47)	157 (39)

Abbreviations: *TTM* Trans Telephonic Monitoring, patient activated event recorder, *HM* Holter Monitoring (24-h monitoring), [+]Includes 25 patients with heart disease

tachycardia was found, whereas 30–40% of young patients have no symptoms in AECG monitoring. Thus, one of the primary uses of AECG monitoring in pediatric patients is to exclude an arrhythmia as the cause of palpitations [7]. Recently, the value of transtelephonic monitoring (TTM) in the evaluation of symptoms in young persons has been clearly demonstrated by Saarel et al. [219] in a large cohort of 420 patients with palpitations, 43 with chest discomfort, and 32 with presyncope and syncope. Fifty-two percent ($n = 257$) of patients failed to transmit an ECG while experiencing symptoms. Of 238 symptomatic patients, 35 (15%) had SVT, and all patients with SVT had palpitations. The overall sensitivity of the TTM test was 83% (35 of 42) for detection of SVT, and the NPV was 99% in this patient population. The conclusion was that TTMs are useful for the evaluation of children and adolescents with palpitations but not with isolated chest pain, syncope, or presyncope.

Because of the intermittent nature of transient neurological symptoms such as dizziness, syncope, or near syncope in pediatric patients without structural heart disease, the efficacy of 24-h or 48-h AECG monitoring is low and thus, its ability to clarify patients' symptoms is limited. Therefore, prolonged AECG monitoring is only recommended in those individuals with known heart disease or with exertional symptoms, in whom the presence and significance of an arrhythmia may be increased [220, 221]. An alternative diagnostic tool may be the implanted loop recorder (ILR) in case conventional investigations have failed to identify the cause of syncope or palpitations. In a small series of 4 children with congenital heart disease, who suffered from presyncope ($n = 1$), syncope ($n = 2$), and palpitations ($n = 1$), an ILR was implanted. All patients experienced typical symptoms and activated the device appropriately at a median of 86 days (46–102) after implantation. In 2 of 4 cases, a likely cause for the symptoms was identified, with exclusion of more malignant arrhythmic diagnoses in all patients. The conclusion from this study was that an ILR can be implanted in young children without difficulty and that this device may prove to be very useful for excluding malignant arrhythmias as a cause of symptoms in patients at high risk [222]. Chest pain is a relatively rare symptom, and a cardiac cause is identified in only 5% or less of pediatric patients, so that the primary role of AECG monitoring in these patients may be to exclude rather than diagnose a cardiac cause [7].

1.9.2 Evaluation of Patients with Known Cardiovascular Disease

AECG monitoring may be particularly useful in pediatric patients after surgery for congenital heart disease, but the frequency of recording periods has to be based on the type of defect, ventricular function, and late postoperative arrhythmias. Uncomplicated repairs of simple defects such as atrial or ventricular septal defects or with aortic or pulmonary stenosis have a low incidence of late postoperative arrhythmias, whereas complex repairs or those with residual hemodynamic abnormalities display a high incidence of late postoperative arrhythmia. High grade ambulatory VEA associated with ventricular dysfunction seems to identify patients at an increased risk of late sudden death [223–227]. Major atrial surgery such as Mustard's or Senning's operation for transposition of great arteries or Fontan's operation for functional single ventricle hearts is often associated with sinus node dysfunction and with unusual types of AFl (which is called incisional atrial re-entrant tachycardias = IART). Major ventricular surgeries such as tetralogy of Fallot repair, repair of double outlet right ventricle, etc. may predispose to serious ventricular tacharrhythmias in the long run. In the past, complex VEA or nsVT were considered as risk stratifiers in those patients. However, Cullen et al. [225] showed, at least in patients after repair of Fallot, that after a follow-up of 12 years, asymptomatic VPBs were common and the presence of complex VEA or non-sustained VT were not prognostically significant in this patient group. Nevertheless, if complex ventricular arrhythmias are detected with AECG monitoring in post-operative high-risk pediatric patients with depressed ventricular function, there is a need for further investigation, even in the absence of overt clinical signs or symptoms [228].

A second group of pediatric patients may benefit from periodic AECG monitoring, namely, those with hypertrophic or dilated cardiomyopathy as well as with the congenital long QT syndrome because of the tendency of progression of these diseases and the need to adjust medication doses with growth [7]. The rate of 9–15% of sudden death as a first symptom in young patients with these types of disease is significantly higher than in adults, and AECG monitoring is needed to identify occult arrhythmias that may indicate the need for reevaluation of therapy in asymptomatic patients, though the absence of an arrhythmia during one or several monitoring periods does not necessarily indicate a low risk of arrhythmic sudden death. There is no doubt that unexplained syncope or cardiovascular collapse in young patients with known cardiovascular disease generally requires in-hospital continuous ECG monitoring and sophisticated (e.g., by MRI) or invasive evaluation when the cause of the event is uncertain. But if a cause cannot be established by MRI or invasive methods, AECG monitoring may be used for subsequent surveillance to possibly detect both transient brady- and tachyarrhythmias [7].

1.9.3   Evaluation of Medical Therapy or Intervention

AECG monitoring may be helpful to evaluate both beneficial and potentially harmful effects of pharmacological therapy as well as to detect possible causes of symptoms in patients with pacemakers or after radiofrequency catheter ablation or cardiac surgery, particularly when complicated by transient AV block [229, 230]. Another important indication for AECG monitoring is the evaluation of cardiac rhythm after treatment of incessant tachyarrhythmias, which have been associated with progressive ventricular dysfunction [231]. In this context, the above mentioned technical aspects and limitations of AECG monitoring (e.g., day-to-day variability of arrhythmias, etc.) have to be taken into account.

1.10   Future Perspectives of Ambulatory Monitoring

Further advances in AECG monitoring analysis include better characterization of duration and dispersion of ventricular depolarization (QTI), the detection of T-wave alternans, the identification of different patterns of onset of arrhythmias (short–long–short sequence, tachycardia versus bradycardia dependence of arrhythmias), the computation of heart-rate turbulence indexes, and the evaluation of P wave and QRS-wave morphology including P-wave averaging and late potential analysis, from high-quality AECG signals [232]. By this means, old and new markers derived from AECG monitoring could be integrated to provide a comprehensive noninvasive AECG test, to fully characterize all three components of the triangle of risk factors (❷ Fig. 1.37) that may lead to electrical instability and SCD: the electrophysiologic (arrhythmia) substrate, the triggers for malignant ventricular arrhythmias provoking SCD, and the modulation of the (background) sympatho–vagal balance of the ANS [233].

Thanks to the availability of larger storage capacities, in the near future long-term (weeks–months) continuous high-quality AECG monitoring may become available. Moreover, devices for long-term long-distance telemetric surveillance using transtelephonic transmission of ECG data for high-risk cardiac patients have already become a reality. Some modern digital recorders already have the capability for multichannel (8–12 channels) simultaneous ECG recordings, which might be interesting for ischemia monitoring. Finally, multichannel digital recordings will allow the retrieval of different

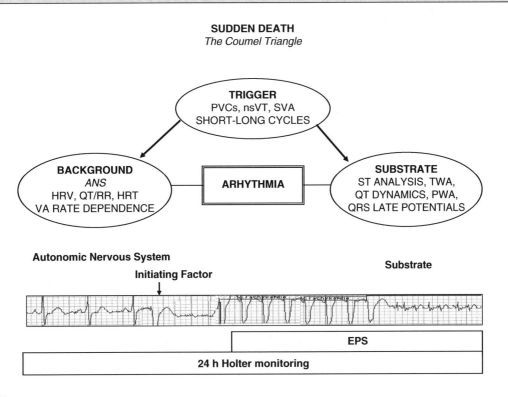

SUDDEN DEATH
The Coumel Triangle

○ Fig. 1.37
Schematic representation of the triangle of risk factors that may lead to electrical instability with subsequent ventricular fibrillation, including the different parameters that can be derived from AECG monitoring: the electrophysiologic substrate, the balance of the ANS, and the triggers of malignant ventricular arrhythmias that provoke SCD. Abbreviations: PVCs: premature ventricular contractions, nsVT: non-sustained VT, SVA: supraventricular arrhythmias, HRV: heart-rate variability, QT/R–R: QT/R–R interval relation, HRT: heart-rate turbulence, VA: ventricular arrhythmias, TWA: T-wave alternans, PWA: P-wave duration from averaged ECG (Modified from Coumel 1990)

biological signals by appropriate sensors, such as arterial pulse pressure, respiratory rate, peripheral oxygen tension, EEG, and others. This will transform AECG monitoring into ambulatory polycardiography that will allow the comprehensive evaluation of patients with complex disorders, such as CHF, cor pulmonale, or sleep apnea syndromes, and the detection and quantification of underlying interactive pathophysiological mechanisms [232].

References

1. Harrison, D.C., J.W. Fitzgerald, and R.A. Winkle, Ambulatory electrocardiography for diagnosis and treatment of cardiac arrhythmias. *N. Engl. J. Med.*, 1976;**294**: 373–380.
2. Hinkle, L.E., Jr., Equipment specifications and analytic techniques: clinical implications, in *Ambulatory Electrocardiographic Recording*, N.K. Wenger, M.B. Mock, and I. Ringqvist, Editors. Chicago, IL: Year Book Medical, 1981, pp. 33–57.
3. Holter, N.J., New method for heart studies: continuous electrocardiography of active subjects over long periods is now practical. *Science*, 1961;**134**: 1214–1220.
4. Kennedy, H.L., *Ambulatory Electrocardiography – Current Clinical Concepts*. Cardiol. Clin.; Philadelphia/London/Toronto/Montreal/Sydney/Tokyo: W.B. Saunders, 1992.
5. Van Keulen. G.J., J. Boter, C.A.A. Hakkenberg Van Gaasbeek, and G.E.P.M. Van Venrooij, *MFI Test "Holter Systems": Long-Term ECG Tape Recorder Systems*. Utrecht: Institute of Medical Physics TNO, 1980.
6. Sheffield, L.T., A. Berson, D. Bragg-Remschell, et al., Recommendations for standards of instrumentation and practice in the use of ambulatory electrocardiography. *Circulation*, 1985;**71**: 626A–636A.

7. Crawford, M.H., S.J. Bernstein, P.C. Deedwania, et al., ACC/AHA guidelines for ambulatory electrocardiography. A report of the American College of Cardiology/American Heart Association Task Force on Practical Guidelines (Commission to Revise the Guidelines for Ambulatory Electrocardiography). *J. Am. Coll. Cardiol.*, 1999;**34**: 912–948.

8. Lanza, G.A., M. Mascellanti, M. Placentino, et al., Usefulness of a third Holter lead for detection of myocardial ischemia. *Am. J. Cardiol.*, 1994;**74**: 1216–1219.

9. Osterhues, H.H., T. Eggeling, M. Kochs, and V. Hombach, Improved detection of transient myocardial ischemia by a new lead combination: value of bipolar lead Nehb D for Holter monitoring. *Am. Heart J.*, 1994;**127**: 559–566.

10. Seeberger, M.D., J. Moerlen, K. Skarvan, et al., The inverse Nehb J lead increases the sensitivity of Holter electrocardiographic monitoring for detecting myocardial ischemia. *Am. J. Cardiol.*, 1997;**80**: 1–5.

11. Cristal, N., M. Gueron, and R. Hoffman, VI-like and aVF-Iike leads for continuous electrocardiographic monitoring. *Br. Heart J.*, 1972;**34**: 696–698.

12. Jenkins, J.M., D. Wu, and R.C. Arzbaecher, Computer diagnosis of supraventricular and ventricular arrhythmias. A new esophageal technique. *Circulation*, 1979;**60**: 977–985.

13. Schnittger, I., I.M. Rodriguez, and R.A.Winkle, Esophageal electrocardiography: A new technology revives an old technique. *Am. J. Cardiol.*, 1986;**57**: 604–607.

14. Rosengarten, M.D., J.F. Leclercq, P. Attuel, and Ph. Coumel, Holter monitoring and cardiac rhythm, in *What's New in Electrocardiography*, H.J.J. Wellens and H.E. Kulbertus, Editors. The Hague: Nijhoff, 1981, pp. 344–365.

15. Bragg-Remschell, D.A., C.M. Anderson, and R.A. Winkle, Frequency response characteristics of ambulatory ECG monitoring systems and their implications for ST segment analysis. *Am. Heart J.*, 1982;**103**: 20–31.

16. Nygards, M.-E., T. Ahren, I. Ringqvist, and A. Walker, Phase correction for accurate ST segment reproduction in ambulatory ECG recording, in *Computers in Cardiology, 1984*, K. Ripley, Editor. Silver Spring, MD: IEEE, 1984, pp. 33–38.

17. Shook, T.L., C.W. Balke, P.W. Kotilainen, et al., Comparison of amplitude-modulated (direct) and frequency-modulated ambulatory techniques for recording ischemic electrocardiographic changes. *Am. J. Cardiol.*, 1987;**60**: 895–900.

18. Nearing, B.D., P.H. Stone, and R.L. Verrier, Frequency response characteristics required for detection of T-wave alternans during ambulatory ECH monitoring. *Ann. Noninvasive Electrocardiol.*, 1996;**1**: 103–112.

19. Kennedy, H.L., S.C. Smith, J. Mizera, et al., Limitations of ambulatory ECG real-time analysis for ventricular and supraventricular arrhythmia accuracy detected by clinical evaluation. *Am. J. Noninvasive Cardiol.*, 1992;**6**: 137–146.

20. Krahn, A.D., G.J. Klein, and V. Manda, The high cost of syncope: cost implications of a new insertable loop recorder in the investigation of recurrent syncope. *Am. Heart J.*, 1999;**137**: 870–877.

21. Krasnow, A.Z. and D.K. Bloomfield, Artifacts in ambulatory ECG monitoring, in *Ambulatory ECG Monitoring*, S. Stern, Editor. Chicago, IL: Year Book Medical, 1978, pp. 171–189.

22. Leclercq, J.F., *L 'Enregistrement Holter en Rhythmologie*. Paris: Labaz, 1980.

23. Quiret, J.C., J.L. Rey, M. Lombaert, and P. Bernasconi. Les artefacts au cours de l'e:nregistrement electrocardiographique continu par la methode de Holter. *Arch. Mal. Coeur Vaiss.*, 1979;**72**: 757–765.

24. Cashman, P.M.M., Methods for tape analysis II. *Postgrad. Med. J.*, 1976;**52**(Suppl. 7): 19–23.

25. Crow, R.S. and R.J. Prineas, Quality control, in *Ambulatory Electrocardiographic Recording*, N.K. Wenger, N.I.B. Mock, and I. Ringqvist, Editors. Chicago, IL: Year Book Medical, 1981, pp. 19–64.

26. Palma Gamitz, J.L., *Electrocardiografia de Holter*. Madrid: Norma, 1983.

27. Corday, E. and T.-W. Lang, Accuracy of data reduction systems for diagnosis and quantification of arrhythmias. *Am. J. Cardiol.*, 1975;**35**: 927–928.

28. Coumel, Ph., P. Attuel, J.F. Leclercq, and D. Flammang, Computerized quantitative evaluation of cardiac arrhythmias, in *Computers in Cardiology. (1977)*. New York: IEEE, 1977, pp. 571–577.

29. Weber, H.S., G. Joskowicz, D. Glogar, K.K. Steinbach, and F. Kaindl, Clinical importance of computer assisted long-term ECG analysis, in *Long-Term Ambulatory Electrocardiography*, J. Roelandt and P.G. Hugenholtz, Editors. The Hague: Nijhoff, 1982.

30. Stern, S. and D. Tzivoni, Early detection of silent ischaemic heart disease by 24-hour electrocardiographic monitoring of active subjects. *Br. Heart J.*, 1974;**36**: 481–486.

31. Cohn, P.F. and W.B. Kannel, Recognition, pathogenesis, and management options in silent coronary artery disease. *Circulation*, 1987;75: II-1.

32. Benhorin, J., F. Badilini, A.J. Moss, et al., New approach to detection of ischemic-type ST segment depression, in *Noninvasive Electrocardiology – Clinical Aspects of Holter Monitoring*, A.J. Moss and S. Stern, Editors. London/Philadelphia/Toronto/Sydney/Tokyo: WB Saunders, 1996, pp. 345–355.

33. Badilini, F., W. Zareba, E.L. Titlebaum, and A.J. Moss, Analysis of ST segment variability in Holter recordings, in *Noninvasive Electrocardiology – Clinical Aspects of Holter Monitoring*, A.J. Moss and S. Stern, Editors. London/Philadelphia/Toronto/Sydney/Tokyo: WB Saunders, 1996, pp. 357–372.

34. Ghuran, A. and M. Malik, Time domain heart rate variability, in *Noninvasive Electrocardiology in Clinical Practice*, W. Zareba, P. Maison-Blanche, and E.H. Locati, Editors. Armonk/New York: Futura, 2001, pp. 145–162.

35. Lombardi, F., Frequency domain analysis of heart rate variability, in *Noninvasive Electrocardiology in Clinical Practice*, W. Zareba, P. Maison-Blanche, and E.H. Locati, Editors. Armonk/New York: Futura, 2001, pp. 163–180.

36. Task Force of the ESC and NASPE, Heart rate variability standards of measurement, physiological interpretation, and clinical use. *Circulation*, 1996;**93**: 1043–1065.

37. Malliani, A., M. Pagani, F. Lombardi, et al., Cardiovascular neural regulation explored in the frequency domain. *Circulation*, 1991;**84**: 482–492.

38. Saul, J.P., Y. Arai, R.D. Berger, et al., Assessment of autonomic regulation in chronic congestive heart failure by heart rate spectral analysis. *Am. J. Cardiol.*, 1988;**61**: 1292–1299.

39. Schmidt, G., M. Malik, P. Barthel, et al., Heart-rate-turbulence after ventricular premature beats as a predictor of mortality after acute myocardial infarction. *Lancet*, 1999;**353**: 1390–1396.

40. Hainsworth, R., Physiology of the cardiac autonomic system, in *Clinical Guide to Cardiac Autonomic Tests*, chapter 1, M. Malik, Editor. London: Kluwer Academic, 1998, pp. 3–28.

41. Voss, A., V. Baier, A. Schymann, et al., Postextrasystolic regulation patterns of blood pressure and heart rate in idiopathic dilated cardiomyopathy. *J. Physiol. (London)*, 2002;**538**: 271–278.

42. Schneider, R., P. Barthel, G. Schmidt, Methods for the assessment of heart rate turbulence in Holter ECGs. *J. Am. Coll. Cardiol.*, 1999;**33**(Suppl. A): 351A.

43. Locati, E.H., QT interval duration and adaptation to heart rate, in *Noninvasive Electrocardiology in Clinical Practice*, W. Zareba, P. Maison-Blanche, and E.H. Locati, Editors. Armonk/New York: Futura, 2001, pp. 71–96.

44. Lepeschkin, E. and B. Surawicz, The measurement of the QT interval of the electrocardiogram. *Circulation*, 1952;**6**: 378–388.

45. Cowan, J.C., K. Yusoff, M. Moore, et al., Importance of lead selection in QT interval measurement. *Am. J. Cardiol.* 1988;**61**: 83–87.

46. Laguna, P., N.V. Thakor, P. Caminal, et al., New algorithm for QT analysis in 24-hour Holter ECG: performance and applications. *Med. Biol. Eng. Comput.*, 1990;**28**: 67–73.

47. Maison-Blanche, P., D. Catuli, J. Fayn, and P. Coumel, QT interval, heart rate and ventricular arrhythmias, in *Noninvasive Electrocardiology – Clinical Aspects of Holter Monitoring*, A.J. Moss and S. Stern, Editors. London/Philadelphia/Toronto/Sydney/Tokyo: WB Saunders, 1996, pp. 383–404.

48. Han, J. and G.K. Moe, Nonuniform recovery of excitability in ventricular muscle. *Circ. Res.*, 1964;**14**: 44–60.

49. Antzelevich, C., W. Shimizu, G.X. Yan, et al., The M cell: its contribution to the ECG and normal and abnormal electrical function of the heart. *J. Cardiovasc. Electrophysiol.*, 1999;**10**: 1124–1152.

50. Sylvén, J.C., B.M. Horacek, C.A. Spencer, et al., QT interval variability on the body surface. *J. Electrocardiol.*, 1984;**17**: 179–188.

51. Zareba, W., A. Nomura, and J. Perkiömäki, Dispersion of repolarization: concept, methodology, and clinical experience, in *Noninvasive Electrocardiology in Clinical Practice*, W. Zareba, P. Maison-Blanche, and E.H. Locati, Editors. Armonk/New York: Futura, 2001, pp. 97–121.

52. Rautaharju, P.M., Why did QT dispersion die? *CEPR*, 2002;**6**: 295–301.

53. Malik, M., QT dispersion: time for an obituary? *Eur. Heart J.*, 2000;**21**: 955–957 (Editorial).

54. Simson, M.B., Use of signals in the terminal QRS complex to identify patients with ventricular tachycardia after myocardial infarction. *Circulation*, 1981;**64**: 235–241.

55. Breithardt, G., M. Cain, N. El-Sherif, et al., Standards for analysis of ventricular late potentials using high-resolution signal-averaged electrocardiography: a statement by a Task Force Committee of the European Society of Cardiology, the American Heart Association, and the American College of Cardiology. *J. Am. Coll. Cardiol.*, 1991;**17**: 999–1006.

56. Kelen, G., R. Henkin, M. Lannon, et al., Correlation between the signal-averaged electrocardiogram from Holter tapes and from real-time recordings. *Am. J. Cardiol.*, 1989;**63**: 1321–1325.

57. Leenhardt, A., P. Maison-Blanche, I. Denjoy, et al., Signal averaging of ventricular late potentials using Holter recordings. *Eur. Heart J.*, 1990;**11**: 402 (Abstract).

58. Kostis, J.B., A.E. Moreyra, M.T. Amendo, J. Di Pietro, N. Cosgrove, and P.T. Kuo, The effect of age on heart rate in subjects free of heart disease. Studies by ambulatory electrocardiography and maximal exercise stress test. *Circulation*, 1982;**65**: 141–145.

59. Bjerregaard, P., Mean 24 hour heart rate, minimal heart rate and pauses in healthy subjects 40–79 years of age. *Eur. Heart J.*, 1983;**4**: 44–51.

60. Bjerregaard, P., Prevalence and variability of cardiac arrhythmias in healthy subjects, in *Cardiac Arrhythmias in the Active Population. Prevalence, Significance and Management*, D.A. Chamberlain, H. Kulbertus, L. Mogensen, and M. Schlepper, Editors. Molndal Sweden: Hassle, 1980, p. 24.

61. Bjerregaard, P., Premature beats in healthy subjects 40–79 years of age. *Eur. Heart J.*, 1982;**3**: 493–503.

62. Djiane, P., A. Egre, M. Bory, B. Savin, S. Mostefa, and A. Serradimigni, L'enregistrement electrocardiographique chez les sujets normaux. *Arch. Mal. Coeur Vaiss.*, 1979;**72**: 655–661.

63. Goulding, L., Twenty-four hour ambulatory electrocardiography from normal urban and rural populations, in *ISAM 1977*, F.D. Stott, E.B. Raftery, P. Sleight, and L. Goulding, Editors. London: Academic, 1978, pp. 13–22.

64. Verbaan, C.J., J. Pool, and J. Van Wanrooy, Incidence of cardiac arrhythmias in a presumed healthy population, in *ISAM 1977*, F.D. Stott, E.B. Raftery, P. Sleight, and L. Goulding, Editors. London: Academic, 1978, pp. 1–5.

65. Brodsky, M., D. Wu, P. Denes, C. Kanakis, and K.M. Rosen, Arrhythmias documented by 24 hour continuous electrocardiographic monitoring in 50 male medical students without apparent heart disease. *Am. J. Cardiol.*, 1977;**39**: 390–395.

66. Armstrong, W.F., J.W. Jordan, S.N. Morris, and P.L. McHenry, Prevalence and magnitude of S-T segment and T wave abnormalities in normal men during continuous ambulatory electrocardiography. *Am. J. Cardiol.*, 1982;**49**: 1638–1642.

67. Quyyumi, A.A., C. Wright, and K. Fox, Ambulatory electrocardiographic ST segment changes in healthy volunteers. *Br. Heart J.*, 1983;**50**: 460–464.

68. Bjerregaard, P., Prevalence and magnitude of ST segment and T-wave abnormalities in healthy adult subjects during continuous ambulatory electrocardiography, in *Ambulatory Monitoring: Cardiovascular System and Allied Applications*, C. Marchesi, Editor. The Hague: Nijhoff, 1984, pp. 114–118.

69. Burckhardt, D., B.E. Luetold, M.V. Jost, and A. Hoffmann, Holter monitoring in the evaluation of palpitations, dizziness and syncope, in *Long-Term Ambulatory Electrocardiography*, J. Roelandt and P.G. Hugenholtz, Editors. The Hague: Nijhoff, 1982, pp. 29–39.

70. Krasnow, A.Z. and D.K. Bloomfield, The relationship between subjective symptomatology and objective findings from ambulatory ECG monitoring studies in a large unselected population, in *Ambulatory ECG Monitoring*, S. Stem, Editor. Chicago, IL: Year Book Medical, 1978, pp. 149–169.

71. Shenasa, M., P.V.L. Curry, and E. Sowton, The relationship between symptoms and arrhythmias during 24-hour ECG recording, in *ISAM 1979*, F.D. Stott, E.B. Raftery, and L. Goulding, Editors. London: Academic, 1980, pp. 39–49.

72. Bass, E.B., E.I. Curtiss, V.C. Arena, et al., The duration of Holter monitoring in patients with syncope: is 24 hours enough? *Arch. Intern. Med.*, 1990;**150**: 1073–1078.

73. Babalis, D., P. Maison-Blanche, J.F. Leclercq, and Ph. Coumel, Interet d'un electrocardiogramme de longue duree chez les patients ayant eu un accident cerebral ischemique. *Arch. Mal. Coeur Vaiss.*, 1984;**77**: 100–105.

74. Fisher, M., Holter monitoring in patients with transient focal cerebral ischemia. *Stroke*, 1978;**9**: 514–516.

75. Reed, R.L., R.G. Siekert, and J. Merideth, Rarity of transient focal cerebral ischemia in cardiac dysrhythmia. *J. Am. Med. Assoc.*, 1973;**223**: 893–895.

76. Tonet, J.L., R. Frank, A. Ducardonnet, et al., L'enregistrement de Holter dans les accidents ischemiques cerebraux. *Nouv. Presse Med.*, 1981;**10**: 2491–2494.

77. Allen, R.D., L.S. Gettes, C. Phalan, and M.D. Avington, Painless ST-segment depression in patients with angina pectoris. Correlation with daily activities and cigarette smoking. *Chest*, 1976;**69**: 467–473.

78. Araki, H., Y. Koiwaya, O. Nakagaki, and M. Nakamura, Diurnal distribution of ST-segment elevation and related arrhythmias in patients with variant angina: a study by ambulatory ECG monitoring. *Circulation*, 1983;**67**: 995–1000.

79. Biagini, A., M.G. Mazzei, C. Carpeggiani, et al., Vasospastic ischemic mechanism of frequent asymptomatic transient ST-T changes during continuous electrocardiographic monitoring in selected unstable angina patients. *Am. Heart J.*, 1982;**103**: 13–20.

80. Gettes, L.S. and S.R. Winternitz, The use of ambulatory ECG monitoring to detect "silent" ischemia, in *Ambulatory ECG Monitoring*, S. Stern, editor. Chicago, IL: Year Book Medical, 1978, pp. 93–105.

81. Sellier, P., F. Proust, P. Dellebarre, J.L. Guermonprez, P. Ourbak, and P. Maurice, l'enregistrement electrocardiographique continu dans l'insuffisance coronarie interet diagnostique. *Arch. Mal. Coeur Vaiss.*, 1978;**71**: 638–644.

82. Stern, S. and D. Tzivoni, Evaluation of ST-T alterations in the ECG by ambulatory monitoring, in *Ambulatory ECG Monitoring*, S. Stern, editor. Chicago, IL: Year Book Medical, 1978, pp. 85–91.

83. Coumel, Ph., D. Milosevic, M. Rosengarten, J.F. Leclercq, and P. Attuel, Interet theorique et pratique du monitoring de Holter dans le bloc sino-auriculaire. *Ann. Cardiol. Angeiol.* 1980;**29**: 19–22.

84. Coumel, Ph., J.-F. Leclercq, P. Attuel, J.-P. Lavalle, and D. Flammang, Autonomic influences in the genesis of atrial arrhythmias: atrial flutter and fibrillation of vagal origin, in *Cardiac Arrhythmias Electrophysiology, Diagnosis and Management*, O.S. Narula, Editor. Baltimore, MD: Williams and Wilkins, 1979, pp. 243–255.

85. Coumel, Ph., P. Attuel, J.F. Leclercq, and P. Friocourt, Arythmies auriculaires d'origine vagale ou catecholergique. Effets compares du traitement Beta-bloquant et phenomene d'echappement. *Arch. Mal. Coeur Vaiss.*, 1982;**75**: 373–387.

86. Anderson, G.J. and M. Greenspan, Ventricular ectopic beats with exit block: a retrospective Holter monitor study. *J. Electrocardiol.*, 1983;**16**: 133–140.

87. Coumel, Ph., J.-F. Leclercq, P. Attuel, J.-P. Lavallee, and D. Flammang, Autonomic influences: sympathetic drive and the genesis of ventricular arrhythmias, in *Cardiac Arrhythmias. Electrophysiology, Diagnosis and Management*, O.S. Narula, Editor. Baltimore, MD: Williams and Wilkins, 1979, pp. 457–473.

88. Lown, B., M. Tykocinski, A. Garfein, and P. Brooks, Sleep and ventricular premature beats. *Circulation*, 1973;**48**: 691–701.

89. Vellani, C.W. and A. Murray, The effect of sinus rhythm on the periodicity and coupling interval of ventricular parasystolic rhythm. *Eur. Heart J.*, 1981;**2**: 429–439.

90. Deedwania, P.C., Ischemia detected by Holter monitoring in coronary artery disease, in *Noninvasive Electrocardiology – Clinical Aspects of Holter Monitoring*, A.J. Moss and S. Stern,

Editors. London/Philadelphia/Toronto/Sydney/Tokyo: WB Saunders, 1996, pp. 331–343.

91. Stone, P.H. and G. MacCallum, ST segment analysis in ambulatory ECG (Holter) monitoring, in *Noninvasive Electrocardiology in Clinical Practice*, W. Zareba, P. Maison-Blanche, and E.H. Locati, Editors. Armonk/New York: Futura, 2001, pp. 97–121.

92. Stone, P.H., B. Chaitman, R.P. McMahon, et al. for the ACIP Investigators, The relationship between exercise-induced and ambulatory ischemia in patients with stable coronary disease. *Circulation*, 1996;**94**: 1537–1544.

93. Tzivoni, D. and S. Stern, Complimentary role of ambulatory electrocardiographic monitoring and exercise testing in evaluation of myocardial ischemia. *Cardiol. Clin.*; in *Ambulatory Electrocardiography – Current Clinical Concepts*, H.L. Kennedy, Editor. Philadelphia/London/Toronto/Montreal/Sydney/Tokyo: W.B. Saunders, 1992, pp. 461–466.

94. Gettes, L.S., Painless myocardial ischemia. *Chest*, 1974;**66**: 612–613 (editorial).

95. Stern, S. and D. Tzivoni, Early detection of silent ischaemic heart disease by 24-hour electrocardiographic monitoring of active subjects. *Br. Heart J.*, 1974;**36**: 481–486.

96. Cohn, P.F., *Silent myocardial ischemia and infarction*. New York: Marcel Dekker, 1986.

97. Cohn, P.F., Silent myocardial ischemia: the early years, in *Silent Myocardial Ischemia*, S. Stern, Editor. London: Martin Dunitz, 1998, pp. 1–5.

98. Stone, P.H. and A.P. Selwyn, The prognostic significance of silent myocardial ischemia, in *Silent Myocardial Ischemia*, S Stern, Editor. London: Martin Dunitz, 1998, pp. 55–66.

99. Deanfield, J.E., A.P. Selwyn, S. Chierchia, et al., Myocardial ischemia during daily life in patients with stable angina: its relation to symptoms and heart rate changes. *Lancet*, 1983;**ii**: 753–758.

100. Chipkin, S.R., D. Frid, J.S. Alpert, et al., Frequency of painless myocardial ischemia during exercise tolerance testing in patients with and without diabetes mellitus. *Am. J. Cardiol.*, 1987;**50**: 61–65.

101. Marchant, B., V. Umachandran, R. Stevenson, et al., Silent myocardial ischemia: role of subclinical neuropathy in patients with and without diabetes. *J. Am. Coll. Cardiol.*, 1993;**22**: 1433–1437.

102. Droste, C. and H. Roskamm, Experimental pain measurement in patients with asymptomatic myocardial ischemia. *J. Am. Coll. Cardiol.*, 1983;**1**: 940–945.

103. Droste, C. and H. Roskamm, Pain perception and endogenous pain modulation in angina pectoris. *Adv. Cardiol.*, 1990;**37**: 142–149.

104. Rosen, S.D., E. Paulsen, P. Nihoyannopoulos, et al., Silent ischemia as a central problem: regional brain activation compared in silent and painful myocardial ischemia. *Ann. Intern. Med.*, 1996;**124**: 1006–1008.

105. Rocco, M.B., E.G. Nabel, S. Campbell, et al., Prognostic importance of myocardial ischemia detected by ambulatory monitoring in patients with stable coronary artery disease. *Circulation*, 1988;**78**: 877–884.

106. Tzivoni, D., A. Gavish, D. Zin, et al., Prognostic significance of ischemic episodes in patients with previous myocardial infarction. *Am. J. Cardiol.*, 1988;**62**: 661–664.

107. Hedblad, B., S. Juul-Möller, K. Swensson, et al., Increased mortality in men with ST segment depression during 24h ambulatory

long-term ECG recording. Results from prospective population study "Men born in 1914" from Malmo, Sweden. *Eur. Heart J.*, 1989;**10**: 149–158.

108. Deedwania, P.C. and E.V. Carbajal, Silent ischemia during daily life is an independent predictor of mortality in stable angina. *Circulation*, 1990;**81**: 748–756.

109. Raby, K.E., L. Goldman, E.F. Cook, et al., Long-term prognosis of myocardial ischemia detected by Holter monitoring in peripheral vascular disease. *Am. J. Cardiol.*, 1990;**66**: 1309–1313.

110. Yeung, A.C., J. Barry, J. Orav, et al., Effects of asymptomatic ischemia on long-term prognosis in chronic stable coronary disease. *Circulation*, 1991;**83**: 1598–1604.

111. Deedwania, P.C. and E.V. Carbajal, Usefulness of ambulatory silent myocardial ischemia added to the prognostic value of exercise test parameters in predicting risk of cardiac death in patients with stable angina pectoris and exercise-induced myocardial ischemia. *Am. J. Cardiol.*, 1991;**68**: 1279–1286.

112. Quyumi, A.A., J.A. Panza, J.G. Diodati, et al., Prognostic implications of myocardial ischemia during daily life in low risk patients with coronary artery disease. *J. Am. Coll. Cardiol.*, 1993;**21**: 700–708.

113. Moss, A.J., R.E. Goldstein, J. Hall, et al., Detection and significance of myocardial ischemia in stable patients after recovery from an acute coronary event. *JAMA*, 1993;**269**: 2379–2385.

114. de Marchena, E., J. Asch, J. Martinez, et al., Usefulness of persistent silent myocardial ischemia in predicting a high cardiac event rate in men with medically controlled, stable angina pectoris. *Am. J. Cardiol.*, 1994;**73**: 390–392.

115. Madjilessi-Simon, T., M. Mary-Krause, F. Fillette, et al., Persistent transient myocardial ischemia despite beta-adrenergic blockade predicts a higher risk of adverse cardiac events in patients with coronary artery disease. *J. Am. Coll. Cardiol.*, 1996;**27**: 1586–1591.

116. Gill, J.B., J.A. Cairns, R.S. Roberts, et al., Prognostic importance of myocardial ischemia detected by ambulatory monitoring early after acute myocardial infarction. *N. Engl. J. Med.*, 1996;**334**: 65–70.

117. Pepine, C.J., P.F. Cohn, P.C. Deedwania, et al., Effects of treatment on outcome in mildly symptomatic patients with ischemia during daily life: the Atenolol Silent Ischemia Study (ASIST). *Circulation*, 1994;**90**: 762–768.

118. Rogers, W.J., M.G. Bourassa, T.C. Andrews, et al., Asymptomatic Cardiac Ischemia Pilot (ACIP) study: outcome at 1 year for patients with asymptomatic cardiac ischemia randomized to medical therapy or revascularization: the ACIP Investigators. *J. Am. Coll. Cardiol.*, 1995;**26**: 594–605.

119. Dargie, H.J., I. Ford, and K.M. Fox, Total Ischaemic Burden European Trial (TIBET): effects of ischmaemia and treatment with atenolol, nifedipine SR and their combination on outcome in patients with chronic stable angina: the TIBET Study Group. *Eur. Heart J.*, 1996;**17**: 104–112.

120. von Arnim, Prognostic significance of transient ischemic episodes: response to treatment shows improved prognosis: results of the Total Ischemic Burden Bisoprolol Study (TIBBS) follow-up. *J. Am. Coll. Cardiol.*, 1996;**28**: 20–24.

121. Bailey, J.J., A. Berson, H. Handelsman, and M. Hodges, Utility of current risk stratification tests for predicting major arrhythmic events after myocardial infarction. *J. Am. Coll. Cardiol.*, 2001;**38**: 1902–1911.

122. Moss, A.J., W.J. Hall, D.S. Cannom, et al., Improved survival with an implanted defibrillator in patients with coronary disease at high risk for ventricular arrhythmia: Multicenter Automatic Defibrillator Implantation Trial Investigators. *N. Engl. J. Med.*, 1996;**335**: 1933–1940.

123. Denes, P., A.M. Gillis, Y. Pawitan, et al., Prevalence, characteristics and significance of ventricular premature complexes and ventricular tachycardia detected by 24-hour continuous electrocardiographic recording in the Cardiac Arrhythmia Suppression Trial. CAST Investigators. *Am. J. Cardiol.*, 1991;**68**: 887–896.

124. Ruberman, W., E. Weinblatt, J.D. Goldberg, et al., Ventricular premature complexes and sudden death after myocardial infarction. *Circulation*, 1981;**64**: 297–305.

125. Olson, H.G., K.P. Lyons, P. Troop, et al., The high-risk acute myocardial infarction patient at 1-year follow-up: identification at hospital discharge by ambulatory electrocardiography and radionuclide ventriculography. *Am. Heart J.*, 1984;**107**: 358–366.

126. Mukharji, J., R.E. Rude, W.K. Poole, et al., Risk factors for sudden death after myocardial infarction: two-year follow-up. *Am. J. Cardiol.*, 1984;**54**: 31–36.

127. Kostis, J.B., R. Byington, L.M. Friedman, et al., Prognostic significance of ventricular ectopic activity in survivors of acute myocardial infarction. *J. Am. Coll. Cardiol.*, 1987;**10**: 231–242.

128. Verzoni, A., S. Romano, L. Pozzoni, et al., Prognostic significance and evolution of late ventricular potentials in the first year after myocardial infarction: a prospective study. *Pacing Clin. Electrophysiol.*, 1989;**12**: 41–51.

129. Gomes, J.A., S.L. Winters, M. Martinson, et al., The prognostic significance of quantitative signal-averaged variables relative to clinical variables, site of myocardial infarction, ejection fraction and ventricular premature beats: a prospective study. *J. Am. Coll. Cardiol.*, 1989;**13**: 377–384.

130. Richards, D.A., K. Byth, D.L. Ross, et al., What is the best predictor of spontaneous ventricular tachycardia and sudden death after myocardial infarction? *Circulation*, 1991;**83**: 756–763.

131. Farrell, T.G., Y. Bashir, T. Cripps, et al., Risk stratification for arrhythmic events in postinfarction patients based on heart rate variability, ambulatory electrocardiographic variables and the signal-averaged electrocardiogram. *J. Am. Coll. Cardiol.*, 1991;**18**: 687–697.

132. de Cock, C.C., F.C. Visser, M.J. van Eenige, et al., Independent prognostic value of supraventricular arrhythmias on 24-h ambulatory monitoring following myocardial infarction. *Eur. Heart J.*, 1991;**12**: 1070–1075.

133. Steinberg, J.S., A. Regan, R.R. Sciacca, et al., Predicting arrhythmic events after acute myocardial infarction using the signal-averaged electrocardiogram. *Am. J. Cardiol.*, 1992;**69**: 13–21.

134. Bigger, J.T., Jr, J.L. Fleiss, R.C. Steinman, et al., Frequency domain measures of heart rate period variability and mortality after myocardial infarction. *Circulation*, 1992;**85**: 164–171.

135. Pedretti, R., M.D. Etro, A. Laporta, et al., Prediction of late arrhythmic events after acute myocardial infarction from combined use of noninvasive prognostic variables and inducibility of sustained monomorphic ventricular tachycardia. *Am. J. Cardiol.*, 1993;**71**: 1131–1141.

136. McClements, B.M. and A.A. Adgey, Value of signal-averaged electrocardiography, radionuclide ventriculography, Holter monitoring and clinical variables for prediction of arrhythmic events in survivors of acute myocardial infarction in the thrombolytic era. *J. Am. Coll. Cardiol.*, 1993;**21**: 1419–1427.

137. Kuchar, D.L., C.W. Thorburn, and N.L. Sammel, Prognostic implications of loss of late potentials following acute myocardial infarction. *Pacing Clin. Electrophysiol.*, 1993;**16**: 2104–2111.

138. Hohnloser, S.H., P. Franck, T. Klingenleben, et al., Open infarct artery, late potentials, and other prognostic factors in patients after acute myocardial infarction in the thrombolytic era: a prospective trial. *Circulation*, 1994;**90**: 1747–1756.

139. Hermosillo, A.G., V. Araya, J.M. Casanova, et al., Risk stratification for malignant arrhythmic events in patients with an acute myocardial infarction: role of an open infarct-related artery and the signal-averaged ECG. *Coron. Artery Dis.*, 1995;**6**: 973–983.

140. El-Sherif, N., P. Denes, R. Katz, et al., Definition of the best prediction criteria of the time domain signal-averaged electrocardiogram for serious arrhythmic events in the postinfarction period. *J. Am. Coll. Cardiol.*, 1995;**25**: 908–914.

141. La Rovere, M.T., J.T. Bigger Jr, F.I. Marcus, et al., Baroreflex sensitivity and heart-rate variability in prediction of total cardiac mortality after myocardial infarction. ATRAMI (Autonomic Tone and Reflexes After Myocardial Infarction) Investigators. *Lancet*, 1998;**351**: 478–484.

142. Hohnloser, S.H., T.K. Klingenleben, M. Zabel, and O. Mauss, Prevalence, characteristics, and prognostic value during long-term follow-up of nonsustained ventricular tachycardia after myocardial infarction in the thrombolytic era. *J. Am. Coll. Cardiol.*, 1999;**33**: 1895–1902.

143. Kleiger, R.E., J.P. Miller, J.T. Bigger, et al., Decreased heart rate variability and its association with increased mortality after acute myocardial infarction. *Am. J. Cardiol.*, 1987;**59**: 256–262.

144. Odemuyiwa, O., M. Malik, T. Farrell, et al., Comparison of the predictive characteristics of heart rate variability index and left ventricular ejection fraction for all-cause mortality, arrhythmic events and sudden death after acute myocardial infarction. *Am. J. Cardiol.*, 1991;**68**: 434–439.

145. Zuanetti, G., J.M. Neilson, R. Latini, et al., Prognostic significance of heart rate variability in post-myocardial infarction patients in the fibrinolytic era. The GISSI-2 results. Gruppo Italiano per lo Studio della Sopravvivenza nell'Infarto Miocardio. *Circulation*, 1996;**94**: 432–436.

146. Copie, X., K. Hnatkova, A. Staunton, et al., Predictive power of increased heart rate versus depressed left ventricular ejection fraction and heart rate variability for risk stratification after myocardial infarction. Results of a two-year follow-up study. *J. Am. Coll. Cardiol.*, 1996;**27**: 270–276.

147. Lanza, G.A., V. Guido, M.M. Galeazzi, et al., Prognostic role of heart rate variability in patients with a recent acute myocardial infarction. *Am. J. Cardiol.*, 1998;**82**: 1323–1328.

148. Katz, A., I.F. Liberty, A. Porath, et al., A simple bedside test of 1-minute heart rate variability during deep breathing as a prognostic index after myocardial infarction. *Am. Heart J.*, 1999;**138**: 32–38.

149. Malik, M., A.J. Camm, M.J. Janse, et al., Depressed heart rate variability identifies postinfarction patients who might benefit from prophylactic treatment with amiodarone: a substudy of EMIAT (The European Myocardial Infarct Amiodarone Trial). *J. Am. Coll. Cardiol.*, 2000;**35**: 1263–1275.

150. Mäkikallio, T.H., P. Barthel, R. Schneider, et al., Prediction of sudden cardiac death after acute myocardial infarction: role of Holter monitoring in the modern treatment era. *Eur. Heart J.*, 2005;**26**: 762–769.

151. Bauer, A., P. Guzik, P. Barthel, et al., Reduced prognostic power of ventricular late potentials in post-infarction patients of the reperfusion era. *Eur. Heart J.*, 2005;**26**: 755–761.

152. Schmidt, G. and Malik, M., Heart rate turbulence, in *Noninvasive Electrocardiology in Clinical Practice*, W. Zareba, P. Maison-Blanche, and E.H. Locati, Editors. Armonk/New York: Futura, 2001, pp. 207–215.

153. Kjekshus, J., Arrhythmias and mortality in congestive heart failure. *Am. J. Cardiol.*, 1990;**65**: 421–428.

154. Gradman, A., P. Deedwania, R. Cody, B. Massie, M. Packer, B. Pitt, and S. Goldstein, Predictors of total mortality and sudden death in mild-to-moderate heart failure. Captopril-Digoxin Study Group. *J. Am. Coll. Cardiol.*, 1989;**14**: 564–570.

155. Fletcher, R.D., G.B. Cintron, G. Johnson, J. Orndorff, P. Carson, and J. Cohn for the V-HeFT VA Cooperative Studies Group, Enalapril decreases prevalence of ventricular tachycardia in patients with chronic congestive heart failure. *Circulation*, 1993;**87**(Suppl.): VI-49–55.

156. Doval, H.C., D.R. Nul, H.O. Grancelli, et al., Nonsustained ventricular tachycardia in severe heart failure: independent marker of increased mortality due to sudden death. GESICA-GEMA Investigators. *Circulation*, 1996;**94**: 3198–3203.

157. Fei, L., P.J. Keeling, J.S. Gill, Y. Bashir, D.J. Statters, J. Poloniecki, W.J. McKenna, and A.J. Camm, Heart rate variability and its relation to ventricular arrhythmias in congestive heart failure. *Br. Heart J.*, 1994;**71**: 322–328.

158. Hoffman, J., W. Grimm, V. Menz, and B. Maisch, Heart rate variability and major arrhythmias in patients with idiopathic dilated cardiomyopathy. *Pacing Clin. Electrophysiol.*, 1996;**19**: 1841–1844.

159. Yi, G., J.H. Goldman, P.J. Keeling, M. Malik, and W.J. McKenna, Heart rate variability in idiopathic dilated cardiomyopathy: relation to disease severity and prognosis. *Heart* 1977;**77**: 108–114.

160. Fauchier, L., D. Babuty, P. Cosnay, M.L. Autret, and J.P. Fauchier, Heart rate variability in idiopathic dilated cardiomyopathy: characteristics and prognostic value. *J. Am. Coll. Cardiol.*, 1997;**30**: 1009–1014.

161. Ponikowski, P., S.D. Anker, T.P. Chua, et al., Depressed heart rate variability as an independent predictor of death in chronic congestive heart failure secondary to ischemic or idiopathic dilated cardiomyopathy. *Am. J. Cardiol.*, 1997;**79**: 1645–1650.

162. Szabo, B.M., D.J. van Veldhuisen, N. van der Veer, J. Brouwer, P.A. De Graeff, and H.J.G.M. Crijns, Prognostic value of HRV in chronic congestive heart failure secondary to idiopathic or ischemic dilated cardiomyopathy. *Am. J. Cardiol.*, 1997;**79**: 978–980.

163. Boveda, S., M. Galinier, A. Pathak, et al., Prognostic value of heart rate variability in time domain in congestive heart failure. *J. Intervent. Card. Electrophysiol.*, 2000;**5**: 181–187.

164. Bilchik, K.C., B. Fetics, R. Djoukeng, et al., Prognostic value of heart rate variability in chronic congestive heart failure (Veterans Affair's Survival Trial of Antiarrhythmic Therapy in Congestive Heart Failure). *Am. J. Cardiol.*, 2002;**90**: 24–28.

165. Aronson, D., M.A. Mittleman, and A.J. Burger, Measures of heart period variability as predictors of mortality in hospitalized patients with decompensated congestive heart failure. *Am. J. Cardiol.*, 2004;**93**: 59–63.

166. La-Rovere, M.T., G.D. Pinna, R. Maestri, et al., Short-term heart rate variability strongly predicts sudden cardiac death in chronic heart failure patients. *Circulation*, 2003;**107**: 565–570.

167. Guzzetti, S., M.T. La-Rovere, G.D. Pinna, et al., Different spectral components of 24 h heart rate variability are related to different modes of death in chronic heart failure. *Eur. Heart J.*, 2005;**26**: 357–362.

168. Adamson, P.B., A.L. Smith, W.T. Abraham, et al., Continuous autonomic assessment in patients with symptomatic heart failure: prognostic value of heart rate variability measured by an implanted cardiac resynchronization device. *Circulation*, 2004;**110**: 2389–2394.

169. Koyama, J., J. Watanabe, A. Yamada, et al., Evaluation of heart rate turbulence as a new prognostic marker in patients with chronic heart failure. *Circ. J.*, 2002;**66**: 902–907.

170. Kawasaki, T., A. Azuma, S. Asada, et al., Heart rate turbulence and clinical prognosis in hypertrophic cardiomyopathy and myocardial infarction. *Circ. J.*, 2003;**67**: 601–604.

171. Grimm, W., J. Sharkova, M. Christ, et al., Prognostic significance of heart rate turbulence following ventricular premature beats in patients with idiopathic dilated cardiomyopathy. *J. Cardiovasc. Electrophysiol.*, 2003;**14**: 819–824.

172. McKenna, W.J., S. Chetty, C.M. Oakley, et al., Arrhythmia in hypertrophic cardiomyopathy: exercise and 48 hour ambulatory electrocardiographic assessment with and without beta adrenergic blocking therapy. *Am. J. Cardiol.*, 1980;**45**: 1–5.

173. Maron, B.J., D.D. Savage, J.K. Wolfson, et al., Prognostic significance of 24 hour ambulatory electrocardiographic monitoring in patients with hypertrophic cardiomyopathy: a prospective study. *Am. J. Cardiol.*, 1981;**48**: 252–257.

174. McKenna, W.J., C.M. Oakley, D.M. Krikler, et al., Improved survival with amiodarone in patients with hypertrophic cardiomyopathy and ventricular tachycardia. *Br. Heart J.*, 1985;**53**: 412–416.

175. Fanapazir, L., A.C. Chang, S.E. Epstein, et al., Prognostic determinants in hypertrophic cardiomyopathy. *Circulation*, 1992;**86**: 730–740.

176. McKenna, W.J. and E.R. Behr, Hypertrophic cardiomyopathy: management, risk stratification, and prevention of sudden death. *Heart*, 2002;**87**: 169–178.

177. Counihan, P.J., L. Fei, Y. Bashir, et al., Assessment of heart rate variability in hypertrophic cardiomyopathy: association with clinical and prognostic features. *Circulation*, 1993;**88**: 1682–1690.

178. Elliott, P.M., J. Poloniecki, S. Dickie, et al., Sudden death in hypertrophic cardiomyopathy: identification of high risk patients. *J. Am. Coll. Cardiol.*, 2000;**36**: 2212–2220.

179. Von Olshausen, K., F. Schwarz, J. Apfelbach, N. Rohrig, B. Kriimer, and W. Kiibler, Determinants of the incidence and severity of ventricular arrhythmias in aortic valve disease. *Am. J. Cardiol.*, 1983;**51**: 1103–1109.

180. Chesler, E., R.A. King, and J.E. Edwards, The myxomatous mitral valve and sudden death. *Circulation*, 1983;**67**: 632–639.

181. Jeresaty, R.M., Sudden death in the mitral valve prolapse-click syndrome. *Am. J. Cardiol.*, 1976;**37**: 317–318.

182. Leclercq, J.F., M.C. Malergue, D. Milosevic, M.D. Rosengarten, P. Attuel, and Ph. Coumel, Troubles du rythme ventriculaires et prolapsus mitral. A propos de 35 observations. *Arch. Mal. Coeur Vaiss.*, 1980;**73**: 276–287.

183. Winkle, R.A., M.G. Lopes, R.L. Popp, and E.W. Hancock, Life-threatening arrhythmias in the mitral valve prolapse syndrome. *Am. J. Med.*, 1976;**60**: 961–967.

184. Kannel, W.B., A.L. Dannenberg, and D. Levy, Population implications of electrocardiographic left ventricular hypertrophy. *Am. J. Cardiol.*, 1987;**60**: 85I–93I.

185. Levy, D., K.M. Anderson, D.D. Savage, et al., Risk of ventricular arrhythmias in left ventricular hypertrophy: the Framingham Heart Study. *Am. J. Cardiol.*, 1987;**60**: 560–565.

186. Bikkina, M., M.G. Larson, and D. Levy, Asymptomatic ventricular arrhythmias and mortality risk in subjects with left ventricular hypertrophy. *J. Am. Coll. Cardiol.*, 1993;**22**: 1111–1116.

187. Singh, J.P., M.G. Larson, H. Tsuji, et al., Reduced heart rate variability and new-onset hypertension: insights into the pathogenesis of hypertension. *Hypertension*, 1998;**32**: 293–297.

188. Liao, D., J. Cai, R.W. Barnes, et al., Association of cardiac autonomic function and the development of hypertension: the ARIC Study. *Am. J. Hypertens.*, 1996;**9**: 1147–1156.

189. Kohara, K., W. Nishida, M. Maguchi, et al., Autonomic nervous function in nondipper essential hypertensive subjects: evaluation by power spectral analysis of heart rate variability. *Hypertension*, 1995;**26**: 808–814.

190. Ewing, D.J., I.W. Campbell, B.F. Clarke, et al., The natural history of diabetic autonomic neuropathy. *QJ Med.*, 1980;**49**: 95–108.

191. Malpas, S.C. and T.J. Maling, Heart rate variability and cardiac autonomic function in diabetes. *Diabetes*, 1990;**39**: 1177–1181.

192. Ewing, D.J., J.M. Neilson, C.M. Shapiro, et al., Twenty four hour heart rate variability: effects of posture, sleep, and time of day in healthy controls and comparison with bedside tests of autonomic function in diabetic patients. *Br. Heart J.*, 1991;**65**: 239–244.

193. Bellavere, F., I. Balzani, G. De Masi, et al., Power spectral analysis of heart-rate variations improves assessment of diabetic cardiac autonomic neuropathy. *Diabetes*, 1992;**41**: 633–640.

194. D'Elia, J.A., L.A. Weinrauch, R.E. Gleason, et al., Application of the ambulatory 24-hour electrocardiogram in the prediction of cardiac death in dialysis patients. *Arch. Intern. Med.* 1988;**148**: 2381–2385.

195. O'Kelly, B., W.S. Browner, B. Massie, et al., Ventricular arrhythmias in patients undergoing noncardiac surgery: the Study of Perioperative Ischemia Research Group. *JAMA*, 1992;**268**: 217–221.

196. Huikuri, H.V., S. Yli-Mayry, U.R. Korhonen, et al., Prevalence and prognostic significance of complex ventricular arrhythmias after coronary arterial bypass graft surgery. *Int. J. Cardiol.*, 1990;**27**: 333–339.

197. DiMarco, J.P. and J.T. Philbrick, Use of ambulatory electrocardiographic (Holter) monitoring. *Ann. Intern. Med.*, 1990;**113**: 53–68.

198. Sami, M., H. Kraemer, D.C. Harrison, N. Houston, C. Shimasaki, and R.I. De Busk, A new method for evaluating antiarrhythmic drug efficacy. *Circulation*, 1980;**62**: 1172–1179.

199. Sami, M., D.C. Harrison, H. Kraemer, N. Houston, C. Shimasaki, and R.F. De Busk, Antiarrhythmic efficacy of encainide and quinidine: validation of a model for drug assessment. *Am. J. Cardiol.*, 1981;**48**: 147–156.

200. Burkart, F., M. Pfisterer, W. Kiowski, et al., Effect of antiarrhythmic therapy on mortality in survivors of myocardial infarction with asymptomatic complex ventricular arrhythmias: Basel Antiarrhythmic Study of Infarct Survival (BASIS). *J. Am. Coll. Cardiol.*, 1990;**16**: 1711–1718.

201. Ceremuzynski, L., E. Kleczar, M. Krzeminska-Pakula, et al., Effect of amiodarone on mortality after myocardial infarction: a double-blind, placebo-controlled pilot study. *J. Am. Coll. Cardiol.*, 1992;**20**: 1056–1062.

202. Doval, H.C., D.R. Nul, H.O. Grancelli, et al., Randomised trial of low-dose amiodarone in severe congestive heart failure: Grupo

de Estudio de la Sobrevida en la Insufficiencia Cardiaca en Argentina (GESICA). *Lancet*, 1994;**344**: 493–498.

203. The CASCADE Investigators, Randomised drug therapy in survivors of cardiac arrest (the CASCADE Study). *Am. J. Cardiol.*, 1993;**72**: 280–287.

204. Julian, D.G., A.J. Camm, G. Frangin, et al., Randomised trial of effect of amiodarone on mortality in patients with left-ventricular dysfunction after recent myocardial infarction: EMIAT, European Myocardial Infarct Amiodarone Trial Investigators. *Lancet*, 1997;**349**: 667–674.

205. Cairns, J.A., S.J. Conolly, R. Roberts, et al., Randomised trial of outcome after myocardial infarction in patients with frequent or repetitive ventricular premature depolarisations: CAMIAT, Canadian Amiodarone Myocardial Infarction Arrhythmia Trial Investigators. *Lancet*, 1997;**349**: 675–682.

206. Singh, S.N., R.D. Fletcher, S.G. Fisher, et al., Amiodarone in patients with congestive heart failure and asymptomatic ventricular arrhythmias: Survival Trial of Antiarrhythmic Therapy in Congestive Heart Failure. *N. Engl. J. Med.*, 1995;**333**: 77–82.

207. Lampert, S., B. Lown, T.B. Graboys, et al., Determinants of survival in patients with malignant ventricular arrhythmia associated with coronary artery disease. *Am. J. Cardiol.*, 1988;**61**: 791–797.

208. Hallstrom, A.P., H.L. Greene, and M.L. Huther, The healthy responder phenomenon in non-randomized clinical trial. CAST Investigators. *Stat. Med.*, 1991;**10**: 1621–1631.

209. Mason, J.W., A comparison of electrophysiologic testing with Holter monitoring to predict antiarrhythmic-drug efficacy for ventricular tachyarrhythmias: Electrophysiologic Study Versus Electrocardiographic Monitoring Investigators. *N. Engl. J. Med.*, 1993;**329**: 445–451.

210. Morganroth, J. and C.M. Pratt, Prevalence and characteristics of proarrhythmia from moricizine (ethmozine). *Am. J. Cardiol.*, 1989;**63**: 172–176.

211. Kennedy, H.L., Late proarrhythmia and understanding the time of occurrence of proarrhythmia. *Am. J. Cardiol.*, 1990;**66**: 1139–1143.

212. Balasubramanian, V., M.W. Millar Craig, A.B. Davies, and E.B. Raftery, Verapamil therapy in variant angina: assessment by high-fidelity frequency modulated ambulatory ECG. *Am. Heart J.*, 1981;**101**: 849–850.

213. Dick, M., II, D. McFadden, D. Crowley, et al., Diagnosis and management of cardiac rhythm disorders by transtelephonic electrocardiography in infants and children. *J. Pediatr.*, 1979;**94**: 612–615.

214. Porter, C.J., P.C. Gillette, and D.G. McNamara, Twenty-four-hour ambulatory ECGs in the detection and management of cardiac arrhythmias in infants and children. *Pediatr. Cardiol.*, 1980;**1**: 203–208.

215. Fyfe, D.A., D.R. Holmes, S.A. Neubauer, et al., Transtelephonic monitoring in pediatric patients with clinically suspected arrhythmias. *Clin. Pediatr.*, 1984;**23**: 139–143.

216. Goldstein, M.A., P. Hesslein, and A. Dunningan, Efficacy of trans-telephonic electrocardiographic monitoring in pediatric patients. *Am. J. Dis. Child.*, 1990;**144**: 178–182.

217. Hoyel, L., A. Fournier, S. Centazzo, et al., Use of transtelephonic electrocardiographic monitoring in children with suspected arrhythmias. *Can. J. Cardiol.*, 1992;**8**: 741–744.

218. Karpawich, P.P., D.L. Cavitt, and J.S. Sugalski, Ambulatory arrhythmia screening in symptomatic children and young adults: comparative effectiveness of Holter and telephone event recordings. *Pediatr. Cardiol.*, 1993;**14**: 147–150.

219. Saarel, E.V., C.B. Stefanelli, P.S. Fischbach, et al., Transtelephonic electrocardiographic monitors for evaluation of children and adolescents with suspected arrhythmias. *Pediatrics*, 2004;**113**: 248–251.

220. Seliem, M.A., D.W. Benson, J.F. Strasburger, et al., Complex ventricular ectopic activity in patients less than 20 years of age with or without syncope, and the role of ventricular extrastimulus testing. *Am. J. Cardiol.*, 1991;**68**: 745–750.

221. Driscoll, D.J., S.J. Jacobsen, C.J. Porter, et al., Syncope in children and adolescents. *J. Am. Coll. Cardiol.*, 1997;**29**: 1039–1045.

222. Sanatani, S., A. Peirone, C. Chiu, et al., Use of an implantable loop recorder in the evaluation of children with congenital heart disease. *Am. Heart J.*, 2002;**143**: 366–372.

223. Wolfe, R.R., D.J. Driscoll, W.M. Gersony, et al., Arrhythmias in patients with valvular aortic stenosis, valvular pulmonary stenosis, and ventricular septal defect: results of 24-hour ECG monitoring. *Circulation*, 1993;**87**(Suppl. I): I-89–I-101.

224. Garson, A., Jr, M. Bink-Boelkens, P.S. Heslein, et al., Atrial flutter in the young: a collaborative study of 380 cases. *J. Am. Coll. Cardiol.*, 1985;**6**: 871–878.

225. Cullen, S., D.S. Celermajer, R.C. Franklin, et al., Prognostic significance of ventricular arrhythmia after repair of tetralogy of Fallot: a 12-year prospective study. *J. Am. Coll. Cardiol.*, 1994;**23**: 1151–1155.

226. Chandar, J.S., G.S. Wolff, A. Garson, Jr, et al., Ventricular arrhythmias in postoperative tetralogy of Fallot. *Am. J. Cardiol.*, 1990;**65**: 655–661.

227. Garson, A., Jr, Ventricular arrhythmias after repair of congenital heart disease: who needs treatment? *Cardiol. Young*, 1991;**1**: 177–181.

228. Paul, T., C. Marchal, and A. Garson, Jr, Ventricular couplets in the young: prognosis related to underlying substrate. *Am. Heart J.*, 1990;**119**: 577–582.

229. Krongrad, E., Prognosis for patients with congenital heart disease and postoperative intraventricular conduction defects. *Circulation*, 1978;**57**: 867–870.

230. Fenelon, G., A. d'Avila, T. Malacky, et al., Prognostic significance of transient complete atrioventricular block during radiofrequency ablation of atrioventricular node reentrant tachycardia. *Am. J. Cardiol.*, 1995;**75**: 698–702.

231. Packer, D.L., G.H. Bardy, S.J. Worley, et al., Tachycardia-induced cardiomyopathy: a reversible form of left ventricular dysfunction. *Am. J. Cardiol.*, 1986;**57**: 563–570.

232. Locati, E.H., Advances in modern electrocardiographic equipment for long-term ambulatory monitoring. *Card. Electrophysiol. Rev.*, 2002;**6**: 185–189.

233. Coumel, P., Noninvasive exploration of cardiac arrhythmias. *Ann. NY Acad. Sci.*, 1990; 312–328.

2 The Pre-Hospital Electrocardiogram

Johan Herlitz · Leif Svensson · Per Johansson

P. W. Macfarlane et al. (eds.), *Specialized Aspects of ECG*, DOI 10.1007/978-0-85729-880-5_2,

2.1 Background

2.1.1 Historical Background

The first mobile coronary care unit was reported by Frank Pantridge in 1967 [1]. He described 352 patients with presumed acute myocardial infarction who were treated prior to hospital admission. Ten of them were successfully resuscitated following an out-of-hospital cardiac arrest. In 1970, electrocardiographic telemetry from ambulances was first described [2]. At that stage, only rhythm strips were transmitted. However, in the 1980s, at the time of the introduction of fibrinolysis, many ambulance organizations started to routinely record a 12-lead electrocardiogram (ECG). This was originally done with the sole purpose of detecting ST-segment elevation, thereby starting treatment with fibrinolysis prior to hospital admission. However, when this research area was in its infancy, it was thought that all patients with an impending myocardial infarction could perhaps benefit from this treatment [3] and the need for a prehospital ECG was therefore not obvious [4].

In an important meta-analysis published in 1993 [5], it was clearly shown that patients who would benefit from fibrinolysis were those with ST-segment elevation or left bundle branch block and that the earlier the treatment started, the better it would be. This important finding put the 12-lead prehospital ECG in focus. However, in large screening studies, it was shown that only a minority of patients with acute chest pain, who were transported by ambulance, had these changes on their prehospital ECG [6]. At this early stage, it was shown that other ECG changes, such as ST depression, were also an alarming ECG sign, but the prehospital treatment for these changes was not established.

During the last few years, the use of the prehospital ECG has become more and more widespread, with the aim not only of starting prehospital fibrinolysis but also improving the prehospital triage of patients with acute chest pain. Parallel to this, research on out-of-hospital cardiac arrest has been going on for the past 3 decades. In this case, the prehospital ECG is the most important tool when it comes to advising optimal treatment. During the last decade, ECG research has focused on the opportunity to predict the outcome of defibrillation in ventricular fibrillation based on wave-form analysis.

2.1.2 Ideological Background

Two major pathophysiological considerations constitute the principal background for the need for a prehospital ECG when a heart attack is suspected: (1) "Time is saved myocardium" and (2) the occurrence of life-threatening arrhythmias in myocardial ischemia and myocardial infarction, which is most common in the very early phase.

1. The opportunity to limit myocardial damage with early medication was first described in dogs in 1971 [7]. These findings have been followed by a very large number of studies in humans, showing that early treatment with medical [8] or mechanical [9] reperfusion and with antiplatelet [10] and anti-ischemic agents [11] will improve the outcome in a threatening myocardial infarction.

   Although we lack absolute proof of the value of prehospital initiated aspirin versus aspirin started after hospital admission [12–14], for example, our current knowledge strongly indicates that the earlier the various interventions in acute coronary syndrome are started, the better it would be. The question of whether to start treatment prior to or after hospital admission is more a cost-benefit issue. Based on such thinking, the most optimal solution for every single patient with any suspicion of acute coronary syndrome should be that he or she has an ECG recorded prior to hospital admission.

2. The fact that life-threatening arrhythmias are most frequent in the early phase of acute coronary syndrome and nearly half the deaths from ischemic heart disease occur outside hospital (mostly as sudden deaths) underlines the importance of research in this area [15]. More knowledge on the information that is hidden in the electrocardiogram in this scenario might improve the outcome for these patients.

3. At present, we do not know whether a prehospital ECG might be of benefit in other clinical scenarios in the prehospital setting. Theoretically, there are conditions such as stroke [16].

2.1.3   Three Major Objectives

The three major objectives for a prehospital ECG are:

1. Detection of myocardial ischemia/infarction.
2. Detection of arrhythmias.
3. Remaining objectives, of which little is known, but heart rate variability and stroke are interesting aspects.

In what follows, these three objectives will be evaluated in more detail.

2.1.4   Symptoms that Indicate a Prehospital ECG

The indications for a prehospital ECG should be liberal, since a variety of symptoms might be caused by an acute coronary syndrome. These symptoms are listed in ❷ Table 2.1. Although the typical symptom in acute coronary syndrome is acute chest pain, the disease can present with pain in other locations and various other symptoms. The symptoms that are listed in the table often appear in combination.

2.1.5   Benefits

The principle behind the proposed benefit of using a prehospital ECG is shown in ❷ Table 2.2. The detection of the presence or absence of ECG abnormalities will improve the triage in patients in whom it is used. In selected patients, this will result in the earlier treatment of myocardial ischemia/infarction or arrhythmias, which are associated with hemodynamic consequences. It is to be hoped that this will then result in an improved outcome.

2.2   Detection of ECG Abnormalities

The various ECG abnormalities (excluding arrhythmias) that the ambulance crew or other health-care providers should look for in the prehospital setting are shown in ❷ Table 2.3. The percentage of patients with an abnormal or

❏ Table 2.1

Symptoms that indicate a prehospital ECG

Suspicion of Ischemia/Infarction
Typical symptoms
Pain/oppression in chest
Atypical symptoms
Dyspnea
Pain in arms
Pain in back
Pain in stomach
Pain in neck
Unexplained tiredness
Nausea
Suspicion of arrhythmias
Palpitation
Syncope
Vertigo

▢ Table 2.2

Aspects on mechanisms of how the introduction of a prehospital ECG might improve outcome in acute chest pain

1. Detection of electrical abnormalities
(a) Myocardial ischemia/infarction
(b) Arrhythmia
(c) Other (for example decreased heart rate variability)
2. Improved triage
(a) Direct transport to coronary care unit
(b) Direct transport to catheterization laboratory
(c) Direct transport to a remote hospital
3. Earlier start of treatment
(a) Earlier start of fibrinolysis
(I) Prior to hospital admission
(II) In hospital
(b) Earlier start of percutaneous coronary intervention (PCI)
(c) Earlier start of other antiplatelet agents
(d) Earlier start of other anti-ischemic agents
(e) Earlier start of antiarrhythmic treatment
4. Improved outcome
(a) Reduced mortality?
(b) Reduced morbidity?

▢ Table 2.3

ECG abnormalities to look for when a prehospital ECG is recorded

Acute ischemia/infarction
ST elevation
ST depression
T-wave inversion
Q wave
Bundle branch block
Other abnormalities
Pacemaker ECG
Left ventricular hypertrophy
QRST signs indicating previous myocardial damage

pathological ECG depends on the study population. Reported studies have comprised patients who call for an ambulance due to acute chest pain or other symptoms raising suspicion of an acute coronary syndrome [17–19]. In these reports, a high percentage have an abnormal ECG (❷ Fig. 2.1). It is important to stress that patients who call for an ambulance represent a population with high comorbidity and a high likelihood of underlying cardiac pathology as compared with other chest pain populations [20–22]. So, if a prehospital ECG was recorded among patients who visited a general practitioner because of acute chest pain, the percentage of patients with a pathological ECG could be expected to be lower, since these patients are less likely to have a cardiac pathology [23]. The most common ECG abnormalities in the prehospital ECG among patients with acute chest pain are those indicating myocardial ischemia/infarction and various rhythm abnormalities.

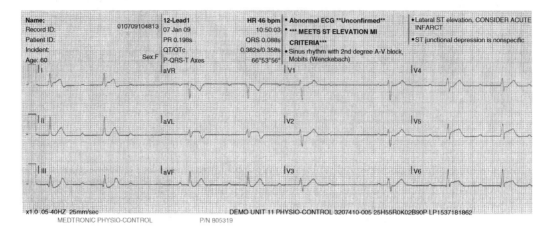

Fig. 2.1

A 12-lead ECG report from a Lifepak15. This simulated example shows ST elevation that is correctly detected and highlighted

2.2.1 Myocardial Ischemia/Infarction

Myocardial ischemia/infarction have been reported in about 50% of patients who called for an ambulance due to acute chest pain and in whom a prehospital ECG was recorded [17–19, 24]. Signs of myocardial ischemia/infarction include ST-segment deviation, Q waves and T-wave inversion. The relative importance of these changes will be described separately. In overall terms, when any of these are present in association with acute chest pain, the likelihood of a fresh myocardial infarction is high and the presence of any of them are mostly equivalent to an acute coronary syndrome. The presence of ECG changes indicating acute ischemia/infarction is also an alarming sign with regard to the risk of early death [25].

Difficulties in interpretation arise when a complete left bundle branch block is present. If this abnormality is new, it could indicate an extensive myocardial infarction and is therefore an indication for early reperfusion [5]. However, there are difficulties in the prehospital setting when it comes to determining whether the left bundle branch block is new or not, as no previous ECG is generally available for comparison. Similar difficulties might also arise for other ECG indicators of myocardial ischemia/infarction.

2.2.2 Arrhythmias

The rate of occurrence of various arrhythmias is entirely dependent on the study population. Among patients with acute chest pain who call for an ambulance, life-threatening arrhythmias leading to cardiac arrest are found, but only among a small percentage [19, 24]. On the other hand, among patients found in cardiac arrest and in whom resuscitation was attempted, about one third are found in ventricular fibrillation [26]. However, in such a study population, particularly if there is a cardiac etiology, a much higher percentage (about 80%) is thought to have ventricular fibrillation at the onset of cardiac arrest [26].

Supraventricular arrhythmias, such as atrial fibrillation, during ambulance transport have been reported to occur in about 10% of patients with acute chest pain [24] and in less than 10% of patients with ST-elevation acute myocardial infarction [27–29]. The occurrence of various arrhythmias during continuous ECG monitoring will be described later in this chapter.

2.2.3　Other

Other ECG abnormalities suggesting a cardiac pathology, including signs of a previous acute myocardial infarction, pacemaker ECG, and signs of left ventricular hypotrophy, are frequently seen in patients transported by ambulance with acute chest pain (between 10% and 20%) [18, 19]. It was recently reported that, among patients with trauma, the evaluation of heart rate variability in the prehospital setting might improve triage, if information on the Glasgow Coma Score (the degree of consciousness) was not available [30] and also independent of the Glasgow Coma Score [31].

2.3　Improved Triage

To date, the prehospital ECG has primarily resulted in the improved triage of patients with an acute coronary syndrome and patients with various arrhythmias. This improvement will have a number of consequences.

2.3.1　Direct Transport to Coronary Care Unit

Information on the percentage of patients with acute coronary syndrome or ST-elevation acute myocardial infarction, who are directly transported to a coronary care unit, bypassing the emergency department, is limited. In one previous study, it was reported that 67% of patients transported by ambulance fulfilled these criteria and that these patients had improved survival [32]. Experience from Sahlgrenska University Hospital in Göteborg, Sweden, indicates that among ambulance transported patients, 50% of patients with ST-elevation myocardial infarction have been directly transported to a coronary care unit and that this has been associated with a marked improvement in long-term survival [33].

2.3.2　Direct Transport to Catheterization Laboratory

Today in urban areas, there are single ambulance organizations which can transport the vast majority of patients with ST-elevation acute myocardial infarction directly to the catheterization laboratory with a median delay between the onset of symptoms and the start of percutaneous coronary intervention (PCI) of less than 2 h (unpublished observations). If the nearest hospital has facilities for PCI, effective collaboration can increase the opportunity for very early coronary intervention.

2.3.3　Direct Transport to Remote Hospital

Since primary coronary intervention is currently regarded as the preferred treatment strategy in ST-elevation acute myocardial infarction, it has been suggested that these patients should be transported to hospitals with these facilities, even if the transport time is prolonged [34]. It has been stated that patients admitted to noninterventional hospitals should be immediately transferred to interventional hospitals for primary coronary intervention, if the time from the first medical contact to balloon inflation is kept at less than 90 min [35–38]. Recent data indicate that an even longer delay might be acceptable [39].

In previous studies, patients have waited between 30 min and more than 1 h at local hospitals before being transferred to the intervention hospitals [37, 38, 40]. This local hospital delay may be reduced or even eliminated by prehospital diagnosis if a combined strategy of rerouting patients directly to an intervention hospital is implemented. However, limited evidence is available about the benefit, safety and feasibility of this kind of re-routing strategy. However, programs to further evaluate the possible benefits of such a procedure have been described [35].

2.4   Earlier Start of Treatment

2.4.1   Earlier Start of Fibrinolysis

2.4.1.1   Prior to Hospital Admission

A number of studies have shown that, if a 12-lead prehospital ECG is recorded and is followed by prehospital fibrinolysis, the potential time saved with regard to the start of fibrinolysis varies between 45 and 125 min [3, 6, 28, 29, 41–47]. In a national perspective (Sweden) it has been shown that treatment can start $\leqslant$2 h after the onset of symptoms in half of patients [27]. However, such figures will vary between countries due to local facilities. It has been suggested that more patients can be treated at an early stage in urban areas compared with rural areas [48].

2.4.1.2   In Hospital

It has also been shown that a prehospital ECG reduces the in-hospital delay to the start of fibrinolysis (door-to-needle time) [49]. A systematic review in which 1,283 citations were identified and five studies met the inclusion criteria [50] indicated that the introduction of a 12-lead prehospital ECG and advanced emergency department notification reduced the mean door-to-needle time by 36 min (95% confidence limits 9–63 min).

   In a national registry of acute myocardial infarction in the USA, the mean door to in-hospital drug time was reduced from 35 to 25 min with a prehospital ECG (p < 0.0001) [51]. A meta-analysis comprising four studies (99 patients) from an original 2,129 publications revealed a shortening of the in-hospital delay to reperfusion by 25 min (95% confidence limits 17–37 min) with the introduction of a prehospital ECG [52].

2.4.2   Earlier Start of Percutaneous Coronary Intervention (PCI)

A study from North Carolina revealed that prehospital wireless transmission of an ECG to a cardiologist's hand-held device reduced the median door-to-reperfusion time (PCI) by about 50 min [53]. In a national survey in Sweden, it was shown that, among patients who were transported by ambulance and had ST-elevation acute myocardial infarction, those who did not have a prehospital ECG had a delay between the onset of symptoms and reperfusion (PCI) of 240 min as compared with 181 min among patients with a prehospital ECG (p < 0.0001) (a time saving of 59 min) [54]. In the National Registry of Acute Myocardial Infarction in the USA, it was shown that, with a prehospital ECG, the in-hospital delay time to PCI was reduced from 1 h 49 min to 1 h 34 min [51]. A number of studies performed during the last few years have further confirmed these data, strongly suggesting a clear reduction in delay to PCI in ST-elevation acute myocardial infarction where a prehospital ECG is used and communicated to hospital appropriately [55–59].

2.4.3   Earlier Start of Antiplatelet and Antithrombotic Therapy

Various antiplatelet agents such as aspirin [60] and clopidogrel [61] and various antithrombotic agents such as heparin [62] have been shown to improve the prognosis in acute coronary syndrome. A prehospital ECG improved the opportunity to start this treatment prior to hospital admission. Aspirin treatment can then start as early as 1–2 h after the onset of symptoms. Similar findings have been reported for heparin and low molecular weight heparin [63].

2.4.4   Earlier Start of Anti-Ischemic Therapy

Beta-blockers have been shown to improve the prognosis in acute myocardial infarction [11], and intravenous treatment with beta-blockers, started prior to hospital admission, has been shown to relieve pain [24]. A prehospital ECG increases the opportunity to select the right patients for this treatment in the prehospital setting.

2.4.5   Earlier Start of Antiarrhythmic Therapy

Based on findings in the prehospital ECG, a number of antiarrhythmic drugs are of potential value in the prehospital setting when it comes to treating supraventricular and ventricular arrhythmias [64]. They include adenosine [65, 66], verapamil [67], diltiazem [68], and amiodarone [69].

2.5   Improved Outcome

2.5.1   Reduced Mortality

A systematic review found one study that revealed a nonsignificant reduction in all-cause mortality from 15.5% to 8.4% associated with the introduction of a prehospital ECG and advanced emergency department notification as compared with no such intervention [50].

In an observational study in Sweden on patients who had ST-elevation acute myocardial infarction, were transported by ambulance, and were treated with percutaneous coronary intervention, it was shown that a prehospital ECG was an independent predictor of reduced 30-day mortality [54]. Field triage of patients with ST-elevation acute myocardial infarction has also been shown to reduce mortality in Australia [70]. A similar trend was also found in the USA [71].

2.5.2   Reduced Morbidity

We are not aware of any study evaluating morbidity (various complications associated with the disease) changes associated with the introduction of a prehospital ECG. It can be assumed that there are subsets of patients in whom the duration of hospital stay (number of days in hospital) might be shortened. In a recent report, field triage with a prehospital electrocardiogram was associated with a preserved left ventricular function [70].

2.5.3   Health Economy

The use of health-economic analyses to assess the value of medical technologies is well established, but these analyses have been under-used in studies of ECG. One article [72] has outlined a general framework for the economic evaluation of the ECG and applied these methods to the development of an economic analysis protocol for assessing the economic attractiveness of the wireless transmission of ECG data to the cardiologist making the treatment decision.

2.6   Negative Consequences

There are two major negative consequences of the prehospital ECG.

2.6.1   Increase in Delay

The delay to arrival at hospital will increase, particularly among patients in whom the ECG does not show any pathological changes. However, it has been shown that the on-scene time is not dramatically prolonged by the recording of a 12-lead ECG [73, 74]. A systematic review revealed that the on-scene time increased by 1.2 min (95% confidence limits 0.8–3.2 min) [50].

2.6.2   False Information

The second major negative consequence is that ECG abnormalities may mimic myocardial infarction, but may in fact be caused by other conditions [75]. It has been reported that, among patients with chest pain and ST elevation in the prehospital setting [76] and at the emergency department [77], 85% and 51% respectively had diagnoses other than myocardial infarction. Conditions in which misinterpretation has occurred and in which fibrinolytic treatment can be detrimental include intracranial hemorrhage [75] and aortic dissection [78].

Negative consequences associated with technical problems will be dealt with in the implementation part of this chapter.

2.7   Implementation

2.7.1   Education and Training

There is currently a wide range of teaching techniques that can be used to train healthcare professionals in the use of 12-lead ECG-monitoring equipment and ECG interpretation.

The methods identified range from

1. Traditional teaching methods including (a) books, (b) lectures, (c) videos, (d) hospital placements (using patients), and (e) practical laboratory sessions (using volunteers) to
2. Advanced teaching methods including (a) PC-based ECG software packages (b) 12-lead ECG signal generators, and (c) advanced training mannequins (patient simulators) [79].

The traditional teaching methods have some disadvantages in terms of patient or volunteer consent and discomfort and also in terms of teaching effectiveness. The more advanced teaching methods make use of simulation which can be either screen based (computer software) or physical (realistic models or mannequins).

There are a number of ECG simulators on the market that can be connected to an ECG machine. Various models of ECG simulators that are connected to a mannequin are also available.

2.7.2   Technical Problems

The transmission of ECGs is the most common technical problem associated with the use of a prehospital ECG. With a few exceptions, the transmission of an ECG is associated with problems at the start. Most EMS systems experience a learning curve when a 12-lead ECG transmission technology is first implemented. One study reported a 33% failed transmission rate after initiating the system, but it had been reduced to 11% 6 months later [74].

2.7.3   Practical Implementation

Implementing a prehospital ECG program represents a significant investment in terms of time, effort, personnel and resources. The implementation has three phases: (1) phase I is a retrospective baseline analysis; (2) phase II is a feasibility and safety assessment; and (3) phase III involves the implementation of the accurate and routine prehospital identification of candidates for various aspects of treatment of an acute coronary syndrome, such as candidates for treatment with fibrinolysis or percutaneous coronary intervention [80]. Eligibility for fibrinolysis or percutaneous coronary intervention can be determined by means of a check list, the results of which can be sent to either the base or the receiving physician [81]. A written protocol including clinical algorithms for prehospital personnel should be established [80]. Finally, an effective quality assurance and improvement program should be initiated before implementing a prehospital ECG program [81].

Prehospital 12-lead ECG programs should be strongly considered by all EMS systems with advanced life support capability. Prehospital 12-lead ECG programs should be implemented through a systematic process that encompasses every facet of the EMS system [82].

2.7.4 Process Monitoring

One of the principal aims of the introduction of a prehospital ECG is to reduce the time to reperfusion in ST-elevation myocardial infarction. In order to evaluate the impact on this important end point, the delay from the first medical contact to the start of reperfusion either with fibrinolysis or with percutaneous coronary intervention must be continuously monitored. Although, as previously stated, the short-term impact on delay to reperfusion with a clear-cut reduction is impressive, the results in the long-term perspective are less well described. It is to be hoped that, in the long term, the teamwork between prehospital and in-hospital health-care providers will improve with a successive decline in the time to reperfusion over the years.

However, the results so far are disappointing. In a recent 10-year survey, it was shown that the delay from door to primary coronary intervention was not sustained [83]. In the first year of the intervention (including the implementation of the prehospital ECG), the time from hospital arrival to primary coronary intervention was 80 min. In years 2, 3, and 4, this delay was 93, 85, and 94 min, respectively. In 2003, 10 years after the intervention, the delay had increased to 113 min [83].

Experience from the Swedish registry on heart intensive care indicates that the time between admission to hospital and the start of reperfusion has remained unchanged during the last few years [84].

2.8 Interpretation

The category of health care professionals who interpret the prehospital ECG varies markedly. They include cardiologists, emergency physicians, anesthesiologists, general practitioners, nurses, semi-nurses (nursing assistants), paramedics, and emergency technicians. The educational levels of these various categories vary considerably. So, when discussing the problem of interpreting the prehospital ECG, each category of health-care professionals must be discussed separately, and separate educational programs should probably be implemented for these various groups.

There are different ways to interpret the prehospital ECG.

2.8.1 In-Field Interpretation

2.8.1.1 By Health-Care Providers

In-field interpretation by health-care providers without assistance requires a high educational level. This type of interpretation is most common when a physician is on board the ambulance or when a general practitioner sees the patient prior to the arrival of the ambulance. In several countries such as France, this is the most common way of interpreting the prehospital ECG. However, it has been suggested that highly trained paramedics in an urban EMS system can identify patients with ST-elevation acute myocardial infarction as accurately as blinded physician reviewers [85]. This has been supported by others [86] and it seems as though paramedics as well as CCU nurses can learn to conduct live reperfusion decision making in ST-elevation myocardial infarction [87].

2.8.1.2 With Computer Assistance

Computer algorithms for the diagnosis of ST-elevation myocardial infarction may also be considered [88, 89]. This strategy has, however, previously been restricted to the diagnosis of large ST-elevation myocardial infarctions with cumulative ST elevation above 600–1,000 μ V [90, 91]. Interpretation in the field with computer assistance has been reported to be a relatively safe procedure [92]. Recently, a new acute coronary syndrome computer algorithm for interpreting prehospital ECGs was suggested [93]. The results demonstrated that, with the assistance of the new algorithm, the emergency physician and cardiologist improved their sensitivity when it came to interpreting acute myocardial infarction by 50% and 26% respectively, without any loss of specificity. The patients' age and gender were taken into consideration in the algorithm. However, it was recently suggested that a correction should be made to obtain optimal results in the automated analysis of ECGs [94].

2.9   Wireless Transmission

2.9.1   To Nearest Hospital

The in-field transmission of the prehospital ECG to the emergency department, coronary care unit, another hospital ward, or directly to the on-call cardiologist for interpretation by a more experienced health-care provider is common [53]. This mode of interpretation is more common when the ambulance is manned by a nurse and or a paramedic.

Studies have shown that cardiologists' diagnoses of cardiac abnormalities on a liquid crystal display are very similar to their interpretation of the same ECG displayed on paper [95, 96]. Furthermore, there was no significant difference with regard to cardiologists' decisions to initiate reperfusion therapy when interpreting study-displayed ECGs versus ECGs displayed on a liquid crystal display screen [97]. In many countries, this is a widespread means of communication between the prehospital and in-hospital health-care providers [27].

2.9.2   To Remote Hospital

Even in urban areas, up to 80% of ambulance-transported ST-elevation myocardial infarction patients can be diagnosed prehospitally using telemedicine [98]. In principle, a strategy of this kind could be adapted in any region covered by a mobile phone network and the health-care providers (mostly a physician) responsible for the diagnosis can be located at a central unit serving a large catchment area [34, 35, 98, 99]. It is possible to speculate that primarily low-risk patients (limited ST elevation) will be found to be eligible for prehospital referral directly to an intervention centre [98]. However, the opposite has been found, that is, patients transported directly to the intervention center were those with a more pronounced ST elevation [98]. It is most likely that there is a geographical border, at a certain distance or transport time from the intervention center, beyond which patients may obtain a beneficial effect from prehospital fibrinolysis or even in-hospital fibrinolysis.

An attractive way of solving the problem is to obtain an ECG on the scene for subsequent transmission to the intervention center. A physician on call will evaluate the ECG, phone the ambulance, possibly interview the patient who is in the ambulance and equipped with headphones, and thereby establish the prehospital diagnosis [34]. An ECG could also be sent to an attending cardiologists mobile telephone for rapid triage and transport to a primary PCI center [100].

2.9.3   Elsewhere

The in-field transmission of the ECG to an advanced mobile phone outside hospital was recently described [101]. This is an alternative when a helicopter is very far from the hospital, and an emergency medical service physician capable of interpreting the ECG is at a shorter distance, for example. He can then view the ECG on his advanced phone and give recommendations about fibrinolysis or other treatment alternatives. A novel approach is to use a cell phone with a camera feature. This method will allow transfer of ECG images to the local hospital and the PCI center [102].

2.10 ECG Indicators for Myocardial Ischemia/Infarction and Adverse Outcome

More than 10 years ago, it was shown that, in the prehospital setting, a pathological ECG was a strong predictor and was associated with a fourfold increase in the risk of a cardiac pathology as the etiology of acute chest pain [17]. It has also been shown that, if the patient has chest pain and/or other symptoms indicating acute coronary syndrome, signs of myocardial ischemia (including new ST-T wave changes or Q waves) are associated with a marked increase in 30-day and 1-year mortality, particularly if there is simultaneous elevation of biochemical markers prior to hospital admission [25].

2.10.1 ST Elevation

Among patients with chest pain and/or other symptoms of acute coronary syndrome, the presence of ST elevation in the prehospital ECG has been reported to increase the likelihood of acute myocardial infarction nearly 50 times when simultaneously considering other risk indicators including the elevation of biochemical markers [103].

2.10.2 ST Depression

It is important to stress that, from ECG studies in which the ECG was recorded directly after hospital admission, ST depression in the ECG among patients with symptoms indicating acute coronary syndrome has been reported to be associated with an adverse long-term prognosis [104, 105]. Among patients with chest pain or other symptoms of acute coronary syndrome, the presence of ST depression in the prehospital ECG has been reported to be associated with a fourfold increase in the risk of acute myocardial infarction [103].

Although by tradition patients with ST elevation or (presumed) new left bundle branch block have formed the group demanding urgent revascularisation in acute coronary syndrome, there are subsets among patients showing ST depression who also suffer from a critical coronary stenosis or occlusion and who therefore most likely would benefit from a similar treatment strategy. These include patients with marked ST depression in anterior leads and those with extensive ST depression where a large number of leads is involved.

A gender perspective has been found. If there are symptoms of acute coronary syndrome, the presence of ST depression in the prehospital ECG appears to be more strongly associated with acute myocardial infarction in men than in women [106].

2.10.3 T-Wave Inversion

Although the presence of T-wave inversion without simultaneous changes in the ST segment might indicate myocardial ischemia [107], these changes are less frequently associated with an ongoing acute myocardial infarction [103].

2.10.4 Other Changes

Needless to say, the presence of Q waves might also indicate acute myocardial infarction [103, 106]. However, as things stand, it is not possible in the prehospital setting to make comparisons with previous ECG findings and a Q wave in isolation without concomitant ST-T wave changes might therefore be a sign of an old myocardial infarction. Other ECG abnormalities found in the prehospital ECG, such as pacemaker ECG, bundle branch block, and signs of left ventricular hypertrophy, are less specific for acute myocardial infarction but are, on the other hand, often indicators of an adverse outcome in a long-term perspective [25].

2.11 Prehospital Continuous ECG Monitoring

2.11.1 Background

Little is known about the natural course of myocardial ischemia and the development of arrhythmias in the prehospital phase of acute coronary syndrome. Small pilot studies indicate a relatively high prevalence of tachyarrhythmias during prehospital ECG monitoring as compared with the first ECG recording in hospital [19]. Recent reports suggest that prehospital ECG monitoring should have the potential to detect myocardial ischemia in the prehospital phase much more frequently than a standard 12-lead ECG [108].

2.11.2 Method Development

This has been done in particular by Drew et al. [19]. A system was developed that: (1) synthesizes a 12-lead ECG from five electrodes, (2) measures ST amplitudes in all 12 leads every 30 s and (3) automatically transmits an ECG to the target emergency department if there is a change in ST amplitude of 200 μ V in one lead or more or 100 μ V in two contiguous leads or more lasting 2.5 min.

2.11.3 Occurrence of Arrhythmias

Among all the patients involved in the first part of a randomized clinical trial [19] (the ST SMART Study; n = 433), one third overall (33%) had some arrhythmias during continuous prehospital ECG monitoring as compared with 29%, according to the initial hospital ECG diagnosis among patients with chest pain – anginal equivalent (p < 0.001). The corresponding figure for patients with acute coronary syndrome was 30% versus 26% (p < 0.001). In overall terms, more tachyarrhythmias (sinus tachycardia, atrial fibrillation/flutter, supraventricular tachycardia of unknown mechanism and sustained ventricular tachycardia) were observed in continuous prehospital ECG monitoring, whereas more bradyarrhythmias (complete heart block, sinus arrest with junctional or ventricular escape rhythm) were observed in the first hospital ECG.

2.11.4 Wide QRS Complex

Among patients with acute coronary syndrome, 15% had a rhythm with a wide QRS complex and secondary repolarization abnormalities that confound the diagnosis of myocardial ischemia. These ECG confounders included left bundle branch block (6%), right bundle branch block (6%) and ventricular pacing rhythm (3%) [19].

2.11.5 Advantages of Continuous Prehospital ECG Monitoring

In the area of early reperfusion with percutaneous coronary intervention in acute coronary syndrome, a rerouting strategy may result in some patients being transported longer distances without any accompanying staff skilled in the diagnosis and treatment of malignant arrhythmias. Continuous real-time, one-lead ECG transmission from ambulance to hospital may then allow physicians to support ambulance personnel in the treatment of arrhythmias during this kind of transportation [98]. Furthermore, continuous prehospital ST monitoring indicates that patients with ST-elevation myocardial infarction are heterogeneous and various types of dynamic change in the prehospital setting might indicate a more favorable or a more adverse prognosis [109]. A pre-specified ST-monitoring classification may therefore be useful for stratifying patients at the time of percutaneous coronary intervention into groups with a low, intermediate, and high-risk profile [109].

2.11.6 Number of Electrodes for Detection of Myocardial Ischemia/Infarction

The optimal number of electrodes that should be used in the diagnosis of myocardial infarction/ischemia has been debated over the years [110]. An alternative to the 12-lead ECG, such as the five-electrode-derived EASI ECG, has been tested in the prehospital setting [111, 112]. It offers the advantages of using only five electrode positions (four active and one ground) over easy-to-locate, bony structures on the torso. The E electrode is therefore placed on the lower extreme of the sternum, the A and I electrodes in the left and right mid-axillary lines respectively and at the same transverse level as the E electrode, and the S electrode on the sternal manubrium.

The five-electrode-derived EASI ECG has been compared with the paramedic-acquired 12-lead ECG using Mason–Likar limb lead configuration in patients with chest pain [111, 112]. Both appear to produce a similar difference compared with standard ECGs in terms of wave forms. It has been suggested that either method can be used as a substitute for standard ECGs for monitoring, but neither should be regarded as being equivalent to the standard ECG for diagnostic purposes [111].

Parallel to this research, studies have been performed using 80-lead prehospital ECG mapping [113]. In these studies, the sensitivity has increased to 80% as compared with 57% for a 12-lead ECG [113]. The specificity remained unchanged (92%) for an 80-lead ECG versus 94% for a 12-lead ECG [113].

2.12 Different Technical Models

2.12.1 Medtronic Lifepak

The *Medtronic Lifepak15* (❯ Fig. 2.2) is a traditional system transmitting a standard 12-lead ECG and is capable of defibrillation. The principle for this system is that it registers a snapshot ECG. This procedure can be repeated if the patient's symptoms change during transportation to hospital. One Lifepak version is able to transmit continuous ST monitoring while using a reduced number of electrodes [114].

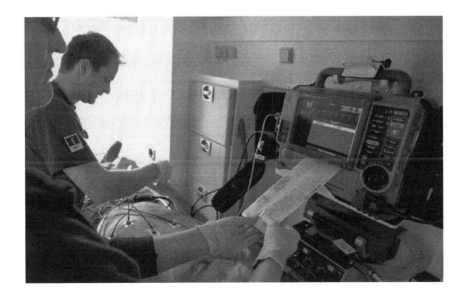

◻ Fig. 2.2
The Lifepak15 in use. The ECG (cf ❯ Fig. 2.1) report is produced directly from the machine as shown
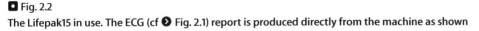

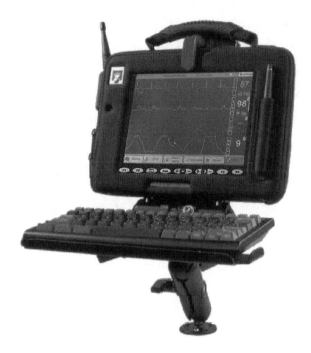

☐ Fig. 2.3
The Ortivus Mobimed

☐ Table 2.4
Clinical determinants of patient instability

Altered mental status
Significant hypotension
Pulmonary edema
Ischemic chest pain
Ischemic electrocardiographic changes (or other evidence of significant hypoperfusion)

2.12.2   Ortivus Mobimed

Ortivus Mobimed (❯ Fig 2.3) is a prehospital concept presenting data in a Windows setup. This system is able to transmit a 12-lead ECG, continuous vector trends, or ST analysis and collect data such as patient files. This system requires a separate defibrillator.

2.12.3   Other

Several other manufacturers offer equipment for prehospital ECG recording and defibrillation. There are variations between countries in respect of choice of machine and a complete review is not appropriate here.

2.13   Various Types of Arrhythmia

The use of the prehospital ECG to detect various arrhythmias is particularly important when there are signs of clinical instability [64]. These signs are listed in ❯ Table 2.4.

2.13.1 No Cardiac Arrest

2.13.1.1 Bradyarrhythmias

Limited data are available on the occurrence of various bradyarrhythmias and the value of various treatments such as atropine and the use of pacemakers in these conditions. Continuous ECG monitoring among patients with chest pain indicated that 2% had sinus bradycardia (heart rate < 50 beats/min), 0.7% had heart block, and 0.7% had sinus arrest with ventricular escape rhythm during ambulance transport [19].

2.13.1.2 Tachyarrhythmias

Paroxysmal Supraventricular Tachycardia
Paroxysmal supraventricular tachycardia is usually a regular narrow-complex tachyarrhythmia caused by a reentry, which may or may not be accompanied by underlying cardiovascular disease. Many of these patients are clinically stable and in these patients a prehospital ECG will be a support for improved triage rather than improved treatment. Among patients with acute chest pain, supraventricular tachycardia (unknown mechanism) was reported to occur in 2% [19].

Atrial Fibrillation/Flutter
Because the disorder is not commonly seen by emergency medical system providers (the reported incidence among ambulance-transported patients ranges from only 0.2–0.7%) [58], there is no consensus on the optimal prehospital therapy. Among patients with acute chest pain, continuous ECG monitoring in the prehospital phase revealed atrial fibrillation flutter in 11% of cases [19]. Almost every patient with rapid atrial fibrillation has another underlying disease, such as heart failure, chronic obstructive pulmonary disease, or ischemic heart disease.

Perfusing Ventricular Tachycardia
Hemodynamically stable monomorphic ventricular tachycardia can be treated either pharmacologically or with synchronized cardioversion [58]. Cardioversion is the therapy of choice for unstable patients and for those with marginal blood pressure in whom there may not be enough time or stability to allow for drug infusion. Among patients with chest pain who underwent continuous ECG monitoring during transport, sustained ventricular tachycardia was reported to occur in 0.2% of cases [19].

2.13.2 Cardiac Arrest

Every year, between 40 and 50 patients per 100,000 inhabitants suffer an out-of-hospital cardiac arrest, and in such cases, it is regarded as meaningful to attempt resuscitation [115]. The prehospital ECG is used most importantly in order to distinguish patients with a shockable rhythm from those without. However, detection of ST elevation immediately after return of spontaneous circulation, has also been shown to reflect the presence of acute myocardial infarction as the underlying etiology behind cardiac arrest [116].

2.13.2.1 Ventricular Fibrillation

The percentage of patients found in ventricular fibrillation among cardiac arrest victims has been reported to have decreased during the last 2 decades [117, 118]. The mechanism behind this decrease is unclear. The earlier a prehospital ECG is recorded, the more likely is it to find the patients in a shockable rhythm. Out-of-hospital cardiac arrest has therefore been regarded by many as a community problem rather than an ambulance problem, as the ambulance frequently reaches the patient too late in the course of events. Over the years, a strong relationship has been reported between the delay from cardiac arrest and defibrillation, that is, the earlier the patient is defibrillated, the higher the likelihood of survival [26].

2.13.2.2   Pulseless Electrical Activity

The percentage of patients suffering an out-of-hospital cardiac arrest in whom resuscitation was attempted and who were found in pulseless electrical activity has been reported to be about 20% [119]. These patients have been reported to have a low chance of survival (1–2%). However, other studies have shown more encouraging results, indicating that some of these patients can be successfully resuscitated [120, 121]. The data do not indicate a strong relationship between the delay from cardiac arrest to the arrival of the rescue team and survival [119].

2.13.2.3   Asystole

The percentage of patients suffering an out-of-hospital cardiac arrest in whom resuscitation was attempted and who were found in asystole has been reported to be about 50% [122]. The longer the delay from cardiac arrest to ECG recording, the greater the likelihood of finding the patients in asystole. In one study, it was reported that, the earlier the mobile coronary care unit arrived at the patient's side, the greater the likelihood of survival [122].

2.14   Electrocardiographic Factors Associated with Outcome in Cardiac Arrest

2.14.1   Ventricular Fibrillation

2.14.1.1   Waveform Analysis

The determination of the optimal time for delivering a defibrillatory shock has focused on the ventricular fibrillation wave form in many studies [123–128]. It has been suggested that a characteristic pattern of median frequency could be used to estimate the duration of ventricular fibrillation [124, 125]. Eftestøl et al. described a combination of spectral features in the ventricular fibrillation wave form from which they developed a probability function for successful defibrillation in a study of ventricular fibrillation in cardiac arrest patients [129]. They were subsequently able to confirm their findings in an independent data set [130].

Following these findings, wavelet transform methods of ventricular fibrillation that could be useful in identifying patients for whom shocks would be ineffective were described [131, 132]. Further support for ECG analysis in order to predict outcome in ventricular fibrillation was given by Snyder et al. [133].

It was recently reported that the accuracy of shock outcome prediction could be further increased by using filtered ECG features from higher ECG subbands instead of features derived from the main ECG spectrum [134].

A new method, based on the roughness of the ventricular fibrillation waveform, called the logarithm of the absolute correlation, has been suggested to better predict the duration of ventricular fibrillation and thereby the chance of successful defibrillation [135].

By calculating the mean slope of the electrocardiogram it has been possible to estimate the association between the time without chest compression and the probability of return of spontaneous circulation [136].

By calculating the median slope of the electrocardiogram, a new indicator of a chest compression quality measurement has been developed [137]. The configuration of the waveform has also been shown to be helpful in the identification of acute myocardial infarction as the underlying etiology behind ventricular fibrillation [138].

It has been hypothesized that interventions with thrombolytic therapy in ventricular fibrillation will change the wave form with increased amplitude and thereby increase the chance of successful defibrillation [139].

2.14.2   Pulseless Electrical Activity

Previous ECG studies performed in animals and patients demonstrated a progression of ECG characteristics in pulseless electrical activity with the time from the onset of anoxia. In a retrospective study comprising 503 patients whose prehospital initial rhythm was pulseless electrical activity, Aufderheide et al. found that patients who were successfully resuscitated had significantly higher initial heart rates, a higher incidence of p-values, and shorter average QRS and QT intervals than patients who did not respond to therapy [140]. It has been suggested that pulseless electrical activity often follows prolonged untreated ventricular fibrillation and that the characteristics of initial post-countershock pulseless electrical activity may predict the resuscitation outcome [141].

In animals, it has been shown that those with post-countershock pulseless electrical activity, which were converted to spontaneous circulation, had fewer shocks prior to the onset of initial post-countershock pulseless electrical activity, greater ventricular fibrillation wavelet amplitude prior to initial post-countershock pulseless electrical activity, and short QRS intervals and a higher heart rate [141]. It is therefore possible that various ECG characteristics among patients suffering from pulseless electrical activity might be used in order to predict outcome in these patients.

2.15 Use of a Prehospital Electrocardiogram in a Global Perspective

2.15.1 Use and Transmission of a Prehospital ECG

This information is based on rough estimations by leading authorities in the field. One exception is the USA, where data are collected from a reference [142]. The use of or response to a prehospital ECG is mainly dependent on the level of education among the EMS personnel who are in charge of the EMS vehicle. In cases where there is a physician in the ambulance (as in Spain and France), ECGs are usually interpreted on line by a doctor and there is usually no need for ECG transmission from the patient/ambulance to the hospital. However, in cases where a paramedic or a registered nurse (as is mostly the case in Scandinavia, Canada, and the USA) is in charge of the ambulance, the ECG must be transmitted to a nearby hospital. Printable copies of the ECG can be transmitted to the hospital emergency department, coronary care unit, or intensive care unit through a cellular phone or using the patient's regular phone. The doctor on call and the EMS personnel can then jointly discuss the ECG findings, patient symptoms, and risk profile. In some countries (like the Netherlands), an effective computerized algorithm is used to support the nurse when assessing the patient.

This estimation of the global use of prehospital ECG is unfortunately restricted to Europe and North America. In a large US survey among patients suffering from myocardial infarction 172,059 patients used the ambulance. Among them, only 6% had a prehospital ECG recorded. In a large database in the USA, it was recently shown that among 12,097 patients with ST-elevation myocardial infarction 59% used EMS and among them 27% had a prehospital ECG [71]. In contrast to these data, the 200-City survey in the USA previously reported that 67% of all emergency medicine service organizations do have a 12-lead ECG system (❯ Table 2.5) [142]. Thus, with regard to the USA there is some uncertainty of the actual proportion of ambulance organizations using a prehospital ECG. The estimation indicates that, in overall terms, a prehospital ECG is implemented in the routine prehospital care of patients with a presumed acute coronary syndrome more frequently in Europe than in North America. However, the proportion of patients with presumed acute coronary syndrome in whom a prehospital ECG is recorded is not known.

2.15.2 Important Prehospital ECG Research Projects

Perhaps the most important ongoing clinical trial of the use of a prehospital ECG is the ST SMART trial in the USA [114]. This is an ongoing study which aims to evaluate the impact of implementing prehospital ST monitoring with the automatic mobile telephone transmission of ST events to the target hospital. It is a prospective, randomized trial using these ST data for real-time clinical decision-making. The first patient had been randomized by November 1, 2003 and randomization should continue for 5 years. All subjects calling 911 for chest pain or anginal equivalent symptoms receive prehospital, synthesized, 12-lead, ST-segment monitoring with the manual transmission of an initial ECG and the automatic transmission of subsequent ST-event ECGs to the target hospital. The experimental group of patients has incoming ECGs from the field conveyed to clinical staff at the hospital, heralded by an audible voice message and printed out at the emergency department. The control group of patients have no field ECGs printed out and the first ECG is recorded after hospital admission. It is to be hoped that this study will document the value of prehospital ECG monitoring in a presumed acute coronary syndrome.

◘ Table 2.5

Use of prehospital ECG in a global perspective[a]

Country	Overall prehospital ECG use %	Transmission	Comments
Norway	>90%	Yes	Mostly no physician – 1
Sweden	>90%	Yes	No physician – 2
Denmark	>90%	Yes	Mostly no physician – 3
Spain	>90%	No	Physician operating – 4
Netherlands	>90%	No/Yes	No physician but online computerized ECG – 5
France	>90%	No	Physician operating – 6
Canada	25%	Yes	No physician – 7
USA	67%[b]	Yes	Williams D JEMS 2005;30:42–60

[a] Personal communication with: (1) Hans Morten Lossius, (2) Leif Svensson, (3) C Juhl Terkelsen, (4) Fernando Rosell, (5) Evert Lamfers, (6) Patrick Goldstein, and (7) Laurie Morrison

[b] In ref [71], it was reported that only 27% of EMS transported patients with ST-elevation myocardial infarction received a prehospital ECG in 2007 in the USA

2.16 Future Perspective

A number of important implementation and research issues remain to be addressed in the near future with regard to the prehospital ECG. The most important one is to implement a prehospital ECG in all EMS systems. The use of a prehospital ECG is probably the most important part of the prehospital care of patients suffering a heart attack. It seems as though the speed of this process varies in different parts of the world. It remains to be proved whether continuous ECG monitoring will improve the prehospital care in a presumed acute coronary syndrome as compared with a single 12-lead ECG recording on the arrival of the rescue team.

The optimal number of electrodes for use in the prehospital ECG has not been clarified. Should we use a 12-lead ECG or should we reduce or increase the number of electrodes? Wave-form analysis in ventricular fibrillation could perhaps be improved still further in order to optimize the timing of defibrillation. Finally, we need to decide whether there is hidden information in the ECG among patients suffering a cardiac arrest and pulseless electrical activity, which could guide us in the management of these patients.

But, most likely, the most important challenge for the future is to overcome barriers to the implementation and integration of the prehospital electrocardiogram into systems of care for acute coronary syndrome [143, 144].

References

1. Pantridge, J.F., Manning mobile intensive-care units. *Lancet*, 1967;**2**(7521): 888.
2. Uhley, H.N., Electrocardiographic telemetry from ambulances. A practical approach to mobile coronary care units. *Am. Heart J.*, 1970;**80**: 838–842.
3. Risenfors, M., G. Gustavsson, L. Ekström, M. Hartford, J. Herlitz, B.W. Karlson, R. Luepker, K. Swedberg, B. Wennerblom, and S. Holmberg, Prehospital throm-bolysis in suspected acute myocardial infarction: results from the TEAHAT Study. *J. Intern. Med.*, 1991;**229**(suppl 1): 3–10.
4. Herlitz, J., B.W. Karlson, T. Karlsson, M. Dellborg, M. Hartford, and R.V. Luepker, Diagnostic accuracy of physicians for identifying patients with acute myocardial infarction without an electrocardiogram. Experiences from the TEAHAT trial. *Cardiology*, 1995;**86**: 25–27.
5. Fibrinolytic Therapy Trialists' (FTT) Collaborative Group, Indications for fibrinolytic therapy in suspected acute myocardial infarction: collaborative overview of early mortality and major morbidity results from all randomised trials of more than 1000 patients. *Lancet*, 1994;**343**: 311–322.
6. Weaver, W.B., M.S. Eisenberg, J.S. Martin, et al., Myocardial infarction triage and intervention project – Phase I: Patient characteristics and feasibility of pre-hospital initiation of thrombolytic therapy. *J. Am. Coll. Cardiol.*, 1990;**15**: 925–931.

7. Maroko, P.R., J.K. Kjekshus, B.E. Sobel, T. Watanabe, J.W. Covell, J. Ross, and E. Braunwald, Factors influencing infarct size following experimental coronary artery occlusions. *Circulation*, 1971;**43**: 67–82.

8. Gruppo Italiano per lo Studio della Streptochinasi nell'Infarto Miocardico (GISSI), Effectiveness of intravenous thrombolytic treatment in acute myocardial infarction. *Lancet*, 1986;**1**: 397–401.

9. Grines, C.L., K.F. Browne, J. Marco, et al., A comparison of immediate angioplasty with thrombolytic therapy for acute myocardial infarction. *N. Engl. J. Med.*, 1993;**328**: 673–679.

10. ISIS-2 (Second International Study of Infarct Survival) Collaborative Group, Randomised trial of intravenous streptokinase, oral aspirin, both or neither among 17.187 cases of suspected acute myocardial infarction: ISIS-2. *Lancet*, 1988;**2**: 349–360.

11. Hjalmarson, Å., D. Elmfeldt, J. Herlitz, S. Holmberg, I. Málek, G. Nyberg, L. Rydén, K. Swedberg, A. Vedin, F. Waagstein, A. Waldenström, J. Waldenström, H. Wedel, L. Wilhelmsen, and C. Wilhelmsson, Effect on mortality of metoprolol in acute myocardial infarction. A double-blind randomised trial. *Lancet*, 1981;**ii**: 823–827.

12. Freimark, D., S. Matetzky, J. Leor, V. Boyko, I.M. Barbash, S. Behar, et al., Timing of aspirin administration as a determinant of survival of patients with acute myocardial infarction treated with thrombolysis. *Am. J. Cardiol.*, 2002;**89**: 381–385.

13. Barbash, I.M., D. Freimark, S. Gottlieb, H. Hod, Y. Hasin, A. Battler, et al., Outcome of myocardial infarction in patients treated with aspirin is enhanced by pre-hospital administration. *Cardiology*, 2002;**98**: 141–147.

14. Zijlstra, F., N. Ernst, M.J. deBoer, E. Nibbering, H. Suryaparanata, J.C.A. Hoorntje, et al., Influence of prehospital administration of aspirin and heparin on initial patency of the infarct-related artery in patients with acute ST elevation myocardial infarction. *JACC*, 2002;**39**: 1733–1737.

15. Chambless, L., U. Keil, A. Dobson, M. Mähönen, K. Kuulasma, A.M. Rajakangas, and H. Löwel, Tunstall-Pedoe H for the WHO MONICA project. Population versus clinical view of case fatility from acute coronary heart disease. Results from the WHO MONICA project 1985–1990. *Circulation*, 1997;**96**: 3849–3859.

16. Vingerhoets, F., J. Bogousslavsky, F. Regli, and G. Van Melle, Atrial fibrillation after acute stroke. *Stroke*, 1993;**24**: 26–30.

17. Grijseels, E.W.M., J.W. Deckers, A.W. Hoes, J.A.M. Hartman, E. Van der Does, E. Van Loenen, and M.L. Simoons, Pre-hospital triage of patients with suspected myo-cardial infarction. Evaluation of previously developed algorithms and new proposals. *Eur. Heart J.*, 1995;**16**: 325–332.

18. Svensson, L., C. Axelsson, R. Nordlander, and J. Herlitz, Elevation of biochemical markers for myocardial damage prior to hospital admission in patients with acute chest pain or other symptoms raising suspicion of acute coronary syndrome. *J. Int. Med.*, 2003;**253**: 311–319.

19. Drew, B.J., C.E. Sommargren, D.M. Schindler, J. Zegre, K. Benedict, and M.W. Krucoff, Novel electrocardiogram configurations and transmission procedures in the prehospital setting: effect on ischemia and arrhythmia determination. *J. Electrocardiol.*, 2006;**39**: S157–S160.

20. Herlitz, J., Å. Hjalmarson, S. Holmberg, A. Richter, and B. Wennerblom, Mortality and morbidity in suspected acute myocardial infarction in relation to ambulance transport. *Eur. Heart J.*, 1987;**8**: 503–509.

21. Herlitz, J., B.W. Karlson, A. Bång, and J. Lindqvist, Characteristics and outcome for patients with acute chest pain in relation to whether or not they were tran-sported by ambulance. *Eur. J. Emerg. Med.*, 2000;**7**: 195–200.

22. Canto, J.G., R.J. Zalenski, J.P. Ornato, W.J. Rogers, C.I. Kiefe, D. Magid, et al., Use of emergency medical services in acute myocardial infarction and subsequent quality of care: observations from the National Registry of Myocardial Infarction 2. *Circulation*, 2002;**106**: 3018–3023.

23. Erhardt, L., J. Herlitz, L. Bossaert, M. Halinen, M. Keltai, R. Koster, C. Marcassa, T. Quinn, and H. van Weert, Task force report. Task force on the management of chest pain. *Eur. Heart J.*, 2002;**23**(15): 1153–1176.

24. Gardtman, M., M. Dellborg, C.h. Brunnhage, J. Lindqvist, L. Waagstein, and J. Herlitz, Effect of intravenous metoprolol before hospital admission on chest pain in suspected acute myocardial infarction. *Am. Heart J.*, 1999;**137**(5): 821–829.

25. Svensson, L., C. Axelsson, R. Nordlander, and J. Herlitz, Prognostic value of biochemi-cal markers, twelve lead ECG and patients characteristics among patients calling for an ambulance due to a suspected acute coronary syndrome. *JIM*, 2004;**255**: 469–477.

26. Holmberg, M., S. Holmberg, and J. Herlitz, Incidence, duration and survival of ventricular fibrillation in out-of-hospital cardiac arrest patients in Sweden. *Resuscitation*, 2000;**44**: 7–17.

27. Svensson, L., T. Karlsson, R. Nordlander, M. Wahlin, C. Zedigh, and J. Herlitz, Implementation of prehospital thrombolysis in Sweden. Components of delay until delivery of treatment and examination of treatment feasibility. *Int. J. Cardiol.*, 2003;**88**: 247–256.

28. Weaver, W.D., M. Cerqueira, A.P. Hallstrom, P.E. Litwin, J.S. Martin, P.J. Kudenchuk, et al., Prehospital-initiated vs hospital-initiated thrombolytic therapy. The myocardial infarction triage and intervention trial. *JAMA*, 1993;**270**: 1211–1216.

29. The European Myocardial Infarction Project Group, Prehospital fibrinolytic therapy in patients with suspected acute myocardial infarction. *N. Engl. J. Med.*, 1993;**329**: 383–389.

30. Cooke, W.H., J. Salinas, V.A. Convertino, D.A. Ludwig, D. Hinds, J.H. Duke, F.A. Moore, and J.B. Holcomb, Heart rate variability and its association with mortality in prehospital trauma patients. *J. Trauma*, 2006;**60**: 363–370.

31. Batchinsky, A.I., L.C. Cancio, J. Salinas, T. Kuusela, W.H. Cooke, J.J. Wang, M. Boehme, V.A. Convertino, and J.B. Holcomb, Prehospital loss of R-to-R interval complexity is associated with mortality in trauma patients. *Trauma*, 2007;**63**: 512–518.

32. Steg, P.G., J.P. Cambou, P. Goldstein, et al., Bypassing the emergency room reduces delays and mortality in ST-elevation myocardial infarction: the USIC 2000 registry. *Heart*, 2006;**92**: 1378–1383.

33. Bång, A., L. Grip, J. Herlitz, S. Kihlgren, T. Karlsson, K. Caidahl, and M. Hartford, Lower mortality after prehospital recognition and treatment followed by fast tracking to coronary care compared with admittance via emergency department in patients with ST-elevation myocardial infarction. *Int. J. Cardiol.*, 2008;**129**: 325–332.

34. Terkelsen, C.J., B.L. Nørgaard J.F. Lassen J.C. Gerdes J.P. Ankersen, F. Rømer, T.T. Nielsen, and H.R. Andersen, Telemedicine used for remote prehospital diagnosing in patients suspected of acute myocardial infarction. *J. Intern. Med.*, 2002;**252**: 412–420.

35. Terkelsen, C.J., B.L. Nørgaard, J.F. Lassen, and H.R. Andersen, Prehospital evaluation in ST-elevation myocardial infarction patients treated with primary percutaneous coronary intervention. *J. Electrocardiol.*, 2005;**38**: 187–192.

36. Dalby, M., A. Bouzamondo, P. Lechat, and G. Montalescot, Transfer for primary angioplasty versus immediate thrombolysis in acute myocardial infarction: a meta-analysis. *Circulation*, 2003;**108**: 1809.

37. Andersen, H.R., T.T. Nielsen, K. Rasmussen, L. Thuesen, H. Kelbaek, P. Thayssen, et al., A comparison of coronary angioplasty with fibrinolytic therapy in acute myocardial infarction. *N. Engl. J. Med.*, 2003;**349**: 733.

38. Widimsky, P., et al., on behalf of the PRAGUE Study Group Investigators, Multicentre randomized trial comparing transport to primary angioplasty vs immediate thrombolysis vs combined strategy for patients with acute myocardial infarction presenting to a community hospital without a catheterization laboratory. The PRAGUE study. *Eur. Heart J.*, 2000;**21**: 823.

39. Stenestrand, U., J. Lindbäck, Wallentin L for the RIKS-HIA Registry, Long-term outcome of primary percutaneous coronary intervention vs prehospital and in-hospital thrombolysis for patients with ST-elevation myocardial infarction. *JAMA*, 2006;**296**: 1749–1756.

40. Grines, C.L., J. Westerhausen, L.L. Grines, J.T. Hanlon, T.L. Logemann, M. Niemela, et al., A randomized trial of transfer for primary angioplasty versus on-site thrombolysis in patients with high-risk myocardial infarction: the air primary angioplasty in myocardial infarction study. *J. Am. Coll. Cardiol.*, 2002;**39**: 1713.

41. Aufderheide, T.P., D.J. Kereiakes, W.D. Weaver, W.B. Gibler, and M.L. Simoons, Planning, implementation and process monitoring for prehospital 12lead ECG Diagnostic programs. *Prehosp. Disaster Med.*, 1996;**11**(3): 162–171.

42. Rawles J on Behalf of the GREAT Group, Halving of mortality at 1 year by domiciliary thrombolysis in the Grampian Region Early Anistreplase Trial (GREAT). *J. Am. Coll. Cardiol.*, 1994;**23**: 1–5.

43. Aufderheide, T.P., M.H. Keelan, G.E. Hendley, et al., Milwaukee prehospital chest pain projekct – Phase I: Feasibility and accuracy of prehospital thrombolytic candidate selection. *Am. J. Cardiol.*, 1992;**3**: 41–46.

44. Gibler, W.B., D.J. Kereiakes, E.N. Dean, et al., Prehospital diagnosis and treatment of acute myocardial infarction: north-south perspective. *Am. Heart J.*, 1991;**121**: 1–11.

45. Castaigne, A., C. Herve, A. Duval-Moulin, et al., Prehospital use of APSAC: Results of a placebo-controlled study. *Am. J. Cardiol.*, 1989;**64**: 30A–33A.

46. Schofer, J., J. Buttner, G. Geng, et al., Pre-hospital thrombolysis in acute myocardial infarction. *Am. J. Cardiol.*, 1990;**66**: 1429–1433.

47. Aufderheide, T.P., W.C. Haselow, G.E. Hendley, et al., Feasibility of pre-hospital r-TPA therapy in chest pain patients. *Ann. Emerg. Med.*, 1992;**21**: 379–383.

48. Svensson, L., T. Karlsson, R. Nordlander, M. Wahlin, C. Zedigh, and J. Herlitz, Safety and delay time in prehospital thrombolysis of acute myocardial infarction in urban and rural areas in Sweden. *Am. J. Emerg. Med.*, 2003;**21**(4): 263–270.

49. Kereiakes, D.J., W.D. Weaver, J.C.L. Anderson, et al., Time delays in the diagnosis and treatment of acute myocardial infarction: A tale of eight cities. Report from the Prehospital Study Group and the Cincinnati Heart Project. *Am. Heart J.*, 1990;**120**: 773–780.

50. Morrison, L.J., S. Brooks, B. Sawadsky, A. McDonald, and P.R. Verbeek, Prehospital 12-lead electrocardiography impact on acute myocardial infarction treatment times and mortality: A systematic review. *Acad. Emerg. Med.*, 2006;**13**: 84–89.

51. Currtis, J.P., E.L. Portnay, Y. Wang, R.L. McNamara, J. Herrin, E.H. Bradley, D.J. Magid, M.E. Blaney, J.G. Canto, and H.M. Krumholz, The pre-hospital electrocardiogram and time to reperfusion in patients with acute myocardial infarction 2000–2002. *J. Am. Coll. Cardiol.*, 2006;**47**: 1544–1552.

52. Brainard, A.H., W. Raynovich, D. Tandberg, and E.J. Bedrick, The prehospital 12-lead electrocardiogram's effect on time to initiation of reperfusion therapy: a systematic review and meta-analysis of existing literature. *Am. J. Emerg. Med.*, 2005;**23**: 351–356.

53. Adams, G.L., P.T. Campbell, J.M. Adams, D.G. Strauss, K. Wall, J. Patterson, K.B. Shuping, C. Maynard, D. Young, C. Corey, A. Thompson, B.A. Lee, and G.S. Wagner, Effectiveness of prehospital wireless transmission of electrocardiograms to a cardiologist via hand-held device for patients with acute myocardial infarction (from the Timely Intervention in Myocardial Emergency, NorthEast Experience [TIME-NE]). *Am. J. Cardiol.*, 2006;**98**: 1160–1164.

54. Björklund, E., U. Stenestrand, J. Lindbäck, L. Svensson, L. Wallentin, and B.A. Lindahl, Pre-hospital diagnostic strategy reduces time to treatment and mortality in real life patients with ST-elevation myocardial infarction treated with primary percutaneous coronary intervention. *JACC*, 2006;**47**(4) (Suppl A): 192A.

55. Brown, J.P., E. Mahmud, J.V. Dunford, and O. Ben-Yehuda, Effect of prehospital 12-lead electrocardiogram on activation of the cardiac catheterization laboratory and door-to-ballon time in ST-segment elevation acute myocardial infarction. *Am. J. Cardiol.*, 2008;**101**: 158–161.

56. Sillesen, M., M. Sejersten, S. Strange, S. Loumann-Nielsen, F. Lippert, and P. Clemmensen, Referal of patients with ST-segment elevation acute myocardial infarction directly to the catheterization suite based on prehospital teletransmission of 12-lead electrocardiogram. *J. Electrocardiol.*, 2008;**41**: 49–53.

57. Sejersten, M., M. Sillesen, P.R. Hansen, S. Loumann-Nielsen, H. Nielsen, S. Trautner, D. Hampton, G.S. Wagner, and P. Clemmensen, Effect on treatment delay of prehospital teletransmission of 12-lead electrocardiogram to a cardiologist for immediate triage and direct referral of patients with ST-segment elevation acute myocardial infarction to primary percutaneous coronary intervention. *Am. J. Cardiol.*, 2008;**101**: 941–946.

58. Eckstein, M., W. Koenig, A. Kaji, and R. Tadeo, Implementation of speciality centers for patients with ST-segment elevation myocardial infarction. *Prehosp. Emerg. Care*, 2009;**13**: 215–222.

59. Eckstein, M., E. Cooper, T. Nguyen, and F.D. Pratt, Impact of paramedic transport with prehospital 12-lead electrocardiography on door-to-balloon times for patients with ST-segment elevation myocardial infarction. *Prehosp. Emerg. Care*, 2009;**13**: 203–206.

60. Patrono, C., F. Bachmann, C. Baigent, C. Bode, et al., Expert consensus document on the use of antiplatelet agents. The task force on the use of antiplatelet agents in patients with atherosclerotic cardiovascular disease of the European society of cardiology. *Eur. Heart J.*, 2004;**25**: 166–181.

61. Yusuf, S., F. Zhao, S.R. Mehta, S. Chrolavicius, G. Tognoni, and K.K. Fox, The Clopidogrel in unstable angina to prevent recurrent events trial investigators. Effects of Klopidogrel in addition to aspirin in patients with acute coronary syndromes without ST-segment elevation. *N. Engl. J. Med.*, 2001;**345**: 494–502.

62. Fragmin-During-Instability-In-Coronary-Artery-Disease-Study-Group, Low-molecular-weight heparin during instability in coronary artery disease. *Lancet*, 1996;**347**: 561–568.

63. Wallentin, L., P. Goldstein, P.W. Armstrong, C.B. Granger, et al., Efficacy and safety of tenecteplase in combination with the low-molecular-weight heparin enoxaparin or unfractionated heparin in the prehospital setting: the Assessment of the Safety and Efficacy of a New Thrombolytic Regimen (ASSENT)-3 PLUS randomized trial in acute myocardial infarction. *Circulation*, 2003;**108**: 135–142.

64. Slovis, C.M., P.J. Kudenchuk, M.A. Wayne, R. Aghababian, and E.J. Rivera-Rivera, Prehospital management of acute tachyarrhythmias. *Prehosp. Emerg. Care*, 2003;7: 2–12.

65. Lozano, M. Jr., B.A. McIntosh, and L.M. Giordano, Effect of adenosine on the management of supraventricular tachycardia by urban paramedics. *Ann. Emerg. Med.*, 1995;**26**: 691–696.

66. Gausche, M., D.E. Persse, T. Sugarman, et al., Adenosine for the prehospital treatment of paroxysmal supraventricular tachycardia. *Ann. Emerg. Med.*, 1994;**24**: 183–189.

67. Madsen, C.D., J.E. Pointer, and T.G. Lynch, A comparison of adenosine and verapamil for the treatment of supraventricular tachycardia in the prehospital setting. *Ann. Emerg. Med.*, 1995;**25**: 649–655.

68. Wang, H.E., R.E. O'Connor, R.E. Megargel, et al., The use of dilitiazem for treating rapid atrial fibrillation in the out-of-hospital setting. *Ann. Emerg. Med.*, 2001;**37**: 38–45.

69. Kudenchuk, P.J., L.A. Cobb, M.K. Copass, et al., Amiodarone for resuscitation after out-of-hospital cardiac arrest due to ventricular fibrillation. *N. Engl. J. Med.*, 1999;**341**: 871–878.

70. Sivagangabalan, G., A.T.L. Ong, A. Narayan, N. Sadick, P.S. Hansen, G.C.I. Nelson, M. Flynn, D.L. Ross, S.C. Boyages, and P. Kovoor, Effect of prehospital triage on revascularization times, left ventricular function, and survival in patients with ST-elevation myocardial infarction. *Am. J. Cardiol.*, 2009;**103**: 907–912.

71. Diercks, D.B., M.C. Kontos, A.Y. Chen, C.V. Pollack, S.D. Wiviott, J.S. Rumsfeld, D.J. Magid, W.B. Gibler, C.P. Cannon, E.D. Peterson, and M.T. Roe, Utilization and impact of prehospital electrocardiograms for patients with acute ST-segment elevation myocardial infarction. *J. Am. Coll. Cardiol.*, 2009;**53**: 161–166.

72. Eisenstein, E.L., Conducting an economic analysis to assess the electrocardiogram's value. *J. Electrocardiol.*, 2006;**39**: 241–247.

73. Grim, P.S., T. Feldman, and R.W. Childers, Evaluation of patients for the need of thrombolytic therapy in the prehospital setting. *Ann. Emerg. Med.*, 1989;**18**: 483–488.

74. Aufderheide, T.P., G.E. Hendley, J. Woo, et al., A prospective evaluation of prehospital 12-lead ECG application in chest pain patients. *J. Electro-cardiol.*, 1992;**24**(suppl): 8.

75. Musuraca, G., F. Imperadore, C. Cemin, C. Terraneo, C. Vaccarini, P. Giuseppe De Girolamo, and G. Vergara, Electrocardiographic abnormalities mimicking myocardial infarction in a patient with intracranial haemorrhage: a possible pitfall for prehospital thrombolysis. *J. Cardiovasc. Med.*, 2006;7: 434–437.

76. Otto, L.A. and T.P. Aufterheide, Evaluation of ST-segment elevation criteria for the prehospital electrocardiographic diagnosis of acute myocardial infarction. *Ann. Emerg. Med.*, 1994;**23**: 17–24.

77. Brady, W.J., A. Perron, and E. Ullman, Errors in emergency physician interpretation of ST-segment elevation in emergency department chest pain patients. *Acad. Emerg. Med.*, 2000;7: 1256–1260.

78. Eriksen, U.H., H. Ölgaard, J. Ingerslev, and T.T. Nielsen, Fatal haemostatic complications due to thrombolytic therapy in patients falsely diagnosed as acute myocardial infarction. *Eur. Heart J.*, 1992;**13**: 840–843.

79. Alinier, G., R. Gordon, C. Harwood, and W.B. Hung, E.C.G. 12-lead, training: the way forward. *Nurse Educ. Today*, 2006;**26**: 87–92.

80. Aufderheide, T.P., Prehospital 12-lead electrocardiography and evaluation of the patient with chest pain, in *Emergency Cardiac Care*, W.B. Gibler and T.P. Aufterheide, Editors. St Louis, MO: Mosby Year Book, 1994, pp. 38–65.

81. Garvey, J.L., B.A. MacLeod, G. Sopko, and M.M. Hand, Prehospital 12.lead electrocardiography programs. A call for implementation by emergency medical services systems providing advanced life support – national heart attack alert program (NHAAP) coordinating committee; National Heart, Lung and Blood Institute (NHLBI); National Institutes of Health. *J. Am. Coll. Cardiol.*, 2006;**47**: 485–491.

82. Voluntary Guidelines for Out-of-Hospital Practices, A joint policy statement of PREP between the American College of Emergency Physicians, the National Association of Emergency Medical Services Physicians, and the National Association of State Emergency Medical Services Directors. June 2001. Policy # 400305.

83. Vaught, C., D.R. Young, S.J. Bell, C. Maynard, M. Gentry, S. Jacubowitz, P.N. Leibrandt, D. Munsey, M.R. Savona, T.C. Wall, and G.S. Wagner, The failure of years of experience with electrocardiographic transmission from paramedics to the hospital emergency department to reduce the delay from door to primary coronary intervention below the 90-minute threshold during acute myocardial infarction. *J. Electrocardiol.*, 2006;**39**: 136–141.

84. RIKS-HIA. www.ucr.uu.se/rikshia/

85. Feldman, J.A., K. Brinsfield, S. Bernard, D. White, and T. Maciejko, Real-time paramedic compared with blinded physician identification of ST-segment elevation myocardial infarction: results of an observational study. *Am. J. Emerg. Med.*, 2005;**23**: 443–448.

86. Trivedi, K., J.D. Schuur, and D.C. Cone, Can paramedics read ST-segment elevation myocardial infarction on prehospital 12-lead electrocardiograms? *Prehosp. Emerg. Care*, 2009;**13**: 207–214.

87. McLean, S., G. Egan, P. Connor, and A.D. Flapan, Collaborative decision-making between paramedics and CCU nurses based on 12-lead ECG telemetry expedites the delivery of thrombolysis in ST-elevation myocardial infarction. *Emerg. Med. J.*, 2008;**25**: 370–374.

88. Bouten, M.J.M., M.L. Simoons, J.A.M. Hartman, A.J.M. van Miltenburg, E. van der Does, and J. Pool, Prehospital thrombolysis with alteplase (rt-PA) in acute myocardial infarction. *Eur. Heart J.*, 1992;**13**: 925–931.

89. Lamfers, E.J.P., A. Schut, D.P. Hertzberger, T.E.H. Hooghoudt, P.W.J. Stolwijk E. Boersma, M.L. Simoons, and F.W.A. Verheught, Prehospital versus hospital fibrinolytic therapy using

automated versus cardiologist electrocardiographic diagnosis of myocardial infarction: abortion of myocardial infarction and unjustified fibrinolytic therapy. *Am. Heart J.*, 2004;**147**: 509–515.

90. Grijseels, E.W.M., M.J.M. Bouten, T. Lenderink, J.W. Deckers, A.W. Hoes, J.A.M. Hartman, E. van der Does, and M.L. Simoons. Prehospital thrombolytic therapy with either alteplace or streptokinase. Practical applications, complications and long-term results in 529 patients. *Eur. Heart J.*, 1995;**16**: 1833–1838.

91. Lamfers, E.J.P., A. Schut, T.E.H. Hooghoudt, D.P. Hertzberger, E. Boersma, M.L. Simoons, and F.W.A. Verheught, Prehospital thrombolysis with reteplase: the Nijmegen/Rotterdam study. *Am. Heart J.*, 2003;**146**: 479–483.

92. Kudenchuk, P.J., M.T. Ho, W.D. Weaver, P.E. Litwin, J.S. Martin, M.S. Eisenberg, A.P. Hallstrom, and L.A. Cobb, Kennedy JW for the MITI project investigators. Accuracy of computer-interpreted electrocardiography in selecting patients for thrombolytic therapy. *J. Am. Coll. Cardiol.*, 1991;**17**: 1486–1491.

93. Xue, J., T. Aufderheide, R.S. Wright, J. Klein, R. Farrell, I. Rowlandson, and B. Young, Added of new acute coronary syndrome computer algorithm for interpretation of prehospital electrocardiograms. *J. Electrocardiol.*, 2004;**37S**: 233 (Suppl).

94. Eskola, M.J., K.C. Nikus, L.M. Voipio-Pulkki, H. Huhtala, T. Parviainen, J. Lund, T. Ilva, and P. Porela, Comparative accuracy of manual versus computerized electrocardiographic measurement of J-, ST- and T-wave deviations in patients with acute coronary syndrome. *Am. J. Cardiol.*, 2005;**96**: 1584–1588.

95. Pettis, K.S., M.R. Savona, P.N. Leibrandt, C. Maynard, W.T. Lawson, K.B. Gates, and G.S. Wagner, Evaluation of the efficacy of hand-held computer screens for cardiologists' interpretations of 12.lead electrocardiograms. *Am. Heart J.*, 1999;**138**: 765–770.

96. Leibrandt, P.N., S.J. Bell, M.R. Savona, K.S. Pettis, R.H. Selvester, C. Maynard, R. Warner, and G.S. Wagner, Validation of cardiologist's decisions of initiate reper-fusion therapy for acute myocardial infarction using electrocardiograms viewed on liquid crystal displays of cellular telephones. *Am. Heart J.*, 2000;**140**: 747–752.

97. Nallamothu, B.K., Y. Wang, D. Magid, R.L. McNamara, J. Herrin, E.H. Bradley, E.R. Bates, C.V. Pollack, and H.M. Krumholz, Relation between hospital specialization with primary percutaneous coronary intervention and clinical outcomes in ST-segment elevation myocardial infarction. National Registry of Myocardial Infarction-4 Analysis. *Circulation*, 2006;**113**: 222–229.

98. Terkelsen, C.J., J.F. Lassen, B.L. Nørgaard, J.C. Gerdes, S.H. Poulsen, K. Bendix, J.P. Ankersen, L.B. Gøtzsche, F.K. Rømer, T.T. Nielsen, and H.R. Andersen, Reduction of treatment delay in patients with ST-elevation myocardial infarction: impact of pre-hospital diagnosis and direct referral to primary percutaneous coronary intervention. *Eur. Heart J.*, 2005;**26**: 770–777.

99. Rokos, I.C., D.M. Larson, T.D. Henry, W.J. Koenig, M. Eckstein, W.J. French, C.B. Granger, and M.T. Roe, Rationale for establishing regional ST-elevation myocardial infarction receiving center (SRC) networks. *Am. Heart J.*, 2006;**152**: 661–667.

100. Sejersten, M., M. Sillesen, P.R. Hansen, S. Loumann Nielsen, H. Nielsen, S. Trautner, D. Hampton, G.S. Wagner, and P. Clemmensen, Effect on treatment delay of prehospital teletransmission of 12-lead electrocardiogram to a cardiologist for immediate triage and direct referral of patients with ST-segment elevation acute myocardial infarction to primary percutaneous coronary intervention. *Am. J. Cardiol.*, 2008;**101**: 941–946.

101. Väisänen, O., M. Jäkijärvi, and T. Silfvast, Prehospital ECG transmission: comparison of advanced mobile phone and facsimile devices in an urban emergency service system. *Resuscitation*, 2003;**57**: 179–185.

102. Carmody, B.J., A novel approach to transmission of the out-of-hospital ECG in patients with ST segment elevation myocardial infarction. *Ann. Emerg. Med.*, 2008;**52**: 183–184.

103. Svensson, L., L. Isaksson, C. Axelsson, R. Nordlander, and J. Herlitz, Predictors of myocardial damage prior to hospital admission among patients with acute chest pain or other symptoms raising a suspicion of acute coronary syndrome. *Coron. Artery Dis.*, 2003;**14**(3): 225–231.

104. Lee, H.S., S.J. Cross, J.M. Rawles, and K.P. Jennings, Patients with suspected myocardial infarction who present with ST-depression. *Lancet*, 1993;**342**: 1204–1207.

105. Brady, W.J., A.D. Perron, S.A. Syverud, C. Beagle, R.J. Riviello, C.A. Ghaemmaghami, E.A. Ullman, B. Erling, A. Ripley, and C. Holstege, Reciprocal ST-segment depression: impact on the electrocardiographic diagnosis of ST-segment elevation acute myocardial infarction. *Am. J. Emerg. Med.*, 2002;**20**: 35–38.

106. Svensson, L., R. Nordlander, C. Axelsson, and J. Herlitz, Are predictors for myocardial infarction the same for women and men when evaluated prior to hospital admission? *Int. J. Cardiol.*, 2006;**109**: 241–247.

107. Karlson, B.W., J. Herlitz, O. Wiklund, A. Richter, and Å. Hjalmarson, Early prediction of acute myocardial infarction from clinical history, examination and electrocardiogram in the emergency room. *Am. J. Cardiol.*, 1991;**68**: 171–175.

108. Drew, B.J., M.M. Pelter, E. Lee, J. Zegre, D. Schindler, and E. Fleischmann, Designing prehospital E.C.G systems for acute coronary syndromes. Lessions learned from clinical trials involving 12-lead ST-segment monitoring. *J. Electrocardiol.*, 2005;**38**: 180–185.

109. Terkelsen, C.J., B.L. Nørgaard, J.F. Lassen, S.H. Poulsen, J.C. Gerdes, K. Bendix, J.P. Ankersen, L.B. Gøtzsche, F.K. Rømer, T.T. Nielsen, and H.R. Andersen, Reduction of treatment delay in patients with ST-elevation myocardial infarction: impact of pre-hospital diagnosis and direct referral to primary percutaneous coronary intervention. *Eur. Heart J.*, 2005;**26**: 770–777.

110. Herlitz, J., L. Sillfors, and Å. Hjalmarson, Experiences from the use of 24 precordial chest leads in suspected acute myocardial infarction. *J. Electrocardiol.*, 1986;**19**(4): 381–388.

111. Sejersten, M., O. Pahlm, J. Pettersson, S. Zhou, C. Maynard, C.L. Feldman, and G.S. Wagner, Comparison of EASI-derived 12-lead electrocardiograms versus paramedic-acquired 12-lead electrocardiograms using Mason-Likar limb lead configuration in patients with chest pain. *J. Electrocardiol.*, 2006;**39**: 13–21.

112. Feldman, C.L., S.Z. Milstein, D. Neubecker, B.K. Underhill, E. Moyer, S. Glumm, M. Womble, J. Auer, C. Maynard, R.K. Serra, and G.S. Wagner, Comparison of the five-electrode-derived EASI electrocardiogram to the Mason Likar electrocardiogram in the prehospital setting. *Am. J. Cardiol.*, 2005;**96**: 453–456.

113. Owens, C.G., A.J.J. McClelland, S.J. Walsh, B.A. Smith, A. Tomlin, J.W. Riddell, M. Stevenson, and A.A.J. Adgey, Prehospital 80-Lad mapping: does it add significantly to the diagnosis of acute coronary syndromes? *J. Electrocardiol.*, 2004;**37**: 223–232.

114. Drew, B.J., E.D. Dempsey, T.H. Joo, C.E. Sommargren, J.P. Glancy, K. Benedict, and M.W. Krucoff, Prehospital synthesized 12-lead ECG ischemia monitoring with transtelephonic transmission in acute coronary syndromes. *J. Electrocardiol.*, 2004;**37**(Suppl 1): 214–221.

115. Hollenberg, J., A. Bång, J. Lindqvist, J. Herlitz, R. Nordlander, L. Svensson, and M. Rosenqvist, Difference in survival after out of hospital cardiac arrest between the two largest cities in Sweden – a matter of time? *JIM*, 2005;**257**: 247–254.

116. Müller, D., L. Schnitzer, J. Brandt, and H.R. Arntz, The accuracy of an out-of-hospital 12-lead ECG for the detection of ST-elevation myocardial infarction immediately after resuscitation. *Ann. Emerg. Med.*, 2008;**52**: 658–664.

117. Kuisma, M., J. Repo, and A. Alaspää, The incidence of out of hospital ventricular fibrillation in Helsinki Finland from 1994 to 1999. *Lancet*, 2001;**358**: 473–474.

118. Herlitz, J., J. Engdahl, L. Svensson, M. Young, K.A. Ängquist, and S. Holmberg, Decrease in the occurrence of ventricular fibrillation as the initially observed arrhythmia after out-of-hospital cardiac arrest during 11 years in Sweden. *Resuscitation*, 2004;**60**: 283–290.

119. Engdahl, J., A. Bång, J. Lindqvist, and J. Herlitz, Factors affecting short and long-term prognosis among 1069 patients with out-of-hospital cardiac arrest and pulseless electrical activity. *Resuscitation*, 2001;**51**: 17–25.

120. Pepe, P.E., R.L. Levine, R.E. Fromm, P.A. Curka, P.S. Clark, and B.S. Zachariah, Cardiac arrest presenting with rhythms other than ventricular fibrillation: contribution of resuscitative efforts toward total survivorship. *Crit. Care Med.*, 1993;**21**: 1838–1843.

121. Stratton, S.J. and J.T. Niemann, Outcome from out-of-hospital cardiac arrest caused by nonventricular arrhythmias: contribution of successful resuscitation to overall survivorship supports the current practice of initiating out-of-hospital ACLS. *Ann. Emerg. Med.*, 1998;**32**: 448–453.

122. Engdahl, J., A. Bång, J. Lindqvist, and J. Herlitz, Can we define patients with no and those with some chance of survival when found in asystole out of hospital? *Am. J. Cardiol.*, 2000;**86**(6): 610–614.

123. Weaver, W.D., L.A. Cobb, D. Dennis, et al., Amplitude of ventricular fibrillation waveform and outcome after cardiac arrest. *Ann. Intern. Med.*, 1985;**102**: 53–55.

124. Brown, C.G., R. Dzwoncyk, and D.R. Martin, Physiologic measurement of the ventricular fibrillation ECG signal: esitimating the duration of ventricular fibrillation. *Ann. Emerg. Med.*, 1993;**22**: 70–74.

125. Brown, C.G. and R. Dzwoncyk, Signal analysis of the human electrocardiogram during ventricular fibrillation: frequency and amplitude parameters as predictors of successful countershock. *Ann. Emerg. Med.*, 1996;**27**: 184–188.

126. Noc, M., M.H. Weil, W. Tang, et al., Electrocardiographic prediction of the success of cardiac resuscitation. *Crit. Care Med.*, 1999;**27**: 708–714.

127. Strohmenger, H.U., T. Eftestol, K. Sunde, et al., The predictive value of ventricular fibrillation electrocardiogram signal frequency and amplitude variables in patients with out-of-hospital cardiac arrest. *Anesth. Analg.*, 2001;**93**: 1428–1433.

128. Ahmann, A., U. Achleitner, H. Antretter, et al., Analysing ventricular fibrillation ECG-signals and predicting defibrillation success during cardiopulmonary resuscitation employing N(alpha)-histograms. *Resuscitation*, 2001;**50**: 77–85.

129. Eftestøl, T., K. Sunde, S.O. Aase, et al., Probability of successful defibrillation as a monitor during CPR in out-of-hospital cardiac arrested patients. *Resuscitation*, 2001;**48**: 245–254.

130. Eftestøl, T., H. Losert, J. Kramer-Johansen, et al., Independent evaluation of a defibrillation outcome predictor for out-of-hospital cardiac arrested patients. *Resuscitation*, 2005;**67**: 55–61.

131. Watson, J.N., N. Uchaipichat, P.S. Addison, et al., Improved prediction of defibrillation success for out-of-hospital VF cardiac arrest using wavelet transform methods. *Resuscitation*, 2004;**63**: 269–275.

132. Watson, J.N., P.S. Addison, G.R. Clegg, et al., Practical issues in the evaluation of methods for the prediction of shock outcome success in out-of-hospital cardiac arrest patients. *Resuscitation*, 2006;**68**: 51–59.

133. Snyder, D.E., R.D. White, and D.B. Jorgenson, Outcome prediction for quidance of initial resuscitation protocol: Shock first or CPR first. *Resuscitation*, 2007;**72**: 45–51.

134. Neurauter, A., T. Eftestøl, J. Kramer-Johansen, B.S. Abella, V. Wenzel, K.H. Lindner, J. Eilevstjønn, H. Myklebust, P.A. Steen, F. Sterz, B. Jahn, and H.U. Strohmenger, Improving countershock success prediction during cardiopulmonary resuscitation using ventricular fibrillation features from higher ECG frequency bands. *Resuscitation*, 2008;**79**: 453–459.

135. Sherman, L.D., T.D. Rea, J.D. Waters, J.J. Menegazzi, and C.W. Callaway, Logarithm of the absolute correlations of the ECG waveform estimates duration of ventricular fibrillation and predicts successful defibrillation. *Resuscitation*, 2008;**78**: 346–354.

136. Gundersen, K., J.T. Kvaløy, J. Kramer-Johansen, P.A. Steen, and T. Eftestøl, Development of the probability of return of spontaneous circulation in intervals without chest compressions during out-of-hospital cardiac arrest: an observational study. *BMC Med.*, 2009;**7**: 6.

137. Gundersen, K., J. Nysaether, J.T. Kvaløy, J. Kramer-Johansen, and T. Eftestøl, Chest compression quality variables influencing the temporal development of ROSC-predictors calculated from the ECG during VF. *Resuscitation*, 2009;**80**: 177–182.

138. Olasveengen, T.M., T. Eftestøl, K. Gundersen, L. Wik, and K. Sunde, Acute ischemic heart disease alters ventricular fibrillation waveform characteristics in out-of hospital cardiac arrest. *Resuscitation*, 2009;**80**: 412–417.

139. Lederer, W., C.J. Schlimp, T. Niederklapfer, and A. Amann, Altered electrical activity of fibrillation process following thrombolytic therapy in out-of-hospital cardiac arrest patients with sustained ventricular fibrillation. *Med. Hypotheses*, 2006;**67**: 3313–335.

140. Aufderheide, T.P., R.K. Thakur, H.A. Stueven, et al., Electrocardiographic characteristics in EMD. *Resuscitation*, 1989;**17**: 183–193.

141. Fang, X., W. Tang, S. Sun, J. Wang, L. Huang, and M.H. Weil, The characteristics of post countershock pulseless electrical activity may indicate the outcome of CPR. *Resuscitation*, 2006;**69**: 303–309.

142. Williams, D. in collaboration with Fitch and associates, JEMS 200-City survey. *JEMS Feb.*, 2005;**30**: 42–60.

143. Ting, H.H., H.M. Krumholz, E.H. Bradley, D.C. Cone, J.P. Curtis, B.J. Drew, J.M. Field, W.J. French, W.B. Gibler, D.C. Goff,

A.K. Jacobs, B.K. Nallamothu, R.E. O'Connor, and J.D. Schuur. Implementation and integration of prehospital ECG:s into systems of care for acute coronary syndrome. *Circulation*, 2008;**118**: 1066–1079.

144. Frendl, D.M., S.T. Palmeri, J.R. Clapp, D. Hampton, M. Sejersten, D. Young, B. Drew, R. Farrell, J. Innes, J. Russell, G.I. Rowlandson, Y. Purim-Shem-Tov, B.K. Underhill, S. Zhou, and G.S. Wagner, Overcoming barriers to developing seamless ST-segment elevation myocardial infarction care systems in the United States: recommendations from a comprehensive prehospital 12-lead electrocardiogram working group. *J. Electrocardiol.*, 2009;**42**: 426–431.

3 Heart Rate Variability

Maciej Sosnowski

P. W. Macfarlane et al. (eds.), *Specialized Aspects of ECG*, DOI 10.1007/978-0-85729-880-5_3,
© Springer-Verlag London Limited 2012

Introduction

Changes of pulse rate and rhythm have attracted the attention of physicians since the earliest stages of medicine. Only recently, with the advance of computer techniques that allow for parsing heart rate variability (HRV) into components, which potentially yield information about the autonomic nervous control of cardiac activity, has there been an increased clinical interest. The technical advances, however, have not resulted in bedside application of HRV methods and evidence of their usefulness in real-world clinical practice is still limited. Moreover, from the point of view of the physician, complex approaches to HRV phenomena and the use of complicated mathematical formulae may have a rather limited implementation in everyday practice. In this chapter, several aspects of HRV are thoroughly reviewed giving priority to their physiological and pathophysiological meanings in order to render HRV more clinically useful. For that reason, technical descriptions are limited to providing only the necessary background information.

3.1   Historical Note

Fluctuations in heart rate were first recorded by ancient physicians. Disturbances of heart rate due to changes in psycho-emotional state were revealed by Erastratos, an Alexandrian physician, in the third century B.C. [1]. Similarly, a description of pulse-shift in relation to emotion or illness is ascribed to Galen (129–199 A.D.) [1]. A decrease in heart rate variation was recognized by the Chinese physician Wang Shuhe (265–317 A.D.) as a sign which could predict the onset of death [2] (❷ Fig. 3.1). Later, many physicians raised the examination of the pulse rate to the level of an art. An excellent example of this is given by Józef Struś, Polish physician to Zygmunt August, King of Poland, in his work "*Sphigmicae Artis*" (Basel 1555) [3].

The fundamentals of current knowledge are usually credited to the observations of Stephen Hales (1733) and Carl Ludwig (1847). Hales first found, in the horse, that the pattern of blood pressure was dependent on respiration [4, 5]. Ludwig, armed with the smoked kymograph, recorded a quickening of the pulse rate with inspiration and a slowing with expiration in the dog [5]. He is credited with the term *respiratory sinus arrhythmia (RSA)* [5, 6]. Two decades later, F.C. Donders (1868) followed up this research to describe the role of the vagus nerve in RSA. Traube (1865) advised on the importance of the medullary respiratory centers in modulating the brainstem nuclei controlling heart rate. Hering (1871) put forward an alternate explanation for RSA, namely the consequence of a reflex modulation of the central oscillator by pulmonary afferent feedback [5]. A few years later, Mayer (1877) established that longer-wave oscillation in blood pressure was due to vasomotor tone. Continuing these efforts, Hering (1910) first stated that the function of vagi could be quantified in humans by means of RSA [6]. Next, in 1920 Bainbridge reported on the effects of thoracic pressure changes with respiration and their association with RSA [6]. German psychiatrists Eppinger and Hess (1915) focused on the clinical application of RSA as a measure of vagal tone and first made observations on the effects of cholinergic agents [6]. This was further emphasized by the study of Samaan (1935) in which stimulation of a section of vagus nerve abolished RSA [7].

With the advent of electrocardiography (ECG), accurate and continuous recording of the electrical activity of the heart became possible. Not surprisingly, the first recording of RSA was made in the first decade of the twentieth century by Samojloff in 1909. Schlomka, in 1936, provided the first quantitative measures of RSA from short-term ECG tracings. He also reported on an age-dependency of RSA and the reduction of RSA in patients with advanced heart failure (After [8]).

The seminal works listed in ❷ Table 3.1 have provided a solid grounding for the current knowledge and application of HRV in cardiology. Interestingly, well before HRV analysis was appreciated in cardiology, its usefulness had been documented in obstetrics and psychology [5, 6, 10, 11].

3.2   Definitions, Synonyms, Abbreviations

Heart rate (HR) – frequency of the heart beating usually calculated as the average of four or more consecutive heartbeats, expressed in beats per minute (bpm).

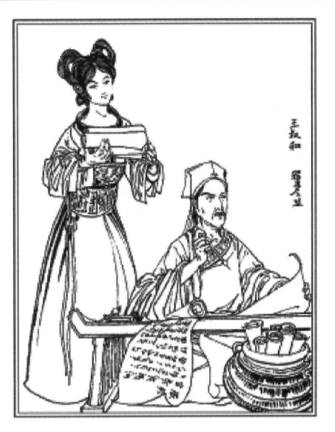

◻ Fig. 3.1

HRV and an ancient medicine (From [2])

Instantaneous heart rate (HRi) – heart rate confined to a given sinus cycle duration on a beat-to-beat manner (60/R–R interval).

Intrinsic heart rate (iHR) – heart rate after cessation of the autonomic influences (pharmacological or surgical denervation), i.e., in situ heart rate.

Heart period (HP) – the duration of a given cardiac cycle, usually calculated as a period between two consecutive R-waves or P-waves, expressed in seconds (s) or milliseconds (ms). Unless indicated otherwise, cardiac cycle is defined as a presumed sinus (in origin) cycle irrespective of the polarity of the P-waves. Sometimes, if the signal is acquired using a technique other than the ECG, heart period is referred to as a *pulse interval* or an *interbeat interval* (IBI).

R–R interval – description of heart period based on detection of the R-wave instead of the P-wave. The "R" labeling is used in short-term ECG recordings and assumes sinus origin of the heartbeat. However, in a few studies such a labeling indicates any depolarizations, irrespective of their origin (usually noted).

N-N interval – description of heart period for long-term ECG recordings, where sinus (supraventricular) origin of the heartbeat is assumed and labeled as normal (N).

Heart rate variability (HRV) – a variation in the duration of HP (which might not be consecutive). It can be quantified using various methods in the time, frequency, and nonlinear dynamics domains.

Heart period variability (HPV) – a term similar to HRV.

Time-domain analysis – an analytical approach to HRV quantification in which the sequence of heartbeats is generally ignored. It usually gives information about the magnitude of heart beat variation around its mean value.

Respiratory sinus arrhythmia (RSA) – heart period fluctuations due to breathing. RSA can be quantified preferably by using spectral analysis; however, time-domain analysis and other approaches are possible.

⬛ Table 3.1

Historical background of contemporary HRV analysis

Author[s]	Year	Issue discovered/solved	Ref.
Samaan A	1935	Various influence of separate and joined vagal-sympathetic stimulation upon heart rate	[7]
Anrep et al.	1936	First extensive and systematic study of RSA as a function of respiration	[9]
Lacey & Lacey	1958	RSA as a trait of behavioral response	[10]
Hon/Lee	1963	RR interval variation monitoring in prediction of a fetus death	[11]
Schneider/Costiloe	1965	Relationship of RSA to age and its prognostic significance in ischemic heart disease	[A34]
Wolf S	1967	Brain-heart link contribution to sudden cardiac death	[13]
Katona et al.	1970	Evaluation of the carotid baroreflex	[14]
Levy MN	1971	Description of the accentuated angiotensin	[15]
Hinkle et al.	1972	Association of chronotropic incompetence with adverse outcome in middle-aged man	[16]
Sayers	1973	First spectral analysis of HRV Detection of lower frequency components; association with vasomotor tone	[17]
Wheeler/Watkins	1973	Description of diabetic autonomic neuropathy	[18]
Wolf et al.	1978	First report on a prognostic significance of a reduced RSA in acute MI	[19]
Akselrod et al.	1981	Documentation of autonomic and humoral background of HRV	[20]
Kobayashi/Musha	1982	Nonlinear dynamics applied to HR data	[21]
Ewing et al.	1984	Usefulness of HRV for diagnosis of diabetic autonomic neuropathy	[22]
Pomeranz et al.	1985	Spectral analysis for physiological stimuli assessment in humans	[23]
Kleiger et al.	1987	Independent prognostic value of SDNN in AMI patients	[24]
Camm et al.	1998	First EBM-study that used HRV as the inclusion criterion	[25]

Spectral analysis – an analytical approach for decomposition of frequency components in a signal time series, which requires strict maintenance of R – R interval sequence. A graphical presentation is usually given as a plot of the amplitude of variation (cycle, bpm, s, or ms), variance or power (cycle^2, bpm^2, s^2, or ms^2), or power spectral density (cycle^2/beat, bpm^2/Hz, s^2/Hz, or ms^2/Hz) against various period or frequency ranges (beats/min, Hz).

High frequency component (HF) – part of the power spectrum that (in adult humans) is contained within the arbitrary frequency band between 0.15 and 0.40 Hz (or higher). The HF component represents short-term (2.5–6.0 s) heartbeat variation within the frequency of respiration. Its relative contribution to the total power decreases exponentially as duration of a time series is increasing; it is also cited as the RSA-related or vagally-related power.

Low frequency component (LF) – part of the power spectrum within the frequency band from 0.04 (0.05) to 0.15 Hz (*in humans*) and represents medium-term (6–25 s) heartbeat variation within the frequency of Mayer waves of blood pressure. Its relative contribution to the total power decreases exponentially as the duration of a time series is increasing.

Very low frequency component (VLF) – part of the power spectrum that (*in humans*) is contained within the frequency band between 0.003 and 0.04 Hz and represents long-term (> 25 s) heartbeat variation. Its relative contribution to the total power decreases as the duration of a time series is increasing.

Ultra low frequency component (ULF) – part of the power spectrum that (*in humans*) is contained within the frequencies below 0.003 Hz and represents very long-term (> 5 h) heartbeat variation. It cannot be reliably evaluated from a short time series. It constitutes the main contribution to the total power from a 24-h signal recording. Day–night difference is the most prominent oscillation within the ULF component.

Nonlinear dynamics – a field applying a variety of analytical approaches to the study of R – R interval variations that are not linearly related, and presumed not to be random. These approaches allow evaluating different properties of heartbeat variation in terms of its determinism, predictability, sequence, scale-invariant similarity, patterns, complexity, information flow, and other features.

Abbreviations related to HRV analysis

ACI–Acceleration change index
A_I–Asymmetry index
AIF–Autonomic information flow
ApEn–Approximate entropy
AR–Autoregressive modeling
BRS–Baroreflex sensitivity
CIPA–Cardiac index of parasympathetic activity
CE–Compressed entropy
CWA–Continuous wavelet analysis
CV–Coefficient of variation
CSI–Cardiac sympathetic index
CVI–Cardiac vagal index
DC–Deceleration capacity
DI–Deceleration index
$D_{iff}I$–Differential index
DFA–Detrended fluctuation analysis
EMD–Empirical mode decomposition
FFT–Fast Fourier transform
HR6%–Number of consecutive HRi periods that differ by > 6% from the preceding one
HRT–Heart rate turbulence
HRVF–Heart rate variability fraction (%)
HRVI–Heart rate variability index (St.George's index, absolute units)
HT–Hilbert transform
HHT–Huang-Hilbert transform
LLE–Largest Lyapunov exponent
MIF–Mutual information function
MSE–Multiscale entropy
MSSD–Mean sum of the squared difference between adjacent intervals
NL–Noise limit
(p)NN50–(percentage) Number of consecutive NN (RR) intervals that differ by > 50 ms
PLF–Prevalent low frequency
PLM–Power-law model
RQA–Recurrence quantification analysis
RLS–Recursive least-squares estimation
RMSSD–Root mean square of the successive difference between consecutive NN (RR) intervals
SampEn–Sample entropy
SD1–Standard deviation of interbeat intervals over minor axis of scatterplot
SD2–Standard deviation of interbeat intervals over major axis of scatterplot
SDNN (SDRR)–Standard deviation of the mean NN (RR) intervals
SDANN–Standard deviation of the averaged NN intervals over a pre-specified period (typically a 5-min period)
SDNNI–The average of the standard deviation of N – N intervals over a pre-specified period (typically a 5-min period)
SDyn–Symbolic dynamics
STFT–Short-term Fourier transform
TCA–Temporal cumulative approach
TINN–Triangular interpolation index
TO–Turbulence onset
TS–Turbulence slope
WVD–Wigner-Ville distribution

VR–Variation range, i.e., the difference between the longest and the shortest interval
%DET–Percent of determinism

Other abbreviations in the chapter

ACE–Angiotensin converting enzyme
ACEIs–ACE inhibitors
Ang–Angiotensin
ACh–Acetylcholine
AF–Atrial fibrillation
AFl–Atrial flutter
ANS–Autonomic nervous system
AVN–Atrio-ventricular node
ARBs–Angiotensin receptor blockers
BB–Beta-blockers (beta-adrenolytics)
BNP–Brain natriuretic peptide
BP–Blood pressure (*SBP* – systolic, *DBP* – diastolic, *MBP* – mean)
bpm–Beats per minute
CABG–Coronary artery by-pass grafting
CAD–Coronary artery disease (atherosclerotic)
CI–Confidence interval
CRT–Cardiac resynchronisation therapy
DAN–Diabetic autonomic neuropathy
dB–Decibel(s)
DM–Diabetes mellitus
DVN–Dorsal motor nucleus of the vagus nerve
E–Epinephrine
ECG–Electrocardiogram, electrocardiography, electrocardiographic (depending on a context)
HF–Heart failure (CHF – congestive heart failure)
Hz–Hertz
ICC–Intra-class coefficient
ICD–Implantable cardioverter-defibrillator
LOA–Limit of agreement
LVEF–Left ventricular ejection fraction
MI–Myocardial infarction
ms–Millisecond(s)
NA–Nucleus ambiguous
NE–Norepinephrine
NO–Nitric oxide
NYHA–New York Heart Association
OSAS–Obstructive sleep apnea syndrome
PEB(s)–Premature ectopic beat(s)
PNS–Parasympathetic nervous system
PSD–Power spectrum density
s–Second(s)
SAN–Sino-atrial node
SIDS–Sudden infant death syndrome
SCD–Sudden cardiac death
SNR–Signal-to-noise ratio
SNS–Sympathetic nervous system

SR–Sinus rhythm
VF–Ventricular fibrillation
VT–Ventricular tachycardia

3.3   Methods for HRV Assessment

Heart beat variation can be examined by replacing the complex waveform of an individual heartbeat recorded in the ECG with the time of occurrence of the contraction as a single number. Thus, the sequence of heartbeat duration can be expressed as a function of its duration (*tachogram*) (Time series derived from the occurrence time of the R-wave. The term is applicable also for cardiac events series, interval tachogram, interval function, instantaneous heart rate, heart timing signal, and low-pass filtered event series.). Sometimes, by interpolating and resampling the R – R sequence, the HRV signal can be presented as a function of time. Since the presence of sinus rhythm is formally defined as the onset of normally oriented P-waves, heartbeat variation assessment should ideally be based on a calculation of time-intervals between consecutive P-waves. Because the shape of the P-wave is unfavorable for its automated detection with currently used commercial equipment (difficulties in fiducial point determination, relatively low SNR), two important assumptions are made [26]. First, that the detection of the P-wave can be replaced by the detection of the R-wave, and second, that interbeat duration between consecutive R waves equals that of consecutive P waves. Since the variability of the P – R interval is approximately — two to three orders lower than that of the P–P or R–R intervals [27], it is assumed that the P–R interval variability does not influence the HRV measurements. Thus, in practice the QRS complex (R-wave) is commonly used to determine the time period between consecutive heartbeats.

3.3.1   Time Domain HRV Analysis

Techniques used in time-domain analysis provide the simplest measures of heartbeat variation over time. These measures are simple to calculate and relatively easy to understand. Time-domain methods describe the overall magnitude of R–R interval fluctuation around its mean value. One class is the statistical descriptors of beat-to-beat intervals (not necessarily consecutive) or of differences in the duration between adjacent heartbeats. Another class is the geometrical method (frequency distribution representations).

3.3.1.1   Statistical Methods

The earliest quantitative indices for HRV (RSA) have been described in studies by Schlomka et al. and Schäfers et al. (after [8]) in the 1930s, as the difference between the sum of the — three to four longest and — three to four shortest R–R intervals either as absolute values (*arrhythmia magnitude*) or as normalized data for the mean HR (percentage of the mean, *arrhythmia index*). Similar measures are still in use and referred to as the *variation range* (*VR, absolute*) and *coefficient of variation* (*CV, normalized*). Simple measures of cardiac vagal activity from standard ECG recordings have been described recently [28, 29].

The most widely used time-domain measure is the standard deviation (*SDNN or SDRR*) (❷ Table 3.2), which is equal to the square root of the variance of all normal-to-normal or R–R intervals, respectively [30]. Depending on data-length and signal representation (HRi, HP) various SD-based measures are in use. This simple HRV measure can be drawn from a time series of any duration.

From 24-h ECG recordings, two other measures allow the quantification of the average N–N interval or SD changes over predefined periods, usually of 5-min duration (SDANN and SDNNI, respectively) [30]. If a permutation of SD is applied to the differences between consecutive N–N (R–R) intervals, a widely used and recommended index is derived, referred to as the *RMSSD* [30] (❷ Table 3.2). The SD-based measures represent a coarse quantification of overall variation, while RMSSD represents a more accurate quantification of short-term beat-to-beat variation. More recently, a new index has been derived which is the ratio SD/RMSSD [31].

◘ **Table 3.2**

Time-domain HRV measures from short- and long-term ECG recordings

Parameter	Units	Description
SDRR	ms	Standard deviation of all quantifiable R–R intervals over a period of recording
CV	%	Coefficient of variation, i.e., SDNN normalised for mean RRI
VR	ms	Variation range, i.e., difference between the longest and shortest RRI over a period of recording
DSCL	ms	Maximal difference between two consecutive R–R intervals (sinus cycles) over a period of recording
AAD	ms	Average absolute difference, i.e., the average of the differences between successive R–R intervals ignoring their sign
SDSD	ms	Standard deviation of differences between successive R–R intervals
RMSSD	ms	Root mean square of successive differences in R–R intervals, i.e., the square root of the mean squared differences of successive R–R intervals
CIPA	units	Cardiac index of parasympathetic activity
SDNN	ms	Standard deviation of all quantifiable N–N intervals
SDANN	ms	Standard deviation of the averages of N–N intervals in all quantifiable 5-min epochs of the entire recording
SDNNI	ms	Mean of the standard deviations of all N–N intervals for all quantifiable 5-min epochs of the entire recording
RMSSD	ms	The square root of the mean squared differences of successive N–N intervals
NN50 count		Absolute number of pairs of successive R–R intervals that differ by more than 50 ms; three variants are possible counting all such R–R interval pairs or only pairs in which the first or the second interval is longer
pNN50	%	Percentage of pairs of successive N–N intervals that differ by more than 50 ms, i.e., NN50 count divided by the total N–N intervals' number
HR6%	%	Number of consecutive heartbeats that differ in their instantaneous heart rate by more than 6%

A separate type of statistical analysis is based on counting of events defined as the occurrence of consecutive heartbeats that differs above a pre-selected (arbitrary) limit of values or bins (absolute or relative). The index NN50+ expresses the number ("counts") of consecutive heartbeats that differ by 50 ms or more [22, 30]. Conventionally 6% bpm (HR6%) or 50 ms difference (NN50 or pNN50) is used. However, those arbitrary cut-off values represent only one of a family of possible statistics (NNx) [32]. The unfavorable statistical properties of count-derived indices (❯ Fig. 3.2) has led experts to advise against their use [4]. Logarithmic transformation of the pNN50 was proposed to improve count-derived index statistics and their reproducibility. A novel proposal that may help to overcome statistical limitations suggests the expression of the pNN50 after the logit transformation (logit50) [33]. The Logit50 = Ln [pNN50/(100-pNN50)] is the natural logarithm of the odds of the occurrence of preset R–R interval differences >50 ms (❯ Fig. 3.2).

Statistical measures are the most commonly used method despite their sensitivity to extreme values (such as true or false) and which requires time-consuming review of the data-series to obtain reliable values [34]. Dependence on the duration of recording excludes comparisons of short-term and long-term data, even if they are closely correlated [4]. It might also influence the reproducibility of the statistical measures. As these indices provide only crude information, they do not allow different HRV patterns (or dynamics) to be distinguished. Moreover, various patterns of HRV with similar statistical properties can be erroneously gathered into one class of HRV [35].

3.3.1.2 Geometric Methods

Graphic representations of event distribution and their quantitative evaluation can be obtained by plotting the frequency of occurrence of values in selected ranges or bins. This is referred to as a *histogram*. Classic descriptors of such representation are skewness and kurtosis, which quantify symmetry and peakness, respectively. Such descriptors are frequently used in HRV studies [36].

A histogram of time series can be analyzed using the absolute or relative number of "frequencies" within bins [37]. The most frequent bin is termed the mode of the histogram and its "height" can be measured as the number of R–R intervals with modal duration. The area of the histogram is equal to all R–R intervals. Assuming that the major peak of

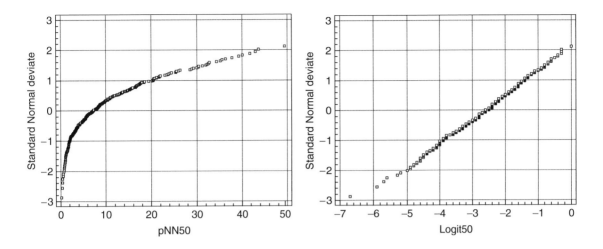

◘ Fig. 3.2
Unfavorable distribution of pNN50 (*left plot*) and its improvement if expressed as the Logit50 values. Data from 290 healthy subjects (Author's data)

the histogram is a triangle, the simplest measure of any HRV geometric method can be derived. It is referred to as the *HRV Triangular index (HRVI)* [37, 38]. Here, if the number of intervals in the *i*th bin centered at t_i is represented as $b(t_i)$, then HRVI is defined as (3.1):

$$\text{HRVI} = \frac{\sum_{i=1}^{Nb} b(t_i)}{\max_i b(t_i)} = \frac{N-1}{\max_i b(t_i)} \tag{3.1}$$

where N_b is the number of bins (❯ Fig. 3.3). Usually, a constant bin is used with a width of $1/fs = 7.8125$ ms, where *fs* is the sampling frequency. A selection of bin widths is critical for HRVI and other histogram-derived indices [39].

A modification of the HRVI, less dependent on the sampling frequency, is the *Triangular Interpolation Index* (TIRR or TINN depending on whether the selected intervals are R–R or N–N), which is the base of a triangle that approximates the highest peak of the sample density histogram by means of the minimum square difference interpolation [40] (❯ Fig. 3.4). Generally, a uniform distribution representing large variability gives large values and a distribution with a single large peak provides small values.

The HRVI and TINN are dependent on the distribution of R–R intervals and are suitable for a reliable HRV estimation only if one dominant peak is present. Such a pattern is usual in a stable in-hospital environment. In ambulant patients and in normal subjects a bimodal distribution is more common, therefore, the HRVI or TINN underestimates the global HRV.

Similar approaches can be applied to data derived from the differences between successive heartbeats (*differential histogram*). Interestingly, a negative exponential interpolation of a differential histogram (specifically the slope of the interpolation curve) appears to be a robust method that is useful for the automatic assessment of HRV [41].

Another technique of differential histogram analysis referred to as a *sample asymmetry analysis* quantifying R–R interval deviations from the median (or mean) values has been proposed recently [42]. Two quantities representing the sum of the weighted deviation to the left (R1(α), HR accelerations) and to the right (R2(ß), HR decelerations) can be calculated, where α and β are parameters describing the degree of weighting from the median value (α = β = 2 are chosen). The ratio of R2/R2 represents the sample asymmetry. For a symmetric histogram, R1 and R2 are equal.

The *differential index* ($D_{iff}I$), obtained from a differential histogram, defined as the width of the base of a triangle constructed by using the width of the histogram at 10,000 R–R intervals and at 1,000 intervals, plotted on a semilogarithmic scale [43]. Data for healthy subjects and the prognostic value in subjects with angina pectoris have been obtained by using 16 ms bins [43, 44].

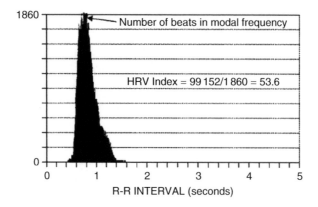

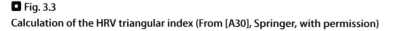

◘ Fig. 3.3
Calculation of the HRV triangular index (From [A30], Springer, with permission)

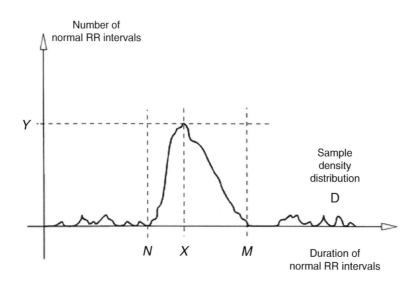

◘ Fig. 3.4
Calculation of the TINN index. For the computation of the TINN measure, the values *N* and *M* are established on the time axis and a multilinear function q constructed such that $q(t) = 0$ for $t \leqslant N$ and $t \geqslant M$ and q(X) = Y, and such that the integral $\int_0^{+\infty} (D(t) - q(t))^2 dt$ is the minimum among all selections of all values *N* and *M*. The TINN measure is expressed in milliseconds and given by the formula TINN = $M - N$ (From [4])

In general, histogram-based methods require a sufficient data length, so they are less applicable to a short data-series. They are also sensitive to the sampling frequency.

3.3.1.3   Return Map Evaluation

This geometric method is based on a *return map* (Plot of a time series as a function of the current and of the previous values. Known also as a Lorenz plot, scatterplot and less appropriately as a Poincaré plot.), which is a plot of each R–R interval (RR_n) (on the abscissa) against the following interval (RR_{n+1}) (on the ordinate) (❷ Fig. 3.5). The first approaches

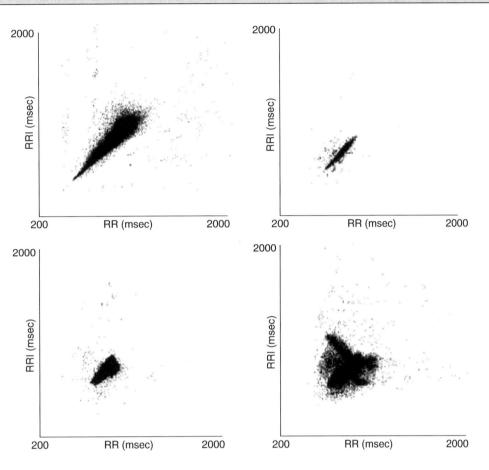

◘ Fig. 3.5

Examples of patterns of a return map. Upper panel, comet (*left*) and torpedo (*right*) pattern (usual in healthy subjects), lower panel, fan (*left*) and complex (*right*) pattern (usually abnormal) (From [47] with permission)

based on the return map for ventricular rhythm assessment in atrial fibrillation were reported by Arnoldi (1927) and Soderstrom (1950) [45]. Nakanishi et al. were the first to use this method for HRV analysis [46].

In this section, time-domain measures that can be drawn from the return map are described. Possible nonlinear approaches are discussed in a later section.

A qualitative evaluation of the return map is based on the overall shape of distribution (❯ Fig. 3.5) [47]. The shape of the return map can be classified into several pattern-based categories, such as a comet or torpedo in healthy humans, while fan-like or more complex patterns may occur in patients with certain cardiovascular pathologies or after autonomic blockade. The use of qualitative evaluation is limited because of the subjective nature of evaluation and there is a probability of a misleading interpretation. However, a qualitative approach remains a unique and valid method for the assessment of the quality of the ECG recordings [4]. Recently, a subject-independent method for scatterplot pattern recognition has been proposed [47].

Several measures for return map quantification have been proposed. To be reliably calculated, longer ECG recordings are usually necessary. However, solutions for quantifying return maps from short-term recordings have been reported [46, 48–50].

The simplest measures can be derived from the regression line (slope, intercept, or correlation coefficient). The slope or the intercept of the regression line does not seem to have any advantage over simple max–min R–R interval difference or mean RRI itself. The Pearson correlation coefficient of the return map was shown to correlate with short-term variation

[50, 51]. Successive Pearson correlation coefficients calculated for each 1-min return map from long-term ECG recordings were proposed to reveal distinct patterns of sleep–wake states (❷ Fig. 3.6) [52].

The most frequently used quantitative analysis of the return map includes calculation of its width- and length-derived parameters [53–60]. Schechtman et al. applied those parameters for HRV analysis in newborns with aborted SIDS [54–56]. They proposed calculating all following intervals for the given percentile value of the preceding R–R intervals, specifically at the 10th and 90th percentile [53]. Alternative methods were proposed by Kamen et al. [57] and Tulpo et al. [58] (❷ Fig. 3.7). The derived indices *SD1* (standard deviation of intervals over the minor axis), *SD2* (standard deviation of intervals over the major axis), and their ratio *SD1/SD2*, all enable the approximate estimation of autonomic cardiac control [54–56]. Toichi et al. [59] calculated the length of the return map over transverse T and longitudinal L axes and derived two indices, referred to as the *Cardiac Vagal Index* ($CVI = \log 10(L^*T)$) and the *Cardiac Sympathetic Index* ($CSI = L/T$) (❷ Fig. 3.8). They showed that only 100 R–R intervals (~2 min.) were necessary for a reliable calculation of those indices. Copie et al. [60] manually determined both L and T of the scatterplot in order to calculate the scatterplot area. Another variant of HRV partitioning has recently been proposed [61]. Unfortunately, in the presence of more complex patterns of the return map, width and length-related metrics cannot be used.

The introduction of a "z" coordinate as the next time lag (i.e., $R - R_{n+2(or>)}$) was proposed for evaluating the return map in 3D space [62]. Such an approach gives a novel insight into the complexity of heartbeat dynamics, yet no clinically useful index has been proposed.

Another proposal is to represent the number of pairs (RR_n, RR_{n+1}) that lie within predefined bins, related to the percentiles [55], sampling interval (usually 7.8 ms) [63] or R–R ranges [64], equally spaced in "x" and "y" axes. In this way, a "z" axis represents a density function and a pseudo-3D graphic presentation can be obtained. In this proposal, for

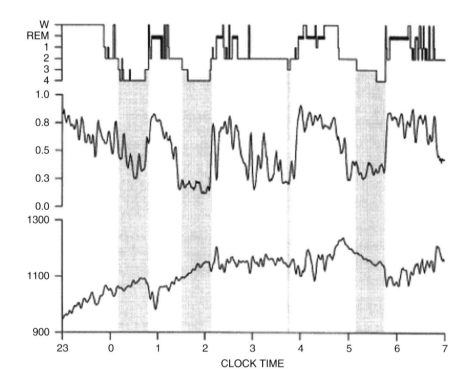

◨ Fig. 3.6
Return map coefficients use to follow transitory changes following various sleep stages. Profiles of 1-min interbeat autocorrelation coefficient rRR (*middle panel*) and of R – R interval (*lower panel*) together with sleep pattern (*upper panel*). Slow wave sleep (stage 3 and 4) lies in shaded areas. rRR and RR curves smoothed using the moving average method over a 5-point span (From [52])

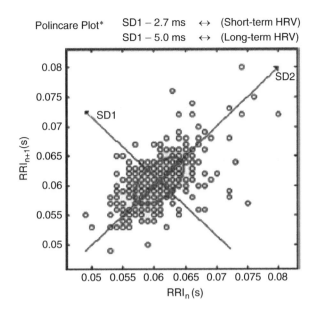

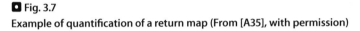

Fig. 3.7
Example of quantification of a return map (From [A35], with permission)

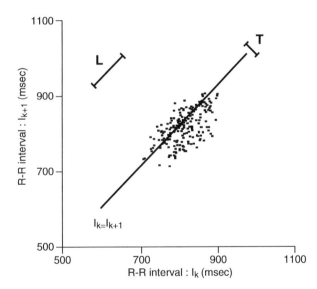

Fig. 3.8
Quantitative assessment of the return map from short-term recordings. The length of the transverse axis, T, and the length of the longitudinal axis, L, can be determined. The derived indices of vagal (CVI) and sympathetic (CSI) are proposed and can be calculated as simple product (decimal log) or ratio of the L and T (From [59]).

each rectangular area of the plot, the relative number of RR_n/RR_{n+1} samples is determined. Then, the maximum density of samples for each size of the area of the plot is calculated. Schechtman et al. found this approach useful for studying the changeable pattern over sleep–wake states in neonates [55]. Hnatkova et al. have proposed the logarithmic integral of the density function to express numerically the compactness of the plot in post-infarct patients (the *Compactness Index*) (❯ Fig. 3.9) [63].

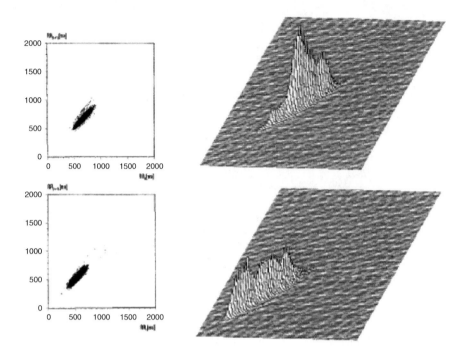

⬛ Fig. 3.9

Three-dimensional representation of the return map from long-term ECG recordings. Two examples of 3-D return map (*right panel*) of low (*upper panel*) and high risk (*lower panel*) post-infarct patients clearly mark differences between both cases with nearly identical 2-D return map (*left panel*) (From [63])

Sosnowski et al. proposed a simplified method for 3D return map evaluation [64, 65]. The distribution of pairs of neighboring heartbeats (counts) within R–R interval ranges with 100 ms resolution (bins) is presented (❷ Fig. 3.10). Then, the density of counts in the two highest grid boxes (the area for each grid box being $0.01\,\mathrm{s}^2$) can be determined by applying a 16×16 array to the scatterplot between 200 and 1,800 ms. Such a 3D view of the return map allows for an easy determination of the density function in normal subjects, patients with sinus rhythm (❷ Fig. 3.11), with premature beats and atrial fibrillation. The derived index of HRV referred to as the *HRV Fraction (HRVF)* is calculated according to the following formula (3.2):

$$\mathrm{HRVF} = \left[1 - \frac{\mathrm{RR}_1 + \mathrm{RR}_2}{\mathrm{RR} - \mathrm{RR50}}\right] * 100[\%] \tag{3.2}$$

where RR_1 and RR_2 represent two highest counts (from squares that are not necessarily adjacent), RR (total beat number) and RR50 (the number of intervals that differ from a succeeding interval by 50 ms or more).

The HRVF possesses unique properties that make it useful for HRV quantification irrespective of heart rhythm [65]. Actually, the HRVF is the only time-domain index allowing for HRV assessment in the presence of AF (❷ Fig. 3.11). Significantly, a similar range of normal and abnormal HRV can be applied for subjects with sinus rhythm and atrial fibrillation [66]. The HRVF is normally distributed (as HR itself). This makes any statistical performance straightforward, contrary to most time-domain statistical measures, which frequently require transformation (usually logarithmic) before any statistical analysis (❷ Fig. 3.12). In addition, its calculation is not affected by the distribution of data-points, so it can be applied to more complex patterns of the return maps. Physiological meaning of the HRVF as a global HRV index appears to be similar to that of other global HRV measures (i.e., SDNN). At present, only the author has evidence of the potential clinical utility of this method.

Moraes et al. have presented a somewhat different approach to return map construction [67]. A plot of RRI (on the x axis) against $\mathrm{RR}_i - \mathrm{RR}_{i+1}$ (on the y axis) and number of pairs within the bin of 7.2 ms duration (on the z axis) can be

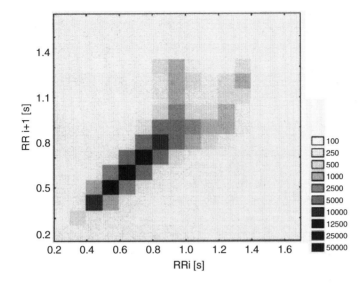

◘ Fig. 3.10
Simplified 2-D view of a return map of RR against RR_{i+1}. The boxes with two highest number of RR interval pairs is easily seen as black boxes lying between 0.6 and 0.8 s. These two numbers are RR1 and RR2 in the HRV Fraction equation. All heartbeats in the range of 0.2–1.8 s are included, irrespective of their origin (normal, supra-ventricular or ventricular) (From [64])

obtained. The derived index MN is the product of parameters derived from the three axes (**◐** Fig. 3.13). Its clinical utility remains unknown.

3.3.1.4   Time-Domain Analysis for Parsing Frequency Components

Peak-to-valley ("*peak-to-trough*") statistics is the time-domain method introduced for distinguishing respiratory-related oscillation from nonrespiratory periodic components [5, 6, 49, 68]. Accordingly, the RSA is quantified as the average difference between the shortest sinus cycle associated with inspiration and longest sinus cycle within expiration. This method is vulnerable to artifacts associated with low frequencies. In addition, a separate measure of respiration is required. This method has become popular in psychological studies [5, 6, 68, 69].

The second time-domain method that allows for HRV distinction within specified frequency bands is the *moving polynominal method* [69]. By using this method, the statistical variance of the data within the respiratory frequency is obtained. However, it requires epochs of data points before and after the analytical time series to "prime" the polynominal filter. This method and other variants are extensively used in psychological studies [5, 6, 68–71].

Repeated calculations of the coefficient of return maps with increasing time-lag (RR_n vs. RR_{n+i}, i = 1–6) can reflect the RSA pattern from relatively short-term recordings (~2,000 heartbeats) [72]. Even shorter epochs (~70 heartbeats) are reported to be suitable for quantifying the pattern underlying RSA [73].

3.3.1.5   Time-Domain Analysis of the HR-HRV Relationship

Only a few attempts have been made to quantify the relationship between HR and HRV from long-term ECG recordings. The HRV Fraction is one example, as the probability of a certain value strongly depends on the mean RRI [65]. The most recent attempt is referred to as the *HRV Footprint*, which is a plot of heart rate against SDANN. This plot renders the likelihood (or density) of a particular HRV change occurring at each intrinsic HR over a 24-h period. The

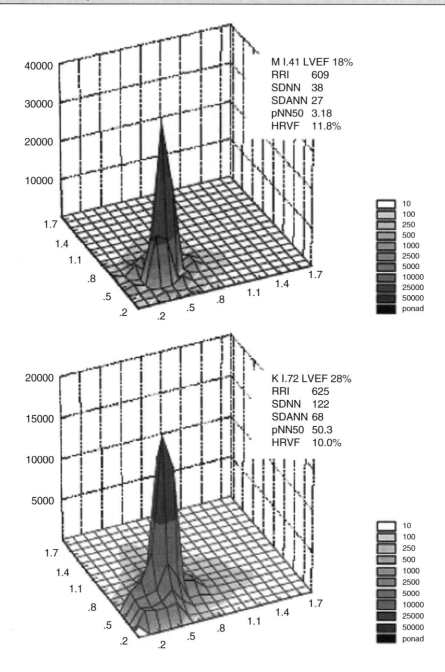

◻ Fig. 3.11

3D return map view in a patient with sinus rhythm and in a patient with atrial fibrillation. Two examples of R − R interval distribution in patients with depressed LV systolic function. Upper graph from a patient with sinus rhythm, lower – with AF. Values of HRV Fraction, as well as mean R − R interval are comparable, while SDNN was three times higher in AF-patient, reaching value far above the lower normal limit (Author's data)

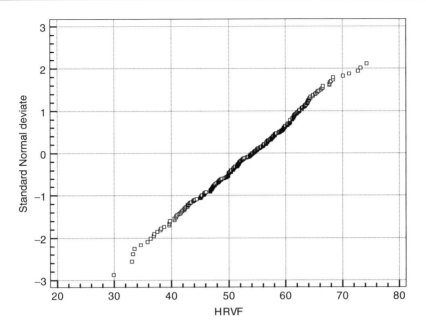

□ Fig. 3.12
Plot of HRVF values distribution in healthy subjects against standard normal deviate (Author's data)

footprint-area is calculated and expressed as a percentage. An example of the HRV Footprint in a patient with heart failure is shown in ❷ Fig. 3.14. [74]. Its usefulness has recently been documented in HF-patients with implantable cardiac resynchronization devices [74, 75].

3.3.2 Frequency-Domain Analysis

Time series collected from biological signals may be considered as a sum of oscillations (usually overlapping). Different mathematical analytical techniques used for the conversion of time series representation from time-domain to frequency-domain present the opportunity to quantify various amplitude and distinct frequencies that contribute to the underlying signal [4, 5, 17, 20, 23, 76–82].

Such a representation is termed *spectral analysis* and displays the distribution of the amplitude of each oscillation (usually a sine wave) as a function of its frequency. The squared contribution of each frequency is actually the *power* of that particular frequency contribution to the total power spectrum. The duration of the recording should be at least ten times the wavelength of the lowest frequency band of the investigated spectral component. According to *Parceval's theorem* (Parceval's theory states that the sum of squares measured among the time samples is equal to the sum of squares of the Fourier transform results, when frequency samples are included from zero to the sampling frequency (f_s).), the total power spectrum, defined as the area under the curve of the power spectrum, equals the variance irrespective of data length. For physiological and clinical information to be obtained, a post-processing of the power spectral density spectra is necessary.

The power spectrum of heartbeat variation in healthy humans consists of three or four major frequency peaks depending on the duration of data recordings (usually 5-min or 24-h period). Although they do not have fixed periods and the central frequencies may vary considerably, by convention [4, 5] these peaks lie within the following ranges: *high frequency* (HF) 0.15–0.4Hz (cycle length 2.5–6 s), *low frequency* (LF) 0.04–0.15 Hz (6–25 s), and *very low frequency* (VLF) <0.04 Hz (>25 s) (❷ Fig. 3.15).

In 24-h recordings the VLF is subdivided into the VLF component 0.003–0.04 Hz (25 s–6 min) and the *ultra-low frequency* (ULF) component <0.003 Hz (cycle length > 5 h).

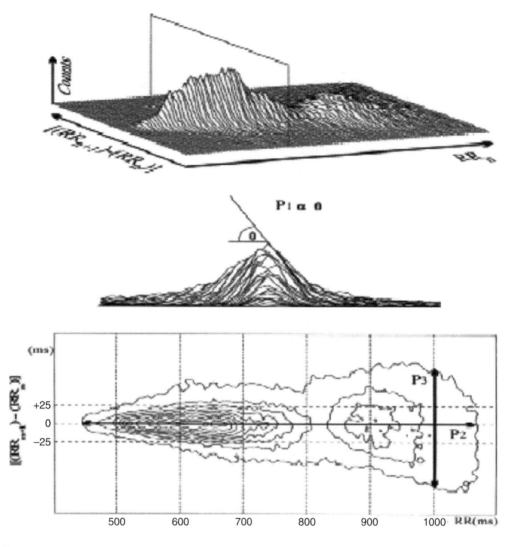

◘ Fig. 3.13
Presentation of 3-D distribution of RRI. The plane (*upper graph*) depicted intercept the distribution across maximum density (counts). The P1 (*middle graph*) is measured at maximum density taking into account the tangent of the angle. Other parameters (P2,P3, *lower graph*) are simply maximum longitudinal and transverse ranges. An MN index is a product of P1, P2 and P3 ($\times 10^{-3}$) (From [67])

The power of an individual frequency component is the area under the proportion of the curve related to each component. The power of the ULF, VLF, LF, and HF components is usually expressed as square milliseconds and the PSD is expressed as milliseconds per Hertz. The ratio between LF and HF components (LF/HF ratio) is commonly calculated [4, 5, 79, 81]; however, it has not been resolved whether absolute or normalized values should be included for the LF/HF calculation.

The relative LF and HF power can be expressed in normalized units (or percentages) by dividing the power of the LF and HF components (in ms²) by the total power from which the power <0.04 Hz is subtracted and multiplying by 100 [79–81]. The normalization procedure tends to minimize the effect of changes in total power on the HF and LF components. However, is seems important *to quote both the absolute and normalized values* in order to describe the distribution of power within the spectral components completely.

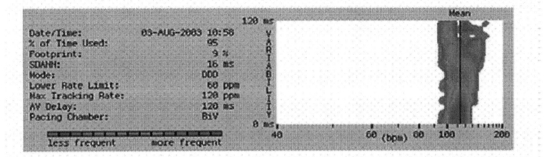

◻ Fig. 3.14
HRV footprint. A graphical representation of SDANN scatter occurring at each intrinsic sinus rate over a 24-h period. Colors indicate the frequency of HR and SDANN occurrence (third dimension, i.e., density) (From [75])

Because of statistical properties, the absolute values of the total power spectrum (or PSD) and their components are usually reported after logarithmic conversion (either natural or decimal) [79].

The spectral measures of HRV are most widely applied in current clinical investigations. Their prognostic power is fully documented in a variety of populations [4, 5, 79–81].

A new index called *prevalent low frequency* (PLF, Hz) has been proposed by the St. George's Hospital Investigators Group [83]. Here, with 1/60 Hz resolution, the LF band contains seven power spectrum values at frequencies of 0.033, 0.050, 0.067, 0.083, 0.100, 0.117, and 0.133 Hz. In each spectrum, local peaks (spectral position with the PSD greater than both adjacent power spectral densities) are detected within the LF band, and the greatest powered peak is included in the PLF computation. Frequencies of all maximum peaks ($\leqslant 1$ per each 5-min segment) are averaged over the entire Holter recording to obtain the single value of PLF. Detectable peaks in $\geqslant 10$ segments are necessary for valid PLF calculation. At present, only the authors have found evidence of the potential clinical use of this method [83].

3.3.2.1 Nonparametric Spectral Analysis

Nonparametric methods are traditionally used for the evaluation of rhythmic events presented in a signal. The Fourier transform is the most common method for the decomposition of the signal. It provides an evaluation of the contribution of all frequencies, irrespective of whether its frequency components show specific spectral peaks or broadband powers. Thus, FFT techniques include all data independent of their deterministic or stochastic properties. These frequencies are multiples (harmonics) of the basic frequency, which is a reciprocal of time series data-length. For a reduction of the number of computations, the fast (a discrete) Fourier transform (FFT) is commonly employed [79, 84, 85]. The fast Fourier transform allows for obtaining the PSD of a signal directly from the time series by means of *periodogram* (Estimate of power spectral density on the basis of the modulus squared Fourier transform.) (see 3.3):

$$\text{PSD}(f) = \left| \frac{1}{N\Delta t} \Delta t \sum_{k=0}^{N-1} y(k) \exp(-j2\pi k f \Delta t) \right|^2 = \frac{1}{N\Delta t} |Y(f)| \tag{3.3}$$

where Δt is the sampling period, N is the number of samples, and $Y(f)$ is the discrete Fourier transform of $y(k)$.

The FFT method uses a relatively simple algorithm with high-speed processing. It requires strict periodicity and stationarity (Property of a time series in which probability distributions involving values of the time series are independent of time translations.) of data. Also, the length of data for an FFT requires to be long enough (at least 256–512 consecutive heartbeats) for a reliable PSD estimation [79, 84].

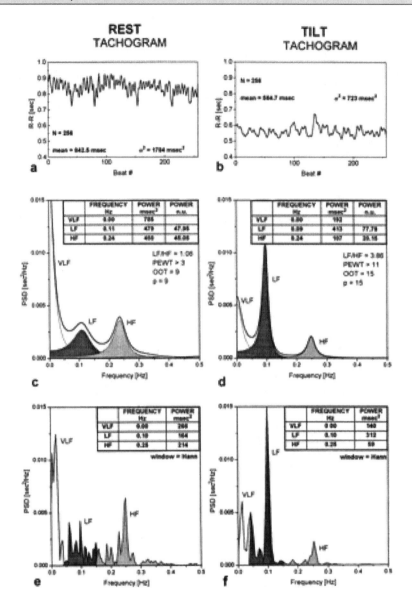

Interval tachogram of 256 consecutive RR values in a normal subject at supine rest (**a**) and after head-up tilt (**b**). The HRV spectra are shown, calculated by parametric autoregressive modeling (**c** and **d**) and by a fast Fourier transform-based non-parametric algorithm (**e** and **f**). Mean values (m), variances (s²), and the number (N) of samples are indicated. For **c** and **d**, VLF, LF, and HF central frequency, power in absolute value and power in normalized units (n.u.) are also indicated together with the order p of the chosen model and minimal values of the prediction error whiteness test (PEWT) and optimal order test (OOT) that satisfy the tests. In e and f, the peak frequency and the power of VLF, LF, and HF were calculated by integrating the power spectral density (PSD) in the defined frequency bands. The window type is also specified. In c through f, the LF component is indicated by dark shaded areas and the HF component by light shaded areas (From [4])

Since the FFT is theoretically defined on an infinite time series, its application to real data of finite length leads to unavoidable errors. The assumption of zero-value of the data outside the recording window is necessary and results in a *spectral leakage* (Spectral leakage is the effect whereby power is removed from the correct frequency and distributed in the neighboring frequencies. This is a case when periodicities are not precise factors of the epoch length.) in the PSD. Therefore, different window functions are used to connect the side samples to zero smoothly. The rectangular, triangular (Bartlett), cosine, Han, Hamming, Blackman-Harris, Lanczos, and Welch, window tapers are among the most popular. Spectra which are better formed are obtained at the expense of *frequency resolution* (Spectral resolution is related to the number of discrete harmonic components, each of which is separated in frequency by a given range (i.e., 0.0005 Hz). If the frequency difference between adjacent components is small, the power is distributed amongst more components, each of which must therefore be smaller.) [4, 79, 80].

A further reduction in the frequency resolution can be reached by smoothing the rapid oscillation of the spectrum [79, 80]. Different procedures of averaging and overlapping are used. One of the most popular methods is the Welch periodogram (Periodogram estimate is based on the splitting of the time series in overlapped segments multiplied by data windows, and on the ensemble average of periodograms computed in each data window.). In this method, data segments are allowed to overlap by 50% or 70%, and each data segment is weighted with a window function before calculating the periodogram. Sometimes it is necessary to approximate a periodogram more closely, which can be done by using the zero padding procedure [79, 85]. Zero padding actually interpolates the values of the measured spectrum at additional frequencies, producing a smoother spectrum.

Rüdiger et al. [86] proposed a new approach for the FFT use based on trigonometric regression. This method, similar to the cosinor method [87], creates the kth rhythmic part with amplitude a_k, frequency ω_k, and a phase shift φ_k as a regressively estimated function by using the method of least squares in the form (see 3.4):

$$u_k(t_i) = a_k * \sin(\omega_k t_i + \varphi_k) \tag{3.4}$$

This method provides a clear separation of rhythmic from nonrhythmic information. It is robust and does not require interpolation for artificial or missing segment deviations. Oscillations with a variance part $\varepsilon < 1\%$ are stored as general residual variance. Estimation of the residual variance (nonrhythmic component) in four frequency bands from the FFT analysis showed that the total variance within each frequency band contains a substantial amount of the residual variance, especially in the VLF range (~13–17%) and in the HF range (~6–10%) [86]. The clinical usefulness of this method remains unknown (❯ Fig. 3.15).

3.3.2.2 Parametric Spectral Analysis

Autoregressive modeling (AR) uses a raw signal to identify a best fitting model from which the spectrum is derived [78–81, 88–92]. AR modeling is based on the assumption that each value of the series depends on a weighted sum of the previous values of the same series with noise.

AR models are completely independent of the characteristics of the biological system, simply representing the "black-box" approach. The AR methods are suitable for identifying the central frequency driven by a fixed-rate oscillator. Thus, the AR method allows concentration on the most significant peaks, excluding noise-related frequencies. As a result, the AR analysis provides a better spectral resolution, where the components are smoother and easier for post-processing. AR enables spectral estimation from shorter time periods than the FFT approach [79, 89].

In the AR model, a priori choice of the structure and the order of the model are crucial. The order is usually empirically selected based on the investigator's expertise or by comparing the AR power spectra with those computed from other techniques. Too low a model order results in a low resolution power spectrum and too high a model order can generate false peaks in the spectrum [90].

Different criteria may help to determine the value of the order of the model (*Akaike, Rissanen, Parzen*) [79, 80, 90–92]. A correct identification of the model is required by using a posteriori tests of reliability. Changing the model order across different physiological conditions may introduce a new variable into the computation of the power spectrum. A fixed model order seems to be a practical rule for AR spectral estimation. This approach, although attractive in its

■ **Table 3.3**

Classification of time-frequency methods (After Cerutti et al. [78])

Linear decomposition of the signal	Short-time Fourier Transform Wavelet Transform
Quadratic energy distributions	Spectrogram Scalogram Wigner-Ville Transform Cohen's class of time-frequency distribution
Adaptive parametric models	Time-variant parametric models Adaptive filters

simplicity, is criticized as unrealistic as it assumes the same model for all subjects, independent of their clinical characteristics and physiological conditions, as well as of signal sampling rate and SNR [90]. Moreover, in contrast to the FFT-based estimation, the amplitude of AR peaks does not faithfully reflect the actual power of the associated spectral component [89].

Many algorithms are proposed for obtaining estimates of AR parameters, for example, methods based on estimation of the Yule-Walker autocorrelation sequence, the Burg algorithm, and the Kay-Marple least squares linear prediction algorithms (including the modified covariance method) [79, 80, 85, 92]. There are also adaptive algorithms such as mean or recursive least square (*RLS*) which permit updating the parameter estimates as a new data sample becomes available [91].

3.3.3   Time-Frequency Spectrum Analysis

An evaluation of the power spectral density for short time series when the stationarity is met and subsequent repetition through the entire recording allows changes in signal variation over time to be quantified in a continuous manner. Several time-varying spectral approaches have been proposed [93–105]. These methods are particularly suitable for evaluating power and frequency transient alterations over time in response to physiological (body movement, exercise, mental tasks, sleep), pathophysiological (ischemic episodes, cardiac arrhythmias), or treatment (drugs, interventions) stimuli. However, the patterns of signal variation that are present across the entire spectrum, including long-range control mechanisms, are hidden with time-variant spectral analysis. A classification of time-frequency methods is given in ❷ Table 3.3 [93]. Most of these methods use frequency bands corresponding to those arbitrarily chosen in the frequency domain analysis. Only those that have a clinical application are described below. More in-depth review of these methods is beyond the scope of this chapter (see references [93, 94, 98]).

3.3.3.1   Nonparametric Methods

Short-Time Fourier Transform

The short-time Fourier transform (STFT) is a linear time frequency representation of changes in the signal that vary with time. The Fourier transform does not explicitly show the time location of the frequency components, but some form of time location can be obtained by using a suitable pre-windowing $g(s)$. The STFT can be defined for $x(t)$ as a local spectrum of the signal $x(s)$ around the analysis time as (see 3.5):

$$S_x^g(t, \omega) = \int x(s)g(s-t)e^{-j\omega s}ds \qquad (3.5)$$

The time-frequency resolution of the STFT is limited by the time-frequency product, that is, having a small time resolution means poor frequency resolution, or vice versa. The resolution is also constant as a function of the frequency, which is due to the window chosen for the STFT. Also, it depends on the bandwidths of the analysis functions and the length of the window, which are unlikely to be optimally chosen [99–101].

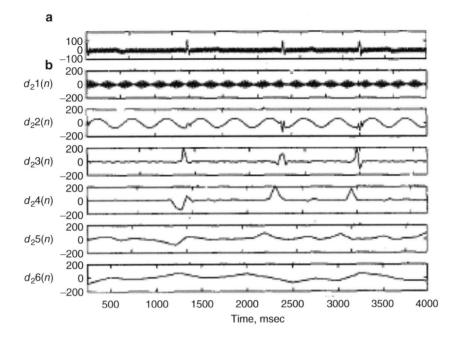

◘ Fig. 3.16
Wavelet analysis of HRV. **(a)** A theoretical example of wavelet analysis, **(b)** Wavelet analysis applied to HRV signal. For explanation see text and ref [103]

Wavelet Analysis

Continuous wavelet analysis (CWA) is another method that provides time–frequency decomposition of a continuous signal. This method is usually devoted to the analysis of non-stationary signals [98, 102, 103]. Conversely to STFT, CWA allows temporal evolution of the spectrum of frequencies contained in the signal to be followed.

A basic function of CWA is the wavelet (Wavelet – wave of finite duration and finite energy, which is correlated with the signal.) function, denoted as $m\psi(t)$. This function, used to decompose the analyzed signal in the time–frequency plane, is localized both in time and in frequency (and must have the spectral pattern of a band-pass filter). The initial function should be adequately regular and is the localized "mother" wavelet. There are a number of mother functions (Daubechies's fourth coefficient wavelet, Haar wavelet, Morlet wavelet). Starting from the mother wavelet, a family of wavelets is set by scaling (contracting or dilating) and shifting in time (❯ Fig. 3.16). The resulting wavelets coefficients indicate the evolution of the correlation between the signal $x(t)$ and the mother wavelet in different time-intervals and frequency-levels. Particular wavelets are defined as (3.6):

$$\psi_{k,j}(t) = a_0^{-\frac{1}{2}}\,\psi\left(a_0^{-j}\left(t - ka_0^j T\right)\right) \tag{3.6}$$

where a_0 is the dilation factor, j and k are integers that determine dilation (scale) and the time-position of the wavelet, respectively, and T is the sampling interval. The corresponding wavelet coefficients are (see 3.7):

$$C_{k,j} = \int x(t)\psi_{j,k}^*(t)\mathrm{d}t \tag{3.7}$$

By using CWA, the signal can be analyzed in different scale levels. Low scale levels (small j value) correspond to rapidly changing details (i.e., high frequency), whereas high scale levels (higher j values) correspond to slow changes (i.e., low frequency).

Wigner-Ville Technique

The energy distribution of the signal in the time and the frequency domain can be obtained simultaneously if the PSD of the signal is evaluated by Fourier transformation of the instantaneous autocorrelation function (central covariance function) [95, 97]. Obtaining the time–frequency distribution is known as the Wigner-Ville distribution (WVD) (see 3.8):

$$\text{WVD}(t,f) = \int_{-\infty}^{+\infty} x\left(t - \frac{\tau}{2}\right) x * \left(t + \frac{\tau}{2}\right) e^{-j2\pi f \tau} dt \tag{3.8}$$

It preserves the time t and frequency f shift of the signal. The time (of frequency) integral corresponds to the signal's instantaneous power (or power spectrum). The instantaneous frequency can also be estimated.

As the WVD introduces the cross-term interference due to nonlinearity of the transformation, the *kernel function* (Gaussian (known as Choi-Williams), Bessel, korn-shaped, and others) is used to remove this interference, obtaining the Cohen's class. The kernel performs a 2D filtering (in both domains) and determines the properties of the distribution. However, its choice influences the time and frequency resolution and optimal selection of the kernel requires knowledge about the signal. For the analysis of HRV data, the *smoothed pseudo-Wigner-Ville transform* (SPWV) has largely been used. It introduces time and frequency windows which determine SPWV resolution [97, 101].

Huang-Hilbert Transform

By using the *Huang-Hilbert transform* (HHT), an analyzed signal is represented in the time–frequency domain by combining the *empirical mode decomposition* (EMD) with the Hilbert transform (HT). The first step uses EMD [104]. This procedure decomposes the signal into so-called *intrinsic mode function* (IMF) (IMF defines an oscillating wave if the number of extrema and the number of zero crossings differ only by one and the local average is zero.). A finite number of IMFs can be obtained from a real data-series. The IMFs are produced sequentially with each subsequent IMF being derived from the residual (i.e., the portion of the initial signal not represented by a previous IMF) initial signal. The iterative algorithm is called *sifting*. The first IMF is defined as $c_l(t)$. Having separated $c_l(t)$ from $x(t)$, one has the residual signal $r_l(t) = x(t) - c_l(t)$. After several iterations (until the residual part becomes a monotonic function or a constant), the $x(t)$ can be expressed as the combination of $c_i(t)$ and $r_n(t)$ (3.9):

$$x(t) = \sum_{i=1}^{n} c_i(t) + r_n(t) \tag{3.9}$$

Then, the Hilbert transform (HT), given by (3.10),

$$H[x(t)] = y(t) = \frac{1}{\pi} \int_{-\infty}^{\infty} \frac{x(\tau)}{t - \tau} dt \tag{3.10}$$

is performed on the $c_i(t)$, and yields the instantaneous amplitude $a_i(t)$ and phase $\vartheta_i(t)$ (3.11):

$$a_i t = \sqrt{[c_i(t)]^2 + H[c_i(t)]^2}; \qquad \vartheta_i t = \tan^{-1}\left\{\frac{H[c_i(t)]}{c_i(t)}\right\} \tag{3.11}$$

The instantaneous frequency is given by (3.12).

$$\omega(t) = \frac{d\vartheta_i(t)}{d(t)}. \tag{3.12}$$

Thus, the Huang-Hilbert transform of $x(t)$, denoted as HHT(t,ω), can be expressed as (3.13):

$$\text{HHT}(t, \omega) = \sum_{i=1}^{n} a_i(t, \omega) \tag{3.13}$$

The HHT is adaptively data-driven and possesses higher time and frequency resolution than STFT, WVD, and CWA [102].

3.3.3.2 Parametric Methods

Recursive Autocorrelation

The recursive autocorrelation, also referred to as time-variant spectral estimation, is based on modeling of signal changes [93–97]. Spectral modification of a signal is realized by calculation of a new set of a model parameter $a(t)$ from the preceding one $a(t-1)$ and from the prediction error (3.14):

$$a(t) = a(t-1) + K(t)[y(t) - \hat{y}(t)], \tag{3.14}$$

where $y(t) - \hat{y}(t)$ is the *prediction error* estimated by the model through the coefficients evaluated at time $t-1$ and $K(t)$ is the *gain* of the algorithm. $K(t)$ contains a forgetting factor μ that exponentially weighs the past of the signal (the length of the past signal that really contributes to the change). Thus, the most recent terms contribute significantly to changes in a new sample, while the oldest one are progressively forgotten. The gain of the algorithm determines its adaptation and sensitivity to the signal changes. Many algorithms have been proposed for the $K(t)$ calculation (*RLS, smoothed Kalman filter, directional, Fortesque*). The sequence of spectra can be represented as a contor plot or a spectral array [93–97]. The recursive implementation of the AR models allows monitoring of the spectral components in real time. The advantage of this method is related to its possibility for multiple signal systems analyses for cross-correlation (*time and phase coherence*) evaluation.

Temporal Cumulative Approach (TCA)

This relatively simple approach uses a PSD calculation over the frequency range of interests within short-epochs and reconstruction of its cumulative plot against time. This method allows instability in PSD to be overcome from neighboring epochs and reduces the effects of noisy data. The temporal cumulative approach enables temporal changes of interesting spectral components to be tracked, especially those with a relatively undisputable physiological background, i.e., the HF component. The cumulative plot is constructed by summing the PSD of the HF component versus time. This plot is then analyzed by a stepwise linear regression procedure (least squares) that helps time segments with consistent parasympathetic tone to be isolated. The length of these segments is determined automatically in order to find a minimal number of segments that describes the cumulative plot. The intensity of parasympathetic tone at each time-segment is defined by the slope of power units per minute [106].

3.3.4 Nonlinear/Chaos-Derived Methods

The majority of biological systems exhibit nonlinear behavior (e.g., the baroreceptor reflex, Starling curve, hemoglobin dissociation, lung hysteresis on a pressure–volume curve, etc.). Attempting to explain such a behavior using linear models does not seem sufficient or even appropriate. Thus, it is not surprising that over the last decade many nonlinear methods have been developed and postulated for HRV evaluation [107–115]. They can be classified according to the main features that they evaluate (❏ Table 3.4.) [107]. Overall, a valid and reliable assessment of HRV nonlinear behavior requires relatively long-term ECG recordings. Some mathematical formulae are provided below and physical meanings are only summarized as necessary. A more in-depth description of these methods does not seem to be of interest to clinicians. However, researchers with an interest are invited to explore more extensive reviews [107–112].

To become familiar with nonlinear methods knowledge and understanding of both the mathematical and physical background are required. Unfortunately, advanced mathematics and physics are areas of limited understanding for the vast majority of physicians. In addition, chaos-theory or nonlinear dynamics derived methods are actually far removed from a definite physiological explanation or interpretation. A statement such as "broken fractal" means little to a physician. Thus, despite being introduced into clinical studies, these methods still remain research tools, and will be unlikely to be commonly used at the bedside. Nevertheless, by providing insight into many aspects of cardiac (heart rate) behavior, their employment (despite being experimental) might widen our understanding of cardiovascular system control [116–120], and in some cases, these techniques might find a practical application [118]. In other words, some of the gaps between science and practice can be demonstrated with HRV analysis. Fortunately, mathematicians, physicists, and

◼ Table 3.4

Nonlinear complexity mechanisms and phenomena in physiology: partial list of possible contenders (From [107]. With permission)

Abrupt changes	Scale-invariance
• Bifurcations • Intermittent bursting • Bistability, multistability • Phase transitions	• Fractal and multifractal scaling • Long-range correlations • Self-organized criticality • Diffusion limited aggregation
Hysteresis	Nonlinear waves: spirals; scrolls; solitons
Nonlinear oscillations • Limit cycles • Phase-resetting • Entrainment • Pacemaker annihilation	Complex periodic cycles and quasiperiodicities
Complex networks	Stochastic resonance and related noise-modulated mechanisms
Alternans phenomena	Time irreversibility
Deterministic chaos	Emergent properties

manufacturers have convinced physicians to employ these methods, albeit with their "black box" meaning remaining unresolved.

3.3.4.1 Scale Invariant/Fractal Analysis

The scale invariant self-similar nature is a property of *fractals* (Fractal, derived from the Latin word *fractus*, meaning broken or fragmented.), which are geometric structures that have no fixed length [21, 107, 113–115, 121–127]. Their length increases with increased precision (magnification) of measurement, a property that confers a non-integer dimension to all fractals (*fractal dimension* (Geometric dimension of an object which includes fractal objects (Hausdorff dimension D_H).)). With respect to time series, the pattern of variation appears to be the same at different scales (i.e., magnification of the pattern reveals the same pattern). The self-similar pattern can be recognized in either spatial or temporal aspects (❷ Fig. 3.17).

Power-Law Behavior (1/f Fluctuation)

Kobayashi and Musha first reported the dependence of the spectral power on the frequency of the R–R interval fluctuations [21]. Further to this, different methods for a scale-invariant (self-similar) relationship between the magnitude of the effect and its frequency distribution (❷ Fig. 3.18) have been developed [102–105, 118–120].

The power relationship is described by (3.15):

$$f = aE^{\beta}, \tag{3.15}$$

where E is the amount of variation (e.g., spectral power), f is the frequency of observations, and α and β are constants. Taking the logarithm of both sides the equation gives (3.16):

$$\log(f) = \log(\alpha) + \beta(\log(E)). \tag{3.16}$$

Plotting a graph of log(f) against log(E) reveals an almost straight line in the range of 10^{-2} to 10^{-4} Hz with β *as an exponent factor* (slope) and *log* (α) referred to as the intercept. The range of log–log representation is consistent with the size and duration of the system. Some authors also calculate the squared coefficient of correlation (r^2), referred to as the *coefficient of determination*.

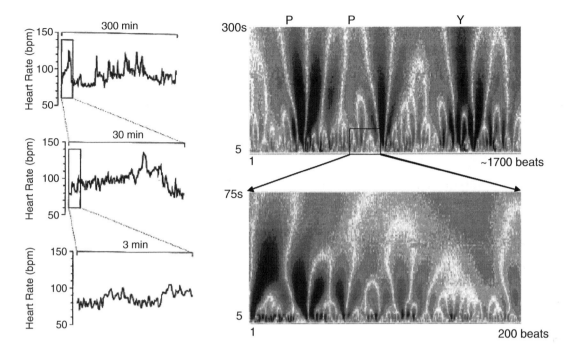

◘ Fig. 3.17
Fractal nature of heart rate variability. On the left graph heart rate variation appears to have no clear scale, as similar temporal pattern can be seen irrespective of time series data length. Right side graph shows distribution of wavelets in heartbeat series of different length. Pattern similarity is clearly seen between both epochs (From [107])

The value of β *exponent* is around -1 in healthy subjects (❷ Fig. 3.19). An altered β *exponent* was reported in patients after MI [126] and with CHF [127].

In contrast to a relatively stationary long time series (thousands of heartbeats) used for a reliable power-law behavior assessment, a model based on *HRi* calculation over a short time series (5 min) has been proposed [106]. Accordingly, the squared deviation from the mean heart rate is plotted on a 20-bin histogram with a bin size that equals 1/20 of the largest squared difference from the mean HR. A frequency distribution calculated from the histogram is plotted in the decimal log–log space. A regression line is fitted to the 20 data points and r^2, slope and intercept are derived. Although interesting results can been obtained in a selected population [128], this method is susceptible to the presence of non-stationarities or artifacts. In addition, a relatively long ECG recording is necessary for its reliable calculation.

Rescaled Range (R/S)
Fractal properties of data series can be measured by characterizing the divergence of data defined as the range (R) of the sum of deviations from the mean divided by sample standard deviation (S). For some processes that exhibit a long-range dependence (*persistence*), the R/S is proportional to a power of T (duration of the data sample) (see 3.17):

$$\frac{R}{S} = T^H. \tag{3.17}$$

The exponent H is called *Hurst exponent* [108, 109, 123, 124].

Given a time series $x(n)$, $n = 1, \ldots N$, H can be estimated by taking the slope of the plot of (R/S) vs. n on a log–log scale. H is related to the fractal dimension $D_{(h)}$. For 1D signals, $H = 2D_{(h)}$ [123].

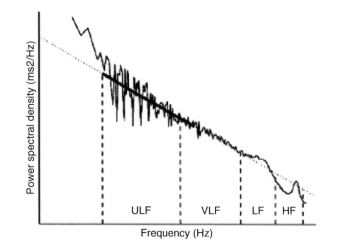

◻ Fig. 3.18

l/f scaling behavior of HRV spectrum. The slope of a plot of power against frequency is almost straight in the range of 10^{-2} and 10^{-4} Hz. Two measures can be taken from 1/f relationship: intercept and slope of this line (referred to as scaling index β) (From [A32])

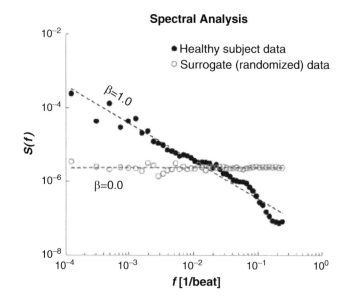

◻ Fig. 3.19

Scaling properties of power spectrum. Fractal scaling analyses for two 24-h inter-beat interval time series. The solid black circles represent data from a healthy subject, whereas the open red circles are for the artificial time series generated by randomizing the sequential order of data points in the original time series. Exponent β in healthy indicates for the presence of long-range correlation (1/f noise). Loss of correlation properties is consistent with uncorrelated random time series (white noise) and β-exponent equals zero (From [107])

Detrended Fluctuation Analysis

A distinction between a local variation generated by external stimuli and intrinsic fluctuations from a complex system has been proposed to be feasible with *detrended fluctuation analysis (DFA)* [124]. These intrinsic fluctuations are presumed to exhibit a long-range scale-invariant (i.e., fractal) relationship. The DFA is a robust method for studying fractal (or self-similar) behaviors of systems from which the originating signal exhibits an absence of characteristic temporal and/or spatial scale.

The calculation of DFA includes several steps. At first, heartbeat signals are represented as an integrated time series, following the equation (3.18):

$$y(k) = \sum_{i=1}^{N} (NN_i - NN_{ave}),$$ (3.18)

where $y(k)$ represents an evaluation of trends, NN_i is the difference between individual inter-beat intervals, and NN_{ave} is the average interval of the total number of heartbeats N. The trend function $y(k)$ is then separated into equal nonoverlapping boxes of length n, where $n = N/$(total number of boxes). In each box, the local trend $y_n(k)$ is calculated using the least square method (❷ Fig. 3.20). By subtracting the local trend $y_n(k)$ from the trend function $y(k)$ ("detrending") for all possible length of boxes n, the function $F(n)$ is calculated as the root mean square of the integrated and detrended series (3.19):

$$F(n) = \sqrt{(1/N)\Sigma_{k=1}^{N}\left[y(k)^2 - y_n(k)^2\right]}$$ (3.19)

Graphic presentation of the relationship between $F(n)$ and n on a bi-logarithmic scale provides a regression line (❷ Fig. 3.21). The slope of this line is termed the *scaling exponent* α. It may vary from 0.5 (uncorrelated random data or white noise) to 1.5 (random walk or Brownian noise). If the signal obeys the power-law behavior, that is, corresponds to the $1/f$ noise, the α exponent equals 1 (❷ Fig. 3.16) [124]. The exponent α of this power relation defines

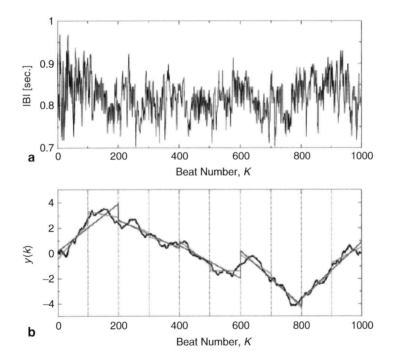

◼ Fig. 3.20
Illustration of the DFA algorithm to test for scale-invariance and long-range correlations. (a) Interbeat interval (IBI) time series from a healthy young adult. (b) The solid black curve is the integrated time series, $y(k)$. The vertical dotted lines indicate boxes of size n 100 beats. The red straight line segments represent the "trend" estimated in each box by a linear least squares fit. The blue straight line segments represent linear fits for box size n 200. Note that the typical deviation from the $y(k)$ curve to the red lines is smaller than the deviation to the blue lines (From [107], Nat Acad Sci USA, with permission)

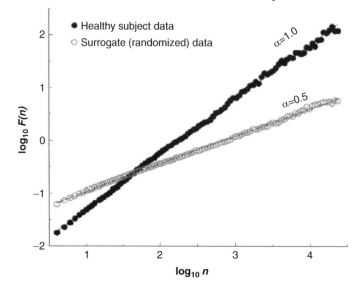

Detrended Fluctutaion Analysis

□ Fig. 3.21
Bi-logarithmic presentation of the relationship between F(n) and n. The slope of the line is referred to as α-exponent and in healthy subjects varies around 1 (1/f noise). For white noise or uncorrelated random data α -exponent equals 0.5 (From [107])

a pertinent parameter called the *self-similarity parameter* (when applicable it is related to the *Hurst exponent H* by $\alpha = H + 1$).

Applying this analysis to real-life data-series, the scaling exponent shows two distinct linear segments that depend on *n* values. Depending on a crossover phenomenon, arbitrary cutoffs for the *n*-values are initially proposed ($n = 4$–16 and $n = 16$–64) [122–127]. This yields two scaling exponents, α_1 and α_2, referred to as the short and intermediate-term exponents, respectively. However, in the most commonly applied variant of DFA, the *n*-values for α_1 and α_2 exponents range between 4–11 and 12–400, respectively [103, 110]. Thus, in contrast to $1/f$ scaling methods, the DFA allows the determination of a scale-invariant property over a relatively short data-series (~8,000 heartbeats). A loss of fractal-like HR dynamics has been shown to characterize patients with cardiovascular disease [112].

DFA is a mono-fractal technique, assuming that the scaling properties of the system are the same throughout the entire signal. In addition, only normal-to-normal heartbeats are included. As all of these assumptions may be flawed, another technique has been developed, namely multi-fractal analysis [129–132]. Multi-fractal DFA may help to detect changes of scaling behavior with time, providing the multiple scaling exponent $D(h)$ (❯ Fig. 3.22).

Multi-fractality in heartbeat dynamics raises the possibility that many nonlinear control mechanisms are actually involved with coupled cascades of feedback loops in a system operating far from equilibrium. A loss of such dynamics was reported in patients with heart failure [132].

Correlation Dimension
Correlation dimension is an alternative procedure for the calculation of the fractal dimension (although it is not strictly the same) [133, 134]. It is also considered as a measure of degrees of freedom stimulated by a system, thus expressing the complexity of a system. From a defined data vector (y_i, $i = 1,\ldots, N$) with *N* points, an *m*-dimensional phase-space of dimension *p* (*embedding dimension* (Number of axes of a return map sufficient to describe the properties of the corresponding phase space)) is constructed according to *Takens theorem* (A delay embedding theorem gives the

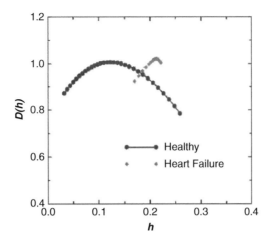

Fig. 3.22
Multifractal properties of heartbeat variation (From [107])

conditions under which a chaotic dynamic system can be reconstructed from a sequence of observations of the state of a dynamic system.) [113], obtaining (3.20):

$$\vec{x}_t \equiv \left(y_t, y_{t+\tau}, y_{t+2\tau}, \ldots, y_{t+(m-1_\tau)} \right), \tag{3.20}$$

for $t = 1, \ldots, N - (m - 1)\tau$, where τ is the time delay or lag. Grassberger and Procaccia [136] have developed the basic algorithm which consists of computing the fraction of pairs of points in the *embedded space* that lie within a distance ε of each other with the dimension d (also referred to as D_2) (3.21):

$$d = \lim_{6 \to 0} \left[\frac{log_2 \left(C_m(\varepsilon) \right)}{log_2(\varepsilon)} \right], \tag{3.21}$$

where $C_m(\varepsilon)$ is the correlation integral which measures the number of points x_j that are correlated with each other in a sphere of radius ε around the points x_t. This algorithm is also known as *sphere (box) counting method*. Thus, in the phase-space, the correlation integral $C_m(\varepsilon)$ is defined (3.22):

$$C_m(\varepsilon) = \frac{1}{N \cdot (N-1)} \cdot \Sigma_{i \neq j} \theta \left(\varepsilon - |Z_i - Z_j| \right), \tag{3.22}$$

where $\Theta(z)$ is the Heaviside function: $\Theta(z) = 0$, if $z \leqslant 0$ and $\Theta(z) = 1$, if $z > 0$, and $|z_i - z_i|$ is the distance between a pair of points within the *attractor* (Attractor – an object to which the time series in a phase space is attracted.).

When $log_2 C_m(\varepsilon)$ is plotted versus $log_2(\varepsilon)$, the slope of the resulting straight line, determined by linear regression at lower ε, yields the dimension D_2. Several $C_m(\varepsilon)$ are computed for increasing values of the embedding dimensions m, and the slopes are determined from a *scaling region* of the log–log plot, as shown in ❷ Fig. 3.23a, obtaining a sequence of $d(m)$. As m is increased, $d(m)$ tends to a constant value of saturation (the D_2 value) shown in ❷ Fig. 3.23b [137]). The D_2 value is obtained by considering the points where $d(m)$ values remain constant (high values of m). A variance of the D_2 calculation, the point estimate of the heartbeat D_2, has also been proposed [138].

3.3.4.2 Entropy Analysis

Entropy H, as a physical term, is an energy that dissipates with time, as embodied by the Second Law of Thermodynamics. The concept of entropy was introduced into the theory of information by Shannon [139]. Applying entropy analysis to

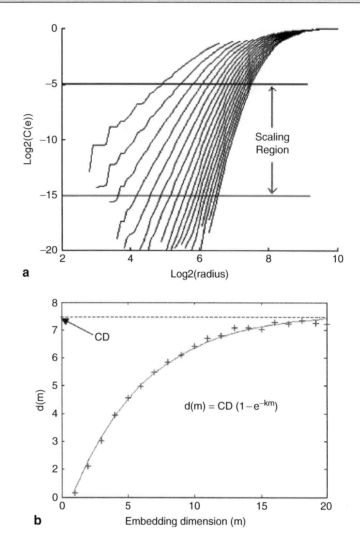

⬛ Fig. 3.23
(a) Correlation integral as a function of the sphere radius (r) for each embedding dimension showing the scaling region. (b). Correlation dimension (D2, here CD) as a function of the embedding dimension *m* with a fitted exponential curve

a real time series is based on its ability to measure order (regularity) and disorder (irregularity/randomness) and the probability *p* of these states.

Approximate Entropy (ApEn)

Approximate entropy analysis exhibits the rate of generation of new information within a biological signal (similar to the classic Kolmogorov-Sinai entropy).

To calculate *ApEn* [140], a data series is evaluated for the presence of recurrent patterns. First, a length *m* of data sequences is defined and the likelihood of similarity with other sequences of length *m* with a *tolerance r* is determined. Vector sequences $x(i)$ of consecutive data-points $u(i)_{(i=1,2,3...N)}$ of length *m* are derived. Then, the distance $d(x(i),x(j))$ is defined, as the maximum difference between two vector components $x(i)$ and $x[j]$. If this difference is within tolerance *r*, the vectors are considered similar.

The frequency $(C_i^m(r))$ of occurrence of similar vectors Nj of sequences with length m and tolerance r throughout the data set is calculated (3.23):

$$C_i^m(r) = N_j \in d(x[i], x[j] \leqslant r)/(N - m - 1), \tag{3.23}$$

where $j \leqslant (N - m - 1)$. Then, the relative occurrence of repetitive patterns $\Phi_{m(r)}$ of length m within the tolerance r is obtained (3.24):

$$\Phi m(r) = \sum_i \ln C_i^m(r)(N - m - 1), \tag{3.24}$$

where Σ_i is a sum from $i = 1$ to $(N - m - 1)$. Finally, the approximate entropy ApEn is calculated, following the equation (3.25):

$$\text{ApEn}(m, r, N) = \Phi_{m(r)} - \Phi_{m+1(r)}, \tag{3.25}$$

Thus, the ApEn(m, r, N) measures the logarithmic frequency (probability) that runs of patterns (within the tolerance r) of length m remain similar when the length m of the run is increased by 1. Small values of the ApEn indicate regularity, given that increasing the data sequence of a length m by 1 does not decrease the value of $\Phi m(r)$ significantly (i.e., regularity connotes that $\Phi_{m(r)} \approx \Phi_{m+1(r)}$). The value of ApEn ($m$, r, N) is expressed as a difference, but in essence it represents a ratio, as the $\Phi_{m(r)}$ is a logarithm of the averaged $C_i^m(r)$ and the ratio of logarithms is equivalent to their difference. Although the ApEn can be calculated from relatively short data-series, the length of ECG recordings influences the value of ApEn (similarly to the SDNN). In healthy subjects, the ApEn is found to be slightly over or around 1 [141]. In pathological conditions, ApEn was found to be higher [112, 142] indicating the existence of more unpredictable patterns.

As with many other HRV measures, the ApEn requires data to be stationary and noise-free (without artifacts). In addition, relatively long ECG recordings are required for the ApEn to be measured reliably. Also, ApEn includes a spurious contribution from "self-matching".

A variant of ApEn in which self-matching is not included, referred to as the *sample entropy (SampEn)* has been proposed [143]. SampEn describes the conditional probability that two sequences for m data points (with a tolerance r) remain within r of each other (similar) at the next point. The SampEn converges to a consistent value for a considerably lower r and N than the ApEn [143]. A reduced *SampEn* was described in neonates prior to the clinical diagnosis of sepsis [144] and before the onset of atrial fibrillation [145].

As biological systems are structured on multiple spatial-temporal scales, a description of their dynamics using the ApEn or SampEn, which evaluate regularity on one scale only, might provide conflicting results. Thus, the so-called *multi-scale entropy (MSE)* evaluation has been proposed in which the SampEn is calculated for the coarse-grained data for a range of scales (e.g., $\tau = 1$ to $\tau = 20$ [146]). The MSE is applicable to a data-series of finite length (~30,000). Increased regularity irrespective of variability (decreased or increased) was found to characterize pathological states. A reduced MSE, depending on the scale of reduction, distinguishes patients with CHF, AF, or diabetes from healthy subjects [146, 147].

Another variant is *compression entropy (CE)*. It quantifies the extent to which the data-series can be compressed, depending on the occurrence of repeated sequences [148]. CE reduction was documented in patients with CHF and malignant ventricular arrhythmia [149]. The reliability of this method depends on sampling rate, the window length, buffer size, and integer numbers [148].

Symbolic Dynamics

The absolute value of parameters is seldom of importance for diagnostic (classification) purposes, while the relative orders or qualitative values (above or below a threshold) are significant. In such instances, a great simplification in the form of *symbolic dynamics (SDyn)* can be applied [150–152]. SDyn is based on coarse graining and involves the transformation of the original time series into a series of a limited amount of discretized symbols that are processed to extract important information about the system generating the process.

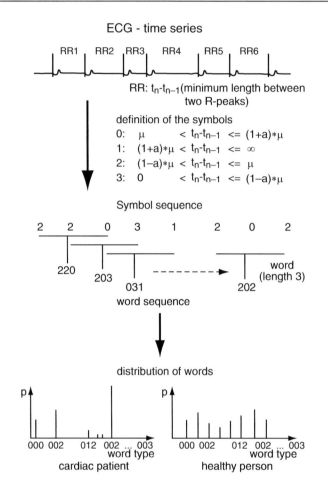

⬛ Fig. 3.24
Illustration of symbolic analysis method. R – R interval series is uniformly spread on pre-determined levels. Each level is described by symbol (number) and 3-symbols patterns (words) are constructed (From [A37])

A variant of the SDyn approach has been proposed to describe short-term HRV dynamics [151]. First, the data series is transformed into a sequence of symbols. These symbols are simply the alphabet A = (0,1,2,3...) and permit the classifying of various patterns and monitoring of their occurrence and changes with time (❷ Fig. 3.24). At least three symbols (*strings*) are necessary to characterize short-time dynamics. The resulting data are expressed as the probability of distribution of each single word (3 symbols) within a word sequence. A modified procedure of SDyn that permits a shortened data series (~300 heartbeats) to be analyzed has been proposed [151]. This method naturally results in a considerable compression of the data with a subsequent loss of detailed information. It also improves the sensitivity to noise. However, the presence of artifact influences the symbol strings.

To quantify low-variability data epochs, a parameter called *POLVAR10* has been proposed [152]. It is calculated on the basis of the most simplified transformation of differences of 10 ms or more (symbol:1) or less (symbol:0) between successive heartbeats. Only words of six unique symbols (all 1 or all 0) are counted. The POLVAR10 represents the probability of occurrence of the word "000000," which indicates severely depressed variability [152].

The *acceleration change index (ACI)*, an index that can be obtained from the sign (1 for HR deceleration, 0 for acceleration) of the beat-to-beat difference, which characterizes the dynamics of zero-crossing, has been proposed [141].

A series of sign changes (SC) is generated. Then, the differentiation of SC (*DSC*) is calculated and the ACI is defined as (3.26):

$$\text{ACI} = \frac{k}{M},$$ (3.26)

where k is the number of times that the DSC time series equals 1, and M is the total number of samples in the DSC series. Therefore, the ACI is the proportion of times that a local maximum (or minimum) is followed immediately by a local minimum (or maximum) by the total number of local maxima and minima. Despite the method being simple and robust, the ACI quantifies similar changes of a different length (increase or decrease by 20 or 40 ms for example, and so on). Arif and Aziz have proposed the *threshold-based* (indicating the necessary change to be signed) *acceleration index* (TACI). The TACI allows better classification of patients with specific diseases [154]. However, its clinical applicability is not proven and the threshold value has to be chosen empirically.

Information Entropy

The entropy of a random variable is defined in terms of its probability distribution and can be considered as a good measure of randomness (or uncertainty). This is the basis of the so-called *Shannon entropy* (or *measure of uncertainty*) [155].

Consider a stationary time series $\{x(n)\}_{n=1}^{N}$ that is characterized by the discrete probability distribution $\{S_i\}_{i=1}^{K}$ with the marginal distribution $p_i = \sum_i S_i$. Then, for the discrete probability distribution $\{p_i\}$, the Shannon information measure is defined (3.27) as:

$$H_x = -\sum_i p_i \log_2 p_i$$ (3.27)

For HRV complexity measurements, the Shannon entropy can be applied for time series transformed into symbol sequences (see symbolic dynamics). Thus, having the W^k set of all words ω of length k, the H_k calculated from the distribution of probability of words $p(\omega)$ is given by (3.28):

$$H_k = -\sum_{\omega \in W^k, p(\omega) > 0} p_\omega \log p_\omega$$ (3.28)

Larger values of *Shannon's entropy* H_k indicate a higher complexity. Among various "words" there are some that never or only seldom occur. These "words" are called "forbidden". Counting the forbidden words in the distribution of words (of length 3 symbols), regular or irregular behavior in the data series can be distinguished (with a high or low number, respectively).

If the data series contains negative values, one informative measure, which allows negative values in the distribution is *Renyi's entropy* described as (3.29):

$$H_\alpha = \frac{1}{1 - \alpha} \log_2 \left\{ \sum_{k=1}^{N} p_k^\alpha \right\}$$ (3.29)

where α is order ($\alpha > 0$, $\alpha \neq 1$). The result produced by this measure is expressed in *bits*: if one elementary signal yields zero bits of information, then two well-separated elementary singles will yield one bit of information, four well-separated elementary singles will yield two bits of information, and so on. Thus, for different cardiac signals, Renyi's entropy in the time–frequency domain is different [155].

Mutual information function (MIF) is an informative approach analogous to the cross-correlation or the autocorrelation function. For two stationary data series *x(n)* and *y(n)* the Shannon H_k can be calculated (H_x and H_y, respectively). Then, the MIF is given by (3.30):

$$MI_{xy} = H_x + H_y - H_{xy} = \sum_{ij} S_{ij} \log_2 \frac{S_{ij}}{p_i q_j}$$ (3.30)

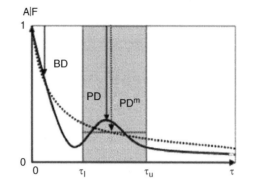

◼ Fig. 3.25
Scheme of Autonomic Information Flow (AIF) as function of the time scale τ. The AIF value at $\tau = 1$ heartbeat quantifies the information flow to the successive heartbeat. The respective loss of the signal inherent information (AIF normalised to 1 at $\tau = 0$) is quantified by the AIF decay measure BD (beat decay at $\tau = 1$ heart beat). Correspondingly, the loss of information over a longer time scale τ, such as the vagal or respiratory sinus arrhythmia rhythms, which can appear as peak in AIF (full line), can be assessed as PD (peak decay). In cases of nonappearing peaks, the decay with regard to the mean AIF of appropriate time scale range (PD^m, dashed lines) are used as robust measure. The lower boundary τ_l and the upper boundary τ_u of the time scale range is chosen according to the corresponding frequency band boundaries f by $\tau = 1/(2f)$ (From [A 36])

The MIF measures the average information in $x(n)$ on $y(n)$ in units of "bit". MIF is symmetrical ($MI_{xy} = MI_{yx}$), non-negative, and bounded from above by min $\{H_x, H_y\}$. MIF vanishes if the time series are statistically independent. Thus, the $x(n)$ (almost surely) determines $y(n)$ only if $MI_{xy} \geqslant H_y$.

On the basis of the MIF, the *autonomic information flow (AIF)* has been proposed by Hoyer et al. [156]. In this method, all statistical dependencies are considered as *information flow* within the time series. AIF is independent of signal amplitudes and allows the predictability and regularity of a signal to be quantified.

A typical AIF is sketched in ❷ Fig. 3.25. The amplitude at $\tau = 0$ (normalized to 1) represents the entire information of a time series. The decay of this function over a prediction time τ (which is considered as a time scale) represents the loss of information (here, over one heartbeat interval). In the case of a highly complex interval series, the next RRI is poorly predictable and consequently the decay of the AIF curve (information loss) is high (large BD, beat decay). In the opposite case of a confidently predictable heartbeat series, the AIF decay is low and consequently the BD is small. Predominant rhythms (such as vagal oscillations) can be assessed by the information loss over respective prediction time horizons (= time scales) corresponding to the well-known autonomic rhythms. The resulting measure is called *peak decay* [156]. Various time scales of AIF can improve prognostication in patients with multiple organ dysfunction syndrome and after cardiac arrest.

3.3.4.3 Methods for Chaos and Determinism Analysis

(Chaos – a property of a system that looks random being in fact deterministic (albeit irreversible and unpredictable). Determinism–this means that points close to each other in phase space at a time t will probably be close to each other at a time $t + \Delta t$. Thus, determinism implies that evolving from time t_0 to t_1, and then from t_1 to t_2, is the same as evolving from t_0 to t_2 *(known as Chapman-Kolmogorov law)*.)

Many biological phenomena which look like a random (stochastic) process (atrial fibrillation, ventricular fibrillation) are in fact related to many factors (the number of degrees of freedom (Mathematically, the number of degrees of freedom (or the dimension of state space) equals the number of first-order differential equations necessary to describe the system.), usually not known exactly) that determine their nonlinear dynamics (behavior) [108, 109, 111]. Dynamical

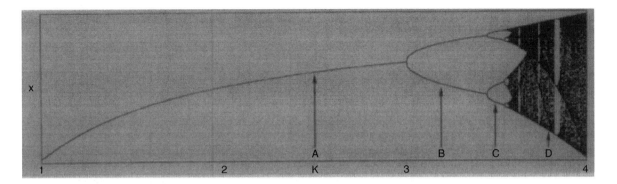

◘ Fig. 3.26
Bifurcation diagram of logistic map (From [108])

(biological) systems (continuous) usually consist of phase space (M) and map (evolution, flow, F). Typically, there are at best *differential equations* (Differential equation is a mathematical equation for an unknown function of one or several variables that relates the values of the function itself and its derivatives of various orders.) to express the evolution of the system. For exploratory reasons, the continuous system behavior is evaluated after discretization (i.e., "time" is given as a set of points 1,2,3. . ...F). For a 1D system, a nonlinear behavior can be characterized by means of a so-called *logistic map* (Logistic map – a polynomial mapping of chaotic behavior can arise from very simple nonlinear dynamic equations.) (3.31):

$$x_{n+1} = a x_n \left(1 - x_n\right),$$ (3.31)

where x_{n+1} is the point (state) after time 1, x_n is the initial point (state), and a is the bifurcation parameter. When a increases, the system switches to higher periodicities (so-called *period-doubling bifurcations*) until at a certain value of a the system exhibits chaotic behavior (period-doubling route to chaos) (❯ Fig. 3.26) [108, 109]. The transition from regular (periodic) to chaotic behavior takes place via a quasi-periodicity, sub-criticality, or intermittency. All possible dynamics have been observed with respect to cardiac arrhythmias (i.e., ventricular fibrillation [116–120]).

Consider two initial states of $x(t)$ and $y(t)$ at time $t = 0$. If the tendency is to diverge at an exponential rate with time ($\gamma > 0$), then the system exhibits chaotic dynamics (3.32)

$$\left|x\left(t\right) - y\left(t\right)\right| \approx \left|x\left(0\right) - y\left(0\right)\right| e^{\gamma t},$$ (3.32)

which define a property of chaotic dynamics, that is, the sensitivity of the evolution of the system to the initial condition [157].

Largest Lyapunov Exponent

The Lyapunov exponent (λ) is a quantitative measure of the sensitive dependence on initial conditions [109, 157]. It defines the average rate of divergence of two neighboring trajectories. An exponential divergence of infinitesimally close trajectories in phase space, coupled with a folding of trajectories to ensure that the solutions will remain finite, is the general mechanism for generating deterministic randomness and unpredictability. A negative exponent implies that the orbits approach a common fixed point. A zero exponent means that the orbits maintain their relative positions – they are on a stable attractor. Finally, a positive λ implies that the orbits are on a chaotic attractor. Thus, Lyapunov exponents allow the discrimination between periodicity and chaotic dynamics. Amongst all possible λ, the largest Lyapunov exponent (LLE) is of particular interest. Its positivity is presumed to be a "gold standard" for chaos in "deterministic" time series.

Wolf et al. [158] have proposed the algorithm for LLE calculation from time series. For a given time series $x(t)$ and the nearest to initial point $x(t0)$, the average exponential rate of divergence is characterized by (3.33):

$$\lambda = \frac{1}{t_M - t_o} \sum_{k=1}^{M} \log_2 \frac{L(t_k)}{L(t_{k+1})},$$ (3.33)

where L indicates the distance between these two points. To calculate the LLE, the following set of parameters must be chosen: m – the embedding dimension, τ – the delay, evaluation time t_{k-1}, t_{k+1}, as well as separation points and maximum orientation error. For LLE calculation for ECG data series, an m between 5–20 and a time delay of 1 is indicated. However, a reliable calculation of LLE requires a relatively long and uncorrupted data series. In addition, it remains controversial whether LLE per se allows sufficient proof of chaos or provides a quantitative measure of chaos intensity.

Poincaré Sections
This is a way of obtaining a discrete $(n-1)$ dimensional dynamic from an n-dimensional continuous space-phase. For a 3D orbit, it is possible to intersect the orbit in a discrete set of points $x(t_k)$ with a suitably oriented plane P (Poincaré section). Then, the points where the orbit intersects the plane from the same side (from behind) can be chosen. Therefore, a two-dimensional discrete dynamics $x_{k+1} = G(x_k)$ in the plane P can be determined [108, 116, 117].

Noise Limit Titration
The presence of noise in real (experimental) data series is the main factor that limits the reliability of various methods that are proposed for the detection of deterministic chaos. Poon and Barahona [159] have proposed an analytical technique called *noise titration*. Instead of removing or separating noise from the data, artificially generated random noise is added to the quantitatively titrate chaos. White (or linearly correlated) noise of increasing standard deviation (δ) is added to the data until its nonlinearity goes undetected by a particular *indicator* at a limiting value of δ = *noise limit (NL)* (noise ceiling of the signal) and at a limiting condition (equivalence point). An NL value > 0 indicates chaos, and its given value estimates its relative intensity. If NL = 0, the data-series can be considered either nonchaotic or the background noise (so-called noise floor) neutralizes the chaotic component. The power of the numerical titration technique depends critically on the choice of a suitable *nonlinear indicator*, which has to be specific (to nonlinear dynamics) and tolerant (to measurement noise). One verified method is the *Volterra-Wiener algorithm* [159]. The titration procedure is highly sensitive and specific to chaos, immune to noise, relatively simple and robust. Its ability to distinguish healthy young and elderly people from CHF-patients has recently been reported [160]. However, its clinical significance still remains unexplored.

3.3.4.4 Nonlinear Prediction (Forecasting)

A characteristic feature of a dynamic system with deterministic chaos is that the prediction of its behavior is possible with some degree of confidence only in the short term. Thus, with some knowledge about a part of system dynamics (so-called *library*), it is possible to try to predict its behavior several steps into the future. These assumptions provide a basis for the development of methods for HRV predictability (forecasting) [161, 162].

Correlation Coefficients
Sugihara and May [161] have arbitrarily proposed dividing a given time series into two equal parts, using the first half as a library, from which the behavior of the second half can be predicted. By constructing an m-dimensional vector (called *the predictee*) $X_t = (x_t, x_{t+1} \ldots x_{t-(m-1)})$ from the first half of the time series, it is then possible to make a numerical prediction for the parts immediately following the elements of the predictee. Denoting these predicted values by x'_{t+p} for $p = 1, 2, \ldots . p_{max}$, it is then possible to plot the x'_{t+p} against the values x_{t+p} actually occurring in the time series. By repeating this procedure for many m-dimensional vectors drawn from the second half of the series, it is feasible to compute the correlation coefficient ρ for the predicted and actual values as a function of p, the number of time-steps into the future.

S-map (Sequential Locally weighted Global Linear Maps)

A locally weighted map can provide a simple test for nonlinearity in a time series [156]. Suppose there is an embedding of the actual time series $X_t \in R^{m+1}$ where $X(t) \equiv 0$, and the time step Tp forward is $X_{t+Tp}(1)$, then the forecast at Tp is given by (3.34):

$$\widehat{Y}_t = \sum_{j=0}^{m} C_t(j)X_i(j).$$ (3.34)

3.3.4.5 Irreversibility/Asymmetry Analysis

Time irreversibility analysis is a nonlinear dynamics technique that produces temporal *asymmetries* in statistical properties that are different when the series are observed after time reversal. Thus, if a stationary time series is considered to be time reversible, then the probability of the vector $(z_n, .. z_{n+k-1})$ is equal to the probability of the vector $(z_{n+k-1}, .. z_n)$ for all k and n [163]. *For* a time-reversible segment, it follows that the return map $R - R_{n+1}$ versus $R - R_n$ is symmetrical with respect to the line of identity. Thus, the irreversibility is defined by the asymmetry of the distribution of the difference of consecutive intervals with respect to zero. The simplest test statistic used for detection of deviations from time reversibility is the *skewness of the differences of R−R intervals* [163].

Costa et al. [164] have proposed a so-called multi-scale time asymmetry index A_I that is based on methods derived from basic physics assumptions. First, data-series are transformed into binary sequences of HR accelerations and decelerations. Then, a set of coarse-graining time series y_τ is constructed by taking the average inside the moving window with a different scale factor τ. The difference between the probability of energy distribution for HR accelerations and decelerations provides the estimator of time reversal asymmetry $\widehat{A}(\tau)$ (3.35):

$$\widehat{A}(\tau) = \frac{\Sigma_{y_\tau > 0} P(y_\tau) \ln[P(y_\tau)]}{\Sigma_{y_\tau} P(y_\tau) \ln[P(y_\tau)]} - \frac{\Sigma_{y_\tau < 0} P(y_\tau) \ln[P(y_\tau)]}{\Sigma_{y_\tau} P(y_\tau) \ln[P(y_\tau)]},$$ (3.35)

where $P(y)$ denotes the probability of y_τ. For a range of time scales τ, the *multi-scale time asymmetry index* (A_I) is calculated as the summation of the asymmetry values $\widehat{A}(\tau)$ obtained for each time scale (3.36):

$$A_t = \sum_{\tau=1}^{L} \widehat{A}(\tau).$$ (3.36)

The A_I values are significantly higher for young healthy adults than for the elderly and subjects with CHF or AF. Interestingly, highly irregular time series of AF and less variable (compared to healthy subjects) time series of patients with CHF tend to be more symmetric [164]. Thus, A_I can be considered as a measure that can be applied irrespective of heart rhythm.

Many simple tests for time-irreversibility that are based on return map evaluation have been proposed by Ehlers et al. [165], Guzik et al. [166], and Porta et al. [167]. The distribution of R−R intervals (or differences) with respect to the main diagonal of the return map is quantified as the number of points (or distances) below or above the diagonal.

The clinical significance of time-irreversibility remains unresolved. However, evidence of a link between autonomic control and the asymmetry index has been found [168]. Recently, Porta et al. have described a method for distinguishing various types of nonlinearities over different temporal scales [169].

3.3.4.6 Phase-Rectified Signal Averaging Method

Periodicities in HR signals are usually contaminated by the presence of noise and artifacts, which may cause a reset of the periodicities (quasi-periodicities). These "new" quasi-periodicities can be determined by means of a phase-rectified averaging method (❯ Fig. 3.27) [170]. First, the so-called anchor points (Anchor points correspond to increases (or decreases) of the signal.) in the phase of deceleration or acceleration are determined (❷ Fig. 3.27). The averages over anchor points are calculated within a segment (window) containing signals close to them (usually two intervals for each side). Differences in PRSA over increasing and decreasing parts of the signal indicate a loss of time-reversal symmetry. The derived index called *deceleration capacity* (DC) has been shown to be helpful in risk stratification in post-MI patients [171], especially in those with preserved left ventricular function [172].

3.3.4.7   Recurrence Quantification Analysis

Recurrence quantification analysis (*RCA*) is a method for quantification of determinism in a time series [173]. This method is especially useful for transient behavior far from equilibrium (RQA software (Webber & Zbilut), can be downloaded from the following URL: http://homepages.luc.edu/$\sim$cwebber/.). Basically, the difference in the embedding dimension $z_n - z_m$, which constitute the *recurrence matrix* $R_{n,m}$ can be calculated. Points of the recurrence matrix are designated "recurrent" if the difference between paired vectors is below a cut-off value. Recurrent points are plotted as darkened pixels at corresponding n, m coordinates (❷ Fig. 3.28) [174]. If the signal is regular, its deterministic nature will show regular patterns. A quantitative description is given by the parameter percent of determinism (%DET) (among others proposed), which is about zero for the stochastic process and approximately 100 for a deterministic signal. %DET provides information about the intrinsic structure of the signal [174]. Although the RCA also allows for the determination of the LLE and Shannon entropy, this method has been found to be of limited clinical interest [175].

3.3.4.8   Stochastic Resonance

The presence of noise might not necessarily be considered harmful. In fact, under certain circumstances, an "extra dose" of noise can help the performance of the system [176]. The noise component can be calculated by means of several methods, with the most popular being the *signal-to-noise ratio (SNR)* [176]. The geometric mean of the average distribution values below and above the signal bandwidth has been proposed for its calculation. The SNR of the RRIs (SNR_{RRI}) can be calculated as a ratio of $(D_{S+N} - D_S)/D_N$, where D_{S+N} is a distribution of the recorded signal (signal *[s]* + noise *[n]*), and D_S is a distribution of the true signal over a prespecified bandwidth. For transient changes to be examined, a robust locally weighted regression can be used to smooth varying SNR temporally [177].

3.3.5   Methods for Qualifying and Quantifying HRV Relationship with Other Biological Signals

Important information provided by HRV analysis extracted from a single time series cannot enhance other time series. Therefore, the interaction between two (or more) physiological (sub)systems might be necessary. Sometimes, a single ECG time series can provide data regarding breathing rate though the respiratory function is not recorded [177, 178]. In addition, other ECG-derived parameters that might be related to heart rate control can be obtained, estimated, and correlated with the HRV signal [179].

Usually, simultaneously recorded time series for each system are required. Hence, many bivariate or multivariate techniques have been developed that aim to quantify the imprint of the physiological interaction between the two or more systems. Apart from the detection of interrelations, some of these techniques are designed to assess causal relationships between the signals.

3.3.5.1   Time-Domain Method

Time-domain approaches for quantifying a relationship between any two signals (HR and respiration or SBP or other) are based on the simultaneous measurement of changes of the two parameters and the calculation of the correlation of their

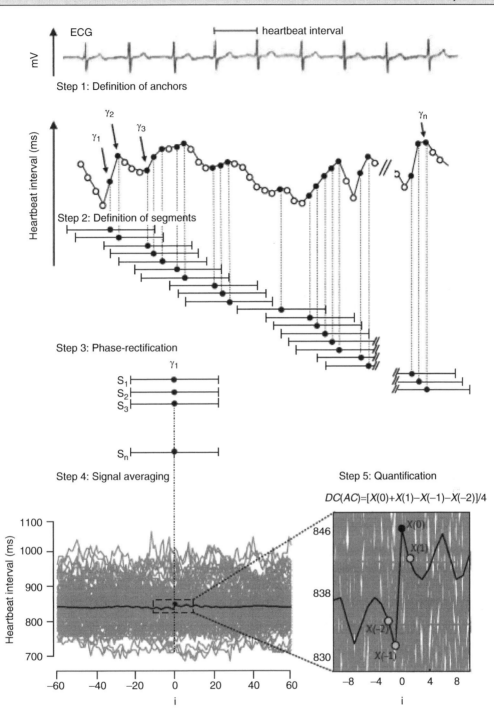

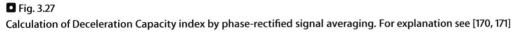

Fig. 3.27

Calculation of Deceleration Capacity index by phase-rectified signal averaging. For explanation see [170, 171]

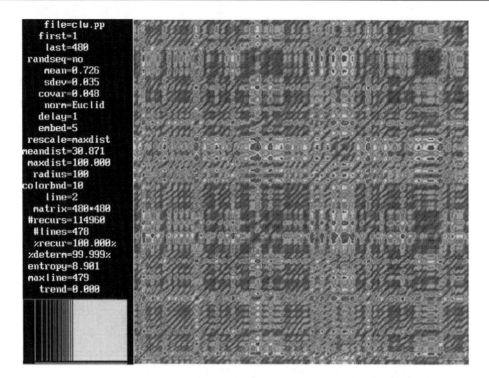

◼ Fig. 3.28

Recurrence plot. The various color s reflect different Euclidean distances between trajectories and are analogous to geographical relief maps. Five RQA variables are computed (%recurrence, %determinism, information entropy, maximum diagonal line length, state trend) which have relevancy as nonlinear markers of changes in dynamical systems and physiological states. If the signal is regular, its deterministic nature will show regular patterns (From http://homepages.luc.edu/$\sim$cwebber/ withpermission)

linear regression. Accordingly, the change of a signal $x(t) - x(t + i)$ is plotted against the change of a signal $y(t)-y(t + i)$. The slope of a linear regression describes the magnitude of the relation. This relatively simple approach forms the basis of some clinical tests, like the RSA deep breathing test, Valsalva or Muller test, tilt test, and BRS evaluation.

Time-dependent occurrence of the signal changes with another signal may help to investigate coordination and synchronization. The simplest example is the relation of the P-wave to the QRS complex. If the relation is given by the number 2, it simply indicates the presence of a II° A-V block Mobitz I with a 2:1 pattern. A similar approach can be applied in studying coordination of HRV and respiration or blood pressure changes. In addition, nonlinear phenomena that can mimic AV block patterns (i.e., bifurcations) cycle-multiplying (i.e., periodicities including alternans) can also be examined.

3.3.5.2 Cross-Spectrum

The *coherence* is a complex function of the frequency and estimates a degree of linear correlation between two signals [180–187]. If $S_{xx}(f)$ and $S_{yy}(f)$ are spectra of xx and yy signals, and $S_{xy}(f)$ is a cross-spectrum of the signal $x(t)$ and $y(t)$, then the coherence $K(f)$ is given as:

$$K(f) = \frac{S_{xy}[f]}{\sqrt{S_{xx}[f] * S_{xyy}[f]}}$$

(3.37)

The coherence is commonly represented as the squared modulus $K^2(f)$, which at any frequency band is an index between 0 and 1 of the amount of squared correlation. Values above 0.5 are considered significant (❯ Fig. 3.29).

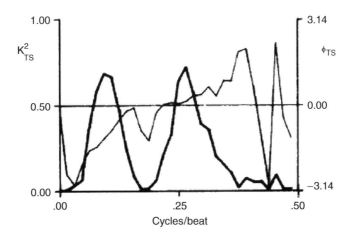

■ Fig. 3.29
Bivariate analysis of BP-HR variation in a healthy subject. Thick line – squared coherence spectrum, thin line – phase spectrum (From [185])

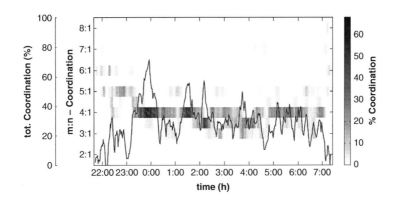

■ Fig. 3.30
Example of a coordination diagram. The coordination diagram indicates changes in the relative number of coordinated R-peaks as a respective m:n ratio (see text). In this example the cardiorespiratory coordination is oscillating with the 4:1 pattern's predomination. The absolute maximum of 68% of coordinated R-peaks (left *y* axis) is reached at midnight. Amount of coordination regardless of m:n ratio is depicted by the line of the %coordination (right *y* axis) (From [195])

Availability of the cross-spectrum allows also the calculation of the phase relationship in the range of $-180°$ and $+180°$ or $-\pi$rad to $+\pi$rad, with a positive angle for a leading x(t), and a negative angle for a leading y(t). The phase relationship is commonly represented as the *phase spectrum* ($\varphi(f)$).

The relationship between two signals, which are the input and output of the system, can also be described by the *transfer function*, which is given as:

$$H(f) = \frac{S_{xy}[f]}{S_{xx}[f]} \qquad (3.38)$$

The cross-spectrum can be calculated from spectra obtained by means of parametric or nonparametric methods, including the Fourier Transform, autoregressive modeling, wavelet transform and others [185, 186].

3.3.5.3   Nonlinear Methods

Phase Coordination and Synchronization

The term *coordination* means that there is some kind of temporal or phase incidence between HRV (the time of the R-wave) and another signal (e.g., onset of respiration, maximum blood pressure). The term *synchronization* means that there is a real physiological coupling between signals [187, 188].

In order to obtain coordination and synchronization indexes, signals (x, y) have to be recorded simultaneously and continuously and presented as time series $x(i)$ ($i = 1, \ldots m(x)$) and $y(j)$ ($j = 1, \ldots n(y)$. The absolute (t) or relative (φ) distance between the $y(j)$ and the preceding $x(i)$ or successive $x(i)$ can be calculated. This allows for presentation of the so-called synchrogram (or post-event time series) that illustrates variety in how the mth $x(t)$ corresponds with the nth $y(t)$ (i.e., *m:n coupling*) [187].

Hildebrandt et al. and Kenner et al. have provided the first description of methods for continuous measurement of the phase relation between HR and respiration [189, 190]. They found an intermittent coordination between the onset of inspiration and the preceding R-wave. In addition, the ratio of HR and respiratory rate has been suggested as a simple measure of cardiorespiratory coordination [191]. Many advanced approaches to cardio-respiratory coordination have been proposed (e.g., state-space correspondence, phase synchronization λ, phase recurrence, information flow, distribution) [192–194]. The performance of these methods depends on the time-window used. Cysarz and coworkers have recently shown (❯ Fig. 3.30) that the largest number of coordinated R-peaks and coordinated sequences was detected by the phase recurrence approach [195]. As the clinical usefulness of these methods has not been thoroughly validated [196], all the proposed methods seem to be valid for research purposes only.

Nonlinear Prediction

Nonlinear predictability of one $x(n)$ of two series given from samples of another series $y(n)$ is used to define directional coupling. This approach is suitable for short and noisy data, frequently present in physiological series (artefacts, transitions etc.), which contains local constants, local linear parts and nonlinearities. The predictability can be quantified by using the cross-predictability and the predictability improvement calculation. The degree of predictability can be calculated as the squared coherence between the original and predicted values. Nonlinear prediction methods are especially useful for investigating HRV-BPV causal relationships in many clinical states [192].

Stochastic Resonance

The stochastic resonance analysis might be more helpful for the analysis of interactions between various systems (e.g., heart rate and blood pressure) [197]. Its analysis might open new possibilities for the understanding of physiological and pathological phenomena associated with HR control [198]. At present, data accumulated for its application is limited, being anecdotal for clinical use [199].

3.3.5.4   Baroreflex Sensitivity

Analysis of baroreflex sensitivity (BRS) enables the quantification of the reflex circulatory effects of arterial baroreceptor activation or deactivation at the sinus node level through changes in vagal and sympathetic activity [77, 82, 182, 183, 186, 200, 201]. It has to be borne in mind that HR changes are only a part of the complex circulatory response to short (sensitivity) and long-term (resetting) blood pressure fluctuations, in which the systemic vascular resistance control seems to be the main target. Various methods can be used for BRS assessment [202]. All of them are based on the measurement of the extent of R–R interval change (ms) per unit (mmHg) change in systolic blood pressure. Assuming that the relationship between SBP and R–R interval in response to a rapid BP change is linear, the quantitative measure of BRS is provided by the slope of the regression line fitting changes in SBP against the second succeeding R–R interval (one-beat delay) [186, 201]. Usually, a significant relationship is required to accept the BRS value obtained. However, the BRS value calculated on a linear fit with a lack of a significant correlation is allowed if an adequate increase in SBP (>20 mmHg) is obtained [186].

Invasive Approach (External Stimuli)

Vasoconstrictor agents are normally used to explore the vagal component of the baroreflex sensitivity. Phenylephrine, a pure α-adrenergic agonist, is administered intravenously during the continuous recording of ECG (R–R interval) and BP (beat-to-beat arterial pressure) [203]. The latter can be performed either invasively, mainly in experiments on animals, or noninvasively, by using the finger-cuff method, which provides overestimation of BP variability [204], largely within the lower frequency bands [205]. After a bolus dose of 1–2 ug/kg, incremental doses of 25–50 ug are given until a SBP increase of 20–30 mmHg is reached. In normal subjects, the average values of 15 ms/mmHg have been reported [186]. In certain clinical settings, the BRS values close to zero, or even a negative BRS, can be observed [206]. Vasodilating agents are normally used to explore the sympathetic component of the BRS [207]. Nitroglycerine, a direct vasodilator, is given via the injection of 100–200 μg to obtain a rapid and progressive fall in SBP of 20 mmHg. The BRS values after administration of vasodilators are lower, indicating that the use of both vasoactive agents allows for a more comprehensive assessment of BRS. Alongside, a "steady-state" method for estimating BRS has been proposed [208], in which either phenylephrine or nitroglycerine is administered in order to obtain the step-wise increase or reduction of blood pressure.

Methods that use vasoactive agents are criticized because of their nonselective actions leading to the introduction of changes that alter the baroreceptor reflex at various levels (e.g., central effects, direct action on sinus node). On the other hand, these methods allow the initiation of an integral response, irrespective of the mechanisms contributing to the reflex.

Mechanical maneuvers, like the neck chamber technique or lower body negative pressure, represent other approaches to studying BRS. In the neck chamber technique, either positive or negative pressure is applied to the neck region inducing a decrease or increase in SBP with corresponding changes in R–R intervals [209]. The negative pressure ranges from −7 to −40 mmHg and HR response is observed over three heartbeats following the maneuver. The BRS is defined as a slope of R–R interval over neck pressure. A modified method of the neck chamber method has been proposed that allows both for activation or for deactivation of carotid baroreceptors [210]. The lower body negative pressure that imitates a reduction in circulating blood volume can be helpful in an evaluation of sympathetic activation and HR response [211]. However, in contrast to direct carotid baroreceptor stimulation/inhibition, this method provides information regarding cardiopulmonary reflexes [211]. Methods based on mechanical manipulations should be used in a specifically designed research laboratory and for particular pathophysiological purposes [212, 213].

Noninvasive Approach (Internal Stimuli)

Noninvasive methods of BRS analysis represent alternatives to invasive techniques in that they use internal stimuli that can be simply induced (e.g., Valsalva or Muller maneuver, head-up, or downward tilt) or that they occur spontaneously (❯ Fig. 3.26).

(a) The Valsalva maneuver

The Valsalva maneuver is a forced expiratory effort against a closed airway. The Muller maneuver is the reverse. There are four phases of these tests, and among them, phase IV is commonly used for the BRS assessment purposes. The BRS

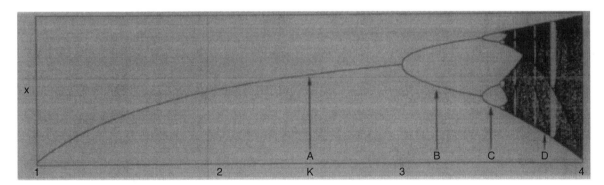

⬛ Fig. 3.31

The relation between the changes in systolic blood pressure increase and corresponding RR interval lengthening during downward tilting (From [216], Elsevier, with permission)

is calculated using linear regression of instantaneous R–R intervals and corresponding SBP values. Kautzner et al. have proposed calculating the BRS index, which is the ratio of the differences between maximum and minimum R–R interval and SBP during the so-called overshoot period of the maneuver [214]. Unfortunately, reliable measurements cannot be obtained in a large proportion of normal and post-infarction patients [215]. In addition, the correlation coefficients with invasive methods vary between 0.27 and 0.91 [214].

(b) Tilt testing

A body movement introduces changes in blood pool compartments and venous return, with corresponding BP and HR changes. Takahashi et al. have proposed a method for BRS evaluation during a rapid downward tilting from an upright to a supine position, which provides values comparable to the phenylephrine test [216].

(c) Time-domain (sequence) method

The sequence method is based on the spontaneous presence of concurrent R–R interval and systolic blood pressure changes (increase or decrease) over at least three consecutive heartbeats (sequence) [217]. For each sequence, the linear correlation between R–R intervals and SBP values is fitted. The average of individual slopes of sequences that are significant (r >0.8) and reach predefined minimum change (1 mmHg and 4–6 ms for SBP and interbeat duration respectively) is taken as the BRS measure. Usually, lower BRS values have been observed in comparison with the phenylephrine test [78]. Simplified variants of the sequence method have been proposed. Among them, the measurement of R–R interval variation over a 5-min period of controlled breathing at 0.1 Hz, that allows SBP changes to be ignored, has been documented as useful for distinguishing normal subjects (77 ms) from patients with heart failure (31 ms) [218].

(d) Spectral ratio (alpha-index)

Spectral ratio (gain, alpha-index) provides an estimate of the sensitivity of the baroreceptor-heart rate reflex based on frequency-domain analysis of the spontaneous variability of SBP and HR [77, 78, 82, 203]. The method is based on a high degree of linear correlation between systolic blood pressure and heart rate at the respiratory frequency and at 0.1 Hz in normal subjects, and on the assumption that that correlation is due to the baroreflex coupling [82].

First, the spectra of systolic blood pressure and RR-interval series, and their squared-coherence modulus, are computed. If the coherence at 0.1 Hz and at the respiratory frequency is sufficiently high (i.e., greater than a threshold usually set at 0.5), the spectra of systolic blood pressure and RR-interval are integrated over the 0.1 Hz peak, giving the SBP_{LF} and RR_{LF} powers, and over the respiratory peak, giving the SBP_{HF} and RR_{HF} powers. Then the square-root ratio of RR and SBP powers at low and high frequencies is computed:

$$\alpha_{LF} = \sqrt{\frac{RRI_{LF}}{SBP_{LF}}} \quad \text{and} \quad \alpha_{HF} = \sqrt{\frac{RRI_{HF}}{SBP_{HF}}} \tag{3.39}$$

A close correlation of α-coefficients with the phenylephrine methods has been reported in a small-number of initial studies. Larger studies have revealed a moderate linear association between the two techniques with a relatively high limit of agreement ($\sim$ 5 ms/mmHg in normal subjects and hypertensives and $\sim$13 mmHg in post-infarct patients) [218–221]. These observations indicate limitations of the BRS assessment using frequency-domain methods. Despite these limitations, a noninvasive approach provides BRS estimation of a short-term liability coming from complex and redundant reflexes with no procedural (apart from laboratory conditions) requirements.

3.3.5.5 Heart Rate Turbulence

A short-term fluctuation in sinus cycle duration after a ventricular premature beat forms the basis for introducing another noninvasive method that is related to the baroreflex control of HR, and is referred to as heart rate turbulence (HRT) [222–226] for explanation see text and ref. [294] (❯ Fig. 3.27). Interestingly, the description of this method has been forced by

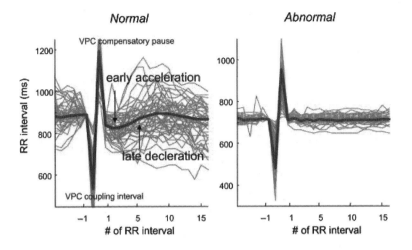

◙ Fig. 3.32

Normal (*left*) and abnormal (*right*) ventricular premature contractions tachograms used for the heart rate turbulence

simultaneous evidence of its usefulness in risk stratification after myocardial infarction [222], while the pathophysiological background that might help to explain the strength of HRV as a risk stratifier [112, 222, 226, 227] using this method is not known.

The HRT is quantified by two measures termed turbulence onset (TO) and turbulence slope (TS). The turbulence onset is a measure of immediate initial R–R interval shortening following a ventricular premature beat and is calculated using the equation (3.40):

$$TO\,[\%] = \frac{(RR_1 + RR_2) - (RR_{-2} + RR_{-1})}{(RR_{-2} + RR_{-1})} * 100 \qquad (3.40)$$

where RR_{-2} and RR_{-1} are sinus cycles preceding a ventricular premature beat, and RR_1 and RR_2 are the two intervals following the compensatory pause. TO is calculated for each single premature beats and then averaged. TO > 0 means deceleration, TO < 0 means acceleration of the sinus rhythm.

The turbulence slope (ms/beat) is a measure of subsequent deceleration phase and is calculated as the maximum slope of a regression line assessed over any sequence of five subsequent sinus-rhythm RR intervals within the first 20 (15) sinus-rhythm intervals after a ventricular premature beat and is assessed in the average HRT tachogram.

HRT cannot be calculated in the presence of interpolated ventricular premature beats without compensatory pauses. Also, a minimum number of five premature beats is necessary to obtain a reliable pattern. However, a recommendation for TO and TS calculation in the presence of only a single premature beat can be found [226, 228]. The HRT measure depends on heart rate itself, and the coupling interval (prematurity) of ventricular beats [226, 229]. Considering HRT as a specific noninvasive measure of BRS, it is necessary to keep in mind that the sinus rate response to premature ventricular beats depends also on intact SAN function and the post-extrasystolic potentiation phenomenon [226, 230].

3.4 Methodological Considerations

3.4.1 Ideal HRV Method and Index

The complexity of heart rate fluctuation *a priori* excludes an ideal HRV method or index to be identified. However, such an attempt can be made for a particular purpose of HRV assessment. The requirements and characteristics of the index or method that can meet the purposes of an HRV study are presented in ❷ Table 3.5 and discussed below.

Criteria for an ideal HRV index that have to be met for the index to be applicable for the assessment of cardiac autonomic control in physiological and pathophysiological studies, proposed by Goldberger et al. [231], are listed as follows:

1. The ideal index should behave in a comparable manner in various subjects in response to stimulating or inhibiting maneuver s that lead to changes in cardiac autonomic balance or in its main components
2. Between-subject variability of the index at the same conditions should be minimal
3. The ideal HRV index should be explicable on the basis of physiological or pathopysiological mechanisms contributing to vagal-sympathetic interactions

For the reasons above, only short-term HRV analysis (and derived indices) seems to be applicable if cardiac autonomic control is to be explored (❷ Table 3.6).

From a clinical point of view, an ideal HRV index should possess quite different features, while the association between HRV and cardiac autonomic control might not necessarily be so tight. Considering these issues, the criteria for a clinically useful HRV index might be proposed as follows:

1. The ideal HRV index should be an independent prognostic measure of the risk of death, especially if sudden (unexpected)
2. The ideal HRV index should have the potential to be applied in a wide population (without exception for cardiac rhythm disturbances)
3. Common applicability in clinical practice requires the ideal HRV index to be as simple as possible in order to be understandable to physicians
4. The ideal HRV method should be implemented in available analytical systems, allowing for its practical use in large populations
5. Normal limits defined as limits of agreement (LOA) should be established in a local (geographically or race-homogenous) population.

For these reasons, long-term HRV analysis (and derived indices) can be considered more suitable, as they cover most mechanisms related to the HRV phenomenon (❷ Table 3.7). However, the interpretation of the meaning of these indices on the basis of cardiac autonomic control does not seem to be appropriate.

The common HRV measures also suffer from other limitations, including the non-normal distribution that requires mathematical transformation (usually natural logarithm), and a lack of standardization.

There is still a place for an ideal method and index from the mathematical, physical and technical point of view. The implementation of ideas that come from other areas or phenomena might prove to be fruitful. However, their physiological (Goldberger criteria) or clinical (clinical criteria) meaning should be tested each time. This requires close cooperation between inventors and clinicians. Otherwise, methods can proliferate without solving any important physiological or clinical issues, and simply add "scientific-like" noise.

3.4.2   Data Acquisition

3.4.2.1   Integration of the Signal

The basic cardiac signal, generally in the form of the electrocardiogram, is required to be digitized by a computer in order to obtain a series of R−R intervals. However, sometimes the R−R-interval series can be derived from analog systems. Also, a use of plethysmography or blood pressure recordings can provide the opportunity to derive pulse intervals.

Ideally, a raw ECG record should be preserved to check for the integrity of the signal, the presence of non-sinus beats and for editing artefacts [4, 5]. Accurate on- and off-line analysis depends primarily on the integrity of the signal. However, for HRV analysis purposes, the digitization rate (sampling frequency) is crucial for the detection of small variations of cardiac rhythm. Several types of errors and their solutions are presented in ❷ Table 3.8.

3.4.2.2   Errors Relating to Digitization Rate

A sampling frequency of 250–500 Hz has been recommended [4, 5]. However, in many studies the sampling frequency is not reported. Others considered a digitization rate of 500–1000 Hz, which would provide a basic resolution of 1–2 ms

◼ Table 3.5

Characteristics of HRV index/method used in various kinds of studies (purpose-oriented)

Purpose/ Requirements	Index or method	Universality (no exclusions)	Availability (common)	Robustness (high)	Reproducibility	Intersubjects variation	Physiological meaning	Diagnostic value
Epidemiological studies Fundamental requirements: HRV index calculable from short time series (routine ECG?) Controlled study conditions	Mean RRI (or HR)	Yes	Yes	Yes	High	Small	Sympatho-vagal balance	Prognostic value proven in many studies
	SDRR CV RMSSD CIPA	No	Yes	No	Relatively high	Large	Respiratory/ vagally related	Screening for DAN Screening for early atherosclerosis ? Outcome prediction
Physiological studies Fundamental requirements: HRV index calculable from short time series (1–5 min) Controlled study conditions	Mean RRI (or HR)	Yes	Yes	Yes	High	Small	Sympatho-vagal balance	Unspecific
	SDRR RMSSD	No	Yes	No	Relatively high	Large	Respiratory/ vagally related	Detection of sinus node dysfunction Screening for DAN ? Screening for early atherosclerosis ?
Multi-signal recordings recommended	Spectral/ cross-spectral analysis	No	Yes	No	Modest or unknown	Large	Ambiguous, (various in different frequency-band)	
	Time-variant spectral analysis					Large	Contradictory data	
	Nonlinear methods	No	No	Various or unknown	Fair or unknown	Large or unknown	Unknown	
Clinical outcome studies Fundamental requirements: HRV index calculable from 24-h ECG recordings	SDNN	No	Yes	No	Relatively high	Large	Multifactorial Unexplainable	Prognostic value proven in many studies
	HRVI	No	Yes	Yes	High	Relatively small		
	HRVF	Yes	No	Yes	High	Relatively small		Prognostic value proven in one study
	DC	No	No	Yes	Unknown	Unknown		
	Nonlinear methods	No	No	Various or Unknown	Fair or unknown	Unknown		Prognostic value proven in many studies

◘ Table 3.6

Short-term HR and HRV measures characteristics from an "ideal" HRV requirements view

Requirements	HR (RRI)	SDRR	SDSD	CV	VLF	LF	HF	Fractal measures	Others
Comparable (in direction) change in response to a defined stimulating or inhibiting maneuvers in various subjects	+++	+	+/−	+	+/−	+/−	+	+/−	NA
Minimal between-subjects variability	+++	+	+	+	+/−	+/−	+	+/−	NA
Explanation on basis of physiology and pathophysiology	+++	+	++	+	+/−	+/−	++	+/−	NA

+++ highly predictable/consistent data, ++ moderately predictable/exceptions reported, + marginally predictable/high variation, +/− unpredictable/conflicting data exists, NA - not assessed

◘ Table 3.7

Long-term HR and HRV measures characteristics from an "ideal" HRV requirements view

Requirements	HR (NNI)	SDNN	SDANN	RMSSD	HRVI	HRVF	Fractal measures	HRT	BRS
Independent risk factor/marker of death/sudden death	+++	+	+/−	+/−	++	+	++	++	+++
Applicability to a wide range population	+++	+/−	++	+/−	+	++	+/−	+/−	−
Comprehensible for physician/bedside use	+++	+	+	+/−	+/−	+	−	+	+
Implementation on a commercial system	+++	+++	+++	+++	+/−	−	−	−	−
Normal limits with a LOA defined	+++	+	−	+	+/−	+/−	−	+/−	+/−

+++ well documented/consistent data, ++ moderately documented/consistent data, + moderately documented/inconsistent data, +/− less well documented/conflicting data exists, − undefined/lack of data/experimental tool as yet

[232–237]. A higher sampling frequency might be necessary to gain small variations in the amplitude of cardiac rhythm, especially in pre-term newborns and after heart transplantation. Most of the studies of HRV have gathered data using 24-h ECG systems with a nonoptimal sampling frequency of 128 Hz (~ 8 ms resolution), despite a resolution of at least 4 ms (250 Hz) suggested for adequate RSA quantification [4, 5, 235]. The noise introduced by an insufficient sampling rate can be overcome by the use of template matching or an interpolation algorithm. A digitization rate below 100 Hz is not considered acceptable [4, 5].

A low sampling frequency can cause a jitter in the determination of the fiducial points of the QRS complex, thus creating an error in the RR interval measurements [237]. The jitter-error is a source of additional high frequency content, and thereby affects the reliable determination of short-term variation.

Conventional Holter systems influence parameters estimating short-term, high frequency variation (RMSSD, NN50, pNN50). The R wave detection error using conventional systems can make spectral HRV analysis inaccurate and too low a sampling rate can influence high-frequency components irrespective of the spectral analysis methods used [236–238].

▫ Table 3.8

Errors in ECG data (unedited and edited)

Type of R–R interval distortion	QRS pattern	Mechanisms	Influence on HRV assessment	Solution	Limitation
True Premature ectopic beats (PEBs)	Supraventricular normal pattern	Abnormal automaticity or delayed potentials	Significant error in short-term statistical descriptors, spectral analysis unreliable	Rejection of epochs with beats which duration differ from neighbor by more than 20%	Inappropriate in the presence of long-coupled (late) PEBs
	Ventricular abnormal pattern			Rejection if frequent, interpolation procedures if sporadic	Ignores effects of PEBs on the autonomic milieu, introduces a sort of technical error
Parasystolic (allorhythmic) ectopic beats	Normal or abnormal	Constant coupling between repetitive PEBs	Presence of a separate oscillation	Unsolved, usually treated as PEBs	Introduces a sort of technical error
Normal sinus beats with abnormal connotation	Abnormal pattern	Abnormal intraventicular conduction (i.e., BBB)	"Jitter" error, may influence short-term spectral measures	Unsolved, usually treated and managed as ventricular PEBs	Introduces a sort of technical error
Spurious premature beats	Normal or abnormal	External noise, baseline shifting	None if recognised	Correct skin-electrode contact	Sometimes impossible due to sweating, body motion
		Low sampling rate		Appropriate sampling rate	Less possible in commercial long-term ECG recordings
		Large P- or T-wave amplitude		Appropriate threshold for QRS detection	Not always possible in commercial systems
Missed beats	None, RRI is doubled or a multiple of the preceding average	External noise, baseline shifting	Significant error in short-term statistical descriptors, spectral analysis unreliable	Correct skin-electrode contact, manual correction, splitting into equivalent R–R intervals, interpolation algorithms	Sometimes impossible due to sweating, body motion, introduces a sort of technical bias
		Low R-wave amplitude		Appropriate threshold for QRS detection, manual correction	Not always possible in commercial systems
Pauses	None, RRI is doubled or a multiple of the preceding average	Post-ectopic beats	Significant error in short-term statistical descriptors, spectral analysis unreliable	Rejection if frequent, interpolation algorithms if sporadic, splitting into equivalent R–R intervals	Ignores effects of or on the autonomic milieu, introduces a sort of technical bias
		Sinus arrest/high grade sino-atrial block			
		A-V block			

An error of up to 4% in the RMSSD and HF power has been reported when systems with conventional (8 ms) and high resolution (1 ms) timing accuracy have been compared [237]. These errors have been even greater in patients after MI, reaching 7.1% and 8%, respectively. A higher sampling rate leads to a reduction in the HF power. As a result, significant error is introduced with a sampling rate of 128 Hz not only to the HF power, but also to the LF/HF ratio with an error of up to 14%. Tapanainen et al. observed a large error in post-MI patients reaching 22.6% in those with low HRV and 17.5% in those with normal HRV. A 5% error of short-term components of the return map (SD1) has been shown to be due to a low sampling rate. Voss et al. reported a 2% error in the nonlinear symbolic RR interval dynamics in normal subjects, when a conventional system had been compared to a high resolution system with a sampling frequency of 2 kHz [235]. A similar range of error has been observed in the short-term scaling exponent $\alpha 1$ (DFA) in subjects with normal HRV. However, the error increased to 5% in post-MI patients with a reduced HRV. A marked difference (11%) between low (~8 ms) and high (1 ms) resolution has been observed for the approximate entropy (ApEn). The error was more pronounced in post-MI patients with low HRV or faster HR (17.6% and 15.0%, respectively) [237]. The magnitude of all these differences grew proportionately when the overall heart HRV diminished. Thus, *the measurement of the nonlinear dynamics parameters should preferably be done with a sampling frequency higher than the conventional 128 Hz.*

The sampling frequency does not seem to affect long-term (RRI, SDNN, SDANN) or low-frequency HRV components (VLF, LF).

Sampling frequency is more important in the accurate detection of IBI short-term fluctuations if the RR interval series are shorter or smaller in amplitude [235]. Most prognostic studies on post-AMI patient populations, however, are based on the SDNN calculation. It is unlikely that the results of these studies would change with a higher sampling rate. However, *for experimental studies in physiology, psychophysiology and pathophysiology, the minimum sampling rate of 250 Hz should be mandatory.*

3.4.2.3 Errors Introduced by Noise

A rigorous recording method should be used in order to minimize noise, which usually interferes with the signal and results in an overlapping with the true R-wave amplitude [34, 239–242]. This can lead to *spurious R-wave* timing due to variation in peak amplitude and makes the use of simple maxima-based peak-finding algorithms unreliable. However, smoothing or filtering of the digitized signal, template or derivate matching and interpolation procedures can help to solve this problem. If the heartbeat signal is obtained from continuous BP recordings, where the fiducial point detection is more problematic due to a lack of clearly defined peaks, a template-matching approach is considered most appropriate.

Another consequence of noisy recordings is the identification of artifactual waves as *spurious R-waves*. Such erroneous R-waves might be harder to eliminate through the above mentioned algorithms. A careful visual investigation of a series of data is necessary. It is quite easy for short-term ECG recordings. However, for a 24-h recording it can be achieved through an automatic class (template) ascertainment of accuracy, by the visual checking of R–R interval (or differential) distribution histograms' tails, or step-by-step correction using a full disclosure option available in commercial systems. These procedures are time-consuming and may require up to 45 min for thorough analysis, labeling and editing.

3.4.2.4 Errors Related to the QRS-Wave Detectors

Another set of *spurious R-waves* results from an inappropriate threshold for R-wave detection. If the threshold is too low, an R–R interval would be subdivided into additional inter-event intervals due to the detection of T-waves (usually peaked with a relatively high amplitude, not infrequently in normal subjects), or more rarely, due to P-waves (usually when the amplitude of the R-waves is small, a frequent feature in patients with an advanced heart failure). If the threshold is set too high, R-waves of smaller amplitudes would be undetected and an exceptionally long IBI that merges two or more normal R–R interval would be recorded. These undetected beats are referred to as *missing beats* [239–242]. Their presence introduces sizeable and dramatic biases in estimates of HRV that can result in errors of up to 80% for SDNN, 25% for HF power and above 200% within lower frequencies [242].

◨ Table 3.9

Steps to avoid non-stationarity in ECG recordings

1	Minimize non-stationarities in data through conditions control
2	Use filtering procedures for the removal of slow trends
3	Avoid unnecessarily long analytical epochs
4	Test for non-stationarities if appropriate
5	Omit (or remove) highly non-stationarity data segments
6	Use approaches explicitly designed for non-stationarity data evaluation

Another type of error is related to the identification of abnormal (either ectopic or artifactual) beats as normal. As the data-series containing abnormal heartbeats could be rejected from further analysis, leaving *mistakenly labeled R-waves* introducing a significant error especially in spectral estimates, particularly within the HF bands [34, 239–242].

Instabilities of the isoelectric line (baseline) with extreme upwards or downwards shifts due to a poor electrode-skin contact, and following rapid changes in impedance, would result in *missing beats* even if the technical requirements are fulfilled. Some aspects of these sources of errors are discussed in other chapters (Ambulatory ECG, Signal averaging etc.).

3.4.2.5 Errors Relating to the Presence of True Ectopic Beats

The presence of a few premature ectopic beats (PEBs) is a normal feature of long-term ECG recording in healthy subjects. The number of ectopic beats increases with age and in patients with CVD. In such cases, they can also appear in a short-time series. Irrespective of data length, their presence introduces an error that is related to a sudden shortening of the sinus fulfill cycle preceding the PEB (coupling interval) and a compensatory prolongation of the subsequent cycle (compensatory pause). As a result, a significant error in time-domain and especially in frequency domain measures is introduced [34, 238, 240–242]. In an excellent paper, Berntson and Stowell showed that the presence of only one ectopic PEB in a 2-min recording introduced an error in the SDNN of up to 50%, in the HF of around 10% and in the LF of approximately 80% [242]. Interpolation procedures for the replacement of PEBs with interpolation-derived heartbeats do not necessarily prevent these errors. The use of a filter function to interpolate for heartbeats preceding and following PEBs can help to solve this problem. However, it may lead to a disruption of the continuity of data.

3.4.2.6 Non-Stationarity as a Source of Errors

Stationarity is defined as the invariance of distributional characteristics of data-series in all moments over time. In a controlled laboratory setting, when short-time data series are subjected to evaluation, ECG signal non-stationarity might reflect the physiological properties of complex heart rate control. If long-term ECG recordings are used for HRV assessment, occurrence of sudden changes in sinus cycles related to internal or external stimuli is frequent. Also, sustained trends can reflect physiological control mechanisms. They may distort spectral frequencies and usually are subject to detrending procedures [243]. These procedures provide technically valid data-series, but at the cost of a loss of information. Another way to fit stationarity of data is the use of linear or polynominal trend removal or bandpass filters to isolate the periodicities of interests and minimize the effects of non-stationarities. For the stationarity of the time series to fit, the simplest way is to maintain test and subject conditions stable throughout the recording period and to minimize the length of recordings. If non-stationary epochs cannot be removed or extracted from prolonged data-series, multiple short-epochs, in which stationarity is satisfied, should be analyzed to examine the dynamics of the signal over time. Otherwise, *the analysis of relatively stable short-time series with appropriate methods (e.g., discrete FFT, time-frequency analysis) seems to be more advisable than the use of detrending algorithms.* Steps necessary to solve the stationarity issue are listed in ❷ Table 3.9.

3.4.2.7   Management with Errors Relating to the Presence of Ectopic, Spurious and Missed Beats

In acute studies, when the ECG signal recorded is of only a few minutes duration, continuous visual inspection is required. *Only data that does not contain any abnormal beats should be extracted for further analysis.* For short-term recordings, it seems advisable to acquire time series somewhat longer than the period assumed for further analysis as it increases the probability for taking undisturbed portions of a required length from the entire recordings. In any other cases, the studies have to be repeated or rejected [4, 5, 34, 242, 243].

Less strict approaches are proposed for 24-h ECG recordings [4, 5, 34, 242, 243]. For time-domain methods, data can be passed through various filters that eliminate annotated heartbeats other than the normal (dominant) beat. Additional logical conditions are imposed to eliminate the preceding and post-ectopic heartbeats. If the sequence of heartbeats is required to be sustained (e.g., for spectral analysis), various solutions are proposed. However, there are no specific recommendations regarding the cut-off of absolute or relative frequency of abnormal heartbeats. Many authors use different criteria.

If the number of abnormal heartbeats is considered insignificant, algorithms that allow the correction (substitute) of abnormal (usually ectopic) heartbeats could be applied. A variety of algorithms have been proposed and reviewed in depth elsewhere.

The duration of the compensatory pause depends in a complex manner on the coupling interval and the mean IBI before PEBs. Thus, PEBs can occur as interposed, compensated or phase-shifted extrasystoles, so simple replacement using interpolation procedures is not reliable. Also, the annotated PEBs may in fact represent either true physiological phenomena, especially in healthy young people, or true pathological phenomena related to SAN dysfunction. Most algorithms ignore the fact that ventricular PEB occurrence is associated with changes in the autonomic milieu.

All errors in QRS detection and IBI measurements are of special significance in individuals with low HRV, where the same level of error is associated with much greater influence upon a true signal. These errors are more likely to be found in persons with PEBs as well as intraventricular conduction disturbances. Guidelines indicate the necessity for a clear description of the specific procedures for interpolation or data rejection and for a discussion of their contribution to the results [4, 5, 242]. Even so, *if the data is corrupted, the analysis should be limited to more robust time domain statistics.*

3.4.3   Data Length

The duration of the R–R interval recording for HRV analysis is not a priori limited. However, for comparison between different studies, the data is required to be of similar length. The total variance of IBI increases with the length of recordings. From a physiological point of view, a fundamental issue is the duration of the cycle of a certain phenomenon (wavelength) considered for analysis, assuming a relative selectivity of various periodicities (spectral analysis). It is required that the R–R interval recording time be ten times longer than the wavelength of certain oscillatory phenomena. A recording of at least 1 min is necessary to assess reliably short-term vagally mediated respiratory-related HR variation, and of 2 min for longer-term variation attributed in part to sympathetic control. For cycles recognized as VLF (~0.0033 Hz), it is necessary to prolong recording time periods to approximately 1 h.

A standard recording period of 5 min is recommended for clinical purposes [4, 5]. However, it has been shown that very short ECG recordings of 8–10 s duration covering no more than two to three respiratory cycles, can efficiently estimate the vagal tone (i.e., CIPA) [28, 29]. In addition, for certain purposes (e.g., psychological, exercise studies), a 5-min period may be too long to meet stationarity requirements. It would be ideal to use time-frequency approaches if shorter data-length is required to be analyzed.

With the use of a nonlinear dynamics approach, nonlinearities in time series are apparently the true subject of analysis. For the calculation of nonlinear measures, more prolonged time series is advised. However, attempts have been made to calculate these measures from short-term recordings.

For long-term recording, it is necessary to present data regarding a true period of analysis since there are some methodical differences in data selection. These differences are related to the definition of prematurity of non-sinus heartbeats (>30% or >20% deviation from the previous heartbeat interval or >10% of an interpolated beat interval), pause detection (usually >125% of averaged local means or 120% of running time), minimum duration of recordings (from 12 h including 6 night hours, to 22 h) and at least 50–90% normal (sinus) heartbeats. Also, data substitution varies with different equipment where non-sinus beats, together with the neighboring one to two heartbeats, are either eliminated or interpolated with a range of algorithms. The differences in these procedures influence time-domain HRV measurements by no more than 10%, while for spectral-measures, it can be expected to be even higher. However, this has not yet been calculated.

3.4.4 Data Presentation

Although IBI is usually employed for HRV analysis, heart rate and counts are also used as a basic metric in studies of cardiac rhythm. It is important, as a distinct relationship exists between vagal activation and HR or IBI, whereas the relationship between sympathetic activation and HR or IBI seems to be nonlinear. As the range of vagal control is considerably greater than that of the sympathetic branch and fundamentally influences the latter itself, IBI presentation has advantages over HR for the analysis of cardiac rhythms. However, if HR is employed on a beat-to-beat manner and referred to as an instantaneous HR (iHR), analyses based on iHR may not necessarily produce a similar pattern of results as for heart period analyses. Janssen et al. showed that various data presentations influenced the magnitude of HF power and LF/HF ratio, which could differ up to 37% depending on the method used [244]. Normalization procedure (dividing of observed values by their corresponding average values) has recently been proposed [245].

The HRV signal can be presented as a function of beat number. Such a presentation is referred to as the R–R *interval tachogram*. Interpolating and resampling the heartbeat series allow HRV to be expressed in a common time scale [4, 5, 77].

Successive R–R intervals are spaced unevenly in time. However, time series analyses require the data to be sampled at equal time intervals. Resampling procedures are necessary to derive the R–R series suitable for spectral analyses. Various methods have been proposed and discussed in the literature [4, 5, 77, 79].

As indicated by the guidelines, it is preferable to use a sampling approach in which the value at a given point represents a weighted average of the beats that fall within the sample interval [4, 5]. The resampling rate seems to be crucial in order to avoid aliasing. The sampling rate is recommended to be at least twice the lowest resolvable frequency. A sampling rate of 4 times the target frequency is considered most appropriate. Thus, the higher the mean heart rate, the higher is the sampling frequency required. For studies in adult humans, it is at least 2 Hz, whereas in children or individuals with higher heart rates it would be more prudent to use 4 Hz. For animal studies, a higher sampling frequency is needed [246].

3.4.5 Universality of HRV Analysis

Ideally, HRV measurement should be applied to all subjects. This requirement is referred to as *universality*. Current recommendations necessitate the presence of sinus rhythm in order to evaluate HRV qualitatively (high, normal, low or normal/abnormal pattern) and quantitatively. For this reason, heartbeats are labeled as normal (N) and IBIs as normal-to-normal (N-N or NN-intervals) [4, 5]. In fact, the American Heart Association/American College of Cardiology Task Force for Ambulatory Monitoring listed the presence of *sinus rhythm as an a priori inclusion criterion for standard HRV analysis* [247]. Such a statement excludes a substantial proportion of more severely diseased patients with a higher risk of an unfavorable outcome from studies on the clinical use of HRV, especially HF and older patients in whom the presence of frequent ectopic PEBs or atrial fibrillation is not uncommon.

A detailed analysis of the methodological descriptions of the most important studies indicates that standard HRV methods cannot be applied to 6–55% of study populations (❷ Table 3.10). In addition, newer proposed measures based on spectral analysis or nonlinear techniques, including HRT, cannot be used in 17–35% of patients (❷ Tables 3.10 and ❷ 3.11). The reasons for rejecting patients from HRV studies are varied and only rarely reported. In a small number of studies in which the reasons for exclusion are listed, the presence of artefact or insufficient data length accounts for 10–65% of exclusions, while the presence of cardiac arrhythmias/pacemakers is the reason for 10–100% of exclusions.

The clinical consequences of these assumptions and recommendations are critical in a high risk population with frequent ventricular premature beats and atrial flutter/fibrillation, in whom the opportunity for HRV analysis is abandoned (❷ Table 3.10). Farrel et al. reported a significantly higher total mortality rate (19.7%) and arrhythmic events rate (12.3%) in acute MI patients excluded from the HRV study, compared to 11.3% and 5.7% in those who entered the study [248]. The clinical course of acute MI in the rejected group was worse, with higher Killip classes and a higher proportion of

▣ Table 3.10

Applicability of HRV analysis in clinical outcome studies

Author/year	Population (included)	HRV measure (most prognostic)	% rejected[a] Overall	For the presence of artefacts	For the presence of cardiac arrhythmias	Clinical significance/comments
Farrell et al. 1991 [40]	416 post AMI St George's Hospital	HRVI	14.6	NR	NR	Total mortality: rejected vs analyzed 19.7% vs 11.3%, arrhythmic events: 12.3% vs 5.7%
Cripps et al. 1991 [38]	177 post AMI St George's Hospital	HRVI	23	NR	NR	Total mortality: rejected vs analyzed 21% vs 6% Among rejected more frequently previous MIs, more common Killip >2
Odemuyiva et al. 1991 [A1]	385 post AMI St George's Hospital	HRVI	19.3	NR	NR	Not reported
Bigger et al. 1992 [A2]	715 post MI MPIP population	ULF power	8.8		2.6 (for AF)	Not reported
Bigger et al. 1993 [122]	331 post AMI MPIP population	SDANN	6.0	4.2	1.4	Similar characteristics, outcome not reported
Vainshav et al. [A3]	226 post AMI OCS[b]	SDNN	11.7	7.8	0.8	Not reported
Touboul et al. [A4]	383 post AMI OCS	SDNN	18.7	–	–	Not reported
Huikuri et al. [127]	446 post AMI	α_1–fractal index	31.9	–	–	Not reported
Tsuji et al. 1994 [A5]	1028 Framingham elderly cohort	Log LF 100s avgs	26.8	15.6	7.4	Similar outcome in excluded for arrhythmia/artefacts/medication use
Algra et al. 1993 [362]	245 SCD victims 268 controls	SDNNI SDANNI	19.6 / 14.1	– / –	– / –	90% survival rate in included 88% survival rate in excluded
Zuanetti et al. 1996 [346]	567 AMI GUSTO participants	NN50+	~50	NR	NR	Similar clinical characteristics Outcome not reported
Lanza et al. 1998 [348]	239 AMI OCS[b]	VLF	34	NR	NR	Not reported

Study	Sample	Measure				Comments
Nollo et al. 2001 [A6]	324 AMI GISSI-3 participants	LF power	13.4	NR	13.4 (non-sinus rhythm)	Not reported
Bilchick et al. 2002 [360]	179 CHF-STAT participants	SDNN	29.1	2.7	19.6	Not reported
Carnethon et al. 2002 [249]	9267 ARIC participants	SDNN 2 min	13.3 25.6^d	NR	NR	Rejected subjects older, more frequently females, obese. Worse outcome among rejected (higher MI and fatal CHD rate compared to included sample)
Forslund et al. 2002 [A7]	641 CAD APSIS participants		20.7	NR	NR	Not reported
Sosnowski et al. 2002 [64]	298 PMI patients OCS	HRVF	<1	0	<0.5^b	^{b}Implanted pacemaker and paroxysmal tachyarrhythmias among excluded
Sajadieh et al. 2003 [524]	643 Copenhagen Holter Study healthy	SDNN	17%	NR	NR	Technically best continuous period of 24 h selected from the 48-h Holter recordings
Abildstrom et al. 2003 [706]	366 BEAT Study screening phase participants	SDNN	23.9	NR	NR	Not reported
Lampert et al. 2003 [A8]	184 BHAT participants	HF pNN50	40.5	NR	NR	A significant proportion of patients excluded for insufficient data length
La Rovere et al. 2003 [A9]	202/242 CHF (derivation/ validation sample)	LF power (AR)	50.9	9.6	26 (AF or pace-maker)	15.3% clinically unstable patients among excluded
Jokinen V et al. 2003 [A10]	600 AMI/416 PMI MRFAT – OCS	α_1 – fractal index	11.1	NR	NR	Not reported

◻ **Table 3.10** (Continued)

Author/year	Population (included)	HRV measure (most prognostic)	% rejected[a] Overall	For the presence of artefacts	For the presence of cardiac arrhythmias	Clinical significance/comments
Schroeder EB et al. 2003 [A11]	6931 ARIC participants	RMSSD (2–6 min)	2.3	NR	NR	Not reported
Aronson et al. 2004 [361]	255 decompensated CHF, PRECEDENT participant	SDNN	22.0	NR	NR	Not reported
Stein Pk et al. 2004 [A12]	830 CAST participants		11.4		4.3	Not reported
Wichterle D et al. 2004 [83]	663 EMIAT participants	Time Spectral PLF	6.5 4.1 17.9	NR	NR	Not reported
Carpeggiani C et al. 2004 [A13]	413 AMI MCS[c]	LF power (AR)	9.2	NR	NR	Not reported
Jokinen V et al. 2005 [578]	41 elderly subjects longitudinal FU study		35.9		14 (AF)	Not reported
Rashba EJ et al. 2006 [250]	274 DEFINITE participants	SDNN	23.0	NR	16 (AF) 7 (frequent PEBs)	Worst outcome in patients excluded from the study ($p < 0.02$)
Casaleggi et al. 2007 [A14]	200 HF patients	SDNN	54.9	NR	23.9 (AF or pacemaker)	Not reported
Huikuri et al. 2009 [352]	312 CARISMA participants	SDNN HRT TWA	NR	NR	NR	HRV available in 252 (80.8%), HRT in 243 (77.9%), TWA in 215 (68.9%); outcome in those without HRV/HRT/TWA not reported

[a] Patients rejected due to exclusion criteria not included

[b] OCS – one centre study

[c] MCS – multi-centre study

[d] in standing position TM – total (all-cause) mortality, CVM – cardio-vascular mortality, AE – arrhythmic events, AMI – acute myocardial infarction, PMI – previous myocardial infarction, AF- atrial firbillation, PEB– premature ectopic beats, NR- not reported

◻ Table 3.11

Applicability of HRT, BRS or combined cardiac autonomic control measures in clinical outcome studies

Author/year	Population (included)	HRV measure (most prognostic)	% rejected Overall	% rejected For the presence of artefacts	% rejected For the presence of cardiac arrhythmias	Clinical significance/comments
Schmidt et al. 1999 [222]	577 MPIP 614 EMIAT	HRT (TS+TO)	19 [MPIP] 17.4 [EMIAT]	NR	NR	Outcome in excluded patients not reported AF among a priori criteria of exclusion
Ghuran et al. 2002 [226]	1212 ATRAMI	SDNN HRT BRS All 3	9.8 19.1 7.6 22.7	NR	NR	Similar survival in patients with and without HRT AF among a priori criteria of exclusion
Barthel et al. 2003 [A15]	1455 ISAR-HRT	HRVI HRT	NR	NR	NR	HRT calculation impossible in 29.1% Outcome in these patients as good as in patients with normal HRT
Bauer at al. 2006 [170]	608 EMIAT	HRT (TD)	58.8	NR	NR	Outcome in excluded patients not reported AF among a priori criteria of exclusion
Exner et al. 2007 [A16]	332 AMI REFINE	SDNN HRT BRS	49.0	NR	20 (for AF) 6 (ICD)	Outcome in excluded patients not reported
Stein PK et al. 2008 [365]	1197 CHS (>65 YOA)	DFA1 HRT	16.2	NR	6.1	Clinical characteristics of initial 1429 eligible subjects similar, outcome not reported AF among a priori criteria of exclusion
Mäkikallio et al. 2006 [A17]	2130 AMI FINGER	SDNN HRT (TS) DFA1	NR	NR	NR	NR AF among a priori criteria of exclusion
Klingenheben et al. 2008 [A18]	114 HF Frankfurt DCM	SDNN HRT BRS	2 10 25	NR	NR	23% with and ICD implanted AF among a priori criteria of exclusion

patients with previous MI. In an epidemiological study (The ARIC Study), excluded subjects were older, more frequently females and obese, and their outcome was worse with a higher MI/fatal CHD rate compared to HRV study participants [249]. Observations from the DEFINITE trial indicate that patients excluded due to the presence of frequent ventricular PEBs or atrial fibrillation have a lower survival rate than patients in whom HRV analysis is possible [250].

A new promising index of HRV, i.e., *deceleration capacity* (DC), has been shown to be applicable to almost all patients in sinus rhythm. However, the presence of atrial fibrillation still limits its applicability to the entire spectrum of patients [171].

The index that possesses the potential for HRV global description in patients either in sinus rhythm or in atrial fibrillation is the HRV Fraction [65]. A uniquely low exclusion rate (less than 1%) with HRVF use has been observed in the post-MI population [66]. Unfortunately, this index has not achieved wider interest. The HRVF can be applied extensively but not to ECG recordings with long periods of atrial flutter/tachycardia or very frequent PEBs (>25% of all heartbeats) or with a pacemaker-driven rhythm. Interestingly, the author's investigations indicate very similar properties for the SDANN (*unpublished*). However, systematic studies are necessary to justify its usefulness in nonselected populations of patients with and without arrhythmias. Nevertheless, documented data on risk prediction with the use of the SDANN, indicates its superiority compared to the SDNN [252–254], as does our own data. More intensive use of the SDANN in clinical outcome studies is awaited.

3.4.6   Robustness

Robustness is one of the most important properties of indices of HRV methods, mainly because the necessity for time-consuming manual editing of the data-series can be minimized [4, 5, 34]. Results of HRV analysis with the use of a robust index/method are similar irrespective of the presence of noisy data (artefacts, non-stationarities, PEBs, AF). The use of a less robust index/method requires noisy data to be eliminated. The latter procedure, however, might lead to a loss of significant information. From data provided in ❷ Table 3.10, it can be concluded that the standard time- and spectral HRV indices are sensitive to artefacts and sudden IBI changes of either physiological or pathological origins. The robustness of nonlinear indices is rather moderate and strongly depends on the method used. However, for most such indices, their robustness is unknown. The HRV index (St. George's index) was the first introduced to improve robustness. However, the HRVI is critically sensitive to the distribution of data and cannot be reliably determined in the presence of a bimodal distribution [38]. HRVF and DC are indices with high robustness, which are also independent of the distribution of IBIs [65, 171].

3.4.7   Biological Variations

Variation in HR reflects the adjustment to changeable metabolic demands of key vital organs in response to internal and external stimuli in a specific neuro-humoral milieu, and any of the HRV measures obtained at a given time varies accordingly. In a controlled environment (the same time of recording, mental and physical activity, drugs and so on), this variation is still present in an individual subject and between individuals. This variation is referred to as *biological variation*. The biological variation is always present as most of the factors (genetics, race, age, gender etc.) that determine HRV cannot be controlled in any way. Biological variation differs from other sources of HR variation which are related to investigator biases (intra- and inter-observer errors) and technical precision of measurements (❷ Fig. 3.28). However, it has to be stressed that in an individual subject or a population sample, the biological variation can be much greater than reported as the average. The study population (healthy subjects, patients with certain diseases), conditions of examinations, like breathing (spontaneous, controlled, deep breathing, Valsalva maneuver), body position (supine, standing), exercise (treadmill, bicycle) or other testing (head-up or head-down tilting, mental stressing, cold pressor test, and so on) might be an important determinant of intra- and inter-individual reproducibility. Importantly, errors due to the foregoing might have a different contribution on the overall measurements in patients with an already reduced HRV. Lastly, use of various periods of ECG recordings (second, minutes, hours) or different algorithms for traditional spectral HRV measures (AR, FFT) might be in part responsible for differences in quantification of the degree of such errors. Thus, a purpose-specific use of different HRV methods requires the determination of predictable errors (possibly drawn from

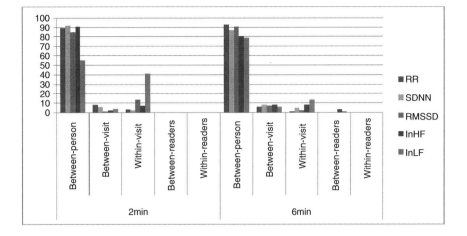

Fig. 3.33

Measurement errors of common HRV measures: components by length of short-term recordings. The main source of HRV errors can attribute to inter-individual variation, except for spectral HRV measures, where between- and within-visit changes may play a significant role (i.e., lnLF, lnHF). Importantly, readers' errors are entirely negligible. However, there is a space for within-visit errors if spectral HRV is aimed to be measured (According to data provided by Schroder et al. [255])

former validation studies) and a proper calculation of the sample in order to detect a significant change of a particular HRV measure [255].

3.4.7.1 Intra-Individual Variation

The determination of intra-individual variation of HRV indices requires the definition of their range in the setting of controlled conditions in the same subject. Within the same visit, variation attributed to intra-individual short-term variation accounted for 5–14% for SDRR, 2–7% for RMSSD, 8–28% for HF power and 14–41% for LF power [256]. The contribution of intra-individual variation decreases with prolongation of recording length (● Table 3.12). Also, between-measurement period duration influences the contribution of intra-individual variation on the measurements (● Table 3.12). If more repeated measurements on different visits are performed, the contribution of intra-individual variation between visits appears to be even lower. It accounted for 0.5–7% for SDRR, 2–7% for RMSSD, 3–8% for HF power and 4–6% for LF power [256]. In contrast, the contribution of intra-individual variation increases with prolongation of recording length and can reach 30% for a certain HRV measures. Intra-individual variations might be of importance for studies in which the effects of internal or external stimuli are to be examined. The intra-individual variation can be in part a source of measurement error of HRV indices calculated from long-term recordings. However, strict estimates of these errors have not yet been provided.

Intra-individual variation range provides limits beyond which HRV changes can be considered significant and interpreted as a true effect of interventions or changes in study conditions. It is of importance since intra-individual variation might be even greater than inter-individual variation [256].

3.4.7.2 Inter-Individual Variation

Inter-individual variation defines the range of HRV in a population. The determination of between-subject variation is necessary when population (or subpopulation) studies are going to be undertaken in order to detect effects of various interventions. Awareness of inter-individual variations is necessary with the interpretation of changes of the mean

▣ Table 3.12

Intra-individual variability of HRV measures in healthy subjects (Coefficient of variation)

Author[s] Source/Year	Subjects	Condition[s]	RRI [or HR]	SDRR	RMSSD	LF	HF	Comments
Kanters et al. 1996 [A19]	12 healthy adults 6F, 6M Age 31 (25–38)	Supine Free breathing	3.7%	11.7%	NR	20.3%	35.2%	3 separate days 3 h FFT
Sinnreich et al. 1998 [269]	70 healthy adults 38F, 32M Age 49 (31–67)	Supine Free breathing	NR	6.0%	8.0%	11.5%	12.1%	2 months apart 5 min AR [16 order]
		Supine Metronome 15/min	NR	6.1%	7.4%	10.7%	10.5%	
Schroeder et al. 2004 [255]	63 healthy adults 31F, 32M Age 52 (45–64)	Supine Free breathing	8.6%	5.8%	6.7%	6.3%	8.0%	1–2 weeks apart 6 min FFT
Højgaard et al. 2005 [266]	14 healthy adults 5F, 9M Age 31 (22–38)	Supine Free breathing	6.0%	NR	NR	27%	28%	Day-to-day 1024 s (~17 min) FFT
		Head-up tilt of 60°	5.0%	NR	NR	26%	32%	
Zollei et al. 2007 [A20]	10 healthy adults 3F, 7M Age 25 ± 2	Supine Free breathing	7.1%	22.5%	32.8%	61.8%	63.7%	10 consecutive days 5 min, FFT
		Metronome 6/min	6.4%	17.3%	24.3%	36.5%	50.4%	
Kobayashi et al. 2007 [A21]	73 healthy males Age 20–61	Supine	5.0%[HR]	NR	NR	21.2%	19.5%	4–8 sessions 1 day 204.8 s (~3 min) FFT
		Standing	4.7%	NR	NR	23%	20.1%	

or median values. This is also an ultimate condition for the determination of normal limits and the definition of abnormal HRV.

Between-subject variation is the main source of measurement error. For time-domain HRV indices, it contributes 86 to 91% of the entire error and was shown to be independent of data length [256] (❷ Table 3.13). For spectral HRV indices (HF and LF power), its contribution ranges from 69 to 81% and 55 to 79%, respectively, being greater for a longer data-length [256].

3.4.7.3   Intra and Inter-Observer Errors

Measurement errors define the range of subjective assessment of data-series. Intuitively, this depends on the robustness of the HRV method or index. If manual editing and visual inspection is necessary, the differences both between measurements performed by the same investigator (intra-observer error) and by two investigators within the same data-series (inter-observer error) can be assumed to be greater compared to a robust method/index, which is calculated automatically without any investigator's management of the data-series [34, 256].

Intra-observer errors for HRV short-term recordings have been shown to account for less than 0.1% of total measurements errors. Inter-observer errors for short-term HRV were estimated to account for less than 0.1% of the measurement error for time-domain indices and less than 3% for spectral indices [256]. In the ARIC study, the intra- and inter-observer variance of 2-min SDNN has been reported to reach $0.04\ ms^2$ (0.6%) and $3.24\ ms^2$ (5.3%) [258]. The inter-observer error relates also to the condition of analysis (manual, automatic, pre-defined fixed frequency) [259], being lower in the latter setting. The inter-observer error has been reported to be greater in a study on patients with chronic stable CAD, where the respective data for 5-min and 40-min recordings ranged between 0.2–6.0% and 0.1–1.2% [260] The longer the data-series analyze d, the greater the errors on the part of the observers. Kroll et al. noticed the inter-observer errors reaching 8% as a result of inaccurate labeling of heartbeats, especially PEBs, in intentionally selected patients with aortic regurgitation [261]. The SDANN index proved to be least sensitive to the inter-observer error [261, 262].

Only one study addressed this issue in children [263]. In the Bogalusa Heart Study, in which 20 children aged 10–16 years old had been included, the inter-observer errors in the estimation of time-domain and frequency-domain measures did not exceed 1% and 4%, respectively [263].

The intra- and inter-observer errors depend in part on technical characteristics of available instruments. The use of different devices influences the level of agreement for either short-time frequency-domain or long-term time-domain indices [257, 263, 264].

3.4.7.4   Reproducibility

Reproducibility characterizes the summarized effect of intra-individual, inter-individual, intra-observer and inter-observer errors, as well as precision accuracy, assuming similar length and conditions of HRV recordings. In addition, the use of different devices influences the comparisons of different interventions and their reproducibility. A high reproducibility can be defined by various measures, like the coefficient of variation (as being <10%), intra-class coefficient (>0.79), limits of agreement (LOA, 75–125%) and others [256]. Values of CV, ICC and LOA that indicate acceptable (minimum) reproducibility are <30% and >0.60 and 60–140%, respectively.

❷ Tables 3.14 and ❷ 3.15 provide results of selected studies that addressed this issue in healthy subjects. The results of reproducibility in patients with specific CV diseases are presented in ❷ Tables 3.16 and ❷ 3.17.

Murray et al. showed a poor to moderate reproducibility of 5-min HRV measurements repeated 2–3 min apart with LOA between 61% and 157% for SDNN in a wide age-range sample (21–77 years) [265]. Similarly, minute-to-minute reproducibility of spectral HRV indices was found to be moderate in young subjects in a study of Højgaard et al. [266]. The CV was lowest for HF and LF/HF (27–28%), However, a great inter-individual variability range was noticed (2–75%). On the contrary, in middle-aged subjects, Pikkujämsä et al. found the SDNN very highly reproducible if evaluated by means of a CV of 2% [141].

Moderate or poor day-to-day reproducibility of short-term HRV measures has been reported for various spectral indices (mean CV between 27–39%) in young adults [266] and even poorer in children with a CV range of 35–97% [267].

■ Table 3.13

Inter-individual variability of HRV measures (Reliability coefficient)

Author[s] Year	Subjects	Condition[s]	RRI [or HR]	SDRR	RMSSD	LF	HF	Comments
Kanters et al. 1996 [A19]	12 healthy adults 6F, 6M Age 31 (25–38)	Supine Free breathing	0.96	0.86	NR	0.94 (AU)	0.89 (AU)	3 separate days 3 h FFT
Sinnreich et al. 1998 [268]	70 healthy adults 38F, 32M Age 49 (31–67)	Supine Free breathing	NR	0.77	0.75	0.68	0.76	2 months apart 5 min AR [16 order]
		Supine Metronome 15/min	NR	0.78	0.78	0.75	0.82	
Schroeder et al. 2004 [255]	63 healthy adults 31F, 32M Age 52 (45–64)	Supine Free breathing	0.93	0.87	0.91	0.79 (ln)	0.81 (ln)	1–2 weeks apart 6 min FFT

◼ Table 3.14

Reproducibility of HRV measures from long-term ECG recordings in healthy subjects

Author[s]/ Source/Year	No of examined subjects	Between-measurement period	Parameter	Mean difference between recordings	Statistics	Results
Kleiger et al. 1991 [A22]	14 healthy adults	3–65 days	NNI SDNN SDNNI RMSSD pNN50 lnTP [FFT] lnLF lnHF	–	ICC (mean, ±3 SEM)	0.90, 297 ms 0.70, 54 ms 0.90, 24 ms 0.90, 24 ms 0.90, 12% 0.89, 4025 ms^2 0.91, 1042 ms^2 0.84, 1042 ms^2
Pitzalis et al. 1996 [296]	20 healthy adults Mean age 28 ± 2	Day-to-day 2 weeks and 7 months	NNI SDNN pNN50 RMSSD	NA	ICC	0.75 0.57 0.78 0.79
Nolan et al. 1996 [276]	19 healthy adults 44 ± 13 years	13 ± 9 days	pNN50	1.15%	ICC	0.97
Sosnowski M et al. 2005 [65]	165 healthy adults 49.5 ± 6 years	Day-to-day	RRI SDNN SDANN pNN50 HRVI HRVF	17.8 ms −2.8 ms −4.4 ms 0.78% −0.02 U −0.72%	LOA	−79 – 112.5 ms −41 – 35 ms −57 – 48 ms −4.79 – 6.35% −12.9 – 12.9U −13.4 – 11.9%
Huikuri et al. 1990 [284]	20 healthy males 20–40 years	7 days	SDNNI	–	CV (intraindividual) CV (interindividual)	7 ± 6% 24%
		Day-to-day (recalculated)	SDNNI	–	CV (intraindividual)	4.2 ± 2.9%

Table 3.14 (Continued)

Author[s]/ Source/Year	No of examined subjects	Between-measurement period	Parameter	Mean difference between recordings	Statistics	Results
Hohnloser et al. 1992 [281]	17 healthy adults Mean age 24±2.5 years	Day-to-day, 1 week and 1 month	SDNN pNN50 RMSSD	NA	CV	13.7 ± 6.8% 23.5 ± 14.6% 18.5 ± 12.6%
Ziegler D et al. 1997 [580]	17 healthy subjects 7M/10F 26–45 years	Median 29 weeks	SDNNI RMSSD pNN50 CV HRVI lnHF lnLF lnVLF CV-SA CV-LA	–	CV	6.8% 10.6% 14.8% 4.2% 1.9% 11.1% 11.9% 10.5% 7.9% 13.0%
Van Hoogenhuyze et al. 1991 [277]	33 healthy adults Mean age 34 years	Day-to-day	SDANN SDNNI SDNNI-CV	12.3 ± 11.7% 7.8 ± 6.9% 5.7 ± 4.3%	VR	0.2–46% 0.4–25.9% 0–16%

ICC (intraclass coefficient), ≥0.6 acceptable, ≥0.8 high, LOA (limit of agreement) 75–125% high, 60–140% acceptable, CV (coefficient of variation)=(SD$_{within}$/mean$_{between\ measurements}$)*100%, <30% acceptable, VR (variation range), <30% acceptable

Table 3.15

Reproducibility of HRV measures from short-term ECG recordings in healthy subjects

Author[s], Source/Year	Subjects	Duration of ECG recordings / Between-measurements period	HRV measures	Statistics	Results
Intraclass coefficient (ICC, ≥0.6 acceptable, ≥0.8 high)					
Pitzalis et al. 1996 [296]	20 young adults 10F, 10M Aged 28 ± 2 SB / CB 16 breaths/min	10 min 2 weeks 7 months	RRI SDRR pNN50 rMSSD LF [FFT] HF LF/HF LF [AR12] HF LF/HF	ICC (mean) SB / CB	0.37 / 0.35 0.56 / 0.27 0.40 / 0.43 0.23 / 0.20 0.77 / 0.60 0.48/0.65 0.20 / 0.36 0.70 / 0.60 0.15 / 0.70 0.06 / 0.48
Carrasco et al. 2003 [300]	11 healthy adults 6F, 5M Age 23.1± 1.3 SB / CB 12 breaths/min	5 min 3 sessions 5 day period	HR SDHR rMSSD [HR] CV [HR] HF [AR, order?] HF [N.U.] LF LF [N.U]. LF/HF	ICC (mean) SB / CB	0.82 / 0.81 0.93 / 0.94 0.92 / 0.94 0.91 / 0.94 0.86 / 0.93 0.77 / 0.88 0.86 / 0.92 0.79 / 0.88 0.85 / 0.88
Lobnig et al. 2003 [297]	7 healthy adults Age 20–28 CB 12 breaths/min	5 min 3 sessions (2 in supine position) 4 days	Ln LF [FFT] Ln HF	ICC (range of means)	0.66–0.69 0.76–0.81
Kowalewski, Urban 2004 [A23]	26 healthy males Age 22 ± 1 SB	10 min 3 pairs of tests, 3 days initially, 6 months, 24 months, Long-term (0', 6 and 24 months)	TP [FFT] LF HF LF/HF	ICC (95%CI)	0.73–0.89 0.66–0.85 0.72–0.89 0.54–0.75

Table 3.15 (Continued)

Author[s]. Source/Year	Subjects	Duration of ECG recordings Between-measurements period	HRV measures	Statistics	Results
Schroeder et al. 2004 [255]	63 adults* 31F, 32M Age 45–64 SB	10 sec, 2 min, 6 min 1–2 weeks	RRI SDNN RMSSD HF [FFT] LF HF(N.U.) LF (N.U.).	ICC (95%CI)	0.78–0.96 0.22–0.92 0.30–0.95 0.79–0.93 0.65–0.89 0.48–0.85 0.48–0.85
Guijt et al. 2007 [302]	26 healthy adults 18F, age 28 ± 6 8M, age 34 ± 12 SB	7 min lying down, night 2nd and 4th 10 min light exercise (cycling)	SDNN RMSSD SDNN RMSSD	ICC 95%CI SEM	0.50–0.94 0.51–0.99 12.35–13.95 2.01–10.37
Zollei et al. 2007 [A20]	10 healthy adults 3F, 7M Age 25 ± 2 SB / CB 6 breaths/min	5 min supine 10 consecutive days	RRI SDNN RMSSD LF (ms2)(FFT) HF	ICC (mean) SB / CB	0.961 / 0.961 0.967 / 0.979 0.968 / 0.977 0.873 / 0.974 0.964 / 0.970
Maestri et al. 2007 [268]	42 healthy adults 21F, 21M Age 38 (26–56)	5 min supine Day-to-day	RRI SampEn DFA HDF SD21 nCCE other nonlinear¶	ICC (mean, 95%CI)	0.76 (0.59–0.87) 0.54 (0.28–0.72) 0.68 (0.47–0.82) 0.69 (0.49–0.82) 0.78 (0.62–0.88) 0.67 (0.46–0.82) 0.18–0.72 (–0.13–0.84)

Study	Population	Protocol	Measures	Statistic	Values
Murray et al. 2001 [265]	50 healthy adults 19F, 31M Age 21–77 SB	5 min 2–3 minutes apart	CIPA RMSSD SDNN ln HF ln LF	LOA	72–140% 68–153% 61–157% 76–133% 77–131%
Sandercock et al. 2004 [295]	29 healthy adults 9F, aged 29 ± 11 20M, aged 35 ± 13 SB / CB 12 breaths/min	5 min 7 ± 3 days apart	RRI SDNN RMSSD LF (FFT) HF	LOA For CB Absolute values	−147–147 −49.5–44.6 −73.8–63.9 −968–749 −1803–1670
Maestri et al. 2007 [268]	42 healthy adults 21F, 21M Age 38 (26–56) SB	5 min supine Day-to-day	RRI SampEn DFA HDF SD21 nCCE	LOA Absolute values	−162–162 −0.59–0.59 −0.45–0.45 −0.29–0.29 −1.48–1.48 −0.16–0.16
Coefficient of variation (CV, <30% acceptable)					
Kanters et al. 1996 [A19]	12 adults 6F, 6M Age range 25–38 SB	3 hour periods 3 separate days	RRI SDRR HF [a.u.][FFT] LF [a.u.] CorrDim	CV (mean)	3.7% 11.7% 35.3% 20.3% 12.5%
Sinnreich et al. 1998 [269]	70 healthy adults 38F, 32M Age 31–67 SB / CB 15 breaths/min	5 min 2 month apart	Ln SDRR Ln RMSSD Ln TP [AR16] Ln LF LnHF	CV (mean)	6.0%/6.1% 8.0%/7.4% 7.0%/6.7% 11.5%/10.7% 12.1%/10.5%
Lord et al. 2001 [271]	21 healthy adults Mean age 37 CB 10 breaths/min	5 min 3 sessions 3 separate days (one week apart)	lnLF [FFT]	CV (mean)	45%

Table 3.15   (Continued)

Author[s], Source/Year	Subjects	Duration of ECG recordings / Between-measurements period	HRV measures	Statistics	Results
Pikkujämsa et al. 2001 [141]	50 healthy adults 25F, 25 M Age 40–59	5 min One session, two separate periods from 13 min recording	SDNN LF (ms²)[AR20] HF (ms²)	CV (recalculated, mean)	2% 10% 14%
Gerritsen J 2003 [599]	36 healthy adults Age 50–75	3 min 3 consecutive days 2 sessions one day	RRI SDNN HF LF LF/(LF+HF)	CV (mean)	8% 30% 71% 76% 22%
Winsley et al. 2003 [267]	12 healthy children Age 11–12 Controlled breathing 12 breath/min	5 min Day-to-day	SDNN RMSSD pNN50 HF (ms2) HF (N.U.) LF (ms2) LF (N.U.) LF/HF	CV (mean)	31% 37% 81% 84% 35% 97% 38% 83%
Højgaard MV et al. 2005 [266]	14 healthy adults 5F, 9M Age 22–38 years	5 min Day-to-day 4 sessions	RRI TP [FFT] LF HF LF/HF	CV (mean, range)	4% (0–10) 36% (9–93) 39% (2–73) 27% (2–75) 28% (2–60)
		5 min, 17 min (1024 s) 2 weeks apart, 3 sessions	RRI TP (FFT) LF HF LF/HF	CV (mean, short/long)	5 / 6% 25 / 24% 29 / 27% 31 / 28% 20 / 18%
Koskinen et al. 2009 [576]	43 healthy adults Age 24–39 CB 15 breaths/min	3 min supine 131 ± 4 days	SDNN RMSSD TP (FFT) LF HF LF/HF	CV	5.3% 7.1% 5.9% 8.1% 6.8% 11.5%

□ Table 3.16

Reproducibility of HRV measures from short-term ECG recordings in patients

Author[s], Source/Year	Subjects	Duration of ECG recordings Between-measurements period	HRV measures	Statistics	Results
Stein et al. 1995 [280]	15 CHF-patients Aged 52 ± 9 CB 6 breaths/min	30 s 2 weeks	RSA (peak-to trough, CB)	ICC	0.70
Ponikowski et al. 1996 [733]	16 CHF-patients Aged 60 ± 8	5-, 10-, 20 and 40 min from two 60-min recordings 25 days (mean)	RRI SDNN pNN50 Spectral *(FFT)*	CV (%)	*8% 25.3–30.2% 70–139% 45–111%*
Freed et al. 1994 [274]	15 CHF-patients	2 adjacent 10-min Pre- and post-operative 2 periods	TP *(FFT)* LF HF	CV (%) Pre/Post	9/6 15/12 11/9
Salo TM et al. 1999 [270]	15 hypertensive patients with OSAS Aged 47 ± 10 SB/CB 6 breath/min	5 min/2 min > 3 weeks apart 4 recordings	HR RMSM (~SDNN) CV RMSSD HF (AR) HF [N.U.] LF LF [N.U.] LF/HF	CV_{SD} (mean)	*9.3%/8.3% 33.9%/21.8% 32.8%/21.4% 56.7%/30.4% 97.3%/56.3% 13.9%/3.3% 92.7%/59.5% 13.9%/3.3% 71.3%/48.6%*
Haas et al. 2000 [272]	158 AMI-patients 39F, 119M Aged 60 ± 12 SB (39) and CB (n=83) 10 breaths/min	5 min One session, 2 measurements (5 min in between) 1 week	SDRR [ms] VR [bpm]	Pearson's r	0.87/0.88 0.87/0.95
			SDRR [ms] VR [bpm]	LOA	−14.12 − 11.64 ms −8.87 − 7.98 bpm
Parati et al. 2001 [299]	8 hypertensive females Age 29–54 CB 18 breaths/min	15 min 1 month	PI (IBI) SD(PI) VLF *(FFT)* LF HF	VC (SB/CB)	5 ± 1/5 ± 4 19 ± 8/18 ± 15 6 ± 4/6 ± 5 5 ± 4/6 ± 9 12 ± 8/6 ± 8
Lord SW et al. 2001 [271]	21 HTX-patients Mean age 55 CB 10 breaths/min	5 min 3 sessions 3 separate days (1 week apart)	LF *(FFT)*	CV (%)	76

◻ **Table 3.16**   (Continued)

Author[s], Source/Year	Subjects	Duration of ECG recordings Between-measurements period	HRV measures	Statistics	Results
Chemla et al. 2005 [275]	12 DM-patients Aged 49 ± 12	5 min 3 measurements 5 s apart (overlapping) Day-by-day	RRI SDRR TP (*FFT*) LF HF LF/HF TP (*AR*) LF HF LF/HF	CV (%) or bias error (%)*	2 ± 11* 17 ± 41* 8 ± 5 10 ± 6 5 ± 6 10 ± 5 7 ± 9 47 ± 55 6 ± 6 44 ± 55
Tarkiainen et al. 2005 [260]	89 stable CAD-patients 21F, 68M Aged 67 ± 8 (40–83) SB and CB (12 breaths/min)	5 min 3–4 months	RRI SDNN RMSSD lnLF (*FFT*) lnHF ln (LF/HF)	CV (%) (SB/CB)	6.1/6.0 29.9/37.1 48.9/52.1 11.3/16.5 14.7/14.9 11.5/16.1
	Spontaneous breathing + controlled breathing + exercise test + recovery period	40 min 3–4 months	NNI SDNN RMSSD lnVLF (*FFT*) lnLF lnHF ln(LF/HF)	CV (%) (all protocols)	5.1 16.7 31.1 4.9 8.6 11.0 7.3

The evidence for reproducibility of nonlinear HRV measures is sparse. In a study by Maestri et al. [268], only a ratio of SD1 to SD2 from a return map has been shown to be reproducible (❯ Table 3.14). The DFA and SampEn were shown to be moderately reproducible. Reproducibility of other nonlinear HRV measures has been reported to be rather poor [268].

In several studies, measurement errors were quantified for a longer period between repeated investigations. It was found that the long-term reproducibility of short-term HRV indices appears better than that of the shorter term reproducibility. Sinnreich et al. found the CV values of logarithmically transformed HRV indices to be between 6–12.1% [269]. In their study, the SDNN, RMSSD, total and VLF power were highly reproducible while the HF and LF power were only moderately reproducible. Interestingly, controlled breathing did not improve their reproducibility. Reported ICC values for LF vary from 0.66 to 0.87 with FFT and 0.70–0.86 with AR. Similarly, for HF, the ICC values are between 0.48–0.96 (FFT) and 0.15–0.86 (AR). The largest differences of the ICC related to LF/HF with the worst reported being 0.06 (sic)(AR) and the best being 0.85 (AR). For very short registrations (10 s), the ICC values ranged between 0.41 and 0.57 [255]. Increasing the number of repeated measurements seems to improve reproducibility of short-term HRV measures (❯ Table 3.14).

Thus, 5-min recordings provide most (moderate in fact) of the reproducible data for standard indices. However, in healthy subjects, their relative changes between examinations can reach 30% (overall), which should be considered as independent of biological and measurement variation.

Many studies have addressed the issue of reproducibility of HRV indices from 24-h ECGs in healthy subjects (❯ Table 3.15). In the largest one, 165 healthy adults were included [65]. For the time-domain HRV indices the ICC was found to be good or high (>0.7) if compared from day-to-day. However, individual subjects showed a high range of variation explored by means of LOA. Thus, if significant changes of HRV indices are defined as lying beyond LOA, significant (independent from biological and measurement variation) changes of SDNN

■ Table 3.17

Reproducibility of HRV measures from long-term ECG recordings in patients

Author[s], Source/Year	Subjects	Between-measurements period	HRV measures	Statistics	Results
Bigger et al. 1992 [278]	40 PMI-patients (20 CAPS, 20 ESVEM participants)	Day-to-day	ULF (FFT) other spectral	ICC (CAPS/ESVEM)	0.79/0.89 > 0.85/ > 0.79
Van Hoogenhuyze et al. 1991 [277]	22 CHF-patients (CAD) NYHA II-III 4F, 18M Aged 59 ± 7	Day-to-day	RRI SDNNI SDANN	ICC (recalculated from data)	0.95 0.96 0.87
Stein et al. 1995 [280]	17 CHF-patients NYHA II-III, EF 12F, 5M Aged 52 ± 9	2 weeks	HR NNI SDNN SDANN SDNNI RMSSD pNN50 TP (ln) ULF (ln) VLF (ln) LF(ln) HF (ln)	ICC	0.95 0.88 0.91 0.88 0.87 0.49 0.23 0.91 0.90 0.91 0.88 0.86
Nolan et al. 1996 [276]	67 CAD-patients 58 ± 7	2–16 weeks	pNN50	ICC CR	0.94 41%
Anastasiou-Nana et al. 2001 [282]	14 CHF-patients NYHA II-IV, EF 13± 6% 2F, 12M Aged 52 ± 11 (25–65)	14 consecutive days > 18 h of analyzable data	SDNN SDANN SDNNI RMSSD pNN50 LF HF	ICC (mean ± SD)	0.87 ± 0.01 0.85 ± 0.02 0.82 ± 0.02 0.44 ± 0.05 0.31 ± 0.05 0.80 ± 0.02 0.66 ± 0.03
Kautzner J et al. 1995 [275]	33 AMI-patients 5F, 28M Aged 55 ± 11	Day-to-day (48-h recordings)	SDNN SDANN SDNNI RMSSD pNN50 HRVI TINN	Absolute relative errors (range)	1–27% 2–30% −2–23% −8–37% 0–90% 2–36% −1–38%
Weber et al. 1998 [283]	421 CAD-patients 45F, 376M Aged 56,6 (31–78)	Day-to-day	SDNN SDANN pNN50	Maximum value relative to base-line/Pearson's correlation coefficient	35.8/0.86 40.4/0.84 53.5/0.91
Burger et al. 1997 [A24]	23 DM1-type patients 8F, 15M Aged 37 ± 10	3, 6, 9, and 12 months	Time-domain Spectral-domain	Pearsons's correlation coefficient	0.35–0.98 0.47–0.93

would be considered if its value was reduced by 41 ms or increased by 35 ms (for the mean SDNN of 140 ms changes need to be less than 99 ms or greater than 175 ms) in an individual subject. This corresponds to a change of 25–30% from the initial value. Similarly, a change of at least 25% is necessary to consider significant difference for time-domain indices, including HRVI and HRVF. This finding is consistent with observations made by others for short-term recordings.

The reported CV of SDNN from 24-h ECG recordings in healthy subjects varies from 4.2 to 10.3% on a day-to-day basis, and 9.6% for a 6-month period between repeated measurements. Thus, *the difference of approximately 10% from the initial SDNN value can be considered statistically significant if the time-distance from repeated measurements is longer than 6 months*. The pNN50 was found to be least reproducible in some studies and highly reproducible in others (❷ Table 3.15).

Reproducibility of the HRV indexes may play a greater role in patients with a reduced HRV, in whom a similar range of absolute differences between measurements makes the relative differences even greater. However, a simple comparison between data from healthy subjects and patients with certain diseases cannot be conclusive, as various data-length and reproducibility measures have been used.

Studies in which a comparison between normal subjects and patients has been performed are scarce. Short-term HRV reproducibility has been found to be poorer in hypertensive patients with OSAS in a study of Salo et al. [270] (❷ Tables 3.14 and ❷ 3.16). In another study in patients after heart transplantation, the coefficient of variation of the LF component reached 76%, being greater than in healthy controls [45%] [271]. According to the dots-data (from the figure) provided in a report by Haas et al. in post-MI patients [272], the mean value of short-term (5-min) SDNN of around 20 ms was associated with the LOA of measurement being −14 to 12 ms, accounting for −70 to 160%, indicating rather a poor reproducibility. In a comparable study of Sinnreich et al. in healthy subjects, the recalculated mean value of 5-min SDNN of 37 ms has been associated with a 6% coefficient of variation (i.e., ± 17% range) [269].

A poor or moderate reproducibility of short-term HRV measures has been reported in patients with CHF (❷ Table 3.16) with the CV range between 25 and 139% for time-domain, and 45–115% for frequency domain HRV indices in a study of Ponikowski et al. with a between-measurement period of 7–56 days [273]. In contrast, Freed et al. found a good short-term variability between two adjacent 10-min periods in CHF [274] with the CV range between 9–12% for LF and HF (FFT). Much better reproducibility of short-term HRV has been reported in the largest study in patients with stable CAD [260] with the CV range being between 11.3–29.9% for all measured indices, except for RMSSD with a CV value of 48.9%. Also in patients with diabetes mellitus, the day-to-day reproducibility has been moderate or high for SDNN (mean bias 17%) and moderate for FFT-derived spectral measures (mean bias 2–39%), while reproducibility for AR-derived spectral measures has been poor (27–102%) [275].

Thus, short-term HRV reproducibility seems to be lower in patients than in healthy subjects. Accordingly, a greater change of particular HRV measures is necessary to detect the true effect of interventions in patients with autonomic neuropathies or certain diseases. As yet, there are no indications from standards, statements or reviews. A magnitude of necessary change (absolute or relative) considered to be significant should be pre-defined taking into account the age of the population examined and the methods used.

There are independent studies in which normal subjects and patients with a certain disease have been compared simultaneously to evaluate reproducibility of 24-h HRV measures (❷ Table 3.17). Nolan et al. analyzed the NN50+ index in 67 patients with CAD [276]. The ICC reached 0.94 (similar to 0.97 in healthy subjects). However, there was a much poorer CR (0.41) than in healthy subjects (0.21). In a sample of 87 diabetic patients in the same study, the ICC values have varied between 0.80–0.91 depending on between-measurement interval whereas the CR values were unacceptably large (0.61–0.98) [276]. Day-to-day variation of 24-h HRV has been found to be moderate in patients with CHF in a study of van Hoogenhuyze et al. [277]. The mean values of differences ranged from 8.5–13.8% (SDNNI and SDANN), However, individual variations have been observed of up to 50.6% and 28.2%, respectively [277]. Recalculated ICC values ranged from 0.87–0.95 (❷ Table 3.17). Also, a high reproducibility for all 24-h spectral measures with an ICC>0.79 has been reported by Bigger's group [278] in post-AMI patients. Time-domain (SDNN, SDANN and SDNNI, geometric) measures have been found reproducible in a sample of post-AMI patients [279] and in HF studies [280–282]. However, reproducibility of the pNN50 has been shown to be poor in these studies (❷ Table 3.17).

In the largest study on long-term HRV reproducibility in CAD patients, Weber et al. reported a maximum change of ~36 ms for SDNN in stable angina (~25% of the average) [283]. Comparing this value with the corresponding values reported by Hohnloser et al. [281] and Sosnowski et al. [65], the range of variation between examinations in cardiac patients appeared to be similar to that in healthy subjects (~30%).

Thus, whereas the reproducibility in patients with cardiac disease can be seen to be significantly lower with short-term HRV (~ twice than that in healthy subjects), in long-term recordings a similar reproducibility with long-term HRV examination can be assumed both in normal subjects and in patients with known cardio-vascular disease.

There is little data on the stability of diurnal variation of HRV measures. Huikuri et al. found the diurnal variation of HRV indices to be very stable in 20 normal persons on two consecutive days and then at 1-week intervals. However, neither results of rhythm analysis nor its reproducibility was reported [284]. A more detailed cosinor-based analysis [87] in patients with stable CAD has been provided by Hayano et al. [285], who repeated 48-h ECG recordings in 40 patients aged 58 years (38–72). The mesor (corresponding to the median values) of SDNN, LF (ms), HF (ms) and LF/HF were shown to be highly reproducible with ICC values ranging between 0.8–0.89. The values of the amplitude (the magnitude of change from the mesor) varied between 0.63–0.73, and of the acrophase (the time of maximum amplitude) varied between 0.76–0.95 [285]. These results may indicate that the use of a highly reproducible, understandable and robust cosinor-based circadian rhythm analysis may offer more than other statistical analyses to evaluate the effects of interventions. However, one has to bear in mind that the period of recording has to be longer than one day.

Noninvasive baroreflex sensitivity (BRS) reproducibility has been reported as being moderate to poor with a range of CVs of about 8–40% if the BRS is calculated using spontaneous approaches [266, 286–290]. However, some studies indicate a high reproducibility [291, 292]. The reproducibility of BRS is affected by the specific methodological features [289, 291, 293], age, health status, mean arterial pressure and period between measurements and the failure rate [287, 290, 291, 293]. The 95% limit of agreement varies between 1.7 ms/mmHg up to 10.6 ms/mmHg [287, 291] depending on the mean BRS value in the sample examined. Transfer function BRS and cross-spectral BRS appear to be applicable to most subjects, and calculated sample size to detect a change of 15% varies between 20 and 80 subjects [291, 292]. Within-subject variability seems to be responsible for a substantial proportion of reproducibility [287, 293]. The use of logarithmically-transformed HRV measures might improve the reproducibility [293]. However, the net results are similar. As pharmacologic and mechanical intervention-based methods are rarely used and restricted to highly specialized laboratory centres, the issue of the reproducibility of these methods is of marginal importance. However, in any laboratory study, the validity of the method of study still remains a fundamental requirement.

Heart rate turbulence (HRT) reproducibility (i.e., turbulence onset, turbulence slope, turbulence dynamics) has never been explored despite significant support in some investigators' teams for their superiority over traditional HRV measures (SDNN and HRVI only) [222, 226, 227]. A lack of reproducibility studies on HRT has been observed in recently published standards [294].

3.4.7.5   Reclassification Rate

Reproducibility of a specific HRV measure influences the categorization of its value as normal or abnormal depending on the cut-off values defined *a priori* (from the literature or guidelines) or *a posteriori* (from the distribution of values in the studied sample, i.e., mean or median, 10th, 25th, or 33rd percentile).

For the SDANN cut-off of 90 ms, the day-to-day variation in the SDANN calculation in data from van Hoogenhuyze et al. [277] caused a change in classification from normal to abnormal in 4 out of 22 CHF-patients (18%) and from abnormal to normal in 2 (9%). The overall reclassification rate achieved was 27% (6/22). Similar values for a cut-off of 100 ms resulted in a lower rate of reclassification (overall 2/22, 9%, from normal to abnormal 2/6, 30%), while with a cut-off value of 50 ms, only 1 out of 4 cases with SDANN<50 ms moved into the normal category (5% overall, 25% of abnormal). In 33 normal middle-aged (35 years) subjects, the reclassification rate from normal to abnormal (cut-off <100 ms) was 3 out of 29 (10%) and from abnormal to normal was 1 out of 4 (25%). Overall, there was a 6/33 (18%) rate of change in category for SDANN<120 ms, 4/33 (12%) for SDANN<100 ms and 3/33 (10%) for SDANN<90 ms.

From data of Haas et al. [272], the reclassification rate of 10.2% (4 out of 39 AMI-patients) can be calculated for 5-min SDRR with cut-off defined as values below 20 ms, and of 8 (9.6%) out of 83 for VR < 10 bpm. A detailed analysis of figures (1 and 2) from the paper of Stein et al. [280] on the stability of HRV indexes in CHF patients indicates that despite a high ICC of 24h-SDNN (= 0.91), the reclassification rate dichotomized at 70 ms regarding 6/17 patients (35%!), including 3 out of 5 with an abnormal value in the first recording and normal in the second visit. The SDANN categorization changes within two visits appeared similar (1 out of 3 (33%) changed from abnormal to normal).

Reclassification rate might be of importance in some clinical syndromes, which use an HRV analysis for their diagnosis, for example, diabetic autonomic neuropathy, sinus node dysfunction and obstructive sleep apnea syndrome. As yet, studies that address this issue are lacking.

3.4.8   Selection of Method for HRV Analysis

The choice of HRV method to be applied in a specific study is dictated by the purposes and conditions of the study. From a clinical point of view, it is important that the HRV measure is normally distributed (like LV ejection fraction), thereby providing results which can be easily expressed and understood as raw values rather than log-transformed measures (❯ Fig. 3.34). If the distribution is not normal, data should be transformed for statistical calculation. However, the presentation of results requires re-transformation.

A fraction of abnormality, i.e., the proportion of abnormal range and total range, would also be informative (❯ Fig. 3.35). Within a restricted limit of abnormality (98%CI) that is based on distribution of the results, there was nobody (neither healthy nor post-MI-patients) with the SDNN value <20 ms, whereas 13% of CAD patients were recognized on the basis of HRVF evaluation. For less restricted limits, there was still a significant difference in the proportion of CAD-patients with abnormal results (i.e., 5. % for SDNN vs 36.7%), albeit the cut-off points lay below the 2.5th percentile. This indicates that the definition of abnormal values is strongly affected by the normality of distribution of an HRV measure.

The duration of HRV recordings seems to play a crucial role in the applicability of HRV analysis. Studies on clinical outcome and risk factor association with HRV, in which HR had been used as an independent measure of the autonomic balance, were undertaken in tens of thousands of people. Meanwhile, in other studies in which short- or median-time HRV analysis was used, smaller populations, around a tenth of the size, were gathered. While 24-h HRV analysis was applied, the number of subjects studied was reduced by a further factor of 10 (❯ Fig. 3.41).

If the HRV analysis is going to be performed in a large sample population, as in epidemiological studies and registries, the use of simple statistical methods from short-term recordings seems to be most appropriate (❯ Fig. 3.37). HRV from routine ECG recordings lasting 8–10 s can be applied taking into account that each index derived from routine ECG strips (VR, SDRR, CIPA, CV) reflects vagally-mediated respiratory HR modulation. As short epochs are characterized by a relatively great biological variation, the reproducibility of individual measures should be assessed or simple HR used as an index of sympathovagal balance of greatest reproducibility. Otherwise, the duration of EGC recordings should last 5 min, because there is a relatively large experience with the use of HRV from 5-min epochs. However, as there is an inverse relationship between the statistical power of a study and the reliability of an HRV measure for a given sample size, it is necessary to calculate sample size on the basis of *a priori* defined change of an HRV index to be detected and of *a priori* or *a posterior* defined reproducibility [285].

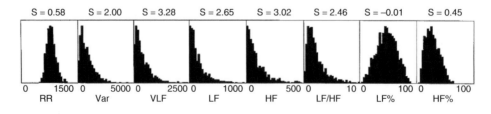

◼ Fig. 3.34

Frequency distribution and estimated skewness (S) of the commonly used HRV measures. Data from 1,070 healthy subjects. The SDNN (Var) and spectral HRV measures are characterized by a nonnormal distribution, so the logarithmic transformation is necessary. Normal distribution is present for the RRI, HF [N.U.] and LF [N.U.], however the latter two (HF, LF expressed as %) do not have an explanation on physiological or pathophysiological basis (From [324])

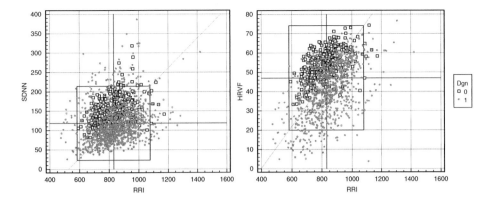

◘ Fig. 3.35

Comparison of the distribution of normal and abnormal SDNN and HRVF in respect to health status. Median values of the 24-h mean R – R interval (RRI = 830 ms), SDNN (119 ms) and HRVF (47%) in the entire cohort (805 subjects) are depicted by the vertical or horizontal lines (respectively). These values constitute approximately 30% and 60% of the total ranges, respectively. If one considers abnormally low HRV values on basis of a population distribution, only few normal subjects have SDNN and HRVF below the lower normal limit (here: 89 ms and 35%), however these values constitute various percentile of the total range (here: 23% and 46%). The open boxes indicate the 98% CI of prediction of the normal/abnormal result. Each value of RRI, SDNN and HRV that lies outside the boxes are definitively abnormal. Interestingly, there are none subjects (normal or post-MI) with SDNN<98%CI (22 ms), whereas 67 patients (13%) (exclusively from the postMI-cohort) had abnormal value (i.e., HRVF<20%). If we turn into established cut-off of SDNN (<50 ms) and HRVF (<30%), the respective proportions reach 27/515 (5.2%) for SDNN and 187/515 (36.7%) for HRVF again exclusively form the CAD cohort. Open squares indicate healthy subjects (n = 290) and circles indicate patients after myocardial infarction (with/without sinus rhythm, n = 515) (Author's data)

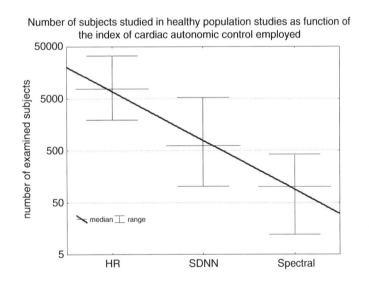

◘ Fig. 3.36

An exponential relationship between simplicity of available indices of cardiac autonomic tone and examined population. Data from 94 studies in normal population (either selectively healthy or random sample). A magnitude of 10 is a scaling factor for this relationship. Thus, HR as a crude sympathovagal balance index can be employed in largest population, whereas spectral analysis seems to be applicable to 100 times lower samples (Author's data)

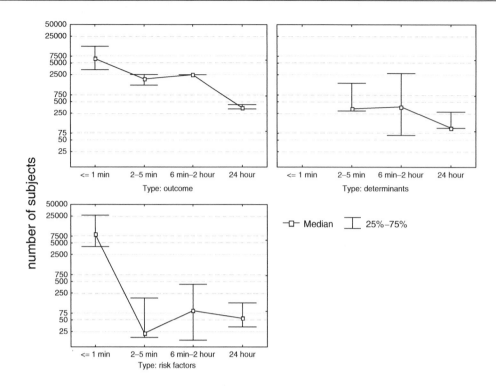

⬤ Fig. 3.37
Reportable size of population samples as a function of HRV indices and length of ECG recordings chosen. Data from 94 studies that employed HR and/or different time- and spectral HRV measures for clinical outcomes, HR and HRV associations with risk factors and HRV determinants evaluation. (Author's data)

If HRV analysis is to be used for physiological, psychological, and pathophysiological reasons, either short-time or long-term time series could be appropriate. However, a prolongation of HRV recordings for these purposes reduces the number of factors that can be controlled during a study.

Cumulated experience indicates that long-term HRV analysis appears to be a useful tool for clinical outcome studies. It is necessary to be aware of the contribution of the autonomic control of HR to the entire HRV over a 24-h period, which is less than 10% of total variance [80]. Thus, in clinical outcome studies, it is not advisable to search for an association between clinical events and sympathetic and vagal activity as well as their balance. However, most global HRV measures certainly require the autonomic system to mediate their influences. The uses of various HRV methods/indices for different purposes are summarized in ❷ Table 3.18.

3.4.8.1   Reliability

Homogeneity in the evaluation of the effects of interventions and in agreement with other methods determines the reliability of various HRV indices as noninvasive measures of cardiac autonomic control. There are several methods that allow the determination of HRV reliability.

For short-term HRV reliability assessment, simple maneuvers are used (controlled breathing, body position change from supine to standing, head-up tilt, exercise, mental stress) for which changes in cardiac autonomic control are well established. ❷ Tables 3.19–3.21 summarize the results of selected studies that have addressed this issue.

The reproducibility of 5-min SDNN and spectral HRV indices in response to a head-up tilt has been shown to be poor or moderate [266, 295, 296]. Data are conflicting regarding the reproducibility of HRV in response to active standing.

◼ **Table 3.18**

HRV methods used in population studies depending on their type and objectives

Authors, acronym of the study (if exists)	Year	Total sample (% men)	Age (range)	Length of recording	HRV method/ index	Specific purposes
Macfarlane et al. The WOSCOPS Study [A25]	2007	6596 (100%)	45–65 years	8–10 s	CIPA	Outcome prediction
Dekker et al. The Zutphen Study [A26]	1997	1763	40–85 years		SDRR	Outcome prediction (CHD mortality)
De Bruyne et al. The Rotterdam Study [650]	1999	5272 (40%)	⩾ 55 years	10 s	SDRR	Outcome prediction (Cardiac mortality)
Liao et al. The ARIC Study [248]	1995	1984 (46%)	45–64 years	2 min	LF, HF, LF/HF	Determinants of HRV
Liao et al. The ARIC Study [649]	1997	2252 (45%)			SDNN, LF, HF, LF/HF	
Dekker et al. The ARIC Study [258]	2000	856 (45%)			SDNN	Outcome prediction (CHD, mortality)
Carnethon et al. The ARIC Study [249]	2002	9267 (40.5%)			SDNN, LF, HF	
Kageyama et al. [817]	1997	282 (100%)	21–49 years	3 min	LF, HF	
Korkushko et al. Population-based [555/A27]	1991	354 (50%)	3 months to 89 years	4 min	LF, HF	Determinants of HRV in population
Sinnreich et al. Cross-sectional study [1998]	1998	294 (50%)	35–65 years	5 min	SDNN, LF, HF, LF/HF	
Kuo et al. Healthy volunteers [324]	1999	1070 (44%)	40–79 years		SDNN, LF, HF, LF/HF	
Agelink et al. [335]	2001	309 (49%)	18–77 years		LF, HF, LF/HF	
Kuch et al. [648]	2001	286 (52%)	56 years mean		LF, HF	
Ryan et al. [A28]	1994	67 (60%)	20–90 years	8 min	LF, HF, LF/HF	
Hotta et al. The LILAC Study [A29]	2005	298 (40%)	> 75 years	10 min	Nonlinear (a2, DFA)	Outcome prediction
Fagard et al. [654]	1999	424 (48%)	25–89 years	15 min	SDNN, LF, HF, LF/HF	
Huikuri et al. [323]	1996	374 (50%)	40–60 years	30 min	SDNN, LF, HF, LF/HF	
Tsuji et al. Framingham offspring [251]	1996	2722 (45%)	21–93 years	2 h	SDNN, LF, HF, LF/HF	Determinants of HRV in population, outcome study

Salo et al. [270] reported an unacceptably high CV for RMSSD and all spectral measures (42–83%), while Lobing et al. observed low ICC of LF and HF (0.57 and 0.33, respectively) using a very complicated protocol [297]. On the contrary, an excellent reproducibility has been reported by others (❷ Table 3.19). In a study in children, Dietrich et al. observed good reproducibility of standing LF and HF (natural logarithms). However, differences in these measures have been found to be highly unpredictable (❷ Table 3.19) [298].

In a head-to-head comparison of FFT and AR spectral HRV indices in analysis of controlled breathing, Pitzalis et al. showed a moderate ICC for the LF and HF, and a poor reproducibility (ICC<0.6) for TP and LF/HF in 20 young healthy subjects [296], while a moderate reproducibility was found for SDNN and RMSSD. Limitations of the reliability of spectral HRV measures for evaluation of the effect of controlled respiration have been confirmed in many studies (❷ Table 3.20). On the other hand, positive studies confirming good reliability of HRV in the examination of the effects of respiration do exist (❷ Table 3.20) [256, 269, 297, 299, 300]. Tarkiainen et al. reported that logarithmic transformation

◘ Table 3.19

Reproducibility of HRV in response to body movement (active standing or head-up tilt (HUT))

Author	Intervention	Test for reproducibility	HR/RRI	SDRR	RMSSD	TP	LF	HF	LF/HF	Comments
Pitzalis 1996 [296]	Head-up tilt 70°	ICC > 0.6 accept.	0.44	0.30	0.30	0.59 / 0.57	0.65 / 0.65	0.59 / 052	0.36 (FFT) / 0.09 (AR)	FFT, AR12 / 10 min
Salo 1999 Hypertensive [270]	Standing	CV_{SD} [%] < 30 accept.	6.6	26.3	41.7	83.2	75.3	56.3	75.1	FFT? 5 min
Sandercock 2004 [295]	Standing	ICC	0.87–0.93	0.67–0.85	0.86–0.91	–	0.77–0.94	0.79–0.92	0.71–0.82	3 different instruments, FFT, 5 min
Hojgaard 2005 [?]	Head-up tilt 60°	CV [%](intra) < 30 accept	5/5	–	–	33/25	28/26	33/32	18/23	FFT, 300s/1024s
Carrasco 2003 [300]	Standing	ICC	0.89	0.95	0.93	0.94	0.94	0.91	0.90	AR bpm2 5 min
Kowalewski Urban 2004 [A23]	Standing	ICC	–	–	–	0.73–0.91	0.69–0.86	0.71–0.89	0.68–0.85	FFT, 10 min 3 x 2 x 3periods
Lobnig 2003 [297]	Standing + CB 12/min	ICC	–	–	–	–	0.567	0.326	–	FFT (coarse-graining), ln values, 5 min 4 x 4–5 days
Kobayashi 2007 [A21]	Standing	Intra CV Inter CV	5 / 14.9	–	–	–	21.2 / 48.2	19.5 / 41.4	–	FFT bpm2 204.8 s (~3')
Dietrich A 2007 Children [298]	Standing Change from supine	CV	9.4 / 36.2	–	–	–	6.2 / 315.3	7.7 / 44.6	– / –	DFT 3 min

Table 3.20

Reproducibility of HRV in response to controlled breathing

Author	Controlled breathing	Test for reproducibility	HR/RRI	SDRR	RMSSD	TP	LF	HF	LF/HF	Comments
Pitzalis 1996, healthy [296]	16/min	ICC > 0.6 accept.	0.35	0.27	0.20	0.52 0.55	0.60 0.65	0.65 0.70	0.36 (FFT) 0.48 (AR)	FFT, AR12 10 min
Salo 1999, hypertensive [270]	6/min	CV$_{SD}$ [%] < 30 accept.	8.3	21.8	30.4	58.2	59.5	56.3	48.6	FFT? 5 min
Sandercock 2004, healthy [295]	12/min	ICC	0.84–0.92	0.72–0.83	0.69–0.91	–	0.83–0.87	0.47–0.82	0.64–0.82	3 different instruments, FFT, 5 min
Sinnreich 1998 Healthy [530]	15/min	CV [%]	–	6.1	7.4	6.7	10.7	10.5	–	AR16 5 min
Parati 2001 Hypertensives [299]	18/min	CV [%]	5	18	–	–	6	6	–	FFT, 15 min
Jauregi-Renaud 2001, healthy [301]	12/min	CR < 30 accept.	6.33	–	–	–	–	40.8 (NU)	3.59	AR, 5 min
Carrasco 2003, healthy [300]	12/min	ICC	0.81	0.94	0.94	0.94	0.92	0.93	0.88	AR bpm^2 5 min
Lobnig 2003 Healthy [297]	12/min	ICC	–	–	–	–	0.66–0.69	0.71–0.81	–	FFT (coars-graining), ln values, 5 min, 4x4–5days
Tarkiainen 2005 CAD [260]	12/min	CV [%]	6 5.6 – –6.3	37.1 35.0–39.5	52.1 49.1–55.4	9.9 [ln] 9.3–10.5	16.5 [ln] 15.5–17.5	14.9 [ln] 14.0–15.8	16.1 [ln] 15.2–17.2	FFT 5 min
Lord 2001 Healthy [271]	10/min	CV [%]	–	–	–	–	–	0.45	–	FFT 5 min

◻ Table 3.21

Reproducibility of HRV in response to other interventions

Author	Intervention	Test for reproducibility CV$_{SD}$ [%]	HR/RRI	SDRR	RMSSD	TP	LF	HF	LF/HF	Comments
Salo 1999 Hypertensive [270]	Exercise	CV$_{SD}$ [%]	6.6	26.3	41.7	76.2	80.0	131.6	54.0	FFT?
	Cold pressor test	< 30 accept	10.1	29.4	57.9	101.6	100.6	145.3	79.1	5 min
Carrasco 2003 [300]	Exercise 80W	ICC	0.86	0.85	0.79	0.91	0.92	0.88	0.87	AR/ bpm^2 5 min
Jauregi-Renaud 2001 [301]	Cold pressor test+CB 12/m	CR	17.1	–	–	–	–	37.9 (NU)	2.87	AR, 2 min
Guijt 2007 [302]	Sleep	ICC	–	0.79/0.85 0.54–0.94	0.94/0.98 0.86–0.99	–	–	–	–	2 x 1 h
	Exercise 50W	ICC	–	0.85 0.70–0.93	0.84 0.67–0.92	–	–	–	–	15 min

of the standard HRV measures (RMSSD, TP, LF, HF) improved the reliability of evaluation of HRV response to controlled breathing [260]. The reliability of HRV in response to other maneuvers is shown in ❱ Table 3.21 [270, 300–302]. In general, the reliability of HRV measures in evaluating the effects of the aforementioned interventions seems to be unsatisfactory [256].

Other methods of reliability evaluation are related to the pharmacological action of agents that exert either direct or indirect stimulatory or inhibitory effects upon the vagus or sympathetic branch or both. Unfortunately, data on reliability of HRV analysis in such settings are extremely rare. Cloarec-Blanchard et al. examined the effects of nitroglycerin infusion on LF components in ten healthy volunteers 1 week apart and found it to be reproducible [303]. Moderate to good reproducibility (CV between 4 to 30%) of HRV has been reported by Piepoli et al. in heart failure patients under dobutamine infusion [304].

For long-term HRV reliability assessment, quite different approaches are in use. Physical training or body mass changes are assumed to be associated with HRV changes, but unfortunately, studies addressing HRV reliability in this area are lacking.

3.4.8.2 Explicitness

Ideally, the HRV index changes should be caused by a specific alteration in cardiac autonomic control. Effects of an intervention, like vagus nerve intersection, which results in almost total reduction of IBI variation [305], should be universally observed. Similar effects should be observed by a muscarinic receptor blockade in any examined subject [23]. Data from studies by the Goldberger group [231] indicates that cholinergic blockade with a high dose of atropine results in elimination of RSA and HRV in almost every subject examined. However, parasympathetic stimulation does not necessarily result in uniform HRV changes [231]. As indicated by an early study of Anrep et al. in dogs, blood pressure increment beyond a certain level (associated with a reflex parasympathetic excitement) results in a reduction of VR of HR [3]. A suppression of HRV (SDNN, LF and HF) as a result of the phenylephrine-induced activation of parasympathetic branch of the ANS has been found in normal humans [231]. However, changes of certain HRV spectral measures in response to parasympathetic baroreflex-related stimulation have been observed to depend on the initial level of HRV, because a reduction in those with a high basal HRV and an increase in those with a low basal HRV, despite slowing of HR, was found in each case [231]. A possible explanation for such a discrepancy is the phenomenon of saturation (see part 3.5), where the effects of inspiration and expiration-induced vagal activity can be rather diminished [231].

The situation is even more complicated if the effects of sympathetic inhibition or stimulation are considered. Alpha-adrenergic stimulation with phenylephrine in a setting of a so-called total autonomic blockade (atropine 0.04/kg + propranolol 0.2/kg [306]) has not been found to have an effect on either time or spectral HRV indices in healthy subjects, while a significant reduction of HRV has been observed in subjects with an intact activity of both branches of the ANS [231]. It indicates that inhibition of ß1-adrenergic and M1-muscarinic receptors prevents the effect of action of α-adrenergic-mediated stimulation, or that these effects are truly negligible [231].

The effects of beta-adrenergic stimulation or inhibition on HRV strongly relate to the choice of stimulus/inhibitor. For instance, a large increase of LF power in response to up-right body movement is accompanied by a significant reduction in total HRV [307]. Such an LF power increase has been observed to be lower in a setting of parasympathetic blockade [231]. In addition, the use of different sympathomimetics elicits various effects. Exogenous epinephrine has been shown to reduce HRV (SDNN) with variable changes (increase, no change or a decrease) in the LF power in healthy subjects, while isoproterenol infusion has exerted more of an inhibitory effect on LF power. Interestingly, the HF power has been simultaneously reduced with isoproterenol, in contrast to epinephrine [307].

Such experimental circumstances are rather unique in clinical settings. Changes in a specific physiologically explainable R–R variation (e.g., RSA, LF power) need not follow changes in the entire HRV [308]. Thus, *a reduction or an increase of heartbeat variation cannot definitively indicate its cause.*

For instance, in a patient with an acute MI, a reduction of HRV can be attributed to various mechanisms, which can depend on factors such as age of the MI, its location and size, LV function, drugs, interventions, coexisting diseases (e.g., diabetes, respiratory system disease, depression), and finally complications and adverse events such as malignant ventricular arrhythmia, stroke, cardiac tamponade, loss of blood, etc. In addition, the magnitude of

HRV reduction is pre-determined by the pre-event level of cardiac autonomic control (age, sex, coexisting diseases). For such a complex clinical entity, the detection of a specific alteration in the cardiac autonomic control is *a priori* impossible.

However, if an effect of a specific intervention with known patho-mechanism(s) contributing to a certain HRV measure is to be studied, a link between them can be explored. Again, the control of many factors is necessary to draw an explicit interpretation. The more sophisticated and mathematically complex the method used for HRV assessment, the less likely is its unequivocal explanation.

Actually, none of the currently used HRV measures can help to explain what specific alteration (in terms of level and location) is responsible for HRV changes in any physical condition or in cardiac and noncardiac diseases.

3.4.8.3   Redundancy and Inter-Changeability Among Different Methods and Measures

The variety of HRV measures determined in different domains has, in fact, a similar complex physiological and pathological background. Current guidelines indicate that some HRV measures are most useful, but actually only very few are commonly applied in clinical settings [309]. A plethora of methods and derived indices have been proposed for which the advantages over standard HRV measures have been justified in terms of a better description of underlying physiological and pathological processes and in prediction of hard end-points or their surrogates [310]. As a result, researchers and physicians are faced with a dilemma of choosing the most appropriate method and indices that would help to meet the purpose of their studies. From this point of view, it is important to know the meaning of particular HRV measures, but also their redundancy and inter-changeability, as well as differences between the methods used for obtaining their measurements. Simple comparisons of techniques for HRV analysis are given in ❱ Table 3.22 [after 310].

There are relationships between HRV indices from the same or different domains (time, spectral, nonlinear) that permit them to be used as a substitute for one another, or to interpret (within a limited credibility) simple time-domain or complex nonlinear measurements on the basis of the known background of spectral components. The higher the correlation between different indices, the higher is their inter-changeability. The most significant relationships among HRV indices in various domains are shown in ❱ Table 3.23. [4, 11, 311, 312].

Time-domain measures are least dependent on the algorithms used for their determination and the main differences between means are related to the duration of recording. However, spectral estimates are not necessarily similar if obtained using the two most popular methods, namely FFT and AR modeling.

In a comparative study of FFT and AR spectral techniques for LF and HF components of the HRV power spectrum, Pichon et al. found a significant bias between these two methods meaning that they are not interchangeable. For the 265 s ECG registrations, the bias calculated from FFT and AR [16th order] has been measured and reached -132 ms^2 for LF and -111 ms^2 for HF with the lower LOA of -1442 and -469 ms^2 for LF and HF respectively and the upper LOA of 1176 and 246 ms^2, respectively [313]. Even greater bias was found after body position movement, where LOA (lower and upper) lie far from the mean values [313]. Similar observations have been reported by Chemla et al. [275]. They found that the fast Fourier transform and AR analysis provided quite different estimates of spectral HRV in diabetic patients. Moreover, they stated that these methods are not interchangeable at all and in this specific patient population, the FFT method provided spectral estimates of TP, HF and LF in all patients contrary to the AR method which was unable to produce spectral peaks in almost half of the diabetic patients [275]! They observed that in subjects in whom spectral peaks could be detected by means of either method, spectral estimates within frequency bands were similar. Also, the FFT appeared less dependent on the minor changes (5%) in the timing of the onset of the analysis. In a former head-to-head study of Pitzalis et al., the power spectrum of LF and HF was 20–30% lower if assessed by means of AR [12th order] than that obtained by means of FFT [296]. Also, in a study of Sinnreich et al. in 398 healthy subjects [269], the AR [16th order] LF and HF spectral powers [mean of LF of 221 and HF of 151 ms^2 in males and 126 and 128 ms^2 in females, respectively] were clearly lower than those reported by Pikkujämsa et al. in 50 healthy subjects of similar age [mean LF of 520 and mean HF of 375 ms^2] calculated by using 5-min AR [20th order]. They were even lower than in diabetic patients (5-min) [275] and similar (with respect to LF components) to the mean 24-h value estimated in patients in the early phase of acute MI by means of AR [10th

□ Table 3.22

Comparison of techniques of HRV analysis (Modified after [310] and [111])

HRV analysis	Description	Advantages	Limitations	Universality
Time-domain	Statistical	Simple, easy to calculate, proven clinical utility, gross distinction of high and low frequency variation	Sensitive to artefact; requires stationarity, fails to discriminate distinct signals	SDNN most widely used, SDANN most widely applicable (also in AF)
	Frequency distribution	Visual representation of data, can fit to normal or log-normal distribution	Lacks widespread clinical application, arbitrary number of bins	Undetermined
	Geometric	Visual representation of data, does not requires stationarity, relatively robust, can be also used for nonlinear analysis	Fails to discriminate distinct signals, requires relatively large datasets	HRVI most widely used HRVF most widely applicable (also in AF)
Frequency-domain	Frequency spectrum representation	Visual and quantitative representation of frequency contribution to waveform, useful to evaluate relationship to mechanisms, widespread HRV evaluation	Requires stationarity and periodicity for validity, sensitive to artifacts, altered by posture, sleep, activity	Only in subjects with sinus rhythm
Fractal analysis	Power law	Ubiquitous biologic application, characterization of signal with single linear relationship, enables prognostication	Requires stationarity and periodicity, requires large datasets, vulnerable to artifacts	1/f slope of power law most widely applicable (also in AF)
	Detrended fluctuation analysis	Indentifies intrinsic variations to system (versus external stimuli), does not required stationarity, enables prognostication	Requires large datasets (>8000 data points), dependence on artifacts	Undetermined (only in sinus rhythm?)
Entropy	Measures the degree of disorder (information or complexity)	Unique representation of data, requires fewest data points	Needs to be complemented by other techniques, stationarity is required	Undetermined (only in sinus rhythm?)

Abbreviations see ❷ Table 3.2 and ❷ Sect. 3.1

order] modeling (299 and 270 ms^2 respectively) [316]. A comparison of the corresponding means of AR-spectral indices reported in a study of 50 age-comparable healthy subjects (LF of 520 ms^2 and HF of 375 ms^2) [141] and in those with diabetes (similar age range) (LF and HF of 222 ms^2 and 485 ms^2) in a study by Chemla et al. [275] might indicate that there is either a problem with the determination of a proper order for AR modeling or that it might not be [empirically] a reliable method for HRV spectral assessment.

There are also data indicating that the so-called sympatho-vagal balance, indicated by means of the LF/HF power ratio, is not interchangeable while using either FFT or AR for estimation. Apart from controversies regarding the rationale and background of the use of this index, the comparability of the LF/HF ratio is low either in normal subjects, namely 3.84

◼ **Table 3.23**

Inter-changeability diagram of various HRV measures

Analytic method		Frequency-range			
		<0.033 Hz	0.033-0.04 Hz	0.04-0.15 Hz	0.15-0.40 Hz
Analytic method	Time-domain	SDNN, SDANN		SDNNI	RMSSD, pNN50(20)
	geometric	HRVI, HRVF, SD2			SD1
	Frequency-domain	ULF	VLF	LF	HF
		TP (long-term)			TP*
	Non-linear dynamics	1/f slope			Symbolic dynamics ApEn*
				DFA α₂	
					DFA α₁*
				SampEn*	
	HRT		TS		
				TO	

Abbreviations as in ❷ Sect. 3.1. On basis of data provided by HRV Standards [4], Voss A et al. [111], Stein KM et al. [311], Cygankiewicz I et al. [312].
* short-term

in AR[12] modeling in normal young subjects, 4.11 in AR[16] modeling in middle-aged subjects and around 5 in AR[20] modeling in a similar sample [269, 275, 313].

The accumulated data also indicates that cut-off values of prognostic values of spectral HRV estimates stated in the Standards [4] should not be applied in studies in which AR modeling is to be applied. This might also imply that the use of the fast Fourier transform, despite its limitations [see 3.4], should be preferred for short-term HRV assessment in laboratory settings. If the AR modeling is to be used, referencing of previous studies should be limited and should include studies in which other methods (FFT in particular) had been applied.

3.4.9 Normal Limits and Abnormal HRV

The successful application of HRV analysis to clinical medicine is critically dependent on the definition of normal limits and abnormal values. Guidelines [4] provide standard HRV measurements in a healthy population. However, they might be useful only as a reference for comparison with population samples with known characteristics (e.g., prevalence of CAD, mean age, mean RRI, etc.). HRV analysis, like other diagnostic methods, should take into account the prevalence of the disease and its influence on the performance of a particular HRV index. As yet, in almost all studies, the positive predictive value of HRV indices has been reported ignoring the prevalence of a disease in a population (if normal persons had been comparators). The author's studies, confirmed by others, clearly indicates that examination of a sample of a population is necessary to determine normal limits and to define abnormal values [64, 65]. As there are significant age-, gender-, race-, HR-, respiration-, and distribution-related differences among various populations, normal limits as well as abnormal and risk-predictive values should therefore be determined in a sample of a "regional" population rather than be drawn from the literature [315, 316]. Also, even if they can be controlled for the constitutional factors, a skewed distribution of most standard HRV measures (❷ Fig. 3.34) prevents use of their standard deviation value for setting normal limits. Thus, the use of data provided by the Standards [4] does not seem to be justified at present. It should be remembered that there have been specific technical limitations (>12 h with at least 6 night hours and >50% sinus heartbeats) for HRV analysis in the study of Bigger et al. [317] from which data cited in the Standards [4] have had been drawn. Currently, these data cannot be used further in terms of the same Standards, which indicates requirement for at least 18 h of acceptable data. Nevertheless, researchers might need to compare results of their studies to the corresponding data of others. Also, if population sample characteristics cannot be established accurately, the use of published normative values might be helpful.

Thus, reported values of traditional long-term and short-term HRV indices are provided (❷ Tables 3.24 and ❷ 3.25). In addition, if nonlinear HRV measures are to be more commonly used, then reported values (not references) of either

Table 3.24

Reported values of 24-h HRV time-domain indices (average population ranges)

Author(s) Year	No sbs	Age (mean/range)	% males	Normal value Mean/median	SD	Normal ± 1,96SD or 95% CI* limits	Normal value Mean/median	SD	Normal ± 1,96SD or 95% CI* limits
RRI (NNI) [ms] (only from papers on HRV)							**RMSSD [ms]**		
Standards 1996 [4] (Bigger 1995 [122])	274	40–63	73	–	–	–	27	12	NR
Mølgaard 1991 [318]	140	40–77	64	812	NR	645–1089*			
Ramaekers 1998 [319]	276	18–71	51	784	89	610–958			< 610
Pikkujämsa 1999 [320]	394	1–82	49	891	131	629–1153			
Grimm 2003 [366]	110	21–77	68	817	96	640–1055*	42/339	50	12–158
Bonnemeier 2003 [321]	166	20–70	51	789	86		32.6	16.9	NC
Sosnowski 2005 [65]	296	18–63	82	799	94	636–1005 (2–98%)/648–1024*	611–636		< 611
SDNN [ms]							**HRVI [A.U]**		
Standards 1996 [4]	274	40–63	73	141	39	63–219	37	15	NR
Mølgaard 1991 [318]	140	40–77	64	139	NR	78–231			
Umetani 1998 [322]	167	30–79	50	131	29	76–211			
Raemaekers 1998 [319]	276	18–71	51	148	37	86			
Grimm 2003 [366]	110	21–77	68	154	44	83–272			
Bonnemeier 2003 [321]	196	20–70	51	149	40	NR	40.5	11.9	17.2–63.8
Sosnowski 2005 [65]	296	18–63	82	142	33	86–221 (2–98%)/89–220 (5–95%)	35.7	8.1	19.2–52.2 [2–98% CI]
SDANN [ms]							**HRVF [%]**		
Standards 1996 [4]	274	40–63	73	127	35	58–196			
Raemaekers 1998 [319]	276	18–71	51	140	37	78–209 (5–95%)			
Pikkujämsa 1999 [320]	58	40–82	59	153	36	84–223			
Bonnemeier 2003 [321]	196	20–70	51	135	38				
Sosnowski 2005 [65]	296	18–63	82	135	39	74–230 (2–98%)/79–212 (5–95%)	53	9	35–70 [2–98% CI]

Abrreviations see ❷ Table 3.1 and ❷ Sect. 3.1

Table 3.25

Spectral HRV indices from a short-term ECG (supine) as reported in literature (average population ranges)

Author[s], year number, age range	Total power (ms²) ln/raw			LF power (ms²) ln/raw			HF power (ms²) ln/raw			Method
	Mean/median	SD	Normal limits	Mean/median	SD	Normal limits	Mean/median	SD	Normal limits	FFT/AR [order]
Standards 1996 [4]	8.15 3466	1018	NR	7.06 1170	416	NR	6.88 975	203	NR	NR
Molgaard 1994 104, 40–77 [577]	–	–	–	6.18 484	–	3.99–7.60 56–2007	3.86 48	–	2.30–5.66 10–286	AR [?], 5min over 24h
Huikuri 1996 374, 40–60 [323]	–	–	–	6.42 613	526	NR	5.76 317	2.56 347	NR	AR [?], 512 heartbeats (~12')
Sinnreich 1998 294, 35–65 [530]	6.57 713	–	5.95–7.29*	5.37 215	–	4.61–6.20*	4.79 120	–	4.04–4.99*	AR [16], 5min * [25–75%]
Kuo 1999 1070, 40–79 [324]	6.48 652	1.92	NR	4.60 99	1.92	NR	4.06 58		NR	FFT (288s, 2048 Datapoints)
Pikkujämsa 2001 389, 40–59 [320]	–	–	–	6.14 654	0.81 652	NR	5.41 383	1.00 580	NR	AR [20], 13min ECG
Pikkujämsa 2001 50, 40–59 [320]	–	–	–	6.23 512	396	NR	5.91 368	289	NR	AR [20], 5min ECG
Šlachta 2002 216, 12–70 [325]	7.46 1737	1.03	NR	6.08	1.14	NR	6.60	1.34	NR	FFT (300s, CGSA)
Laitinen 2004 63, 23–77 [326]	7.54 1888	441	NR	6.13 459	120	NR	6.62 752	280	NR	FFT (300s, triangular averaging)

Abbreviations see ⊘ Table 3.2 and ⊘ Sect. 3.1

□ Table 3.26

Reported data on nonlinear HRV measures

Author(s), year ECG duration	Age	N	1/f (ß)	DFA α1	DFA α2	ApEn	SD1/SD2
Pikkujämsa 1999 24-h ECG [320]	< 15	27	−1.15 ± 0.18	1.06 ± 0.11	0.98 ± 0.06	1.26 ± 0.12	–
	15–39	29	−1.12 ± 0.19	1.15 ± 0.16	1.00 ±0.08	1.21 ± 0.14	–
	40–60	29	−1.32 ± 0.14	1.19 ± 0.14	1.07 ± 0.07	1.01 ± 0.16	–
	> 60	29	−1.38 ± 0.17	1.19 ± 0.16	1.14 ± 0.07	0.88 ± 0.16	–
Acharya 2004 20-min ECG [327]	10 ± 5	25	–	2.01 ± 0.33	0.58 ± 0.35	1.90 ± 0.35	0.51 ± 0.19
	25 ± 10	50	–	1.83 ± 0.15	0.41 ± 0.20	2.07 ± 0.18	0.53 ± 0.24
	40 ± 15	40	–	1.67 ± 0.21	0.14 ± 0.21	1.88 ± 0.35	0.43 ± 0.19
	60 ± 5	35	–	1.71 ± 0.22	0.22 ± 0.32	1.68 ± 0.41	0.61 ± 0.29
				CD	LLE	ApEn	–
Kuo 2002 5-min ECG [328]	40–79	480	–	1.83 ±0.04	0.063 ± 0.003	0.303 ± 0.012	–

For abbreviations see ❷ Table 3.2 and ❷ Sect. 3.1

short-term or long-term HRV studies need to be provided as has been done (❷ Table 3.26.). Strong dependence of HRV on age indicates that reference values require either age-adjustment or that age-related references need to be considered (❷ Table 3.27). Separate data on HRV measures (not references) in children is presented in ❷ Table 3.28.

A multitude of factors influencing HRV prevents the determination of normal limits for short-term measures. Lower normal limits (2.5 percentile) of 5-min spectral indexes have been published (❷ Table 3.29) [335]. However, these values can be considered as reference only if a similar method (FFT, 1 kHz sampling rate) is used. Thus, the use of other techniques or algorithms requires data from a control group with comparable characteristics and recordings made under similar examination conditions.

An apparently abnormal result from any HRV measurement has to be interpreted in the light of the known statistical performance (i.e., sensitivity, specificity, predictive value, likelihood etc.) of the measure. For HRV measures, a relative paucity of well defined normal limits excludes a wider use of values <2.5 percentile and >97.5 percentile in practice. Therefore, it is necessary to be aware of whether an apparently abnormal value is defined as population-driven or as an arbitrarily set cut-off value based on statistical performance (❷ Table 3.30).

In fact, there are only a few studies in which the HRV value, thought to be abnormal on the basis of its distribution in a healthy sample, has been used in diagnosing patients with diabetic autonomic neuropathy (DAN) [336], sinus node dysfunction (SND) [337] or in risk-prognostication in patients after a myocardial infarction [64, 315]. By using a range of 2.5%–97.5% of the normal values, the specificity of the selected HRV index is 97.5% both for abnormally low and high results. The respective sensitivities of such a defined abnormal result have reached 88% [336], 70% [337] and 25% [64, 315]. Some authors have proposed defining three categories of results, i.e., abnormal, borderline, and normal for DAN detection [339–341] or in patients with diagnosed cardiovascular disease [342]. This message has already come from Standards [4], which have cited HRV values indicating severe (SDNN<50 ms, HRVI<15a.u.) and moderate (SDNN<100, HRVI<20s.u.) abnormality. It has also been proposed that for HRV indices with normal distributions, the values lower or higher than 2SD from the mean could be considered as pathologic, those between −1 SD and −2 SD or +1 SD and +2 SD as moderately changed and those within the mean ± 1 SD as normal [342]. For HRV indices with other than normal distribution, it has been suggested that the values lower than 2.3 percentile or higher than 97.7 percentile could be considered to be pathologic, those between 2.3–15.9 percentiles and 84.1–97.7 percentiles to be moderately changed and those between 15.9–84.1 percentiles to be normal [32]. An almost similar categorization of HRV data has been used in the ATRAMI study [343].

In another proposal, a categorical distinction of a low, moderate and high HRV has been made on the basis of a calculation of the mean and 1 SD value. Therefore, a low HRV is defined as < mean −1 SD, a high HRV as > mean +1 SD, and moderate HRV as a result in between [283]. In patients with stable angina pectoris, the corresponding 24-h SDNN values were <106 ms, >178 ms and 106–178 ms, for the SDANN, they were <94, >164 and 94–164 ms, and for RMSSD they

□ Table 3.27
Reported normative data of 24-h HRV time-domain indices in respect to age

Author[s]/year	Age range	No of sbs.	SDNN		SDANN		RMSSD		HRVI	
			Mean ± SD	± 1.96 SD / 95%CI	Mean ± SD	± 1.96 SD / 95%CI	Mean ± SD	± 1.96 SD / 95%CI	Mean ± SD	± 1.96 SD / 95%CI
Bonnemeier 2003 [321]	20-29	47	177 ± 37	105–250	158 ± 37	85–231	46 ± 18	10.5–81.5	49 ± 11	27–71
	30-39	34	148 ± 34	81–214	133 ± 32	70–196	36 ± 15	6.5–65.5	41 ± 12	17–65
	40-49	28	141 ± 36	70–213	127 ± 33	62–192	26 ± 9	8.3–43.7	37 ± 11	15–59
	50-59	32	135 ± 34	68–202	130 ± 38	56–204	24 ± 11	2.3–45.7	35 ± 7	21–49
	60-70	25	118 ± 27	65–170	107 ± 26	56–156	19 ± 7	5.2–32.8	32 ± 7	18–46
Umetani 1998 [322]	10-19	30	176 ± 38	101 – 279	159 ± 35	85 – 261	53 ± 17	25–103		
	20-29	42	153 ± 44	93 – 257	137 ± 43	79 – 241	43 ± 19	21–87		
	30-39	39	143 ± 32	86 – 237	130 ± 33	73 – 223	35 ± 11	18–74		
	40-49	65	132 ± 30	79 – 219	116 ± 31	67 – 206	31 ± 11	15–63		
	50-59	22	121 ± 27	73 – 202	106 ± 27	63 – 190	25 ± 9	13–53		
	60-69	20	121 ± 32	68 – 186	111 ± 31	58 – 176	22 ± 6	11–45		
	70-79	21	124 ± 22	62 – 172	114 ± 20	53 – 163	24 ± 7	9–38		
	80-89	21	106 ± 23	57–159/53–147*	95 ± 24	49–151 (45–140)*	21 ± 6	8–32/7–28	HRVF	
Sosnowski 2002 [689]	18-34	31	189	115 – 289	161	96 – 260	–	–	55	50 – 72
	35-44	89	152	91 – 218	141	79 – 211	–	–	50	38 – 70
	45-54	122	143	89 – 216	133	79 – 213	–	–	47	26 – 65
	55-63	54	133	89 – 190	126	76 – 195	–	–	45	33 – 62

◻ Table 3.28

Reported normative data of HRV time-domain indices in children in respect to age

Author[s], year	Age	No of sbs.	SDNN Mean ± SD / 95%CI	SDANN Mean ± SD / 5–95%CI	RMSSD Mean ± SD / 5–95%CI	HRVI Mean ± SD / 5–95%CI	ECG duration
Newborns	1–7 days						
Mehta 2002, 2000 [329]		96	47 ± 12 / 30 – 75	35 ± 9 / 21 – 51	22 ± 6 / 14 – 33	14 ± 4 / 8 – 22	24-h
Longin 2005 [330]		80	50 ± 22 / 23 – 95	–	20 ± 15 / 8 – 62	–	10-min
Infants							
Massin 1998, 1997 [331]	2 week	Each data-group of 10 subjects	52 ± 13				24-h
	1 month		59 ± 15				
	3 month		74 ± 19				
	6 month		85 ± 22				
	1 year		97 ± 25				
Pre-school childhood	1–5 years						
Massin 1998, 1997 [331]			134 ± 34				
Silvetti 2001 [332]		23	102 ± 21	83 ± 18	53 ± 25		24-h
Young childhood	6–10						
Silvetti 2001 [332]		28	147 ± 33	115 ± 26	89 ± 60		24-h
Lenard 2004 [333]		34	64 ± 45	–	64 ± 68		10-min
Early-adolescence	11–14						
Silvetti 2001 [332]		37	169 ±	139 ± 40	74 ± 24		24-h
Faulkner 2003 [334]		43	174 ± 37	140 ± 37	55 ± 18	–	24-h
Lenard 2004 [333]		37	61 ± 48	–	55 ± 60		10-min
Late-adolescence	15–17						
Silvetti 2001 [332]		15	194 ± 62	174 ± 30	71 ± 22		24-h
Faulkner 2003 [334]		15	150 ± 30	133 ± 29	50 ± 13		24-h
Lenard 2004 [333]		35	81 ± 70		77 ± 93		10-min
Young adulthood	18–22						
Faulkner 2003 [334]		12	152 ± 37	127 ± 37	55 ± 16		24-h
Lenard 2004 [333]		31	72 ± 55		70 ± 76		10-min

◨ **Table 3.29**

Lower normal limits of standard 5-min HRV spectral indices (2.5 percentile) in respect to age and gender

Index/age	15	20	25	30	35	40	45	50	55	60	65
Women (n = 158)											
LF	230	193	161	135	113	94	79	66	55	46	39
HF	194	154	122	97	77	62	49	39	31	25	20
Men (n = 151)											
LF	362	300	249	207	172	142	118	98	81	68	56
HF	236	185	145	113	89	69	54	42	33	26	20

Data from Agelink et al. 2001 [335]. Spectral analysis using a Fast Fourier Transform (5 min, 1,000 Hz, discrete signal of 1,024 datapoints)

were <15, >41 and 15–41 ms [283]. However, the use of standard deviation as a determinant of limits should be cautioned as its value is influenced by outliers (from a statistical point of view) and by the age range of the sample (important for HRV indices). On the other hand, use of percentiles requires a relatively larger number of subjects in order to be reliably calculated. Also, a wide or narrow range of age may produce different 2.5 and 97.5 percentile values.

In most studies on HRV, the abnormal results indicating optimal statistical performance are drawn from the distribution of a particular index, with either median, tercile or quartile values defining a cut-off point. Such an attempt is commonly justified by the need to find the cut-off value of a particular index with the highest positive predictive power [338]. Actually, these values should not be considered "pure abnormal" since they do not necessarily correspond to an HRV index distribution in a population and might show a significant variation (❯ Table 3.30). It might be suggested that the term "risk predictive value" (RPV) should be used.

It is necessary to be even more prudent when an index like the HRT-derived turbulence slope (TS) or onset (TO) is in use, as it is difficult (*a priori*) to determine normal limits and abnormal values in a sample of population since this requires either ventricular PEBs to be present or induced in persons without diagnosed cardiac disease. Even so, normal limits have been calculated in healthy volunteers with mean TO values ranging from −2.7% to −2.3% and mean TS from 11.0–19.2 ms/RRI [294]. Grimm et al. found the 95% percentile range for HRT slope to be 11.78–17.69 and HRT onset of −0.033 to −0.009 [366]. A bias regarding the presence of atrial PEBs conducted with intra-ventricular aberration should be noted, as many Holter systems detect abnormal ventricular PEBs only on the basis of the QRS duration [367].

In most clinical studies, TS<0% and TS>2.5 ms/RRI are considered normal. However, it should be noted that despite these values not being close to normal limits in normal persons cited above (of whatever calculation method), there is still a significant proportion of subjects with abnormal HRT results, especially for the HRT onset, reaching almost 20% [366]. Both descriptors of the HRT are in use for categorical classification, where an HRT category of 0 means that both TO and TS are normal, 1 means that either TO or TS is abnormal, while 2 is used if both TO and TS are abnormal. Importantly, those with no or too few suitable VES are considered to have an HRT category of 0 [294].

As the baroreflex sensitivity examination is limited to laboratory centers, normal and abnormal data are not provided, despite some efforts to define normal limits having been undertaken [368–371]. Various methods for the BRS (analogous to the frequency-domain HRV) exclude an indication of unified normal data. It would be helpful if definitive normal values could be agreed by the laboratories working in this field.

3.4.10 Physicians' Compliance with HRV Measures

The familiarity of physicians with HRV phenomena and currently available methods for its evaluation is generally poor. Such a statement seems to be justified by reviewing, in depth, the details from most of the so-called evidence-based studies in internal medicine and cardiology in particular. As a result, it can be stated that a fundamental clinical sign such as heart rate is frequently missed. Thus, it should not be expected that its variation (HRV) would attract greater attention. A simplified comparison of the proportion of real-life and scientific-life awareness of the importance of HRV and related phenomena (❯ Table 3.31) indicates that the HRV contribution to knowledge regarding such important fields like

◼ Table 3.30

Risk predictive values (RPV) of HRV measures (abnormal values) in selected outcome studies

Author[s], year	HRV index	RPV	Choice of cut-off value	Method of verification
Acute myocardial infarction/Coronary artery disease				
Standards 1996 [4]	SDNN	50 ms	Statistical/arbitrary/post hoc	Highest statistical discrimination (Cox hazard)
	RMSSD	20 ms		
	HRVI	15 a.u.		
Kleiger et al. MPIP 1987 [24]	SDNN	50 ms	Arbitrary/post hoc	Mean – 1SD
Rich et al. 1988 symptomatic Emergency coronary angiography [344]	SDANN	50 ms	Arbitrary/post hoc	Univariate analysis
Farrell et al. 1991 [40]	SDNN	50 ms	Arbitrary/a priori	Mean – 1SD
	HRVI	16 a.u.		
Cripps et al. 1991 [38]	HRVI	25 a.u.	Statistical/post hoc	Highest statistical discrimination (ROC)
Odemuyiwa et al. 1994 [345]	HRVI	20 a.u.		Highest statistical discrimination (long-rank survival)
Zuanetti et al. GISSI-2 1996 [346]	SDNN	70		Highest statistical discrimination (ROC)
	RMSSD	17.5		
	NN50+	200		
Copie et al. 1996 [347]	HRVI	18 a.u.		
Lanza et al. 1998 [348]	SDNN	55		Highest statistical discrimination (Cox hazard)
	SDNNI	20		
	SDANN	50		
	RMSSD	23		
La Rovere et al. ATRAMI 1998 [343]	SDNN	70	Arbitrary/a priori	< 15th percentile (~1SD)
	BRS	3 ms*mmg		
Huikuri et al. DIAMOND 2000 [127]	SDNN	65	Statistical/post hoc	Highest statistical discrimination (long-rank survival) within 10–70 percentiles
	HRVI	16		
	DFA α1	0.75		
	ß (1/f)	–1.5		
Whang/Bigger MPIP 2003 [249]	SDNN	50		Highest statistical discrimination (ROC)
Balanescu et al. 2004 [350]	SDNN	50	Arbitrary/ a priori	Reference-drawn
	RMSSD	20		
Stein PK et al. CAST 2005 [351]	SD1/SD2	0.55	Statistical/post hoc	Highest statistical discrimination (univariate Cox hazard)
	SDNN	70	Arbitrary/ a priori	Reference-drawn

⬛ Table 3.30   (Continued)

Author[s], year	HRV index	RPV	Choice of cut-off value	Method of verification
Acute myocardial infarction/Coronary artery disease				
Huikuri et al. CARISMA 2009 [352]	SDNN	70	Arbitrary/a priori	Reference-drawn
	DFA α1	0.75		
	TS (HRT)	< 2.5 ms/RRI		
Heart Failure				
Stein KM et al. 1993 [353]	SDANN	decrease by 47ms	Arbitrary/a priori	mean-1SD
Szabó et al. 1995, 1997 [354]	SDNN	108	Arbitrary/post hoc	Median value
		50	Arbitrary a priori	Reference-drawn
Ponikowski et al. 1997 [355]	SDNN	100	Arbitrary/a priori (post hoc)	Median value (also a high association with cardiac death (Cox))
Nolan et al. UK-Heart Study 1998 [356]	SDNN	93	Arbitrary/a priori	Lower tercile
		117		Median value
		100	Arbitrary/ post hoc	Reference value
Fauchier et al. 1999 IDC [357]	SDNN	100	Arbitrary/a priori	
Galinier et al. 2000 [358]	SDNN	67 ms	Arbitrary/Lower tercile/ post hoc	Highest statistical discrimination (likelihood ratio)
Mäkikallio et al. DIAMOND-CHF 2001 [359]	SDNN	67	Statistical/post hoc	Highest log-rank survival estimate within 10–70 percentiles
	HRVI	22		
	DFA α1	0.9		
Bilchick et al. 2002 [360]	SDNN	65.3ms	Arbitrary/a priori	Lowest quartile
Aronson et al. 2004 Acute decompensated HF [361]	SDNN	44	Statistical/post hoc	Highest statistical discrimination (Cox hazard)
	SDANN	37		
Rashba et al. DEFINITE 2006 [250]	SDNN	81	Arbitrary/a priori	Lower tercile
General population				
Algra et al. 1993 Symptomatic patients with a 24-h ECG [362]	NN50+	3%	Arbitrary/a priori	Lower tercile
	SDNNI (1min)	25		
	SDANN (1min)	8		
Huikuri et al. 1998 Elderly subjects [363]	SDNN B (1/f)	120 −1.5	Statistical/post hoc	Highest statistical discrimination (Cox hazard)
Sajadieh et al. 2006 [364]	SDNN SDNNI pNN50	100 34 0.8%	Arbitrary/a priori	Lowest quartile
Stein PK et al. 2008 Elderly subjects CHS [365]	SDNN DFA α1 TS (HRT)	Continuous 1 < 3 ms/RRI	Arbitrary/a priori Arbitrary/a priori Arbitrary/post hoc	Highest statistical discrimination (Cox hazard)

◨ Table 3.31

Proportion of studies on HRV/BRS or HRT use in myocardial infarction and heart failure as indicated by number of citations in various databases

Database	PubMed	CINAHL	Scopus	Cochrane	Google Scholar
Searched term[s]	N [%]	N [%]	N [%]	N [%]	N [%]
MI	154197 [100]	21112 [100]	167616 [100]	10672 [100]	~930, 000 [100]
MI + HRV	727 [0.47]	134 [0.63]	2368 [1.41]	98 [0.92]	~18, 900 [2.03]
MI + EF	7698 [4.99]	700 [3.31]	12917 [7.71]	1081 [10.13]	~91, 900 [9.88]
MI + HRV + EF	162 [0.11]	17 [0.08]	750 [0.45]	19 [0.18]	~6, 670 [0.72]
MI + BRS	165 [0.11]	25 [0.12]	681 [0.41]	20 [0.19]	~5, 290 [0.57]
MI + BRS + EF	43 [0.03]	4 [0.02]	276 [0.16]	3 [0.03]	~ 1, 900 [0.20]
MI + HRT	63 [0.04]	18 [0.09]	142 [0.08]	3 [0.03]	~839 [0.09]
MI + HRT + EF	26 [0.02]	11 [0.05]	80 [0.05]	3 [0.03]	~469 [0.05]
	N [%]	N [%]	N [%]	N [%]	N [%]
HF	102357 [100]	16452 [100]	147756 [100]	6857 [100]	~1, 460, 000 [100]
HF + HRV	600 [0.59]	97 [0.59]	2970 [2.01]	107 [1.56]	~17, 500 [1.20]
HF + EF	9612 [9.39]	1652 [10.0]	22234 [15.05]	1635 [23.84]	~109, 000 [7.47]
HF + HRV + EF	157 [0.15]	26 [0.16]	1141 [0.72]	35 [0.51]	~6, 730 [0.46]
HF + BRS	144 [0.14]	13 [0.08]	767 [0.52]	22 [0.32]	~5, 350 [0.36]
HF + BRS + EF	39 [0.04]	3 [0.02]	287 [0.18]	8 [0.12]	~1, 930 [0.13]
HF + HRT	30 [0.03]	12 [0.07]	118 [0.08]	3 [0.04]	~688 [0.05]
HF + HRT + EF	15 [0.015]	6 [0.04]	72 [0.05]	3 [0.04]	~424 [0.03]

MI – myocardial infarction, HF – heart failure, HRV – heart rate variability, EF – ejection fraction. Terms present in titles, abstracts or keywords. ? HRT

myocardial infarction (past epidemic) or heart failure (future epidemic) is between 0.5–2.0%. Meanwhile, the contribution of studies, in which ventricular function is investigated, reaches 10% on average (range 5–~25%).

Some reasons for a such situation are related to the multiplicity of methods, variety of algorithms within the same method, different number of confounding factors, use of complicated measures sometimes (or commonly) completely unintelligible for physicians, and inconsistency of data.

It would greatly improve matters if members of the next Task Force setting new Standards could unequivocally establish a basic protocol for HRV analysis. In addition, recommendations for minimum requirements for investigation reports would be helpful.

Some methodological suggestions that present an opportunity for a wider use of HRV in clinical practice are listed in ❷ Table 3.32. As the investigators' and clinicians' interests might not appear to converge, a close cooperation between clinicians and technicians or physicists would seem to be mandatory.

3.5 Physiological Basis of Heart Rate Fluctuations

Changes in heart rate have to be considered in the context of changes in the entire cardiovascular system, as well as in extra-cardiac body compartments, mainly within key vital organs. Hence, the physiological and pathophysiological interpretation of HR variation cannot be restricted to HR control itself. For clinical use, it would be necessary to separate HR changes that are functional (reflex or compensatory) from those which are related to true neuropathies.

The primary assumption usually taken is that the function of the sino-atrial node (SAN) is intact. Really, this holds true mainly in physiological states. In certain settings, it might not be unusual that heartbeat formation is compromised. The common clinical syndrome of heart failure may serve as an example [306], according to the early observation of

🔲 **Table 3.32**

Methodological guide for clinical HRV studies

1	Use a method explicable to physicians not familiar with HRV phenomenon
2	For global HRV estimates it is required (not obligatory) to:

2.
1. Calculate the number of subjects necessary to be examined on basis of reproducibility of the HRV measure going to be used
2. Look on data regarding reproducibility of chosen HRV measures in previous studies or provide results of a separate pilot-study
3. Be familiar with the prevalence of abnormal HRV within an examined sample (as it influences sensitivity of detection of abnormal HRV in a planned study)
4. Not rely on references' data that come from a limited (usually unsatisfactory) number of examined subjects
5. Be aware that there may be a substantial number of subjects (10–25%) with other than normal HRV indexes behavior
6. Do not rely on data obtained from a healthy population if the examined subjects suffer from any disease that is associated with HRV abnormality
7. Be sure that changes in HRV measures are really a result of an intervention and not contaminated by errors
8. Use devices with the lowest possible technical-related errors
9. Be familiar with the errors relating to characteristics of devices used
10. Balance gender proportion

3	For HRV estimates of certain [patho]physiological explanation (i.e., respiratory-related (=cardiac vagal tone), arterial pressure-related (= baroreflex (LF, HRT), vasomotor-tone related (VLF), day–night difference, activity (ULF, TP), baroreflex sensitivity, heart rate turbulence, it is required (not obligatory) to:

3.
1. Be sure that chosen method truly complies with an examined phenomenon
2. Be aware of reproducibility of chosen method or provide coefficient of variation in a sample of examined population
3. Carefully observe conditions of study for all examined persons (i.e., the same time of study for short-term HRV, similar diurnal activity for long-term HRV)
4. Balance gender proportion or perform separate investigation in females and males
5. Perform investigation in a few groups of different ages instead of a single study in large age-range group
6. Use a control group (nested-study design)
7. Comprehensively check for outliers
8. Include individual data if a small number of subjects is examined
9. Use a reference method (if exists) if a new method or a modification of an established method is introduced
10. Provide data regarding other significant determinants of HRV phenomenon (age, gender, race, HR, BP, respiratory rate, usual physical activity)
11. Provide data regarding important clinical entities (for example in AMI-patients: time-to-reperfusion (successful or failed), door-to-balloon time, infarct extension (CKMB mass, cardiac troponins), functional status (Killip class), hemodynamic data LVEF), use of drugs that interfere with HRV, etc.)
12. Avoid inclusion of subjects with various ANS derangement (i.e., diabetics, post-CABG) or with other confounding factors into a single group with subjects with a presumed intact ANS (no neuropathy), instead perform an investigation in separate groups

4.	Carefully follow the HRV Standards or the other Statements' requirements (if applicable)

Wollenberger in 1939. In this syndrome, pacemaker function is compromised and the responsiveness of the SAN to sympathetic over-activity is attenuated (so-called *chronotropic incompetence* (A term indicating inadequacy between heart rate and requirements, i.e. impaired HR adjustment for functional needs (usually metabolic))) [372], despite the resting HR being accelerated and the HRV reduced. Moreover, changes in intrinsic SAN properties appear before the overt HF syndrome [306]. The importance of intrinsic SAN should also be considered in such syndromes like hyperthyroidism, inappropriate sinus tachycardia, postural orthostatic tachycardia, and also in subjects with a high-vagal tone (endurance athletes) [306, 373, 374]. Also, in the model of high renin systemic arterial hypertension, an increased intrinsic firing of the SAN has been observed [374].

One the other hand, SAN abnormalities may be responsible for the inadequate response to proper neural stimuli leading to pacemaker desynchronization and irregular heart rate fluctuation. This can be observed experimentally in transgenic knock-in mice without the expression of cardiac connexin $Cx40^{-/-}$ and in the clinical setting in patients with sinus node disease [375, 376].

The second assumption usually taken is that heart period changes reliably reflect changes in sinus node firing. As parallel changes are normally seen in physiology and pathophysiology, sporadically this assumption is false. Overdrive stimulation of the SAN may lead to the so-called exit block [377, 378]. In such settings, the surface ECG shows a prolongation of heart period, while a series of SAN depolarization can actually be recorded from intra-cardiac electrodes.

The examples mentioned are given to emphasize the fact that heart period variation should be interpreted with caution when making conclusions about cardiac autonomic control of SAN activity. In fact, significant progress in the understanding of mechanisms of heartbeat formation, briefly described below, makes a detailed evaluation of the contribution of the autonomic nervous system and other modulators to heart period variation even more difficult.

3.5.1 Ionic Mechanisms of Heart Beat Formation

The self-excitability of specialized cardiac cells is related to the function of ionic channels that carry ionic currents responsible for *spontaneous diastolic depolarization* (The fourth phase of action potential of specialised cardiac myocytes involved in the impulse propagation.). The most important currents in this phase of the action potential are inward calcium currents (I_{CaL}, I_{CaT}), outward potassium currents (I_{Kr},I_{Ks},$I_{K[ACh]}$, $I_{K[Ca]}$) and inward hyperpolarization-activated cyclic nucleotide-gated (HCN) current I_f (*funny current* (Funny current means a current having a combined property aimed at distinct ion transportation)) [379, 380]. The latter current plays a major role in the generation and control of pacemaker activity (*pacemaker current* (An ionic current specific to self-excitable cardiomyocytes, not present in other working myocardial cells)) [380]. The I_f activation range varies largely from cell to cell, being more negative at peripheral areas. The I_f channels are uniquely activated by a direct binding of cyclic AMP (cAMP) molecules to the intracellular aspect of the channels. This property means that a funny-channel can be voltage-gated, as well as being a cyclic-nucleotide-gated (CNG) channel – part of a superfamily of CNG channels of sensory neurons (for review see [380]). Four isoforms of molecular components of f-channels have been cloned forming a family of HCN channels. In the heart, HCN4 is the major component in the pacemaker region. Accumulated data suggests that HCN2 prevents the diastolic membrane potential from becoming too negative and HCN4 is the major channel mediating sympathetic stimulation of the pacemaker activity. Recent studies indicate that a manipulation in HCN components was able to modify the spontaneous rate of pacemaker cells, thus opening an area for a clinical application of the so-called "biological" pacemakers [380].

Experimental studies have shown that I_f is a common effector of muscarinic and β-adrenergic activation through an allosteric conformation of the α-subunit of G-protein, a trimer protein coupled with a membrane GTP-ase [380]. It is suggested that this interaction depends on a lipid composition of the P-cells plasma membrane [381]. Experimental data also indicates an involvement of the sodium channel in the generation of sinus arrhythmia. A low concentration of tetrodotoxin reduces sinus rate and increases its variability [382]. The accumulated experimental and clinical data strengthen the role of the I_f current in heartbeat formation and opens an area for the clinical use of drugs that inhibits I_f currents (so-called HR-lowering drugs) [383].

3.5.2 Cellular Mechanisms

3.5.2.1 Pacemaker Cells

Sinus beat formation is the result of a *synchronisation* (Forced rate by a dominant pacemaker over neighboring P-cells, which generate diverse rates of spontaneous depolarisation while uncoupled.) of a group of spontaneously depolarizing cells, referred to as pacemaker cells (P-cells, pale, pacemaker, primitive) [384]. The highest density of P cells is to be found in the central region. However, they are also sparsely scattered in the right atrium. Each isolated P-cell possesses a similar self-excitable property. However, the frequency of beating is varied, even among neighboring P-cells due to the stochastic nature of channels opening and closing. A synchronized rate of firing is possible thanks to the between-cell communication related to the presence of gap junctions [384]. The common rate of a group of P-cells (synchronization) is based on a phenomenon called *phase resetting* (Changes in the frequency of depolarisation usually through recruitment of a new dominant pacemaker or alteration of the dominant pacemaker's rate.) due to mutual entrainment [385].

3.5.2.2 Sino-Atrial Node and Sino-Atrial Pacemaker Complex

That cardiac beats have their origin within the heart's own "substance" was initially proposed by Galen centuries ago. This "substance" had been discovered by Keith and Flack in 1907 as a fine subendocardial structure lying within the anterolateral part of the right atrium near the superior vena cava orifice (sino-atrial node, SAN). The proof of its role in heartbeat formation was provided by Lewis in 1910 [after 386]. However, electrophysiological studies in humans with the use of multisite mapping demonstrated that consecutive sinus beats of various lengths could appear in different sites that functionally might lie well beyond the anatomically defined SAN. This functional region, referred to as the *sino-atrial pacemaker complex*, spreads from the upper portion of the right atrium to the orifice of the inferior vena cava [387]. Pacemaker recruitment (a group of P-cells) with shortening cycle length appears more cranially, while when it moves caudally, a cycle length prolongation is observed due to the different sensitivity of P-cells to norepinephrine and acetylcholine depending on their location within the SAN and right atrium [388]. This phenomenon is referred to as *pacemaker shift* (A movement of a dominant pacemaker.) [381]. Apart from the different sensitivity of the P-cells to NA and ACh, a nonuniform autonomic innervation is thought to constitute an anatomical basis for the pacemaker shift, as evidenced by pharmacological interventions and SAN-specific autonomic nerve stimulation [389]. The pacemaker shift phenomenon is basically responsible for changeable sinus cycle length through variation in *sino-atrial conduction time* (Electrophysiological term (SACT, ms), indicates the time between the first depolarisation within the pacemaker complex (usually SAN) and the first depolarisation within atrial tissue (usually onset of the P-wave).). Changes in the chemical and physical environment could modulate this phenomenon, as happens with temperature changes, hypoxia, acidosis or hyperkalemia [390, 391].

3.5.3 Neuromediators and Hormones

3.5.3.1 Acethylcholine

Acethylcholine (ACh) is a key neurotransmitter of the parasympathetic branch of the autonomic nervous system [389]. ACh acts through the activation of ligand-gated ion channels (nicotinic receptors) or G-protein-coupled receptors (muscarinic receptors). With respect to heart rate autonomic control, nicotinic α-7 subunits mediate fast synaptic transmission in ganglia supplying the heart and muscarinic M_2 receptors mediate vagal stimulation in the SAN [389]. In addition, ACh modulates central pre-motor vagal activity [392].

ACh concentration at the SAN neuroeffector junction depends primarily on its kinetics. Tonic [DC] and phasic [AC] "net" vagal activity modulates ACh release from efferent cardiac vagal motorneurons endings [389]. In addition, ACh release is controlled by other mechanisms, including automodulation (pre-synaptic inhibition by ACh), transneuronal (pre-synaptic inhibition by NE through alfa1-adrenoceptor and NPY) and trans-synaptic (via prostaglandin PGE1 and adenosine) modulations [393]. Pre-synaptic automodulation is discussed as a possible mechanism involved in paradoxical HR slowing after low doses of atropine, an M_2-receptor antagonist [394].

The ionic mechanisms of ACh action depends on its local concentration. Small amounts of ACh inhibit I_f current, while larger (20-fold) amounts inhibit I_{CaL} and stimulates $I_{K[ACh]}$. The I_f inhibition is achieved through the stimulation of M_2-cholinergic receptor-coupled inhibitory G-protein G_i, that results in cAMP levels reduction and a negative shift of the I_f activation curve, thereby modulating its gating properties. It was also shown that a reduction of intracellular cAMP leads to a reduction of L-type Ca^{2+} current. The latter requires M_2-receptor coupling to $G_{\alpha 0}$ subunit and seems necessary to opposite effects of β-adrenergic stimulation [395].

Clearance properties depend on the rate of ACh hydrolysis by acetylcholinesterase. Its washout from the junction determines the actual local *effective concentration* of ACh [389]. Other factors, like the size of the release store terminal and diffusion to distant receptors, also influence the effective ACh concentration. ACh action on the P-cells is related to the number of M_2-receptors and their *saturation* (Lack of changes in sinus cycle duration in response to a certain increment or reduction in stimulation frequency above or below breakpoints. In a clinical setting, saturation denotes a lack of changes in heart beat variation with alteration in heart period duration. Such a phenomenon may be observed either in an extreme heart period prolongation or shortening.). The binding of ACh to M_2-receptors is necessary for its inhibitory effect on P-cell activity. This action modulates the intrinsic diastolic depolarization rate and antagonizes simultaneous sympathetic effects. In an *in vitro* study on isolated rabbit pacemaker cells, a superperfusion with ACh increases cycle length and its variation exponentially and interdependently [396]. However, in earlier experiments with vagal stimulation, a linear relationship has been observed [397]. Within a physiological (and pathophysiological) range of sinus cycle length, a linear relationship with vagal stimulation can also be seen in studies that advocate nonlinear relationships (❯ Fig. 3.38) [398]. Saturation at a longer sinus cycle length does not allow further prolongation to be linearly related, as an increase in stimulation frequency of the vagus does not result in a further substantial increase in ACh concentration (❯ Fig. 3.38 inset) [398]. A clinical study supporting such experimental data has been published [399]. Thus, two parts of a relationship can be observed, one within the usual range of the sinus cycle, where such a relationship is linear and a second within prolonged sinus cycles, where such a relationship is also linear but flat. In an extreme case, further increase in the frequency of vagal stimulation would result in significant sinus cycle prolongation. However, nonlinearities in the SAN response to stimulation of the vagus may, sporadically, result in sudden cycle shortening [377, 378]. Experimental studies have shown that under normal physiological conditions maximal diastolic potential and threshold potential are actually not affected by neural activation. However, this may not hold true in a pathological setting [396].

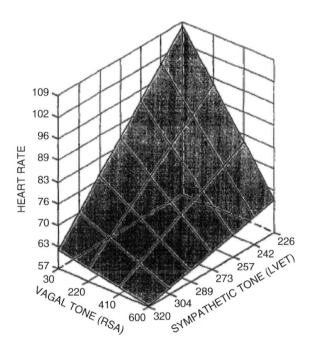

◻ Fig. 3.38
Dependency of pacemaker cycle length on the rate of vagal neural activity. Nonlinear relationship between the frequency of vagal stimulation and sinus cycle length in a rabbit pacemaker cells. Note, within physiological rate the relationship is linear. Inset: a plot of ACh concentration against the frequency of vagal stimulation indicating a phenomenon of saturation (From [396])

3.5.3.2   Norepinephrine and Epinephrine

Norepinephrine (NE) is a catecholamine released from sympathetic nerve terminals, while epinephrine (Epi) is a circulating hormone synthesized in and released from the suprarenal medulla. These substances accelerate the spontaneous diastolic depolarization of the pacemaker cells via stimulation of the β-adrenergic receptors (βAR) coupled to the stimulatory G-protein G_s, with activation of adenylate cyclase and increase in cAMP levels [393, 398]. Subsequently, a shift of the I_f activation curve to a more positive voltage occurs and heart rate accelerates. In certain conditions, activation of I_{CA} and I_K channels mediates NE effects on pacemaker cells [400]. Although NE and Epi act mainly through activation of βAR, their effects depend on the specific properties and pathways of various types of βAR, as well as on the action on α-adrenergic receptors (αAR) [401, 402].

3.5.3.3   Neuropeptide Y

Neuropeptide Y (NPY) represents one of various neuropeptides that act in addition to the "classical" neurotransmitters. NPY coexists with NE in cardiac sympathetic nerve terminals. Dense population of NPY-immunoreactive nerves is found in the SAN region [403]. The NPY-nerves also form synapses on the soma and dendrites of vagal preganglionic neurons within NA [404]. Upon a direct sympathetic stimulation, NPY is co-released with NE within the α-adrenoceptor [404]. Some data suggests that NPY inhibits ACh release from pre- and postganglionic parasympathetic neurons, thereby attenuating cardiac vagal action [404–407].

3.5.3.4   Nitric Oxide

Nitric oxide (NO) is a signaling molecule that mediates vasomotor tone, ATP production and cardiac contractility. Recently, its role as a mediator of the peripheral autonomic control of the heart has been extensively studied [408–418]. The presence of endothelial NO synthase (eNOS) in human cardiomyocytes [413] and neuronal NO synthase (nNOS) in cholinergic and sympathetic nerve terminals, as well as NO-sensitive neurons in the stellate and intrinsic cardiac ganglia argues for a role for NO in heartbeat control [408, 409, 411, 412]. Neuronal NOS is present in the central nervous system nuclei contributing to vasomotor and cardiac control, like the solitary tract nucleus (STN), nucleus ambiguous, dorsal nucleus of vagus, ventrolateral zona reticularis in the medulla oblongata, and in the periphery in carotid bodies [409, 410].

NOS inhibition has been shown to block the negative chronotropic effects of cholinergic agonists and prevent cholinergic inhibition of I_{CaL} in sympathetically activated pacemaker cells *in vitro* [414]. In a study with a nNOS inhibitor, a dose-dependent profound bradycardia has been found in parallel with a large increase in heart rate variability and, at larger doses, vasoconstriction [415]. The effects of NO donors and inhibitors on HR control are thought to be indirect, consistent with a presynaptic modulation of vagal neurotransmission and ACh release during vagal activation. A significant post-synaptic action via ACh-M_2 receptor coupling to eNOS has also been reported. The post-synaptic action of NO (HR acceleration via I_f activation) has been shown to be opposite to that of pre-synaptic action (HR slowing via a facilitation of the ACh release). However, data are not consistent. The importance of NO action seems to be more pronounced with age and adrenergic activation [408, 410–412].

Nitric oxide can also interfere with β-adrenergic signaling. This action can be mediated through cAMP degradation (either via activation of phosphodiesterase activity or inhibition of Ca channels) and the inhibition of NE release (via NO-cGMP and, independently, K_{ATP}–channel mechanisms) [408]. Additionally, NO contributes to the metabolic breakdown of NE and provides a barrier for diffusion of the NE into the bloodstream. NO can also inhibit central sympathetic neurotransmission [411, 412]. The central part of NO contribution to CV control includes the modulation of aortic and carotid mechanoceptor reflexes, reduction in the sensitivity of cardiac baroreflex and augmentation of tonic vagal activity [410].

Recent studies indicate that NO action on the cardiac vagus might have a clinical perspective [416, 418]. In an experimental study, targeted nNOS gene transfer enhancing nNOS expression resulted in a rapid increase in parasympathetic activity. In a study in patients with heart failure, those who were homozygous for the T/C polymorphism of the e-NOS promoter had a more advanced imbalance of the autonomic cardiac control [421] in spite of better left ventricular function.

As vagal stimulation is thought to be cardioprotective [419] and might increase the probability of survival after myocardial infarction [420], the importance of vagal modulation through NO donors [418] or NOS expression manipulations [416] awaits clinical verification.

3.5.3.5 Serotonin (5-Hydroxytryptamine)

All central brain nuclei that are involved in cardiovascular control are innervated by fibers containing serotonin and have direct or indirect synaptic contact with cardiac vagal preganglionic fibers that are likely to originate from within the brainstem [422]. Some vagal afferents also contain 5-HT. In addition, these regions express a wide range of 5-HT receptors. The blockade of 5-HT1A receptors attenuates the bradycardic response evoked by baroreceptor and cardiopulmonary receptor afferents stimulation. However, the number of 5-HT receptors and variable effects of their activation/inhibition limits understanding of their functional roles [422].

3.5.3.6 Neuregulins

Neuregulins are growth factors that are required for the maintenance of ACh receptor-inducing activity of nicotinic receptors. A recent observation in an experimental study in mice with neuregulin-1 gene deletion supports a role for neuregulins in maintaining normal parasympathetic modulation of excess β-adrenergic stimulation of the heart [423]. It might be of clinical importance in patients treated with cardiotoxic drugs that are known to suppress neuregulins signaling. Such drugs, i.e., doxorubicine, can lead to the development of cardiac impairment that is accompanied by a reduction in parasympathetic activity that may even precede the occurrence of overt heart failure [424].

3.5.4 Local Tissue Factors

Locally released mediators, mainly neuropeptides, may generally act as neurotransmitters, neuromodulators or neurohormones. Substances, like vasoactive intestinal peptide, somatostatin, substance P, neurotensin, phenyl-histidin-isoleucine, dynorphine or melatonin-stimulating hormone are released from neuronal endings within the SA node or from interconnecting neurons in peri-nodal ganglia. Peptides synthetized locally in the endothelium of coronary microcirculation or in the SA node, atrial or ventricular myocytes, can modulate sinus beat formation [425, 426]. Positive chronotropic action was observed after stimulation with adreno-medulline, angiotensin II (via AT1 receptor), atrial natriuretic peptide C and endothelin (via ET_A receptor), while a negative chronotropic effect was observed in response to bradykinin, somatostatin and endothelin (via ET_B receptor) [425, 426]. Other peptides (ANP, BNP, substance P) are considered as cardiac rhythm modulators. However, evidence for their direct actions are conflicting [427]. Cholinergic and sympathetic neuron activity can also be modulated by several amino acids, purine derivates, and free radicals [428]. A role for all of these local factors is probably limited in a normal physiological state.

3.5.5 Mechanical-Electrical Feedback

Active and passive changes in the mechanical load of the heart, either physiological or pathological, can influence the initiation and propagation of cardiac electrical excitation via pathways that are intrinsic to the heart itself. This cross-talk between mechanical and electrical activity is referred to as contraction-excitation or mechanical-electrical feedback (MEF) [429]. Processes involved in the MEF include stretch-activated ion channels in cardiomyocytes, changes in calcium handling, interaction with other mechano-sensitive non-myocyte cells, or stimulation of protein expression, local peptides secretion, and biochemical changes [430, 431]. Mechanical factors are believed to be involved in heartbeat triggering during the early stages in embryogenesis [432]. The mechanical contribution to HRV can be observed in heart transplant patients, in whom a small (2–8% of normal) RSA has been recorded [433]. Similar findings have been reported in individuals after brain death [434].

3.5.6   Vascular Factors (Endothelium)

In general, the ANS and endothelium play opposite roles in controlling vascular tone through their action on the vascular smooth muscle layer, which lies between the two [435]. There is evidence that the ANS directly influences the endothelial cell function due to the presence of α_2- and β-adrenoceptors and muscarinic receptors. The activation of α_2-adrenergic and muscarinic receptors results in eNO release and subsequent vasodilation. In addition, sympathetic activation can stimulate the release of endothelium-derived contracting factors. The effect of ANS stimulation can be observed despite the presence of major conduit vessels that do not receive direct innervation. On the other hand, the endothelium may affect the extent of ANS-mediated vascular tone mainly through the changes in NO production and release [435]. The role of the endothelium in mediating ANS effects increases in clinical entities, in which endothelial dysfunction is a common feature (e.g., diabetes mellitus, hypertension).

3.5.7   Hormonal, Inflammatory and Other Humoral Factors

3.5.7.1   Renin–Angiotensin–Aldosterone System

The renin-angiotensin-aldosterone system (RAAS) interacts with the autonomic control of the heart at both central and peripheral levels [425]. Angiotensin II (AngII), a key hormone of RAAS, enhances central sympathetic tone and facilitates the NE release from sympathetic nerve terminals [436]. The net effect of RAAS activation is related to the entire circulatory response (circulating AngII level), cardiac local AngII action, and central local interaction within cardiovascular and respiratory centers [425, 437]. The magnitude of RAAS-ANS interactions depends on genetic variations (polymorphisms) within RAAS [438, 439]. In addition, the response of the RAAS blockade (with either ACEI or ARBs) varies, as different agents of these classes have been shown to exhibit divergent effects on autonomic function [440–442]. In addition, these effects depend on the initial status (before treatment) of the autonomic balance, with negligible changes in healthy persons or significant, albeit not uniform, changes in patients with hypertension or heart failure [440–442]. Sympathoexcitatory action of aldosterone (central or peripheral) both directly or via an inhibition of nitric oxide synthesis [443], together with the involvement of bradykinin, with its direct chronotropic effects [444, 445], further complicate explanation of the effects of RAAS activation or inhibition on cardiovascular autonomic control.

3.5.7.2   Hypothalamic–Pituitary–Adrenal System

Corticotropin-releasing hormone (CRH) is the principal regulatory neuropeptide that mediates stress-related biological responses as a physiologic regulator of adrenal epinephrine secretion [425, 446]. Neuroanatomical studies show a projection of CRH-fibers linked directly to autonomic regulatory nuclei in the brainstem [447, 448]. There is little experimental evidence of its sympathotonic effect. This action depends on a heterogeneous distribution of CRH-receptor subtypes between ANS brain centres and the heart and vasculature [447–449]. Recent studies have shown the presence of endogenous agonist for CRH2-receptor, referred to as urocortin, which mediates many actions previously attributed to CRH [450]. Interestingly, the results of a study in CRH2-receptor-deficient rodents suggest that CRH may act on a long time scale, i.e., h, thereby influencing the circadian rhythm of HR and its variation [451]. Adrenocorticotropin and cortisol actions are very complex and diverse, depending on the magnitude and length of stressful conditions [452]. Although they are involved in circadian and ultradian (12-h, 90-min) circulatory oscillations, short-term fluctuations (3-min) have been observed [453]. An increased vagal HR control has been reported in a clinical setting such as hypercortisolemia [454].

3.5.7.3 Insulin-Leptin-Adiponectin and Inflammatory Cytokines

Insulin leads to an acute hyperpolarization of the plasma membranes. With respect to excitable cardiac conduction tissue, this may result in an attenuation of the firing response to stimulation and desensitization of HRV during euglycemic hyperinsulinemia in subjects with intact autonomic control [455–459]. Insulin also affects the sensitivity of arterial baroreceptors. Insulin exerts its action indirectly through adrenergic activation that is expressed as a centrally-mediated stress reaction, an increase in the firing rate of adrenergic nerves and a shift in the sympathovagal balance in the HRV power spectrum [456–459]. These effects are age-dependent [460].

Insulin action, like other trophic factors (growth hormone, tumor necrosis factor α, transforming growth factor β), might be also related to the modification of M_2R expression via transcriptional regulation and M_2R downregulation. These changes may lead to parasympathetic withdrawal [459, 461]. Clinical studies suggest that parasympathetic modifications can occur early on in the development of obesity and diabetes and are concomitant with a greater variation in plasma insulin levels [460, 461] and insulin sensitivity or resistance [462, 463].

Leptin, the adipose tissue hormone, plays a crucial role in body weight control. A release of leptin is under tonic feedback control by the sympathetic nervous system. Adrenergic neurotransmitters exert an inhibitory effect on leptin release and synthesis [464]. Actually, leptin itself might influence the sympathetic neural drive and either acutely or chronically increase HR. This action can be completely reversed by a combined adrenergic blockade [465]. The significance of leptin-sympathetic activity in normal subjects is not clear, as a greater correlation with HR alone than with sympathetic nerve traffic has been reported. However, gender differences have been observed [466]. Recently, an association of leptin circadian and ultradian rhythms with a very-low oscillation of HR has been reported [467]. Also, the G/A polymorphism in the human leptin receptor gene influences sympathovagal balance.

Adiponectin is an adipocyte derived hormone which acts on the CNS to control autonomic function, energy and cardiovascular homeostasis [468, 469]. It acts as an insulin-sensitizing hormone and its circulating concentration is inversely related to adipose tissue mass [468]. Adiponectin receptors have been found in brain nuclei, playing a central role in the integration of cardiac autonomic control where it interacts with neuropeptide-Y neurons [470, 471]. Low serum adiponectin has been shown to negatively correlate with a sympathovagal index in patients with type-2 diabetes [472]. Hypoadiponectinemia has also been reported to be associated with sympathetic overactivity in obstructive sleep apnea syndrome [473].

Inflammatory cytokines are normally produced by the immune system. However, their excessive expression can in some circumstances lead to damage of various tissues, as they are involved in chronic inflammatory diseases, including atherosclerosis among others [474]. Experimental and clinical evidence indicates that stimulation of parasympathetic activity (via the nicotinic receptor) can result in anti-inflammatory action via inhibition of the production of some cytokines, like tumor necrosis factor α, interleukin-1, interleukin-6 and interleukin-8 [475]. Activated macrophages and lymphocytes also express specific receptors for other neurotransmitters released by the autonomic and central nervous system, including those mentioned above [475].

On the other hand, there are many clinical reports on the association of noninvasive measures of cardiac autonomic control (on the basis of HRV analysis) with the most commonly examined inflammatory substances, like C-reactive protein, interleukin-6 and TNF-α. However, negative observations also exist [370, 476, 477].

3.5.7.4 Gonadal Hormones

Accumulating evidence suggests that gonadal hormones, especially oestrogen, have significant effects on the brain, peripheral efferent nerves and signaling pathways of effector organ/cells that respond to neurotransmitters [478]. Gonadal hormone signals are mediated through binding of steroids to cytoplasmic/nuclear receptors (genomic actions) and membrane receptors (non-genomic actions). Nuclear oestrogen receptor and membrane binding sites for oestrogen, progestrone and testosterone have been identified in brain nuclei involved in the regulation of cardiovascular function [478].

The central action of oestrogen includes increased vagal tone via stimulation of choline uptake and ACh synthesis and suppressed sympathetic efferent activity via the stimulation of catalytic activity of catechol-0-methyltransferase and monamino oxidase. On the contrary, testosterone increases sympathetic activity via the stimulation of the synthesis of

NE and neuropeptide Y and the inhibition of NE clearance. Oestrogen increases the density and affinity of muscarinic receptors. In the periphery, the actions of gonadal hormones are similar to those acting centrally. Under experimental conditions, exogenous oestrogen and progesterone increases the density of β-adrenergic and muscarinic receptors in the heart, while testosterone stimulates choline uptake and thyrosine hydroxylase (catecholamine synthetase). Some effects of gonadal hormones are mediated through nitric oxide [478].

There are differences in the parasympathetic and sympathetic responsiveness in females and males - the parasympathetic response is greater in females and the sympathetic response greater in males. There is more pronounced bradycardia after vagal stimulation. Apart from experimental data, there are concordant data indicating the positive correlation between oestrogen level and cardiac vagal activity that can be observed during either the menstrual cycle or the menopausal period [479–482]. Some of these changes can be related to the action of endogenous progesterone-related steroids, which inhibits muscarinic receptors probably via their allosteric conformation and increases central NE release [478]. The attenuation of HRV has also been observed during progestogen-containing replacement therapy [483]. However, in a randomized trial on hormone replacement therapy in postmenopausal women, multiple 24-h HRV indices remained unchanged [484]. However, it has to be noted that the approach used in this trial is too crude to explore cardiac autonomic control.

3.5.8   Thermoregulation

Heart rate (or pulse rate) changes with hyper- or hypothermia are easy to detect. In some disease states (e.g., typhoid fever), a lack of heart rate acceleration, or even HR slowing in spite of increasing body temperature, has been considered to be an ominous sign by attending physicians.

Thermoregulation is a complex integrative process generating patterns of autonomic, motor, endocrine and behavioral changes in response to endogenous and environmental challenges. By considering the impact of thermoregulation on cardiac autonomic control, both circadian variation of body temperature balancing over a core temperature "set-point" and reactivity to cold or heat exposure can be investigated.

Circadian variation of body temperature is related to the central pacemaker located in suprachiasmatic nuclei, acting upon hypothalamic centres modulating the set point, and altering the thresholds for cutaneous vasodilatation and sweating [485, 486]. This circadian rhythm is involved in the regulation of the sleep–wake cycle together with pineal melatonin rhythm, and the responsiveness of the circadian pacemaker to light. From this point of view, thermoregulation is associated with the circardian rhythm of heart rate and its variation, being similar to sympathetic rhythm and opposite to cardiac vagal rhythm. There is neuroanatomical and neurochemical evidence linking central sympathetic activity with the sleep-wake clock and temperature rhythm [487].

The potentiation of cardiac vagal action in response to cold and vagal inhibitory effects during heat stress has been reported [488–490]. Also, thermogenic-related changes within cardiac autonomic control have been studied in response to various meals [491]. Variations in the frequency of the thermal component of HRV has been shown to arise from variations in the time delay in response to a periodic thermal stimulus and has been referred to as thermal entrainment [492].

3.5.9   Architecture of Cardiac Autonomic Control

3.5.9.1   Anatomical Basis for Cardiac Autonomic Control

Efferent Limb of Cardiac Vagal Control

Inhibitory vagal motorneurons originate in the dorsal vagal nucleus (DVN) and nucleus ambiguous (NA). The preganglionic motor neurons in the DVN and NA may exert preferential control over separate populations of neurons within the intrinsic cardiac ganglionated nervous system [493]. Their activity is characterized by tonic discharges modulated in phase with respiration. However, they are not able to generate spontaneous activity. Instead, their action potential generation rate follows the impulsation of glutaminergic neurones from the solitary tract nucleus (STN) in the dorsal medulla, where all afferent autonomic fibers are terminated. The importance of diverse cardiac vagal efferents may lie in the fact that an intact DVN is not necessary for an efficient baroreceptor reflex, while other cardiopulmonary reflexes are critically-dependent on an intact DVN [494, 495].

Vagal efferent motorneurons sprouting to the mediastinum form the anterior and posterior cardiac plexus. Aside from presynaptic parasympathetic fibers, these plexi also contain presynaptic sympathetic fibers, intermediate puriner-gic neurons and autonomic ganglia [496]. Postsynaptic fibers of the vagi preferentially innervate SAN and AVN regions and atrial muscles [497]. Parasympathetic innervation of the ventricle is rather sparse and, accordingly, the ACh concentration in ventricular tissue is lower, achieving approximately ¼ of its concentration in the atria. Although a weak inhibitory action of parasympathetic stimulation on LV hemodynamics can be observed in experiments, espe-cially when the sympathetic drive is augmented (*accentuated antagonism*), such an effect seems to be negligible in physiology [498].

The main effect of vagal stimulation is a reduction of sinus node rate. The magnitude of sinus cycle prolongation is greater after stimulation of the right vagus nerve, while the left vagus nerve exerts a stronger inhibitory action on the impulse conduction through the AV junction. A negative chronotropic action of vagal stimulation is phase and frequency-dependent. The SAN response to vagal stimulation is rapid, with a latency period less than 400 ms, and is sustained for less than 5 s after cessation of stimulation [396, 498]. Since the relationship between the frequency of vagal stimulation and slowing HR is nonlinear, changes in the heart period (sinus cycle) seem to be a better indicator of vagal influences [396]. However, it has to be remembered that the time-delay of the vagally-mediated response can vary significantly not only in healthy people, but even more so in patients with cardiac disease [499].

Efferent Limb of Cardiac Sympathetic Control

Pre-motor sympathetic neurons are located in clusters in four topographically defined nuclei in the intermediate gray matter on either side of the spinal cord (mainly intermediolateralis thoraco-lumbalis pars funiculus) [500]. Presynaptic sympathetic stimulating fibers spread like the sympathetic nerves into the thoracic sympathetic ganglia. Postsynap-tic fibers from these ganglia travel by two pathways: firstly as sympathetic nerves directly to intrathoracic extra- and intra-cardiac plexi, further innervating atrial and myocardial muscle, and secondly, as sympathetic fibers of the stellate ganglions joining the vagi, traveling to specialized cardiac self-excitable and conducting tissue [500]. The sympathetic fibers traveling with the vagus nerve may contribute to the axo-axonal synapses that have been observed to lie between these nerves, providing a morphological basis for the observed vagal-sympathetic interaction [501].

Afferent Limb of Cardiac Autonomic Control

In general, cardiovascular afferent neurons are divided as those that are sensible to mechanical deformation in the region of their sensory endings (mechanosensors) and those that detect alteration in chemical milieu surrounding their sensory neurites (chemosensors) [397]. Anatomical and functional data indicate that most of afferent neurons can simultaneously transmit mechanical and chemical signals [502]. Also, the distribution of neural somata of different sensors is similar throughout nodose, dorsal root, intrathoracic and cardiac ganglia.

Mechanosensors localized in the right ventricular papillary muscle transmit RV loading or pressure in a linear and reciprocal manner. Those distributed throughout the outflow tract of the right and left ventricles sense development of chamber pressure, but their exponential activation patterns vary. Significant populations of mechanosensors along the adventitia of the inner arch of the thoracic aorta and the base of both venae cavae precisely detect phasic mechanical changes that are undergone during each systolic and diastolic event.

There is a limited population of chemosensors, which are activated when exposed to an altered concentration of a variety of local chemicals. Most local mechanical and chemical stimuli sensed by the neuronal endings are transmitted to adjacent neurons that form local circuit interconnections at cardiac and intrathoracic ganglia. These functional linkages are relevant to short-loop cardio-cardiac and vascular-cardiac reflexes. Sensory information arising from the heart and major vessels initiate central and peripheral reflexes that control the activity of extracardiac (long- and short-loop) and intrinsic cardiac motorneurons (ultra short-loop) [496, 503].

The direct measurement of vagal nerve activity is usually employed in experimental settings. However, the invasive nature, need for anesthesia and limited functional and behavioral contexts restrict the utility of the direct approach. Occasionally, direct recordings can be made from cervical vagal afferents and their stimulation can be applied to humans [504].

3.5.9.2   Local Cardiovascular-Cardiac Reflexes

Cardiac mechanosensory reflexes characterize short-tem latency due to a relatively short distance to the first synapse. The short-term scaling properties are responsible for the cardiac motorneurons' differential activation at any phases of the cardiac cycle [505]. Cardiac mechanosensitivity seems to be related to an expression of titin [506]. Some intrathoracic efferent neurons display activation reflecting initiation of the aortic and carotid baroreflex. In addition, the stretching of vena cava mechanosensors (which can be found with venous congestion) trigger intrathoracic reflexes.

Cardiac chemosensory reflexes modulate large numbers of cardiac motorneurons over longer timescales and multiple cardiac cycles. They also lead to the resetting of cardiac motorneuron activity for a period considered to be long enough to indicate the retention of information (*memory* (Biological phenomenon of determinism in which future events are causally set by past events)) [507].

3.5.9.3   Accentuated Antagonism

The nonlinear nature of autonomic interactions within the sino-atrial pacemaker complex is emphasized when both arms of autonomic cardiac control are activated. Levy et al. found that the cardiac pacemaker response to the vagus nerve stimulation is greater with a rise in sympathetic activity (*accentuation*) in spite of their opposite action (*antagonism*) [15, 498] (❯ Fig. 3.39). Such a phenomenon, referred to as *accentuated antagonism*, can be seen in very fit humans. In older people, and in certain clinical pathophysiological settings, this phenomenon cannot be observed easily, as the vagal activity or inhibitory effects of its stimulation are usually depressed. Pyetan et al. [508] found an increase in power at respiratory frequency in a healthy young adult with a high level of cardiac vagal tone subjected to a relatively large cumulative dose

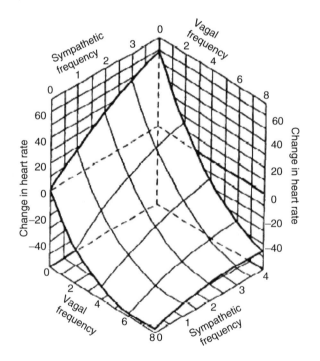

◻ **Fig. 3.39**

Sympathetic-parasympathetic accentuated antagonism. Changes in HR in response to various vagal and sympathetic stimulation. Vagal inhibition is greater when sympathetic activity increases, sympathetic stimulation is much less when vagi are active. The formed exemplifies synergism, the latter antagonism (From [A31])

of atropine. They interpreted such a response as a feature of the reduction of sympathetic influence accompanying vagal effector inhibition.

3.5.10 Nonregulatory Reflexes Involving Co-Activation of ANS

Classic reciprocal action between sympathetic and parasympathetic outflows represents a highly simplified description of cardiac autonomic control. The presence of the accentuated antagonism between two branches of the ANS in physiologic and pathophysiologic settings can find further support in some protective reflexes that are accompanied by excitation of both autonomic outflows [509].

Among reflexes that are accompanied by the co-activation of both ANS branches, the peripheral chemoreflex, diving response, oculocardiac reflex, defense response, and somatic nociception response are considered [509]. The common functional significance of these reflexes/responses is considered to coordinate the relationship between ventricular contractility and heart rate with sympathetic and vagal activation targeting the ventricular myocardium and SAN, respectively. This may be of special importance during a prolonged and deep hypoxia (diving response), when the bradycardic response causes a substantial fall in ventricular function via a nonneural mechanism (So-called Bowdich effect.) and sympathetic co-activation may serve as a compensatory response to maintain stroke volume, as well as blood flow and oxygen delivery to the heart through action upon coronary arterioles via β-adrenoceptor stimulation. Another possible significance is related to vagally-mediated tachycardia, when both branches of the ANS act synergistically. It is suggested that this paradoxical feature is related to ACh release in the intrinsic cardiac ganglia neurons along with activation of chromafine cells to release catecholamines. Alternative explanations include the muscarinic receptor mediated release of neurotransmitters co-localizing cardiac vagal fibers, which may have the same effect as NE of increasing HR.

3.5.10.1 Peripheral Chemoreceptor Reflex

In experimental settings, activation of carotid body chemosensors resulted in the transient increase in cardiac vagal and sympathetic activity reflected by a profound bradycardic response. Co-activation of branches of the ANS can also be elicited by a mild prolonged hypercapnia and mild hypoxia, whereas a co-inhibition occurs in response to hypocapnia.

3.5.10.2 Diving Reflex

Vagally-mediated bradycardia is a major feature of the diving response in humans and other mammals. It is suggested that facial or nasopharyngeal stimulation is responsible for this reflex. Coincidence of sympathetic activation during the diving reflex is expressed as the occurrence of ventricular arrhythmias, including polymorphic VT, and shortening of the QT interval, that can be prevented by β-adrenoceptor blockade with propranolol.

3.5.10.3 Oculocardiac Reflex

The stimulation of trigeminal nerve endings triggers a reflex that produces vagally-mediated bradycardia and which in extreme cases may lead to cardiac arrest. Historically, this reflex has been used as a manual procedure for the termination of paroxysmal tachycardia (Aschner) by putting pressure on the ocular bulbs (more precisely on the corneal surface). A sympathetic component of this reflex is expressed as increased outflow to the ventricles and, subsequently the occurrence of ventricular ectopic beats.

3.5.10.4 Defence Responses

Experimental stimulation of different discrete hypothalamic areas evokes various possible patterns of ANS activation (sympathetic activation/vagal inhibition or co-activation or co-inhibition). In the case of centrally-mediated ANS co-activation, HR follows vagal changes. The defence-like response may also occur in the response to alerting-eliciting acoustic stimuli (startle reflex). Despite these stimuli provoking a small transient tachycardia, a pronounced negative chronotropic effect of sympathetic blockade suggests a role of vagal co-activation. Interestingly, the vagal response rapidly habituates with repeated stimuli, while sympathetic activation persists.

3.5.10.5 Somatic Nociception Response

Stimulation of somatic nociceptors typically leads to tachycardia, increase in blood pressure and hyperpnea in animals and humans. Direct cardiac vagal nerve recording has shown that the nociception response involves augmentation in the activity of cardiac vagal outputs. It is postulated that this complex response is centrally-mediated and modulated by central respiratory activity. Nociception-evoked tachycardia seems to be vagally-mediated and can be attenuated by atropine. However, a combined blockade is necessary to abolish this chronotropic response completely.

3.5.11   Brain–Heart Interactions

It is well recognized that sympathetic and parasympathetic neurons play a regulatory role in modulating cardiac dynamics. This regulatory role is achieved through a very complex structural and functional interplay between afferent neurons localized in different cardiac regions and within vascular beds (mainly intrathoracic and cervical) and efferent neurons localized in the cerebral cortex, brain stem nuclei, medulla oblongata, spinal cord, paravertebral cervical, and thoracic ganglia, as well as pericardial and intrinsic cardiac ganglia. Spatially overlapping afferent neurons differentially transduce regional cardiac and vascular events throughout each cardiac cycle directly or indirectly (via interconnecting neurons) allowing for temporally organized reflexes. All constitutive parts are redundant and stabilize the whole cardiac behavior [507].

In pathological settings, overactivity of the autonomic nervous system plays a critical role in myocardial damage and mortality [13, 510]. Therefore, abnormal cardiac rhythm oscillations can be seen in patients with stroke, subarachnoid hemorrhage, epilepsy, and head trauma [510–513]. Brain-heart interactions are also important in the pathogenesis of (a) sudden unexpected death in adults and infants, in specific circumstances (for example status asthmaticus, alcohol-withdrawal, drug abuse) [56, 510], and (b) cardiac dysfunction in tako-tsubo cardiomyopathy and phaeochromocytoma, in which altered fluctuations of heart rate can be detected [514–516].

3.6   Determinants of HRV

3.6.1   Genetic Factors

There is accumulating data confirming the role of genetic factors in HR and HRV control. Early data suggested that genetic variance can determine the arrhythmia index, the measure of RSA introduced by Schlomka, which has been reported by Fuller in 1951 in purebred dogs [517]. Kreutz et al. were the first group to identify HR-determining gene location on the rat chromosome 3 [518]. Since that time, other genes which contribute to heart rate have been described [519–523].

Martin et al. [519] performed the variance decomposition linkage analysis for genomic screening in 2209 individuals and found that the heritability of the resting HR was around 26%. In their study, HR linkage on chromosome 4 (4q28.2) was observed. Interestingly, in this region, linkages have also been found for insulin, blood pressure, abdominal subcutaneous fat, as well as for type 4 long QT syndrome, associated with bradycardia [after 519]. Similar heritability (24–27%), as well as HR linkage to chromosome 4 has been reported among hypertensives [520]. A heritability of 36% for HR and 20% for BP responses to exercise training has been found in another set of patients with high blood pressure [521] and various candidate genes have been proposed [522]. A recent meta-analysis of genome wide scans indicates the location of a gene influencing HR on chromosome 5p13–14 [523].

The attempts that explore the HR genetic basis do not necessarily explain the genetic background of HRV. The results of the Copenhagen Holter Study indicate a significant association of a reduced HRV with the familial predisposition to premature heart attack [524]. Using a genome-wide scan in participants from the Framingham Heart Study, Singh et al. have provided evidence of linkage of the LF power to chromosome 2 and of the VLF power to chromosome 15, although the linkage odds scores have not exceeded the threshold for significant linkage on a genome-wide level [525]. Interestingly, around the region of interest (chromosome 2), a candidate gene for KCNJ3, a human gene encoding the G-protein activated inwardly rectifying potassium channel, known to be involved in HR regulation [526], has been identified. Also, candidate genes for human neuronal nicotinic cholinergic receptors have been reported on chromosome 15 [527].

The combined results of the Framingham Heart Study and Framingham Off-Spring Study (1151 subjects) indicate the presence of a significant correlation among standard HRV parameters in siblings (between 0.21 and 0.26), compared to spouses (0.01–0.19) [528]. Genetic factors seem to be responsible for substantial inter-individual variations in HRV that reached 23% in the Framingham cohort. However, after the adjustment for HR, this proportion is reduced to 9–22%, suggesting an involvement of similar genetic factors that determine both the HR and HRV [528]. Genes account for 13–23% of the variation among spectral HRV measures in this population [529]. Heritability estimates of 0.41–0.45 for SDNN and of 0.39–0.45 for RMSSD from 5-min ECG recordings have been reported to be independent of breathing mode (spontaneous vs controlled) [530].

Associations between HRV and genetics are frequently explored in twins [531–539]. In a small sample of twins, Piha et al. found that both ANS branches were strongly related to genetic factors independently of body mass [531]. In a larger sample of 160 twins, the RSA appeared to be determined by stable genetic factors and variable environmental components [532]. Snieder et al. have estimated a genetic contribution to RSA of 31% at rest and between 28% and 43% at four different stress task conditions [533], independently of respiratory rate. A genetic contribution to the mean ambulatory SDNN index (ranging from 35% to 47%) and the mean ambulatory RMSSD (ranging from 40% to 48%) has been reported [534]. Short-term vagally-related HRV measures (RMSSD and HV power) at rest and under stress have been found to be largely influenced by the same gene [535]. An association of reduced HRV and depression has been found to be genetically-predetermined [536]. Also, the dipper-pattern of the blood pressure has been found to be heritable [537]. Importantly, HRV-related familiarity can be detected already in newborns. However, environmental influences seem to play a greater role than genetic factors early in life [538].

In a recent study, an association of parasympathetic activity with the variation in the choline transporter, a component of ACh neurotransmission, has been reported. Subjects having any T-allele (TT or GT genotype) had greater HF power and lower LF power and LF/HF ratio, compared to subjects with GG genotype [539]. Studies that compared HRV in relation to known genetic polymorphisms (ACEI, angiotensinogen, uncoupling proteins) complement evidence for a genetic background of HRV [540, 541]. Furthermore, an experimental investigation has confirmed the importance of G-protein heritability for HR autonomic control [542].

3.6.2 Constitutional Factors

3.6.2.1 Age

Heart rate and its variation is critically dependent on age, especially if one considers the period of the entire lifespan [322]. Within the lifespan, two distinct phases are present with distinct HRV behavior. The first phase is a period of development and maturation, and the second starts early in adulthood and is related to aging and senescence. Therefore, in studies in which the age-range is limited (e.g., a young adult cohort or middle-aged subjects) the possibility of detection of significant HRV changes with age is *a priori* reduced. Also, data on the age-dependence of HRV is generally obtained from cross-sectional studies. To evaluate within-person age-related changes, longitudinal observations seem to be more appropriate.

Autonomic Control Changes During Development

Detectable variation in heart rate can already be observed in fetuses [543]. Mechanisms underlying these variations are largely unknown. An intrinsic rhythmicity of the SAN seems to determine HR changes early in gestation (9–15 weeks), albeit cholinesterase activity can be detected at the eighth gestational week. With the advance of gestation, parasympathetic effects become evident [543]. More data is available regarding maturation of cardiac autonomic control from infancy to adolescence. A dominating role of maturation of central parasympathetic signal processing has been suggested [544].

HRV Changes During Development

The main component of HRV is attributed to RSA, which is detectable at around 33 weeks gestational age, and remains a predominant component of HRV in neonates [330–332, 545]. An earlier occurrence of HR fluctuation in the LF range (<20 week of gestational age) has been documented. However, it seems to be secondary to maternal HR and BP variation [546]. A clear dependency of all time- and frequency domain measures on gestational age has been shown [547, 548]. It has to be pointed out that, in fetuses and neonates, the spectral HRV component may have different ranges, i.e., 0.025–0.07 Hz for VLF, 0.07–0.13 Hz for LF and 0.13–1.0 Hz for HF [549]. Global HRV changes from 3 h to 7 days of post-natal life have not been consistently observed [550]. It might also be difficult to assess spectral HRV indices in this period of life, since the influence of various factors may lead to misinterpretation of HRV data [551]. A significant increase in SDNN (+20%) and MSSD (+42%) between the first and third month, with a prominent increase in SDNN following awakening (+72%) in spite of a shortening of mean RR interval, has been reported [552]. In a study by Massin and von Bernuth in 210 healthy children aged 3 days to 14 years, 24-h SDNN values were found to have almost doubled between 1 month and 1 year, and tripled at 5–6 years (tab.3.28) [331]. Further increases of SDNN and SDANN from long-term ECG recordings with maxima at a late adolescence period have been reported [332, 334]. Meanwhile, RMSSD has been found to reach a maximum value already in early childhood [332]. This is in accordance with the findings of Finley and Nugent, who have observed maxima of both short- and long-term spectral HRV indices at about 5–6 year of age [553, 554]. The maxima of short-term HF and LF power have been observed at late adolescence in another study [555]. The difference between both studies might be as a result of different data presentation (instantaneous HR vs RR), length of ECG recordings and the use of different algorithms (FFT vs AR). The significance of data presentation and length as well as choice of algorithm for HRV power spectrum estimation is discussed in 3.4.

3.6.2.2 Cardiac Autonomic Control Changes Related to Aging

Aging is associated with complex and diverse changes in cardiovascular structure and changes [556]. The most important variations are listed in ❱ Table 3.33.

Some of these changes gain a special importance when HRV is considered. A reduced responsiveness of the SAN to adrenergic stimuli and an increased responsiveness to vagal stimulation is the most relevant [397, 556–560]. As intrinsic properties of the SAN are altered, leading to the partial uncoupling of P-cells [561], an increase in the level of sympatho-excitatory hormones is detected (increasing plasma NE) as well as central sympathetic discharge (increasing efferent sympathetic nerve activity in microneurographic studies) [562]. This is accompanied by a reduction in a high affinity state β_1-adrenergic receptor density, with changes in the proportion of β_1AR to β_2AR from 4:1 to 2.5:1, mimicking that observed in heart failure [558]. A 30% reduction in the amount of activated adenyl cyclase in response to Gs-mediated β_2AR stimulation has been reported [557, 558]. As a net result, although aging is associated with sympathetic over-activity, HR and age has not been correlated in the majority of studies.

On the other hand, muscarinic receptor density is increased in older subjects in spite of a surprisingly increased responsiveness to vagal stimulation [556, 564]. This seems to indicate that a reduced central vagal outflow can play a greater role in tonic cardiac parasympathetic control changes with age than SAN responsiveness to ACh itself [556, 564]. However, these changes are not consistently observed, and even the opposite has been reported [557, 558]. In terms of M_2-R mRNA concentration and muscarinic/β-adrenergic mRNA proportion, the heart does not age as a unit: age-related changes are focused on the SA node area [564]. Among possible mechanisms leading to a reduced vagal tone in elderly people, a reduced baroreflex sensitivity mainly due to increased arterial wall thickening and stiffness, and a reduced arterial wall distensibility together with endothelial dysfunction (mainly a reduction in NO) are of greatest importance

◻ **Table 3.33**

Factors affecting ANS control and HRV measures associated with aging (Modified after Ferrari et al. [550, 556])

Level of integration	Morphological changes	Functional changes	Consequences (regarding HRV)
Cellular/subcellular			
cardiomyocytes *non-muscle cells* *adrenergic receptors* *muscarinic receptors*	Increased dimension/number Increase in collagen cross-linking Altered β_1/β_2 density ratio Up-regulation	Reduced responsiveness to stimuli Increased responsiveness to stimuli	Altered SAN responsiveness
Cardiac tissue			
Sino-atrial node	Reduced P cells: all cells ratio P-cells uncoupling	Altered pacemaker shifting Reduced SAN-respiratory coupling	Altered SAN responsiveness
Organ			
Heart	Increase in heart weight, LV hypertrophy/ fibrosis Decreased sympathetic innervation	Reduced lusitropic properties/ diastolic function	Altered mechano-electrical coupling/reflexes
Circulation			
Endothelium	Reduced NO synthesis/release Reduced SOD activity VSMC migration	Endothelial dysfunction Increased oxidative stress Increased total peripheral resistance	Reduced baroreflex sensitivity
Arteries	Increased subendothelial collagen Increased intima-media thickness VSMC proliferation Reduced elastin Increased elastin fragmentation	Increased total peripheral resistance Decreased arterial distensibility Increased pulse wave velocity Reduced cardioacceleration after baroreceptor deactivation (delayed response)	Reduced baroreflex sensitivity
Hormones/ mediators	Increased level of vasoconstrictive peptides Increased ANP/BNP synthesis/release Increased inflammatory mediators level	Endothelial dysfunction Increased oxidative stress	Reduced baroreflex sensitivity
Brain			
ANS	Loss of neurons Pigments accumulation Neurotransmitters activity changes	Altered responsiveness to afferent inputs	Central control alteration

[556, 565]. Only a few studies systematically addressed the issue of cardiopulmonary reflexes in aging and the evidence is in favor of a blunting of the hemodynamic and humoral components of cardiopulmonary responses. However, evidence to the contrary does exist [556].

Consistently observed age-related reduction in vagal tone measures should not simply be interpreted as signs of vagal neuropathy or an impaired parasympathetic control. Instead, reduced afferent signals coming from peripheral sensors may lead to a reduced central vagal outflow, irrespective of an altered SAN responsiveness. Moreover, age related autonomic innervation changes can appear relatively early in adulthood (>35 years of age) [557] mainly as a reduction in sympathethic nerve endings [566]. Generally, aging is associated with alterations in cardiac autonomic control that, not surprisingly, lead to consistent observations on a reduction of HRV with age. However, other factors not necessarily directly connected to autonomic modulation, are also changed in ways that actually are associated with a reduced HRV, especially over a 24-h period.

HRV Changes Related to Aging

An age-dependent reduction in the RSA from short-term ECG tracings has been reported as early as 1940 by Schlomka et al. [after 8]. Further studies in adults consistently reported a reduction in time-domain HRV measures with aging

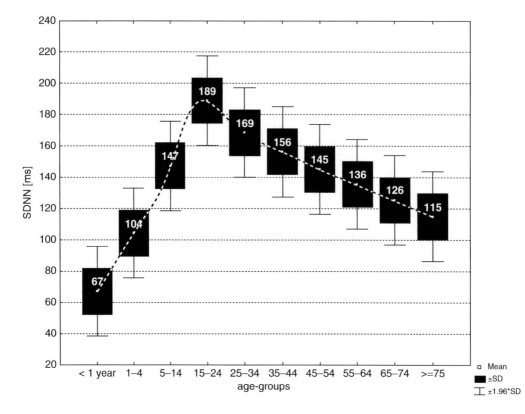

◻ Fig. 3.40

Age-dependence of the SDNN from 24-h ECG in healthy subjects. A combined data from 18 studies in children and adults. HRV reaches its maximum in late adolescence or early adulthood. Thereafter HRV reduces gradually. Confidence limits (1.96 SD) shown do not mean the normal limits (Author's data)

[567–570]. Interestingly, the RSA assessment over five heartbeats has originally been proposed to estimate "cardiac age" [570]. Similarly, the estimation of "cardiac age" has been proposed by others, though, by using a more sophisticated approach [571]. Actually, there is only one alternative method for "cardiac age" estimation, namely coronary artery calcium scoring on cardiac computed tomography [572].

The rates of HRV decline at different stages in the life course vary with different traditional HRV measures and the times of recordings. For the HRV indices that are acknowledged to strongly relate to vagal tone (RMSSD or pNN50 from 24-h recording and almost all statistical descriptors from short-term recordings) the decline is exponential and occurs early in adulthood, beginning usually well before the fourth decade of age [321, 322]. At the sixth decade of life, pNN50 and RMSSD reach values that are 25% and 50% of that observed in young adults. Over the following decades, these indices do not change significantly. In 4% to 12% of people after 65 years of age, these values can be as low as cut-off values indicating an increased risk of CV mortality [322].

The 24-h SDNN and SDANN decline more gradually. According to the accumulated data from 18 Holter-based studies, SDNN is reduced by approximately 25% in middle-aged persons (compared to young persons), and by ~40–50% in the elderly (>75 years of age) (❷ Fig. 3.40) [64, 320–322]. There is still a small reduction of SDNN in senescence [322] (❷ Table 3.27). Importantly, the lowest SDNN and SDANN values in subjects ⩾65 years old sporadically achieve the level indicating an increased risk for all-cause or CV death. Reported 24-h SDNNI values decline almost linearly from their maximum at 20–30 years of age achieving a 25% reduction in the elderly compared to young adults with a significant proportion (25%) below the cut-off value for being at risk [322].

Data from studies on HRV analysis from shorter ECG recordings show a similar trend. In the Framingham Heart Study in 2,722 subjects with an age range of 21–93 years, the 2-h SDNN has been reported to decline by 25% in middle-aged persons and by 40% in subjects older than 70 years as compared to young persons [573]. In another cross-sectional study in subjects aged between 35 and 65 years, the reduction of the median values of 5-min SDRR and RMSSD has reached 17% to 25% from the fourth to fifth decade of age and 7% to 11% from fifth to sixth decade, respectively [269]. In another cross-sectional study in 373 healthy Japanese (16–67 years old), the rate of short-term SDRR decrease from the third to fifth decade was greater in females (–35%) than in males (–17%), and was similar from the fifth to seventh decade (17% and 15%, respectively) [574]. Agelink et al. reported a smaller rate of the 5-min RMSSD of 33% and 22% over 3 decades in men and women, respectively [335]. In a large prospective within-persons study (1,999 participants, 29% females, mean age 55.6 ± 6.0 years) over the 5-year follow-up period, the mean 5-min SDRR decrease of 2.3% after 55 years of age was observed only in males, in contrast to a mean increase of 3.9% in females [575].

The power of the HF component declines exponentially from the maximum value usually between the age of 16–20 with almost 50% reduction over next 2 decades [555]. In a longitudinal investigation of 1,780 young Finnish children re-examined at the ages of 24–39 years, the short-term (3 min) lower 2.5% reference limit of HF power decreased by more than 50% from young adulthood to middle-age consistently for three heart rate strata [576]. Thereafter, the 24 h-HF power reduced at a rate of 10–15% per decade [317, 577]. After 65 years of age, variations of HF power are smaller or insignificant [317, 577]. In a longitudinal within-persons study the power of 24-h HF was unchanged over 15 years in a small sample of elderly persons [578]. In another longitudinal study, a 6% reduction of the short-term HF power over 5 years of follow-up has been observed only in males [579]. At the same time, the lower normal limit of the 24-h HF power diminishes with age, being highest in subjects who are 20 years old, decreasing by 50% at 40 years of age, with a further reduction to 20% of the maximum values at 65 years of age [580].

The power of the LF component decreases more gradually from the maximum value at 20–30 years of age, with a rate of ~20% per decade [317, 320]. A similar rate of LF power decrease with age has been reported in a cross-sectional study on short-term HRV [335]. A steeper decline of ~30–35% per decade was found in the Framingham Heart Study population [573]. Biphasic changes with 50% reduction between the fourth and fifth decade and 10% between the fifth and sixth decade [269], as well as oppositely directed changes with a rate of 20% reduction between 35 and 55 and of ~50% from 55 to 65 years of age have been reported [574]. In a longitudinal study in young adults, the LF power diminished by 50% between 24- and 39-year-old persons [576], while in another longitudinal study in the elderly followed over 16 years, a continuous decrement of the LF power was noted [578]. A significant reduction of 11.3% in older males and an increase of 4.1% in older females has been reported over a 5-year period of follow-up [575]. There is also a report in which the LF power in subjects ⩾ 60 years was comparable to that of younger people (<35 years old) despite a significant 40% reduction in cardiac NE turnover and peripheral MSNA over 2 decades [581].

The VLF and ULF power are almost linearly age-related. A rate of VLF power reduction of 12% per decade from the base value at age 40 years has been observed [317, 320]. A decrease of ULF power is less distinct and in persons ⩾ 60 years of age, the ULF power represents ~ 90% of initial values [320].

Geometrical HRV measures are also age-dependent [64, 321, 580]. The highest value of HRVI is observed in young adults, and then it declines exponentially, reaching values of ~60% of maximum (overall 40% over 4 decades) in the seventh decade [321]. The mean HRVF decreases more gradually, from 55% at age 25 years to 45% at age 60 (overall decrease of 20% over 4 decades). Interestingly, there are distinct rates of reduction of the lower and the higher normal limits. They change from the third to sixth decade by 33% and 15%, respectively [64].

Results of investigations on age-dependence of nonlinear HRV measures are far from consistent. The DFA $\alpha 1$ index has been shown to increase with age in several studies [320, 584, 585], decrease [327, 583], or remain unchanged [582, 586]. However, in longitudinal studies in young and elderly persons, DFA $\alpha 1$ has been consistently found to decrease with age [578, 579]. In various reports, the DFA $\alpha 2$ index increases [320, 583, 584], decreases [327] or remains stable over various age ranges [582, 586]. The beta-coefficient (slope of 1/f power) becomes steeper with age [574, 578, 579], although in the elderly it remains stable [579]. Two distinct behaviors of the beta-coefficient have been reported depending on the frequency break-point [587]. There are other inconsistent data regarding other scale-invariant measures [583, 586].

Results of cross-sectional studies indicate a gradual decrease of the approximate entropy [320, 327, 583]. However, in a longitudinal observation, no change of ApEn has been seen [578]. Investigations on other entropy measures provide inconclusive data [582, 588]. In addition, aging-related alteration of the largest Lyapunov exponent has been found to differ in magnitude and direction in cross-sectional studies [327, 582, 583, 586, 588].

Multilevel influences of aging on cardiac autonomic control are reflected by changes in the baroreflex sensitivity (❷ Table 3.33). An inverse effect of the aging process on BRS has been reported in several cross-sectional studies [589–594]. This age-association reduction has been confirmed in a number of investigations using various experimental techniques providing information on separate aspects of the BRS [595]. In a cross-sectional study, the BRS assessed by means of the Valsalva maneuver decreases by ~33% in middle-aged subjects (from 17.8 ± 1·8 to 11.9 ± 1·3 ms/mmHg), and by ~60% in older subjects (7.1 ± 0.6) [592]. A similar reduction has been found for the phenyleprhine method (19.5 ± 1.4, 10.7 ± 1.2 and 6.0 ± 0.6 ms/mmHg, respectively) [593].

The vagally-related arm of the BRS loop declines by a rate of 10% per decade, while sympathetic-related BRS reduces at a rate of 5% per decade [594]. The α-index of high- and low-frequency has been shown to reduce by ~33% and ~45% over 3 decades, respectively, as estimated by means of the spectral method and by 50% as estimated by means of the phenylephrine method [595]. Reduction in the BRS with age resulted in the occurrence of abnormal risk-predictive values in a significant proportion of elderly persons (30–50%). However, the proportion of abnormal BRS depends on the technique used for its assessment, with the mean BRS of 4.5 ms/mmHg with the Valsalva method (50% abnormal), 7.8 ms/mmHg with a vasopressor agent (phenylephrine, 37% abnormal) and 5.6 ms/mmHg with vasodilator (sodium nitroprusside, 30% abnormal) based techniques [596]. Cumulative data indicates that in subjects older than 50 years, it is almost impossible to differentiate whether the reduction of BRS is related to the aging process or the presence of other risk-factors, with systemic hypertension being amongst the most important [590, 597, 598]. However, spontaneous BRS during controlled breathing has been shown to linearly decrease from 50 to 75 years of age [599]. In one reported longitudinal study, the aging effect on spectral BRS has been evaluated in 205 men (36 ± 10 years at entry) over a mean 5-year period [600]. The rate of BRS decrease of 3.6% per year until 45 years of age has been observed. In the oldest group (46–50 years at baseline), no significant change over the 5-year follow-up was observed.

Age-associated changes of cardiac autonomic control are also reflected by the effect of age on heart rate turbulence. The TO increases with age, while the TS appears to remain stable [601]. These relationships strongly depend on the duration of the preceding sinus cycle at younger ages, and the influence of the basic HR attenuation as age increases [601]. On the contrary, in another study, an inverse relation of TS with age and no relation between age and TO has been reported [366]. In a study of healthy children, lower TS has been found in those with pre-pubertal status compared to those during puberty, while TO has been found to be age-independent [602]. Thus, conclusive statements on the age-relationship cannot be established as yet.

3.6.2.3 Gender

Gender differences in cardiac autonomic control are multi-factorial and originate not only from differences in hormonal status, but also from distinctive heart rate, blood pressure and respiratory control, constitutional and demographic factors, life-style and psycho- behavioral factors, as well as intrinsic central and peripheral nervous system features. Some of these factors with their possible influences upon HRV are presented in ❷ Table 3.34. These factors may have a different role to play at various points throughout life, and in many studies the differences between women and men actually disappear.

Gender related differences in the time and frequency domain variables are the subject of diverse opinions. In most studies, some HRV measures are reported to be gender-related whereas others are not. Age and race (where applicable) are only rarely added as the covariate [248, 269, 315, 615, 616]. In a small number of studies, heart rate has been analyzed as a covariate or a separate analysis for various heart rate strata has been performed [319, 573, 576]. A combination of reported relationships between HRV and gender is schematically presented in ❷ Table 3.35. More detailed data from short-term and long-term HRV studies are shown in ❷ Tables 3.36 and ❷ 3.37.

Clearly, these results indicate that global HRV measures and LF power are either comparable or lower in females, while the respiratory-related HRV measures are either similar or higher. Interestingly, time-domain short-term variation measures (RMSSD, pNN50) from 24-h ECG recordings, which are known to be closely correlated with HF power, have been found to be either similar [65, 316, 319, 321, 332], higher [619], or lower [319, 322] in women. Some authors prefer using the relative powers of LF and HF for their superiority in detecting the effect of gender [323, 324]. However, these relative spectral indices have the least well defined or even no physiological background. Evidence for lower values of HRV measures in females might be of clinical importance, although in some instances, normal limits remain to be established. For example, Gerritsen et al. proposed separate reference values of 3-min LF power for women and men, while proposing HF power and SDRR normal limits for the entire population [599].

◻ Table 3.34

Factors associated with gender differences in HRV. See ❯ Table 1.2 for list of abbreviations

Factor[s]	Difference	Mechanisms	Effect on HRV
Blood pressure	Lower	Baroreflex gain changes	Reduction
HR	Faster	Closer HRV-HR relationship	Reduction
Intrinsic HR	Faster	Intrinsic SAN properties	Reduction
Respiratory pattern	Thoracic	Greater intra-thoracic pressure changes	Increase (RSA)
Breathing frequency	Faster	Smaller intra-thoracic pressure changes	Reduction (RSA)
Physical fitness	Usually lower	Lower cardiac autonomic tone	Reduction
Smoking habits	Less frequent	Lower sympathetic activation	Reduction (LF)
Alcohol abuse	Less frequent	Greater cardiac vagal activity	Increase (RSA)
Psycho-behavioral factors	Multiple	Greater sympathetic activation, lower vagal sympatho-inhibitory actions	Reduction
Personality type	More complex	Multiple	Reduction
Nor/epinephrine level	Lower	Lower response to sympathetic activation Lower adrenal medullary content of Epi Higher epinephrine clearance rate Lower neuronal/extraneuronal uptakes	Reduction
Central control	Multiple	Less sensitive to excitatory stimuli and more sensitive to inhibitory stimuli, varies with oestral and menstrual cycles	Not studied
Noradrenergic neurotransmission	Higher	Increased presynaptic α_2-adrenoceptors number/activity varies with oestral and menstrual cycles	Not studied

◻ Table 3.35

Patterns of HR and HRV differences in females (versus males) from short-term ECG recordings

HR	SDRR (or TP)	HF power	LF power
↑	↔	↔	↓
		↑	↓
	↓	↔	↓
↔	↔	↑	↔
			↓
		↔	↔
	↓	↔	↔

Variability in patterns depends on age, race, algorithms used, and statistical adjustment.

Differences between women and men have also been studied in terms of nonlinear dynamics. Gender differences of fractal dynamics measures vary depending on methods and duration of registration. In short-term HRV studies, the β-exponent has been found to be less steep in women than in men [481, 574], contrary to long-term study findings, where a steeper β-exponent or no difference has been observed in females [320, 583]. Short-term and long-term DFA α1 coefficients have been found to be lower in females, with no differences in DFA α2 [141, 320, 583]. Higher approximate entropy in women has been observed in some HRV studies [141, 328, 583], but not confirmed by others [320]. Other indices have only rarely been studied (❯ Tables 3.36 and ❯ 3.37).

Actually, accumulated data indicates that gender-related differences should be taken into account or a proper statistical method should be applied for a valid interpretation to be drawn, irrespective of the duration of HRV recordings.

■ Table 3.36
Gender-differences in HRV measurements from short-term ECG recordings

Author, year	Sample	Parameter	Differences in women	Methodical issues
Korkushko et al. 1991 [555]	354 subjects 3 months – 89 years	LF HF	Higher/lower* Higher/lower ¶	4 min, FFT * > 40 years of age ¶ > 20 years of age
Ryan et al. 1994 [A28]	67 subjects 20–90 years	LF HF LF/HF	Lower Higher Higher	8 min FFT
Huikuri HV et al. 1996 [323]	374 subjects 40–60 years	HR* SDRR pNN50* HF (ms2)*/ HF (n.u.) LF (n.u.) LF/HF	Slower Lower Higher Higher Lower Lower	512 heartbeats AR 20 order * sitting posture
Tsuji H et al. 1996 [251]	2,722 subjects 21–93 years	SDNN* LF* HF*	Higher Lower Higher	2 h AECG 100s epochs, FFT * Ln transformed values Marginal effects of gender
Sosnowski et al. 1996 Author's data	228 healthy volunteers 8–67 years	RRI/ SDRR HF LF* LF/HF	No difference Higher Lower Lower	512 heartbeats FFT * standing position/no difference in supine
Liao et al. 1997 [649]	2252 subjects 45–64 years	SDNN LF HF LF/HF	Lower Lower Higher Higher	2 min FFT
Sinnreich R et al. 1998 [269]	294 subjects 35–65 years	SDRR*/ TP* RMSSD*/ HF* VLF*/ LF*/LF/HF*	No difference Higher Lower	5 min AR 16 order *age-adjusted
Fagard et al. 1998 [614]	424 subjects 25–89 years	SDNN LF HF LF/HF	Lower Lower No difference Lower/No difference*	15 min * in older subjects

Study	Subjects	Parameters	Result	Notes
Kuo TB et al. 1999 [324]	1070 healthy volunteers 40–79 years	RRI/ TP*/ VLF*/LF* LF% HF* HF% LF/HF*	No difference Lower Higher/No difference¶ Higher Lower/Higher¶	288 s FFT * Ln transformed spectral measures ¶ > 60 years of age
Dishman et al. 2000 [611]	92 healthy volunteers 20–59 years	HR SDNN LF HF LF/HF	Faster Lower Lower No difference Lower	5 min FFT
Agelink et al. 2001 [335]	309 healthy volunteers 18–77 years	LF HF LF/HF	Lower No difference Lower	5 min FFT
Kuch B et al. 2001 [648]	286 subjects 45–65 year	TP* LF(ms², n.u.)* HF(ms², n.u.)*	No difference Lower Higher	5 min AR 16 order * age-adjusted
Pikkujämsä et al. 2001 [141]	392 subjects† 40–60 years	RRI SDNN HF (n.u.) LF (n.u.)* LF/HF* ApEN¶* fractal exponent α1 ¶	No difference Lower Higher Lower Lower Higher Lower	5 min AR 20 order * sitting posture/ no difference in supine ¶13 min † the same as in Huikuri 1996
Evans et al. 2001 [481]	20 volunteers 25 ± 1 year	All spectral parameters HF/total (VLF+LF)/HF β–slope	No difference Higher Higher Less rapid	20 min Welch periodogram, Coarse graining

☐ **Table 3.36**   (Continued)

Author, year	Sample	Parameter	Differences in women	Methodical issues
Colhoun et al. 2001 [615]	163 healthy subjects 30–55 years	HR All spectral parameters*	No difference No difference	5 min AR * Age-adjusted
Kuo TB et al. 2002 [328]	480 healthy volunteers 40–79 years	RRI SDRR LLE[†] CD* ApEn¶	No difference No difference No difference Higher Higher	5 min † largest Lyapunov exponent *Correlation dimension ¶Approximate entropy
Gerritsen J et al. 2003 [599]	631 subjects 50–75 years	SDRR HF LF	No difference No difference Lower	3 min FFT
Laitinen T et al. 2004 [326]	63 HUT-negative subjects 23–77 years	All spectral parameters	No difference	5 min FFT
Neumann SA et al. 2005 [539]	378 subjects 30–54 years	LF HF LF/HF	Lower Higher Lower	5 min AR

Spectral parameters expressed as power (ms^2) either raw or log-transformed unless other metrics noted (i.e., normalized units, n.u.).

⬛ Table 3.37

Gender-differences in HRV measures from long-term ECG recordings

Author, year	Sample	Parameter	Differences in women	Methodological issues
Van Hoogenhuyze et al. 1991 [277]	33 subjects Mean age 33 years	SDANN/SDNNI SDNNI-CV	Lower No difference	
Mølgaard et al. 1991 [318]	140 subjects 40–77 years	SDNN*	Lower	* during night-time
Mølgaard et al. 1994 [577]	104 subjects 40–77 years	RRI/HF/HFsqrt power/ LF	No difference Lower	
Jensen-Urstad et al. 1997 [617]	101 subjects 20–69 years	SDNN LF/HF, HF LF/HF	Lower Lower Lower/higher*	* >40 years of age
Yamasaki et al. 1996 [618]	105 subjects 20–78 years	LF HF	No difference/higher* Lower	* > 50 years
Umetani et al. 1998 [322]	176 volunteers/outpatients 10–49 years	HR SDNN, SDANN/SDNNI RMSSD*, pNN50*	Faster Lower Lower	* difference only below 30 years of age
Ramaekers et al. 1998 [319]	276 healthy volunteers 18–71 years	HR SDNN/ SDANN/ TP RMSSD* pNN50/ HF LF, LF(n.u.), LF/HF HF (n.u.)	Faster Lower Lower No difference Lower Higher	TP 0.1–1.0Hz * difference disappeared after HR-adjustment
Silvetti et al. 2001 [332]	104 healthy children/adolescents 1–20 years	HR SDNN/SDANN SDNNI/ RMSSD/pNN50	Faster Lower* No difference	* higher in 16–20 years old females
Bonnemeier et al. 2003 [321]	166 healthy volunteers 20–70 year	HR SDNN/ SDANN/SDNNI NN50+/ RMSSD/HRVI	Faster Lower No difference	
Grimm et al. 2003 [366]	110 healthy volunteers 21–71 years	HR SDNN RMSSD/ pNN50	No difference Lower No difference	
Antelmi et al. 2004 [619]	653 subjects free of heart disease 14–82 years	SDNN/SDANN SDNNI/ LF, VLF, LF/HF RMSSD,pNN50/HF	No difference Lower Higher	
Sosnowski et al. 2005 [65]	210 healthy volunteers 50 ± 6 years	HR SDNN, SDANN, HRVI, HRVF pNN50	Faster Lower No difference	

The influence of gender on baroreceptor reflex control of heart rate in humans is controversial. Baroreceptor sensitivity has been found to be gender-related in some studies, being lower in women compared to men [323, 593, 621–624], whereas other studies have indicated similar BRS in females and males [625–627]. The discrepancy of BRS-dependence on gender is related to various methods used, age-difference, number of examined subjects (usually small, except for [323, 593, 623]) and training status. In a study of Adbel-Rahman et al. the gender-related differences in BRS were found to depend on the pattern of the rise in blood pressure, being significant with a brief increase (53% lower BRS in females) and undetectable with sustained BP [621]. Women have been found to exhibit greater inter-individual variation [593, 626], to have a shift of the BRS with lower blood pressure [626], and to require a lower infusion rate of phenylephrine in order to increase SBP by 20 mmHg from baseline [625]. Also, the age-dependence of BRS has not been found in females in some studies [623, 627], while it has been observed in others [593]. Interestingly, many of these findings come from studies which had a negative result in assessing gender-BRS interaction [625, 626].

Effect of gender on heart rate turbulence is poorly recognized. Only one study aimed at examining HRT differences between women and men [601]. In women, a greater age-dependence of TO and a lower age-dependence of TS along with a weaker TS relationship with preceding R–R interval was found [601].

3.6.2.4   Ethnicity

Ethnic differences in heart rate response to heat were reported more than half of century ago [628]. Since then, epidemiological, physiological and clinical evidence has been accumulated confirming the importance of ethnicity in the mortality and morbidity from certain cardiovascular causes [629–631]. Ethnic-related variations in the resting ECG have been reported, but with negligible clinical relevance [632].

The evidence of ethnic differences in HRV is sparse and inconclusive. Lower long-term and similar short-term heart rate variations have been reported in the fetuses of African American or Caribbean women when compared to the fetuses of white women of European-ethnic origin [633]. A smaller post-stimulus deceleration of R–R interval and smaller acceleration following four cycles has already been found in black newborns compared to white newborns [634].

Deep-breathing RSA changes in response to atropine have been found to be similar in two ethnic groups [635]. Blunting sympathetic neural modulation as indicated by a lower 24-h LF normalized power and LF/HF ratio in Afro-Caribbean American hypertensives compared to CA hypertensives has been suggested [636]. In the same study, the 1/f power β-coefficient was found to be similar in both ethnic groups [636]. African Americans (AA) have been found to have a lower LF and higher HF compared to Caucasian Americans (CA) in an epidemiological study by Liao et al. [248]. Also, the I/D polymorphism of the ACE genotype may play a greater role in parasympathetic cardiac control in AA hypertensives [637]. In a study in American- and European American youth, a greater age- and HR-adjusted short-term RMSSD and HF power indicates an increased parasympathetic influence on the heart in blacks [638]. AA have around a 3.5 times greater probability of having depressed ULF power, compared to CA [639]. It has also been suggested that higher HRV may buffer AA from the deleterious effects of ethnic-related stress [640]. The HF power and BRS have been found to be lower in young AA males compared to age-matched non-AA males. However, the latter was a heterogeneous group (55% CA, 31% Asian, 15% Hispanic) [641]. In addition, spontaneous BRS assessed by means of sequence method has been found to be lower in AA than in non AA [641]. In another study, resting spontaneous BRS and its change in response to lower body negative pressure were comparable in AA and CA [642].

Results accumulated from cross-sectional comparisons suggest that there is a more parasympathetic predominance in young AA, a similar autonomic balance in middle-aged AA and CA, and greater sympathetic influences in older AA than CA.

Some ethnic HRV differences can result from environmental influences. Data from a study on Caucasian lowlanders and Himalayan Sherpas show higher values of respiratory-related indices (HF and VLF) in CA lowlanders, interpreted as a lower stability in breathing control in Caucasians compared to Sherpas [643].

In general, ethnicity should be taken into account if an HRV study is going to be undertaken in a multiethnic population.

3.6.2.5   Body Mass

There are no consistent data regarding the relationship or causality between body mass and HRV, despite a basic study indicating that dietary-induced weight gain is accompanied with a reduction in M_2-muscarinic gene expression, signaling modifications and density [644]. Moreover, the importance of circulating insulin, leptin and free fatty acids, known to interact with cardiac autonomic control in obesity, have been acknowledged [458, 462, 465–467, 645].

The differences in reported correlations are related to the various HRV measures used and the lack of adjustment for the variety of co-factors (age, gender, ethnics and others). Population size and characteristics examined vary in different studies (healthy volunteers, sample of general population, hypertensives, diabetics and others). Additionally, in a seminal study on HRV determinants, BMI was not included among potentially significant co-factors [573].

In a study of healthy children/adolescents, a significant correlation between BMI and age and gender adjusted 24-h pNN50 and RMSSD has been reported [332]. A similar observation has been reported in normotensive obese school children [646]. In healthy adolescents and young adults (15–31 years), neither BMI nor waist circumference was found to impact significantly on a statistical model of determinants of short-term HRV (30 sec) [647]. In a small sample of young women, BMI was graded as the second factor, after age, influencing overall HRV, but not pNN50 or RMSSD [608]. An approximate 5% contribution of BMI to the total HRV spectral power has recently been reported in a large sample of young adults [576].

In a population-based study, a significant correlation of BMI with age and HR adjusted short-term spectral HRV measures was found in middle-aged males, whereas a similar relationship was not present in females [648]. The contribution of BMI was found to be marginal (5% in males), although in certain conditions it clearly surpasses the effects of age and heart rate [315]. In the ARIC studies on a large cohort of middle-aged subjects, the BMI relationship with short-term HRV was not observed [649]. In a prospective HRV study in middle-aged adults, a higher BMI has been found to increase the probability of being at the worst quartile of age and gender adjusted 5-min HR and HRV over a 5-year follow-up period [575]. In contrast, in middle-aged normal persons, the BMI coefficient of determination relating to the age and gender adjusted total power of spectral HRV was found to be less than 5% [615].

There are conflicting data regarding the relationship of BMI with HRV in the elderly. The lowest short-term SDNN quartile has been found to be associated with a higher BMI in a large population-based cohort of the Rotterdam Study [650]. In a study across four European populations, a higher BMI was found to be associated with a lower HF and higher LF in one population, whereas no association was present in the other countries [651]. Also, in wide age range samples of population, insignificant or negligible contributions of BMI to HRV metrics were reported [580, 619, 652–655]. In the SAPALDIA study, the time and frequency domain HRV indices adjusted for many variables have been shown to correlate negatively with BMI in subjects >50 years old [609]. Also, in the CARLA study, the waist–hip ratio was inversely associated with HRV [655]. In contrast, observations from a longitudinal study in a small sample of the elderly did not produce evidence of a relationship between BMI change and standard HRV measures, while a significant correlation was found for the DFA $\alpha 1$ coefficient [578].

Despite the majority of data indicating that body mass contributes only marginally to HRV, in an individual case, the influence of weight gain or loss might be of importance as indicated by the more concordant data that come from studies in obesity. Both weight gain and its reduction have been found to be associated with a significant change of certain HRV indices [656–661]. Longitudinal studies also provide some evidence regarding the influence of body mass changes on HRV [647]. An impressive amount of data has come from a study in obese patients who were treated surgically for extreme obesity. In these patients with a mean weight loss of 32 kg (28%) over a 1-year follow-up, the mean NNI decreased by 8%, while SDANN and SDNNI increased by 5% and 24%, respectively [658]. Spectral HRV measures also increased by 21% (LF, HF), but a relative increase of 35% for LF and 43% for HF was observed only for daytime, with no changes during night-time. Data on changes in lower frequency components were not reported in that study [658]. In another study in a group of morbidly obese patients treated with bariatric surgery, the average 17% BMI reduction and 13.5 kg fat mass loss 3 months after surgery was associated with 39–49% increase of 24-h SDNN, RMSSD, HRVI and TINN, while the pNN50 values doubled. Further weight loss over the next 9 months (−33% BMI and −28.7 kg fat mass at 12 months after surgery) were not found to be associated with further increase in HRV. On the contrary, a small decrease of 5–16% (SDNN, HRVI, pNN50 and RMSSD) was observed, while the TINN remained unchanged [661]. Changes in HRV have been found to be independent of improvement in insulin resistance [661]. Even a small weight loss (~10%) after dietary restrictions has been found to result in an increase of 24-h HRV in the time and frequency domains [659]. Conversely, a 10% increase in body weight has been associated with HR acceleration and a reduction of short-term respiratory-related HR power [656].

A lower baroreflex sensitivity resulting from increasing body mass and visceral fat in resting conditions and under stress challenges [662–664] was reported to be related in part to sympathetic overactivity in obese subjects [657]. Body weight reduction was found to be associated with a restoration of BRS [665]. This effect has been observed both in young and old obese subjects [666].

In the only study that addresses HRT changes in obese normotensive subjects without co-morbidities, no difference was observed between normal and obese subjects. However, there were limitations in the methods, e.g., allowing calculation of HRT from one ventricular PEB [667].

In general, body mass influences HRV and BRS, but in large-sample studies, its contribution to measured indices is marginal, albeit sometimes significant, and can usually be neglected. However, in an individual, gain or loss in body mass contributes substantially to changes of heart rate and its variation that can surpass the effects of established factors (age, gender).

3.6.2.6   Heart Rate

Heart rate is one of the main factors that always has to be considered for the understanding and interpretation of HRV. Consequently, a lack of knowledge about HR (or RR interval) *a priori* excludes a reliable assessment of its variation. Although HR would be expected to be considered, this fundamental requirement has not necessarily been met in many clinical studies [e.g., 314, 343, 346, 350, 351, 352]

Coumel et al. listed reasons for which HR itself cannot be ignored: (1) HR is probably the best and simplest measure of the ANS balance, (2) HRV indices are influenced by HR itself, and (3) the HR and HRV relationship does have a physiological significance and this perfect harmony between HR and HRV should not be overlooked [668]. This harmony is related to the so called sympathovagal balance, and can be derived from the classical Rosenblueth-Simeone model, describing the net effect of combined vagal and sympathetic stimulation upon SAN [669]. In their model, an actual HR is a function of intrinsic HR and sympathetic and parasympathetic influence:

$$aHR = IHR^* m^* n, \tag{3.41}$$

where *aHR* is actual (resting) HR, *IHR* is an intrinsic HR, *m* is a sympathetic factor, and *n* is a parasympathetic factor [669]. This multiplicative relationship (m^*n) is in concordance with the phenomenon of accentuated antagonism [15]. The m^*n product may be regarded as the sympatho-vagal balance [670]. Simply, $m^*n>1$ indicates a predominance of sympathetic activity (net HR acceleratory influence), while with $m^*n < 1$ there is vagal predominance (net inhibitory effect). Since IHR cannot be simply measured, and there is no HRV index that explicitly describes "m" or "n" factor, the measurement of actual HR remains still the most useful crude estimate of ANS balance. Corroborative observations can be found in a series of studies by investigators in Chicago [671–675], who proposed to replace the m^*n product by the term VSE (vagal-sympathetic effect): VSE = RR interval/intrinsic RR interval [231] or simply aHR/IHR [676].

Intrinsic Heart Rate
A spontaneous firing of the cardiac pacemaker can be easily seen in the heart removed from a body of an experimental animal, when central and circulatory factors controlling heartbeat formation are disrupted. The rate of this spontaneous heartbeat activity is referred to as *intrinsic heart rate* (IHR) [677]. In humans, the IHR can be assessed after pharmacological denervation by means of a combined M_2 and β_1AR (double blockade), with the use of weight-adjusted doses of atropine (0.04 mg/kg) and propranolol (0.2 mg/kg) [677–679]. Despite some limitations owing to the use of a high dose of atropine (nicotine-receptor partial blockade with a subsequent inhibition of the NE release, antagonism with 5-HT and histamine) and propranolol (nonspecific membrane action, negative inotropic effects) and actually incomplete autonomic blockade (with no effects on α-adrenoceptor or humoral factors) [393, 676], this approach is the only one available in physiological and clinical studies.

In healthy subjects the mean IHR is approximately 80–125 bpm [306, 679, 680]. The mean IHR of 128 ± 24 bpm has been reported in seven healthy children [681]. The IHR does not seem to be dependent on gender [306, 680, 682]. The importance of IHR for understanding heartbeat variation is related to its age, ventricular function and autonomic tone dependencies. Age-dependence on IHR is recognized by the inclusion of age into the regression equation ($r^2 = 0.42$) proposed by Jose and Collison 4 decades ago [306]:

$$IHR = 118.1 - 0.56^* age \pm k \tag{3.42}$$

where the constant k is 14% for subjects aged <45 and 18% for subjects aged ⩾45 years.

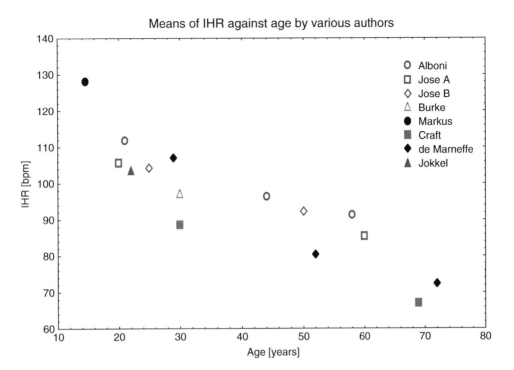

Means of IHR against age by various authors

Legend:
○ Alboni
□ Jose A
◇ Jose B
△ Burke
● Markus
■ Craft
◆ de Marneffe
▲ Jokkel

■ **Fig. 3.41**
Scatterplot of reported means of the intrinsic heart rate against means of age of examined group in various studies. Data from studies in which IHR has been assessed by means of double autonomic blockade using muscarinic antagonist + beta2-adrenergic agents

In a study of Alboni et al., the mean IHR of 103 ± 13 bpm in subjects 45 years of age or younger and of 93 ± 8 in subjects > 45 years was observed [680]. Their data indicate that IHR is additionally related to aHR (resting baseline). Thus, the recalculated equation (r^2 = 0.61) would be:

$$IHR = 90 - 0.57^{*}age + 0.41^{*}aHR \pm 7\ bpm. \tag{3.43}$$

❯ Figure 3.41 shows a plot summarizing age-effect on the IHR in several studies that examined this relationship [306, 679–684].

A dependence of IHR on ventricular function was firstly reported by Wollenberger and Jehl in a model of cardiopulmonary function [685]. This relationship has been corroborated by others, indicating also that a reduction of IHR precedes the occurrence of overt heart failure [306, 678, 679]. An intact innervation of the SAN is a key factor for IHR, as indicated by experimental studies with extrinsic or SAN selective parasympathectomy and pericardial effusion [686, 687]. In clinical settings, it might play a role in patients after open heart surgery [688, 689], coronary artery by-pass surgery [690–692] pericarditis and myocarditis, including chronic Chagas' disease [693, 694], as well as after ablation procedures [695, 696]. In patients, following mitral valve replacement, a reduced HRV with an erratic spectrum can be detected [689], comparable to that seen in SAN dysfunction (❯ Fig. 3.42) [697] and in patients after heart transplantation [433, 698]. An increase in IHR can be observed in patients with hyperthyroidism [306], inappropriate sinus tachycardia and postural orthostatic tachycardia [373]. There is also evidence that increased parasympathetic tone may result in a compensatory increase of IHR in renal hypertension [374]. In addition, temperature changes and atrial stretching might influence the intrinsic SAN firing [676, 699]. Thus, *the presence of changes in IHR in a number of settings indicates that RR interval may vary irrespective of cardiac autonomic tone.*

The change in mean RR interval (or ratio between the longest and shortest RRI) after parasympathetic blockade with atropine is used as an index of the relative basal vagal tone ($\bar{V}$), while the difference in mean RR interval (or ratio between longest and shortest RRI) after sympathetic withdrawal and subsequent vagal blockade with atropine, can serve as an

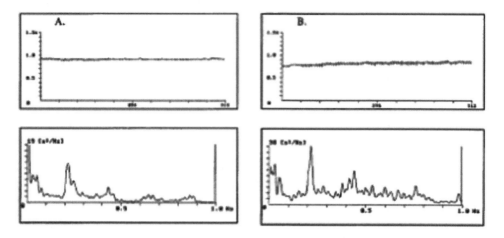

�‌ Fig. 3.42
Patterns of abnormal HRV power spectra in patients with sinus node disease. Tachograms (*upper panel*) in two patients after double autonomic blockade (atropine+propranolol), power spectra (lower panel) show residual contents with abnormal distribution which are resemble harmonics or erratic variation over mean value (From [697])

index of the absolute vagal tone [700, 701]. Similarly, an index of the relative and absolute sympathetic influences can be derived from RRI after adrenergic blockade and after atropine and subsequent propranolol administration, respectively. An alternative approach of autonomic control of the heart based on the analysis of HR recovery from exercise has been reported [702].

Actual Heart Rate (Resting)

Heart rate and HRV can be considered as factors that limit their ranges. Accordingly, at a certain actual HR, the HRV varies within some limits (depending mainly on age). However, a reverse relationship is possible, that is, ANS and other influences reflected by an actual HRV establishes HR limits. This can be easily seen when the circadian variation of heart rate and HRV is examined [284, 318, 321, 703]. Indices of short-term variation (RMSSD and pNN50) follow an RRI circadian pattern, while the index of long-term HRV (SDANN) behaves in a reciprocal manner [321]. Accordingly, circadian rhythm of 24-h HF power mimics the rhythm of RRI, while circadian rhythm of 24-h LF power shows the reciprocal reflection of RRI [703]. A significant negative correlation ($r^2 = 0.74$) of SDNN on day-night RRI difference described in healthy subjects emphasizes the importance of HR itself [318]. In older healthy subjects, similar relationships might not be observed because of a reduction of most time and frequency domain HRV indices, despite sustenance of circadian rhythm of RRI [321]. Interestingly, circadian rhythm of the SDANN index has been shown to be least affected by aging [321]. It has also been found that at in extreme conditions, both HRV decrease or increase cannot further follow changes in R – R interval (saturation areas) [399, 675]. In healthy persons, two distinct patterns of the HF power changes with RRI interval increment can be detected, i.e., saturated or linear [399]. Despite the authors having described a low-correlated pattern in their healthy subjects, detailed analysis of data provided indicates that these subjects had in fact been hypertensive [399].

In an experimental study on dogs with myocardial infarction, a low-correlated response to a beta-blockade with atenolol was observed in animals susceptible to sudden death, in contrast to resistant and sham-operated dogs, in which a parallel HR reduction and SDRR increase was found [704]. Actually, a close negative exponential relationship between HR and HRV (◉ Fig. 3.43) and clearly VF-prone experimental dogs is characterized by a simultaneous reduction in HRV and acceleration of the HR, as expected from the HR-HRV relationship (◉ Fig. 3.43 inset). Thus, the same data might bring different conclusions depending on the type of analysis adopted.

A significant relationship between RRI and HRVI on Holter recording has been found for risk prognostication after myocardial infarction [347]. For a wide range of statistical performance (sensitivity and positive predictive accuracy) results from the lower quartile of mean RRI and mean HRVI were comparable. All-cause mortality reached 24.3% and 22.2% over a mean 2-year follow-up, respectively. Post-AMI patients with simultaneous low HRVI (⩽20 U) and shorter

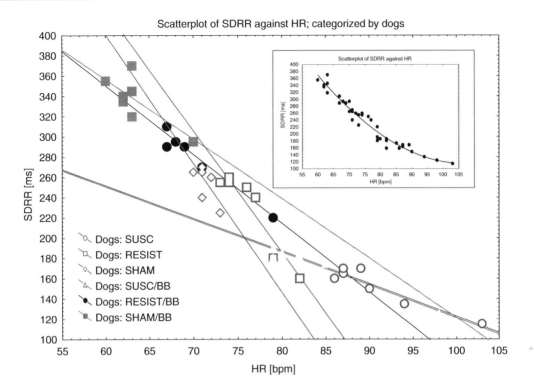

Fig. 3.43

Relationship between HR and SDRR in experimental AMI in dogs. Distinct HR-SDRR relationship is shown in dogs with exper-imental AMI prone to sudden cardiac death (SUSC) before and after beta-blockade (SUSC-BB) as compared to dogs resistant (RESIST) and (RESIST-BB) or sham-operated (SHAM, SHAM-BB). However, an analysis on entire group (inset) indicate that sus-ceptible dogs HR-HRV are simple representing reduced HRV in accordance with a reduced HRV. Plots on basis of data from Adamson et al. [704])

RRI ($\leqslant$736 ms) had the highest all-cause mortality (28.7% over a mean 2-year follow-up). On the contrary, in those in the lowest quartile for HRVI and the highest for RRI, the survival rate was excellent (no deaths) [347]. However, the mortality rate in those with HRVI in the highest quartile and RRI in the lowest quartile was still substantial (16.7%). The impact of a beta-blockade (40% of patients) that might prolong RRI without significant alteration of HRVI was not discussed. It might also be speculated whether a good prognosis in patients with low HRVI and longer RRI overall reflects better survival in patients with sinus node disease [705]. Another outcome of a separate study in patients with acute MI has found evidence that HRV indices do not provide additional prognostic power over that of RRI itself, clearly because of the significant mutual relationship ($r^2 = 0.37$) [706].

The significance of basic RRI for HRV evaluation has been reflected in some investigations that addressed the issue of HRV normal limits [573, 576, 707]. In a recent study, the influence of RRI duration on HRV indices was underlined again [585]. In a short-term HRV study, the most common tests revealed a distinct behavior in RRI and HRV (❷ Fig. 3.44) in healthy subjects and post-MI patients [708].

In certain pathological states (heart failure, sinus node dysfunction) the actual heart rate is different than expected from a concomitant HRV change [709]. As a reduced HRV represents parasympathetic withdrawal in HF patients (with/without sympathetic over-excitation) [710], an R – R interval shortening (faster HR) can be expected. In such cases, an impaired IHR prevents heart rate adjustment. Therefore, a relatively slow HR and a reduced HRV can be observed. The author referred to this feature as the *metronome-like bradycardia* (Metronome-like bradycardia – a specific feature of chronotropic impairment in which slow HR is associated with a significantly reduced HRV.) and found it to be a specific sign of an organic sinus node impairment (in patients not treated with agents that may interfere with SAN function)

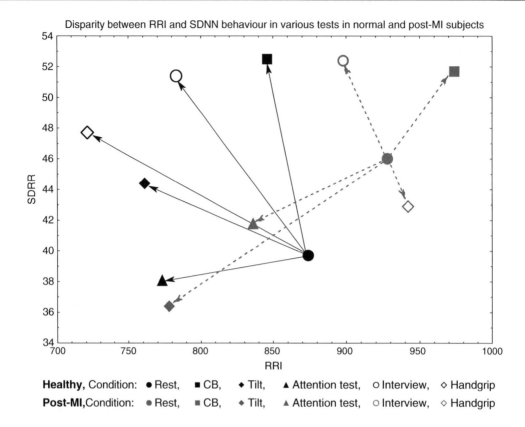

A distinct behavior of HR and HRV in response to various stimuli. Example shows that changes in HRV do not necessarily follow RRI alteration. Also, differences between healthy and post myocardial infarction patients are clearly seen (On basis of data from [708])

[711]. In heart failure, circadian HRV measures have not been found to vary correspondingly to HR changes [712]. Also, in a third of post-AMI patients, a poorly correlated pattern of HF-RRI relationship has been reported [399]. Abnormal HR–HRV relationship can be ascribed to an increased HRV in spite of HR acceleration. Such behavior is seldom observed in heavily trained healthy subjects [709]. More commonly, such behavior can be seen in patients after heart transplantation and with obstructive sleep apnea syndrome [212, 433, 698, 713, 714]. Under these conditions, HRV may be increased due to the rising contribution of mechanical respiratory influences unrelated to cardiac autonomic tone (that is actually shifted towards a sympathetic predominance). A similar feature can be observed in patients with sinus node dysfunction after double autonomic blockade [697]. Therefore, an increase in short-term HRV in patients after heart transplantation cannot be simply interpreted as a sign of re-innervation or increased mechanical load unless sinus node function is reassessed [715, 716]. A higher HRV than expected from actual HR is a frequent feature of SAN dysfunction [337, 697, 711]. Interestingly, a prognostic value of increased HRV has recently been confirmed [53].

Baroreflex sensitivity does not seem to depend on heart rate. Despite a weak negative correlation ($r^2 = 0.06$) between BRS and HR having been found in healthy subjects, the significance of the relationship was lost in multivariate analysis [593]. The BRS–HR relationship was not found in persons $\geqslant 60$ years old even in a univariate analysis [593]. Another study indicated that there might be a gender difference in BRS-HR correlation. However, the small number of subjects examined does not allow a conclusive opinion to be drawn [621]. A lack of correlation between HR and BRS has been reported in most studies in which the BRS had been estimated by means of various methods [595, 600, 627, 629].

Heart rate turbulence parameters are dependent on heart rate in healthy subjects. Turbulence onset and turbulence slope decreases with HR increase [601]. A need for adjustment of the turbulence slope for heart rate was concluded from a study in patients with coronary heart disease [312]. However, the accumulated data is relatively sparse, so a general statement cannot be given.

In summary, heart rate is of the utmost importance in the analysis of HRV. Actually, an interpretation of HRV data without information regarding actual (or mean) HR or RR interval might be inappropriate, diminishing conclusions drawn from such an investigation. Even in a case of seemingly insignificant HR (RRI) differences in comparative studies, HRV measures should be adjusted not only for age, gender and ethnicity, but also for HR (RRI).

3.6.2.7 Respiration

Respiration is one of the most important determinants of short-term heartbeat variation, which is clearly evidenced by a phenomenon referred to as *respiratory sinus arrhythmia* (RSA, Carl Ludwig 1847) [1, 4–6, 9, 20, 23, 717–725]. During normal breathing, the raw (unadjusted) RSA contributes to 30–80% of the total short-term HRV. Respiratory-related short-term HR variation is frequently interpreted as an index of tonic cardiac vagal modulation of heart rate [68, 69, 700, 720, 721]. However, respiratory influences on HRV do extend beyond high frequencies, and in certain settings can affect HRV within low- and very-low frequencies (❷ Fig. 3.45) [296, 717, 722].

The RSA magnitude is significantly related to respiratory parameters both in laboratory conditions and during daily life [6, 9, 718–720]. In an early investigation, Eckberg found that a 50% increase in tidal volume led to only a 15% increase of RSA estimated by means of the peak-valley method [720]. In a study of Grossman et al. with similarly determined RSA, the amount of variance accounted for by frequency of breathing and tidal volume has reached 64% (58–69%) [723]. By dividing RSA by tidal volume (RSA$_{TF}$ [ms/ml]), the greater proportion of HR variance was explained. Additionally, a correction for breathing frequency has been shown to be unnecessary [723]. A need for additional adjustment for arterial partial pressure of CO_2 has also been pointed out, especially while central autonomic drive is affected, i.e., hyperventilation, sleep-related breathing disorders, heart failure [724]. The respiratory HR variation is accentuated during slow (~0.1 Hz) deep breathing [18, 718, 720]. This relationship constitutes the basis for a clinical test [18, 725]. Interestingly, an evolution of this method can still be seen [726].

Respiratory parameters should be obligatorily controlled for in laboratory studies [727]. In clinical settings, some information about respiration (breathing rate) might be extracted from the mean (or median) frequency of HF component of the short-term HRV power spectrum. Unfortunately, respiration parameters are only rarely taken into account in clinical studies both in normal subjects and those with various clinical entities. Meanwhile, the respiratory rate (defined as the frequency of maximum HF power) has been identified as a factor explaining HRV differences between CAD-patients

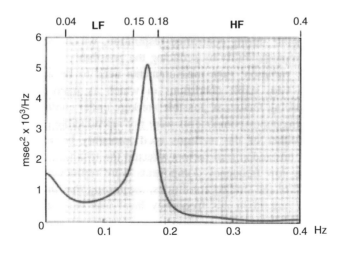

□ Fig. 3.45

Spontaneous slow respiration effect on HRV spectral components. In an example, the power spectrum (AR) shows only one peak that cannot be considered either a LF or HF power (From [296], Oxford Univ Press, with permission)

with preserved and depressed LV systolic function [728]. As respiration influences frequencies lower than that of the HF component [184, 717, 722, 729], its contribution for VLF and LF components should also be considered. It could be of the utmost importance in patients with heart failure and sleep-related breathing disorders in whom chemoreceptor-reflex or centrally-driven changes contribute significantly to HRV [730–734]. Recently, it has been observed that the frequency of respiration influences fractal measures of HRV [735].

The contribution of nonneural influences to short-term HR variation due to lung volume oscillation is usually small under normal conditions (~3%). However, it can be responsible for up to 30% of the HF power in healthy middle-aged persons [730]. It has been shown that a slow deep breathing can provoke R − R interval oscillations of ~120 ms after complete autonomic blockade [717]. In addition, the proportion of nonneural components of RSA has been observed to increase during exercise [736]. The relative contribution of nonneural RSA mechanisms increases even in mild heart failure, and accounts for 15% of the HF power. Importantly, in an individual patient, this mechanical contribution can reach 77% of the HF component [730]. Abnormal breathing patterns that can occur in patients with heart failure during exercise influence lower frequencies [737].

Another form of respiratory contribution to HRV is related to so-called cardio-ventilatory coupling [188, 190, 193–196] and seems to be independent of cardiac autonomic tone, blood pressure variability, and baroreflex sensitivity [738]. The cardioventilatory coupling has been observed in two third of healthy subjects, being most apparent at low breathing rates and associated with high HRV [738]. As reduced cardiorespiratory interactions have been found in patients with a myocardial infarction [196] and is associated with low HRV [738], it might be another mechanism that should be taken into account while interpreting reduced HRV in a number of clinical conditions.

In general, respiratory parameters should be measured and reported in studies on HRV, especially in patients in whom breathing and related disorders play a significant role in pathophysiology and clinical presentation.

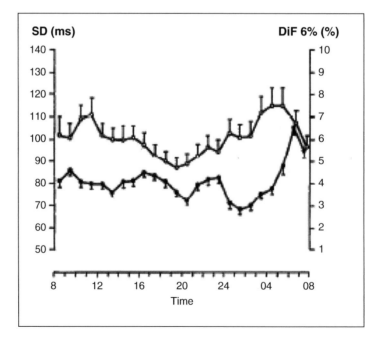

◻ Fig. 3.46

Examples of diurnal fluctuation of long-wave (SD) and short-term (dif 6%) measures of HRV in a healthy subject. (From [318], with permission)

3.6.2.8 Day–Night Rhythm

Diurnal variation of HR and HRV are well recognized [739]. They are related to the circadian rhythm of sleep and activity. Measurement of the global 24-h HRV indices (SDNN, SDANN, HRVI, or HRVF) provides a crude description of the level of circadian rhythm, since the sleep–wake cycle is the strongest determinant of overall HRV (❷ Fig. 3.40). More detailed analysis requires a partitioning of 24-h recordings into day and night periods, or even hourly intervals. In healthy subjects, HRV measures of high frequency variation (pNN50, RMSSD, HF power) reach their maximum early in the morning before awakening (usually about 5 AM) independently of gender and activity [321, 618, 739, 740]. However, a lack of diurnal variation has been reported [318] as has attenuation of cardiac vagal modulation with age [321]. Sleep-related increase in HRV short-term indices has been confirmed in shift workers [741]. Also, cardiorespiratory coupling has been found to exhibit day–night differences [195]. Sleep deprivation has been shown to result in attenuation of parasympathetic and augmentation of sympathetic-related HRV indices [742]. Diminished LF/(LF+HF) ratio during non-REM sleep that mimics sleep deprivation has been found in subjects homozygous for the PER3$^{5/5}$ allele, in contrast to other polymorphisms in this gene encoding circadian clock [743]. Apart from the sleep–wake cycle, there is a role for light–dark rhythm intrinsically coupled with HRV changes over 24-h [744].

In a recent study, Hu et al. investigated intrinsic circadian cardiac dynamics in healthy subjects by adjusting the sleep–wake behavior cycle to 28 h [745]. They found significant circadian changes of DFA scaling exponent α with the average maximum value at ~9–11 am and the average minimum value at ~1 pm. The protocol used in this study forcing a lack of synchrony allowed the detection of the influence of the circadian pacemaker on cardiac dynamics independent of HR circadian rhythm [745].

Early HRV abnormalities can easily be detected in diabetic patients without autonomic test abnormalities and in patients with uncomplicated coronary artery disease in the form of a reduction of night-time (sleep) HF power, whereas daytime values can still be comparable [746, 747]. In diabetic patients with autonomic neuropathy, the HRV diurnal pattern is reduced or even lost, thereby making both daytime and night-time HF and LF power lower compared to healthy subjects [747]. Similar findings have been reported in heart failure patients [277]. Increased night-time SDNN, in spite of a smaller HF increase, has been observed in post acute MI patients [748]. Also, higher pNN50 values during sleep have been reported in hypertensive patients with left ventricular hypertrophy [749]. The absence or reversal of circadian rhythm of a particular HRV measure has been shown to be of prognostic significance in post-MI patients and in survivors of sudden death [750–752]. Last, but not least, the pharmacodynamic effects of certain agents can be tracked by means of circadian HR and HRV analysis [753].

Baroreflex sensitivity also undergoes clear day-night rhythmicity with minimum values during the day [754].

In general, evaluation of HR and HRV circadian rhythms may add information beyond their mean values that may be useful in risk-prognostication. Additionally, diurnal changes of certain HRV measures indicate that measurements of short-term HRV should be performed at similar specific times in the day.

3.6.3 Behavioral Factors

3.6.3.1 Physical Activity

The autonomic nervous system is involved in the complex adjustment of circulatory control to altered demand in response to physical activity. Thus, the effects of short-term exercise or prolonged training can be easily recognized by means of HRV analysis. The autonomic response to exercise or training depends on the type of physical activity (tonic or phasic), its frequency, intensity, and duration. Also, initial physical status should be taken into account. On the contrary, spells of physical inactivity can be studied in the setting of prolonged bed rest.

Physical activity has been listed among the most important determinants of 24-h HRV [318]. Subjects with good fitness levels have a higher power of both HF and LF components [577]. However, conflicting data exists in general population studies. Vigorous self-reported physical activity has been found to be associated with short-term HRV in males. Those men in the highest category of vigorous activity had an 8% higher SDNN, 19% higher LF power, and 23% higher HF power than those men who reported no vigorous activity, after adjustment for age and for light and moderate activity [755]. Similar observations have been reported in healthy adolescents [756] and in middle-aged subjects [757].

Interestingly, in the latter study, moderate and vigorous physical activity has been associated with a higher LF power [757]. In the SAPALDIA study, each hour of heavy physical exercise has been associated with a 2.0% increase in SDNN, a 3.6% increase in the high frequency (HF) range power and a 4.2% increase in LF power [609]. A lower LF power but not HF power has been found in women with a sedentary lifestyle [758]. In contrast, in a large cross-sectional study in an elderly population, no association between physical activity and HRV measures has been reported [655]. In addition, in a cross-sectional study of Byrne et al., physical fitness has not been identified as an independent predictor of HRV, despite univariate associations having been observed [652]. Cumulated data indicate that preserved age-dependent HRV measures can be found in those humans who are physically active over years or decades [759, 760].

Basic physical fitness can be improved by various exercise protocols. However, the effects of training depend on its intensity and duration. Light or moderate physical training that can improve peak VO_2 does not necessarily alter HRV measures [761–763]. More vigorous training has been found to increase parasympathetically-mediated HRV indices irrespective of age [755, 759, 764–766]. Aerobic training at 50% of maximum VO_2 exerts evident influences on HRV in post-menopausal women [767, 768]. An extreme physical loading may exert harmful effects upon HRV [769]. A distinct effect of physical training on various measures of autonomic control (HRV, HR recovery, and HRT) has been discovered recently in patients with heart failure [770].

Increased HF power response to exercise and increased RMSSD during recovery have been associated with a worse prognosis in one study (mainly males) [771], whereas no evidence of prognostic value has been found in another [772]. Differences might result from exercise testing (treadmill test vs bicycle ergometer), gender-differences or intensity of workload. Heavy exercise above the ventilatory threshold has been shown to determine occurrence of increased HF power [773].

The effects of physical fitness and training on baroreflex function are more difficult to evaluate since exercise simultaneously exerts influence on central command, the exercise pressor reflex and the arterial baroreflex. Some harmony between these three components of an integrative response to exercise is required to produce a normal response to exercise [774]. The use of various methods for BRS assessment, different parameters for its description (usually only maximum gain), different intensity, protocols and duration of exercise or training is one reason for data inconsistency. Exercise capacity parameters, like maximum or peak VO_2, have been found not to correlate with BRS changes or their lack of change [593, 624].

Too short a period of physical training, as well as BRS examination by means of baroreceptor unloading, are more frequently reported in studies in which the BRS has been found reduced or unchanged [775–778]. Also, the use of semi-invasive maneuvers results in inconsistent observations, including those usually with unchanged BRS following exercise [779]. In studies with spontaneous BRS estimation, an increase of BRS in response to exercise can be observed more consistently [780–782]. More regular exercise of moderate intensity has been reported to attenuate age-related reduction in BRS [592]. Multi-phasic response to prolonged exercise training has been described with an initial BRS improvement after 3 months, which is sustained for the next few months and followed by a decline after a 1-year period despite markedly increased training [783]. This might be an effect of baroreceptor resetting. However, more detailed analysis of baroreflex function curve and its operative parameters would help to explain the changes described [774].

3.6.3.2 Mental Stress

Mental stressors (anger, mental arithmetic, presentation with/without audience participation, and others) are frequently used in acute psychophysiological studies in which short-term spectral HRV analysis is preferentially employed [5, 6, 10, 784, 785]. Others have investigated more chronic traits, like depression, anxiety disorders, panic disorder, personality types, hostility, mistrust, and work stress, as well as the white-coat effect and post-traumatic stress [785–790]. Also, the effects of anti-stressor behavior (mental distraction, yoga, relaxation training) have been investigated [791]. For the effects of chronic mental stress evaluation, either short-term or long-term HRV analysis is in use [785].

Cardiac vagal withdrawal is evoked by a wide range of stressful states [791]. However, acute stressors induce various effects on HRV sympathetic and parasympathetic-related components that are related to mutual influence on respiration [786]. Anger has been found to induce an increase in both LF and HF components, while anticipation of giving a presentation has been associated with an increase in LF power although HF power has remained unchanged [793, 794]. An increase of LF power and a shift of HF power towards higher frequencies in response to the reaction time task have been associated with a shift of the respiratory spectrum in healthy subjects [784]. Meanwhile, a mental arithmetic test has been shown to induce a large increase in LF power with a reduction of HF power into almost undetectable values, broadening and flattening of the respiratory spectrum and a reduction of the alfa-index of BRS gain [784]. Unfortunately, the changes described have not been adjusted for accompanying HR acceleration and SBP increment. Delaney and Brodie found a shift of the HRV power spectrum towards low frequencies in response to defence-arousal reaction [795]. Decreases in HRV in response to random number generation have allowed the detection of anxiety and depression in apparently healthy subjects, even though basal HRV remained similar in all those in the study [796].

Anxiety traits and disorders are associated with changes in HRV [792]. In phobic disorder, decreased vagal and increased sympathetic cardiac function, have been revealed in a study of HRV by Yeragani et al. [797]. A phobic anxiety self-rating score has been inversely related with age-adjusted SDNN in the Normative Aging Study [798]. In a small case-control study, both 24-h HF and LF powers were found to be lower among subjects with panic disorder as compared to those without [799]. Also, a negative relationship between cardiac vagal indices and anxiety trait has been reported in many studies [see 792 for review], but contradictory data has appeared [800, 801]. Encouraging data on the potential of HRV analysis for evaluation of treatment of anxiety has been reported. These and other studies are reviewed elsewhere [785, 792]. Depression has been found to be another entity in which HRV can be seen as abnormal. Agelink et al. compared short-term HRV in depressive and normal subjects and found a faster HR in moderately and severely depressed subjects, while HF power was lower only in patients with a high Hamilton Depression Score [802].

Some difficulties in interpretation of the cumulated data arise from the lack of information about such fundamental physiological parameters as heart rate or respiration in the majority of studies. In the most frequently cited study of Carney et al., an association between depression and low 24-h HRV in patients with acute MI (the Enhancing Recovery in Coronary Heart Disease (ENRICHD) trial), the average HR in the groups compared has neither been adjusted for nor compared. In addition, more important clinical data have been missed [803]. Interestingly, in a few studies in which HR has been accounted for, the differences in HRV have not been seen. O'Connor et al. found significant differences in HR, but not in RSA, in bereaved and depressed subjects [804]. Similar results have been obtained by others [805]. A significant correlation of anxiety state with HR has been observed in a study by Watkins et al., while RSA and anxiety state were not found to be correlated [806]. These authors also reported that respiratory control did not change this relationship. However, in their multivariate analysis, they did not include heart rate and respiratory rate (despite being measured) into the final model [805]. In addition, respiratory rate and arterial pressure variability have been the most consistently changeable parameters among all those measured in an acute sleep deprivation study. However, conclusions have been drawn on the basis of unadjusted HRV parameters [807].

Generally, accumulated data document the role of mental stressors (acute and chronic) for cardiac autonomic control. However, the effects of heart rate and respiration are required to be considered or at least adjusted for in further investigations in order to draw clinically valid conclusions.

3.6.3.3   Smoking

Smoking is one of the most important determinants of HRV because of the direct effects of nicotine on the autonomic nervous system and the indirect consequences related to the role of smoking on the processes of atherosclerosis, thrombosis and chronic pulmonary diseases.

The association of smoking and increased heart rate is consistent across many reports. Gillum et al. quantified the HR increase of 2.9 bpm and 1.4 bpm in current male and female smokers, as compared to ex-smokers and those who had never smoked [808]. Acute nicotine administration increases HR by 10–25 bpm [809].

The acute effects of smoking in young persons was not reflected in the 5-min SDRR, although RSA was reduced [810]. Heavy chronic smoking (>25 cigarettes per day) can be associated with RSA being reduced to a level observed in sedentary nonsmoking subjects [810, 811]. However, in one study, differences in RSA were not detected in subjects older than 31 years of age [810]. In the ARIC study, a greater reduction of 2-min adjusted SDRR and HF power during active postural changes was noticed in smokers compared to nonsmokers [812]. Blunted changes of unadjusted short-term HRV measures in response to controlled breathing have also been reported [813]. Lower amplitudes of LF and HF components of 24-h HRV have been found in smokers [577]. A diverse influence upon circadian HRV measures has been described, with significant differences between smokers and nonsmokers only within daytime HF power, while LF power has been reduced both during daytime and nighttime in smokers [577]. In another study, the 24-h SDNN and SDANN were found to be lower in smokers only during daytime, while RMSSD was comparable to that of nonsmokers over the whole ECG recording [814]. Also, tobacco use was found to be an independent determinant of global time-domain, but not short-term HRV measures in patients referred for coronary angiography [815].

There are also negative studies in which the relationship between smoking and HRV was not confirmed [816, 817]. The minimal significance of smoking as an HRV determinant has been observed as a lack of influence of smoking as a covariate on the predictive value of reduced SDNN in the Framingham Heart Study and in the ARIC Study [251, 649]. Also, in a study by Kuch et al., smoking was associated with short-term HF power only in women. However, the significance of association was weak and smoking as a determinant of HRV was rejected from the final multivariate models both for the resting state and controlled breathing [648]. The contribution of smoking to the total variance of HF and LF has been accounted for as approximately 3.5% [654]. In a number of studies, smoking habits have not been considered [141, 269, 322, 555, 583, 599]. Also, in the majority of clinical studies, smoking has not been listed among sample characteristics.

3.6.3.4   Other Factors

There are a plethora of reports accounting for the association between HRV and other factors, like anthropometrics (height), biochemical (lipids and glucose, insulin, leptin, adiponectin, uric acid, anemia), inflammatory measures (white blood cell counts, CPR, interleukins), habits (caffeine and alcohol consumption), social status and others [4–6, 521, 609, 655, 785, 816–821]. However, none of these factors has been evaluated reliably without taking into account contributions of all of the more important determinants. It is reasonable to consider the impact of a single factor that might influence HRV measures in certain circumstances. However, in general, the contribution of other factors to HRV seems to be negligible.

3.6.4   General Comments

In any subject, at a certain point of the life-course, HRV seems to be dependent on nonmodifiable determinants, such as heritability, age, gender and ethnicity. These factors should always be considered in any statistical analysis (if an examined population is heterogeneous). However, as indicated by studies in twins, these factors have accounted for less than 60% of explained variation in the HRV [521, 528, 533, 534, 638]. So, there is still a place for the role of other factors.

If short-term HRV examination is to be performed, the significance *of heart rate, respiration, body position and physical fitness* might be of importance, and so these determinants should be controlled apart from nonmodifiable factors. However, these factors have been found to account for no more than 8–15% of explained HRV variation.

If long-term HRV is to be examined, *median HR, day–night difference and sleep–wake cycle*, as well as *diurnal activity*, including work pattern, are of greater importance. Therefore, it seems necessary to check for these determinants in every study in addition to nonmodifiable factors.

Importantly, in longitudinal studies, a change in factor that is known to have only a marginal effect on HRV in the population might be of special interest, as changes in modifiable determinants can influence actual HRV by a factor of at least 10, as compared to their impact in population studies. Thus, if body mass influences HRV by 1–2%, an individual decrease of 10 kg affects HRV by at least 10%. Probably, a similar rule can influence changes in other factors, including physical training, smoking cessation, stress controlling approaches (i.e., yoga), and others. However, it is important to keep in mind that HRV error estimation is necessary to account for differences. As mentioned earlier, changes of at least 25–30% in HRV can be considered significant.

References

1. Hasset, J. and D. Danforth, An introduction to the cardiovascular system, in: *Perspectives in Cardiovascular Psychophysiology*, Cacioppo, J.T. and R.E. Petty, Editors. The Guilford Press: New York/London, 1982, pp. 4–18.

2. Cheng, T.O., Decreased heart rate variability as a predictor for sudden death was known in China in the third century A.D. *Eur. Heart. J.* 2000;**21**: 2081–2082.

3. Struthus, J., Sphygmicae artis tam mille ducentos annos perditae & desierate Libri V. Basel 1955 (Reprinted by the Polish Cardiac Society, Poznan 2004).

4. Task Force of the European Society of Cardiology and the North American Society of Pacing Electrophysiology, Heart rate variability, standards of measurement, physiological interpretation, and clinical use. *Eur. Heart. J.* 1996;**17**: 354–381.

5. Berntson, G.C., J.Tr. Bigger, D.L. Eckberg, P. Grossman, P.G. Kaufmann, M. Malik, H.N. Nagaraja, S.W. Porges, J.P. Saul, P.H. Stone, and M.W. van der Molen, Heart rate variability: origins, methods and interpretative caveats. *Psychophysiology* 1997;**34**: 623–648.

6. Porges, S.W., P.M. McCabe, and B.G. Younge, Respiratory-heart rate interactions: psychophysiological implications for pathophysiology and behavior, in: *Perspectives in Cardiovascular Psychophysiology*, Cacioppo, J.T. and R.E. Petty, Editors. The Guilford Press: New York/London, 1982, pp. 223–264.

7. Samaan, A., The antagonistic cardiac nerves and heart rate. *J. Physiol.* 1935;**83**: 332–340.

8. Holzmann, M., *Klinische Elektrokardiographie*. Georg Thieme Verlag: Stuttgart, 1961, pp. 554–561.

9. Anrep, G.V., W. Pascual, and R. Rössler, Respiratory variations of the heart rate. I. The reflex mechanism of the respiratory arrhythmia. *Proc. R. Soc. Lond. B. Biol. Sci.* 1936;**119B**: 191–217.

10. Lacey, J.I. and B.C. Lacey, Verification and extension of the principle of autonomic response-stereotypy. *Am. J. Psychol.*, 1958;**71**: 50–73.

11. Hon, E.H. and S.T. Lee, Electronic evaluation of the fetal heart rate. *Am. J. Obstet. Gynecol.*, 1963;**87**: 814–826.

12. Camm, A.J. and L. Fei, Clinical significance of heart rate variability, in *Noninvasive Electrocardiology. Clinical Aspects of Holter Monitoring*, Moss, A.J. and S. Stern S, Editors. W.B. Saunders: London, 1996, pp. 225–248.

13. Wolf, S., The end of the rope: the role of the brain in cardiac death. *Can. Med. Assoc. J.*, 1967;**97**: 1022–1025.

14. Katona, P.G., J.W. Poitras, G.O. Barnett, and B.S. Terry, Cardiac vagal efferent activity and heart period in the carotid sinus reflex. *Am. J. Physiol.*, 1970;**218**: 1030–1037.

15. Levy, M.N., Sympathetic-parasympathetic interactions in the heart. *Circ. Res.* 1971;**29**: 437–445.

16. Hinkle, L.E. Jr, S.T. Carver, and A. Plakun, Slow heart rates and increased risk of cardiac death in middle-aged men. *Arch. Intern. Med.*, 1972;**129**: 732–748.

17. Sayers, B.M., Analysis of heart rate variability. *Ergonomics*, 1973;**16**: 17–32.

18. Wheeler, T. and P.J. Watkins, Cardiac denervation in diabetes. *Br. Med. J.*, 1973;**8**: 584–586.

19. Wolf, M.M., G.A. Varigos, D. Hunt, and J.G. Sloman, Sinus arrhythmia in acute myocardial infarction. *Med. J. Aust.*, 1978;**2**: 52–53.

20. Akselrod, S., D. Gordon, F.A. Ubel, D.C. Shannon, A.C. Berger, and R.J. Cohen, Power spectrum analysis of heart rate fluctuation: a quantitative probe of beat-to-beat cardiovascular control. *Science*, 1981;**213**: 220–222.

21. Kobayashi, M. and T. Musha, 1/f fluctuation of heart beat period. *IEEE. Trans. Biomed. Eng.*, 1982;**29**: 456–457.

22. Ewing, D.J., J.M. Neilson, and P. Travis, New method for assessing cardiac parasympathetic activity using 24 hour electrocardiograms. *Br. Heart J.*, 1984;**52**: 396–402.

23. Pomeranz, B., R.J. Macaulay, M.A. Caudill, I. Kutz, D. Adam, D. Gordon, K.M. Kilborn, A.C. Barger, D.C. Shannon, and R.J. Cohen, Assessment of autonomic function in humans by heart rate spectral analysis. *Am. J. Physiol. Heart Circ. Physiol.*, 1985;**248** (1 Pt 2): H151–153.

24. Kleiger, R.E., J.P. Miller, J.T. Jr. Bigger, and A.J. Moss, Decreased heart rate variability and its association with increased mortality after acute myocardial infarction. *Am. J. Cardiol.*, 1987;**59**: 256–262.

25. Camm, A.J., R. Karam, and C.M. Pratt, The azimilide postinfarct survival evaluation (ALIVE) trial. *Am. J. Cardiol.*, 1998;**81**: 35D–39D.

26. Kors, J.A., J.H. Bemmel and C. Zywietz, Signal analysis for ECG interpretation. *Meth. Inf. Med.*, 1990;**29**: 317–329.

27. Forester, J., H. Bo, J.W. Sleigh, and J.D. Henderson, Variability of R–R, P wave-to-R wave, and R wave-to-T wave intervals. *Am. J. Physiol. Heart Circ. Physiol.*, 1997;**273**: H2857–2860.

28. Hamilton, R.M., P.S. Mckenzie, and P.W. Macfarlane, Can cardiac vagal tone be estimated from the 10-second ECG? *Int. J. Cardiol.*, 2004;**95**: 109–115.

29. Teixeira, F.P., D.R. Ricardo, C.L.B. Castro, and C.G.S. Araújo, Evaluating cardiac vagal activity on a conventional electrocardiogram. *Arq. Bras. Cardiol.*, 2007;**88**: 333–337.

30. Kleiger, E., P.K. Stein, M.S. Bosner, and J.N. Rottman, Time-domain measurements of heart rate variability, in *Heart Rate Variability*, Malik, M. and A.J. Camm, Editors. Futura Publishing: Armonk, NY, 1995, pp. 33–45.

31. Balocchi, R., F. Cantini, M. Varanini, G. Raimondi, J.M. Legramante, and A. Macerata, Revisiting the potential of time-domain indexes in short-term HRV analysis. *Biomed. Tech. (Berl).*, 2006;**51**: 190–193.

32. Mietus, J.E., C-K. Peng, I. Henry, R.L. Goldsmith, and A.L. Goldberger, The pNNx files: re-examining a widely used heart rate variability measure. *Heart*, 2002;**88**: 378–380.

33. Burr, R.L., S.A. Motzer, W. Chen, M.J. Cowan, and M.M. Heitkemper Logit50: a nonlinear transformation of pNN50 with improved statistical properties. *J. Electrocardiol.*, 2003;**36**: 41–52.

34. Malik, M., Effect of electrocardiogram recognition artifact on time-domain measurement of heart rate variability, in *Heart Rate Variability*, Malik, M. and A.J. Camm, Editors. Futura Publishing Company, Inc.: Armonk, NY, 1995, pp. 99–118.

35. Kaplan, D.T., The analysis of variability. *J. Cardiovasc. Electrophysiol.*, 1994;**5**: 16–19.

36. Griffin, M.P. and J.R. Moorman, Toward the early diagnosis of neonatal sepsis and sepsis-like illness using novel heart rate analysis. *Pediatrics*, 2001;**107**: 97–104.

37. Malik, M., T. Farrell, T. Cripps, and A.J. Camm, Heart rate variability in relation to prognosis after myocardial infarction: selection of optimal processing techniques. *Eur. Heart J.*, 1989;**10**: 1060–1074.

38. Cripps, T.R., M. Malik, T.G. Farrell, and A.J. Camm, Prognostic value of reduced heart rate variability after myocardial infarction: clinical evaluation of a new analysis method. *Br. Heart J.*, 1991;**65**: 14–19.

39. Scott, D.W., On optimal and data-based histograms. *Biometrika*, 1979;**66**: 605–610.

40. Farrell, T.G., Y. Basir, T. Cripps, M. Malik, J. Poloniecki, E.D. Bennett, D.E. Ward, and A.J. Camm, Risk stratification for arrhythmic events in postinfarction patients based on heart rate variability, ambulatory electrocardiographic variables and the

signal-averaged electrocardiogram. *J. Am. Coll. Cardiol.*, 1991;**18**: 687–697.

41. Scherer, P., J.P. Ohler, H. Hirche, and H.W. Höpp, Definition of a new beat-to-beat-parameter of heart rate variability. *PACE*, 1993;**16**: 939 (abs).

42. Kovatchev, B.P., L.S. Farhy, H. Cao, M.P. Griffin, D.E. Lake, and J.R. Moorman, Sample asymmetry analysis of heart rate characteristics with application to neonatal sepsis and systemic inflammatory response syndrome. *Pediatr. Res.*, 2003;**54**: 892–898.

43. Björkander, I., T. Kahan, M. Ericson, C. Held, L. Forslund, N. Rehnquist, and P. Hjemdahl, Differential index, a novel graphical method for measurements of heart rate varability. *Int. J. Cardiol.*, 2005;**98**: 493–499.

44. Björkander, I., L. Forslund, T. Kahan, M. Ericson, C. Held, P. Hjemdahl, and N. Rehnquist, Differential index: a simple time domain heart rate variability analysis with prognostic implications in stable angina pectoris. *Cardiology*, 2008;**111**: 126–133.

45. Soderstrom N., What is the reason for the ventricular arrhythmia in cases of auricular fibrillation? *Am. Heart J.*, 1950;**40**: 212–223.

46. Nakanishi, A., R. Tabata, and T. Kobayashi, Effect of aging and diseases to fluctuation of the ECG R-R intervals, in *Noise in Physical Systems and 1/f Fluctuations*, T. Musha, S. Sato, and M. Yamamoto, Editors. Ohmsha Ltd., Institute of Physics, 1991, pp. 669–702.

47. Woo, M.A., W.G. Stevenson, D.K. Moser, R.B. Trelease, and R.M. Harper, Patterns of beat-to-beat heart rate variability in advanced heart failure. *Am. Heart J.*, 1992;**123**: 704–710.

48. Esperer, H.D., D. Esperer, and R.J. Cohen, Cardiac arrhythmias imprint specific signatures on Lorenz plots. *Ann. Noninvasive Electrocardiol.*, 2008;**13**: 44–60.

49. Schechtman, V.L., K.A. Kluge,, and R.M. Harper, Time-domain system for assessing variation in heart rate. *Med. Biol. Eng. Comput.*, 1988;**26**: 367–373.

50. Kuo, C.D., G.Y. Chen, Y.Y. Wang, M.J. Hung, J.L. Yang, Characterization and quantification of the return map of RR intervals by Pearson coefficient in patients with acute myocardial infarction. *Auton. Neurosci.I*, 2003;**105**: 145–152.

51. Sosnowski, M., Z. Czyż, T. Petelenz, et al., Repeat return map distinguishes patients in the chronic phase after myocardial infarction with different risk for future cardiac events. *Comput. Cardiol.*, 1995; 285–288.

52. Otzenberger, H., C. Simon, C. Gronfier, and G. Brandenberger, Temporal relationship between dynamic heart rate variability and electroencephalographic activity during sleep in man. *Neurosci. Lett.*, 1997;**229**: 173–176.

53. Stein, P.K., P.P. Domitrovich, N. Hui, P. Rautaharju, and J. Gottdiener, Sometimes higher heart rate variability is not better heart rate variability: results of graphical and nonlinear analyses. *J. Cardiovasc. Electrophysiol.*, 2005;**16**: 954–959.

54. Schechtman, V.L., S.L. Raetz, R.K. Harper, A. Garfinkiel, A.J. Wilson, D.P. Southall, and R.M. Harper, Dynamic analysis of cardiac R-R intervals in normal infants and in infants who subsequently succumbed to the sudden infant death syndrome. *Ped. Res.*, 1992;**31**: 606–612.

55. Schechtman, V.L., R.K. Harper, and R.M. Harper, Development of heart rate dynamics during sleep-waking states in normal infants. *Pediatr. Res.*, 1993;**34**: 618–623.

56. Schechtman, V.L., M.Y. Lee, A.J. Wilson, and R.M. Harper, Dynamics of respiratory patterning in normal infants and

infants who subsequently died of the sudden infant death syndrome. *Pediatr. Res.*, 1996;**40**: 571–577.

57. Kamen, P.W., H. Krum, and A.M. Tonkin, Poincare plot of heart rate variability allows quantitative display of parasympathetic nervous activity in humans. *Clin. Sci.*, 1996;**91**: 201–208.

58. Tulppo, M.P., T.H. Makikallio, T.E. Takala, T. Seppanen, and H.V. Huikuri, Quantitative beat-to-beat analysis of heart rate dynamics during exercise. *Am. J. Physiol. Heart Circ. Physiol.*, 1996;**271**: H244–252.

59. Toichi, M., T. Sugiura, T. Murai, and A. Sengoku, A new method of assessing cardiac autonomic function and its comparison with spectral analysis and coefficient of variation of R-R interval. *J. Auton. Nerv. Syst.*, 1997;**62**: 79–84.

60. Copie, X., J-Y. Le Heuzey, M-C. Iliou, R. Khouri, T. Lavergne, F. Pousset, and L.Guize, Correlation between time-domain measures of heart rate variability and scatterplots in postinfarction patients. *PACE*, 1996;**19**: 342–347.

61. Guzik, P., J. Piskorski, T. Krauze, A. Wykrętowicz, and H. Wysocki, Partitioning total heart rate variability. *Int. J. Cardiol.*, 2009, in press, doi:10.1016/j.ijcardiol 2008.12.151.

62. Schmidt, G. and G.E. Morfill, Nonlinear methods for heart rate variability assessment, in *Heart Rate Variability*, M. Malik and A.J. Camm., Editors. Armonk, NY: Futura Publishing, 1995, pp. 87–98.

63. Hnatkova, K., X. Copie, A. Staunton, and M. Malik, Numeric processing of Lorenz plots of R-R intervals from long-term ECS: comparisons with time-domain measures of heart rate variability for risk stratification after myocardial infarction. *J. Electrocardiol.*, 1995;**28**(Suppl.1): 74–80.

64. Sosnowski, M., P.W. MacFarlane, Z. Czyż, J. Skrzypek-Wańha, E. Boczkowska-Gaik, and M. Tendera, Age-adjustment of HRV measures and its prognostic value for risk assessment in patients late after myocardial infarction. *Int. J. Cardiol.*, 2002;**86**: 249–258.

65. Sosnowski, M., E. Clark, S. Latif, P.W. Macfarlane, and M. Tendera, Heart rate variability fraction—a new reportable measure of 24-hour R-R interval variation. *Ann. Noninvasive. Electrocardiol.*, 2005;**10**: 7–15.

66. Sosnowski, M., P.W. Macfarlane, R. Parma, J. Skrzypek-Wanha, and M. Tendera, Prognostic value of heart rate variability analysis in patients with depressed left ventricular function irrespective of cardiac rhythm. *Comp. Cardiol.*, 2006: 81–84.

67. Moraes, R.S., E.L. Ferlin, C.A. Polanczyk, L.E. Rohde, L. Zaslavski, J.L. Gross, and P. Ribeiro, Three-dimensional return map: a new tool for quantification of heart rate variability. *Autonom. Neurosci.*, 2000;**83**: 90–99.

68. Grossman, P., Respiratory and cardiac rhythms as windows to central and autonomic biobehavioral regulation: selection of window frames, keeping the panes clean and viewing the neural topography. *Biol. Psych.*, 1992;**34**: 131–161.

69. Porges, S.W., Respiratory sinus arrhythmia: an index of vagal tone, in *Psychophysiology of Cardiovascular Control: Models, Methods, and Data*, J.F. Orlebeke, G. Mulder, and L.J.P. Van Domen, Editors. New York: Plenum, 1985, pp. 437–450.

70. Allen, J.J.B., A.S. Chambers, and D.N. Towers, The many metrics of cardiac chronotropy: A pragmatic primer and a brief comparison of metrics. *Biol. Psych.*, 2007;**74**: 243–262.

71. Denver, J.W., S.F. Reed, and S.W. Porges, Methodological issues in the quantification of respiratory sinus arrhythmia. *Biol. Psych.*, 2007;**74**: 286–294.

72. Sosnowski, M., T. Petelenz, and J. Leski, Return maps: a non-linear method for evaluation of respiratory sinus arrhythmia. *Comput. Cardiol.*, 1994; 129–132.

73. Suder, K., F.R. Drepper, M. Schiek, H-H. Abel, One-dimensional, nonlinear determinism characterizes heart rate pattern during paced respiration. *Am. J. Physiol. Heart Circ. Physiol.*, 1998; 275: H1092–1102.

74. Carlson, G., S. Girouard, M. Schlegl, and C. Butter, Three-dimensional heart rate variability diagnostic for monitoring heart failure through an implantable device. *J. Cardiovasc. Electrophysiol.*, 2004;**15**: 506.

75. Gilliam, F.R. IIIrd, J.P. Singh, C.M. Mullin, M. McGuire, and K.J. Chase, Prognostic value of heart rate variability footprint and standard deviation of average 5-minute intrinsic R-R intervals for mortality in cardiac resynchronization therapy patients. *J. Electrocardiol.*, 2007;**40**: 336–342.

76. Penaz, J., J. Roukenz, and H.J. van der Waal, in *Spectral Analysis of Some Spontaneous Rhythms in the Circulation*, H. Drischel and N. Tiedt, Editors. Biokybernetik. Bd I, Karl Marx University, Leipzig, 1968, pp. 223–241.

77. DeBoer, R.W., J.M. Karemaker, and J. Strackee, Beat-to-beat variability of heart rate interval and blood pressure. *Automedica.*, 1983;**4**: 217–222.

78. Parati, G., P. Castiglioni, M. Di Rienzo, S. Omboni, A. Pedotti, and G. Mancia, Sequential spectral analysis of 24-hour blood pressure and pulse interval in humans. *Hypertension*, 1990;**16**: 414–421.

79. Cerutti, S., A.M. Bianchi, and L.T. Mainardi, Spectral analysis of the heart rate variability signal, in *Heart Rate Variability*, M. Malik and A.J. Camm, Editors. Armonk, NY: Futura Publishing 1995, pp. 63–74.

80. Bigger, J.T. Jr., Heart rate variability: frequency domain, in *Non-invasive Electrocardiology. Clinical Aspects of Holter Monitoring*, Moss, A.J. and S. Stern, Editors. London: W.B. Saunders, 1996: 175–198.

81. Malliani, A., M. Pagani, F. Lombardi, and S. Cerutti, Cardio-vascular neural regulation explored in the frequency domain. *Circulation*, 1991;**84**: 482–492.

82. Pagani, M., F. Lombardi, S. Guzzetti, O. Rimoldi R. Furlan, P. Pizzinelli, G. Sandrone, G. Malfatto, S. Dell'Orto, and E. Piccaluga, Power spectral analysis of heart rate and arterial pressure variabilities as a marker of sympatho-vagal interaction in man and conscious dog. *Circ. Res.*, 1986;**59**: 178–193.

83. Wichterle, D., J. Simek, M.T. La Rovere, P.J. Schwartz, A.J. Camm, and M. Malik, Prevalent low-frequency oscillation of heart rate: novel predictor of mortality after myocardial infarction. *Circulation*, 2004;**110**: 1183–1190.

84. Cooley, J.W. and J.W. Tukey, An algorithm for machine cal-culation of complex Fourier series. *Math. Comput.*, 1965;**19**: 297–310.

85. Kay, S.M. and S.L. Marple, Spectrum analysis: a modern perspective. *Proc. IEEE.*, 1981;**69**: 1380–1418.

86. Rüdiger, H., L. Klinghammer, and K. Scheuch, The trigono-metric regressive spectral analysis—a method for mapping of beat-to-beat recorded cardiovascular parameters on to frequency domain in comparison with Fourier transformation. *Comput. Meth. Prog. Biomed.*, 1999;**58**: 1–15.

87. Nelson, W., Y.L. Tong, J.K. Lee, and F. Halberg, Meth-ods for cosinor-rhythmometry. *Chronobiologia.*, 1979;**6**: 305–323.

88. Kitney, R.I., T. Fulton, A.H. McDonald, and D.A. Linkens, Transient interactions between blood pressure, respi-ration and heart rate in man. *J. Biomed. Eng.*, 1985;**7**: 217–224.

89. Di Rienzo, M., P. Castiglioni, G. Mancia G. Parati, and A. Pedotti, 24 hour sequential analysis of arterial blood pressure and pulse interval in free moving subjects. *IEEE. Trans. Biomed. Eng.*, 1989;**36**: 1066–1075.

90. Boardman, A., F.S. Schlindwein, A.P. Rocha, and A. Leite, A study on the optimum order of autoregressive models for heart rate variability. *Physiol. Meas.*, 2002;**23**: 325–336.

91. Lacoss, R.T., Data adaptive spectral analysis methods. *Geophysics* 1971;**36**: 661–675.

92. Marple, S.L., A new autoregressive spectrum analysis algorithm. *IEEE Trans. Acoust., Speech, Signal Process.*, 1980;**28**: 441–454.

93. Cohen, L., Time-frequency distribution. *A. Rev.. Proc. IEEE.*, 1989;**177**: 941–981.

94. Cerutti, S., A.M. Bianchi, and L.T. Mainardi, Advanced spectral methods for detecting dynamic behaviour. *Auton. Neurosci.*, 2001;**90**: 3–12.

95. Pinna, G.D., R. Maestri, and A. Di Cesare, Application of time series spectral analysis theory: analysis of cardiovas-cular variability signals. *Med. Biol. Eng. Comput.* 1996;**34**: 142–148.

96. Novak, P. and V. Novak, Time/frequency mapping of the heart rate, blood pressure and respiratory signals. *Med. Biol. Eng. Comput.*, 1993;**31**: 103–110.

97. Bianchi, A.M., L.T. Mainardi, and S. Cerutti, Time-frequency analysis of biomedical signals. *Trans. Inst. Meas. Control.*, 2000;**22**: 215–230.

98. Mainardi, L.T., On the quantification of heart rate variability spectral parameters using time-frequency and time-varying methods. *Phil. Trans. R. Soc. A.*, 2009;**367**: 255–275.

99. Jason, S., C. Medique, P. Maison-Blanche, N. Montano, L. Meyer, C. Vermeiren, P. Mansier, P. Coumel, A. Malliani, and B. Swynghedaw, Instant power spectrum analysis of heart rate variability during orthostatic tilt using a time/frequency domain method. *Circulation.*, 1997;**96**: 3521–3526.

100. Martinmäki, K., H. Rusko, S. Saalasti, and J. Kettunen, Ability of short-time Fourier transform method to detect transient changes in vagal effects on hearts: a pharmacological block-ing study. *Am. J. Physiol. Heart Circ. Physiol.*, 2006;**290**: H2582–2589.

101. Baillard, C., P. Gonçavales, L. Mangin, B. Swynghedauw, and P. Mansier, Use of time frequency analysis to follow transitory modulation of the cardiac autonomic system in clinical studies. *Autonom. Neurosci.: Basic. Clin.*, 2001;**90**: 24–28.

102. Vigo, D.E., S.M. Guinjoan, M. Scaramal, L.N. Siri, and D.P. Car-dinali, Wavelet transform shows age-related changes of heart rate variability within independent frequency components. *Autonom. Neurosci. Basic. Clin.*, 2005;**123**: 94–100.

103. Pichot, V., J-M. Gaspoz, S. Molliex, A. Antoniadis, T. Busso, F. Roche, F. Costes, L. Quintin, J-R. Lacour, and J-C. Barthélémy, Wavelet transform to quantify heart rate variability and to assess its instantaneous changes. *J. Appl. Physiol.*, 1999;**86**: 1081–1091.

104. Huang, N.E., Z. Shen, S.R. Long, M.L. Wu, H.H. Shih, Q. Zheng, N.C. Yen, C.C. Tung, and H.H. Liu, The empirical mode decomposition and Hilbert spectrum for nonlinear and nonstationary time series analysis. *Proc. Roy. Soc. London. A.*, 1998;**454**: 903–995.

105. Li, M., X-K. Gu, and S-S. Yang, Hilbert-Huang transform based time-frequency distribution and comparison with other three. *Int. J. Circ. Syst. Signal. Proc.*, 2007;**2**: 155–160.

106. Perlstein, I. and A. Hoffman, Cumulative plot of heart rate variability spectrum assesses kinetics of action of cholinergic drugs in rats. *Am. J. Physiol. Heart. Circ. Physiol.*, 2000;**279**: H110–115.

107. Goldberger AL, L.A.N. Amaral, J.M. Hausdorff, P.C. Ivanov, C.K. Peng, and H.E. Stanley Fractal dynamics in physiology: alterations with disease and aging. *Proc. Natl. Acad. Sci. USA.*, 2002;**99**(Suppl 1): 2466–2472

108. Denton, T.A., G.A. Diamond, R.H. Helfant, S. Khan, and H. Karagueuzian, Fascinating rhythm: a prime on chaos theory and its application to cardiology. *Am. Heart. J.*, 1990;**120**: 1419–1440.

109. Elbert, T., W.J. Ray, W.J. Kowalik, K.E.G. Skinner, and N. Birbaumer, Chaos and physiology: Deterministic chaos in excitable cell assemblies. *Physiol. Rev.*, 1994;**74**: 1–47.

110. Goldberger, A.L., Non-linear dynamics for clinicians: chaos theory, fractals, and complexity at the bedside. *Lancet*, 1996;**347**: 1312–1314.

111. Voss, A., S. Schulz, R. Schreoder, M. Baumert, and P. Caminal, Methods derived from nonlinear dynamics for analysis heart rate variability. *Phil. Trans. Roy. Soc. London A.*, 2009;**367**: 277–296.

112. Huikuri, H.V., J.S. Perkiömaki, R. Maestri, and G.D. Pinna, Clinical impact of evaluation of cardiovascular control by novel methods of heart rate dynamics. *Phil. Trans. Roy. Soc. London A.*, 2009;**367**: 1223–1238.

113. Higuchi, T., Approach to an irregular time series on the basis of the fractal theory. *Physica. D.*, 1988;**31**: 277–283.

114. Katz, M., Fractals and the analysis of waveforms. *Comput. Biol. Med.*, 1988;**18**: 145–156.

115. Yamamoto, Y. and R.L. Hughson, Coarse-graining spectral analysis: new method for studying heart rate variability. *J. Appl. Physiol.*, 1991;**71**: 1143–1150.

116. Guevara, M.R. and L. Glass, Phase locking, period doubling bifurcations and chaos in a mathematical model of a periodically driven oscillator: a theory for the entrainment of biological oscillators and the generation of cardiac dysrhythmias. *J. Math. Biol.*, 1982;**14**: 1–23.

117. Chialvo, D.R. and J. Jalife, Non-linear dynamics of cardiac excitation and impulse propagation. *Nature.*, 1987;**330**: 749–752.

118. Garfinkel, A., M.L. Spano, W.L. Ditto, and J.N. Weiss, Controlling cardiac chaos. *Science.*, 1992;**57**: 1230–1235.

119. Weiss, J.N., A. Garfinkel, H.S. Karagueuzian, Z. Qu, and P.S. Chen, Chaos and the transition to ventricular fibrillation: a new approach to antiarrhythmic drug evaluation. *Circulation*, 1999;**99**: 2819–2826.

120. Sato, D., L.H. Xie, A.A. Sovari, D.X. Tran, N. Morita, F. Xie, H. Karagueuzian, A. Garfinkel, J.N. Weiss, and Z. Qu, Synchronization of chaotic early afterdepolarizations in the genesis of cardiac arrhythmias. *Proc. Natl. Acad. Sci. USA.*, 2009;**106**: 2983–2988.

121. Saul, J.P., P. Albrecht, R.D. Berger, and R.J. Cohen, Analysis of long-term heart rate variability: methods, 1/f scaling and implications. *Comput.Cardiol.*, 1987: 419–422. Silver Spring, MD: IEEE Computer Society Press.

122. Bigger, J.T. Jr., R.C. Steinman, L.M. Rolnitzky, J.L. Fleiss, P. Albrecht, and R.J. Cohen, Power law behavior of RR-interval variability in healthy middle-aged persons, patients with recent acute myocardial infarction, and patients with heart transplants. *Circulation*, 1996;**93**: 2142–2151.

123. Schepers, H.E., J.H.G.M. van Beek, and J.B. Bassingthwaighte, Four methods to estimate the fractal dimension from self-affine signals. *IEEE. Eng. Med. Biol.* 1992;**11**: 57–64.

124. Peng, C.K., S. Havlin, H.E. Stanley, and A.L. Goldberger, Quantification of scaling exponents and crossover phenomena in nonstationary heart beat time series. *Chaos*, 1995;**5**: 82–87.

125. Francis, D.P., K. Willson, P. Georgiadou, R. Wensel, L.C. Davies, A. Coats, and M. Piepoli, Physiological basis of fractal complexity properties of heart rate variability in man. *J. Physiol.*, 2002;**542**: 619–629.

126. Ho, K.K., G.B. Moody, C.K. Peng, J.E. Mietus, M.G. Larson, D. Levy, and A.L. Goldberger, Predicting survival in heart failure case and control subjects by use of fully automated methods for deriving nonlinear and conventional indices of heart rate dynamics. *Circulation*, 1997;**96**: 842–848.

127. Huikuri, H.V., T.H. Mäkikallio, C.K. Peng, A.L. Goldberger, U. Hintze, and M. Moller, Fractal correlation properties of R-R interval dynamics and mortality in patients with depressed left ventricular function after an acute myocardial infarction. *Circulation*, 2000;**101**: 47–53.

128. Tibby, S.M., H. Frndova, A. Durward, and P.H. Cox, Novel method to quantify loss of heart rate variability in pediatric multiple organ failure. *Crit. Care. Med.*, 2003;**31**: 2079–2080.

129. Ivanov, P.C., A.N. Amaral, A.L. Goldberger, S. Havlin, M.G. Rosenblum, Z.R. Struzik, and H.E. Stanley, Multifractality in human heart beat dynamics. *Nature*, 1999;**399**: 461–465.

130. Ching, E.S. and Y.K. Tsang, Multifractality and scale invariance in human heart beat dynamics. *Phys. Rev. E. Stat. Nonlin. Soft. Matter. Phys.*, 2007;**76** (4 Pt 1): 041910–04198.

131. Kiyono, K., Z.R. Struzik, N. Aoyagi, S. Sakata, J. Hayano, and Y. Yamamoto. Critical scale- invariance in healthy human heart rate. *Phys. Rev. Lett.*, 2004;**93**: 178103.

132. Kiyono, K., J. Hayano, E. Watanabe, Z.R. Struzik, and Y. Yamamoto, Non-Gaussian heart rate as an independent predictor of mortality in patients with chronic heart failure. *Heart Rhythm.*, 2008;**5**: 261–268.

133. Cerutti, S., D. Hoyer, A. Voss, Multiscale, multiorgan and multivariate complexity analysis of cardiovascular regulation. *Phi. Trans. Roy. Soc. London A.*, 2009;**367**: 1337–1358.

134. Batzel, J., G. Baselli, R. Mukkamala, and K.H. Chon, Modelling and disentangling physiological mechanisms: linear and nonlinear identification techniques for analysis of cardiovascular regulation. *Phil. Trans. Roy. Soc. London A.*, 2009;**367**: 1377–1391.

135. Takens, F., Detecting strange attractors in turbulence, in *Dynamical Systems and Turbulence, Lecture Notes in Mathematics*, vol. 898, D.A. Rand and L-S. Young, Editors. Berlin: Springer-Verlag, 1981; pp. 366–381.

136. Grassberger, P. and I. Procaccia, Measuring the strangeness of strange attractors. *Physica. D.*, 1983;**9**: 189–208.

137. Carjaval, R., N. Wessel, M. Vallverdu, P. Caminal, and A. Voss, Correlation dimension analysis of heart rate variability in patients with dilated cardiomyopathy. *Comput. Meth. Prog. Biomed.*, 2005;**78**: 133–140.

138. Skinner, J.E., C.M. Pratt, and T. Vybiral, A reduction in the correlation dimension of heart beat intervals precedes imminent ventricular fibrillation in human subjects. *Am. Heart. J.*, 1993;**125**: 731–734.

139. Shannon, C.E. and W. Weaver, *The Mathematical Theory of Information*. University of Illinois Press, 1949.

140. Pincus, S.M. and W.M. Huang, Approximate entropy: statistical properties and applications. *Commun. Stat. Theory. Meth.*, 1992;**21**: 3061–3077.

141. Pikkujämsä, S.M., T.H. Mäkikallio, K.E. Airaksinen, and H.V. Huikuri, Determinants and interindividual variation of R-R interval dynamics in healthy middle-aged subjects. *Am. J. Physiol. Heart. Circ. Physiol.*, 2001;**280**: H1400–1406.

142. Mäkikallio, T.H., T. Seppänen, N. Niemelä, K.E. Airaksinen, M. Tulpo, H.V. Huikuri, Abnormalities in beat to beat complexity of heart rate dynamics in patients with a previous myocardial infarction. *J. Am. Coll. Cardiol.*, 1996;**28**: 1005–1011.

143. Richman, J.S. and J.R. Moorman, J.R Physiological time-series analysis using approximate entropy and sample entropy. *Am. J. Physiol. Heart. Circ. Physiol.*, 2000;**278**: H2039–2049.

144. Lake, D.E., J.S. Richman, M.P. Griffin, and J.R. Moorman, Sample entropy analysis of neonatal heart rate variability. *Am. J. Physiol. Regul. Integr. Comp. Physiol.*, 2002;**283**: R789–797.

145. Tuzcu, V., S. Nas, T. Borklu, and A. Ugur, Decrease in the heart rate complexity prior to the onset of atrial fibrillation. *Europace.*, 2006;**8**: 398–402.

146. Costa, M., A.L. Goldberger, and C.K. Peng, Multiscale entropy analysis of complex physiological time series. *Phys. Rev. Lett.*, 2002;**89**: 068–102.

147. Javorka, M., Z. Trunkvalterova, I. Tonhajzerova, J. Javorkova, K. Javorka, and M. Baumert Short-term heart rate complexity in reduced in patients with type 1 diabetes mellitus. *Clin. Neurophysiol.*, 2008;**119**: 1071–1081.

148. Baumert, M., V. Baier, J. Hauesian, N. Wessel, U. Meyerfeldt, A. Schirdewan, and A. Voss, Forecasting of life threatening arrhythmias using the compression entropy of heart rate. *Meth. Inf. Med.*, 2004;**43**: 202–206.

149. Treubner, S., I. Cygankiewicz, R. Schreoder, M. Baumenrt, M. Vallverdú, P. Caminal, R. Vazquez, A. Bayés de Luna, and A. Voss, Compression entropy contributes to risk stratification in patients with cardiomyopathy. *Biomed. Tech. (Berl.)* 2006;**51**: 77–82.

150. Bai-Lin, H., *Elementary Symbolic Dynamics and Chaos in Dissipative Systems*. Singapore: World Scientific, 1989.

151. Kurths, J., A. Voss, P. Saparin, A. Witt, H.J. Kleiner, and N. Wessel, Quantitative analysis of heart rate variability. *Chaos*, 1995;**5**: 88–94.

152. Wessel, N., C. Ziehmann, J. Kurths, U. Meyerfeldt, A. Schirdewan, and A. Voss, Short-term forecasting of life-threatening cardiac arrhythmias based on symbolic dynamics and finite-time growth rates. *Phys. Rev. E.*, 2000;**61**: 733–739.

153. García-Gonzáles, M.A., J. Ramos-Castro, and M. Fernández-Chimeno, A new index for the analysis of heart rate variability dynamics: characterization and application. *Physiol. Meas.*, 2003;**24**: 819–832.

154. Arif, M. and W. Aziz, Application of threshold-based acceleration change index (TACI) in heart rate variability analysis. *Physiol. Meas.*, 2005;**26**: 653–665.

155. Porta, A., S. Guzzetti, N. Montano, R. Furlan, M. Pagani, A. Malliani, and S. Cerutti, Entropy, entropy rate and pattern classification as tools to typify complexity in short heart period variability series. *IEEE. Trans. Biomed. Eng.*, 2001;**48**: 1282–1291.

156. Hoyer, D., H. Friedrich, U. Zwiener, B. Pompe, R. Baranowski, K. Werdan, U. Müller-Werdan, and H. Schmidt. Prognostic impact of autonomic information flow in multiple organ dysfunction syndrome patients. *Int. J. Cardiol.*, 2006;**108**: 359–369

157. Eckmann, J.P. and D. Ruelle, Ergodic theory of chaos and strange attractors. *Rev. Mod. Phys.* 1985;**57**: 617–656.

158. Wolf, A., J.B. Swift, L.H. Swinney, J.A.Vastano, Determining Lyapunov exponent from a time series. *Physica. D.* 1985;**16**: 285–317.

159. Poon, C-S. and M. Barahona, Titration of chaos with added noise. *Proc. Natl. Acad. Sci. USA.* 2001;**98**: 7107–7112

160. Wu, G-Q., N.M. Arzeno, L-L. Shen, D-K. Tang, D-A. Zheng, N-Q. Zhao, D.L. Eckberg, and C-S. Poon, Chaotic signature of heart rate variability and its power spectrum in health, aging and heart failure. *PLoS. ONE.* 2009;**4**: e4323.

161. Sugihara, G. and R. May, Nonlinear forecasting as a way for distinguishing chaos from measurement error in a data series. *Nature* (London), 1990;**344**: 734–741.

162. Sugihara, G., Nonlinear forecasting for the classification of natural time series. *Phil. Trans. R. Soc. A.* 1994;**348**: 477–495.

163. Braun, C., P. Kowalik, A. Freking, D. Hadeler, K.D. Kniffi, and M. Messmann, Demonstration of non-linear components in heart rate variability of healthy persons. *Am. J. Physiol. Heart. Circ. Physiol.* 1998;**275**: H1577–H1584.

164. Costa, M., A.L. Goldberger, C-K. Peng, Broken asymmetry of the human heart beat: loss of time irreversibility in aging and disease. *Phys. Rev. Lett.* 2005;**95**: 198102.

165. Ehlers, C.L., J. Havstad, D. Prichard, and J. Theiler, Low doses of ethanol reduce evidence for nonlinear structure in brain activity. *J. Neurosci.* 1998;**18**: 7474–7486.

166. Guzik, P., J. Piskorski, T. Krauze, A. Wykrętowicz, and H. Wysocki, Heart rate asymmetry by Poincare' plots of RR intervals. *Biomed. Tech.* 2006;**51**: 272–275.

167. Porta, A., S. Guzzetti, N. Montano, T. Gnecchi-Ruscone, R. Furlan, and A. Malliani, Time reversibility in short-term heart period variability. *Comp. Cardiol.* 2006;**33**: 77–80.

168. Porta, A., K.R. Casali, A.G. Casali, T. Gnecchi-Ruscone, E. Tobaldini, N. Montano, S. Lange, D. Geue, D. Cysarz, and P. van Leeuwen, Temporal asymmetries of short-term heart period variability are linked to autonomic regulation. *Am. J. Physiol. Regulatory. Integrative. Comp. Physiol.* 2008;**295**(2): R550–557.

169. Porta, A., G. D'Addio, T. Bassani, R. Maestri, and G-D. Pinna, Assessment of cardiovascular regulation through irreversibility analysis of heart period variability: a 24 hours Holter study in healthy and chronic heart failure populations. *Phil. Trans. R. Soc. A.* 2009;**367**: 1359–1375.

170. Bauer A., J.W. Kantelhardt, A. Bunde, M. Malik, R. Schneider, and G. Schmidt Phase-rectified signal averaging detects quasi-periodicities in non-stationary data. *Physica. A.* 2006;**364**: 423–434.

171. Bauer, A., J.W. Kantelhardt, P. Barthel, R. Schneider, T. Mäkikallio, K. Ulm, K. Hnatkova, A. Schömig, H. Huikuri, A. Bunde, M. Malik, Schmidt G. Deceleration capacity of heart rate as a predictor of mortality after myocardial infarction: cohort study. *Lancet* 2006;**367**: 1674–1681.

172. Bauer, A., P. Barthel, R. Schneider, K. Ulm, A. Müller, A. Joeinig, R. Stich, A. Kiviniemi, K. Hnatkova, H. Huikuri, A. Schömig, M. Malik, G. Schmidt, Improved stratification of autonomic regulation for risk prediction in post-infarction patients with

preserved left ventricular function (ISAR-Risk). *Eur. Heart. J.* 2009;**30**: 576–583.

173. Eckmann, J.P., S.O. Kamphorst, and D. Ruelle, Recurrence plots of dynamical systems. *Europhys. Lett.* 1987;**4**: 973–977.

174. Webber, C.L. and J.P. Zbilut, Dynamical assessment of physiological systems and states using recurrence plot strategies. *J. Appl. Physiol.* 1994;**76**: 965–973.

175. Giuliani, A., G. Piccirillo, V. Marigliano, and A. Colosimo, A nonlinear explanation of aging-induced changes in heart beat dynamics. *Am. J. Physiol. Heart. Circ. Physiol.* 1998;**275**: H1455–1461.

176. Gammaitoni, L., P. Hänggi, P. Jung, and F. Marchesoni, Stochastic resonance. *Rev. Mod. Phys.* 1998;**70**: 223–287.

177. Moody, G.B., R.G. Mark, A. Zoccola, S. Mantero, J.T. Bigger, and J.L. Fleiss, Derivation of respiratory signals from multi-leads ECGs. *Comput. Cardiol.* 1985;**12**: 113–116.

178. Sosnowski, M., J. Skrzypek-Wańha, Z. Czyż, M. Petelenz, and M. Tendera, Importance of respiration for non-invasive assessment of cardiac autonomic control in patients with ischemic left ventricular dysfunction. *Wiad. Lek.*, 1999;**52**: 230–237.

179. Sosnowski, M., Z. Czyż, and M. Tendera, Scatterplots of RR and RT interval variability bring evidence for diverse non-linear dynamics of heart rate and ventricular repolarization duration in coronary heart disease. *Europace*, 2001;**3**: 39–45.

180. Challis, R.E. and R.I. Kitney, Biomedical signal processing (in four parts). Part 3 The power spectrum and coherence function. *Med. Biol. Eng. Comput.*, 1991;**29**: 225–241.

181. Porges, S.W., R.E. Bohrer, M.N. Cheung, F. Drasgow, P.M. McCabe, and G. Keren, New time-series statistic for detecting rhythmic co-occurrence in the frequency domain: the weighted coherence and its application to psychophysiological research. *Psychol. Bull.*, 1980;**88**: 580–587.

182. Kirchheim, H.R., Systemic arterial baroreceptor reflexes. *Physiol. Rev.*, 1976;**56**: 100–176.

183. Smyth, H.S., P. Sleight, and G.W. Pickering, Reflex regulation of arterial pressure during sleep in man. A quantitative method of assessing baroreflex sensitivity. *Circ. Res.*, 1969;**24**: 109–121.

184. Taylor, J.A. and D.L. Eckberg, Fundamental relations between short-term RR interval and arterial pressure oscillations in humans. *Circulation*, 1996;**93**: 1527–1532.

185. Baselli, G., S. Cerutti, S. Civardi, and D. Liberati. Spectral and cross-spectral analysis of heart rate and arterial blood pressure variability signals. *Comput. Biomed. Res.*, 1986;**19**: 520–553

186. La Rovere, M.T., A. Mortara, and P.J. Schwartz, Baroreflex sensitivity. *J. Cardiovasc. Electrophysiol.*, 1995;**6**: 761–774.

187. Bettermann, H., D. Amponsah, D. Cysarz, and P. Van Leeuwen, Musical rhythms in heart period dynamics – a cross-cultural and interdisciplinary approach to cardiac rhythms. *Am. J. Physiol.*, 1999;**277**: H1762–H1770.

188. Galletly, D.C. and P.D. Larsen, Cardioventilatory coupling in heart rate variability: methods for qualitative and quantitative determination. *Br. J. Anaesth.*, 2001;**87**: 827–833.

189. Engel, P., G. Hildebrandt and H.G. Scholz, Die Messung der Phasenkopplung zwischen Herzschlag und Atmung beim Menschen mit einem Koinzidenzmessgerät. *Pflugers. Arch.*, 1967;**298**: 259–270.

190. Kenner, T., H. Pessenhofer, and G. Schwaberger, Method for the analysis of the entrainment between heart rate and ventilation rate. *Pflugers. Arch.*, 1976;**363**: 263–265.

191. Hoyer, D., O. Hader, and U. Zwiener, Relative and intermittent cardiorespiratory coordination. *IEEE. Eng. Med. Biol. Mag.*, 1997;**16**: 97–104.

192. Nollo, G., L. Faes, R. Antolini, and A. Porta, Assessing causality in normal and impaired short-term cardiovascular regulation via nonlinear prediction methods. *Philos. Transact. A. Math. Phys. Eng. Sci.*, 2009;**367**: 1423–1440.

193. Schäfer, C., M.G. Rosenblum, J. Kurths, and H.H. Abel, Heart beat synchronized with ventilation. *Nature*, 1998;**392**: 239–240.

194. Seidel, H. and H. Herzel, Analyzing entrainment of heart beat and respiration with surrogates. *IEEE. Eng. Med. Biol. Mag.*, 1998;**17**: 54–57.

195. Cysarz, D., H. Bettermann, S. Lange, D. Geue, P. van Leeuwen. A quantitiative comparison of different methods to detect cardiorespiratory coordination during night-time sleep. *Biomed. Eng. OnLine*, 2004;**3**: 44

196. Cysarz, D., D. von Bonin, P. Brachmann, S. Buetler, F. Edelhäuser, K. LaederachHofmann, and P. Heusser, Day-to-night time differences in the relationship between cardiorespiratory coordination and heart rate variability. *Physiol. Meas.*, 2008;**29**: 1281–1291.

197. Hidaka, I., S-I. Ando, H. Shigematsu, K. Sakai, S. Setoguchi, T. Seto, Y. Hirooka, A. Takeshita, and Y. Yamamoto, Noise-enhanced heart rate and sympathetic nerve responses to oscillatory lower body negative pressure in humans. *J. Neurophysiol.*, 2001;**86**: 559–564.

198. Schmid, G., I. Goychuk, and P. Hänggi, Stochastic resonance as a collective property of ion channel assemblies. *Europhys. Lett.*, 2001;**56**: 22–28.

199. Chang, K.L., K.J. Monahan, P.M. Griffin, D. Lake, and J.R. Moorman, Comparison and clinical application of frequency domain methods in analysis of neonatal heart rate time series. *Ann. Biomed. Eng.*, 2001;**29**: 764–774.

200. Smyth, H.S., P. Sleight, and G.W. Pickering, Reflex regulation of arterial pressure during sleep in man: a quantitative method of assessing baroreflex sensitivity. *Circ. Res.*, 1969;**24**: 109–121.

201. DeBoer, R.W., J.M. Karemaker, and J. Strackee, Hemodynamic fluctuations and baroreflex sensitivity in humans: a beat-to-beat model. *Am. J. Physiol.*, **253** (Heart Circ Physiol) 1987;**22**: 680–689.

202. Laude, D., L-J. Elghozi, A. Girard, E. Bellard, M. Bouhaddi, P. Castiglioni, C. Cerutti, A. Cividjian, M. Di Rienzo, J-O. Fortrat, B. Janssen, J.M. Karemaker, G. Lefthériotis, G. Parati, P.B. Persson, A. Porta, L. Quintin, J. Regnard, H. Rüdiger, and H.M. Strauss, Comparison of various techniques used to estimate spontaneous baroreflex sensitivity (the EuroBaVar study). *Am. J. Physiol. Regulatory. Integrative. Comp. Physiol.*, 2004;**286**: R226–231.

203. Robbe, H.W.J., L.J.M. Mulder, H. Rudel, W.A. Langewitz, J.B.P. Veldman, and G. Mulder, Assessment of baroreceptor reflex sensitivity by means of spectral analysis. *Hypertension*, 1987;**10**: 538–543.

204. Hartikainen, J.E., K.U.O. Tahvanainen, M.J. Mantysaari, P.E. Tikkanen, E.O. Lansimies, and K.E.J. Airaksinen, Simultaneous invasive and noninvasive evaluations of baroreflex sensitivity with bolus phenylephrine technique. *Am. Heart. J.*, 1995;**130**: 296–301.

205. Pinna, G.D., M.T. La Rovere, and R. Maestri, Estimation of arterial blood pressure variability by spectral analysis: comparison

between Finapres and invasive measurements. *Physiol. Meas.*, 1996;**17**: 147–169.

206. Mortara, A., M.T. La Rovere, G.D. Pinna, A. Prpa, R. Maestri, O. Febo, M. Pozzoli, C. Opasich, and L. Tavazzi, Arterial baroreflex modulation of heart rate in chronic heart failure: clinical and hemodynamic correlates and prognostic implications. *Circulation*, 1997;**96**: 3450–3458.

207. Osculati, G., G. Grassi, C. Giannattasio, G. Seravalle, F. Valagussa, A. Zanchetti, and G. Mancia, Early alterations of the baroreceptor control of heart rate in patients with acute myocardial infarction. *Circulation*, 1990;**81**: 939–934.

208. Korner, P.I., M.J. West, J. Shaw, and J.B. Uther, "Steady-state" properties of the baroreceptor-heart rate reflex in essential hypertension in man. *Clin. Exp. Pharmacol. Physiol.*, 1974;**1**: 65–76.

209. Eckberg, D.L., M.S. Cavanaugh, A.L. Mark, and F.M. Abboud, A simplified neck suction device for activation of carotid baroreceptors. *J. Lab. Clin. Med.*, 1975;**85**: 167–173.

210. Ludbrook, J., G. Mancia, A. Ferrari, and A. Zanchetti, The variable-pressure neck-chamber method for studying the carotid baroaflex in man. *Clin. Sci. Mol. Med.*, 1977;**53**: 165–171.

211. Sundlof, G. and B.G. Wallin, Effect of lower body negative pressure on human muscle sympathetic nerve activity. *J. Physiol.*, 1978;**278**: 525–532.

212. Bernardi, L., B. Bianchini, G. Spadacini, S. Leuzzi, F. Valle, E. Marchesi, C. Passino, A. Calciati, M. Viganó, M. Rinaldi, L. Martinelli, G. Finardi, and P. Sleight, Demonstrable cardiac reinnervation after human heart transplantation by carotid baroreflex modulation of RR interval. *Circulation*, 1995;**92**: 2895–2903.

213. Sleight, P., M.T. La Rovere, A. Mortara, G. Pinna, R. Maestri, S. Leuzzi, B. Bianchini, L. Tavazzi, and L. Bernardi, Physiology and pathophysiology of heart rate and blood pressure variability in humans: is power spectral analysis largely an index of baroreflex gain? *Clin. Sci.* (Colch), 1995;**88**: 103–109.

214. Kautzner, J., Noninvasive provocations of baroreflex sensitivity, in *Dynamic Electrocardiography*, M. Malik and A.J. Camm, Editors. London: Blackwell Futura Publishing, 2004, pp. 162–169.

215. Raczak, G., M.T. la Rovere, G.D. Pinna, R. Maestri, and G. Swiatecka, Assessment of baroreflex sensitivity in patients with preserved and impaired left ventricular function by means of the Valsalva manoeuvre and the phenylephrine test. *Clin. Sci.* (Lond)., 2001;**100**: 33–41.

216. Takaashi, N., M. Nakagawa, and T. Saikawa, Noninvasive assessment of the cardiac baroreflex response to downward tilting and comparison with the phenylephrine method. *J. Am. Coll. Cardiol.*, 1999;**34**: 211–215.

217. Di Rienzo, M., G. Bertinieri, G. Mancia, and A. Pedotti, A new method for evaluating the baroreflex role by a joint pattern analysis of pulse interval and systolic blood pressure series. *Med. Biol. Eng. Comput.*, 1985;**23**: 313–314.

218. Davies, L.C., H. Colhoun, A.J. Coats, M. Piepoli, and D.P. Francis, A noninvasive measure of baroreflex sensitivity without blood pressure measurements. *Am. Heart. J.*, 2002;**143**: 441–447.

219. James, M.A., R.B. Panerai, and J.E. Potter, Applicability of new techniques in the assessment of arterial baroreflex sensitivity in the elderly: a comparison with established pharmacological methods. *Clin. Sci.*, 1998;**94**: 245–253.

220. Maestri, R., G.D. Pinna, A. Mortara, M.T. La Rovere, and L. Tavazzi, Assessing baroreflex sensitivity in post-myocardial

infarction patients: comparison of spectral and phenylephrine techniques. *J. Am. Coll. Cardiol.*, 1998;**31**: 344–351.

221. Pitzalis, M.V., F. Mastropasqua, A. Passantino, F. Massari, L. Ligurgo, C. Forleo, C. Balducci, F. Lombardi, and P. Rizzon, Comparison between noninvasive indices of baroreceptor sensitivity and the phenylephrine method in post-myocardial infarction patients. *Circulation*, 1998;**97**: 1362–1367.

222. Schmidt, G., M. Malik, P. Barthel, R. Schneider, K. Ulm, L. Rolnitzky, A.J. Camm, J.T. Jr Bigger, and A. Schomig, Heart-rate turbulence after ventricular premature beats as a predictor of mortality after acute myocardial infarction. *Lancet*, 1999;**353**: 1390–1396.

223. Mrowka, R., P.B. Persson, H. Theres, et al., Blunted arterial baroreflex causes "pathological" heart rate turbulence. *Am. J. Physiol. Regul. Integr. Comp. Physiol.*, 2000;**279**: R1171–1175.

224. Lin, L.Y., L.P. Lai, J.L. Lin, C.C. Du, W.Y. Shay, H.L. Chan, Y.Z. Tsend, S.K.S. Huang, Tight mechanism correlation between heart rate turbulence and baroreflex sensitivity: sequential autonomic blockade analysis. *J. Cardiovasc. Electrophysiol.*, 2002;**13**: 427–431.

225. Davies, L.C., D.P. Francis, P. Ponikowski, M.F. Piepoli, and A.J. Coats, Relation of heart rate and blood pressure turbulence following premature ventricular complexes to baroreflex sensitivity in chronic congestive heart failure. *Am. J. Cardiol.*, 2001;**87**: 737–742.

226. Ghuran, A., F. Reid, M.T. La Rovere, et al., Heart rate turbulence-based predictors of fatal and nonfatal cardiac arrest (the Autonomic Tone and Reflexes After Myocardial Infarction substudy). *Am. J. Cardiol.*, 2002;**89**: 184–190.

227. Cygankiewicz, I., W. Zareba, R. Vazquez, M. Vallverdu, J.R. Gonzalez-Juantey, M. Valdes, J. Almendral, J. Cinca, P. Caminal, A. Bayes de Luna and MUSIC Investigators, Heart rate turbulence predicts all-cause mortality and sudden death in congestive heart failure patients. *Heart. Rhythm.*, 2008;**5**: 1095–1102.

228. Schneider, R., P. Barther, and M. Watanabe, Heart rate turbulence on Holter, in *Dynamic Electrocardiography*, M. Malik and A.J. Camm, Editors. London: Blackwell Futura Publishing, 2004, pp. 190–193.

229. Watanabe, M.A., J.E. Marine, R. Sheldon, et al., Effects of ventricular premature stimulus coupling interval on blood pressure and heart rate turbulence. *Circulation*, 2002;**106**: 325–330.

230. Voss, A., V. Baier, J. Hopfe, et al., Heart rate and blood pressure turbulence– marker of the baroreflex sensitivity or consequence of postextrasystolic potentiation and pulsus alternans? *Am. J. Cardiol.*, 2002;**89**: 110–111.

231. Goldberger, J. and A.H. Kadish, Influence of sympathetic and parasympathetic maneuvers on heart rate variability, in: *Noninvasive Electrocardiology. Clinical Apects of Holter Monitoring*, A.J. Moss and S. Stern, Editors. London: WB Saunders, 1996, pp. 207–223.

232. Merri, M., D.C. Farden, J.G. Mottley, and E.L. Titlebaum, Sampling frequency of the electrocardiogram for spectral analysis of the heart rate variability. *IEEE. Trans. Biomed. Eng.*, 1990;**37**: 99–106.

233. Hilton, M.F., J.M. Beattie, M.J. Chappell, and R.A. Bates, Heart rate variability: measurement error or chaos. *Comp. Cardiol.*, 1997: 125–128.

234. Bianchi, A.M., L.T. Mainardi, E. Petrucci, M.G. Signorini, M. Mainardi, and S. Cerutti, Time-variant power spectrum analysis for the detection of transient episodes in HRV signal. *IEEE. Trans. Biomed. Eng.*, 1993;**40**: 136–144.

235. Voss, A., N. Wessel, A. Sander, H. Malberg, and R. Dietz, Requirements on sampling rate in Holter systems for analysis of heart rate variability. *Clin. Sci. (Lond).*, 1996;**91** (Suppl): 120–121.

236. Hejjel, L. and E. Roth, What is the adequate sampling interval of the ECG signal for heart rate variability analysis in the time domain? *Physiol. Meas.*, 2004;**25**: 1405–1411.

237. Tapanainen, J.M., T. Seppänen, R. Laukkanen, A. Loimaala, and H.V. Huikuri, Significance of the accuracy of RR interval detection for the analysis of new dynamic measures of heart rate variability. *Ann. Noninvas. Electrocardiol.*, 1999;**4**: 10–18.

238. Merri, M., D.C. Farden, J.G. Mottley, and E.L. Titlebaum, Sampling frequency of the electrocardiogram for spectral analysis of the heart rate variability. *IEEE. Trans. Biomed. Eng.*, 1990;**37**: 99–106.

239. Xia, R., O. Odemuyiwa, J. Gill, M. Malik, and A.J. Camm, Influence of recognition errors of computerised analysis of 24-hour electrocardiograms on the measurement of spectral components of heart rate variability. *Int. J. Biomed. Comput.*, 1993;**32**: 223–235.

240. Sapoznikov, D., M.H. Luria, Y. Mahler, and M.S. Gotsman, Computer processing of artifact and arrhythmias in heart rate variability analysis. *Comput. Methods. Progr. Biomed.*, 1992;**39**: 75–84.

241. Salo, M.A., H.V. Huikuri, and T. Seppänen, Ectopic beats in heart rate variability analysis: effects of editing on time and frequency domain measures. *Ann. Noninvasive. Electrocardiol.*, 2001;**6**: 5–17.

242. Berntson, G.G. and J.R. Stowell, ECG artifacts and heart period variability: don't miss a beat! *Psychophysiology*, 1998;**35**: 127–132.

243. Clifford, G.D., ECG statistics, noise, artifacts, and missing data, in *Advanced Methods for ECG Analysis*, G.D. Clifford, F. Azuaje, and P.E. McSharry, Editors. London: Artech House, 2006.

244. Janssen, M.J., C.A. Swenne, J. de Bie, O. Rompelman, and J.H. van Bemmel, Methods in heart rate variability analysis: which tachogram should we choose? *Comput. Meth. Prog. Biomed.*, 1993;**41**: 1–8.

245. Sacha, J. and W. Pluta, Different methods of heart rate variability analysis reveal different correlation of heart rate variability spectrum with average heart rate. *J. Electrocardiol.*, 2005;**38**: 47–53.

246. Borell von, E., J. Langbein, G. Després, S. Hansen, C. Leterrier, J. Marchant-Forde, R. Marchant-Forde, M. Minero, E. Mohr, A. Prunier, D. Valance, and I. Veissier, Heart rate variability as a measure of autonomic regulation of cardiac activity for assessing stress and welfare in farm animals — A review. *Physiol. Behav.*, 2007;**92**: 293–316.

247. Crawford, M.H., S.J. Bernstein, P.C. Deedwania, J.P. DiMarco, K.J. Ferrick, A. Jr. Garson, L.A. Green, H.L. Greene, M.J. Silka, P.H. Stone, C.M. Tracy, R.J. Gibbons, J.S. Alpert, K.A. Eagle, T.J. Gardner, G. Gregoratos, R.O. Russell, T.H. Ryan, S.C. Jr. Smith, ACC/AHA Guidelines for Ambulatory Electrocardiography. A report of the American College of Cardiology/American Heart Association Task Force on Practice Guidelines (Committee to Revise the Guidelines for Ambulatory Electrocardiography). Developed in collaboration with the North American Society for Pacing and Electrophysiology. *J. Am. Coll. Cardiol.*, 1999;**34**: 912–948.

248. Liao, D., R.W. Barnes, L.E. Chambless, R.J. Jr. Simpson, P. Sorlie, and G. Heiss, Age, race, and sex differences in autonomic cardiac function measured by spectral analysis of heart rate variability– the ARIC study. Atherosclerosis Risk in Communities. *Am. J. Cardiol.*, 1995;**76**: 906–912.

249. Carnethon, M.R., D. Liao, G.W. Evans, W.E. Cascio, L.E. Chambless, W.D. Rosamond, and G. Heiss, Does the cardiac autonomic response to postural change predict incident coronary heart disease and mortality? The Atherosclerosis Risk in Communities Study. *Am. J. Epidemiol.*, 2002;**155**: 48–56.

250. Rashba, E.J., N.A. Estes, P. Wang, A. Schaechter, A. Howard, W. Zareba, J.P. Couderc, J. Perkiomaki, J. Levine, and A. Kadish, for the Defibrillators in Non-Ischemic Cardiomyopathy Treatment Evaluation (DEFINITE) Investigators. Preserved heart rate variability identifies low-risk patients with nonischemic dilated cardiomyopathy: Results from the DEFINITE trial. *Heart. Rhythm.*, 2006;**3**: 281–286.

251. Tsuji, H., M.G. Larson, F.J. Jr. Venditti, E.S. Manders, J.C. Evans, C.L. Feldman, and D. Levy, Impact of reduced heart rate variability on risk for cardiac events: the Framingham heart study. *Circulation*, 1996;**94**: 2850–2855.

252. Bigger, J.T. Jr., J.L. Fleiss, R.C. Steinman, L.M. Rolnitzky, R.E. Kleiger, and J.N. Rottman. Correlations among time and frequency domain measures of heart period variability two weeks after myocardial infarction. *Am. J. Cardiol.*, 1992;**69**: 891–898.

253. Binder, T., B. Frey, G. Porenta, G. Heinz, M. Wutte, G. Kreiner, H. Gossinger, H. Schmidinger, R. Pacher, and H. Weber, Prognostic value of heart rate variability in patients awaiting heart transplantation. *PACE*, 1992;**15** (P.II): 2215–2220.

254. Frey, B., G. Heinz, T. Binder, M. Wutte, B. Schneider, H. Schmidinger, H. Weber, and R. Pacher, Diurnal variation of ventricular response to atrial fibrillation in patients with advanced heart failure. *Am. Heart. J.*, 1995;**129**: 58–65.

255. Schroeder, E.B., E.A. Whitsel, G.W. Evans, R.J. Prineas, L.E. Chambless, and G. Heiss, Repeatability of heart rate variability measures. *J. Electrocardiol.*, 2004;**37**: 163–172.

256. Sandercock, G., P. Bromley, and D. Brodie, The reliability of short-term measurements of heart rate variability. *Int. J. Cardiol.*, 2005;**103**: 238–247.

257. Radespiel-Tröger, M., R. Rauh, C. Mahlke, T. Gottschald, and M. Mück-Weymann, Agreement of two different methods for measurement of heart rate variability. *Clin. Auton. Res.*, 2003;**13**: 99–102.

258. Dekker, J.M., R.M. Crow, A.R. Folsom, P.J. Hannan, D. Liao, C.A. Sweene, and E.G. Schouten, Low heart rate variability in a 2-minute rhythm strip predicts risk of coronary heart disease and mortality from several causes. The ARIC study. *Circulation*, 2000;**102**: 1239–1244.

259. Van Schelven, L.J., P.L. Oey, I.H.I. Klein, M.G.W. Barnas, P. Blankstein, and G.H. Wieneke, Observer variations in short spectral analysis of heart period variability. *J. Auton. Nerv. Syst.*, 2000;**79**: 144–148.

260. Tarkiainen, T.H., K.L. Timonen, P. Tittanen, J.E.K. Hartikainen, J. Pekkanen, G. Hoek, A. Ibald-Mulli, and E.J. Vanninen, Stability over time of short-term heart rate variability. *Clin. Auton. Res.*, 2005;**15**: 394–399.

261. Kroll, D.J., L.A. Freed, K.M. Stein, J.S. Borer, and P. Kligfield, Rhythm annotation and interobserver reproducibility of measures of heart rate variability. *Am. J. Cardiol.*, 1996;**78**: 1055–1057.

262. Pardo, Y., C.N. Bairey Merz, P. Paul-Labrador, I. Velasquez, J.S. Gottdiener, W.J. Kop, D. Krantz, A. Rozanski, J. Klein, and T. Peter, Heart rate variability reproducibility and stability using commercially available equipment in coronary artery disease with daily life myocardial ischemia. *Am. J. Cardiol.*, 1996;**78**: 866–870.

263. Batten, L.A., E.M. Urbina, and G.S. Berenson, Interobserver reproducibility of heart rate variability in children (The Bogalusa Heart Study). *Am. J. Cardiol.*, 2000;**6**: 1264–1266.

264. Jung, J., A. Heisel, D. Tscholl, R. Fries, H. Schiefer, and C. Ozbek, Assessment of heart rate variability by using different commercially available systems. *Am. J. Cardiol.* 1996;**78**: 118–120.

265. Murray, P.G., R.M. Hamilton, P.W. Macfarlane, Reproducibility of a non-invasive real-time measure of cardiac parasympathetic acitivity. *Physiol. Meas.*, 2001;**22**: 661–667.

266. Højgaard, M.V., N-H.Holstein-Athlou, E. Agner, and J.K. Kanters, Reproducibility of heart rate variability and baroreceptor sensitivity during rest and head-up tilt. *Blood Pres. Monit.*, 2005;**10**: 19–24.

267. Winsley, R.J., N. Armstrong, K. Bywater, and S.G. Fawkner, Reliability of heart rate variability measures at rest and during light exercise in children. *Br. J. Sports. Med.*, 2003;**37**: 550–552.

268. Maestri, R., G.D. Pinna, A. Porta, R. Balocchi, R. Sassi, M.G. Signorini, M. Dudziak, and G. Raczak, Assesing nonlinear properties of heart rate variability from short-term recordings: are these measurements reliable? *Physiol. Meas.*, 2007;**28**: 1067–1077.

269. Sinnreich, R., J.D. Kark, Y. Friedelanger, D. Sapoznikov, and D. Luria, Five minute recordings of heart rate variability for population studies: repeatability and age-sex characteristics. *Heart*, 1998;**80**: 156–162.

270. Salo, T.M., L-M. Voipio, J.O. Jalonen, H. Helenius, J.S.A. Viikari, and I. Kantola, Reproducibility of abnormal heart rate variability indices: the case of hypertensive sleep apnoea syndrome. *Clin. Physiol.*, 1999;**19**: 258–268.

271. Lord, S.W., R.R. Senior, M. Das, A.M. Whittam, A. Murray, and J.M. McComb, Low-frequency heart rate variability: reproducibility in cardiac transplant recipients and normal subjects. *Clin. Sci.*, 2001;**100**: 43–46.

272. Haas, J., A. Liebich, E. Himmrich, and N. Treese, Kurzzeitmessung der Herzfrequenzvariabilitat bei Postinfarktpatienten – Methodik, Reproduzierbarkeit and Stellenwert im Rahmen den Postinfarktdiagnostik. *Hertzschr. Elektrophys.*, 2000;**111**: 102–109.

273. Ponikowski, P., M. Piepoli, A.A. Amadi, T.P. Chua, D. Harrington, M. Volterrani, R. Colombo, G. Mazzuero, A. Giordano, and A.J. Coats, Reproducibility of heart rate variability measures in patients with chronic heart failure. *Clin. Sci. (Lond.)*, 1996;**91**: 391–398.

274. Freed, L.A., K. Stein, M. Gordon, M. Urban, and P. Kiligfield, Reproducibility of power spectral measures obtained from short-term sampling periods. *Am. J. Cardiol.*, 1994;**74**: 972–973.

275. Chemla, D., D. Young, F. Badilini, P. Maison-Blanche, H. Affres, Y. Lecarpetier, and P. Chanson, Comparison of fast Fourier transform and autoregressive spectral analysis for the study of heart rate variability in diabetic patients. *Int. J. Cardiol.*, 2005;**104**: 307–313.

276. Nolan, J., A.D. Flapan, N.E. Goodfield, R.J. Prescott, P. Bloomfield, and J.M. Neilson, Measurement of parasympathetic activity from 24-hour ambulatory electrocardiograms and its reproducibility and sensitivity in normal subjects, patient with symptomatic myocardial ischemia, and patients with diabetes mellitus. *Am. J. Cardiol.*, 1996;**77**: 154–158.

277. Van Hoogenhuyze, D., N. Weinstein, G.J. Martin, J.S. Weiss, J.W. Schaad, X.N. Sahyoni, D. Fintel, W.J. Remme, and D.J. Singer, Reproducibility and relation to mean heart rate of heart rate variability in normal subjects and in patients with congestive heart failure secondary to coronary heart disease. *Am. J. Cardiol.*, 1991;**68**: 1668–1676.

278. Bigger, J.T. Jr., J.L. Fleiss, L.M. Rolnitzky, and R.C. Steinman, Stability over time of heart period variability in patients with previous myocardial infarction and ventricular arrhythmias. The CAPS and ESVEM investigators. *Am. J. Cardiol.*, 1992;**69**: 718–723.

279. Kautzner, J., K. Hnatkova, A. Staunton, A.J. Camm, and M. Malik, Day-to-day reproducibility of time-domain measures of heart rate variability in survivors of acute myocardial infarction. *Am. J. Cardiol.*, 1995;**76**: 309–312.

280. Stein, P.K., M.W. Rich, J.N. Rottman, and R.E. Kleiger, Stability of index of heart rate variability in patients with congestive heart failure. *Am. Heart. J.*, 1995;**129**: 975–981.

281. Hohnloser, S.H., T. Klingenheben, M. Zabel, F. Schroder, and H. Just, Intraindividual reproducibility of heart rate variability. *Pacing. Clin. Electrophysiol.*, 1992;**15**: 2211–2214.

282. Anastasiou-Nana, M.I., L.A. Karagounis, J. Kanakakis, N.E. Kouvelas, A. Geramoutsos, K. Chalkis, J. Karelas, and N. Nanas, Correlation and stability of heart rate and ventricular ectopy variability in patients with heart failure. *Am. J. Cardiol.*, 2001;**88**: 175–179.

283. Weber, F., H. Schneider, T. von Arnim, and W. Urbaszek, for the TIBBS investigators group. Heart rate variability and ischemia in patients with coronary artery disease and stable angina pectoris; influence of drug therapy and prognostic value. *Eur. Heart. J.*, 1998;**19**: 38–50.

284. Huikuri, H.V., K.M. Kessler, E. Terracall, A. Castellanos, M.K. Linnaluoto, and R.J. Myerburg, Reproducibility and circadian rhythm of heart rate variability in healthy subjects. *Am. J. Cardiol.*, 1990;**65**: 391–393.

285. Hayano, J., W. Jiang, R. Waugh, C. O'Connor, D. Frid, and J.A. Blumenthal, Stability over time of circadian rhythm of variability of heart rate in patients with coronary artery disease. *Am. Heart. J.*, 1997;**134**: 411–418.

286. Dawson, S.L., T.G. Robinson, J.H. Youde, M.A. James, A. Martin, P. Weston, R. Panerai, and J.F. Potter, The reproducibility of cardiac baroreceptor activity assessed noninvasively by spectral techniques. *Clin. Auton. Res.*, 1997;**7**: 279–284.

287. Davies, L.C., D. Francis, P. Jurak, T. Kara, M. Piepoli, and A.J. Coats, Reproducibility of methods assessing baroreflex sensitivity in normal controls and in patients with chronic heart failure. *Clin. Sci. (Lond.)*, 1999;**97**: 515–522.

288. Iellamo, F., J.M. Legramante, G. Raimondi, F. Gastrucci, M. Massaro, G. Perizzi, Evaluation of spontaneous baroreflex sensitivity at rest and during laboratory tests. *J. Hypertens.*, 1996;**14**: 1099–1104.

289. Laude, D., J-L. Elghozi, A. Girard, E. Bellard, M. Bouhaddi, P. Castiglioni, C. Cerutti, A. Cividjian, M. Di Rienzo, J-O. Fortrat, B. Janssen, J.M. Karemaker, G. Georges Lefthériotis, G. Gianfranco Parati, B. Pontus, P.B. Persson, A. Porta, L. Quintin, J. Regnard, H. Rüdiger, H.M. Stauss, Comparison of various techniques used to estimate spontaneous baroreflex sensitivity (the EuroBaVar study). *Am. J. Physiol. Regul. Integr. Comp. Physiol.*, 2004;**286**: R226–231.

290. Gao, S.A., M. Johansson, A. Hammaren, M. Nordberg, and P. Friberg, Reproducibility of methods assessing beroreflex sensitivity and temporal QT variability in end-stage renal disease and healthy subjects. *Clin. Auton. Res.*, 2005;**15**: 21–28.

291. Wichterle, D., V. Melenovsky, L. Necasova, J. Kautzner, and M. Malik, Stability of the noninvasive baroreflex sensitivity

assessment using cross-spectral analysis of heart rate and arterial blood pressure variabilities. *Clin. Cardiol.*, 2000;**23**: 201–204.

292. Herpin, D. and S. Ragot, Mid- and long-term reproducibility of noninvasive measurements of spontaneous arterial baroreflex sensitivity in healthy volunteers. *Am. J. Hypertens.*, 1997;**10**: 790–797.

293. Lord, S.D., R.H. Clayton, M.C.S. Hall, J.C. Gray, A. Murray, J.M. McComb, and R.A. Kenny, Reproducibility of three different methods of measuring baroreflex sensitivity in normal subjects. *Clin. Sci.*, 1998;**95**: 575–581.

294. Bauer, A., M. Malik, G. Schmidt, P. Barthel, H. Bonnemeier, I. Cygankiewicz, P. Guzik, F. Lombardi, A. Muller, A. Oto, R. Schneide, M. Watanabe, D. Wichterle, and W. Zareba, Heart rate turbulence: standards of measurements, physiological interpretation, and clinical use: International Society for Holter and Noninvasive Electrophysiology Consensus. *J. Am. Coll. Cardiol.*, 2008;**52**: 1353–1365.

295. Sandercock, G.R.H., P. Bromley, and D.A. Brodie, Reliability of three commercially available heart rate variability instruments using short-term (5-min) recordings. *Clin. Physiol. Funct. Imaging.*, 2004;**24**: 359–367.

296. Pitzalis, M.V., F. Mastropasqua, F. Massari, C. Folco, M. Di Maggio, A. Passantino, R. Colombo, M. Di Biase, and P. Rizzon Short- and long-term reproducibility of time and frequency domain heart rate variability measurements in normal subjects. *Cardiovasc. Res.*, 1996;**32**: 226–233.

297. Lobnig, B.M., E. Maslowska-Wessel, and R. Bender, Repeatability of heart rate variability measured via spectral analysis in healthy subjects. *J. Clin. Basic. Cardiol.*, 2003;**6**: 29–33.

298. Dietrich, A., J.G.M. Rosmalen, A.M. van Roon, L.J.M. Mulder, A.J. Oldehinkel, and H. Riese, Short-term reproducibility of autonomic nervous system function measures in 10-to-13-year-old children, in PhD Thesis, Dietrich A. University Medical Center, Groningen, 2007.

299. Parati, G., S. Omboni, A. Villani, F. Glavina, P. Castiglioni, M. Di Rienzo, and G. Mancia. Reproducibility of beat-by-beat blood pressure and heart rate variability. *Blood Press. Monit.*, 2001;**6**: 217–220.

300. Carrasco, S., R. González, M.J. Gaitán, and O. Yáñez, Reproducibility of heart rate variability from short-term recordings during five manoeuvres in normal subjects. *J. Med. Eng. Technol.*, 2003;**27**: 241–248.

301. Jáuregui-Renaud, K., A.G. Hermosillo, M.F. Márquez, F. Ramos-Aguilar, M. Hernández-Goribar, and M. Cárdenas, Repeatability of heart rate variability during simple cardiovascular reflex tests on healthy subjects. *Arch. Med. Res.*, 2001;**32**: 21–26.

302. Guijt, A.M., J.K. Sluiter, M.H.W. Frings-Dresen, Test-retest reliability of heart rate variability and respiration rate at rest and during light physical activity in normal subjects. *Arch. Med. Res.*, 2007;**38**: 113–120.

303. Cloarec-Blanchard, L., C. F. Unck-Brentano, M. Lipski, P. Jaillon, and I. Macquin-Mavier, Repeatability of spectral components of short-term blood pressure and heart rate variability during acute sympathetic activation in healthy young male subjects. *Clin. Sci. (Lond).*, 1997;**93**: 21–28.

304. Piepoli, M., A. Radaelli, P. Ponikowski, S. Adamopoulos, L. Bernardi, P. Sleight, and A.J. Coats, Reproducibility of heart rate variability indices during exercise stress testing and inotrope infusion in chronic heart failure patients. *Clin. Sci. (Lond).*, 1996;**91** (Suppl): 87–88.

305. Randall, D., D. Brown, R. Raisch, J. Yinling, and W. Randall, SA nodal parasympathectomy dealineates autonomic control of heart rate power spectrum. *Am. J. Physiol. Heart. Circ. Physiol.*, 1991;**29**: H985–988.

306. Jose, A.D. and D. Collison, The normal range and determinants of the intrinsic heart rate in man. *Cardiovasc. Res.*, 1970;**4**: 160–167.

307. Ahmed, M., A. Kadish, M. Paker, and J. Goldberger, Effect of physiologic and pharmacologic adrenergic stimulation on heart rate variability. *J. Am. Coll. Cardiol.*, 1994;**24**: 1082–1090.

308. Moser, M., M. Lehofer, A. Seminek, M. Lux, H-G. Zapotoczky, T. Kenner, and A. Noordergraaf, Heart rate variability as a prognostic tool in cardiology: a contribution to the problem from a theoretical point of view. *Circulation* 1994;**90**: 1078–1082.

309. Huikuri, H.V., T. Makikallio, K.E.J. Airaksinen, R. Mitrani, A. Castellanos, and R.J. Myerburg, Measurement of heart rate variability: a clinical tool or a research toy? *J. Am. Coll. Cardiol.*, 1999;**34**: 1878–1883.

310. Seely, A.L.E. and P.T. Macklem, Complex system and the technology of variability analysis. *Crit. Care.*, 2004;**8**: R367–384.

311. Stein, K.M., J.S. Borer, C. Hochreiter, P.M. Okin, E.M. Herrold, R.B. Cevereux, and P. Klgfield, Prognostic value and physiological correlates of heart rate variability in chronic severe mitral regurgitation. *Circulation*, 1993;**88**: 127–135.

312. Cygankiewicz, I., J.K. Wranicz, H. Bolinska, J. Zaslonka, and W. Zareba, Relationship between heart rate turbulence and heart rate, heart rate variability and number of premature beats in coronary patients. *J. Cardiovasc. Electrophysiol.*, 2004;**15**: 731–778.

313. Pichon, A., M. Roulaud, S. Antione-Jonville, C. de Bischop, and A. Denjean, Spectral analysis of heart rate variability: interchangeability between autoregressive analysis and fast Fourier transform. *J. Electrocardiol.*, 2006;**39**: 31–37.

314. Valkama, J.O., H.V. Huikuri, K.E.J. Airaksinen, M.L. Linnaluoto, and J.T. Takkunen, Determinants of frequency domain measures of heart rate variability in the acute and convalescent phases of myocardial infarction. *Cardiovasc. Res.*, 1994;**28**: 1273–1276.

315. Kuch, B., T. Parvanov, H.W. Hense, J. Axmann, and H.D. Bolte, Short-period heart rate variability in the general population as compared to patients with acute myocardial infarction from the same source population. *Ann. Noninvas. Electrocardiol.*, 2004;**9**: 113–120.

316. Grimm, W., J. Liedtke, and H-H. Muller, Prevalence of potential noninvasive arrhythmia risk predictors in healthy, middle-aged persons. *Ann. Nonivas. Electrocardiol.*, 2003;**8**: 37–46.

317. Bigger, J.R. Jr., J.L. Fleiss, R.C. Steinman, L.M. Rolnitzky, W.J. Schneider, and P.K. Stein, RR variability in healthy, middle-aged persons compared with patients with chronic coronary heart disease or recent acute myocardial infarction. *Circulation*, 1995;**91**: 1936–1943.

318. Mølgaard, H., K.E. Sørensen, and P. Bjerregaard, Circadian variation and influence of risk factors on heart rate variability in healthy subjects. *Am. J. Cardiol.*, 1991;**68**: 777–784.

319. Ramaekers, D., H. Ector, A.E. Aubert, A. Rubens, and F. van de Werf, Heart rate variability and heart rate in healthy volunteers. Is the female autonomic nervous system cardioprotective? *Eur. Heart. J.*, 1998;**19**: 1334–1341.

320. Pikkujämsä, S.M., T.H. Mäkikallio, L. Sourander, I.J. Räihä, P. Puuka, J. Skyttä, C-K. Peng, A.L. Goldberger, and H.V. Huikuri, Cardiac interbeat interval dynamics from childhood to senescence. Comparison of conventional and new measures based on fractals and chaos theory. *Circulation*, 1999;**100**: 393–399.

321. Bonnemeier, H., U.K.H. Wiegand, A. Brandes, N. Kluge, H.A. Katus, G. Richardt, and J. Potratz, Circadian profile of cardiac autonomic nervous modulation in healthy subjects: differing effect of aging and gender on heart rate variability. *J. Cardiovasc. Electrophysiol.*, 2003;**14**: 791–799.

322. Umetani, K., D.H. Singer, R. McCraty, and M. Atkinson, Twenty-four hour time domain heart rate variability and heart rate: relations to age and gender over nine decades. *J. Am. Coll. Cardiol.*, 1998;**31**: 593–601.

323. Huikuri, H.V., S.M. Pikkujämsä, K.E.J. Airaksinen, M.J. Ikäheimo, A.O. Rantala, H. Kauma, M. Lilja, and Y.A. Kesäniemi, Sex-related differences in autonomic modulation of heart rate in middle-aged subjects. *Circulation*, 1996;**94**: 122–125.

324. Kuo, T.B., T. Lin, C.C.H. Yang, C-L. Li, C-F. Chen, and P. Chou, Effect of aging on gender differences in neural control of heart rate. *Am. J. Physiol. Heart. Circ. Physiol.*, 1999;**277**: H2233–2239.

325. Šlachta, R., P. Stejskal, M. Elfmark, J. Salinger, M. Kalina, and I. Rehova,. Age and spectral analysis of heart rate variability. *J. Auton. Nerv. Syst.*, 2002;**32**: 191–198.

326. Laitinen, T., L. Niskanen, G. Geelen, E. Lansimies, and J. Hartikainen, Age dependency of cardiovascular autonomic responses to head-up tilt in healthy subjects. *J. Appl. Physiol.*, 2004;**96**: 2333–2340.

327. Acharya, R.U., N. Kannanthal, O.W. Sing, L.Y. Ping, and T. Chua, Heart rate analysis in normal subjects of various age groups. *BioMed. Engineering. Online.*, 2004;**3**: 24.

328. Kuo, T.B.J. and C.C.H. Yang, Sexual dimorphism in the complexity of cardiac pacemaker activity. *Am. J. Physiol. Heart. Circ. Physiol.*, 2002;**283**: H1695–1702.

329. Mehta, S.K., D.M. Super, D. Connuck, A. Salvator, L. Singer, L.G. Fradley, R.A. Harcar-Sevcik, L. Kirchner, and E.S. Kaufman, Heart rate variability in healthy neonates. *Am. J. Cardiol.*, 2000;**89**: 50–53.

330. Longin, E., T. Schaible, T. Lenz, and S. König, Short term heart rate variability in healthy neonates: normative data and physiological observations. *Early. Hum. Develop.*, 2005;**81**: 663–671.

331. Massin, M. and G. von Bernuth, Normal ranges of heart rate variability during infancy and childhood. *Pediatr. Cardiol.*, 1997;**18**: 297–302.

332. Silvetti, M.S., F. Drago, and P. Ragonese, Heart rate variability in healthy children and adolescents is partially related to age and gender. *Int. J. Cardiol.*, 2001;**81**: 169–174.

333. Lenard, Z., P. Studinger, B. Merich, L. Kocsis, and M. Kollai, Maturation of cardiovagal autonomic function from childhood to young adult age. *Circulation*, 2004;**110**: 2307–2312.

334. Faulkner, M.S., D. Hathaway, and B. Tolley, Cardiovascular autonomic function in healthy adolescents. *Heart. Lung.*, 2003: **32**: 10–22.

335. Agelink, M.W., R. Malessa, B. Bauman, T. Majewski, F. Akila, T. Zeit, and D. Ziegler, Standardized tests of heart arte variability: normal ranges obtained from 309 healthy humans, and effects of ag, gender, and heart rate. *Clin. Auton. Res.*, 2001;**11**: 99–108.

336. Braune H- and U. Geisendörfer, Measurements of heart rate variations: influencing factors, normal values and diagnostic impact on diabetic autonomic neuropathy. *Diab. Res. Clin. Pract.*, 1995;**29**: 179–187.

337. Bergfeldt, L., M. Rosenquist, H. Vallin, R. Nordlander, and H. Astrom Screening for sinus node dysfunction by analysis of short-term sinus cycle variations on the surface electrocardiogram. *Am. Heart. J.*, 1995;**130**: 141–147.

338. Malik, M., K. Hnatkova, and A.J. Camm, Practicality of postinfarction risk assessment based on time-domain measurement of heart rate variability, in *Heart Rate Variability*, M. Malik and A.J. Camm, Editors. Armonk, NY: Futura Publishing, 1995, pp. 393–405.

339. Ewing, D.J., C.N. Martyn, R.J. Young, and B.F. Clarke, The value of cardiovascular autonomic function tests: 10 years experience in diabetes. *Diab. Care.*, 1985;**8**: 491–498.

340. O'Brien, I.A., J.P. O'Hare, and R.J.M. Corrall, Heart rate variability in healthy subjects: effects of age and the derivation of normal ranges for test of autonomic function. *Br. Heart. J.*, 1986;**55**: 348–354.

341. Howorka, K., J. Pumprla, A. Schabmann, Optimal parameters of short-term heart rate spectrogram for routine evaluation of diabetic cardiovascular autonomic neuropathy. *J. Auton. Nerv. Syst.*, 1998;**69**: 164–172.

342. Miličević, G., N. Lakušić, J. Szirovicza, D. Cerovec, M. Majsec, Different cut-off points of decreased heart rate variability for different groups of cardiac patients. *J. Cardiovasc. Risk.*, 2001;**8**: 93–102.

343. La Rovere, M.T., J.T. Jr. Bigger, F.I. Marcus, A. Mortara, and P.J. Schwartz for the ATRAMI (Autonomic Tone and Reflexes After Myocardial Infarction) Investigators, Baroreflex sensitivity and heart-rate variability in prediction of total cardiac mortality after myocardial infarction. *Lancet*, 1998;**351**: 478–484.

344. Rich, M.W., J.S. Saini, K.E. Kleiger, R.M. Carney, A. teVelde, and K.E. Freedland, Correlation of heart rate variability with clinical and angiographic variables and late mortality afer coronary angiography. *Am. J. Cardiol.*, 1988;**62**: 714–717.

345. Odemuyiwa, O., J. Poloniecki, M. Malik, T. Farrell, R. Xia, A. Staunton, P. Kulakowski, D. Ward, and J. Camm, Temporal influences on the prediction of postinfarction mortality by heart rate variability: a comparison with the left ventricular ejection fraction. *Br. Heart. J.*, 1994;**71**: 521–527.

346. Zuanetti, G., J.M. Neilson, R. Latini, E. Santoro, A.P. Maggioni, and D.J. Ewing, Prognostic significance of heart rate variability in post-myocardial infarction patients in the fibrinolytic era: The GISSI-2 results. *Circulation*, 1996;**94**: 432–436.

347. Copie, X., K. Hnatkova, A. Staunton, L. Fei, A.J. Camm, and M. Malik, Predictive power of increased heart rate versus depressed left ventricular ejection fraction and heart rate variability for risk stratification after myocardial infarction. Results of a two-year follow-up study. *J. Am. Coll. Cardiol.*, 1996;**27**: 270–276.

348. Lanza, G.A., V. Guido, M. Galeazzi, M. Mustilli, R. Natali, C. Ierardi, C. Milici, F. Burzotta, V. Pasceri, F. Tomassini, A. Lupi, and A. Maseri, Prognostic role of heart rate variability in patients with a recent acute myocardial infarction. *Am. J. Cardiol.* 1998;**82**: 1323–1328.

349. Whang, W. and J.T. Jr. Bigger, Comparison of the prognostic value of RR-interval variability after acute myocardial infarction in patients with versus those without diabetes mellitus. *Am. J. Cardiol.*, 2003;**92**: 247–252.

350. Balanescu, S., A.D. Corlan, M. DOrobantu, and L. Gherasim, Prognostic value of heart rate variability after acute myocardial infarction. *Med. Sci. Monit.*, 2004;**10**: CR307–315.

351. Stein, P.K., P.P. Domitrovich, H.V. Huikuri, and R.E. Kleiger for the CAST Investigators, Traditional and nonlinear heart rate variability. Are each independently associated with mortality after myocardial infarction. *J. Cardiovasc. Electrophysiol.*, 2005;**16**: 13–20.

352. Huikuri, H.V., P. Raatikainen, R. Moechr-Joergensen, J. Hartikainen, V. Virtanen, J. Boland, O. Anttonen, N. Hoest, L.V.A. Boersma, E.S. Platou, M.D. Messier, P-E. Bloch-Thomsen, for the Cardiac Arrhythmias and Risk Stratification after Acute Myocardial Infarction (CARISMA) study group, Prediction of fatal or near-fatal cardiac arrhythmia events in patients with depressed left ventricular function after an acute myocardial infarction. *Eur. Heart. J.*, 2009;**30**: 689–698.

353. Stein, K.M., J.S. Borer, C. Hochreiter, P.M. Okin, E.M. Herrold, R.B. Devereux, and P. Kligfield, Prognostic value and physiological correlated of heart rate variability in chronic severe mitral regurgitation. *Circulation*, 1993;**88**: 127–135.

354. Szabó, B.M., D.J. van Veldhuisen, N. van der Veer, J. Brouwer, P.A. De Graeff, H.J.G.M. Crijns, Prognostic value of heart rate variability in chronic congestive heart failure secondary to idiopathic or ischemic dilated cardiomyopathy. *Am. J. Cardiol.*, 1997;**79**: 978–980.

355. Ponikowski, P., S.D. Anker, T.P. Chua, R. Szelemej, M. Piepoli, S. Adamopoulos, K. Webb-Peploe, D. Harrington, A. Banasiak, K. Wrabec, and A.J.S. Coats, Depressed heart rate variability as an independent predictor of death in chronic congestive heart failure secondary to ischemic or idiopathic dilated cardiomyopathy. *Am. J. Cardiol.*, 1997;**79**: 1645–1650.

356. Nolan, J., P.D. Batin, R. Andrews, S.J. Lindsay, P. Brooksby, M. Mullen, W. Baig, A.D. Flapan, A. Cowley, R.J. Prescott, J.M. Neilson, and K.A. Fox, Prospective study of heart rate variability and mortality in chronic heart failure: results of the United Kingdom heart failure evaluation and assessment of risk trial (UK-heart). *Circulation*, 1998;**98**: 1510–1516.

357. Fauchier, L., D. Babuty, P. Cosnay, and J.P. Fauchier, Prognostic value of heart rate variability for sudden death and major arrhythmic events in patients with idiopathic dilated cardiomyopathy. *J. Am. Coll. Cardiol.*, 1999;**33**: 1203–1207.

358. Galinier, M., A. Pathak, J. Fourcade, C. Androdias, D. Curnier, S. Varnous, S. Boveda, P. Massabuau, M. Fauvel, J.M. Senard, and J.P. Bounhoure, Depressed low frequency power of heart rate variability as an independent predictor of sudden death in chronic heart failure. *Eur. Heart. J.*, 2000;**21**: 475–482.

359. Mäkikallio, T.H., H.V. Huikuri, U. Hintze, J. Videbaek, R.D. Mitrani, A. Castellanos, R.J. Myerburg, M. Møller, and DIAMOND Study Group (Danish Investigations of Arrhythmia and Mortality ON Dofetilide), Fractal analysis and time- and frequency-domain measures of heart rate variability as predictors of mortality in patients with heart failure. *Am. J. Cardiol.*, 2001;**87**: 178–182.

360. Bilchick, K.C., B. Fetics, R. Djoukeng, S.G. Fisher, R.D. Fletcher, S.N. Singh, E. Nevo, and R.D. Berger, Prognostic value of heart rate variability in chronic congestive heart failure (Veterans Affairs' Survival Trial of Antiarrhythmic Therapy in Congestive Heart Failure). *Am. J. Cardiol.*, 2002;**90**: 24–28.

361. Aronson, D., M.A. Mittleman, and A.J. Burger, Heasures of heart period variability as predictors of mortality in hospitalized patients with decompensated congestive heart failure. *Am. J. Cardiol.*, 2004;**93**: 59–63.

362. Algra, A., J.G.P. Tijssen, J.R.T.C. Roelandt, J. Pool, and J. Lubsen, Heart rate variability from 24-hour electrocardiography and the 2-year risk from sudden death. *Circulation*, 1993;**88**: 180–185.

363. Huikuri, H.V., T.H. Mäkikallio, K.E. Airaksinen, T. Seppänen, P. Puukka, I.J. Räihä, and L.B. Sourander, Power-law relationship of heart rate variability as a predictor of mortality in the elderly. *Circulation*, 1998;**97**: 2031–2036.

364. Sajadieh, A., O.W. Nielsen, V. Rasmussen, H.O. Hein, and J.F. Hansen, C-reactive protein, heart rate variability and prognosis in community subjects with no apparent heart disease. *J. Intern. Med.*, 2006;**260**: 377–387.

365. Stein, P.K., J.K. Barzilay, P.H.M. Chaves, S.Q. Mistretta, P.P. Domitrovich, J.S. Gottdiened, M.W. Rich, and R.E. Kleiger, Novel measures of heart rate variability predict cardiovascular mortality in older adults independent of traditional cardiovascular risk factors: The Cardiovascular Health Study (CHS). *J. Cardiovasc. Electropysiol.*, 2008;**19**: 1169–1174.

366. Grimm, W., J. Sharkova, M. Christ, R. Schneider, G. Schmidt, and B. Maisch, Heart rate turbulence following ventricular premature beats in healthy controls. *Ann. Noninvas. Electrocardiol.*, 2003;**8**: 127–131.

367. Lindgren, K.S., T.H. Mäkikallio, T. Seppänen, M.J.P. Ratikainen, A. Castellanos, R.J. Myerburg, and H.V. Huikuri, Heart rate turbulence after ventricular and atrial premature beats in subjects without structural heart disease, *J. Cardiovasc. Electrophysiol.*, 2003;**14**: 447–452.

368. Linden, D. and R.R. Diehl, Estimation of baroreflex sensitivity using transfer function analysis: normal values and theoretical considerations. *Clin. Auton. Res.*, 1996;**6**: 157–161.

369. Madden, K.M., W.C. Levy, A. Jacobson, J.R. Stratton, The effect of aging on phenylephrine response in normal subjects. *J. Amer. Aging. Assoc.*, 2003;**26**: 3–10.

370. Wang, Y-P., Y-J. Cheng, and C-L. Huang, Spontaneous baroreflex measurement in the assessment of cardiac vagal control. *Clin. Auton. Res.*, 2004;**14**: 189–193.

371. Cooper, V.L,. M.W. Elliot, S.B. Pearson, C.M. Taylor, and R. Hainsworth, Daytime variability of carotic baroreflex function in healthy human subjects. *Clin. Auton. Res.*, 2007;**17**: 26–32.

372. Lauer, M.S., P.M. Okin, M.G. Larson, J.C. Evans, and D. Levy, Impaired heart rate response to graded exercise: prognostic implications of chronotropic incompetence in the Framingham Heart Study. *Circulation*, 1996;**93**: 1520–1526.

373. Morillo, C.A., D.L. Eckberg, K.A. Ellenbogen, L.A. Beightol, J.B. Hoag, K.U. Tahvanainen, T.A. Kuusela, and A.M. Diedrich, Vagal and sympathetic mechanisms in patients with orthostatic vasovagal syncope. *Circulation*, 1997;**96**: 2509–2513.

374. Machado, B.H. and M.J. Brody, Contribution of neurogenic mechanisms to control of intrinsic heart rate. *Am. J. Physiol.*, 1989;**256** (1 Pt 2): R231–235.

375. Hagendorff, A., B. Schumacher, S. Kirchhoff, B. Luderitz, and K. Willecke, Conduction disturbances and increased atrial vulnerability in connexin40-deficient mice analyzed by transesophageal stimulation. *Circulation*, 1999;**99**: 1508–1515.

376. Dobrzynski, H., M.R. Boyett, and R.H. Anderson, New insights into pacemaker activity: promoting understanding of sick sinus syndrome. *Circulation*, 2007;**115**: 1921–1932.

377. Asseman, P., B. Berzin, D. Desry, D. VIlarem, P. Durand, C. Delmotte, E.H. Sarkis, J. Lekieffre, and C. Thery, Persistent sinus nodal electrograms during abnormally prolonged postpacing atrial pauses in sick sinus syndrome in humans: sinoatrial block vs overdrive suppression. *Circulation*, 1983;**68**: 33–41.

378. Apfel, H. and M. Vassalle, Acetylcholine induces overdrive excitation in sheep Purkinje fibres. *Cardiovasc. Res.*, 1988;**22**: 425–438.

379. Satoh, H., Sino-atrial nodal cells of mammalian hearts: ionic currents and gene expression of pacemaker ionic channels. *J. Smooth. Muscle. Res.*, 2003;**39**: 175–193.

380. Barbuti, A. and D. DiFrancesco, Control of cardiac rate by "funny" channels in health and disease. *Ann. N. Y. Acad. Sci.*, 2008;**1123**: 213–223.

381. Braun, A.P., T.D. Phan, and P.V. Sulakhe, Muscarinic acetylcholine receptors in the sino-atrial node and right atrium of bovine heart. *Eur. J. Pharmacol.*, 1990;**189**: 201–215.

382. Maier, S.K., R.E. Westenbroek, T.T. Yamanushi, H. Dobrzynski, M.R. Boyett, W.A. Catterall, and T. Scheuer, An unexpected requirement for brain-type sodium channels for control of heart rate in the mouse sinoatrial node. *Proc. Natl. Acad. Sci. USA.*, 2003;**100**: 3507–3512.

383. Riccioni, G., Focus on ivabradine: a new heart rate-controlling drug. *Expert. Rev. Cardiovasc. Ther.*, 2009;**7**: 107–113.

384. Jalife, J., D.C. Michaels, and M. Delmar, Mechanisms of pacemaker synchronization in the sinus node. *Prog. Clin. Biol. Res.*, 1988;**275**: 67–91.

385. Guevara, M.R. and H.J. Jongsma, Phase resetting in a model of sinoatrial nodal membrane: ionic and topologic apects. *Am. J. Physiol.*, 1990;**258**: H734–747.

386. Fye, W.B., The origin of the heart beat: a tale of frogs, jelly-fish and turtles. *Circulation*, 1987;**76**: 493–500.

387. Boineau, J.P., R.B. Schuessler, T.E. Canavan, P.B. Corr, M.E. Cain, and J.L. Cox, The human atrial pacemaker complex. *J. Electrocardiol.*, 1989;**22** (Suppl): 189–197.

388. Schuessler, R.B., B.I. Bromberg, J.P. Boineau, Effect of neurotransmitters on the activation sequence of the isolated atrium. *Am. J. Physiol.*, 1990;**258**: H1632–1641.

389. Löffelholz, K. and A.J. Pappano, The parasympathetic neuroeffector junction of the heart. *Pharmacol. Rev.*, 1985;**37**: 1–24.

390. Miyazaki, T. and D.P. Zipes, Presynaptic modulation of efferent sympathetic and vagal neurotransmission in the canine heart by hypoxia, high K+, low pH, and adenosine. Possible relevance to ischemia-induced denervation. *Circ. Res.*, 1990;**66**: 289–301.

391. Boyett, M.R., H. Honjo, and I. Kodama, The sinoatrial node, a heterogeneous pacemaker structure. *Cardiovasc. Res.*, 2000;**47**: 658–687.

392. Jordan, D. and K.M. Spyer, Effects of acetylcholine on respiratory neurones in the nucleus ambiguus-retroambigualis complex of the cat. *J. Physiol.*, 1981;**320**: 103–111.

393. Rand, M.J., H. Majewski, and D.F. Story, Modulation of neuroeffector transmission, in *Cardiovascular Pharmacology*, M. Antonaccio, Editor. New York: Raven Press, 1990, pp. 229–292.

394. Bruck, H., A. Ulrich, S. Gerlach, J. Radke, and O.E. Brodde, Effects of atropine on human cardiac beta 1- and/or beta 2-adrenoceptor stimulation. *Naunyn. Schmiedebergs. Arch. Pharmacol.*, 2003;**367**: 572–577.

395. Valenzuela, D., X. Han, U. Mende, C. Fankhauser, H. Mashimo, P. Huang, J. Pfeffer, E.J. Neer, and M.C. Fishman, G alpha(o) is necessary for muscarinic regulation of Ca2+ channels in mouse heart. *Proc. Natl. Acad. Sci. USA.*, 1997;**94**: 1727–1732.

396. Zaza, A. and F. Lombardi, Autonomic indexes based on the analysis of heart rate variability: a view from the sinus node. *Cardiovasc. Res.*, 2001;**50**: 434–442.

397. Hainsworth, R., Physiological basis of heart rate variability, in *Dynamic Electrocardiography*, M. Malik and A.J. Camm, Editors. London: Blackwell Futura Publishing, 2004, pp. 3–12.

398. Warner, M.R., Time-course and frequency dependence of sympathetic stimulation-evoked inhibition of vagal effects at the sinus node. *J. Auton. Nerv. Syst.*, 1995;**52**: 23–33.

399. Kiviniemi, A.M., A.J. Hautala, T. Seppänen, T.H. Mäkikallio, H.V. Huikuri, and M.P. Tulppo, Saturation of high-frequency oscillations of R-R intervals in healthy subjects and patients after acute myocardial infarction during ambulatory conditions. *Am. J. Physiol. Heart. Circ. Physiol.*, 2004;**287**: H1921–1927.

400. Zhang, H.and M. Vassalle, Mechanisms of adrenergic control of sino-atrial node discharge. *J. Biomed. Sci.*, 2003;**10**: 179–192.

401. Ecker, P.M., .C-C. Lin, J. Powers, B.K. Kobilka, A.N. Dubin, and C. Bernstein, Effect of targeted deletions of β_1- and β_2-adrenrgic-receptor subtypes on heart rate variability. *Am. J. Physiol. Heart. Circ. Physiol.*, 2006;**290**: H192–199.

402. Brown, R.A. and R.G. Carpentier, Alpha-adrenoceptor-mediated effects of norepinephrine on the guinea pig sinus node. *J. Electrocardiol.*, 1988; **21**: 213–217.

403. Allen, J.M., P. Gjörstrup, J.A. Björkman, L. Ek, T. Abrahamsson, and S.R. Bloom, Studies on cardiac distribution and function of neuropeptide Y. *Acta. Physiol. Scand.* 1986;**126**: 405–411.

404. Gray, A.L., T.A. Johnson, J.M. Lauenstein, S.S. Newton, J.L. Ardell, and V.J. Massari, Parasympathetic control of the heart. III. Neuropeptide Y-immunoreactive nerve terminals synapse on three populations of negative chronotropic vagal preganglionic neurons. *J. Appl. Physiol.*, 2004;**96**: 2279–2287.

405. Kilborn, M.J., E.K. Potter, and D.I. McCloskey,. Neuromodulation of the cardiac vagus: comparison of neuropeptide Y and related peptides. *Regul. Pept.*, 1985;**12**: 155–161.

406. Revington, M.L. and D.I. McCloskey, Sympathetic-parasympathetic interactions at the heart, possibly involving neuropeptide Y, in anaesthetized dogs. *J. Physiol.*, 1990;**428**: 359–370.

407. Warner, M.and M.N. Levy, Neuropeptide Y as a putative modulator of the vagal effects on heart rate. *Circ. Res.*, 1989;**64**: 882–889.

408. Balligand, J.L., Regulation of cardiac beta-adrenergic response by nitric oxide. *Cardiovasc. Res.*, 1999;**43**: 607–620.

409. Chowdhary, S. and J.N. Townend, Role of nitric oxide in the regulation of cardiovascular autonomic control. *Clin. Sci. (Lond).*, 1999;**97**: 5–17.

410. Krukoff, T.L., Central actions of nitric oxide in regulation of autonomic functions. *Brain. Res. Rev.*, 1999;**30**: 52–65.

411. Zanzinger, J., Role of nitric oxide in the neural control of cardiovascular function. *Cardiovasc. Res.*, 1999;**43**: 639–649.

412. Sartori, C., M. Lepori, and U. Scherrer, Interactions between nitric oxide and the cholinergic and sympathetic nervous system in cardiovascular control in humans. *Pharmacol. Therap.*, 2005;**106**: 209–220.

413. Feron, O., C. Dessy, D.J. Opel, M.A. Arstall, R.A. Kelly, and T. Michel, Modulation of the endothelial nitric-oxide synthse-caeolin interaction in cardiac myocytes. Implications for the autonomic regulation of heart rate. *J. Biol. Chem.*, 1998;**273**: 30249–30254.

414. Herring, N., S. Golding, and D.J. Paterson, Pre-synaptic NO-cGMP pathway modulates vagal control of heart rate in isolated adult guinea pig atria. *J. Mol. Cell. Cardiol.*, 2000;**32**: 1795–1804.

415. Picker, O., T.W. Scheeren, and J.O. Arndt, Nitric oxide synthases in vagal neurons are crucial for the regulation of heart rate in awake dogs. *Basic. Res. Cardiol.*, 2001;**96**: 395–404.

416. Heaton, D.A., S. Golding, C.P. Bradley, T.A. Dawson, S. Cai, K.M. Channon, and D.J. Paterson, Targeted nNOS gene transfer into the cardiac vagus rapidly increases parasympathetic function in the pig. *J. Mol. Cell. Cardiol.*, 2005;**39**: 159–164.

417. Chowdhary, S., A.M. Marsh, J.H. Coote, and J.N. Townend, Nitric oxide and cardiac muscarinic control in humans. *Hypertension*, 2004;**43**: 1023–1028.

418. Chowdhary, S., S.L. Nuttall, J.H. Coote, and J.N. Townend, L-arginine augments cardiac vagal control in healthy human subjects. *Hypertension*, 2002;**39**: 51–56.

419. Vanoli, E., G.M. De Ferrari, M. Stramba-Badiale, S.S. Jr. Hull, R.D. Foreman, and P.J. Schwartz, Vagal stimulation and prevention of sudden death in conscious dogs with a healed myocardial infarction. *Circ. Res.*, 1991;**68**: 1471–1481.

420. Li, M., C. Zheng, T. Sato, T. Kawada, M. Sugimachi, and K. Sunagawa, Vagal nerve stimulation markedly improves long-term survival after chronic heart failure in rats. *Circulation*, 2004;**109**: 120–124.

421. Binkley, P.F., E. Nunziatta, Y. Liu-Stratton, and G. Cooke, A polymorphism of the endothelial nitric oxide synthase promoter is associated with an increase in autonomic imbalance in patients with congestive heart failure. *Am. Heart. J.*, 2005;**149**: 342–348.

422. Jordan, D., Vagal control of the heart: central serotonergic (5-HT) mechanisms. *Exp. Physiol.*, 2005;**90**: 175–181.

423. Okoshi, K., M. Nakayama, X. Yan, M.P. Okoshi, A.J. Schuldt, M.A. Marchionni, and B.H. Lorell, Neuregulins regulate cardiac parasympathetic activity: muscarinic modulation of beta-adrenergic activity in myocytes from mice with neuregulin-1 gene deletion. *Circulation*, 2004;**110**: 713–717.

424. Hrushesky, W.J., D.J. Fader, J.S. Berestka, M. Sommer, J. Hayes, and F.O. Cope, Diminishment of respiratory sinus arrhythmia foreshadows doxorubicin-induced cardiomyopathy. *Circulation*, 1991;**84**: 697–707.

425. Beaulieu, P. and C. Lambert, Peptidic regulation of heart rate and interactions with the autonomic nervous system *Cardiovasc. Res.*, 1998;**37**: 578–585.

426. Herring, N. and D.J. Paterson, Neuromodulators of peripheral cardiac sympatho-vagal balance. *Exp. Physiol.*, 2009;**94**: 46–53.

427. Woods, R.L., Cardioprotective functions of atrial natriuretic peptide and B-type natriuretic peptide: a brief review. *Clin. Exp. Pharmacol. Physiol.*, 2004;**31**: 791–794.

428. Anja, G., A.G. Teschemacher, and C.D. Johnson, Cotransmission in the autonomic nervous system. *Exp. Physiol.*, 2009;**94**:18–19.

429. Lab, M.J., Mechanosensitivity as an integrative system in heart: an audit. *Prog. Biophys. Mol. Biol.*, 1999;**71**: 7–27.

430. Kohl, P., P. Hunter, and D. Noble, Stretch-induced changes in heart rate and rhythm: clinical observations, experiments and mathematical models. *Prog. Biophys. Mol. Biol.*, 1999;**71**: 91–138.

431. Taggart, P. and P.M. Sutton, Cardiac mechano-electric feedback in man: clinical relevance. *Prog. Biophys. Mol. Biol.*, 1999;**71**: 139–154.

432. Rajala, G.M., J.H. Kalbfleisch, and S. Kaplan, Evidence that blood pressure controls heart rate in the chick embryo prior to neural control. *J. Embryol. Exp. Morphol.*, 1976;**36**: 685–695.

433. Bernardi, L., F. Keller, M. Sanders, P.S. Reddy, B. Griffith, F. Meno, and M.R. Pinsky, Respiratory sinus arrhythmia in the denervated human heart. *J. Appl. Physiol.*, 1989;**67**: 1447–1455.

434. Conci, F., M. Di Rienzo, and P. Castiglioni, Blood pressure and heart rate variability and baroreflex sensitivity before and after brain death. *J. Neurol. Neurosurg. Psychiatr.*, 2001;**71**: 621–631.

435. Harris, K.F. and K.A. Matthews, Interactions between autonomic nervous system activity and endothelial function: a model for the development of cardiovascular disease. *Psychosom. Med.*, 2004;**66**: 153–164.

436. Story, D.F. and J. Ziogas, Interaction of angiotensin with noradrenergic neuroeffector transmission. *Trends. Pharmacol. Sci.*, 1987;**8**: 269–271.

437. Zimmermann, B.G., E.J. Sybertz, and P.C. Wong, Interaction between sympathetic and renin-angiotensin system. *J. Hypertens.*, 1984;**2**: 581–587.

438. Thayer, J.F., M.M. Merrit, J.J. III Sollers, A.B. Zonderman, M.K. Evans, S. Yie, and D.R. Abernethy, Effect of angiotensin-converting enzyme insertion/deletion polymorphism DD genotype on high-frequency heart rate variability in African Americans. *Am. J. Cardiol.*, 2003;**92**: 1487–1490.

439. Ashley, E.A., A. Kardos, S.J. Jack, W. Habenbacher, M. Wheeler, M. Kim, J. Froning, J. Myers, G. Whyte, V. Froelicher, and P. Douglas, Angiotensin-converting enzyme genotype predicts cardiac and autonomic responses to prolonged exercise. *J. Am. Coll. Cardiol.*, 2006;**48**: 523–531.

440. Osterziel, K.J., R. Dietz, W. Schmid, K. Mikulaschek, J. Manthey, and W. Kubler, ACE inhibition improves vagal reactivity in patients with heart failure. *Am. Heart. J.*, 1990;**120**: 1120–1129.

441. Binkley, P.F., G.J. Haas, R.C. Starling, E. Nunziata, P.A. Hatton, C.V. Leier, and R.J. Cody, Sustained augmentation of parasympathetic tone with angiotensin-converting enzyme inhibition in patients with congestive heart failure. *J. Am. Coll. Cardiol.*, 1993;**21**: 655–661.

442. Heusser, K., J. Vitkovsky, R.E. Schmieder, and H.P. Schobel, AT1 antagonism by eprosartan lowers heart rate variability and baroreflex gain. *Auton. Neurosci.*, 2003;**107**: 45–51.

443. Schmidt, B.M., K. Horisberger, M. Feuring, A. Schultz, and M. Wehling, Aldosterone blunts human baroreflex sensitivity by a nongenomic mechanism. *Exp. Clin. Endocrinol. Diabetes.*, 2005;**113**: 252–256.

444. Nakashima, A., J.A. Angus, C.I. Johnston, Chronotropic effects of angiotensin I, angiotensin II, bradykinin and vasopressin in guinea pig atria. *Eur. J. Pharmcol.*, 1982;**81**: 479–485.

445. Tesfamariam, B., G.T. Allen, and J.R. Powell, Bradykinin β_2 receptor-mediated chronotropic effect of bradykinin in isolated guinea pig atria. *Eur. J. Pharmacol.*, 1995;**281**: 17–20.

446. Smagin, G.N., S.C. Heinrichs, and A.J. Dunn, The role of CRH in behavioral responses to stress. *Peptides*, 2001;**22**: 712–724.

447. Grammatopoulos, D.K. and G.P. Chrousos, Functional characteristics of CRH receptors and potential clinical applications of CRH-receptor antagonists. *Trends. Endocrinol. Metab.*, 2002;**13**: 436–444.

448. Nijsen, M.J.M.A., G. Croiset, R. Stam, A. Bruijnzeel, M. Diamant, D. de Wied, and V.M. Wiegant, The Role of the CRH Type 1 receptor in autonomic responses to corticotropin-releasing hormone in the rat. *Neuropsychopharmacology*, 2000;**22**: 388–399.

449. Arlt, J., H. Jahn, M. Kellner, A. Ströhle, A. Yassouridis, and K. Wiedemann, Modulation of sympathetic activity by corticotropin-releasing hormone and atrial natriuretic peptide. *Neuropeptides*, 2003;**37**: 362–368.

450. Parkes, D.G., R.S. Weisinger, and C.N. May, Cardiovascular actions of CRH and urocortin: an update. *Peptides*, **22**: 821–827.

451. Stiedl, O. and M. Meyer, Cardiac dynamics in corticotrophin-release factor receptor subtype-2 deficient mice. *Neuropeptides*, 2003;**37**: 3–16.

452. Schubert, C., M. Lambertz, R.A. Nelesen, W. Bardwell, J-B. Choi, J.E. Dimsdale, Effects of stress on heart rate complexity - a comparison between short-term and chronic stress. *Biol. Psychol.*, 2009;**80**: 325–332.

453. Benton, L.A. and F.E. Yates, Ultradian adrenocortical and circulatory oscillations in conscious dogs. *Am. J. Physiol. Regulatory. Integrative. Comp. Physiol.*, 1990;**258**: R578–590.

454. Fallo, F., P. Maffei, A. Dalla Pozza, M. Carli, P. Della Mea, M. Lupia, F. Rabbia, and N. Sonino, Cardiovascular autonomic function in Cushing's syndrome. *J. Endocrinol. Invest.*, 2009;**32**: 41–45.

455. Muniyappa, R., M. Montagnani, K.K. Koh, and M.J. Quon, Cardiovascular actions of insulin. *Endocr. Rev.*, 2007;**28**: 463–491.

456. Muntzel, M.S., E.A. Anderson, A.K. Johnson, and A.L. Mark, Mechanisms of insulin action on sympathetic nerve activity. *Clin. Exp. Hypertens.*, 1995;**17**: 39–50.

457. Scherrer, U. and C. Sartori, Insulin as a vascular and sympathoexcitatory hormone: implications for blood pressure regulation, insulin sensitivity, and cardiovascular morbidity. *Circulation*, 1997;**96**: 4104–4113.

458. Van De Borne, P., M. Hausberg, R.P. Hoffman, A.L. Mark, and E.A. Anderson, Hyperinsulinemia produces cardiac vagal withdrawal and nonuniform sympathetic activation in normal subjects. *Am. J. Physiol. Regulatory. Integrative. Comp. Physiol.*, 1999;**276**(1): R178–183.

459. Hausberg, M., R.P. Hoffman, V.K. Somers, C.A. Sinkey, A.L.Mark, and E.A. Anderson, Contrasting autonomic and hemodynamic effects of insulin in healthy elderly versus young subjects. *Hypertension*, 1997;**29**: 700–705.

460. Paolisso, G., M. Varricchio, and F. D'Onofrio, Glucose intolerance in the elderly: an open debate. *Arch. Gerontol. Geriatr.*, 1990;**11**: 125–132.

461. Pathak, A., F. Smith, M. Galinier, P. Verwaerde, P. Rouet, P. Philip-Couderc, J.L. Monstastruc, and J.M. Senard, Insulin downregulated M2-muscarinic receptors in adult rat atrial cardiomyocytes: a link between obesity and cardiovascular complications. *Int. J. Obes.*, 2005;**29**: 176–182.

462. Bergholm, R., J. Westerbacka, S. Vehkavaara, A. Seppälä-Lindroos, T. Goto, and H. Yki-Järvinen, Insulin sensitivity regulates autonomic control of heart rate variation independent of body weight in normal subjects. *J. Clin. Endocrinol. Metab.*, 2001;**86**: 1403–1409.

463. Lindmark, S., U. Wiklund, P. Bjerle, and J.W. Eriksson, Does the autonomic nervous system play a role in the development of insulin resistance? A study on heart rate variability in first-degree relatives of Type 2 diabetes patients and control subjects. *Diabet. Med.*, 2003;**20**: 399–405.

464. Rayner, D.V. and P. Trayhurn, Regulation of leptin production: sympathetic nervous system interactions. *J. Mol. Med.*, 2001;**79**: 8–20.

465. Grassi, G., Leptin, sympathetic nervous system, and baroreflex function. *Curr. Hypert. Rep.*, 2004;**6**: 236–240.

466. Flanagan, D.E., J.C. Vaile, G.W. Petley, D.I. Phillips, I.F. Godsland, P. Owens, V.M. Moore, R.A. Cockington, and J.S. Robinson, Gender differences in the relationship between leptin, insulin resistance and the autonomic nervous system. *Regulat. Peptides.*, 2007;**140**: 37–42.

467. Takabatake, N., H. Nakamura, O. Minamihaba, M. Inage, S. Inoue, S. Kagaya, M. Yamaki, and H. Tomoile, A novel pathophysiologic phenomenon in cachexic patients with chronic obstructive pulmonary disease. The relationship between the circadian rhythm of circulating leptin and the very low frequency component of heart rate variability. *Am. J. Respir. Crit. Care. Med.*, 2001;**163**: 1314–1319.

468. Kadowaki, T. and T. Yamauchi, Adiponectin and adiponectin receptors. *Endocr. Rev.*, 2005 May;**26**(3): 439–451.

469. Katagiri, H., T. Yamada, and Y. Oka, Adiposity and cardiovascular disorders: disturbance of the regulatory system consisting of humoral and neuronal signals. *Circ. Res.*, 2007; 101: 27–39.

470. Hoyda, T.D., W.K. Samson, and A.V. Ferguson, Adiponectin depolarizes parvocellular paraventricular nucleus neurons controlling neuroendocrine and autonomic function. *Endocrinology*, 2009;**150**: 832–840.

471. Hoyda, T.D., P.M. Smith, and A.V. Ferguson, Adiponectin acts in the nucleus of the solitary tract to decrease blood pressure by modulating the excitability of neuropeptide Y neurons. *Brain. Res.*, 2009;**1256**: 76–84.

472. Wakabayashi, S. and Y. Aso, Adiponectin concentrations in sera from patients with type 2 diabetes are negatively associated with sympathovagal balance as evaluated by power spectral analysis of heart rate variation. *Diabetes. Care.*, 2004;**27**: 2392–2397.

473. Lam, J.C., A. Xu, S. Tam, P.I. Khong, T.J. Yao, D.C. Lam, A.Y. Lai, B. Lam, K.S. Lam, and S.M. Mary, Hypoadiponectinemia is related to sympathetic activation and severity of obstructive sleep apnea. *Sleep*, 2008;**31**: 1721–1727.

474. Sprague, A.H. and R.A. Khalil, Inflammatory cytokines in vascular dysfunction and vascular disease. *Biochem. Pharmacol.*, 2009;**78**: 539–552.

475. Reyes-García, M.G. and F. García-Tamayo, A neurotransmitter system that regulates macrophage proinflammatory functions. *J. Neuroimmunol.*, 2009;**216**: 20–31

476. Marsland, A.L., P.J. Gianaros, A.A. Prather, J.R. Jennings, S.A. Neumann, and S.B. Manuck, Stimulated production of proinflammatory cytokines covaries inversely with heart rate variability. *Psychosom. Med.*, 2007;**69**: 709–716.

477. Heansel, A., P.J. Mills, R.A. Nelesen, M.G. Ziegler, and J.E. Dimsdale, The relationship between heart rate variability and inflammatory markers in cardiovascular disease. *Psychoneuroendocrinol*, 2008;**33**: 1305–1312.

478. Dart, A.M., X-J. Du, and B.A. Kingwell, Gender, sex hormones and autonomic nervous control of the cardiovascular system. *Cardiovasc. Res.*, 2002;**53**: 678–687.

479. McCabe, P.M., S.W. Porges, and C.S. Carter, Heart period variability during estrogen exposure and withdrawal in female rats. *Physiol. Behav.*, 1981;**26**: 535–538.

480. Saeki, Y., F. Atogami, K. Takahashi, and T. Yoshizawa, Reflex control of autonomic function induced by posture change during the menstrual cycle. *J. Auton. Nerv. Syst.*, 1997;**66**: 69–74.

481. Evans, J.M., M.G. Ziegler, A.R. Patwardhan, J.B. Ott, C.S. Kim, F.M. Leonelli, and C.F. Knapp, Gender differences in autonomic cardiovascular regulation: spectral, hormonal, and hemodynamic indexes. *J. Appl. Physiol.*, 2001;**91**: 2611–2618.

482. Leicht, A.S., D.A. Hirning, and G.D. Allen, Heart rate variability and endogenous sex hormones during the menstrual cycle in young women. *Exp. Physiol.*, 2003;**88**: 441–446.

483. Christ, M., K. Seyffart, H-C. Tillmann, and M. Wehling, Hormone replacement in postmenoupasual women: impact of

progestogens on autonomic tone and blood pressure regulation. *Menopause*, 2002;**9**: 127–136.

484. Fernandes, E.O., R.S. Moraes, E.L. Ferlin, M.C.O. Wender, and J.P. Ribeiro, Hormone replacement therapy does not affect the 24-hour heart rate variability in ostmenopausal women: results of a randomized, placebo-controlled trial with two regimens. *Pacing Clin. Electrophysiol.*, 2005;**28**: S172–177.

485. Benarroch, E.E., Thermoregulation: recent concepts and remaining questions. *Neurology*, 2007;**69**: 1293–1297.

486. Kumar, V.M., R. Vetrivelan, and H.N. Mallick, Noradrenergic afferents and receptors in the medial preoptic area: neuroanatomical and neurochemical links between the regulation of sleep and body temperature. *Neurochem. Int.*, 2007;**50**: 783–790.

487. Weinert, D. and J. Waterhouse, The circadian rhythm of core temperature: effects of physical activity and aging. *Physiol. Behav.*, 2007;**90**: 246–256.

488. Potter, E.K., P. Parker, A.C. Caine, and E.R. Lumbers, Potentiation of cardiac vagal action by cold. *Clin. Sci. (Lond).*, 1985;**68**: 165–169.

489. Lee, K., D.N. Jackson, D.L. Cordero, T. Nishiyasu, J.K. Peters, and G.W. Mack, Change in spontaneous baroreflex control of pulse interval during heat stress in humans. *J. Appl. Physiol.*, 2003;**95**: 1789–1798.

490. Liu, W., Z. Lian, and Y. Liu, Heart rate variability at different thermal comfort levels. *Eur. J. Appl. Physiol.*, 2008;**103**:361–366.

491. Tentolouris, N., C. Tsigos, D. Perea, E. Koukou, D. Kyriaki, E. Kitsou, S. Daskas, Z. Daifotis, K. Makrilakis, S.A. Raptis, and N. Katsilambros, Differential effects of high-fat and high-carbohydrate isoenergetic meals on cardiac autonomic nervous system activity in lean and obese women. *Metabolism*, 2003;**52**: 1426–1432.

492. Kitney, R.I. and O. Rompelman, Thermal entrainment patterns in heart rate variability. *Proc. Physiol. Soc.*, 1977;**270**: 41–42.

493. Kawashima, T., The autonomic nervous system of the human heart with special reference to its origin, course, and peripheral distribution. *Anat. Embryol. (Berl).*, 2005. **209**: 425–438.

494. Wang, J., M. Irnaten, R.A. Neff, P. Venkatesan, C. Evans, A.D. Loewy, T.C. Mettenleiter, and D. Mendelowitz, Synaptic and neurotransmitter activation of cardiac vagal neurons in the nucleus ambiguus. *Ann. NY. Acad. Sci.*, 2001;**940**: 237–246.

495. Cheng, Z., H. Zhang, S.Z. Guo, R. Wurster, and D. Gozal, Differential control over vagal efferent postganglionic neurons in rat intrinsic cardiac ganglia by neurons in the NA and the DmnX: anatomical evidence. *Am. J. Physiol. Regul. Integr. Comp. Physiol.*, 2004;**286**: R625–633.

496. Armour, J.A., D.A. Murphy, B.X. Yuan, S. Macdonald, and D.A. Hopkins, Gross and microscopic anatomy of the human intrinsic cardiac nervous system. *Anat. Rec.*, 1997;**247**: 289–298.

497. Hou, Y., B.J. Scherlag, J. Lin, Y. Zhang, Z. Lu, K. Truong, E. Patterson, R. Lazzara, W.M. Jackman, and S.S. Po, Ganglionated plexi modulate extrinsic cardiac autonomic nerve input: Effects on sinus rate, atrioventricular conduction, refractoriness, and inducibility of atrial fibrillation. *J. Am. Coll. Cardiol.*, 2007;**50**: 61–68.

498. Levy, M.N., Neural control of cardiac function. *Baillieres. Clin. Neurol.*, 1997;**6**: 227–244.

499. Keyl, C., A. Schneider, M. Dambacher, and L. Bernardi, Time delay of vagally mediated cardiac baroreflex response varies with autonomic cardiovascular control. *J. Appl. Physiol.*, 2001;**91**: 283–289.

500. Taylor, W.E., D. Jordan, and J.H. Coote, Central control of the cardiovascular and respiratory systems and the interactions in vertebrates. *Physiol. Rev.*, 1999;**79**: 855–916.

501. Bałkowiec, A. and P. Szulczyk, Properties of postganglionic sympathetic neurons with axons in the right thoracic vagus. *Neuroscience*, 1992;**48**: 159–167.

502. Fu, L.W. and J.C. Longhurst, Regulation of cardiac afferent excitability in ischemia. *Handb. Exp. Pharmacol.*, 2009;**194**: 185–225.

503. Arora, R.C., J.L. Ardell, and J.A. Armour, Cardiac denervation and cardac function. *Curr. Interven. Cardiol. Rep.*, 2000;**2**: 188–195.

504. Kamath, M.V., G. Tougas, D. Fitzpatrick, E.L. Fallen, R. Watteel, G. Shine, and A.R. Upton, Assessment of the visceral afferent and autonomic pathways in response to esophageal stimulation in control subjects and in patients with diabetes. *Clin. Invest. Med.*, 1998;**21**: 100–113.

505. Fahim, M., Cardiovascular sensory receptors and their regulatory mechanisms. *Indian. J. Physiol. Pharmacol.*, 2003;**47**: 124–146.

506. Granzier, H.L. and S. Labeit, The giant protein titin: a major player in myocardial mechanics, signaling, and disease. *Circ. Res.*, 2004;**94**: 284–295.

507. Armour, J.A., Cardiac neuronal hierarchy in health and disease. *Am. J. Physiol. Regul. Integr. Comp. Physiol.*, 2004;**287**: R262–271.

508. Pyetan, E., E. Toledo, O. Zoran, and S. Akselrod, Parametric description of cardiac vagal control. *Auton. Neurosci.*, 2003;**109**: 42–52.

509. Paton, J.F., P. Boscan, A.E. Pickering, and E. Nalivaiko, The yin and yang of cardiac autonomic control: vago-sympathetic interactions revisited. *Brain. Res. Brain. Res. Rev.*, 2005;**49**: 555–565.

510. Samuels, M.A., The brain-heart connection. *Circulation*, 2007;**116**: 77–84.

511. Baron, S.A., Z. Rogovski, and J. Hemli,. Autonomic consequences of cerebral hemisphere infarction. *Stroke*, 1994;**25**: 113–116.

512. Svigelj, V., A. Grad, and T. Kiauta, Heart rate variability, norepinephrine and ECG changes in subarachnoid hemorrhage patients. *Acta. Neurol. Scand.*, 1996;**94**: 120–126.

513. Tomson, T., M. Ericson, C. Ihrman, and L.E. Lindblad,. Heart rate variability in patients with epilepsy. *Epilepsy. Res.*, 1998;**30**: 77–83.

514. Ako, J., K. Sudhir, H.M. Farouque, Y. Honda, and P.J. Fitzgerald, Transient left ventricular dysfunction under severe stress: brain-heart relationship revisited. *Am. J. Med.*, 2006;**119**: 10–17.

515. Dabrowska, B., A. Dabrowski, P. Pruszczyk, A. Skrobowski, and B. Wocial, Heart rate variability before sudden blood pressure elevations or complex cardiac arrhythmias in phaeochromocytoma. *J. Hum. Hypertens.*, 1996;**10**: 43–50.

516. Nguyen, S.B., C. Cevik, M. Otahbachi, A. Kumar, L.A. Jenkins, and K. Nugent, Do comorbid psychiatric disorders contribute to the pathogenesis of tako-tsubo syndrome? A review of pathogenesis. *Congest. Heart. Fail.*, 2009;**15**: 31–34.

517. Fuler, J.L., Genetic variability in some physiological constants of dogs. *Am. J. Physiol.*, 1951;**166**: 20–24.

518. Kreutz, R., B. Struk, P. Stock, N. Hübner, D. Ganten, and K. Lindpaintner, Evidence for primary genetic determination of heart rate regulation: chromosomal mapping of a genetic locus in the rat. *Circulation*, 1997;**96**: 1078–1081.

519. Martin, L.J., A.G. Comuzzie, G.E. Sonnenberg, J. Myklebust, R. James, J. Marks, J. Blangero, and A.H. Kissebah, Major

quantitative trait locus for resting heart rate maps to a region on chromosome 4. *Hypertension*, 2004;**43**: 1146–1151.

520. Wilk, J.B., R.H. Myers, Y. Zhang, C.E. Lewis, L. Atwood, P.N. Hopkins, and R.C. Ellison. Evidence for a gene influencing heart rate on chromosome 4 among hypertensives. *Hum. Genet.*, 2002; 111: 207–213.

521. Rice, T., P. An, J. Gagnon, A.S. Leon, J.S. Skinner, J.H. Wilmore, C. Bouchard, and D.C. Rao, Heritability of HR and BP response to exercise training in the HERITAGE Family Study. *Med. Sci. Sports. Exerc.*, 2002; 34: 972–979.

522. Rice, T., T. Rankinen, Y.C. Chagnon, M.A. Province, L. Pérusse, A.S. Leon, J.S. Skinner, J.H. Wilmore, C. Bouchard, and D.C. Rao, Genomewide linkage scan of resting blood pressure: HERITAGE Family Study. Health, Risk Factors, Exercise Training, and Genetics. *Hypertension*, 2002;**39**: 1037–1043.

523. Laramie, J.M., J.B. Wilk, S.C. Hunt, R.C. Ellison, A. Chakravarti, E. Boerwinkle, and R.H. Myers, Evidence for a gene influencing heart rate on chromosome 5p13–14 in a meta-analysis of genome-wide scans from the NHLBI Family Blood Pressure Program. *BMC. Med. Genet.*, 2006;**7**: 17.

524. Sajadieh, A., V. Rasmussen, H.O. Hein, and J.F. Hansen, Familial predisposition to premature heart attack and reduced heart rate variability. *Am. J. Cardiol.*, 2003;**92**: 234–236.

525. Singh, J.P., M.G. Larson, C.J. O'Donnell, H. Tsuji, D. Corey, and D. Levy, Genome scan linkage results for heart rate variability (the Framingham Heart Study). *Am. J. Cardiol.*, 2002;**90**: 1290–1293.

526. Schoots, O., T. Voskoglou, and H.H. Van Tol, Genomic organization and promoter analysis of the human G-protein-coupled K+ channel Kir3.1 (KCNJ3/HGIRK1). *Genomics*, 1997;**39**: 279–288.

527. Rempel, N., S. Heyers, H. Engels, E. Sleegers, and O.K. Steinlein, The structures of the human neuronal nicotinic acetylcholine receptor beta2- and alpha3-subunit genes (CHRNB2 and CHRNA3). *Hum. Genet.*, 1998;**103**: 645–653.

528. Singh, J.P., M.G. Larson, C.J. O'Donnell, H. Tsuji, J.C. Evans, and D. Levy, Heritability of heart rate variability: the Framingham Heart Study. *Circulation*, 1999;**99**: 2251–2254.

529. Singh, J.P., M.G. Larson, C.J. O'Donnell, and D. Levy, Genetic factors contribute to the variance in frequency domain measures of heart rate variability. *Auton. Neurosci.*, 2001;**90**: 122–126.

530. Sinnreich, R., Y. Friedlander, D. Sapoznikov, and J.D. Kark, Familial aggregation of heart rate variability based on short recordings–the kibbutzim family study. *Hum. Genet.*, 1998;**103**: 34–40.

531. Piha, S.J., T. Rönnemaa, and M. Koskenvuo, Autonomic nervous system function in identical twins discordant for obesity. *Int. J. Obes. Relat. Metab. Disord.*, 1994;**18**: 547–550.

532. Boomsma, D.I., G.C. van Baal, and J.F. Orlebeke, Genetic influences on respiratory sinus arrhythmia across different task conditions. *Acta. Genet. Med. Gemellol. (Roma).*, 1990;**39**: 181–191.

533. Snieder, H., D.I. Boomsma, L.J. Van Doornen, and E.J. De Geus, Heritability of respiratory sinus arrhythmia: dependency on task and respiration rate. *Psychophysiology*, 1997;**34**: 317–328.

534. Kupper, N.H., G. Willemsen, M. van den Berg, D. de Boer, D. Posthuma, D.I/Boomsma, and E.J. de Geus, Heritability of ambulatory heart rate variability. *Circulation*, 2004;**110**: 2792–2796.

535. Wang, X., X. Ding, S. Su, Z. Li, H. Riese, J.F. Thayer, F. Treiber, and H. Snieder, Genetic influences on heart rate variability at rest and during stress. *Psychophysiology*, 2009;**46**: 458–465.

536. Vaccarino, V., R. Lampert, J.D. Bremner, F. Lee, S. Su, C. Maisano, N.V. Murrah, L. Jones, E. Jawed, N. Afzal, A. Ashraf, and J. Goldberg, Depressive symptoms and heart rate variability: evidence for a shared genetic substrate in a study of twins. *Psychosom. Med.*, 2008;**70**: 628–636.

537. Fava, C., P. Burri, P. Almgren, G. Arcaro, L. Groop, U. Lennart Hulthén, and O. Melander, Dipping and variability of blood pressure and heart rate at night are heritable traits. *Am. J. Hypertens.*, 2005;**18**: 1402–1407.

538. Dubreuil, E., B. Ditto, G. Dionne, R.O. Pihl, R.E. Tremblay, M. Boivin, D. Pérusse, Familiality of heart rate and cardiac-related autonomic activity in five-month-old twins: the Québec newborn twins study. *Psychophysiology*, 2003; 40: 849–862.

539. Neumann, S.A., E.C. Lawrence, J.R. Jennings, R.E. Ferrell, and S.B. Manuck, Heart rate variability is associated with polymorphic variation in the choline transporter gene. *Psychosom. Med.*, 2005;**67**: 168–171.

540. Busjahn, A., A. Voss, H. Knoblauch, M. Knoblauch, E. Jeschke, N. Wessel, J. Bohlender, J. McCarron, H.D. Faulhaber, H. Schuster, R. Dietz, and F.C. Luft, Angiotensin-converting enzyme and angiotensinogen gene polymorphisms and heart rate variability in twins. *Am. J. Cardiol.*, 1998;**81**: 755–760.

541. Matsunaga, T., N. Gu, H. Yamazaki, M. Tsuda, T. Adachi, K. Yasuda, T. Moritani, K. Tsuda, M. Nonaka, and T. Nishiyama, Association of UCP2 and UCP3 polymorphisms with heart rate variability in Japanese men. *J. Hypertens.*, 2009;**27**: 305–313.

542. Walther, T., N. Wessel, N. Kang, A. Sander, C. Tschöpe, H. Malberg, M. Bader, and A. Voss, Altered heart rate and blood pressure variability in mice lacking the Mas protooncogene. *Braz. J. Med. Biol. Res.*, 2000 Jan;**33**(1): 1–9.

543. Hirsh, M., J. Karin, and S. Akselrod, Heart rate variability in the fetus, in *Heart Rate Variability*, M. Malik and A.J. Camm, Editors. Armonk, NY: Futura Publishing, 1995, pp. 517–531.

544. Lenard, Z., P. Studinger, B. Mersich, L. Kocsis, and M. Kollai, Maturation of cardiovagal autonomic function from childhood to young adult age. *Circulation*, 2004;**110**: 2307–2312.

545. Thompson, C.R., J.S. Brown, H. Gee, and E.W. Taylor, Heart rate variability in healthy term newborns: the contribution of respiratory sinus arrhythmia. *Early. Hum. Dev.*, 1993;**31**: 217–228.

546. Struijk, P.C., N.T. Ursem, J. Mathews, E.B. Clark, B.B. Keller, and J.W. Wladimiroff, Power spectrum analysis of heart rate and blood flow velocity variability measured in the umbilical and uterine arteries in early pregnancy: a comparative study. *Ultrasound. Obstet. Gynecol.*, 2001;**17**: 316–321.

547. Van Leeuwen, P., D. Geue, S. Lange, W. Hatzmann, and D. Grönemeyer, Changes in the frequency power spectrum of fetal heart rate in the course of pregnancy. *Prenat. Diagn.*, 2003;**23**: 909–916.

548. Lange, S., P. Van Leeuwen, D. Geue, W. Hatzmann, and D. Grönemeyer, Influence of gestational age, heart rate, gender and time of day on fetal heart rate variability. *Med. Biol. Eng. Comput.*, 2005;**43**: 481–486.

549. Metsälä, T.H., J.P. Pirhonen, J.O. Jalonen, R.U. Erkkola, and I.A. Välimäki, Association of abnormal flow velocity waveforms in the uterine artery with frequency-specific fetal heart rate variability. *Early. Hum. Dev.*, 1993;**34**: 217–225.

550. Nagy, E., H. Orvos, G. Bárdos, and P. Molnár, Gender-related heart rate differences in human neonates. *Pediatr. Res.*, 2000;**47**: 778–780.

551. Witte, H. and M. Rother, High-frequency and low-frequency heart-rate fluctuation analysis in newborns: a review of possibilities and limitations 1992. *Basic. Res. Cardiol.*, 1992;**87**: 193–204.

552. Galland, B.C., R.M. Hayman, B.J. Taylor, D.P.G Bolotn, R.M. Sayers, and S.M. Williams. Factors affecting heart rate variability response to tilting in infants aged 1 and 3 months. *Pediatr. Res.*, 2000;**48**: 360–368.

553. Finley, J.P., S.T. Nugent, and W. Hellenbrand, Heart-rate variability in children. Spectral analysis of developmental changes between 5 and 24 years. *Can. J. Physiol. Pharmacol.*, 1987;**65**: 2048–2052.

554. Finley, J.P. and S.T. Nugent, Heart rate variability in infants, children and young adults. *J. Auton. Nerv. Syst.*, 1995;**51**: 103–108.

555. Korkushko, O.V. V.B. Shatilo, Yu.I. Plachinda, and T.V. Shatilo, Autonomic control of cardiac chronotropic function in man as a function of age: assessment by power spectral analysis of heart rate variability. *J. Auton. Nerv. Syst.*, 1991;**32**: 191–198.

556. Ferrari, A.U., A. Radaelli, and M. Centola, Invited review: aging and the cardiovascular system. *J. Appl. Physiol.*, 2003;**95**: 2591–2597.

557. Lakatta, E.G., Deficient neurondocrine regulation of the cardiovascular system with advancing age in healthy humans. *Circulation*, 1993;**87**: 631–636.

558. Brodde, O.E. and K. Leineweber, Autonomic receptor systems in the failing and aging human heart: similarities and differences. *Eur. J. Pharmacol.*, 2004;**500**: 167–176.

559. Kaye, D. and M. Esler, Autonomic control of the aging heart. *Neuromol. Med.*, 2008;**10**: 179–186.

560. Kelliher, G.J. and T.S. Conahan, Changes in vagal activity and response to muscarinic receptor agonists with age. *J. Gerontol.*, 1980;**35**: 842–849.

561. Bouman, L.N. and H.J. Jongsma, Structure and function of the sino-atrial node: a review. *Eur. Heart. J.*, 1986;**7**: 94–104.

562. Rodefeld, M.D., S.L. Beau, R.B. Schuessler, J.P. Boineau, J.E. Saffitz, β-Adrenergic and muscarinic cholinergic receptor densities in the human sinoatrial node: identification of a high β_2-adrenergic receptor density. *J. Cardiovasc. Electrophysiol.*, 1996;**7**: 1039–1049.

563. White, M., R. Roden, W. Minobe, F. Khan,P. Larrabee, M. Wollmering, D. Port, F. Anderson, D. Campbell, A.M. Feldman, and M.R. Bristow,. Age-related changes in β-adrenergic neuroeffector systems in the human heart. *Circulation*, 1994;**90**: 1225–1238.

564. Hardouin, S., F. Bourgeois, M. Toraasson, A. Oubenaissa, J.M. Elalouf, D. Fellmann, T. Dakhli, B. Swynghedauw, and J.M. Moalic, Beta-adrenergic and muscarinic receptor mRNA accumulation in the sinoatrial node area of adult and senescent rat hearts. *Mech. Age. Dev.*, 1998;**100**: 277–297.

565. Kaushal, P. and J.A. Taylor, Inter-relations among declines in arterial distensibility, baroreflex function and respiratory sinus arrhythmia. *J. Am. Coll. Cardiol.*, 2002;**39**: 1524–1530.

566. Gill, J.S., G.J. Hunter, G. Gane, and A.J. Camm, Heterogeneity of the human myocardial sympathetic innervation: in vivo demonstration by iodine 123-labeled meta-iodobenzylguanidine scintigraphy. *Am. Heart. J.*, 1993;**126**: 390–398.

567. Jennett, S. and J.H. McKillop, Observations on the incidence and mechanism of sinus arrhythmia in man at rest. *J. Physiol.*, 1971;**213**: 58–59.

568. Jarisch, W.R., J.J. Ferguson, R.P. Shannon, J.Y. Wei, and A.L. Goldberger, Age-related disappearance of Mayer-like heart rate waves. *Experientia*, 1978;**43**: 1207–1209.

569. Waddington, J.L., M.J. MacCulloch, and J.E. Sambrooks, Resting heartrate variability in man declines with age. *Experientia*, 1979;**35**: 1197–1198.

570. Hrushesky, W.J.M., O. Schmitt, and V. Gilbertsen, The respiratory sinus arrhythmia: a measure of cardiac age. *Science*, 1984; 1001–1004.

571. Colosimo, A., A. Giuliani, A.M. Mancini, G. Piccirillo, and V. Marigliano, Estimating a cardiac age by means of heart rate variability. *Am. J. Physiol. Heart. Circ. Physiol.*, 1997;**273**: H1841–1847.

572. Nasir, K., C. Vasamreddy, R.S. Blumenthal, and J.A. Rumberger, Comprehensive coronary risk determination in primary prevention: an imaging and clinical based definition combining computed tomographic coronary artery calcium score and national cholesterol education program risk score. *Int. J. Cardiol.*, 2006;**110**: 129–136.

573. Tsuji, H., F.J. Venditti, E.S. Emnders, J.C. Evans, M.G. Larson, C.L. Feldman, and D. Levy, Determinants of heart rate variability. *J. Am. Coll. Cardiol.*, 1996;**28**: 1539–1546.

574. Fukusaki, C., K. Kawakubo, and Y. Yamamoto, Assessment of the primary effect of aging on heart rate variability in humans. *Clin. Auton. Res.*, 2000;**10**: 123–130.

575. Britton, A., M. Shipley, M. Malik, K. Hnatkova, H. Hemingway, and M. Marmot, Changes in heart rate and heart rate variability over time in middle-aged men and women in the general population (from the Whitehall II Cohort Study). *Am. J. Cardiol.*, 2007;**100**(3): 524–527.

576. Koskinen, T., M. Kahonen, A. Jula, T. Laitinen, L. Keltikandas-Jarvinen, J. Viikaris, I. Valimaki, and O.T. Raitakari, Short-term heart rate variability in healthy young adults. The Cardiovascular Risk in Young Finns study. *Auton. Neurosci.*, 2009;**145**: 81–88.

577. Mølgaard, H., K. Hermansen, and P. Bjerregaard, Spectral components of short-term RR interval variability in healthy subjects and effects of risk factors. *Eur. Heart. J.*, 1994;**15**: 1174–1183.

578. Jokinen, V., L.B. Sourander, H. Karanko, T.H. Mäkikallio, and K.V. Huikuri, Changes in cardiovascular autonomic regulation among elderly subjects: follow-up of sixteen years. *Ann. Med.*, 2005;**37**: 206–212.

579. Stein, P.K., J.I. Brzilay, P.H.M. Chaves, P.P. Domitrovich, and J.S. Gottdiener, Heart rate variability and its changes over 5 years in older adults. *Age. Ageing*, 2009;**38**: 212–218.

580. Ziegler, D., R. Piolot, K. Strasburger, H. Lambec, and K. Dannehl, Normal ranges and reproducibility of statistical, geometric, frequency domain, and non-linear measures of 24-hour heart rate variability. *Horm. Metab. Res.*, 1999 Dec;31(12):672–679.

581. Kingwell, B.A., J.M. Thompson, D.M. Kaye, G.A. McPherson, G.L. Jennings, M.D. Esler, Heart rate spectral analysis, cardiac norepinephrine spillover, and muscle sympathetic nerve activity during human sympathetic activation and failure. *Circulation*, 1994;**90**: 234–240.

582. Vuksanovic, V. and V. Gal, Nonlinear and chaos characteristics of heart period time series: healthy aging and postural changes. *Auton. Neurosci:. Basic. Clin.*, 2005;**121**: 94–100.

583. Beckers, F., B. Verheyden, and A.E. Aubert, Aging and nonlinear heart rate control in a healthy population. *Am. J. Physiol. Heart. Circ. Physiol.*, 2006;**290**: H2560–2570.

584. Iyengar, N., C.K. Peng, R. Morin, A.L. Goldberger, and L.A. Lipsitz, Age-related alterations in the fractal scaling of cardiac interbeat interval dynamics. *Am. J. Physiol. Regul. Integr. Comp. Physiol.*, 1996;**271**: R1078–1084.

585. Platsia, M.M. and V. Gal, Dependence of heart rate variability on heart period in disease and aging. *Physiol. Meas.*, 2006;**27**: 989–998.

586. Schmitt, D.T. and P.Ch.Ivanov, Fractal scale-invariant and nonlinear properties of cardiac dynamics remain stable with advanced age: a new mechanistic picture of cardiac control in healthy elderly. *Am. J. Physiol. Regul. Integr. Comp. Physiol.*, 2007;**293**: R1923–1937.

587. Sakata, S., J. Hayano, S. Mukai, A. Okada, and T. Fujinami, Aging and spectral characteristics of the nonharmonic component of 24-hour heart rate variability. *Am. J. Physiol. Regul. Integr. Comp. Physiol.*, **276**: R1724–1731.

588. Giulliani, A., G. Piccirillo, V. Marigliano, and A. Coosimo, A nonlinear explanation of aging-induced changes in heart beat dynamics. *Am. J. Physiol. Heart. Circ. Physiol.*, 1998;**275**: H1455–1461.

589. Monahan, K.D., Effect of aging on baroreflex function in humans. *Am. J. Physiol. Regul. Integr. Comp. Physiol.*, 2007;**293**: R3–12.

590. Gribbin, B., T.G. Pickering, P. Sleight, and R. Peto, Effect of age and high blood pressure on baroreflex sensitivity in man. *Circ. Res.*, 1971;**29**: 424–431.

591. Jones, P.P., D.D. Christou, J. Jordan, and D.R. Seals, Baroreflex buffering is reduced with age in healthy men. *Circulation*, 2003;**107**: 1770–1774.

592. Monahan, K.D., F.A Dinenno, H. Tanaka, C.M. Clevenger, C.A. DeSouza, and D.R. Seals. Regular aerobic exercise modulates age-associated declines in cardiovagal baroreflex sensitivity in healthy men. *J. Physiol.*, 2000;**529**: 263–271.

593. Laitinen, T., J. Hartikainen, E. Vanninen, L. Niskanen, G. Geelen, and E. Länsimies, Age and gender dependency of baroreflex sensitivity in healthy subjects. *J. Appl. Physiol.*, 1998;**84**: 576–583.

594. Huang, C.C., P. Sandroni, D.M. Sletten, S.D. Weigand, and P.A. Low, Effect of age on adrenergic and vagal baroreflex sensitivity in normal subjects. *Muscle. Nerve.*, 2007;**36**: 637–642.

595. Piccirillo, G., V. Di Giuseppe, M. Nocco, M. Lionetti, A. Moisè, C. Naso, D. Tallarico, V. Marigliano, and M. Cacciafesta, Influence of aging and other cardiovascular risk factors on baroreflex sensitivity. *J. Am. Geriatr. Soc.*, 2001;**49**: 1059–1065.

596. Milic, M., P. Sun, F. Liu, C. Fainman, J. Dimsdale, P.J. Mills, and M.G. Ziegler, A comparison of pharmacologic and spontaneous baroreflex methods in aging and hypertension. *J. Hypertens.*, 2009;**27**: 1243–1251.

597. Kornet, L., A.P. Hoeks, B.J. Janssen, A.J. Houben, P.W. De Leeuw, and R.S. Reneman, Neural activity of the cardiac baroreflex decreases with age in normotensive and hypertensive subjects. *J. Hypertens.*, 2005;**23**: 815–823.

598. James, M.A., T.G. Robinson, R.B. Panerai, and J.F. Potter, Arterial baroreceptor-cardiac reflex sensitivity in the elderly. *Hypertension*, 1996;**28**: 953–960.

599. Gerritsen, J., B.J. TenVoorde, J.M. Dekker, R. Kingma, P.J. Kostense, L.M. Bouter, and R.M. Heethaar, Measures of cardiovascular autonomic nervous function: agreement,

600. reproducibility, and reference values in middle age and elderly subjects. *Diabetologia*, 2003;**46**: 330–338.

600. Fauvel, J-P, C. Cerutti, I. Mpio, and M. Duchr, Aging process on spectrally determined spontanus baroreflex sensitivity. A 5-year prospective study. *Hypertension*, 2007;**50**: 543–546.

601. Schwab, J.O., G. Eichner, N. Shlevkov, J. Schrickel, A. Yang, O. Balta, T. Lewalter, B. Lüderitz, Impact of age and basic heart rate on heart rate turbulence in healthy persons. *Pacing. Clin. Electrophysiol.*, 2005;**28** (Suppl 1): S198–201.

602. Kowalewski, M., M. Alifier, D. Bochen, and M. Urban, Heart rate turbulence in children–age and heart rate relationships. *Pediatr. Res.*, 2007;**62**: 710–714.

603. Burke, J.H., J.J. Goldberger, F.A. Ehlert, J.T. Kruse, M.A. Parker, and A.H. Kadish, Gender differences in heart rate before and after autonomic blockade: evidence against an intrinsic gender effect. *Am. J. Med.*, 1996;**100** (5): 537–543.

604. Busha, B.F., E. Hage, and C. Hofmann, Gender and breathing route modulate cardio-respiratory variability in humans. *Respir. Physiol. Neurobiol.*, 2009;**166**: 87–94.

605. Aitken, M.L., J.L. Franklin, D.J. Pierson, and R.B. Schoene, Influence of body size and gender on control of ventilation. *J. Appl. Physiol.*, 1986;**60**: 1894–1899.

606. White, D.P., N.J. Douglas, C.K. Pickett, J.V. Weil, and C.W. Zwillich, Sexual influence on the control of breathing. *J. Appl. Physiol.*, 1983;**54**: 874–879.

607. Sato, N., S. Miyake, J. Akatsu, and M. Kumashiro, Power spectral analysis of heart rate variability in healthy young women during the normal menstrual cycle. *Psychosom. Med.*, 1995;**57**: 331–335.

608. Vallejo, M., M.F. Márquez, V.H. Borja-Aburto, M. Cárdenas, and A.G. Hermosillo, Age, body mass index, and menstrual cycle influence young women's heart rate variability –a multivariable analysis. *Clin. Auton. Res.*, 2005;**15**: 292–298.

609. Felber Dietrich, D., C. Schindler, J. Schwartz, J.C. Barthélémy, J.M. Tschopp, F. Roche, A. von Eckardstein, O. Brändli, P. Leuenberger, D.R. Gold, J.M. Gaspoz, U. Ackermann-Liebrich, and SAPALDIA Team, Heart rate variability in an ageing population and its association with lifestyle and cardiovascular risk factors: results of the SAPALDIA study. *Europace*, 2006;**8**: 521–529.

610. Grossman, P., F.H. Wilhelm, I. Kawachi, and D. Sparrow, Gender differences in psychophysiological responses to speech stress among older social phobics: congruence and incongruence between self-evaluative and cardiovascular reactions. *Psychosom. Med.*, 2001;**63**: 765–777.

611. Dishman, R.K., Y. Nakamura, M.E. Garcia, R.W. Thompson, A.L. Dunn, and S.N. Blair, Heart rate variability, trait anxiety, and perceived stress among physically fit men and women. *Int. J. Psychophysiol.*, 2000;**37**: 121–133.

612. Hinojosa-Laborde, C., I. Chapa, D. Lange, and J.R. Haywood, Gender differences in sympathetic nervous system regulation. *Clin. Exp. Pharmacol. Physiol.*, 1999;**26**: 122–126.

613. Insulander, P. and H. Vallin, Gender differences in electrophysiologic effects of mental stress and autonomic tone inhibition: a study in health individuals. *J. Cardiovasc. Electrophysiol.*, 2005;**16**: 59–63.

614. Fagard, R.H., K. Pardaens, J.A. Staessen, and L. Thijs, Power spectral analysis of heart rate variability by autoregressive modelling and fast Fourier transform: a comparative study. *Acta. Cardiol.*, 1998;**53**: 211–218.

615. Colhoun, H.M., D.P. Francis, M.B. Rubens, S.R. Underwood, and J.H. Fuller, The association of heart-rate variability with

cardiovascular risk factors and coronary artery calcification: a study in type 1 diabetic patients and the general population. *Diabetes. Care.*, 2001;**24**: 1108–1114.

616. Sloan, R.P., M.H. Huang, H. McCreath, S. Sidney, K. Liu, O. Dale Williams, T. Seeman, Cardiac autonomic control and the effects of age, race, and sex: the CARDIA study. *Auton. Neurosci.*, 2008;**139**: 78–85.

617. Jensen-Urstad, K., N. Storck, F. Bouvier, M. Ericson, L.E. Lindblad, and M. Jensen-Urstad Heart rate variability in healthy subjects is related to age and gender. *Acta. Physiol. Scand.*, 1997;**160**: 235–241.

618. Yamasaki, Y., M. Kodama, M. Matsuhisa, M. Kishimoto, H. Ozaki, A. Tani, N. Ueda, Y. Ishida, and T. Kamada, Diurnal heart rate variability in healthy subjects: effects of aging and sex difference. *Am. J. Physiol.*, 1996;**271**: H303–310.

619. Antelmi, I., R.S. de Paula, A.R. Shinzato, C.A. Peres, A.J. Mansur, and C.J. Grupi, Influence of age, gender, body mass index, and functional capacity on heart rate variability in a cohort of subjects without heart disease. *Am. J. Cardiol.*, 2004;**93**: 381–385.

620. Barantke, M., T. Krauss, J. Ortak, W. Lieb, M. Reppel, C. Burgdorf, P.P. Pramstaller, H. Schunkert, and H. Bonnemeier, Effects of gender and aging on diffential autonomic responses to orthostatic maneuvers. *J. Cardiovasc. Electrophysiol.*, 2008;**19**: 1296–1303.

621. Abdel-Rahman, A.R., R.H. Merrill, and W.R. Wooles, Gender-related differences in the baroreceptor reflex control of heart rate in normotensive humans. *J. Appl. Physiol.*, 1994;**77**: 606–613.

622. Convertino, V.A., Gender differences in autonomic functions associated with blood pressure regulation. *Am. J. Physiol.*, 1998;**275**: R1909–1920.

623. Ylitalo, A., K.E. Airaksinen, A. Hautanen, M. Kupari, M. Carson, J. Virolainen, M. Savolainen, H. Kauma, Y.A. Kesäniemi, P.C. White, and H.V. Huikuri, Baroreflex sensitivity and variants of the renin angiotensin system genes. *J. Am. Coll. Cardiol.*, 2000;**35**: 194–200.

624. Beske, S.D., G.E. Alvarez, T.P. Ballard, and K.P. Davy, Gender difference in cardiovagal baroreflex gain in humans. *J. Appl. Physiol.*, 2001;**91**: 2088–2092.

625. Luzier, A.B., J.J. Nawarskas, J. Añonuevo, M.E. Wilson, and D.J. Kazierad, The effects of gender on adrenergic receptor responsiveness. *J. Clin. Pharmacol.*, 1998;**38**: 618–624.

626. Tank, J., A. Diedrich, E. Szczech, F.C. Luft, and J. Jordan, Baroreflex regulation of heart rate and sympathetic vasomotor tone in women and men. *Hypertension*, 2005;**45**: 1159–1164.

627. Sevre, K., J.D. Lefrandt, G. Nordby, I. Os, M. Mulder, R.O. Gans, M. Rostrup, and A.J. Smit, Autonomic function in hypertensive and normotensive subjects: the importance of gender. *Hypertension*, 2001;**37**: 1351–1356.

628. Wyndham, CHm., B. Metz, and A. Munro, Reactions to heat of Arabs and Caucasians. *J. Appl. Physiol.*, 1964;**19**: 1051–1054.

629. Cooper, R.S. and J.K. Ghali, Coronary heart disease: black-white differences. *Cardiovasc. Clin.*, 1991;**21**: 205–225.

630. Watson, K.E. and E.J. Topol, Pathobiology of atherosclerosis: are there racial and ethnic differences? *Rev. Cardiovasc. Med.*, 2004;**5** (Suppl 3): S14–21.

631. Saunders, E. and E. Ofili, Epidemiology of atherothrombotic disease and the effectiveness and risks of antiplatelet therapy: race and ethnicity considerations. *Cardiol. Rev.*, 2008;**16**: 82–88.

632. Macfarlane, P.W., S.C. McLaughlin, B. Devine, and T.F. Yang, Effects of age, sex, and race on ECG interval measurements. *J. Electrocardiol.*, 1994;**27** (Suppl): 14–19.

633. Ogueh, O. and P.J. Steer, Ethnicity and fetal heart rate variation. *Obstet. Gynecol.*, 1998;**91**: 324–328.

634. Schachter, J., J.L. Kerr, F.C. 3rd Wimberly, and JM 3rd Lachin, Phasic heart rate responses: different patterns in black and in white newborns. *Psychosom. Med.*, 1975;**37**: 326–332.

635. Du Plooy, W.J. and C.P. Venter, The effect of atropine on parasympathetic control of respiratory sinus arrhythmia in two ethnic groups. *J. Clin. Pharmacol.*, 1995;**35**: 244–249.

636. Guzzetti, S., J. Mayet, M. Shahi, S. Mezzetti, R.A. Foale, P.S. Sever, N.R. Poulter, A. Porta, A. Malliani, and S.A. Thom, Absence of sympathetic overactivity in Afro-Caribbean hypertensive subjects studied by heart rate variability. *J. Hum. Hypertens.*, 2000;**14**: 337–342.

637. Thayer, J.F., M.M. Merritt, JJ 3rd Sollers, A.B. Zonderman, M.K. Evans, S. Yie, and D.R. Abernethy, Effect of angiotensin-converting enzyme insertion/deletion polymorphism DD genotype on high-frequency heart rate variability in African Americans. *Am. J. Cardiol.*, 2003;**92**: 1487–1490.

638. Wang, X., J.F. Thayer, F. Treiber, and H. Snieder, Ethnic differences and heritability of heart rate variability in African- and European American youth. *Am. J. Cardiol.*, 2005;**96**: 1166–1172.

639. Lampert, R., J. Ickovics, R. Horwitz, and F. Lee, Depressed autonomic nervous system function in African Americans and individuals of lower social class: a potential mechanism of race- and class-related disparities in health outcomes. *Am. Heart. J.*, 2005;**150**: 153–160.

640. Utsey, S.O. and J.N. Hook, Heart rate variability as a physiological moderator of the relationship between race-related stress and psychological distress in African Americans. *Cultur. Divers. Ethnic. Minor. Psychol.*, 2007;**13**: 250–253.

641. Zion, A.S., V. Bond, R.G. Adams, D. Williams, R.E. Fullilove, R.P. Sloan, M.N. Bartels, J.A. Downey, and R.E. De Meersman, Low arterial compliance in young African-American males. *Am. J. Physiol. Heart. Circ. Physiol.*, 2003;**285**: H457–462.

642. Franke, W.D., K. Lee, D.B. Buchanan, and J.P. Hernandez, Blacks and whites differ in responses, but not tolerance, to orthostatic stress. *Clin. Auton. Res.*, 2004;**14**: 19–25.

643. Keyl, C., A. Schneider, R.E. Greene, C. Passino, G. Spadacini, G. Bandinelli, M. Bonfichi, L. Arcaini, L. Malcovati, and L. Bernardi, Effects of breathing control on cardiocirculatory modulation in Caucasian lowlanders and Himalayan Sherpas. *Eur. J. Appl. Physiol.*, 2000;**83**: 481–486.

644. Pelat, M., R. Verwaerde, C. Merial, J. Galitzky, M. Berlan, J.L. Montastruc, J.M. Senard, Impaired atrial M(2)-cholinoceptor function in obesity-related hypertension. *Hypertension*, 1999;**34**: 1066–1072.

645. Paolisso, G., D. Manzella, N. Montano, A. Gambardella, and M. Varricchio, Plasma leptin concentrations and cardiac autonomic nervous system in healthy subjects with different body weights. *J. Clin. Endocrinol. Metab.*, 2000;**85**: 1810–1814.

646. Martini, G., P. Riva, F. Rabbia, V. Molini, G.B. Ferrero, F. Cerutti, R. Carra, and F. Veglio. Heart rate variability in childhood obesity. *Clin. Auton. Res.*, 2001;**11**: 87–91.

647. Li, Z., H. Snieder, S. Su, X. Ding, J.F. Thayer, F.A. Treiber, and X. Wang, A longitudinal study in youth of heart rate variability at rest and in response to stress. *Int. J. Psychophysiol.*, 2009;**73**: 212–217.

648. Kuch, B., H.W. Hense, R. Sinnreich, J.D. Kark, A. von Eckardstein, D. Sapoznikov, and H.D. Bolte, Determinants of short-period heart rate variability in the general population. *Cardiology*, 2001;**95**: 131–138.

649. Liao, D., J. Cai, W.D. Rosamond, R.W. Barnes, R.G. Hutchinson, E.A. Whitsel, P. Rautaharju, and G. Heiss, Cardiac autonomic function and incident coronary heart disease: a population-based case-cohort study. The ARIC Study. Atherosclerosis Risk in Communities Study. *Am. J. Epidemiol.*, 1997;**145**: 696–706.

650. De Bruyne, M.C., J.A. Kors, A.W. Hoes, P. Klootwijk, J.M. Dekker, A. Hofman, J.H. van Bemmel, and D.E Grobbee, Both decreased and increased heart rate variability on the standard 10-second electrocardiogram predict cardiac mortality in the elderly: the Rotterdam Study. *Am. J. Epidemiol.*, 1999;**150**: 1282–1288.

651. Stolarz, K., J.A. Staessen, T. Kuznetsova, V. Tikhonoff, D. State, S. Babeanu, E. Casiglia, R.H. Fagard, K. Kawecka-Jaszcz, and Y. Nikitin, European Project on Genes in Hypertension (EPOGH) Investigators. Host and environmental determinants of heart rate and heart rate variability in four European populations. *J. Hypertens.*, 2003;**21**: 525–535.

652. Byrne, E.A., J.L. Fleg, P.V. Vaitkevicius, J. Wright, and S.W. Porges, Role of aerobic capacity and body mass index in the age-associated decline in heart rate variability. *J. Appl. Physiol.*, 1996;**81**: 743–750.

653. Ziegler, D., C. Zentai, S. Perz, W. Rathmann, B. Haastert, C. Meisinger, H. Löwel, and KORA Study Group, Selective contribution of diabetes and other cardiovascular risk factors to cardiac autonomic dysfunction in the general population. *Exp. Clin. Endocrinol. Diabetes.*, 2006;**114**: 153–159.

654. Fagard, R.H., K. Pardaens, and J.A. Staessen, Influence of demographic, anthropometric and lifestyle characteristics on heart rate and its variability in the population. *J. Hypertens.*, 1999;**17**: 1589–1599.

655. Greiser, K.H., A. Kluttig, B. Schumann, C.A. Swenne, J.A. Kors, O. Kuss, J. Haerting, H. Schmidt, J. Thiery, and K. Werdan, Cardiovascular diseases, risk factors and short-term heart rate variability in an elderly general population: the CARLA study 2002–2006. *Eur. J. Epidemiol.*, 2009;**24**: 123–142.

656. Hirsch, J., R.L. Leibel, R. Mackintosh, and A. Aguirre, Heart rate variability as a measure of autonomic function during weight change in humans. *Am. J. Physiol.*, 1991;**261**: R1418–1423.

657. Zahorska-Markiewicz, B., E. Kuagowska, C. Kucio, and M. Klin, Heart rate variability in obesity. *Int. J. Obes. Relat. Metab. Disord.*, 1993;**17**: 21–23.

658. Karason, K., H. Mølgaard, J. Wikstrand, and L. Sjöström, Heart rate variability in obesity and the effect of weight loss. *Am. J. Cardiol.*, 1999;**83**: 1242–1247.

659. Poirier, P., T. Hernandez, K. Weil, T. Shepard, and R. Eckel, Impact of diet-induced weight loss on the cardiac autonomic nervous system in severe obesity. *Obes. Res.*, 2003;**11**: 1040–1047.

660. Nault, I., E. Nadreau, C. Paquet, P. Brassard, P. Marceau, S. Marceau, S. Biron, F. Hould, S. Lebel, D. Richard, and P. Poirier, Impact of bariatric surgery–induced weight loss on heart rate variability. *Metabolism*, 2007;**56**: 1425–1430.

661. Bobbioni-Harsch, E., J. Sztajzel, V. Barthassat, V. Makoundou, G. Gastaldi, K. Sievert, G. Chassot, O. Huber, P. Morel, F. Assimacopoulos-Jeannet, and A. Golay, Independent evolution of heart autonomic function and insulin sensitivity during weight loss. *Obesity*, 2009;**17**: 247–253.

662. Skrapari, I., N. Tentolouris, D. Perrea, C. Bakoyiannis, A. Papazafiropoulou, and N. Katsilambros, Baroreflex sensitivity in obesity: relationship with cardiac autonomic nervous system activity. *Obesity*, 2007;**15**: 1685–1693.

663. Laederach-Hofmann, K., L. Mussgay, and H. Rúddel, Autonomic cardiovascular regulation in obesity. *J. Endocrinol.*, 2000;**164**: 59–66.

664. Beske, S.D., G.E. Alvarez, T.P. Ballard, and K.P. Davy, Reduced cardiovagal baroreflex gain in visceral obesity: implications for the metabolic syndrome. *Am. J. Physiol. Heart Circ. Physiol.*, 2002;**282**: H630–635.

665. Grassi, G., G. Seravalle, M. Colombo, G. Bolla, B.M. Cattaneo, F. Cavagnini, and G. Mancia, Body weight reduction, sympathetic nerve traffic, and arterial baroreflex in obese normotensive humans. *Circulation*, 1998;**97**: 2037–2042.

666. Alvarez, G.E., B.M. Davy, T.P. Ballard, S.D. Beske, and K.P. Davy, Weight loss increases cardiovagal baroreflex function in obese young and older men. *Am. J. Physiol. Endocrinol. Metab.*, 2005;**289**: E665–669.

667. Avsar, A., G. Acarturk, M. Melek, C. Kilit, A. Celik, and E. Onrat, Cardiac autonomic function evaluated by the heart rate turbulence method was not changed in obese patients without co-morbidities. *J. Korean. Med. Sci.*, 2007;**22**: 629–632.

668. Coumel, P., P. Maison-Blanche, and D. Catuli, Heart rate and heart rate variability in normal young adults. *J. Cardiovasc. Electrophysiol.*, 1994;**5**: 899–911.

669. Rosenblueth, A. and F.A. Simeone, The interrelations of vagal and accelerator effects on the cardiac rate. *Am. J. Physiol.*, 1934, **110**: 42–45.

670. Bootsma, M., C.A. Swenne, H.H. Van Bolhuis, P.C. Chang, V.M. Cats, A.V. Bruschke, Heart rate and heart rate variability as indexes of sympathovagal balance. *Am. J. Physiol. Heart. Cric. Physiol.*, 1994;**266**: H1565–1571.

671. Goldberger, J.J., M.W. Ahmed, M.A. Parker, and A.H. Kadish, Dissociation of heart rate variability from parasympathetic tone. *Am. J. Physiol. Heart. Circ. Physiol.*, 1994;**266**: H2152–2157.

672. Ahmed, M.W., A.H. Kadish, M.A. Parker, and J.J. Goldberger,. Effect of physiologic and pharmacologic adrenergic stimulation on heart rate variability. *J. Am. Coll. Cardiol.*, 1994;**24**: 1082–1090.

673. Goldberger, J.J., Y.H. Kim, M.W. Ahmed, and A.H. Kadish, Effect of graded increases in parasympathetic tone on heart rate variability. *J. Cardiovasc. Electrophysiol.*, 1996;**7**: 594–602.

674. Kim, Y.H., M.W. Ahmed, A.H. Kadish, and J.J. Goldberger, Characterization of the factors that determine the effect of sympathetic stimulation on heart rate variability. *Pacing. Clin. Electrophysiol.*, 1997;**20**: 1936–1946.

675. Goldberger, J.J., S. Challapalli, R. Tung, M.A. Parker, and A.H. Kadish, Relationship of heart rate variability to parasympathetic effect. *Circulation*, 2001;**103**: 1977–1983.

676. Opthof, T. and R. Coronel, The normal range and determinants of the intrinsic heart rate in man. *Cardiovasc. Res.*, 2000;**45**: 175–176.

677. Jose, A.D., Effect of combined sympathetic and parasympathetic blockade on heart rate and cardiac function in man. *Am. J. Cardiol.*, 1966;**18**: 476–478.

678. Frick, M.H., J. Heikkilä, and A. Kahanpää, Combined parasympathetic and beta-receptor blockade as a clinical test. *Acta. Med. Scand.*, 1967;**182**: 621–628.

679. Jose, A.D. and R.R. Taylor, Autonomic blockade by propranolol and atropine to study intrinsic myocardial function in man. *J. Clin. Invest.*, 1969;**48**: 2019–2031.

680. Alboni, P., C. Malacarne, P. Pedroni, A. Masoni, and O.S. Narula, Electrophysiology of normal sinus node with and without autonomic blockade. *Circulation*, 1982;**65**: 1236–1242.

681. Marcus, B., P.C. Gillette, and A. Garson, Intrinsic heart rate in children and young adults: an index of sinus node function isolated from autonomic control. *Am. Heart. J.*, 1990;**119**: 911–916.

682. Burke, J.H., J.J. Goldberger, F.A. Ehlert, J.T. Kruse, M.A. Parker, and A.H. Kadish, Gender differences in heart rate before and after autonomic blockade: evidence against an intrinsic gender effect. *Am. J. Med.*, 1996;**100**: 537–543.

683. Craft, N. and J.B. Schwartz, Effects of age on intrinsic heart rate, heart rate variability, and AV conduction in healthy humans. *Am. J. Physiol. Heart. Circ. Physiol.*, 1995;**268**: H1441–1452.

684. Jokkel, G., I. Bonyhay, and M. Kollai, Heart rate variability after complete autonomic blockade in man. *J. Auton. Nerv. Syst.*, 1995;**51**: 85–89.

685. Wollenberger, A. and J. Jehl, Influence of age on rate of respiration of sliced cardiac muscle. *Am. J. Physiol.*, 1952;**170**: 126–130.

686. Evans, J.M., D.C. Randall, J.N. Funk, and C.F. Knapp, Influence of cardiac innervations on intrinsic heart rate in dogs. *Am. J. Physiol. Heart. Circ. Physiol.*, 1990;**258**: H1132–1137.

687. Miyazaki, T., H.P. Pride, and D.P. Zipes, Prostaglandins in the pericardial fluid modulate neural regulation of cardiac electrophysiological properties. *Circ. Res.*, 1990;**66**: 163–175.

688. Marin-Neto, J.A., J.J. Carneiro, B.C. Maciel, A.L. Secches, L. Gallo Jr., J. Terra-Filho, J.C. Manço, E.C. Lima-Filho, W.V. Vicente, A.A. Sader, et al., Impairment of baroreflex control of the sinoatrial node after cardiac operations with extracorporeal circulation in man. *J. Thorac. Cardiovasc. Surg.*, 1983;**86**: 718–726.

689. Sosnowski, M., T. Petelenz, Z. Czyż, S. Woś, B. Białkowska, B. Grzybek, Noninvasive evaluation of autonomic control of heart rate in patients with mitral valvular disease treated surgically (authors' material, Petelenz T [Ed], Mitral valve disease: an old disease and modern medicine, Medical University of Silesia, 1992).

690. Niemelä, M.J., K.E. Airaksinen, K.U. Tahvanainen, M.K. Linnaluoto, and J.T. Takkunen, Effect of coronary artery bypass grafting on cardiac parasympathetic nervous function. *Eur. Heart. J.*, 1992;**13**: 932–935.

691. Petelenz, T., K. Singer, B. Gabrylewicz, T. Twardela, T. Pawłowski, S. Woś, M. Sosnowski, and Z. Nowak, Effect of aorto-coronary by-pass grafting on ventricular function assessed by means of noninvasive evalation in a 2-year follow-up. *Pol. Tyg. Lek.*, 1993;**48**: 681–685 (*in Polish*).

692. Tuinenburg, A.E., I.C. Van Gelder, M.P. Van Den Berg, J.G. Grandjean, R.G. Tieleman, A.J. Smit, R.C. Huet, J.M. Van Der Maaten, C.P. Volkers, T. Ebels, and H.J. Crijns, Sinus node function after cardiac surgery: is impairment specific for the maze procedure? *Int. J. Cardiol.*, 2004;**95**: 101–108.

693. Davila, D.F., C.F. Gottberg, J.H. Donis, A. Torres, A.J. Fuenmayor, and O. Rossell, Vagal stimulation and heart rate slowing in acute experimental chagasic myocarditis. *J. Auton. Nerv. Syst.*, 1988;**25**: 233–234.

694. Gao, X., L. Peng, Q. Zeng, and Z.K. Wu, Autonomic nervous function and arrhythmias in patients with acute viral myocarditis during a 6-month follow-up period. *Cardiology*, 2009;**113**: 66–71.

695. Jinbo, Y., Y. Kobayashi, A. Miyata, K. Chiyoda, H. Nakagawa, K. Tanno, K. Kurano, S. Kikushima, T. Baba, and T. Katagiri, Decreasing parasympathetic tone activity and proarrhythmic effect after radiofrequency catheter ablation–differences in ablation site. *Jpn. Circ. J.*, 1998;**62**: 733–740.

696. Miyanaga, S., T. Yamane, T. Date, M. Tokuda, Y. Aramaki, K. Inada, K. Shibayama, S. Matsuo, H. Miyazaki, K. Abe, K. Sugimoto, S. Mochizuki, and M. Yoshimura, Impact of pulmonary vein isolation on the autonomic modulation in patients with paroxysmal atrial fibrillation and prolonged sinus pauses. *Europace*, 2009;**11**: 576–581.

697. Sosnowski, M., T. Petelenz, and Z. Czyz, Patterns of non-linear heart rate behaviour in sinoatrial node dysfunction: effects of orthostatic test and autonomic blockade. *Comput. Cardiol.*, 1993: 5–8.

698. Bernardi, L., F. Valle, S. Leuzzi, M. Rinaldi, E. Marchesi, C. Falcone, L. Martinelli, M. Viganò, G. Finardi, and A. Radaelli, Non-respiratory components of heart rate variability in heart transplant recipients: evidence of autonomic reinnervation? *Clin. Sci.*, 1994;**86**: 537–545.

699. Jose, A.D., F. Stitt, and D. Collison, The effects of exercise and changes in body temperature on the intrinsic heart rate in man. *Am. Heart. J.*, 1970;**79**: 488–498.

700. Julu, P.O. and R.G. Hondo, Effects of atropine on autonomic indices based on electrocardiographic R-R intervals in healthy volunteers. *J. Neurol. Neurosurg. Psychiatr.*, 1992;**55**: 31–35.

701. Hayano, J., Y. Sakakibara, A. Yamada, M. Yamada, S. Mukai, T. Fujinami, K. Yokoyama, Y. Watanabe, and K. Takata, Accuracy of assessment of cardiac vagal tone by heart rate variability in normal subjects. *Am. J. Cardiol.*, 1991;**67**: 199–204.

702. Pierpont, G.L. and E.J. Voth, Assessing autonomic function by analysis of heart rate recovery from exercise in healthy subjects. *Am. J. Cardiol.*, 2004;**94**: 64–68.

703. Furlan, R., S. Guzzetti, W. Crivellaro, S. Dassi, M. Tinelli, G. Baselli, S. Cerutti, F. Lombardi, M. Pagani, and A. Malliani, Continuous 24-hour assessment of the neural regulation of systemic arterial pressure and RR variabilities in ambulant subjects. *Circulation*, 1990;**81**: 537–547.

704. Adamson, P.B., M.H. Huang, E. Vanoli, R.D. Foreman, P.J. Schwartz, and S.S. Jr.Hull, Unexpected interaction between beta-adrenergic blockade and heart rate variability before and after myocardial infarction. A longitudinal study in dogs at high and low risk for sudden death. *Circulation*, 1994;**90**: 976–982.

705. Rodriguez, R.D. and D.D. Schocken, Update on sick sinus syndrome, a cardiac disorder of aging. *Geriatrics*, 1990;**45**: 26–30, 33–6.

706. Abildstrom, S.Z., B.T. Jensen, E. Agner, C. Torp-Pedersen, O. Nyvad, K. Wachtell, M.M. Ottesen, J.K. Kanters and BEAT Study Group, Heart rate versus heart rate variability in risk prediction after myocardial infarction. *J. Cardiovasc. Electrophysiol.*, 2003;**14**: 168–173.

707. Goto, M., M. Nagashima, R. Baba, Y. Nagano, M. Yokota, K. Nishibata, and A. Tsuji, Analysis of heart rate variability demonstrates effects of development on vagal modulation of heart rate in healthy children. *J. Pediatr.*, 1997;**130**: 725–729.

708. Pagani, M., G. Mazzuero, A. Ferrari, D. Liberati, S. Cerutti, D. Vaitl, L. Tavazzi, and A. Malliani, Sympathovagal interaction

during mental stress. A study using spectral analysis of heart rate variability in healthy control subjects and patients with a prior myocardial infarction. *Circulation*, 1991;**83** (4 Suppl): II43–51.

709. Chiu, H.W., T.H. Wang, L.C. Huang, H.W. Tso, and T. Kao, The influence of mean heart rate on measures of heart rate variability as markers of autonomic function: a model study. *Med. Eng. Phys.*, 2003;**25**: 475–481.

710. Eaton, G.M., R.J. Cody, E. Nunziata, and P.F. Binkley, Early left ventricular dysfunction elicits activation of sympathetic drive and attenuation of parasympathetic tone in the paced canine model of congestive heart failure. *Circulation*, 1995;**92**: 555–561.

711. Sosnowski, M. and T. Petelenz, Heart rate variability. Is it influenced by disturbed sinoatrial node function? *J. Electrocardiol.*, 1995;**28**: 245–251.

712. Panina, G., U.N. Khot, E. Nunziata, R.J. Cody, and P.F. Binkley, Assessment of autonomic tone over a 24-hour period in patients with congestive heart failure: relation between mean heart rate and measures of heart rate variability. *Am. Heart. J.*, 1995;**129**: 748–753.

713. Vanninen, E., A. Tuunainen, M. Kansanen, M. Uusitupa, and E. Länsimies, Cardiac sympathovagal balance during sleep apnea episodes. *Clin. Physiol.*, 1996;**16**: 209–216.

714. Bauer, T., S. Ewig, H. Schäfer, E. Jelen, H. Omran, and B. Lüderitz, Heart rate variability in patients with sleep-related breathing disorders. *Cardiology*, 1996;**87**: 492–496.

715. Heinz, G., M. Hirschl, P. Buxbaum, G. Laufer, S. Gasic, and A. Laczkovics, Sinus node dysfunction after orthotopic cardiac transplantation: postoperative incidence and long-term implications. *Pacing. Clin. Electrophysiol.*, 1992;**15**: 731–737.

716. Scott, C.D., J.H. Dark, and J.M. McComb, Sinus node function after cardiac transplantation. *J. Am. Coll. Cardiol.*, 1994;**24**: 1334–1341.

717. Cohen, M.A. and J.A. Taylor, Short-term cardiovascular osllation in man: measuring and modeling the physiologies. *J. Physiol.*, 2002;**542**: 669–683.

718. Hirsch, J.A. and B. Bishop, Respiratory sinus arrhythmia in humans: how breathing pattern modulates heart rate. *Am. J. Physiol.*, 1981;**241**: H620–629.

719. Grossman, P. and M. Kollai, Respiratory sinus arrhythmia, cardiac vagal tone, and respiration: within- and between-individual relations. *Psychophysiology*, 1993;**30**: 486–495.

720. Eckberg, D.L., Human sinus arrhythmia as an index of vagal cardiac outflow. *J. Appl. Physiol.*, 1983;**54**: 961–966.

721. Hayano, J., Y. Sakakibara, A. Yamada, M. Yamada, S. Mukai, T. Fujinami, K. Yokoyama, Y. Watanabe, and K. Takata, Accuracy of assessment of cardiac vagal tone by heart rate variability in normal subjects. *Am. J. Cardiol.*, 1991;**67**: 199–204.

722. Malpas, S.C., Neural influences on cardiovascular variability: possibility and pitfalls. *Am. J. Physiol. Heart. Circ. Physiol.*, 2002;**282**: H6–20.

723. Grossman, P., F.H. Wilhelm, and M. Spoerle, Respiratory sinus arrhythmia, cardiac vagal control, and daily activity. *Am. J. Physiol. Heart. Circ. Physiol.*, 2004;**287**: H728–734.

724. Houtveen, J.H., S. Rietveld, and E.J. de Geus, Contribution of tonic vagal modulation of heart rate, central respiratory drive, respiratory depth, and respiratory frequency to respiratory sinus arrhythmia during mental stress and physical exercise. *Psychophysiology*, 2002;**39**: 427–436.

725. Ewing, D.J., D.Q. Borsey, F. Bellavere, and B.F. Clarke, Cardiac autonomic neuropathy in diabetes: comparison of measures of R-R interval variation. *Diabetologia*, 1981;**21**: 18–24.

726. Löllgen, D., M. Müeck-Weymann, and R.D. Beise, The deep breathing test: median-based expiration-inspiration difference is the measure of choice. *Muscle. Nerve.*, 2009;**39**: 536–544.

727. Grossman, P., J. Karemaker, and W. Wieling, Prediction of tonic parasympathetic cardiac control using respiratory sinus arrhythmia: the need for respiratory control. *Psychophysiology*, 1991;**28**: 201–216.

728. Sosnowski, M., J. Skrzypek-Wańha, Z. Czyż, B. Korzeniowska, and M. Tendera, Respiratory rate-heart rate interaction is responsible for reduced heart rate variability in patients with coronary heart disease and depressed left ventricular systolic function. *Eur. Heart. J.*, 1997;**18** (Suppl.): 575 (abstr).

729. Saul, J.P., R.D. Berger, M.H. Chen, and R.J. Cohen, Transfer function analysis of autonomic regulation. II. Respiratory sinus arrhythmia. *Am. J. Physiol.*, 1989;**256**: H153–161.

730. El-Omar, M., A. Kardos, and B. Casadei, Mechanisms of respiratory sinus arrhythmia in patients with mild heart failure. *Am. J. Physiol. Heart. Circ. Physiol.*, 2001;**280**: H125–131.

731. Mortara, A., P. Sleight, G.D. Pinna, R. Maestri, A. Prpa, M.T. La Rovere, F. Cobelli, and L. Tavazzi, Abnormal awake respiratory patterns are common in chronic heart failure and may prevent evaluation of autonomic tone by measures of heart rate variability. *Circulation*, 1997;**96**: 246–252.

732. Shiomi, T., C. Guilleminault, R. Sasanabe, I. Hirota, M. Maekawa, and T. Kobayashi, Augmented very low frequency component of heart rate variability during obstructive sleep apnea. *Sleep*, 1996;**19**: 370–377.

733. Ponikowski, P., T.P. Chua, A.A. Amadi, M. Piepoli, D. Harrington, M. Volterrani, R. Colombo, G. Mazzuero, A. Giordano, and A.J. Coats, Detection and significance of a discrete very low frequency rhythm in RR interval variability in chronic congestive heart failure. *Am. J. Cardiol.*, 1996;**77**: 1320–1326.

734. Tateishi, O., T. Shouda, Y. Honda, T. Sakai, S. Mochizuki, and K. Machida, Apnea-related heart rate variability and its clinical utility in congestive heart failure outpatients. *Ann. Noninvasive. Electrocardiol.*, 2002;**7**: 127–132.

735. Perakakis, P., M. Taylor, E. Martinez-Nieto, I. Revithi, and J. Vila, Breathing frequency bias in fractal analysis of heart rate variability. *Biol. Psychol.*, 2009;**82**: 82–88.

736. Casadei, B., J. Moon, A. Caiazza, and P. Sleight, Is respiratory sinus arrhythmia a good index of cardiac vagal activity during exercise? *J. Appl. Physiol.*, 1996;**81**: 556–564.

737. Ponikowski, P., T.P. Chua, M. Piepoli, W. Banasiak, S.D. Anker, R. Szelemej, W. Molenda, K. Wrabec, A. Capucci, and A.J. Coats, Ventilatory response to exercise correlates with impaired heart rate variability in patients with chronic congestive heart failure. *Am. J. Cardiol.*, 1998;**82**: 338–344.

738. Tzeng, Y.C., P.D. Larsen, and D.C. Galletly, Cardioventilatory coupling in resting human subjects. *Exp. Physiol.*, 2003;**88**: 775–782.

739. Fallen, E.L. and M.V. Kamath, Circadian rhythms of heart rate variability, in *Heart Rate Variability*, M. Malik and A.J. Camm, Editors. Armonk, NY: Futura Publishing, 1995, pp. 293–309.

740. Hartikainen, J., I. Tarkiainen, K. Tahvanainen, M. Mäntysaari, E. Länsimies, and K. Pyörälä, Circadian variation of cardiac autonomic regulation during 24-h bed rest. *Clin. Physiol.*, 1993;**13**: 185–196.

741. Freitas, J., P. Lago, J. Puig, M.J. Carvalho, O. Costa, and A.F. de Freitas, Circadian heart rate variability rhythm in shift workers. *J. Electrocardiol.*, 1997;**30**: 39–44.

742. Zhong, X., H.J. Hilton, G.J. Gates, S. Jelic, Y. Stern, M.N. Bartels, R.E. DeMeersman, and R.C. Basner, Increased sympathetic and decreased parasympathetic cardiovascular modulation in normal humans with acute sleep deprivation. *J. Appl. Physiol.*, 2005;**98**: 2024–2032.

743. Viola, A.U., L.M. James, S.N. Archer, and D.J. Dijk, PER3 polymorphism and cardiac autonomic control: effects of sleep debt and circadian phase. *Am. J. Physiol. Heart. Circ. Physiol.*, 2008;**295**: H2156–2163.

744. Vandewalle, G., B. Middleton, S.M. Rajaratnam, B.M. Stone, B. Thorleifsdottir, J. Arendt, and D.J. Dijk, Robust circadian rhythm in heart rate and its variability: influence of exogenous melatonin and photoperiod. *J. Sleep. Res.*, 2007;**16**: 148–155.

745. Hu, K., P.Ch. Ivanov, M.F. Hilton, Z. Chen, R.T. Ayers, H.E. Stanley, and S.A. Shea, Endogenous circadian rhythm in an index of cardiac vulnerability independent of changes in behavior. *Proc. Natl. Acad. Sci. U. S. A.*, 2004;**101**: 18223–18227.

746. Huikuri, H.V., M.J. Niemelä, S. Ojala, A. Rantala, M.J. Ikäheimo, and K.E. Airaksinen, Circadian rhythms of frequency domain measures of heart rate variability in healthy subjects and patients with coronary artery disease. Effects of arousal and upright posture. *Circulation*, 1994;**90**: 121–126.

747. Bernardi, L., L. Ricordi, P. Lazzari, P. Solda, A. Calciati, M.R. Ferrari, I.Vandea, G. Finardi, and P. Fratino, Impaired circadian modulation of sympathovagal activity in diabetes: a possible explanation for altered temporal onset of cardiovascular disease. *Circulation*, 1992;**86**: 1443–1452.

748. Lombardi, F., G. Sandrone, A. Mortara, M.T. La Rovere, E. Colombo, S. Guzzetti, and A. Malliani, Circadian variation of spectral indices of heart rate variability after myocardial infarction. *Am. Heart. J.*, 1992;**123**: 1521–1528.

749. Chakko, S., R.F. Mulingtapang, H.V. Huikuri, K.M. Kessler, B.J. Materson, and R.J. Myerburg, Alterations in heart rate variability and its circadian rhythm in hypertensive patients with left ventricular hypertrophy free of coronary artery disease. *Am. Heart. J.*, 1993;**126**: 1364–1372.

750. Malik, M., T. Farrell, and A.J. Camm, Circadian rhythm of heart rate variability after acute myocardial infarction and its influence on the prognostic value of heart rate variability. *Am. J. Cardiol.*, 1990;**66**: 1049–1054.

751. Burr, R., P. Hamilton, M. Cowan, A. Buzaitis, M.R. Strasser, A. Sulkhanova, and K. Pike, Nycthemeral profile of nonspectral heart rate variability measures in women and men. Description of a normal sample and two sudden cardiac arrest subsamples. *J. Electrocardiol.*, 1994;**27**(Suppl): 54–62.

752. Klingenheben, T., U. Rapp, and S.H. Hohnloser, Circadian variation of heart rate variability in postinfarction patients with and without life-threatening ventricular tachyarrhythmias. *J. Cardiovasc. Electrophysiol.*, 1995;**6**: 357–364.

753. Sarma, J.S., N. Singh, M.P. Schoenbaum, K. Venkataraman, and B.N. Singh, Circadian and power spectral changes of RR and QT intervals during treatment of patients with angina pectoris with nadolol providing evidence for differential autonomic modulation of heart rate and ventricular repolarization. *Am. J. Cardiol.*, 1994;**74**: 131–136.

754. Pagani, M., V. Somers, R. Furlan, S. Dell'Orto, J. Conway, G. Baselli, S. Ceruti, P. Sleight, and A. Malliani, Changes in autonomic regulation induced by physical training in mild hypertension. *Hypertension*, 1988;**12**: 600–610.

755. Seals, D.R. and P.B. Chase, Influence of physical training on heart rate variability and baroreflex circulatory control. *J. Appl. Physiol.*, 1989;**66**: 1886–1895.

756. Henje Blom, E., E.M. Olsson, E. Serlachius, M. Ericson, and M. Ingvar, Heart rate variability is related to self-reported physical activity in a healthy adolescent population. *Eur. J. Appl. Physiol.*, 2009;**106**: 877–883.

757. Rennie, K.L., H. Hemingway, M. Kumari, E. Brunner, M. Malik, and M. Marmot, Effects of moderate and vigorous physical activity on heart rate variability in a British study of civil servants. *Am. J. Epidemiol.*, 2003;**158**: 135–143.

758. Horsten, M., M. Ericson, A. Perski, S.P. Wamala, K. Schenck-Gustafsson, and K. Orth-Gomér, Psychosocial factors and heart rate variability in healthy women. *Psychosom. Med.*, 1999;**61**: 49–57.

759. De Meersman, R.E., Heart rate variability and aerobic fitness. *Am. Heart. J.*, 1993;**125**: 726–731.

760. Galetta, F., F. Franzoni, F.R. Femia, N. Roccella, F. Pentimone, and G. Santoro, Lifelong physical training prevents the age-related impairment of heart rate variability and exercise capacity in elderly people. *J. Sports. Med. Phys. Fitness.*, 2005;**45**: 217–221.

761. Boutcher, S.H. and P. Stein, Association between heart rate variability and training response in sedentary middle-aged men. *Eur. J. Appl. Physiol. Occup. Physiol.*, 1995;**70**: 75–80.

762. Davy, K.P., W.L. Willis, and D.R. Seals, Influence of exercise training on heart rate variability in post-menopausal women with elevated arterial blood pressure. *Clin. Physiol.*, 1997;**17**: 31–40.

763. Verheyden, B., B.O. Eijnde, F. Beckers, L. Vanhees, and A.E. Aubert, Low-dose exercise training does not influence cardiac autonomic control in healthy sedentary men aged 55–75 years. *J. Sports. Sci.*, 2006;**24**: 1137–1147.

764. Melanson, E.L. and P.S. Freedson, The effect of endurance training on resting heart rate variability in sedentary adult males. *Eur. J. Appl. Physiol.*, 2001;**85**: 442–449.

765. Soares-Miranda, L., G. Sandercock, H. Valente, S. Vale, R. Santos, and J. Mota, Vigorous physical activity and vagal modulation in young adults. *Eur. J. Cardiovasc. Prev. Rehabil.*, 2009 Sep 4. [Epub ahead of print].

766. Gamelin, F.X., G. Baquet, S. Berthoin, D. Thevenet, C. Nourry, S. Nottin, and L. Bosquet, Effect of high intensity intermittent training on heart rate variability in prepubescent children. *Eur. J. Appl. Physiol.*, 2009;**105**: 731–738.

767. Jurca, R., T.S. Church, G.M. Morss, A.N. Jordan, and C.P. Earnest, Eight weeks of moderate-intensity exercise training increases heart rate variability in sedentary postmenopausal women. *Am. Heart. J.*, 2004;**147**: e21.

768. Earnest, C.P., C.J. Lavie, S.N. Blair, and T.S. Church, Heart rate variability characteristics in sedentary postmenopausal women following six months of exercise training: the DREW study. *PLoS. One.*, 2008;**3**: e2288.

769. Melo, R.C., R.J. Quitério, A.C. Takahashi, E. Silva, L.E. Martins, and A.M. Catai. High eccentric strength training reduces heart rate variability in healthy older men. *Br. J. Sports. Med.*, 2008;**42**: 59–63.

770. Piotrowicz, E., R. Baranowski, M. Piotrowska, T. Zieliński, and R. Piotrowicz, Variable effects of physical training of heart rate variability, heart rate recovery, and heart rate turbulence in chronic heart failure. *Pacing. Clin. Electrophysiol.*, 2009;**32** (Suppl 1): S113–115.

771. Dewey, F.E., J.V. Freeman, G. Engel, R. Oviedo, N. Abrol, N. Ahmed, J. Myers, and V.F., Froelicher, Novel predictor of prognosis from exercise stress testing: heart rate variability response to the exercise treadmill test. *Am. Heart. J.*, 2007;**153**: 281–288.

772. Leino, J., M. Virtanen, M. Kähönen, K. Nikus, T. Lehtimäki, T. Kööbi, R. Lehtinen, V. Turjanmaa, J. Viik, and T. Nieminen, Exercise-test-related heart rate variability and mortality The Finnish cardiovascular study. *Int. J. Cardiol.*, 2009. [Epub ahead of print].

773. Cottin, F., C. Médigue, and Y. Papelier, Effect of heavy exercise on spectral baroreflex sensitivity, heart rate, and blood pressure variability in well-trained humans. *Am. J. Physiol. Heart. Circ. Physiol.*, 2008;**295**: H1150–1155.

774. Raven, P.B., P.J. Fadel, and S. Ogoh, Arterial baroreflex resetting during exercise: a current perspective. *Exp. Physiol.*, 2006;**91**: 37–49.

775. Raven, P.B., D. ROhm-Young, and C.G. Blomqvist, Physical fitness and cardiovascular response to lower body negative pressure. *J. Appl. Physiol.*, 1984;**56**: 138–144.

776. Mack, G.W., C.A. Thompson, D.F. Doerr, E.E. Nadel, and V.A. Conveertino, Diminished baroreflex control of forearm resistance following training. *Med. Sci. Sports. Exer.*, 1991;**23**: 1367–1374.

777. Lightfoot, J.T., R.P. Claytor, D.J. Torak, T.W. Journell, and S.W. Fortney, Ten weeks of aerobic training do not affect lower body negative pressure response. *J. Appl. Physiol.*, 1989;**67**: 894–901.

778. Bowman, A.J., R.H. Clayton, A. Murray, J.W. Reed, M.M. Subhan, and G.A. Ford, Effects of aerobic exercise training and yoga on the baroreflex in healthy elderly persons. *Eur. J. Clin. Invest.*, 1997;**27**: 443–449.

779. Smith, S.A., R.G. Querry, P.J. Fadel, R.M. Welch-O'Connor, A. Olivencia-Yurvati, X. Shi, and P.B. Raven, Differential baroreflex control of heart rate in sedentary and aerobically fit individuals. *Med. Sci. Sports. Exerc.*, 2000;**32**: 1419–1430.

780. O'Sullivan, S.E. and C. Bell, The effects of exercise and training on human cardiovascular reflex control. *J. Auton. Nerv. Syst.*, 2000;**81**: 16–24.

781. Ueno, L.M. and T. Moritani, Effects of long-term exercise training on cardiac autonomic nervous activities and baroreflex sensitivity. *Eur. J. Appl. Physiol.*, 2003;**89**: 109–114.

782. Pichot, V., F. Roche, C. Denis, M. Garet, D. Duverney, F. Costes, and J.C. Barthélémy, Interval training in elderly men increases both heart rate variability and baroreflex activity. *Clin. Auton. Res.*, 2005;**15**: 107–115.

783. Iwasaki, K., R. Zhang, J.H. Zuckerman, and B.D. Levine, Dose-response relationship of the cardiovascular adaptation to endurance training in healthy adults: how much training for what benefit? *J. Appl. Physiol.*, 2003;**95**: 1575–1583.

784. Pagani, M., D. Lucini, O. Rimoldi, R. Furlan, S. Piazza, and L. Biancardi, Effects of physical and mental stress of heart rate variability, in *Heart Rate Variability*, M. Malik and A.J. Camm, Editors. Armonk, NY: Futura Publishing, 1995, pp. 245–266.

785. Hemingway, H., M. Malik, and M. Marmot, Social and psychosocial influences on sudden cardiac death, ventricular arrhythmia and cardiac autonomic function. *Eur. Heart. J.*, 2001;**22**: 1082–1101.

786. Bernardi, L., J. Wdowczyk-Szulc, C. Valenti, S. Castoldi, C. Passino, G. Spadacini, and P. Sleight, Effects of controlled breathing, mental activity and mental stress with or without verbalization on heart rate variability. *J. Am. Coll. Cardiol.*, 2000;**35**: 1462–1469.

787. Lantelme, P., H. Milon, C. Gharib, C. Gayet, and J.O. Fortrat JO, White coat effect and reactivity to stress: cardiovascular and autonomic nervous system responses. *Hypertension*, 1998;**31**: 1021–1029.

788. Kageyama, T., N. Nishikido, T. Kobayashi, Y. Kurokawa, T. Kaneko, and M. Kabuto, Self-reported sleep quality, job stress, and daytime autonomic activities assessed in terms of short-term heart rate variability among male white-collar workers. *Ind. Health.*, 1998;**36**: 263–272.

789. Cohen, H., J. Benjamin, A.B. Geva, M.A. Matar, Z. Kaplan, and M. Kotler, Autonomic dysregulation in panic disorder and in post-traumatic stress disorder: application of power spectrum analysis of heart rate variability at rest and in response to recollection of trauma or panic attacks. *Psychiatry. Res.*, 2000;**96**: 1–13.

790. Cohen, H., M. Kotler, M. Matar, and Z. Kaplan, Normalization of heart rate variability in post-traumatic stress disorder patients following fluoxetine treatment: preliminary results. *Isr. Med. Assoc. J.*, 2000;**2**: 296–301.

791. Madden, K. and G.K. Savard, Effects of mental state on heart rate and blood pressure variability in men and women. *Clin. Physiol.*, 1995;**15**: 557–569.

792. Friedman, B.H., An autonomic flexibility–neurovisceral integration model of anxiety and cardiac vagal tone. *Biol. Psychol.*, 2007;**74**: 185–199.

793. McCraty, R., M. Atkinson, W.A. Tiller, G. Rein, and A.D. Watkins, The effects of emotions on short-term power spectrum analysis of heart rate variability. *Am. J. Cardiol.*, 1995;**76**: 1089–1093.

794. De Meersman, R.E., S. Reisman, M. Daum, and R. Zorowitz, Vagal withdrawal as a function of audience. *Am. J. Physiol. Heart. Circ. Physiol.*, 1996;**270**: H1381–1383.

795. Delaney, J.P. and D.A. Brodie, Effects of short-term psychological stress on the time and frequency domains of heart-rate variability. *Percept. Mot. Skills.*, 2000;**91**: 515–524.

796. Shinba, T., N. Kariya, Y. Matsui, N. Ozawa, Y. Matsuda, and K.Yamamoto, Decrease in heart rate variability response to task is related to anxiety and depressiveness in normal subjects. *Psychiatry. Clin. Neurosci.*, 2008;**62**: 603–609.

797. Yeragani, V.K., R.B. Pohl, R. Berger, R. Balon, C. Ramesh, D. Glitz, K. Srinivasan, and P. Weinberg, Decreased heart rate variability in panic disorder patients: a study of power spectral analysis of heart rate. *Psychiatr. Res.*, 1993;**46**: 89–103.

798. Kawachi, I., D. Sparrow, P.S. Vokonas, and S.T. Weiss, Decreased heart rate variability in men with phobic anxiety (data from the Normative Aging Study). *Am. J. Cardiol.*, 1995;**75**: 882–885.

799. McCraty, R., M. Atkinson, D. Tomasino, and W.P. Stuppy, Analysis of twenty-four hour heart rate variability in patients with panic disorder. *Biol. Psychol.*, 2001;**56**: 131–150.

800. Asmundson, G.J.G. and M.B. Stein, Vagal attenuation in panic disorder: an assessment of parasympathetic nervous system function and subjective reactivity to respiratory manipulations. *Psychosom. Med.*, 1994;**56**: 187–193.

801. Dishman, R.K., Y. Nakamura, M.E. Garcia, R.W. Thompson, A.L. Dunn, and S.N. Blair, Heart rate variability, trait anxiety, and perceived stress among physically fit men and women. *Int. J. Psychophysiol.*, 2000;**37**: 121–133.

802. Agelink, M.W., C. Boz, H. Ullrich, and J. Andrich, Relationship between major depression and heart rate variability. Clinical consequences and implications for antidepressive treatment. *Psychiatry. Res.*, 2002;**113**: 139–149.

803. Carney, R.M., J.A. Blumenthal, P.K. Stein, L. Watkins, D. Catellier, L.E. Berkman, S.M. Czajkowski, C. O'Connor, P.H. Stone, and K.E. Freedland, Depression, heart rate variability, and acute myocardial infarction. *Circulation*, 2001;**104**: 2024–2028.

804. O'Connor, M.F., J.J. Allen, and A.W. Kaszniak, Autonomic and emotion regulation in bereavement and depression. *J. Psychosom. Res.*, 2002;**52**: 183–185.

805. Moser, M., M. Lehofer, R. Hoehn-Saric, D.R. McLeod, G. Hildebrandt, B. Steinbrenner, M. Voica, P. Liebmann, and H.G. Zapotoczky, Increased heart rate in depressed subjects in spite of unchanged autonomic balance? *J. Affect. Disord.*, 1998;**48**: 115–124.

806. Watkins, L.L., P. Grossman, R. Krishnan, and J.A. Blumenthal, Anxiety reduces baroreflex cardiac control in older adults with major depression. *Psychosom. Med.*, 1999;**61**: 334–340.

807. Zhong, X., H.J. Hilton, G.J. Gates, S. Jelic, Y. Stern, M.N. Bartels, R.E. Demeersman, and R.C. Basner, Increased sympathetic and decreased parasympathetic cardiovascular modulation in normal humans with acute sleep deprivation. *J. Appl. Physiol.*, 2005;**98**: 2024–2032.

808. Gillum, R.F., Epidemiology of resting pulse rate of persons ages 25–74–data from NHANES 1971–74. *Public. Health. Rep.*, 1992;**107**: 193–201.

809. Robertson, D., C.J. Tseng, and M. Appalsamy, Smoking and mechanisms of cardiovascular control. *Am. Heart. J.*, 1988;**115**: 258–263.

810. Hayano, J., M. Yamada, Y. Sakakibara, T. Fujinami, K. Yokoyama, Y. Watanabe, and K. Takata, Short- and long-term effects of cigarette smoking on heart rate variability. *Am. J. Cardiol.*, 1990;**65**: 84–88.

811. Gallagher, D., T. Terenzi, and R. de Meersman, Heart rate variability in smokers, sedentary and aerobically fit individuals. *Clin. Auton. Res.*, 1992;**2**: 383–387.

812. Carnethon, M.R., D. Liao, G.W. Evans, W.E. Cascio, L.E. Chambless, and G. Heiss, Correlates of the shift in heart rate variability with an active postural change in a healthy population sample: the Atherosclerosis Risk In Communities study. *Am. Heart. J.*, 2002;**143**: 808–813.

813. Barutcu, I., A.M. Esen, D. Kaya, M. Turkmen, O. Karakaya, M. Melek, O.B. Esen, and Y. Basaran, Cigarette smoking and heart rate variability: dynamic influence of parasympathetic and sympathetic maneuvers. *Ann. Noninvas. Electrocardiol.*, 2005;**10**: 324–329.

814. Eryonucu, B., M. Bilge, N. Güler, K. Uzun, and M. Gencer, Effects of cigarette smoking on the circadian rhythm of heart rate variability. *Acta. Cardiol.*, 2000;**55**: 301–305.

815. Christensen, J.H., H.A. Skou, L. Fog, V. Hansen, T. Vesterlund, J. Dyerberg, E. Toft, and E.B. Schmidt, Marine n-3 fatty acids, wine intake, and heart rate variability in patients referred for coronary angiography. *Circulation*, 2001;**103**: 651–657.

816. Murata, K., P.J. Landrigan, and S. Araki, Effects of age, heart rate, gender, tobacco and alcohol ingestion on R-R interval variability in human ECG. *J. Auton. Nerv. Syst.*, 1991;**37**: 199–206.

817. Kageyama, T., N. Nishikido, Y. Honda, Y. Kurokawa, H. Imai, T. Kobayashi, T. Kaneko, and M. Kabuto, Effects of obesity, current smoking status, and alcohol consumption on heart rate variability in male white-collar workers. *Int. Arch. Occup. Environ. Health.*, 1997;**69**: 447–454.

818. Hamaad, A., M. Sosin, A.D. Blann, J. Patel, G.Y. Lip, and R.J. MacFadyen, Markers of inflammation in acute coronary syndromes: association with increased heart rate and reductions in heart rate variability. *Clin. Cardiol.*, 2005;**28**: 570–576.

819. Gehi, A., J. Ix, M. Shlipak, S.S. Pipkin, and M.A. Whooley, Relation of anemia to low heart rate variability in patients with coronary heart disease (from the Heart and Soul study). *Am. J. Cardiol.*, 2005;**95**: 1474–1477.

820. Stein, P.K., J.I. Barzilay, P.H. Chaves, J. Traber, P.P. Domitrovich, S.R. Heckbert, and J.S. Gottdiener, Higher levels of inflammation factors and greater insulin resistance are independently associated with higher heart rate and lower heart rate variability in normoglycemic older individuals: the Cardiovascular Health Study. *J. Am. Geriatr. Soc.*, 2008;**56**: 315–321.

821. Liao, D., J. Cai, F.L. Brancati, A. Folsom, R.W. Barnes, H.A. Tyroler, and G. Heiss, Association of vagal tone with serum insulin, glucose, and diabetes mellitus–The ARIC Study. *Diabetes. Res. Clin. Pract.*, 1995;**30**: 211–221.

Appendix 1
List of references cited only in tables and figures

A1. Odemuyiwa, O., M. Malik, T. Farrell, Y. Bashir, J. Poloniecki, and J. Camm, Comparison of the predictive characteristics of heart rate variability index and left ventricular ejection fraction for all-cause mortality, arrhythmic events and sudden death after acute myocardial infarction. *Am. J. Cardiol.*, 1991;**68**: 434–439.

A2. Bigger, J.T. Jr, J.L. Fleiss, R.C. Steinman, L.M. Rolnitzky, R.E. Kleiger, and J.N. Rottman, Frequency domain measures of heart period variability and mortality after myocardial infarction. *Circulation*, 1992;**85**: 164–171.

A3. Vaishnav, S., R. Stevenson, B. Marchant, K. Lagi, K. Ranjadayalan, and A.D. Timmis, Relation between heart rate variability early after acute myocardial infarction and long-term mortality. *Am. J. Cardiol.*, 1994;**73**: 653–657.

A4. Touboul, P., X. Andre-Fouët, A. Leizorovicz, R. Itti, M. Lopez, Y. Sayegh, H. Milon, and G. Kirkorian, Risk stratification after myocardial infarction. A reappraisal in the era of thrombolysis. The Groupe d'Etude du Pronostic de l'Infarctus du Myocarde (GREPI). *Eur. Heart. J.*, 1997;**18**: 99–107.

A5. Tsuji, H., F.J. Venditti Jr., E.S. Manders, J.C. Evans, M.G. Larson, C.L. Feldman, and D. Levy, Reduced heart rate variability and mortality risk in an elderly cohort. The Framingham Heart Study. *Circulation*, 1994;**90**: 878–883.

A6. Nollo, G., M. Del Greco, M. Disertori, E. Santoro, A.P. Maggioni, G.P.Sanna, and GISSI-3 Arrhythmias Substudy Investigators, Absence of slowest oscillations in short term heart rate variability of post-myocardial infarction patients. GISSI-3 arrhythmias substudy. GISSI-3 Arrhythmias Substudy Investigators. *Auton. Neurosci.*, 2001;**90**: 127–131.

A7. Forslund, L., I. Björkander, M. Ericson, C. Held, T. Kahan, N. Rehnqvist, and P. Hjemdahl, Prognostic implications of autonomic function assessed by analyses of catecholamines and heart rate variability in stable angina pectoris. *Heart*, 2002;**87**: 415–422.

A8. Lampert, R., J.R. Ickovics, C.J. Viscoli, R.I. Horwitz, and F.A. Lee, Effects of propranolol on recovery of heart rate variability following acute myocardial infarction and relation to outcome in the Beta-Blocker Heart Attack Trial. *Am. J. Cardiol.*, 2003;**91**: 137–142.

A9. La Rovere, M.T., G.D. Pinna, R. Maestri, A. Mortara, S. Capomolla, O. Febo, R. Ferrari, M. Franchini, M. Gnemmi, C. Opasich, R.G. Riccardi, E. Traversi, and F. Cobelli, Short-term heart rate variability strongly predicts sudden cardiac death in chronic heart failure patients. *Circulation*, 2003;**107**: 565–570.

A10. Jokinen, V., J.M. Tapanainen, T. Seppänen, and H.V. Huikuri, Temporal changes and prognostic significance of measures of heart rate dynamics after acute myocardial infarction in the beta-blocking era. *Am. J. Cardiol.*, 2003;**92**: 907–912.

A11. Schroeder, E.B., D. Liao, L.E. Chambless, R.J. Prineas, G.W. Evans, and G. Heiss, Hypertension, blood pressure, and heart rate variability: the Atherosclerosis Risk in Communities (ARIC) study. *Hypertension*, 2003;**42**: 1106–1011.

A12. Stein, P.K., P.P. Domitrovich, R.E. Kleiger, and CAST Investigators, Including patients with diabetes mellitus or coronary artery bypass grafting decreases the association between heart rate variability and mortality after myocardial infarction. *Am. Heart. J.*, 2004;**147**: 309–316.

A13. Carpeggiani, C., A. L'Abbate, P. Landi, C. Michelassi, M. Raciti, A. Macerata, and M. Emdin, Early assessment of heart rate variability is predictive of in-hospital death and major complications after acute myocardial infarction. *Int. J. Cardiol.*, 2004;**96**: 361–368.

A14. Casaleggio, A., R. Maestri, M.T. La Rovere, P. Rossi, and G.D. Pinna, Prediction of sudden death in heart failure patients: a novel perspective from the assessment of the peak ectopy rate. *Europace*, 2007;**9**: 385–390.

A15. Barthel, P., R. Schneider, A. Bauer, K. Ulm, C. Schmitt, A. Schömig, and G. Schmidt. Risk stratification after acute myocardial infarction by heart rate turbulence. *Circulation*, 2003;**108**: 1221–1226.

A16. Exner, D.V., K.M. Kavanagh, M.P. Slawnych, L.B. Mitchell, D. Ramadan, S.G. Aggarwal, C. Noullett, A. Van Schaik, R.T. Mitchell, M.A. Shibata, S. Gulamhussein, J. McMeekin, W. Tymchak, G. Schnell, A.M. Gillis, R.S. Sheldon, G.H. Fick, H.J. Duff, and REFINE Investigators, Noninvasive risk assessment early after a myocardial infarction the REFINE study. *J. Am. Coll. Cardiol.*, 2007;**50**: 2275–2284.

A17. Mäkikallio, T.H., P. Barthel, R. Schneider, A. Bauer, J.M. Tapanainen, M.P. Tulppo, J.S. Perkiömäki, G. Schmidt, and H.V. Huikuri, Frequency of sudden cardiac death among acute myocardial infarction survivors with optimized medical and revascularization therapy. *Am. J. Cardiol.*, 2006;**97**: 480–484.

A18. Klingenheben, T., P. Ptaszynski, and S.H. Hohnloser, Heart rate turbulence and other autonomic risk markers for arrhythmia risk stratification in dilated cardiomyopathy. *J. Electrocardiol.*, 2008;**41**: 306–311.

A19. Kanters, J.K., M.V. Højgaard, E. Agner, and N.H. Holstein-Rathlou, Short- and long-term variations in nonlinear dynamics of heart rate variability. *Cardiovasc. Res.*, 1996;**31**: 400–409.

A20. Zöllei, E., A. Csillik, S. Rabi, Z. Gingl, and L. Rudas, Respiratory effects on the reproducibility of cardiovascular autonomic parameters. *Clin. Physiol. Funct. Imaging.*, 2007;**27**: 205–210.

A21. Kobayashi, H., Inter- and intra-individual variations of heart rate variability in Japanese males. *J. Physiol. Anthropol.*, 2007;**26**: 173–177.

A22. Kleiger, R.E., J.T. Bigger, M.S. Bosner, M.K. Chung, J.R. Cook, L.M. Rolnitzky, R. Steinman, and J.L. Fleiss, Stability over time of variables measuring heart rate variability in normal subjects. *Am. J. Cardiol.*, 1991;**68**: 626–630.

A23. Kowalewski, M.A. and M. Urban, Short- and long-term reproducibility of autonomic measures in supine and standing positions. *Clin. Sci. (Lond).*, 2004;**106**: 61–66.

A24. Burger, A.J., M. Charlamb, L.A. Weinrauch, and J.A. D'Elia, Short- and long-term reproducibility of heart rate variability in patients with long-standing type I diabetes mellitus. *Am. J. Cardiol.*, 1997;**80**: 1198–1202.

A25. Macfarlane, P.W., J. Norrie, and WOSCOPS Executive Committee, The value of the electrocardiogram in risk assessment in primary prevention: experience from the West of Scotland Coronary Prevention Study. *J. Electrocardiol.*, 2007;**40**: 101–109.

A26. Dekker, J.M., E.G. Schouten, P. Klootwijk, J. Pool, C.A. Swenne, and D. Kromhout, Heart rate variability from short electrocardiographic recordings predicts mortality from all causes in middle-aged and elderly men. The Zutphen Study. *Am. J. Epidemiol.*, 1997;**145**: 899–908.

A27. Korkushko, O.V., V.B. Shatilo, Yu.I. Plachinda, and T.V. Shatilo, Autonomic control of cardiac chronotropic function in man as a function of age: assessment by power spectral analysis of heart rate variability. *J. Auton. Nerv. Syst.*, 1991;**32**: 191–198.

A28. Ryan, S.M., A.L. Goldberger, S.M. Pincus, J. Mietus, and L.A. Lipsitz. Gender- and age-related differences in heart rate dynamics: are women more complex than men? *J. Am. Coll. Cardiol.*, 1994;**24**: 1700–1707.

A29. Hotta, N., K. Otsuka, S. Murakami, G. Yamanaka, Y. Kubo, O. Matsuoka, T. Yamanaka, M. Shinagawa, S. Nunoda, Y. Nishimura, K. Shibata, H. Saitoh, M. Nishinaga, M. Ishine, T. Wada, K. Okumiya, K. Matsubayashi, S. Yano, K. Ichihara, G. Cornélissen, and F. Halberg, Fractal analysis of heart rate variability and mortality in elderly community-dwelling people – Longitudinal Investigation for the Longevity and Aging in Hokkaido County (LILAC) study. *Biomed. Pharmacother.*, 2005;**59** (Suppl 1): S45–48.

A30. Stein, P.K., Assessing heart rate variability from real-world Holter reports. *Card. Electrophysiol. Rev.*, 2002;**6**: 239–244.

A31. Uijtdehaage, S.H.J., and J.F. Thayer. Accentuated antagonism in the control of human heart rate. *Clin. Autonom. Res.*, 2000; **10**: 107–110.

A32. Corino, V.D.A., M. Matteucci, L. Cravello, E. Ferrari, A.A. Ferrari, and L.T. Mainardi. Long-term heart rate variability as a predictor of patient age. *Comp. Meth. Prog. Biomed.*, 2006; **82**: 248–257.

A37. Voss, A., J. Kurths, H.J. Kleiner, A. Witt, N. Wessel, P. Saparin, K.J. Osterziel, R. Schurath, and R. Dietz, The application of methods of nonlinear dynamics for the improved and predictive recognition of patients threatened by sudden cardiac death. *Cardiovasc. Res.*, 1996;**31**: 419–433.

A34. Schneider, R.A. and J.P. Costiloe,. Relationship of sinus arrhythmia to age and its prognostic significance in ischemie heart disease (abstr). *Clin. Res.*, 1965;**13**: 219.

A35. Acharya U.R., K.P. Joseph, N. Kannathal, C.M. Lim, J.S. Suri. Heart rate variability: a review. *Med. Biol. Eng. Comput.*, 2006;**44**: 1031–1051.

A36. Hoyer D, Friedrich H, Zwiener U, Pompe B, Baranowski R, Werdan K, Müller-Werdan U, Schmidt H. Prognostic impact of autonomic information flow in multiple organ dysfunction syndrome patients. *Int J Cardiol.*, 2006;**108**: 359–369.

A37. Akay, M. Wavelets in biomedical engineering. *Ann. Biomed. Eng.*, 1995:**23**: 531–542.

4 Exercise Electrocardiography and Exercise Testing

K. Martijn Akkerhuis · Maarten L. Simoons

P. W. Macfarlane et al. (eds.), *Specialized Aspects of ECG*, DOI 10.1007/978-0-85729-880-5_4,

4.1   Introduction

Exercise testing is a widely used method for diagnosis in patients with suspected ischemic heart disease and for functional evaluation of patients with known heart disease. Throughout the years, most attention has been given to the information obtained from the electrocardiogram during exercise. However, other information that can be obtained during the test is of equal importance. Such information, as listed in ❷ Table 4.1, can be obtained by observation of the patient, measurement of the heart rate and blood pressure responses, measurement or estimation of total body oxygen consumption, and from other noninvasive investigations such as myocardial-perfusion scintigraphy and evaluation of left ventricular function by radionuclide angiography or echocardiography. This chapter focuses on exercise electrocardiography.

Compared with the noninvasive stress imaging tests such as stress echocardiography and myocardial perfusion scintigraphy, exercise testing can be performed at a much lower cost. However, the noninvasive imaging modalities have been increasingly more used in the last decade and have been shown to outperform the standard exercise test in terms of diagnostic accuracy. This does not mean, however, that exercise electrocardiography should be replaced by these imaging modalities. The standard exercise test remains the initial test of choice in many clinical circumstances. However, new technical improvements in the field of the stress imaging tests are expected to further increase their performance and clinical use. Furthermore, new techniques are being developed that permit direct, noninvasive imaging of the coronary arteries (e.g., multislice computed tomography). These developments will require a continuous reassessment of the relative role of all commonly used diagnostic tests and procedures.

The report of an exercise test should contain a summary of the previous history of the patient, his present symptoms, medication, and an interpretation of the ECG at rest. The exercise protocol should be described with the expected performance of a normal subject of the same age, sex, and body size. The reasons for termination of the test should be stated and symptoms which occur during the test should be described, including the workload at which symptoms began, the type of symptoms, their severity, and the duration of the symptoms after exercise has ceased. Heart rate and blood pressure should be reported at rest, at the onset of symptoms, at peak exercise, and after approximately 6 min into the recovery period. A description of the ECG should contain any arrhythmias which may have occurred and changes in the QRS complex and ST segment. Finally, a conclusion should be drawn which answers the clinical questions that were posed before the test. The report should not be limited to words like "positive" or "negative."

4.2   Safety of Exercise Testing, Precautions, and Contraindications

Exercise testing is a well-established procedure that has been in widespread clinical use for many decades. Although exercise testing is generally a safe procedure, both myocardial infarction and death have been reported. A large survey reported

❒ Table 4.1

Information obtained by exercise testing in patients with (suspected) heart disease

Information	Measurement
• Exercise tolerance	• Maximum workload
	• Heart rate response
	• Maximum oxygen consumption
• Limiting symptoms	• Symptoms during test
• Myocardial ischemia	• Angina pectoris
	• ST segment changes
	• Myocardial perfusion scintigraphy
• Left ventricular function	• Maximum workload
	• Blood pressure response
	• Echocardiography (Radionuclide angiography) (Left ventricular filling pressure)
• Arrhythmias	• Electrocardiogram

17 deaths among 712,285 patients tested in three German-speaking countries [1]. In addition, nonfatal ventricular fibrillation occurred at a rate of 1/7,000 tests and nonfatal myocardial infarction at a rate of 1/70,000 tests. Since these risks are not negligible, all stress testing should be done in a setting where emergencies can be treated efficiently and expeditiously. A defibrillator and an emergency kit of appropriate drugs should be immediately available, and the staff of the exercise laboratory should be trained in cardiopulmonary resuscitation [2]. In addition, exercise testing should be supervised by an appropriately trained physician, who should be in the immediate vicinity and available for emergencies [3]. However, the most important safety factors in stress testing are patient selection and good clinical judgment, deciding which patient should undergo exercise testing and knowing when not to start and when to stop a test are essential in reducing the risk of stress testing. Absolute and relative contraindications to exercise stress testing are listed in ❷ Table 4.2 [4].

4.3   Exercise Protocols

Exercise should be performed on a treadmill or a calibrated bicycle ergometer [5, 6]. Other modalities may be used in special situations; for example, in sports medicine a rowing ergometer or a canoe ergometer might be used. The various forms of step tests are outdated, since these do not permit quantification of the work performed. The choice between a bicycle ergometer and a treadmill can be made on the basis of personal preferences or local custom. In general, normal subjects can reach higher heart rates and a higher level of oxygen consumption on a treadmill [7]. Furthermore, virtually all subjects can be exercised on a treadmill, while riding a bicycle requires some skill. On the other hand, the body position is more stable on a bicycle ergometer, resulting in less motion artifacts on the ECG. For studies of left ventricular function during exercise or studies with indwelling catheters, only bicycles can be used, usually with the patient in the supine position. Guidelines for the design of a clinical exercise testing laboratory have been published by the American Heart Association [2].

Exercise should start at a low workload and increment stepwise or continuously, according to a fixed protocol. A large number of treadmill protocols has been described (❷ Fig. 4.1). Probably the most widely used protocol has been described by Bruce [8]. In this protocol, both the grade (slope) of the treadmill and its speed are altered at the end of

❑ **Table 4.2**

Contraindications to exercise testing (Adapted from ACC/AHA 2002 Guideline Update for Exercise Testing [4])

Absolute
• Acute myocardial infarction (within 2 days)
• High-risk unstable angina
• Symptomatic severe aortic stenosis
• Uncontrolled symptomatic heart failure
• Acute pulmonary embolus or pulmonary infarction
• Uncontrolled cardiac arrhythmias causing symptoms or hemodynamic compromise
• Acute myocarditis or pericarditis
• Acute aortic dissection
Relative
• Left main coronary stenosis
• Moderate stenotic valvular heart disease
• Electrolyte abnormalities
• Severe arterial hypertension[a]
• Tachyarrhythmias or bradyarrhythmias
• Hypertrophic (obstructive) cardiomyopathy and other forms of outflow tract obstruction
• Mental or physical impairment leading to inability to exercise adequately
• High-degree atrioventricular block

[a]Systolic blood pressure of >200 mmHg and/or diastolic blood pressure of >110 mmHg, as suggested by the ACC/AHA Committee on Exercise Testing

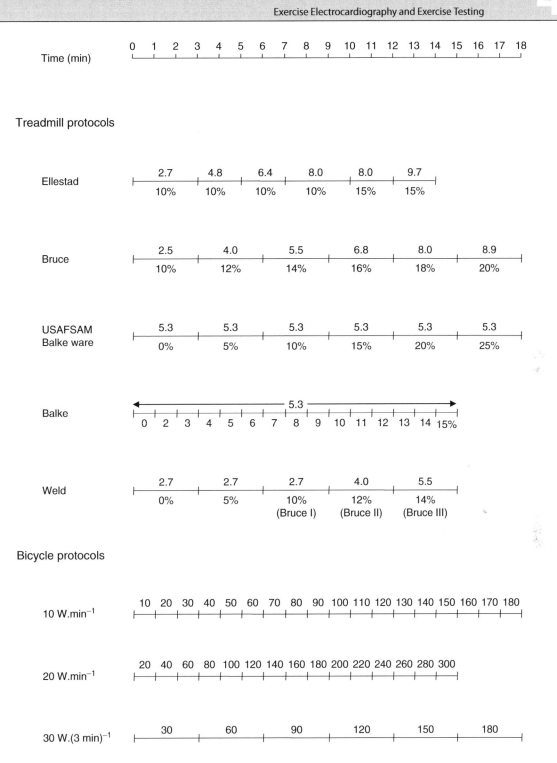

◘ Fig. 4.1

Summary of five treadmill protocols and three bicycle protocols. The figures above the lines of the treadmill protocols represent treadmill speed in kilometers per hour, and the figures below the lines represent the slope. Some treadmill protocols use steps of 3 min each (Bruce, USAFSAM, Weld), while others use steps of 1 min (Balke) or alternating steps of 3 and 2 min (Ellestad). The figures above the lines of the bicycle protocols correspond to workload in Watts. Either 1-min steps or steps of 3 min are used. The value of the divisions marked on these lines is indicated on the *left*

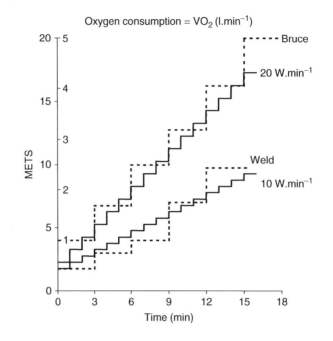

◘ Fig. 4.2
Comparison of oxygen requirements over time for two bicycle protocols (steps of 20 W/min or 10 W/min) and two treadmill protocols (Bruce and Weld) in a 75 kg male subject. The horizontal axis represents time in minutes and the vertical axis represents average oxygen uptake (l/min), which can be equated to metabolic equivalents (*METS*). It should be noted that the actual oxygen consumption of a given patient at a certain level of exercise varies widely and depends on their level of physical condition. Furthermore, oxygen consumption on the treadmill is dependent on body weight

each 3-min stage. In the Ellestad protocol [9], the slope is constant during the first four stages, while the speed increases. At stage five, speed is kept constant while the slope is altered; for stage six, speed is again increased. The Balke protocol and its derivatives maintain a constant speed in the range of 4.8–6.4 km/h with changes of treadmill slope every minute or every 3 min [10]. Modifications of these protocols have been developed for the evaluation of patients prior to discharge from hospital after myocardial infarction. For example, the protocol used by Weld employs two stages with a low treadmill slope prior to the first stage of the Bruce protocol [11].

Workload on a treadmill is dependent on body weight. Accordingly, the workload performed using various protocols can be expressed as ml/kg/min oxygen consumption. In the literature, workload has frequently been expressed in metabolic equivalents (METS) [12, 13]. One MET equals 3.5 ml/kg/min oxygen consumption, which corresponds to the average resting oxygen consumption. In ❷ Fig. 4.2, mean oxygen consumption is given for various protocols and the corresponding METS have been indicated. Oxygen consumption rises more rapidly with the Bruce protocol or the Ellestad protocol than with the USAFSAM modification of the Balke protocol, which uses a speed of 5.3 km/h [14, 15]. The work on a bicycle ergometer is independent of body weight. Frequently used protocols on a bicycle ergometer in the sitting position increase the workload by 10 W/min or 20 W/min. For adult male subjects with average body weight, the metabolic requirement (total body oxygen consumption) of a protocol with 20 W/min workload increments is comparable to the Bruce protocol (❷ Fig. 4.2). Similarly, a protocol with 10 W/min steps is comparable to the Weld protocol for submaximal predischarge tests after myocardial infarction. Predicted normal values for the peak workload for a protocol with steps of 20 W/min are presented in ❷ Table 4.3. In the supine position, lower workload increments are normally used; for example, 20 or 30 W every 3–5 min.

It should be realized that the hemodynamic response to exercise in the supine position differs considerably from the response in the sitting position. In patients with coronary artery disease (CAD), the peak level of exercise in the supine position is approximately 70% of the peak level in the sitting position. Peak heart rate and peak systolic blood pressure

◘ Table 4.3

Predicted normal exercise tolerance (in Watts) using a bicycle ergometer protocol for exercise testing

Age (years)	Exercise tolerance in *women* Height (cm)					Exercise tolerance in *men* Height (cm)				
	160	170	180	190	200	160	170	180	190	200
20	176	192	208	225	241	220	240	261	281	301
25	167	183	199	215	232	209	229	249	269	290
30	158	174	190	206	222	197	217	238	258	278
35	149	165	181	197	213	186	206	226	246	267
40	139	156	172	188	204	174	195	215	235	255
45	130	146	163	179	195	163	183	203	223	244
50	121	137	153	170	186	151	172	192	212	232
55	112	128	144	160	177	140	160	180	201	221
60	103	119	135	151	167	129	149	169	189	209
65	94	110	126	142	158	117	137	157	178	198
70	84	101	117	133	149	106	126	146	166	186

Predicted normal exercise tolerance (in Watts) for women (left) and men (right). These normal values are applicable when a protocol with steps of 20 W/min is used on a bicycle ergometer. The normal range is between 85% and 115% of these values. For example, a 45-year old man with a height of 190 cm has a predicted normal exercise tolerance of 223 W, ranging from 190 to 256 W.

are approximately 10% lower. On the other hand, pulmonary capillary wedge pressure during exercise is higher in the supine position owing to the greater venous return [16–18]. In order to obtain reproducible results, each hospital and laboratory should select one or two protocols which can be applied to all subjects. Reference values for such protocols are readily available as shown in ❯ Fig. 4.3 and ❯ Table 4.3. Nevertheless, each laboratory should verify whether these values are indeed applicable to the local population. Measurement of oxygen consumption is not very useful in a laboratory for exercise electrocardiography. If necessary, oxygen consumption can be estimated from the workload as shown in ❯ Fig. 4.2. The standard deviation of this estimation is between 5% and 10%.

4.4 Exercise Endpoints

For most purposes, exercise can be continued until symptoms occur. It is a fallacy to terminate exercise at an arbitrary percentage (70 or 85%) of the age-adjusted maximum predicted heart rate for a number of reasons. First, the heart-rate response in normal subjects is highly variable [13]. The mean value at each age may be predicted as 220 minus age, or 200 minus age/2. These mean values apply both to men and women up to 70 years of age. However, the standard deviation is large, approximately 10 beats/min. Thus, the 95% confidence interval is between 20 beats below and 20 beats above the predicted mean value [12]. Second, the maximum heart rate reached by patients with severe disease is considerably lower than the heart rate reached by normal subjects. Thus, when heart rate is used as an endpoint for terminating exercise, patients with severe disease may be stressed beyond their limits, while other patients will be unnecessarily prevented from exercising to their true capacity. Finally, the target heart rate approach has additional limitations in patients with heart rate impairment, those with excessive heart rate response, and those receiving medication such as beta-blockers, some calcium antagonists, and specific sinus-node inhibitors [20–23].

Therefore, other endpoints for terminating exercise testing, as summarized in ❯ Table 4.4, are strongly preferred. It should be noted that ST segment elevation developing in leads (other than aVR or V_1) without diagnostic Q-waves of a previous myocardial infarction usually indicates transmural ischemia rather than just a subendocardial problem. It is almost always associated with a high-grade obstruction proximal in the respective coronary artery. If exercise continues, myocardial infarction may be imminent, so that it is necessary to terminate the test and direct the patient to immediate follow-up care including coronary angiography.

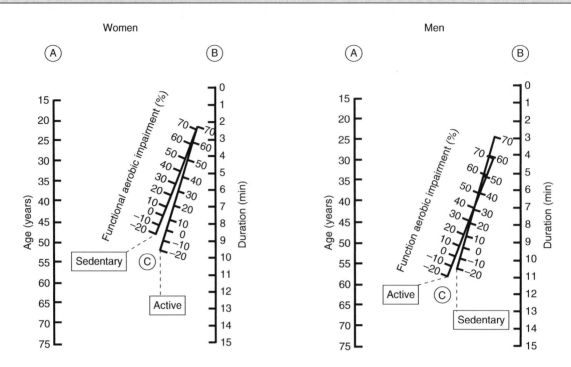

□ Fig. 4.3
Nomogram for assessment of functional aerobic impairment of men and women according to age, duration of exercise by the Bruce multistage procedure, and habitual physical activity status. In order to find functional aerobic impairment (*C*), apply a straight-edge to age (*A*) and duration (*B*) and read intercepts of diagonal (Adapted from Bruce [19])

It is advisable to express symptoms which occur during exercise on a semiquantitative scale, such as the Borg scale (❯ Table 4.5) [24]. The use of rating of perceived exertion scales is often useful in assessment of patient fatigue. Symptom-limited testing with the Borg scale as an aid is very important when the test is used to assess functional capacity. It also permits a comparison of the degree of a patient's symptoms over time.

It has previously been recommended that all medication be stopped one or more days before an exercise test is done. Although this may be useful for some scientific applications, this principle is not generally followed in clinical practice. In patients with stable angina, a period of instability may develop if beta-blockers, nitrates, or calcium antagonists are withdrawn. If the interpretation of the test is significantly hampered by medication, for example, a normal response is obtained in a patient with angina using beta-blockers, the medication may be gradually withdrawn and the test repeated. However, most patients with angina will develop symptoms and ischemic ECG changes in spite of the use of antianginal drugs, albeit at a higher workload than without such drugs [21, 22, 25, 26]. Despite the effect of beta-blockers on maximal exercise heart rate, no differences in test performance were found in a consecutive group of men being evaluated for possible CAD when they were subgrouped according to beta-blocker administration initiated by their referring physician [4, 27]. Therefore, for routine exercise testing, it appears unnecessary for physicians to accept the risk of stopping beta-blockers before testing when a patient exhibits possible symptoms of myocardial ischemia.

4.5   Recording and Computer Processing of the Electrocardiogram

4.5.1   Recording of the Electrocardiogram

It is essential to record a high-quality ECG. Proper ECG quality can be achieved in virtually all patients if skin preparation is meticulous. The skin should be abraded with sandpaper or a special, commercially available, drill. Special electrodes

☐ Table 4.4

Indications for terminating exercise testing (Adapted from ACC/AHA 2002 Guideline Update for Exercise Testing [4])

Sensations felt by *patient*	Observations made by *physician*
Absolute indications	
• Moderate to severe (progressive) angina • Increasing nervous system symptoms (e.g., ataxia, dizziness, or near-syncope) • Subject's desire to stop	• ST-elevation (≥1.0 mm) in leads without diagnostic Q-waves (other than V_1 or aVR) • Technical difficulties in monitoring ECG or systolic blood pressure • Sustained ventricular tachycardia • Drop in systolic BP of >10 mmHg from baseline despite an increase in workload, when accompanied by other evidence of ischemia • Signs of poor perfusion (cyanosis or pallor)
Relative indications	
• Fatigue, shortness of breath, wheezing, leg cramps, or claudication • Increasing chest pain	• Drop in systolic BP of >10 mmHg from baseline despite an increase in workload, in the absence of other evidence of ischemia • ST- or QRS-changes such as excessive ST-depression (>2 mm of horizontal or down-sloping ST segment depression, especially when the magnitude of the ST-depression is increasing rapidly at low workloads) or marked axis shift • Arrhythmias other than sustained ventricular tachycardia, including multifocal PVCs, triplets of PVCs, supraventricular tachycardia, heart block, or bradyarrhythmias • Development of bundle-branch block or IVCD that cannot be distinguished from ventricular tachycardia • Hypertensive response (systolic blood pressure of >250 mmHg and/or diastolic blood pressure of >115 mmHg)[a]

BP, blood pressure; ECG, electrocardiogram; PVCs, premature ventricular contractions; and IVCD, intraventricular conduction delay

[a] As suggested by the ACC/AHA Committee on Exercise Testing

should be used to prevent motion artifacts. Furthermore, the ECG cables should be of special design to prevent artifacts owing to cable motion. As stated, cycle ergometers produce less motion of the upper body resulting in less motion artifacts on the ECG. Finally, ECG amplifiers which meet the American Heart Association standards, and have high input impedance, should be used [2]. If a proper combination of skin preparation, electrodes, cables, and amplifiers is used, a stable baseline can be achieved throughout the test in most subjects.

4.5.2   Computer Processing of the Electrocardiogram

Computerized exercise stress test systems have become the method of choice in most stress testing laboratories. The principles of computer-assisted interpretation of exercise ECGs have been described [28–32] and a review of methods for computer-based resting electrocardiography is also presented elsewhere in this textbook (❷ Chap. 5). A summary of methods for analysis of exercise ECGs is presented here in brief.

■ Table 4.5

Borg scale

Grade	Symptoms
0	Nothing at all
0.5	Extremely weak (just noticeable)
1	Very weak
2	Weak (light)
3	Moderate
4	Somewhat strong
5	Strong (heavy)
6	
7	Very strong
8	
9	Extremely strong (almost maximal)
10	Maximal

The Borg scale for rating of perceptual intensities constructed as a category scale with ratio properties [24]. This can be used for quantitative evaluation of symptoms, for example chest pain

Computer systems for exercise testing regulate the workload of the bicycle or treadmill ergometer according to one of several predefined protocols. The computer systems also maintain a record of time, heart rate, and workload, and display these data on a computer screen together with baseline ECG waveforms [33]. The continuous stream of ECG waveforms, data, and computer measurements are stored and processed online in the system. ECG waveforms are acquired by a process termed analog–digital conversion. Most current digital processing ECG and exercise test systems sample the analog waveforms at the rate of 250 samples/s. A representation of the original analog signal can be obtained by digital–analog reconstruction of the digitized waveform. The computer system subsequently processes the ECG waveforms online to minimize noise and artifactual effects. Especially, at the higher workloads and heart rates, the recorded basic ECG tracings may show so much noise and artifacts from exercising skeletal muscles and respiratory variability that measurements from the original ECG waveforms are unreliable.

The processing involves the steps of QRS-detection, temporal alignment, and signal averaging. The QRS complexes are detected with the aid of a combination of the derivatives of multiple ECG leads. Thus, the characteristic feature used for detection of the QRS complex is the large voltage changes that occur in all leads simultaneously during ventricular activation. The QRS complexes are then classified as normal or abnormal. Abnormal beats may be a result of premature ventricular or supraventricular complexes, or they may be normal beats distorted by excessive noise or baseline drift. The normal beats are then combined into a single representative complex by computation of an average (mean) or median beat. Signal averaging can be performed at preselected intervals, for example, during 20 s of each minute, or continuously. The latter is the method of choice because it permits continuous display of the updated ECG waveform. Since the averaging procedure might be subject to errors in some of the patients, the user should compare the shape of the averaged signal with the original ECG tracings.

From the representative complexes, measurements can be obtained. Since the noise level during exercise is rather high in comparison with resting ECGs, it is not appropriate to take measurements from individual beats as is the case in some resting ECG programs. In commercially available systems, the baseline and ST segment are defined at fixed intervals before and after a single fiducial point in the QRS complex. Therefore, it is necessary to define the proper onset and end of the QRS complex. Such precise definition of QRS-onset and end is only possible if a combination of multiple leads is used [29, 30]. Computerized algorithms for QRS-detection and time alignment are, therefore, more reliable and robust in multichannel recording. Additionally, algorithms are applied that reduce the effect of baseline drift during exercise caused by temperature changes, respiration, and body motion, especially at higher workloads and if there is poor skin–electrode contact.

The processed, online cleaned data allow more accurate measurements of the exercise ECG, especially the low-amplitude signals such as the P-wave, the PR-segment, the junction of the QRS complex and ST segment (J-point), and the ST segment itself [33]. The digital measurements are generally more accurate and reproducible than manual measurements. However, careful overreading to provide quality control for automated choice of onset–offset waveform fiducial markers on the signal-processed data is required to avoid error in interpretation resulting in false-positive test results [4, 33]. Therefore, ECG recordings of the raw, unprocessed ECG data should be available at each stage of the exercise protocol for comparison with the averages that the exercise test monitor generates. Recommendations and standards for the degree of filtering and processing of data have been published [2, 4].

4.5.3 Lead Systems for Exercise Electrocardiography

Various types of lead systems have been developed, studied, and used in the last decades. Bipolar precordial lead systems have been used for a number of years and have produced satisfactory results in patients with suspected CAD and a normal ECG at rest. The two optimal leads for detection of ST segment depression during exercise are the bipolar lead from the right infraclavicular region to the V5 position (CS5 bipolar lead system) and that from the manubrium of the sternum to the V5 position (CM5 bipolar lead system). They have been reported to detect up to 90% of all ST segment depression identified by multiple-lead systems [34–36]. In patients with a previous myocardial infarction, a single-lead system is inadequate and such patients should be tested with a multiple-lead system. Multiple-lead systems that have been evaluated include the pseudo-orthogonal lead system, the corrected orthogonal lead system (with computer-processed Frank leads), the precordial map, the conventional 12-lead ECG system, and systems using a combination of bipolar leads and the standard 12 leads [33–35, 38–41]. The arrival of powerful high-speed microcomputers has allowed the development of systems for continuous online recording and analysis of the standard 12 ECG leads, which has become the norm in most testing facilities today [33]. It should, however, be noted that lead V5 remains by far the most sensitive electrode position that outperforms the inferior leads and the combination of lead V5 with II, because the latter has a relatively high false-positive rate. Therefore, in patients without prior myocardial infarction and with normal resting ECGs, the precordial leads alone are a reliable marker for CAD, and monitoring of inferior limb leads adds little additional diagnostic information. In these patients, exercise-induced ST segment depression confined to the inferior leads is of little value for detection of CAD [4, 42].

4.5.3.1 Right-Sided Chest Leads

In a study of 245 patients, it was shown that the diagnostic accuracy of exercise testing was increased when right ventricular leads were added to the standard 12 ECG leads [43]. By using right-sided chest leads, the sensitivity for the detection of CAD by angiography was comparable to that of myocardial perfusion scintigraphy (92 versus 93%). However, it is important to realize that these data were obtained in a population with a very high prevalence of CAD and might well be less reliable if the prevalence of CAD were to be substantially lower. Therefore, routine clinical use of right-sided chest leads awaits confirmation of these results in differing populations [4].

4.6 Interpretation of the Electrocardiogram

4.6.1 Changes of the ECG During Exercise in Normal Subjects

Normal ECG changes during exercise have been studied in standard chest leads [44], in corrected orthogonal leads [45] and by body-surface mapping [46, 47]. It has been shown that such changes occur gradually in relation to heart-rate changes during stress.

The amplitude of the P-wave increases, without major changes in the waveform. At heart rates over approximately 120 beats/min, this is enhanced by the superposition of the T-wave and the P-wave. At peak exercise with heart rates over 160 beats/min, the P-wave amplitude is on average twice, but in some patients up to five times the amplitude at rest.

Obviously, the PQ-interval shortens, owing to increased sympathetic activity during stress. With the P-wave becoming taller and the Ta-wave (atrial repolarization) increasing, there is a downward displacement of the PQ-junction below the isoelectric line in the resting ECG. This point is considered to be the baseline for terms of measuring ST segment change [33]. Exaggerated atrial repolarization waves during exercise may extend into the ST segment and T-wave and can cause downsloping ST-depression in the absence of ischemia at high peak exercise heart rates [48, 49]. Patients with false-positive exercise tests based on this finding have a high peak exercise heart rate, absence of exercised-induced angina, and markedly downsloping PQ-segments in the inferior leads [4, 48, 49].

QRS-duration does not change significantly during exercise. In one specially designed study, a systematic reduction of QRS-duration of only a few milliseconds was observed [50]. Prolongation of QRS-duration, however, is certainly abnormal. Changes in QRS-morphology have been discussed extensively. At peak exercise, QRS-forces shift toward the right and superiorly. Accordingly, Q-waves in the left precordial leads deepen, R-waves in the left precordial leads decrease, and S-waves become wider and deeper. However, intra-individual variability is large. In standard precordial leads, R-wave amplitude increases frequently at intermediate workloads, with heart rates between 120 and 160 beats/min [44]. This is precisely the heart rate reached by most patients with CAD. At higher heart rates, R-wave amplitude decreases. The situation is even more complex when body-surface maps are analyzed [46, 51]. The position of the maximum amplitude on the chest wall during ventricular depolarization remains located in the left anterior region, but the precise location of the maximum shifted one electrode position or more in seven out of 25 normal subjects studied by Block [46]. No consistent pattern was observed in the changes of the maximum QRS-forces in body-surface maps in normal subjects exercised up to a heart rate of 150 beats/min during maximum exercise. The mechanism of the QRS-changes during exercise is still unclear. It has been claimed that these are related to reduction of end-diastolic volume, which would diminish the effect of the radially oriented depolarization fronts in the left ventricular wall traveling from endocardium to epicardium. However, no reduction in end-diastolic volume was seen in patients studied in the supine position with radionuclide ventriculography [52]. Furthermore, R-wave amplitude variations appeared not to be related to changes in left ventricular volume during experimental myocardial ischemia [53].

The QT-interval shortens during exercise, although it cannot be measured accurately when the T-wave and P-wave overlap at higher heart rates. Usually, there is depression of the J-point followed by an upsloping ST segment. However, the ST segment slope may vary considerably. The T-wave amplitude varies greatly during exercise but increases considerably in most normal subjects immediately after exercise. Generally, the ST segment amplitude 80 ms after the end of the QRS complex remains positive in normal subjects at heart rates around 140 beats/min in the left precordial area, while a minimum develops below the right clavicle. During exercise, depression of the J-point and ST segment are prominent in leads with a lateral and vertical orientation [54]. These changes are far less significant in anterior–posterior and transverse leads. This explains in part the relatively high incidence of so-called false-positive ST segment depressions in these leads. ECG changes in healthy female volunteers are similar to those in males, with the exception of ST segment measurements. Flat or even slightly negative ST segments are present in some of the females at rest. This contributes in part to the false-positive ST segment changes in females [55]. Accordingly, separate criteria were developed for quantitative interpretation of the ECG changes during exercise in females [56].

4.6.2 Changes of the ECG During Exercise in Patients with Coronary Artery Disease

The most prominent electrocardiographic findings associated with CAD are a depression or elevation of the ST segment in the left precordial leads.

4.6.2.1 ST Segment Depression

The probability that a given subject has CAD is higher if the ST segment depression adheres to the following pattern: it develops early during exercise at a low heart rate, is deeper and has a more horizontal, or even downsloping pattern. However, it should be appreciated that, in subjects with a normal ECG at rest, there remains a considerable overlap between ST segment measurements in normal subjects and in patients with CAD. Also, as mentioned, ST segment waveforms in females during exercise differ from males and show a greater tendency towards ST segment depression, particularly in

Bicycle ergometer
Protocol: steps of 20 Watts (W) per minute
ST segment: measured at J-point plus 80 msec (μV)

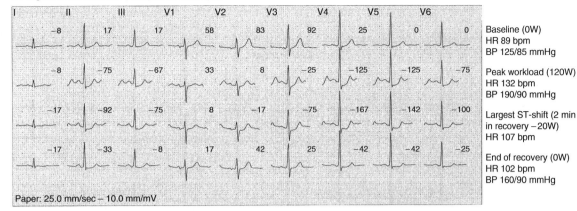

Fig. 4.4
Bicycle exercise stress test in 56-year old male who underwent percutaneous coronary intervention of the left anterior descending artery 10 years earlier for stable angina. He was referred for screening before entering a fitness program. Upon request, he admitted that he had chest pain on exertion. The degree of functional impairment was difficult to assess because of an inactive lifestyle. The patient reached 120 W, whereas the predicted normal value for the peak workload was 174 W. He discontinued the test because of shortness of breath and chest pain. With increasing workload, there is a slow-upsloping ST segment depression up to 1 mm (0.1 mV) in the inferior and left precordial leads, evolving to a downsloping pattern in the recovery phase. The patient was referred for coronary angiography, which revealed a significant stenosis in the left circumflex artery that was subsequently treated by percutaneous coronary intervention

the vertically-oriented leads [54]. In combination with the lower incidence of CAD in females, this results in an increased fraction of false-positive exercise test results in women, as reported in the literature [55, 57–59]. Nevertheless, exercise testing can be used in females when these factors are taken into account [57, 58]. Accordingly, the likelihood of CAD in females is lower than in males for most combinations of age, history, and ST segment depression, as will be discussed later.

Upsloping ST Segment Depression
The significance of upsloping ST segment depression has been studied extensively in the past decades and has generated much controversy. Clearly, downsloping ST segment depression is a stronger predictor of CAD than horizontal depression, and both are more predictive than upsloping depression. However, slowly-upsloping ST segment depression, for example, when the slope is less than 1 mV/s or when the degree of depression at 60–80 ms from the J-point is 1.5 mm (0.15 mV) or more below the baseline level of the PQ-junction, is associated with an increased probability of CAD (❯ Figs. 4.4 and ❯ 4.5) [33, 60–62]. In a study of 70 patients with these ST segment changes, 57% had either two- or three-vessel CAD [33, 61]. On the other hand, junctional depression with a very steep upsloping ST segment is probably not pathological. From this it follows that, if slowly-upsloping ST-depression is considered an abnormal finding, sensitivity of exercise testing is increased, albeit at the cost of decreased specificity resulting in more false-positive test results. In the most recent ACC/AHA guidelines on exercise testing, the use of the more commonly-used definition for a positive test of ≥1 mm (0.1 mV) of horizontal or downsloping ST segment depression is favored [4].

Horizontal and Downsloping ST Segment Depression
The most commonly-used definition for visual interpretation of a positive exercise test result from an electrocardiographic standpoint is ≥1 mm (0.1 mV) of horizontal or downsloping ST segment depression for at least 60–80 ms after the end of the QRS complex (❯ Fig. 4.6 (Continued)) [4]. As stated, downsloping ST segment depression is a stronger predictor of CAD than horizontal depression.

Bicycle ergometer
Protocol: steps of 20 Watts (W) per minute
ST segment: measured at J-point plus 60 msec (µV); ST-slope in mV/sec

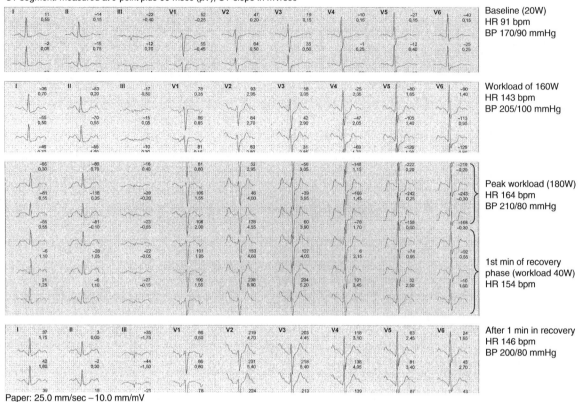

Paper: 25.0 mm/sec – 10.0 mm/mV

◻ Fig. 4.5

A 60-year old male treated for hypercholesterolemia by his general practitioner underwent exercise testing at the request of the specialist in allergy and immunology. He was suspected to have had a severe allergic reaction to the (rare) combination of wheat and exercise. Before planning an exercise test after ingestion of wheat to assess whether an allergic reaction could be provoked, a standard bicycle exercise test was performed as baseline. In daily life, the patient had a good exercise tolerance without any angina-like complaints. He reached 180 W (predicted peak workload 167 W) and discontinued because of fatigue. There were no angina-like symptoms or dyspnea. The baseline ECG was normal. Up to 160 W, there were no significant ST segment changes indicative of myocardial ischemia. From 160 W onward, minimal slow-upsloping ST segment depression developed in the left precordial leads, which got a more horizontal pattern and increased up to 2 mm (0.2 mV) at peak workload. The ST segment depression resolved directly following the discontinuation of exercise. This ECG pattern in which the ST segment becomes abnormal only at high workloads and returns to baseline in the immediate recovery phase may indicate a false-positive test in an asymptomatic subject. A nuclear perfusion scintigraphy using dipyridamole was subsequently performed which showed no signs of myocardial ischemia

Magnitude of ST Segment Depression and Probability of Coronary Artery Disease

❷ Table 4.6 summarizes data from various studies that related the magnitude of ST segment depression at peak exercise to the probability of CAD at coronary angiography [64–67]. It is evident that, for example, horizontal ST segment depression of ≥2 mm (0.2 mV) is highly specific (if only such results were considered abnormal, the specificity would be 99%), but occurs in the minority of patients with CAD (sensitivity would be only 28%). On the other hand, ST segment depression of 0.5 mm (0.05 mV) is nonspecific (sensitivity is 68%, but specificity only 80%), and should, therefore, not be used as a criterion for abnormality. A superior approach is to compute, from the data in ❷ Table 4.6, the ratio of

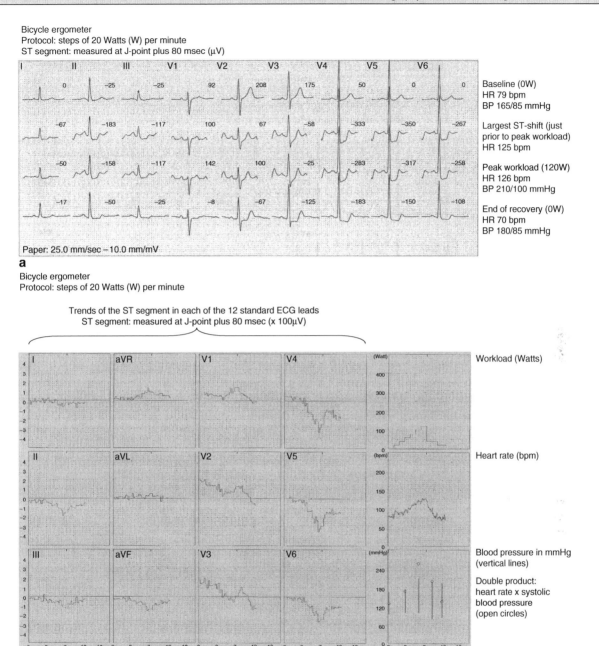

Bicycle ergometer
Protocol: steps of 20 Watts (W) per minute
ST segment: measured at J-point plus 80 msec (μV)

Baseline (0W)
HR 79 bpm
BP 165/85 mmHg

Largest ST-shift (just prior to peak workload)
HR 125 bpm

Peak workload (120W)
HR 126 bpm
BP 210/100 mmHg

End of recovery (0W)
HR 70 bpm
BP 180/85 mmHg

Paper: 25.0 mm/sec –10.0 mm/mV

a

Bicycle ergometer
Protocol: steps of 20 Watts (W) per minute

Trends of the ST segment in each of the 12 standard ECG leads
ST segment: measured at J-point plus 80 msec (x 100μV)

Workload (Watts)

Heart rate (bpm)

Blood pressure in mmHg (vertical lines)

Double product: heart rate x systolic blood pressure (open circles)

b

🔲 Fig. 4.6

(a) Bicycle exercise stress test in 54-year old male with no history of cardiovascular disease who visited the outpatient clinic for angina-like chest pain complaints, class III according to the Canadian Cardiovascular Society [63]. The predicted maximum workload was 175 W. The patient discontinued the test at 120 W because of severe chest pain. Slow-upsloping to horizontal ST segment depression already developed at low workload (80 W) and increased to a maximum of 3.5 mm (0.35 mV) in the left precordial lead V₅ at maximal exertion. The ST segment depression evolved to a downsloping pattern in the recovery phase. Coronary angiography revealed a severe stenosis at the bifurcation of the left anterior descending artery and first diagonal branch, which was subsequently treated by percutaneous coronary intervention with bifurcation stenting according to the culotte technique. (b) Overview of ST segment trends and hemodynamic data of the same exercise test, showing the development of progressive ST segment depression in the inferior and precordial leads with increasing workload

Bicycle ergometer
Protocol: steps of 20 Watts (W) per minute
ST segment: measured at J-point plus 60 msec (μV); ST-slope in mV/sec

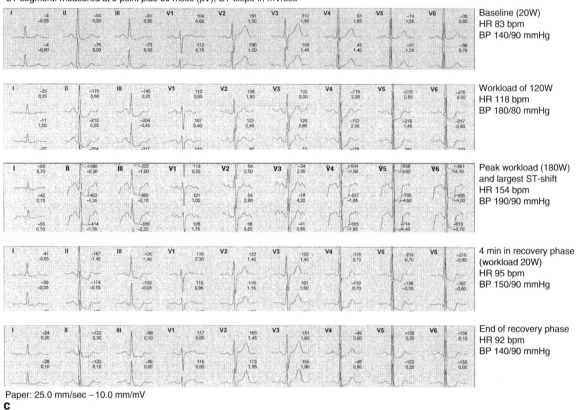

Baseline (20W)
HR 83 bpm
BP 140/90 mmHg

Workload of 120W
HR 118 bpm
BP 180/80 mmHg

Peak workload (180W)
and largest ST-shift
HR 154 bpm
BP 190/90 mmHg

4 min in recovery phase
(workload 20W)
HR 95 bpm
BP 150/90 mmHg

End of recovery phase
HR 92 bpm
BP 140/90 mmHg

Paper: 25.0 mm/sec – 10.0 mm/mV

c

◘ **Fig. 4.6 (Continued)**

(c) The same patient visited the outpatient clinic approximately 1 year after the percutaneous coronary intervention. He indicated that he suffered again from chest pain similar to the complaints he had prior to the revascularization procedure. The only difference was that the chest pain now occurred with more strenuous exertion as compared to the complaints 1 year earlier (functional class II according to the Canadian Cardiovascular Society [63]). The patient reached the predicted workload of 171 W and discontinued the test because of tiredness and shortness of breath. The exercise electrocardiogram again showed marked ST segment depression up to 6 mm (0.6 mV) with a horizontal to downsloping pattern at maximal exertion. Coronary angiography revealed severe in-stent restenosis in the treated segments in the left anterior descending artery and first diagonal. The patient was subsequently successfully treated by repeat percutaneous coronary intervention

the likelihood that a given range of ST segment depression is related to the presence or absence of CAD. This likelihood ratio is 0.4 for ST segment depression up to 0.9 mm (0.09 mV). Only ST segment depression greater than 1 mm (0.1 mV) is clearly associated with CAD. It is apparent that this likelihood increases when the ST segment depression is more pronounced.

Magnitude of ST Segment Depression and the Degree of Anatomical Coronary Artery Disease

Many investigators have attempted to correlate the magnitude of ST segment depression with the degree of anatomical CAD. Initial studies reported that an increased magnitude of ST-depression was associated with an increased degree of ischemia [33, 68]. Later studies have been unable to correlate the ischemia estimated from the magnitude of the ST segment depression in any lead or from the sum of the ST-changes in all leads with either the number of diseased coronary

Bicycle ergometer
Protocol: steps of 20 Watts (W) per minute

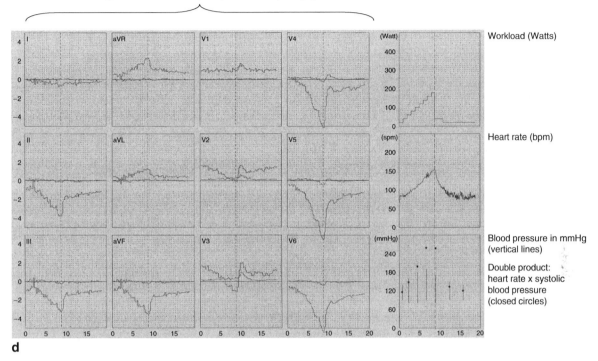

Trends of the ST segment in each of the 12 standard ECG leads
ST segment: measured at J-point plus 60 msec (x 100µV)

d

■ Fig. 4.6 (Continued)
(d) The respective ST segment trends illustrate the marked ST segment depression, predominantly occurring in the inferior and left precordial leads

■ Table 4.6
Probability of CAD in relation to degree of ST segment depression during exercise testing

ST-depression (mV)	Normal subjects (n=225)	Subjects with CAD (n=381)	Specificity (%)	Sensitivity (%)	Likelihood ratio for CAD
< 0.05	181	122			0.4
0.05–0.09	30	19	80	68	0.4
0.1–0.19	11	133	94	63	7.3
> 0.2	3	107	99	28	21.6

Pooled data from four studies [64–67] that provided information on the presence of coronary artery disease (CAD) in relation to the degree of ST segment depression during exercise stress testing. Seventeen patients with ST segment elevation have been excluded from reference [66].

arteries or the size of the area of reversible ischemia observed on myocardial perfusion scintigraphy [33, 69, 70]. As the development of ST segment depression as an electrophysiological phenomenon results from many influences, including those caused by electrolytes, hormones, and hemodynamic, metabolic, as well as anatomical changes, it is unlikely that the magnitude of ST segment depression would correlate well with the coronary anatomy in patients with CAD. Furthermore, the degree of ST-depression at higher workloads also depends on what is used as an indication to terminate exercise. For example, if patients with single vessel disease are encouraged to exercise strenuously or if they have some degree of left

Bicycle ergometer
Protocol: steps of 10 Watts (W) per minute
ST segment: measured at J-point plus 60 msec (μV); ST-slope in mV/sec

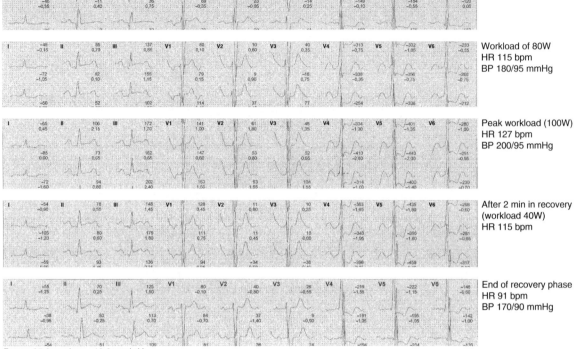

Baseline (10W)
HR 76 bpm
BP 160/95 mmHg

Workload of 80W
HR 115 bpm
BP 180/95 mmHg

Peak workload (100W)
HR 127 bpm
BP 200/95 mmHg

After 2 min in recovery
(workload 40W)
HR 115 bpm

End of recovery phase
HR 91 bpm
BP 170/90 mmHg

Paper: 25.0 mm/sec – 10.0 mm/mV

◻ Fig. 4.7

Bicycle exercise test (10 W/min protocol) in a 77-year old male with angina pectoris complaints, classified as II–III according to the Canadian Cardiovascular Society [63]. His medical history was unremarkable except for poorly controlled arterial hypertension. The resting ECG showed signs of an old inferior myocardial infarction (Q-waves in leads II, III, and aVF), as well as left ventricular hypertrophy with repolarization abnormalities in the left precordial leads (downsloping ST segment with inverted T-wave). With increasing workload, the preexistent ST segment depression increased progressively up to 4 mm (0.4 mV), persisting in the recovery period. Coronary angiography revealed three-vessel coronary artery disease and ventriculography showed a moderately impaired left ventricular systolic function. The patient subsequently underwent coronary artery bypass grafting

ventricular hypertrophy, they may have severe ST-depression (see also ❷ Figs. 4.6 (Continued) and ❷ 4.7). Therefore, the magnitude of ST segment depression at maximum workload may not indicate the severity of CAD.

Time Course of ST Segment Depression

ST segment depression that comes on early during exercise at low workloads is associated with more severe disease and impaired prognosis [33, 68, 71–73]. In a study on the predictive value of the time course of ST segment depression during exercise testing in patients referred for coronary angiography, a direct relationship between the time of onset and offset of ST-depression and the number of diseased coronary arteries was demonstrated [33, 73]. Severe three-vessel CAD was found in 33% of patients with early onset and late offset of the ST-depression, while this increased up to 50% in those with resting ST-depression that increased with exercise [73]. Even ST segment depression occurring at high workloads and with rapid resolution during recovery may be associated with significant CAD, although it may also indicate a false-positive response in an asymptomatic subject (❯ Fig. 4.5).

Furthermore, although ST segment depression during exercise often persists into the recovery phase, it sometimes may not develop until exercise has been terminated (❯ Fig. 4.4). Whereas this phenomenon is still not completely understood, several studies have demonstrated that ST segment depression occurring only during recovery has the same significance as exercise-induced ST-depression in predicting CAD [33, 74, 75].

Adjustment of ST Segment Depression

Subjects with tall R-waves exhibit a greater amount of ST segment depression than those with smaller R-wave amplitude [76]. Accordingly, when the R-wave in the lateral precordial leads is less than 10 mm, the sensitivity of ST-depression for the detection of CAD is low if 1 mm (0.1 mV) of ST-depression is required for a positive test result [77]. Correcting ST-depression for R-wave amplitude has been proposed by dividing the amount of ST segment depression by the R-wave height (both expressed in mm) [78]. The ST/R-ratio may then be used as an alternative to the amount of ST segment depression per se, with 0.1 as a cutoff value for an abnormal test result [33]. In studies, however, adjustment of the amount of ST segment depression by the R-wave height has not been shown to consistently improve the diagnostic value of exercise-induced ST-depression [4].

Several methods of heart rate adjustment have been proposed to increase the diagnostic accuracy of the exercise ECG. The first technique is to derive the maximal slope of the ST segment relative to heart rate (ST/HR slope). The second method, termed the ST/HR index, divides the difference between ST-depression at peak exercise by the delta heart rate (difference between resting and maximum heart rate) [4, 33, 79–82]. The value of ST/HR adjustment in improving diagnostic accuracy has been evaluated in several studies [4, 83–87]. Most studies, however, were limited by work-up bias and enrollment of relatively healthy patients, which presents a limited challenge to the ST/HR index [4, 85–87]. In a large multicenter study without these limitations, the ST/HR slope or index was not found to be more accurate than simple measurement of the ST segment depression [88]. The most recent guidelines on exercise testing take the perspective that the ST/HR adjustment approach in symptomatic patients has at least equivalent accuracy to the standard approach [4]. Although the ST/HR approach might be useful in assessing certain borderline or equivocal ST segment responses during exercise (e.g., ST segment depression associated with a very high exercise heart rate), further validation is required.

ST Segment Depression and the Location of Coronary Artery Disease

In several studies, an attempt has been made to relate the location of ST segment depression during exercise to coronary anatomy. As stated, extensive CAD (three-vessel disease) is more likely to be present in a patient who develops major ST segment depression in multiple leads at low workloads. However, even in patients with single-vessel disease, there is no clear separation between the leads in which ST segment depression develops when either the right coronary artery or the left anterior descending coronary artery is involved [67]. Studies using body-surface mapping indicate that the ST segment depression is most prominent in the precordium. The actual position where the largest ST segment depression occurs varies widely, from the level of the third intercostal space to the tenth intercostal space [46]. However, even analysis of precordial surface maps has not permitted an accurate prediction of the location of CAD [40, 89], although this has previously been claimed [40]. Furthermore, in another study, no relation was found between the spatial orientation of the ST segment vectors during exercise and the location of myocardial ischemia as detected by myocardial perfusion scintigraphy [90].

ST Segment Depression and/or Exercise-Induced Angina

The occurrence of chest pain during stress testing is of equal diagnostic value as the development of ST segment depression [91–93]. Symptoms that cannot be clearly understood during an outpatient clinic visit may be clarified if they occur during the actual exercise procedure and disappear rapidly in the recovery phase. In order to permit optimal comparison between the history of the patient and the observations during the stress test, it is recommended that either the test is performed by the patient's own physician, or that the physician supervising the test reports in detail all the complaints that occur during the test and notes whether these are similar to the complaints that led the patient to the outpatient clinic. In ❯ Fig. 4.8, the incidence of CAD and the number of diseased vessels are presented for ST segment depression with and without angina [92].

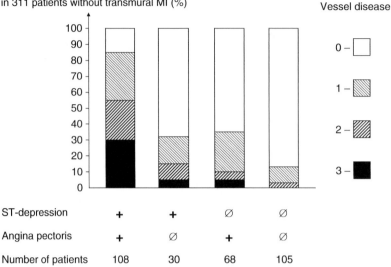

Percentage of one-, two- and three-vessel CAD in 311 patients without transmural MI (%)

ST-depression	+	+	∅	∅
Angina pectoris	+	∅	+	∅
Number of patients	108	30	68	105

■ Fig. 4.8

Incidence of normal coronary arteries (zero-) and one-, two-, or three-vessel disease in 311 patients without a history of transmural myocardial infarction. It should be noted that the incidence of CAD was similar in 30 patients with ST segment depression without symptoms (30%) and in 68 patients with exercise-induced angina without significant ECG changes (36%). ST-depression represents 0.1 mV or greater of ST segment depression in at least one precordial lead (Adapted from Roskamm [92])

4.6.2.2 ST Segment Elevation

ST segment elevation during exercise is observed most frequently in leads with Q-waves in patients with a history of myocardial infarction (❷ Fig. 4.9). The significance of ST segment elevation in areas of Q-waves of an old myocardial infarction is controversial. Some studies have suggested that this ST segment elevation is caused by an area with abnormal wall motion (ventricular akinesia or dyskinesia) [64, 94–97]. However, other studies have shown that in some patients such ST-elevation disappears after coronary bypass surgery, which suggests that the ST-elevation was a result of myocardial ischemia [98]. More recent studies using myocardial perfusion scintigraphy have found such ST-elevation to be a marker of residual viability in the infarcted area [99–101]. Therefore, it seems advisable to consider additional tests such as myocardial perfusion scintigraphy in patients with chest pain complaints after myocardial infarction and ST segment elevation during exercise stress testing.

Exercise-induced ST segment elevation in leads without Q-waves on a normal ECG (other than in aVR or V_1) is very rare and represents severe transmural myocardial ischemia (whereas ST segment depression represents subendocardial ischemia) [94, 102–109]. It is caused by a coronary artery spasm that completely obliterates antegrade flow through the epicardial artery, or a high-grade proximal stenosis in a coronary artery (❷ Fig. 4.10). In patients with variant or Prinzmetal's angina, coronary spasm is most commonly seen at rest, but very occasionally it occurs with exercise, probably indicating the presence of hemodynamically significant coronary atherosclerosis [33, 110, 111]. In contrast to ST segment depression, exercise-induced ST segment elevation is very arrhythmogenic and localizes the ischemic area. When ST segment elevation occurs in leads V_2 through V_4, there is severe anterior wall ischemia with a high-grade stenosis in the proximal left anterior descending coronary artery (❷ Fig. 4.10); in leads II, III, and aVF, there is severe inferior wall ischemia with involvement of a proximal stenosis in a large right coronary artery; and in the lateral leads, the left circumflex or diagonals are involved [4]. As stated previously, this rare finding warrants immediate discontinuation of the stress test and prompt referral for coronary angiography.

Bicycle ergometer
Protocol: steps of 20 Watts (W) per minute
ST segment: measured at J-point plus 60 msec (μV); ST-slope in mV/sec

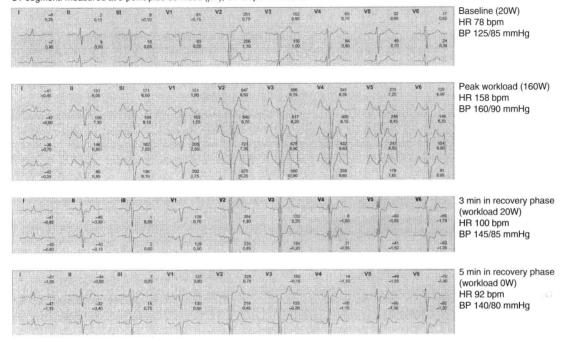

Baseline (20W)
HR 78 bpm
BP 125/85 mmHg

Peak workload (160W)
HR 158 bpm
BP 160/90 mmHg

3 min in recovery phase
(workload 20W)
HR 100 bpm
BP 145/85 mmHg

5 min in recovery phase
(workload 0W)
HR 92 bpm
BP 140/80 mmHg

Paper: 25.0 mm/sec −10.0 mm/mV

◘ Fig. 4.9

Bicycle exercise stress test in a 62-year-old male approximately 1 year after he underwent a primary coronary intervention with recanalization of the occluded left anterior descending coronary artery for an acute anterior myocardial infarction. The result of the intervention was suboptimal because there was no reflow in the infarct-related artery. No intervention was performed on a 50–70% stenosis in the left circumflex coronary artery. Echocardiography showed an impaired systolic left ventricular function with akinesia of the interventricular septum and hypokinesia of the anterior wall and apex. The baseline ECG showed sinus rhythm, a left anterior fascicular block, and a QRS-pattern compatible with an old antero-septal-apical myocardial infarction with QS-complexes in V_1 and V_2, a small R-wave in V_3, as well as a Q-wave in aVL. The patient reached 160 W and discontinued the test because of fatigue. The patient did not experience any anginal complaints or dyspnea during the test. With an increase in workload, there is an increasing level of ST segment elevation in the right precordial leads (V_1–V_3), representing either wall motion abnormalities or residual viability in the infarcted area. Furthermore, the duration of the QRS complex increased. In the recovery phase, minimal 0.5 mm (0.05 mV) downsloping ST segment depression developed in the inferior and left precordial leads

4.6.2.3 Changes of the QRS Complex

R-Wave Amplitude

It has previously been reported that an increase in R-wave amplitude during exercise is a useful indicator of CAD [112]. The first reports on this phenomenon were based on an unusual series of patients with known false-positive or false-negative ST-changes during exercise. Although some studies supported these observations, others found that the R-wave amplitude changes were variable both in patients with CAD and in normal subjects [52–54, 113]. It is possible that the observed differences in R-waves between patients with CAD and normal subjects result in part from differences in heart rate, since most patients stop exercising at heart rates between 120 and 150 beats/min which is the rate at which normal subjects frequently exhibit increased R-wave amplitudes [44]. The mechanisms of these changes also remain unclear. In particular, the hypothesis that the increase in R-wave amplitude would be related to an increase in ventricular volume owing to

Bicycle ergometer
Protocol: steps of 20 Watts (W) per minute
ST segment: measured at J-point plus 60 msec (µV); ST-slope in mV/sec

Baseline (0W) — HR 55 bpm; BP 110/70 mmHg

	I	II	III	V1	V2	V3	V4	V5	V6
line 1	−8 / 0.00	25 / −0.40	33 / −0.45	67 / 0.45	183 / 0.65	108 / 1.25	42 / 0.45	33 / 0.40	25 / 0.40
line 2	0 / 0.00	25 / 0.00	33 / 0.40	75 / 0.85	158 / 2.05	92 / 1.70	42 / 0.85	17 / 0.00	17 / 0.45

Workload of 200W — HR 128 bpm; BP 140/70 mmHg; Symptoms: dyspnea

	I	II	III	V1	V2	V3	V4	V5	V6
line 1	−50 / 0.85	−108 / 0.45	−42 / 0.40	117 / 0.45	25 / 2.10	−158 / 0.45	−183 / 0.45	−167 / 0.00	−125 / 0.40
line 2	−67 / −0.85	−133 / 0.45	−67 / 1.25	192 / 2.50	50 / 2.50	−92 / 1.25	−150 / 0.85	−158 / 0.45	−125 / 0.40
line 3	−100 / −0.40	−183 / 0.00	−83 / 0.85	258 / 2.90	158 / 2.90	−33 / 2.10	−125 / 0.85	−175 / 0.00	−167 / −0.85

Directly after peak workload, in recovery (40W) — HR 105 bpm; BP 140/60 mmHg; Symptoms: angina

	I	II	III	V1	V2	V3	V4	V5	V6
line 1	−0.40	0.40	0.85	2.05	2.90	2.50	1.25	0.85	0.85
line 2	−17 / 0.40	−125 / 0.85	−108 / 0.45	342 / 2.10	575 / 2.50	417 / 2.10	92 / 1.70	−33 / 0.85	−83 / 0.45
line 3	−42 / −0.45	−158 / −0.40	−108 / −0.45	333 / 2.90	542 / 2.10	458 / 2.05	158 / 0.80	8 / 0.40	−75 / 0.00

3 min in recovery phase (workload 20W) — HR 65 bpm; BP 140/80 mmHg

	I	II	III	V1	V2	V3	V4	V5	V6
line 1	−33 / 0.00	−58 / 0.45	−33 / 0.45	−192 / 0.85	250 / 0.85	183 / 0.65	8 / 0.00	−33 / 0.00	−67 / 0.45
line 2	−33 / −0.40	−50 / −0.40	−17 / 0.00	158 / 0.40	208 / 1.25	150 / 0.85	17 / 0.00	−33 / 0.00	−42 / 0.00

9 min in recovery phase — HR 60 bpm; BP 115/65 mmHg

	I	II	III	V1	V2	V3	V4	V5	V6
line 1	0 / 0.00	25 / 0.40	25 / 0.40	92 / 0.45	200 / 2.10	108 / 1.25	42 / 0.85	17 / 0.45	17 / 0.45
line 2	0 / −0.40	25 / −0.40	33 / 0.40	125 / 1.65	200 / 0.85	117 / 0.45	33 / 0.00	8 / 0.00	17 / 0.00

Paper: 25.0 mm/sec −10.0 mm/mV

◼ Fig. 4.10

Bicycle exercise test in a 59-year-old male with no history of cardiovascular disease who underwent stress testing because of complaints of chest pain on exertion suspected for angina pectoris. The predicted maximum workload was 163 W. The test was discontinued at 200 W by the attending physician because of shortness of breath, as well as failure of the blood pressure to rise in the presence of ST segment depression. Starting at 180 W, up to 1.0–1.5 mm (0.1–0.15 mV) of slow-upsloping to horizontal ST segment depression developed in the inferior and left precordial leads, indicating subendocardial ischemia. Directly following discontinuation of exercise, the patient experienced angina-like chest pain. This was attended on the ECG by ST segment elevation and a marked increase in T-wave amplitude in the right precordial leads, suggesting transmural ischemia due to a high-grade stenosis in the proximal left anterior descending artery. Later on in the recovery phase, biphasic T-waves developed in the right precordial leads. At the end of the recovery period, the ECG had returned to normal. The patient was subsequently admitted to hospital. Coronary angiography was performed the same day and revealed, as expected, a severe stenosis in the proximal left anterior descending artery which was treated with stent implantation

myocardial ischemia [114] was not supported by studies in which the volume changes were actually measured [52, 53, 115]. As exercise-induced changes in R-wave amplitude have provided very little, if any, discrimination for myocardial ischemia, the R-wave measurements are not routinely applied in clinical practice.

QRS-Duration

As stated, the duration of the QRS complex during exercise does not increase but may be reduced slightly because conduction velocity is increased by catecholamine release [50, 116]. Although a number of studies have shown that conduction velocity is decreased by myocardial ischemia [61, 117], QRS-duration measurements are not routinely used for the diagnosis of CAD as studies on this phenomenon have had equivocal results [61]. Prolongation of the QRS-duration during exercise was found to be associated with CAD in 330 patients who underwent exercise testing and coronary angiography [118]. The greatest prolongation was found in patients with three-vessel disease. However, the observations could not be used in individual patients to determine the presence or absence of myocardial ischemia as the variations around the mean value were too large [118].

Bundle-Branch Block

Rate-dependent bundle-branch block may become apparent during exercise and the interpretation of such a finding is the same as in rate-dependent bundle-branch block occurring under other circumstances. Rate-dependent left bundle-branch block, right bundle-branch block or left anterior fascicular block may be related to CAD [33, 119]. However, they have also been observed in healthy subjects without myocardial or coronary pathology [33]. The isolated finding of a rate-dependent bundle-branch block should, therefore, not be used as a proof of significant heart disease. On the other hand, the occurrence of a bundle-branch block during exercise should be viewed in light of the other clinical findings in each patient in order to assess the probability that CAD is present. Leftward rotation of the frontal axis with development of a left anterior fascicular block during exercise in a patient *with* CAD usually signifies involvement of the proximal left anterior descending coronary artery or three-vessel CAD [120, 121]. The axis shift associated with left anterior fascicular block may mask the ischemic ST segment changes in the frontal plane and to a lesser extent in the precordial leads.

The significance of ST segment depression as a predictor of ischemia in the presence of right bundle-branch block has been the subject of debate. Exercise-induced ST-depression usually occurs with right bundle-branch block in the anterior chest leads V_1 through V_3, probably because of secondary repolarization changes, and is not associated with ischemia [4, 122]. However, ST segment depression in the left precordial leads (V_5 and V_6) or inferior leads (II and aVF) has the same significance in predicting CAD as exercise-induced ST-depression in a normal resting ECG [123, 124].

Exercise-induced ST-depression usually occurs with left bundle-branch block and has no association with ischemia [125]. Even up to 10 mm of ST-depression occurs in healthy subjects. There is no level of ST-depression that confers diagnostic significance in left bundle-branch block. Therefore, there is a consensus, as stated in the guidelines, that exercise-induced ischemia cannot be diagnosed from the ECG in patients with left bundle-branch block [4].

4.6.2.4 T-Wave Changes

As previously mentioned, the T-wave amplitude varies greatly during exercise but increases considerably in most normal subjects immediately after exercise as a result of an increased stroke volume, which makes up for the lingering metabolic debt after the heart rate has dropped very rapidly. Many patients with flat or inverted T-waves at rest will manifest upright T-waves at the time of exercise. This is particularly true in women. This phenomenon of normalization of inverted T-waves or pseudonormalization of the T-waves is not considered to indicate ischemia. In earlier studies, T-wave normalization was accompanied by significant ST segment depression in 90% of patients with CAD, but by a negative test result based on ST segment criteria in all patients without ischemic heart disease [33, 126]. Similarly, exercise-induced deep T-wave inversion is almost always accompanied by significant ST segment depression and is then associated with a more severe degree of CAD.

4.7   Exercise Testing to Diagnose Coronary Artery Disease

The vast majority of exercise testing is performed in adults with symptoms of known or suspected ischemic heart disease. There has been considerable discussion on the value and use of exercise testing for the diagnosis of CAD and the literature on this subject is extensive. Knowledge of terminology used in describing diagnostic test characteristics and test performance is required for understanding the exercise test literature (❯ Table 4.7).

□ Table 4.7

Diagnostic test characteristics

True-positive test result (TP)	Abnormal test result in subject *with* disease
False-positive test result (FP)	Abnormal test result in subject *without* disease
True-negative test result (TN)	Normal test result in subject *without* disease
False-negative test result (FN)	Normal test result in subject *with* disease
Specificity	Percentage of subjects *without* disease who have a normal test result = TN/(TN + FP)
Sensitivity	Percentage of subjects *with* disease who have an abnormal test result = TP/(TP + FN)
Test accuracy	Percentage of true test results = (TP + TN)/total number of tests performed
Predictive value of a positive test result	Percentage of subjects with abnormal test who have the disease = TP/(TP + FP)
Predictive value of a negative test result	Percentage of subjects with normal test and without disease = TN/(TN + FN)
Formula for calculation of posttest probability (Bayes' theorem):	
Posttest odds (disease present) = pretest odds (disease present) × likelihood ratio (LR) where, odds = probability/(1 − probability) LR = sensitivity/(1 − specificity) in case of an abnormal test result = (1 − sensitivity)/specificity in case of a normal test result	
Posttest odds (disease absent) = pretest odds (disease absent) × likelihood ratio (LR) where, odds = probability/(1 − probability) LR = (1 − specificity)/sensitivity in case of an abnormal test result = specificity/(1 − sensitivity) in case of a normal test result	
The better (very high or very low) the likelihood ratio of the test (determined by sensitivity and specificity), the more discriminant the test is.	

□ Table 4.8

Pretest probability (%) of CAD in patients by age, sex, and chest pain characteristics (Adapted from Diamond and Forrester [127])

Age (years)	Sex	Non-anginal chest pain	Atypical angina	Typical angina
30–39	M	5.2 ± 0.8	21.8 ± 2.4	69.7 ± 3.2
	F	0.8 ± 0.3	4.2 ± 1.3	25.8 ± 6.6
40–49	M	14.1 ± 1.3	46.1 ± 1.8	87.3 ± 1.0
	F	2.8 ± 0.7	13.3 ± 2.9	55.2 ± 6.5
50–59	M	21.5 ± 1.7	58.9 ± 1.5	92.0 ± 0.6
	F	8.4 ± 1.2	32.4 ± 3.0	79.4 ± 2.4
60–69	M	28.1 ± 1.9	67.1 ± 1.3	94.3 ± 0.4
	F	18.6 ± 1.9	54.4 ± 2.4	90.6 ± 1.0

CAD denotes coronary artery disease

4.7.1 Pretest Probability

The pretest probability of obstructive CAD can be estimated from factors such as age, gender, risk factors, and chest pain characteristics [127–129]. The pretest probabilities described in this way by Diamond and Forrester in a series of over 60,000 patients are shown in ❷ Table 4.8 [127]. From this table, it is apparent that exercise testing is not very useful for establishing the diagnosis CAD in a 64-year-old man with typical or definite angina. The pretest probability of CAD is so

■ Table 4.9

Posttest probability (%) of coronary artery disease based on age, sex, symptom classification, and exercise test-induced electrocardiographic ST segment depression

Age	ST-depression (mV)	Typical angina		Atypical angina		Non-anginal chest pain		Asymptomatic	
		M	F	M	F	M	F	M	F
30–39	0.00–0.04	25	7	6	1	1	<1	<1	<1
	0.05–0.09	68	24	21	4	5	1	2	<1
	0.10–0.14	83	42	38	9	10	2	4	<1
	0.15–0.19	91	59	55	15	19	3	7	1
	0.20–0.24	96	79	76	33	39	8	18	3
	>0.25	99	93	92	63	68	24	43	11
40–49	0.00–0.04	61	22	16	3	4	1	1	<1
	0.05–0.09	86	53	44	12	13	3	5	1
	0.10–0.14	94	72	64	25	26	6	11	2
	0.15–0.19	97	84	78	39	41	11	20	4
	0.20–0.24	99	93	91	63	65	24	39	10
	>0.25	>99	98	97	86	87	53	69	28
50–59	0.00–0.04	73	47	25	10	6	2	2	1
	0.05–0.09	91	78	57	31	20	8	9	3
	0.10–0.14	96	89	75	50	37	16	19	7
	0.15–0.19	98	94	86	67	53	28	31	12
	0.20–0.24	99	98	94	84	75	50	54	27
	>0.25	>99	99	98	95	91	78	81	56
60–69	0.00–0.04	79	69	32	21	8	5	3	2
	0.05–0.09	94	90	65	52	26	17	11	7
	0.10–0.14	97	95	81	72	45	33	23	15
	0.15–0.19	99	98	89	83	62	49	37	25
	0.20–0.24	99	99	96	93	81	72	61	47
	>0.25	>99	>99	99	98	94	90	85	76

high that the test result does not substantially change this probability. As shown in ❯ Table 4.9, the likelihood of CAD is 79% if no ST segment depression occurs during the test, while it would be 99% if 2 mm (0.2 mV) of ST segment depression developed. However, the test may still be used to determine the functional impairment of that subject, to measure the blood-pressure and heart rate response, or to estimate the prognosis. Similarly, the diagnostic value of exercise electrocardiography is low in asymptomatic men and women (see also ❯ Fig. 4.11). The greatest diagnostic value of exercise testing is obtained in patients with an intermediate pretest probability of CAD, for example, between 20% and 80%, because the test result has the largest potential effect on diagnostic outcome. If the posttest likelihood is intermediate, another noninvasive (e.g., myocardial perfusion scintigraphy) or invasive test may be applied.

4.7.2 Diagnostic Characteristics and Test Performance

One of the problems with diagnostic tests for CAD is that there is a considerable overlap in the range of measurements for the normal population and those with CAD. Since the depth of exercise-induced ST segment depression and the extent of the myocardial ischemic response can be considered as continuous variables, a certain cutpoint or discriminant value (e.g., 1 mm (0.1 mV) of ST segment depression) cannot completely discriminate patients with CAD from those without

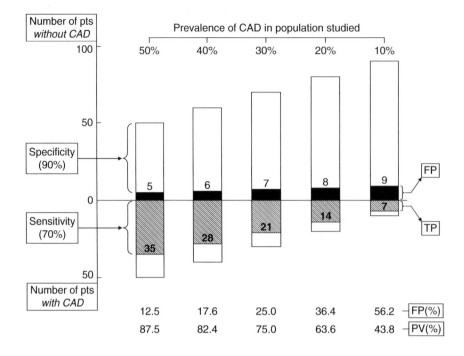

◘ Fig. 4.11
Illustration of the impact of the prevalence of CAD in the population studied on the fraction of false-positive test results and the predictive value of the exercise test. Each bar represents a population of 100 patients. In the left-most bar, 50 patients have CAD, while 50 do not have CAD. In the second bar, 40% has CAD, in the third 30%, in the fourth 20%, and in the right-most bar only 10%. In each theoretical example, the sensitivity for detection of CAD is 70%. Thus, 70% of patients with CAD do indeed have ischemic ST segment depression. On the other hand, the specificity is 90%. Thus, 10% of the patients without CAD exhibit false-positive ST segment depression (black area). In the population with a 50% prevalence of CAD (left-most bar), 40 abnormal tests are found, five of which are false-positive (12.5%). In the population with only a 10% prevalence of CAD (right-most bar), nine false-positive tests occur out of a total of 16 tests with ST segment depression (56.2%). In this latter population, which reflects the prevalence of CAD in many screening conditions, the number of false-positives is higher than the number of correct or true-positive test results. CAD, coronary artery disease; FP, false-positive; PV, predictive value; Pts, patients; and TP, true-positive

disease. A higher discriminant value for ST segment depression improves specificity, but reduces the test's sensitivity. Therefore, sensitivity and specificity are inversely related and determined by the choice of a cutpoint or discriminant value. The positive predictive value (PPV) and negative predictive value (NPV) are also affected by the population tested. The PPV will be higher in a population with a higher prevalence of CAD. Accordingly, PPV is higher in patients with three-vessel CAD and lower in patients with one-vessel CAD. The NPV can be decreased if the test is used in patients in whom false-positive results are more likely such as those with ST segment depression on the resting ECG or left ventricular hypertrophy. ❷ Figure 4.11 illustrates these points.

4.7.3   Probability Analysis

The use of Bayes' theorem of conditional probability can assist in the interpretation of a test result and can also provide a meaningful estimate of the posttest probability in the individual patient. According to this theorem, posttest probability is a function of pretest probability, and the sensitivity and specificity (likelihood ratio) of the test [130].

Under the assumption of the independence of the exercise test result from the clinical (pretest) data, posttest probability can be calculated according to the formula listed in ❯ Table 4.7. Although this calculation is often made intuitively by the clinician, mathematical equations or scores have been developed from multivariate analysis of clinical and exercise test variables (including heart rate at peak exercise, ST segment response, the presence or absence of angina during the test, peak workload, and ST segment slope) that can provide a more accurate estimate of the probability that CAD is present, when compared with use of the ST segment measurements alone [4, 131–135]. However, the use of these statistical models remains limited. Nevertheless, they underline the importance of taking into account all relevant variables when estimating the probability of CAD in a given subject [136–138].

4.7.4 Diagnostic Accuracy of the Standard Exercise Test

A meta-analysis was performed on the diagnostic accuracy of the exercise test based on 147 consecutive published reports involving 24,074 patients who underwent both coronary angiography and exercise testing [139, 140]. There was a wide variability in the reported diagnostic accuracy of the standard exercise test among the studies (❯ Table 4.10). The mean sensitivity was 68% (range 23–100%) and mean specificity was 77% (range 17–100%). This large variability results from the fact that most studies do not fulfill two major criteria that are important when evaluating diagnostic tests [4]. The first concerns the fact that the population studied does not represent the diagnostic dilemma group in clinical practice. In particular, inclusion of patients who most certainly have the disease (e.g., post-myocardial infarction patients) in the test group presents a limited challenge to the diagnostic test. The second cause concerns the presence of work-up bias which refers to the fact that most reported studies were affected to some degree by clinical practice wherein the results of the exercise test were used to decide who would undergo coronary angiography and be included in the study [4]. The reported meta-analysis provides, however, the best estimate of the diagnostic accuracy of the exercise test. When only studies that excluded patients with a previous myocardial infarction were considered, mean sensitivity was 67% and mean specificity 72% (❯ Table 4.10). Only three studies avoided work-up bias and provide an estimate of the diagnostic accuracy of exercise testing in a more general population of patients presenting with chest pain [141–143]. The mean sensitivity and specificity in these studies were 50% and 90%, respectively (❯ Table 4.10).

4.7.5 Electrocardiographic Factors Influencing Sensitivity and Specificity

The influence of left ventricular hypertrophy, resting ST segment depression and use of digoxin on the exercise test characteristics are summarized in ❯ Table 4.10. Left ventricular hypertrophy with repolarization abnormalities is associated

◩ Table 4.10

Meta-analysis of diagnostic performance of exercise test (Adapted from ACC/AHA Practice Guidelines on Exercise Testing [4] and from [139, 140])

(Sub-)Groups	Number of studies	Total number of patients	Sensitivity (%)	Specificity (%)	Predictive accuracy (%)
Meta-analysis of standard exercise test	147	24, 047	68	77	73
Meta-analysis *without* prior MI	58	11, 691	67	72	69
Meta-analysis *without* work-up bias	3	>1,000	50	90	69
Meta-analysis *with* ST-depression	22	9, 153	69	70	69
Meta-analysis *without* ST-depression	3	840	67	84	75
Meta-analysis *with* digoxin	15	6, 338	68	74	71
Meta-analysis *without* digoxin	9	3, 548	72	69	70
Meta-analysis *with* LVH	15	8, 016	68	69	68
Meta-analysis *without* LVH	10	1, 977	72	77	74

LVH left ventricular hypertrophy, *MI* myocardial infarction

with a decreased specificity, but sensitivity is unaffected. If the test result is negative, the probability of CAD is substantially reduced, but additional tests are indicated in patients with an abnormal test result (❷ Fig. 4.7). Although not apparent from ❷ Table 4.10, studies have suggested that digoxin also lowers specificity by producing an abnormal ST segment response to exercise, which occurs in up to 40% of healthy individuals [144, 145]. Resting ST segment depression is associated with a higher prevalence of severe CAD and a higher incidence of adverse cardiac events [4, 146–151]. As shown in ❷ Table 4.10, resting ST-depression lowers specificity of the exercise test. The most recent guidelines on exercise testing state that, if the resting ST segment depression is less than 1 mm (0.1 mV), the standard exercise test may still be the first test because sensitivity is increased [4]. In a retrospective study of male patients with resting ST segment depression, but without prior myocardial infarction, undergoing exercise testing, 2 mm (0.2 mV) of additional exercise-induced ST segment depression, or downsloping ST segment depression of 1 mm (0.1 mV) or more in the recovery phase were found to be important markers for the diagnosis of CAD, with a sensitivity of 67%, a specificity of 80%, and a likelihood ratio of 3.4 [4, 151]. In patients with less than 1 mm (0.1 mV) of resting ST segment depression who are also taking digoxin or have left ventricular hypertrophy, as well as in those with more than 1 mm (0.1 mV) of resting ST segment depression (❷ Fig. 4.7), the diagnostic merits of the standard exercise test may be insufficient and imaging tests such as myocardial perfusion scintigraphy or stress echocardiography are preferred [4].

Finally, as stated, specificity was lowered and sensitivity increased when upsloping ST segment depression was classified as abnormal. Furthermore, the presence of right bundle-branch block does not appear to reduce the diagnostic accuracy of the exercise test for the diagnosis of CAD. On the contrary, exercise testing should not be used for the diagnosis of CAD in patients with complete left bundle-branch block, or in those with pre-excitation (Wolff-Parkinson-White) syndrome, or electronically paced ventricular rhythm [4].

4.7.6 Exercise Electrocardiography Versus Noninvasive Stress Imaging Studies

Although it is beyond the scope of this chapter to include a complete discussion on the comparison of exercise electrocardiography with the noninvasive stress imaging tests for the diagnosis of CAD, some features are presented here in brief. Studies that compared the diagnostic performance between exercise electrocardiography and the noninvasive imaging modalities using pharmacological stress (e.g., stress echocardiography or stress single-photon emission computed tomography (SPECT) myocardial perfusion scintigraphy) indicate that the latter are both more sensitive and more specific for the detection of CAD [152–155]. Furthermore, myocardial perfusion scintigraphy and stress echocardiography permit, to a certain extent, separation of patients with single and multiple vessel CAD and detection of the location of significant coronary artery stenosis [152–156]. This does not mean that exercise electrocardiography should be replaced by these imaging modalities. In many patients, CAD can be effectively ruled out, or diagnosed, by conventional exercise testing. Noninvasive imaging tests may provide additional information if the diagnosis is uncertain after conventional exercise testing, for example, if there is a posttest likelihood of intermediate probability. This likelihood is then considered as the pretest likelihood for the stress imaging test, as shown in ❷ Table 4.11 for myocardial perfusion scintigraphy; a 50% likelihood will reduce to 15% if the scintigram is normal, or increase to 93% if a reversible perfusion defect occurs. Myocardial perfusion scintigraphy and stress echocardiography using pharmacological stress agents can also be a useful alternative to exercise stress protocols in patients who are unable to exercise because of neurological, orthopedic, or peripheral vascular disease, as well as in those patients in whom interpretation of the ECG is hampered [152–158]. For a more complete and detailed overview of the noninvasive imaging modalities and their usefulness in the evaluation of CAD, the reader is referred to the relevant literature and guidelines [152–158].

4.8 Exercise Testing in Patients with Coronary Artery Disease

The value of exercise testing for risk or prognostic stratification must be considered in the light of what is added to that which is already known about the patient's risk status. Most studies on risk assessment in patients with CAD using exercise testing have focused on the relation between test parameters and future survival. The strongest predictor of survival in patients with CAD is the function of the left ventricle. Other important prognostic factors include the anatomic extent

▢ Table 4.11

Calculation of posttest probability of CAD after myocardial perfusion scintigraphy. The pretest probability (*after* exercise testing) can be obtained from the appropriate data in ❷ Table 4.9

Pretest probability (%)	Posttest probability (after nuclear perfusion scintigraphy in %)		
	No defect	Nonreversible defect	Reversible defect
10	2	14	56
20	4	26	74
30	7	38	83
40	10	49	89
50	15	59	92
60	21	68	95
70	29	77	96
80	41	85	98
90	61	93	99

CAD denotes coronary artery disease

and severity of CAD, evidence of a recent acute coronary syndrome resulting from a coronary plaque rupture, and the propensity for the development of ventricular arrhythmias.

4.8.1 Risk Stratification and Assessment of Prognosis with Exercise Testing

In patients with suspected or known CAD and symptoms suggestive of myocardial ischemia, exercise testing is the standard initial test in those with a normal ECG for identification of ischemia and risk assessment [4, 159–161]. In patients with a non-interpretable ECG, exercise testing may still provide useful prognostic information, but cannot be used to identify ischemia. Studies on the prognostic value of the exercise test in symptomatic patients with non-acute CAD identify the maximum exercise capacity to be the strongest and most consistent prognostic factor [4, 162–168]. Maximum exercise capacity can be expressed as maximum exercise duration, maximum workload or MET level achieved, maximum blood pressure, or double (rate-pressure) product and represents at least in part left ventricular function. Markers of exercise-induced ischemia (electrocardiographic and/or clinical) represent the second group of variables that bear adverse prognostic information. In particular, electrocardiographic evidence of myocardial ischemia in patients with a low maximum exercise capacity represents a high-risk population [4, 162, 169].

Using data of 2,842 patients with known or suspected CAD, without prior revascularization or recent myocardial infarction, who underwent exercise testing before coronary angiography, the Duke treadmill score was created [163, 170]. This score is calculated using multiple variables of prognostic importance from the exercise test and can subsequently be converted into an average annual mortality rate [163, 170]. Based on the individual scores, patients can be classified in a high-risk group with a high average annual cardiovascular mortality, an intermediate risk group, or a low-risk group. The Duke treadmill score was shown to independently add prognostic information to the standard clinical data plus the data resulting from cardiac catheterization. The score can also be applied in women, although women have a lower overall risk for any score value than men [171]. Comparable prognostic scores have been developed by other groups [164].

Recently, several studies have identified other parameters from the exercise test to bear important prognostic information. These include chronotropic incompetence, abnormal heart rate recovery, and delayed blood pressure response [172–179]. In one study of almost 10,000, mostly, asymptomatic patients, it was demonstrated that abnormal heart rate recovery and the Duke treadmill score were independent predictors of mortality [4, 177].

Exercise testing is a much stronger predictor of cardiovascular mortality than of nonfatal myocardial infarction. This may, in part, be a result of the fact that myocardial infarctions are mostly caused by rupture of relatively small, vulnerable atherosclerotic plaques that are difficult to detect by exercise testing because of their non-obstructive character, whereas exercise test results are correlated with the presence and severity of obstructive CAD [4, 163, 180].

4.8.2   Exercise Testing to Guide Patient Treatment

The results of exercise testing may be used to guide patient treatment. Patients with a low risk exercise test result and a low predicted average annual mortality rate can be treated medically, whereas patients at higher risk should be referred for additional testing or cardiac catheterization, especially in case of left ventricular dysfunction.

Patients with acute coronary syndromes without persistent ST segment elevation are stratified as low, intermediate, or high risk based on history, physical examination, 12-lead ECG, and cardiac markers of myocardial necrosis [181, 182]. High-risk patients will be scheduled to undergo coronary angiography and subsequent revascularization. In low or intermediate risk patients with unstable angina, exercise or pharmacologic stress testing plays an important part in risk stratification and identification of obstructive CAD. Exercise electrocardiography should be the standard mode of stress testing in patients with a normal resting ECG [4]. In general, stress testing can be performed as soon as the patient has stabilized clinically. Furthermore, studies have shown that exercise testing is safe when used in emergency department chest pain centers to provide risk stratification for chest pain patients believed to possibly have acute coronary disease [4, 183–185]. However, exercise testing in this setting should only be used in low, and intermediate risk patients on the basis of history, physical examination, 12-lead ECG, and markers of myocardial necrosis.

4.9   Exercise Testing after Acute Myocardial Infarction

Exercise testing after acute myocardial infarction can be used for patient management, risk stratification, and prognostic assessment. Treatment strategies for acute myocardial infarction have changed substantially over the past decades. In particular, the advent of reperfusion therapy involving the use of fibrinolytic agents or, more recently, direct or primary percutaneous coronary intervention has led to a marked improvement in the prognosis of patients after myocardial infarction. Contemporary medical treatment with beta-adrenergic blocking agents and angiotensin converting enzyme inhibitors has further improved prognosis. The patient population currently undergoing exercise testing after acute myocardial infarction is, therefore, far different from historical populations before the reperfusion era. The goals and basic principles of exercise testing have, however, not changed dramatically. Therefore, the role of exercise testing must be viewed in the context of the patients who present for exercise testing.

In patients following acute myocardial infarction, exercise testing is frequently performed before hospital discharge to establish the hemodynamic response and functional capacity for exercise prescriptions and cardiac rehabilitation, to detect serious ventricular arrhythmia, and to identify patients with inducible myocardial ischemia [186–191]. Furthermore, it is helpful in reestablishing patients' confidence in their ability to conduct their activities following discharge. Predischarge exercise testing in patients after acute myocardial infarction appears to be safe provided that the proper contraindications are observed [188, 192, 193]. Major contraindications in this patient population include manifest congestive heart failure and postinfarction angina. Predischarge exercise testing has historically been performed between 5 and 26 days following myocardial infarction [188, 192, 194, 196], although studies have suggested that exercise testing can also be performed safely within 3–4 days in patients with an uncomplicated myocardial infarction [196, 197]. Predischarge exercise testing following acute myocardial infarction has traditionally utilized a submaximal protocol that requires the patient to exercise until a target, predetermined workload (e.g., achievement of 5–6 METs or 70–80% of age-predicted maximum) has been reached [198]. However, it has been proposed that symptom-limited exercise testing prior to discharge may be safely performed in patients with an uncomplicated postinfarction course. As opposed to submaximal testing, performance of a symptom-limited test provides a better estimate of peak functional capacity and is associated with an increased detection rate of ischemic ST segment changes and angina pectoris [188, 193, 199].

4.9.1   Exercise Testing in Patient Management

Both in patients treated with thrombolysis and in those who have not received reperfusion therapy, a predischarge standard exercise test remains the test of choice to identify myocardial ischemia and select patients who might benefit from coronary angiography and revascularization. Imaging studies may be helpful for risk stratification and detection of myocardial ischemia in patients who have physical limitations that prevent them from exercising to an adequate workload, or in those with ECG abnormalities that preclude an accurate interpretation of ST segment changes. As expected, patients treated with thrombolytic therapy exhibit exercise-induced angina and ST segment depression less frequently than patients who have not received reperfusion therapy. In patients treated with direct or primary percutaneous coronary intervention, the coronary anatomy is known. If, besides the infarct-related artery, one or more of the other coronary arteries also shows a significant and important coronary obstruction at the time of angiography, additional coronary revascularization may be warranted. If the other coronary lesions found at the time of angiography are of intermediate or equivocal severity and significance, exercise testing or noninvasive stress imaging studies can be used to provoke residual ischemia and select patients who might benefit from additional revascularization, as well as those who can be managed conservatively.

4.9.2 Risk Stratification and Prognostic Assessment

As stated, the prognosis among patients after myocardial infarction has improved significantly, particularly in those who have received thrombolytic therapy or revascularization during hospitalization. Consequently, the low subsequent cardiac event rate associated with this improved treatment and survival substantially reduces the predictive accuracy of early exercise testing. Parameters derived from the exercise test following acute myocardial infarction that are associated with an increased risk of future death or recurrent nonfatal myocardial infarction include inability to perform the submaximal predischarge exercise test, poor exercise capacity, inability to increase - or a decrease in - systolic blood pressure, the development and magnitude of ST segment depression, especially at low workloads, and the development of angina [186, 194, 200–206].

Patients who have not undergone coronary revascularization and are unable to undergo exercise testing have the highest cardiac event rate. This was demonstrated both in trials in the thrombolytic era and in earlier studies in patients not receiving thrombolytic agents [194, 200–204]. In patients who are able to perform the test, exercise capacity is an important predictor of adverse cardiac events [189, 194, 195, 200, 203, 206–209]. Similarly, the hemodynamic response during the exercise test is of prognostic importance. Failure to increase systolic blood pressure by 10–30 mmHg or a decrease in blood pressure during exercise have been shown to be independent predictors of adverse outcome in patients after myocardial infarction [191, 195, 200, 203, 206, 209–211]. In a study in the prethrombolytic era, the degree of blood pressure rise during the exercise test was reported to be the single best predictive measurement [210]. The exercise capacity and the change in systolic blood pressure are, in fact, measures of left ventricular function which is the most important prognostic determinant of mortality following acute myocardial infarction. However, it was demonstrated that the maximum exercise capacity achieved during exercise testing provided an incremental prognostic value in patients with a low (less than 35%) left ventricular ejection fraction by gated radionuclide scintigraphy 1 month after acute myocardial infarction [212].

Exercise-induced ischemic ST segment depression in patients after myocardial infarction is an independent predictor of death or nonfatal myocardial infarction, particularly if the ST segment depression is accompanied by angina, occurs at a low level of exercise or in patients with controlled congestive heart failure [189, 203, 205, 206, 213, 214]. The predictive value of exercise-induced ischemia for adverse outcome is, however, limited by the fact that many patients who have an abnormal test result undergo coronary revascularization, which may alter the natural history of the disease process [193, 194, 201, 208, 215].

Finally, exercise testing can be used for activity counseling after hospital discharge and is an important tool in exercise training as part of a comprehensive cardiac rehabilitation program [4, 198].

4.10 Exercise Testing after Revascularization

4.10.1 Exercise Testing after Coronary Artery Bypass Grafting

The conversion of a positive exercise test result performed before coronary artery bypass grafting (CABG) to a negative postoperative test result is associated with successful revascularization [4, 216]. In patients with recurrent chest pain after

CABG, exercise testing may be used to demonstrate myocardial ischemia, although the exercise ECG is limited in this group of patients by the relatively high frequency of resting ECG abnormalities and the inability to document the site and extent of ischemia, as compared to stress imaging tests [4, 217, 218].

Exercise testing may be used for guiding exercise training as part of cardiac rehabilitation. It has been demonstrated that exercise testing in an asymptomatic individual, who has undergone successful CABG, is not predictive of outcome when the test is performed within the first few years after CABG [219, 220]. Therefore, routine periodic monitoring of asymptomatic patients after CABG is not indicated [4].

4.10.2 Exercise Testing after Percutaneous Coronary Intervention

Several studies that evaluated the diagnostic accuracy of exercise testing for identification of restenosis after percutaneous coronary intervention have shown that the exercise ECG is an insensitive predictor of restenosis [221–226], especially in asymptomatic patients, with sensitivities ranging from 40% to 50%, significantly less than those obtained by stress imaging tests [227, 228]. The insensitivity may be caused by the failure of moderate one-vessel stenoses to lead to significant ischemia on the exercise ECG. Routine, periodic exercise testing of asymptomatic patients after percutaneous coronary intervention without specific indications is therefore not recommended, especially since the prognostic benefit of controlling silent ischemia needs to be proved [4].

4.11 Exercise Testing and Heart Rhythm Disorders

Heart rhythm disorders occur frequently with exercise. The prevalence increases steadily with age, both in patients with heart disease and in normal individuals [229–231]. Increased sympathetic tone with withdrawal of much of the vagal tone, as well as myocardial ischemia may all play a role in the development of cardiac arrhythmias.

4.11.1 Sinus Node Dysfunction

Exercise testing may distinguish subjects with resting bradycardia with a normal increase in heart rate with exercise from those with sinus node dysfunction with a low resting heart rate that fails to accelerate normally with exercise, which is also labeled as chronotropic incompetence [4]. The definition of chronotropic incompetence has varied, the most common definition being failure to achieve 85% of (i.e., more than two standard deviations below) age-predicted maximum heart rate [4, 232]. The mechanisms involved are complex and not yet completely understood [233]. However, studies have confirmed the adverse prognostic implications of chronotropic incompetence [172, 233, 234]. Furthermore, a normal exercise test result does not negate the possibility of sinus node dysfunction.

4.11.2 Supraventricular Arrhythmias

The incidence of any supraventricular arrhythmia during exercise testing varies from 4% to 18% and increases with age. Atrial premature beats regularly occur at lower workloads, disappear as exercise increases and may return in the recovery period. They are considered to be of little clinical significance.

The majority of patients with atrial fibrillation demonstrate an abnormal heart rate response to exercise, which comprises an initial reduction of heart rate followed by delayed acceleration at lower workloads and a subsequent exaggerated increase in heart rate with tachycardia often persisting for a long period of time in the recovery phase [4, 235]. In patients with atrial fibrillation, exercise testing may help to evaluate the efficacy of drug regimens aimed at ventricular rate control. The ST segment changes associated with myocardial ischemia in atrial fibrillation are similar to those observed with sinus rhythm. However, in patients with atrial fibrillation and a very high ventricular response, the very short diastolic intervals may produce subendocardial ischemia because of the inadequate perfusion time in the absence of CAD. Atrial fibrillation initiated by exercise can be associated with CAD, rheumatic heart disease, or cardiomyopathy. However, it is also seen in subjects with no apparent cardiac abnormalities, in whom it may be a prelude to the development of sustained atrial fibrillation at a later stage [33].

Patients with Wolff-Parkinson-White syndrome may exhibit ST segment depression during exercise testing in the absence of CAD. In patients with Wolff-Parkinson-White syndrome, exercise testing may be used to help evaluate the risk of developing rapid ventricular response during atrial arrhythmias. When the pre-excitation disappears during exercise, the antegrade refractory period in the accessory pathway is longer than that in the atrioventricular node and it is unlikely that a rapid ventricular response will occur [4].

4.11.3 Ventricular Arrhythmias

In normal subjects, there is an increase in the incidence of resting premature ventricular contractions (PVCs) of 2–15% with age [236]. It has been demonstrated that, in the absence of overt heart disease, these resting PVCs are usually benign [237]. PVCs are often induced by exercise and the incidence in clinically normal, middle-aged or older subjects during maximum stress testing is about 35%–45%, usually at high workloads [238–240]. In general, exercise-induced ventricular arrhythmias in a large group of subjects without symptoms followed for 5–10 years were found to have no influence on subsequent morbidity and mortality, and appear to be benign [239, 241]. These data are generally believed to apply to all asymptomatic individuals although one study on a large cohort of asymptomatic men suggests that exercise-induced PVCs may have more adverse prognostic implications than previously reported [242].

In patients with CAD, the reported incidence of ventricular arrhythmias during exercise ranges from 40% to 65% [238, 243, 244]. In general, patients with CAD manifest arrhythmias at a lower heart rate than normal subjects. Despite the fact that PVCs are more easily evoked in patients with CAD than in normal subjects, there is too much overlap between those with and without ischemia to allow such arrhythmias to have diagnostic value. Accordingly, the appearance of PVCs, including multiform or repetitive PVCs, should not be interpreted as a sign of myocardial ischemia in diagnostic stress testing [245].

The appearance of frequent, multiform, or repetitive PVCs during exercise is associated with an increased risk of mortality in patients with a previous myocardial infarction, especially apparent in patients with an impaired left ventricular function [246–252]. Most studies suggest that exercise-induced PVCs are also associated with an impaired survival in patients with CAD without a previous myocardial infarction, especially in cases of multiform, repetitive PVCs or (nonsustained) ventricular tachycardia [238, 244, 253–256]. Some reports have disputed such an association, however, at least in low-risk patients with demonstrable stable CAD [245, 257, 258]. Significant multivessel disease is likely to be present in patients with angina and exercise-induced ventricular arrhythmias, especially if ischemic ST segment changes are also present [238, 244, 245, 255, 256]. Although the induction of PVCs by exercise is well recognized, ventricular ectopic activity may also be abolished by exercise in patients with CAD, just as it may be in normal subjects. Therefore, this finding does not exclude the presence of CAD [33, 238, 255].

In general, more arrhythmias are seen on recovery than during exercise. In the recovery period, the imbalance between oxygen supply and demand induced during exercise may be augmented in patients with CAD; peripheral dilatation induced by exercise combined with a reduced venous return caused by cessation of muscular activity may result in reduced cardiac output and coronary flow at a time when myocardial oxygen demand is still high owing to tachycardia. Furthermore, catecholamine levels are considerably elevated [259]. These changes can be minimized by a gradual cool down.

4.11.3.1 Exercise-Induced Sustained Ventricular Tachycardia

Sustained ventricular tachycardia during exercise testing is relatively rare and occurs most frequently in the group of patients with ventricular tachycardia or ventricular fibrillation as their primary complaint. As stated previously, because ventricular tachycardia can deteriorate into ventricular fibrillation, immediate termination of exercise is warranted. Sustained ventricular tachycardia or long runs of non-sustained ventricular tachycardia usually portray serious underlying diseases; either CAD with ischemia or some type of cardiomyopathy should be suspected. Ventricular tachycardia caused by ischemia almost never has a left bundle-branch block pattern.

4.11.3.2 Exercise Testing to Evaluate Spontaneous Ventricular Tachycardia

Exercise testing can play an important role in the workup of patients who survived sudden death, as well as in those with syncope and sustained ventricular tachycardia [4]. The usefulness of exercise-testing in patients with ventricular tachycardia is variable, according to the cause of the tachycardia. In patients with idiopathic right ventricular outflow tract tachycardia, the ventricular tachycardia can be reproducibly induced during stress testing as it is commonly provoked by exercise. During exercise testing, the patients also exhibit many PVCs and coupled PVCs. The ventricular tachycardia has a left bundle-branch block morphology and is more likely to be non-sustained [260].

In adrenergic-dependent ventricular tachycardia, including monomorphic ventricular tachycardia and polymorphic ventricular tachycardia related to long-QT syndromes, exercise testing may supply the circumstances necessary for induction of the ventricular tachycardia and is, therefore, a useful prelude to an electrophysiological study [4]. Furthermore, the occurrence and nature of exercise-induced ventricular ectopy is of prognostic value in these patients [4, 254, 261]. Even in patients at risk of ventricular tachycardia, maximal exercise testing can be conducted safely with the appropriate precautions [4, 262]. The main limitation of exercise testing in patients with ventricular arrhythmias is related to its limited reproducibility so that other testing modalities are also required in the evaluation of these patients [4, 263].

Exercise testing may also be used to unmask pro-arrhythmic responses with development of sustained ventricular tachycardia during exercise in patients receiving anti-arrhythmic therapy.

4.12 Exercise Testing in Valvular Heart Disease

The primary value of exercise testing in valvular heart disease is to objectively assess atypical symptoms, exercise tolerance, and extent of disability to guide decision making with regard to surgical treatment. This is particularly of importance when a patient is thought to be asymptomatic because of inactivity (e.g., as in the elderly) or when a discrepancy exists between the patient's symptom status and the echocardiographic severity of the valvular stenosis or regurgitation. Furthermore, exercise testing can be used in follow-up of asymptomatic patients with valvular heart disease to detect a reduction in exercise capacity over time [4]. Details regarding the uses of exercise testing in patients with valvular heart disease have also been described in the respective guideline for the management of patients with valvular heart disease [264].

4.12.1 Mitral Valve Stenosis and Regurgitation

Exercise testing in mitral valve stenosis is of most value when the patient's symptom status and mitral valve area show discrepancy. When exercise induces excessive heart rate responses to a relatively low level of exercise or hypotension as a sign of a reduction in cardiac output, a more aggressive therapeutic approach aimed at earlier surgery might be considered [264]. In a rare case, exercise may precipitate atrial fibrillation in a patient with mitral valve stenosis.

In patients with mitral valve regurgitation, exercise testing objectively determines the functional capacity of the patient. Patients with severe mitral valve regurgitation commonly demonstrate a reduction in exercise capacity and are usually limited by the development of dyspnea. In patients with moderately-severe mitral valve regurgitation, a combination of exercise testing and assessment of left ventricular function may be useful in documenting occult left ventricular dysfunction and provoking earlier surgery [4, 264, 265]. Furthermore, exercise testing can be used to monitor exercise tolerance over time in these patients.

4.12.2 Aortic Valve Stenosis and Regurgitation

Severe, symptomatic aortic valve stenosis is a contraindication to exercise testing. As aortic valve replacement is not indicated in asymptomatic patients [264], it is important to distinguish those who are truly asymptomatic from patients who are asymptomatic because they are inactive or have adjusted to their functional impairment. In these patients, exercise testing can be used to select a subpopulation of patients who are hemodynamically compromised by aortic valve stenosis and in whom surgery should be considered. Studies in adults with moderate to severe aortic valve stenosis have demonstrated that, with the appropriate precautions, exercise testing can be safely performed in these patients [4, 264, 266, 267]. Adverse hemodynamic responses that advocate aortic valve replacement include profound functional limitation, hypotension during exercise or failure to augment systolic blood pressure with exercise, and a rapid increase in heart rate indicating a fixed stroke volume. In this way, exercise testing can be combined with echocardiography in the follow-up of patients with aortic valve stenosis to help in determining the time at which aortic valve replacement should be performed.

Exercise tolerance is preserved until late in the course of aortic valve regurgitation. Exercise testing is not routinely required to guide treatment as the decision to proceed to valve surgery in chronic aortic regurgitation is primarily based on symptom status, left ventricular systolic (dys)function, and left ventricular size [4, 268].

References

1. Kaltenbach, M., D. Scherer, and S. Dowinsky, Complications of exercise testing. A survey in three German-speaking countries. *Eur. Heart J.*, 1982;**3**: 199–202.

2. Pina, I.L., G.J. Balady, P. Hanson, et al., Guidelines for clinical exercise testing laboratories: A statement for healthcare professionals from the Committee on Exercise and Cardiac Rehabilitation, American Heart Association. *Circulation*, 1995;**91**: 912–921.

3. Schlant, R.C., G.C. Friesinger II, and J.J. Leonard, Clinical competence in exercise testing: A statement for physicians from the ACP/ACC/AHA Task Force on Clinical Privileges in Cardiology. *J. Am. Coll. Cardiol.*, 1990;**16**: 1061–1065.

4. Gibbons, R.J., G.J. Balady, J.T. Bricker, B.R. Chaitman, G.F. Fletcher, V.F. Froelicher, D.B. Mark, B.D. McCallister, A.N. Mooss, M.G. O'Reilly, and W.L. Winters Jr, ACC/AHA 2002 guideline update for exercise testing: A report of the American College of Cardiology/American Heart Association Task Force on Practice Guidelines (Committee on Exercise Testing). 2002.

5. Taylor, H.L., W. Haskell, S.M. Fox, et al., Exercise tests: A summary of procedures and concepts of stress testing for cardiovascular diagnosis and function evaluation, in *Measurement in Exercise Electrocardiography*, H. Blackburn, Editor. Springfield, IL: Thomas, 1969.

6. Sheffield, L.T. and D. Roitman, Stress testing methodology. *Prog. Cardiovasc. Dis.*, 1976;**19**: 33–49.

7. Niederberger, M., R.A. Bruce, F. Kusumi, et al., Disparities in ventilatory and circulatory responses to bicycle and treadmill exercise. *Br. Heart J.*, 1974;**36**: 377–382.

8. Bruce, R.A., Methods of exercise testing. Step test, bicycle, treadmill, isometrics. *Am. J. Cardiol.*, 1974;**33**: 715–720.

9. Ellestad, M.H., Memorial hospital protocol, in *Stress Testing. Principles and Practice*, M.H. Ellestad, Editor. Philadelphia, PA: Davis, 1975, pp. 67–84.

10. Balke, B. and R.W. Ware, An experimental study of physical fitness of Air Force personnel. *US Armed Forces Med. J.*, 1959;**10**: 675–688.

11. Weld, F.M., K.-L. Chu, J.T. Bigger Jr, et al., Risk stratification with low-level exercise testing 2 weeks after acute myocardial infarction. *Circulation*, 1981;**64**: 306–314.

12. Ellestad, M.H., C.G. Blomqvist, and J.P. Naughton, Standards for adult exercise testing laboratories. *Circulation*, 1979;**58**: 421A–430A.

13. Fox, S.M., III, J.P. Naughton, and W.L. Haskell, Physical activity and the prevention of coronary heart disease. *Ann. Clin. Res.*, 1971;**3**: 404–432.

14. Froelicher, V.F., Jr, A.J. Thompson Jr, I. Noguera, et al., Prediction of maximal oxygen consumption. Comparison of the Bruce and Balke treadmill protocols. *Chest*, 1975;**68**: 331–336.

15. Pollock, M.L., R.L. Bohannon, K.H. Cooper, et al., A comparative analysis of four protocols for maximal treadmill stress testing. *Am. Heart J.*, 1976;**92**: 39–46.

16. Lecerof, H., Influence of body position on exercise tolerance, heart rate, blood pressure, and respiration rate in coronary insufficiency. *Br. Heart J.*, 1971;**33**: 78–83.

17. Thadani, U., R.O. West, T.M. Mathew, et al., Hemodynamics at rest and during supine and sitting bicycle exercise in patients with coronary artery disease. *Am. J. Cardiol.*, 1977;**39**: 776–783.

18. Kramer, B., B. Massie, and N. Topic, Hemodynamic differences between supine and upright exercise in patients with congestive heart failure. *Circulation*, 1982;**66**: 820–825.

19. Bruce, R.A., Exercise testing of patients with coronary heart disease: Principles and normal standards for evaluation. *Ann. Clin. Res.*, 1971;**3**: 323–332.

20. Erikssen, J., E. Thaulow, R. Mundal, et al., Comparison of beta-adrenoceptor blockers under maximal exercise (Pindolol v Metoprolol v Atenolol). *Br. J. Clin. Pharmacol.*, 1982;**13**: 201S–209S.

21. Samek, L. and H. Roskamm, Antianginal and antiarrhythmic effects of pindolol in post-infarct patients. *Br. J. Clin. Pharmacol.*, 1982;**13**: 297S.

22. Simoons, M.L., M. Taams, J. Lubsen, et al., Treatment of stable angina pectoris with verapamil hydrochloride: A double blind cross-over study. *Eur. Heart J.*, 1980;**1**: 269–274.

23. Harron, D.W.G., J.G. Riddell, and R.G. Shanks. Alinidine reduces heart rate without blockade of beta-adrenoceptors. *Lancet*, 1981;**1**: 351–353.

24. Borg, G., A. Holmgren, and I. Lindblad, Quantitative evaluation of chest pain. *Acta Med. Scand.*, 1981;Suppl. 644: 43–45.

25. Simoons, M.L., J. Tumraers, H. van Meurs-van Woezik, et al., Alinidine, a new agent which lowers heart rate in patients with angina pectoris. *Eur. Heart J.*, 1982;**3**: 542–545.

26. Simoons, M.L. and K. Balakumaran, The effects of drugs on the exercise electrocardiogram. *Cardiology*, 1981;**68**(Suppl. 2): 124–132.

27. Herbert, W.G., P. Dubach, K.G. Lehmann, et al., Effect of beta-blockade on the interpretation of the exercise ECG: ST level versus delta ST/HR index. *Am. Heart J.*, 1991;**122**: 993–1000.

28. Simoons, M.L., P.G. Hugenholtz, C.A. Ascoop, et al., Quantitation of exercise electrocardiography. *Circulation*, 1981;**63**: 471–475.

29. Wolf, H.K., P.J. MacInnis, S. Stock, et al., Computer analysis of rest and exercise electrocardiograms. *Comput. Biomed. Res.*, 1972;**5**: 329–346.

30. Simoons, M.L., H.B.K. Boom, and E. Smallenburg, On-line processing of orthogonal exercise electrocardiograms. *Comput. Biomed. Res.*, 1975;**8**: 105–117.

31. Bhargava, V., K. Watanabe, and V.F. Froelicher, Progress in computer analysis of the exercise electrocardiogram. *Am. J. Cardiol.*, 1981;**47**: 1143–1151.

32. Pahlm, O. and L. Sornmo, Data processing of exercise ECGs. *IEEE Trans. Biomed. Eng.*, 1987;**34**: 158–165.

33. Ellestad, M.H., *Stress Testing: Principles and Practice*, 5th edn. New York, NY: Oxford University Press.

34. Simoons, M.L. and P. Block, Toward the optimal lead system and optimal criteria for exercise electrocardiography. *Am. J. Cardiol.*, 1981;**47**: 1366–1374.

35. Phibbs, B.P. and L.J. Buckets, Comparative yield of ECG leads in multistage stress testing. *Am. Heart J.*, 1975;**90**: 275–276.

36. Miller, T.D., K.B. Desser, and M. Lawson, How many electrocardiographic leads are required for exercise treadmill tests? *J. Electrocardiol.*, 1987;**20**: 131–137.

37. Simoons, M.L., Optimal measurements for detection of coronary artery disease by exercise electrocardiography. *Comput. Biomed. Res.*, 1977;**10**: 483–499.

38. Mason, R.E., I. Likar, R.O. Biern, et al., Multiple-lead exercise electrocardiography. Experience in 107 normal subjects and 67 patients with angina pectoris, and comparison with coronary cinearteriography in 84 patients. *Circulation*, 1967;**36**: 517–525.

39. Chaitman, B.R., M.G. Bourassa, P. Wagniart, et al., Improved efficiency of treadmill exercise testing using a multiple lead ECG system and basic hemodynamic exercise response. *Circulation*, 1978;**57**: 71–79.

40. Fox, K., A. Selwyn, and J. Shillingford, Precordial electrocardiographic mapping after exercise in the diagnosis of coronary artery disease. *Am. J. Cardiol.*, 1979;**43**: 541–546.

41. Fox, K.M., J. Deanfield, P. Ribero, et al., Projection of ST segment changes on the front of the chest. *Br. Heart J.*, 1982;**48**: 555–559.

42. Miranda, C.P., J. Liu, A. Kadar, et al., Usefulness of exercise-induced ST segment depression in the inferior leads during exercise-testing as a marker for coronary artery disease. *Am. J. Cardiol.*, 1992;**69**: 303–307.

43. Michaelides, A.P., Z.D. Psomadaki, P.E. Dilaveris, et al., Improved detection of coronary artery disease by exercise electrocardiography with the use of right precordial leads. *N. Engl. J. Med.*, 1999;**340**: 340–345.

44. Wolthuis, R.A., V.F. Froelicher, A. Hopkirk, et al., Normal electrocardiographic waveform characteristics during treadmill exercise testing. *Circulation*, 1979;**60**: 1028–1035.

45. Simoons, M.L. and P.G. Hugenholtz, Estimation of the probability of exercise-induced ischemia by quantitative ECG analysis. *Circulation*, 1977;**56**: 552–559.

46. Block, P., J. Tiberghien, I. Raadschelders, et al., Diagnostic value of surface mapping recordings registered at rest and during exercise, in *Computers in Cardiology 1977*, H.G. Ostrow and K.L. Ripley, Editors. New York, NY: IEEE, 1977.

47. Mirvis, D.M., F.W. Keller Jr, J.W. Cox Jr, et al., Left precordial isopotential mapping during supine exercise. *Circulation*, 1977;**56**: 245–252.

48. Sapin, P.M., M.B. Blauwet, G.G. Koch, et al., Exaggerated atrial repolarization waves as a predictor of false positive exercise tests in an unselected population. *J. Electrocardiol.*, 1995;**28**: 313–321.

49. Sapin, P.M., G. Koch, M.B. Blauwet, et al., Identification of false positive exercise tests with use of electrocardiographic criteria: A possible role for atrial repolarization waves. *J. Am. Coll. Cardiol.*, 1991;**18**: 127–135.

50. Bhargava, V. and A.L. Goldberger, New method for measuring QRS duration using high-frequency electrocardiography. *Am. J. Physiol.*, 1982;**242**: H507–H511.

51. Sketch, M.H., S.M. Mohiuddin, C.K. Nair, et al., Automated and nomographic analysis of exercise tests. *Am. Med. Assoc.*, 1980;**243**: 1052–1055.

52. Battler, A., V.F. Froelicher, R. Slutsky, et al., Relationship of QRS amplitude changes during exercise to left ventricular function and volumes and the diagnosis of coronary artery disease. *Circulation*, 1979;**60**: 1004–1013.

53. David, D., M. Naito, C.C. Chen, et al., R-wave amplitude variations during acute experimental myocardial ischemia: An inadequate index for changes in intracardiac volume. *Circulation*, 1981;**63**: 1364–1371.

54. Deckers, J.W., R.V. Vinke, J.R. Vos, et al., Changes in the electrocardiographic response to exercise in healthy women. *Br. Heart J.*, 1990;**64**: 376–380.

55. Cumming, G.R., C. Dufresne, L. Kich, et al., Exercise electrocardiogram patterns in normal women. *Br. Heart J.*, 1973;**35**: 1055–1061.

56. Deckers, J.W., B.J. Rensing, M.L. Simoons, et al., Diagnostic merits of exercise testing in females. *Eur. Heart J.*, 1989;**10**: 543–550.

57. Detry, J.M., B.M. Capita, J. Cosyns, et al., Diagnostic value of history and maximal exercise electrocardiography in men and women suspected of coronary heart disease. *Circulation*, 1977;**56**: 756–761.

58. Val, P.G., B.R. Chaitman, D.D. Waters, et al., Diagnostic accuracy of exercise ECG lead systems in clinical subsets of women. *Circulation*, 1982;**65**: 1465–1474.

59. Barolsky, S.M., C.A. Gilbert, A. Faruqui, et al., Differences in electrocardiographic response to exercise of women and men: A non-Bayesian factor. *Circulation*, 1979;**60**: 1021–1027.

60. Rijneke, R.D., C.A. Ascoop, and J.L. Talmon, Clinical significance of upsloping ST segments in exercise electrocardiography. *Circulation*, 1980;**61**: 671–678.

61. Stuart, R.J. and M.H. Ellestad, Upsloping ST segments in exercise stress testing: Six-year follow-up study of 438 patients and correlation with 248 angiograms. *Am. J. Cardiol.*, 1976;**37**: 19–22.

62. Kurita, A., B.R. Chaitman, and M.G. Bourassa, Significance of exercise-induced ST depression in evaluation of coronary artery disease. *Am. J. Cardiol.*, 1977;**40**: 492–497.

63. Campeau, L., Grading of angina pectoris. *Circulation*, 1975;**54**: 522–523.

64. Simoons, M.L., M. van den Brand, and P.G. Hugenholtz, Quantitative analysis of exercise electrocardiograms and left ventricular angiocardiograms in patients with abnormal QRS complexes at rest. *Circulation*, 1977;**55**: 55–60.

65. Piessens, J., W. van Mieghem, H. Kesteloot, et al., Diagnostic value of clinical history, exercise testing and atrial pacing in patients with chest pain. *Am. J. Cardiol.*, 1974;**33**: 351–356.

66. Bartel, A.G., V.S. Behar, R.H. Peter, et al., Graded exercise stress tests in angiographically documented coronary artery disease. *Circulation*, 1974;**49**: 348–356.

67. Ascoop, C.A., M.L. Simoons, W.G. Egmond, et al., Exercise test, history, and serum lipid levels in patients with chest pain and normal electrocardiograms at rest: Comparison to findings at coronary arteriography. *Am. Heart J.*, 1971;**82**: 609–617.

68. Bogaty, P., et al., Does more ST segment depression on the 12-lead exercise electrocardiogram signify more severe ischemic heart disease. *Circulation*, 1993;**88**(Suppl. 2): 1.

69. Taylor, A.J. and G.A. Beller, Patients with greater than 2 mm of ST depression do not have a greater ischemic burden by thallium-201 scintigraphy. *Circulation*, 1992;**86**(Suppl. II): 138.

70. Husted, R., et al., The failure of multilead ST depression to predict severity of ischemia. *Am. J. Noninvas. Cardiol.*, 1994;**8**: 386.

71. Barlow, J.B., The "false positive" exercise electrocardiogram: Value of time course patterns in assessment of depressed ST segments and inverted T waves. *Am. Heart J.*, 1985;**110**: 1328–1336.

72. Miranda, C.P., K.G. Lehmann, and V.F. Froelicher, Correlation between resting ST segment changes, exercise testing, coronary angiography, and long term prognosis. *Am. Heart J.*, 1991;**122**: 1617–1628.

73. Ellestad, M.H., L. Thomas, R. Ong, et al., The predictive value of the time course of ST depression during exercise testing in patients referred for angiograms. *Am. Heart J.*, 1992;**123**: 904–908.

74. Lachterman, B., K.G. Lehmann, R. Detrano, et al., Comparison of ST segment/heart rate index to standard ST criteria for analysis of exercise electrocardiogram. *Circulation*, 1990;**82**: 44–50.

75. Rywik, T.M., R.C. Zink, N.S. Gittings, et al., Independent prognostic significance of ischemic ST segment response limited to recovery from treadmill exercise in asymptomatic subjects. *Circulation*, 1998;**97**: 2117–2222.

76. Hollenberg, M., M. Go Jr, B.M. Massie, et al., Influence of R-wave amplitude on exercise induced ST depression: Need for a "gain factor" correction when interpreting stress electrocardiograms. *Am. J. Cardiol.*, 1985;**56**: 13–17.

77. Hakki, A.H., A.S. Iskandria, S. Kutalek, et al., R-wave amplitude: A new determinant of failure of patients with coronary heart disease to manifest ST depression during exercise. *J. Am. Coll. Cardiol.*, 1984;**3**: 1155–1160.

78. Ellestad, M.H., R. Crump, and M. Surber, The significance of lead strength on ST changes during treadmill stress tests. *J. Electrocardiol.*, 1992;**25**(Suppl.): 31–34.

79. Elamin, M.S., R. Boyle, M.M. Kardash, et al., Accurate detection of coronary heart disease by new exercise test. *Br. Heart J.*, 1982;**48**: 311–320.

80. Okin, P.M. and P. Kligfield, Computer-based implementation of the ST-segment/heart rate slope. *Am. J. Cardiol.*, 1989;**64**: 926–930.

81. Detrano, R., E. Salcedo, M. Passalacqua, et al., Exercise electrocardiographic variables: A critical appraisal. *J. Am. Coll. Cardiol.*, 1986;**8**: 836–847.

82. Kligfield, P., O. Ameisen, and P.M. Okin, Heart rate adjustment of ST segment depression for improved detection of coronary artery disease. *Circulation*, 1989;**79**: 245–255.

83. Okin, P.M. and P. Kligfield, Heart rate adjustment of ST segment depression and performance of the exercise electrocardiogram: A critical evaluation. *J. Am. Coll. Cardiol.*, 1995;**25**: 1726–1735.

84. Fletcher, G.F., T.R. Flipse, P. Kligfield, et al., Current status of ECG stress testing. *Curr. Probl. Cardiol.*, 1998;**23**: 353–423.

85. Morise, A.P., Accuracy of heart rate-adjusted ST segments in populations with and without posttest referral bias. *Am. Heart J.*, 1997;**134**: 647–655.

86. Okin, P.M., M.J. Roman, J.E. Schwartz, et al., Relation of exercise-induced myocardial ischemia to cardiac and carotid structure. *Hypertension*, 1997;**30**: 1382–1388.

87. Viik, J., R. Lehtinen, and J. Malmivuo, Detection of coronary artery disease using maximum value of ST/HR hysteresis over different number of leads. *J. Electrocardiol.*, 1999;**32**(Suppl.): 70–75.

88. Froelicher, V.F., K.G. Lehmann, R. Thomas, et al., The electrocardiographic exercise test in a population with reduced workup bias: Diagnostic performance, computerized interpretation, and multivariable prediction. Veterans Affairs Cooperative Study in Health Services #016 (QUEXTA) Study Group. Quantitative Exercise Testing and Angiography. *Ann. Intern. Med.*, 1998;**128**: 965–974.

89. Macfarlane, P.W., A. Tweddel, D. Macfariane, et al., Body surface ECG mapping on exercise. *Eur. Heart J.*, 1984;**5**(Suppl. 1): 279.

90. Simoons, M.L., A. Withagen, R. Vinke, et al., ST-vector orientation and location of myocardial perfusion defects during exercise. *Nuklearmedizin*, 1978;**17**: 154–156.

91. Samek, L., H. Roskamm, P. Rentrop, et al., Belastungsprufungen und koronarangiogramm im chronischen infarktstadium. *Z. Kardiol.*, 1975;**64**: 809–814.

92. Roskamm, H., L. Samek, K. Zweigle, et al., Die beziehungen zwischen den befunden der koronarangiographie und des belastungs-ekg bei patienten ohne transmuralen myokardinfarkt. *Z. Kardiol.*, 1977;**66**: 273–280.

93. Fisher, L.D., J.W. Kennedy, B.R. Chaitman, et al., Diagnostic quantification of CASS (Coronary Artery Surgery Study) clinical and exercise test results in determining presence and extent of coronary artery disease: A multivariate approach. *Circulation*, 1981;**63**: 987–1000.

94. De Feyter, P.J., P.A. Majid, M.J. van Eenige, et al., Clinical significance of exercise-induced ST segment elevation. Correlative angiographic study in patients with ischaemic heart disease. *Br. Heart J.*, 1981;**46**: 84–92.

95. Alijarde, M., J. Soler-Soler, J. Perez-Jabaloyes, et al., Significance of treadmill stress testing in transmural myocardial infarction. Correlation with coronary angiography. *Eur. Heart J.*, 1982;**3**: 353–361.

96. Manvi, K.N. and M.H. Ellestad, Elevated ST-segments with exercise in ventricular aneurysm. *J. Electrocardiol.*, 1972;**5**: 317–323.

97. Haines, D.E., G.A. Beller, D.D. Watson, et al., Exercise-induced ST segment elevation 2 weeks after uncomplicated myocardial infarction: Contributing factors and prognostic significance. *J. Am. Coll. Cardiol.*, 1987;**9**: 996–1003.

98. Fox, K.M., A. Jonathan, and A. Selwyn, Significance of exercise induced ST segment elevation in patients with previous myocardial infarction. *Br. Heart J.*, 1983;**49**: 15–19.

99. Margonato, A., C. Ballarotto, F. Bonetti, et al., Assessment of residual tissue viability by exercise testing in recent myocardial infarction: Comparison of the electrocardiogram and myocardial perfusion scintigraphy. *J. Am. Coll. Cardiol.*, 1992;**19**: 948–952.

100. Margonato, A., S.L. Chierchia, R.G. Xuereb, et al., Specificity and sensitivity of exercise-induced ST segment elevation for detection of residual viability: Comparison with fluorodeoxyglucose and positron emission tomography. *J. Am. Coll. Cardiol.*, 1995;**25**: 1032–1038.

101. Lombardo, A., F. Loperfido, F. Pennestri, et al., Significance of transient ST-T segment changes during dobutamine testing in Q wave myocardial infarction. *J. Am. Coll. Cardiol.*, 1996;**27**: 599–605.

102. Dunn, R.F., B. Freedman, D.T. Kelly, et al., Exercise-induced ST segment elevation in leads V_1 or aVL. A predictor of anterior myocardial ischemia and left anterior descending coronary artery disease. *Circulation*, 1981;**63**: 1357–1363.

103. Dunn, R.F., B. Freedman, I.K. Bailey, et al., Localization of coronary artery disease with exercise electrocardiography: Correlation with thallium-201 myocardial perfusion scanning. *Am. J. Cardiol.*, 1981;**48**: 837–843.

104. Waters, D.D., B.R. Chaitman, M.G. Bourassa, et al., Clinical and angiographic correlates of exercise-induced ST segment elevation. Increased detection with multiple ECG leads. *Circulation*, 1980;**61**: 286–296.

105. Waters, D.D., J. Szlachcic, M.G. Bourassa, et al., Exercise testing in patients with variant angina: Results, correlation with clinical and angiographic features and prognostic significance. *Circulation*, 1982;**65**: 265–274.

106. Hegge, F.N., N. Tuna, and H.B. Burchell, Coronary arteriographic findings in patients with axis shifts or ST segment elevations on exercise stress testing. *Am. Heart J.*, 1973;**86**: 603–615.

107. Chahine, R.A., A.E. Raizner, and T. Ishimori, The clinical significance of exercise induced ST segment elevation. *Circulation*, 1976;**54**: 209–213.

108. Longhurst, J.C. and W.L. Kraus, Exercise-induced ST elevation in patients without myocardial infarction. *Circulation*, 1979;**60**: 616–629.

109. Mark, D.B., M.A. Hlatky, K.L. Lee, et al., Localizing coronary artery obstructions with the exercise treadmill test. *Ann. Intern. Med.*, 1987;**106**: 53–55.

110. Prinzmetal, M., A. Ekmekci, R. Kennamer, et al., Variant form of angina pectoris, previously undelineated syndrome. *JAMA*, 1960;**174**: 1794–1800.

111. Detry, J.M., P. Mengeot, M.F. Rousseau, et al., Maximal exercise testing in patients with spontaneous angina pectoris associated with transient ST segment elevation. Risks and electrocardiographic findings. *Br. Heart J.*, 1975;**37**: 897–903.

112. Bonoris, P.E., P.S. Greenberg, M.J. Castellanet, et al., Significance of changes in R wave amplitude during treadmill stress testing: Angiographic correlation. *Am. J. Cardiol.*, 1978;**41**: 846–851.

113. Wagner, S., J.C. Cohn, and A. Selzer, Unreliability of exercise induced R wave changes as indexes of coronary artery disease. *Am. J. Cardiol.*, 1979;**44**: 1241–1246.

114. Brody, D.A., A theoretical analysis of intracavitary blood mass influence on the heart–lead relationship. *Circ. Res.*, 1956;**4**: 731–738.

115. Greenberg, P.S., M.H. Ellestad, R. Berge, et al., Radionuclide angiographic correlation of the R-wave, ejection fraction, and volume responses to upright bicycle exercise. *Chest*, 1981;**80**: 459–464.

116. Froelicher, V.F., Jr, R. Wolthuis, N. Keiser, et al., A comparison of two bipolar exercise ECG leads to V5. *Chest*, 1976;**70**: 611–616.

117. Froelicher, V.F. and J.N. Myers, *Exercise and the Heart*, 4th edn. Philadelphia, PA: W.B. Saunders.

118. Michaelides, A.P., H. Boudoulas, H. Antonakoudis, et al., Effect of number of coronary arteries significantly narrowed and status of intraventricular conduction on exercise-induced QRS prolongation in coronary artery disease. *Am. J. Cardiol.*, 1992;**70**: 1487–1489.

119. Wayne, V.S., et al., Exercise-induced bundle branch block. *Am. J. Cardiol.*, 1983;**52**: 283.

120. Levy, S., R. Gerard, A. Castellanos, et al., Transient left anterior hemiblock during angina pectoris: Coronarographic aspects and clinical significance. *Eur. J. Cardiol.*, 1979;**9**: 215–225.

121. Hegge, F.N., N. Tuna, and H.B. Burchell, Coronary arteriographic findings in patients with axis shifts or ST segment elevations on exercise stress testing. *Am. Heart J.*, 1973;**86**: 603–615.

122. Whinnery, J.E., V.F. Froelicher Jr, M.R. Longo Jr, et al., The electrocardiographic response to maximal treadmill exercise in asymptomatic men with right branch bundle block. *Chest*, 1977;**71**: 335–340.

123. Kattus, A.A., Exercise electrocardiography. Recognition of the ischemic response: False positive and negative patterns. *Am. J. Cardiol.*, 1974;**33**: 721–731.

124. Tanaka, T., M.J. Friedman, R.D. Okada, et al., Diagnostic value of exercise-induced ST segment depression in patients with RBBB. *Am. J. Cardiol.*, 1978;**41**: 670–673.

125. Whinnery, J.E., V.F. Froelicher, and A.J. Stuart, The electrocardiographic response to maximal treadmill exercise in asymptomatic men with left bundle branch block. *Am. Heart J.*, 1997;**94**: 316–324.

126. Aravindakshan, V., W. Surawicz, and R.D. Allen, Electrocardiographic exercise test in patients with abnormal T waves at rest. *Am. Heart J.*, 1977;**93**: 706–714.

127. Diamond, G.A. and J.S. Forrester, Analysis of probability as an aid in the clinical diagnosis of coronary artery disease. *N. Engl. J. Med.*, 1979;**300**: 1350–1358.

128. Fisher, L.D. J.W. Kennedy, B.R. Chaitman, et al., Diagnostic quantification of CASS (Coronary Artery Surgery Study) clinical and exercise test results in determining presence and extent of coronary artery disease. A multivariate approach. *Circulation*, 1981;**63**: 987–1000.

129. Morise, A.P., W.J. Haddad, and D. Beckner, Development and validation of a clinical score to estimate the probability of coronary artery disease in men and women presenting with suspected coronary disease. *Am. J. Med.*, 1997;**102**: 350–356.

130. Altman, X., *Practical Statistics for Medical Research*. London: Chapman and Hall, 1991, pp. 414–417.

131. Detry, J.M., A. Robert, R.R.J. Luwaert, et al., Diagnostic value of computerized exercise testing in men without previous myocardial infarction. A multivariate, compartmental and probabilistic approach. *Eur. Heart J.*, 1985;**6**: 227–238.

132. Pryor, D.B., F.E. Harrell Jr, K.L. Lee, et al., Estimating the likelihood of significant coronary artery disease. *Am. J. Med.*, 1983;**75**: 771–780.

133. Ellestad, M.H., S. Savitz, D. Bergdall, et al., The false positive stress test: Multivariate analysis of 215 subjects with hemodynamic, angiographic and clinical data. *Am. J. Cardiol.*, 1977;**40**: 681–685.

134. Yamada, H., D. Do, A. Morise, et al., Review of studies using multivariable analysis of clinical and exercise test data to predict angiographic coronary artery disease. *Prog. Cardiovasc. Dis.*, 1997;**39**: 457–481.

135. Shaw, L.J., E.D. Peterson, L.K. Shaw, et al., Use of a prognostic treadmill score in identifying diagnostic coronary disease subgroups. *Circulation*, 1998;**98**: 1622–1630.

136. Deckers, J.W., B.J. Rensing, J.G. Tijssen, et al., A comparison of methods of analysing exercise tests for diagnosis of coronary artery disease. *Br. Heart J.*, 1989;**62**: 438–444.

137. Lee, K.L., D.B. Pryor, F.E. Harrell Jr, et al., Predicting outcome in coronary disease: Statistical models versus expert clinicians. *Am. J. Med.*, 1986;**80**: 553–560.

138. Detrano, R., M. Bobbio, H. Olson, et al., Computer probability estimates of angiographic coronary disease: Transportability and comparison with cardiologists' estimates. *Comput. Biomed. Res.*, 1992;**25**: 468–485.

139. Gianrossi, R., R. Detrano, D. Mulvihill, et al., Exercise induced ST depression in the diagnosis of coronary artery disease: A meta analysis. *Circulation*, 1989;**80**: 87–98.

140. Detrano, R., R. Gianrossi, and V. Froelicher, The diagnostic accuracy of the exercise electrocardiogram: A meta analysis of 22 years of research. *Prog. Cardiovasc. Dis.*, 1989;**32**: 173–206.

141. Morise, A.P. and G.A. Diamond, Comparison of the sensitivity and specificity of exercise electrocardiography in biased and unbiased populations of men and women. *Am. Heart J.*, 1995;**130**: 741–747.

142. DelCampo, J., D. Do, T. Umann, et al., Comparison of computerized and standard visual criteria of exercise ECG for diagnosis of coronary artery disease. *Ann. Noninvasive Electrocardiogr.*, 1996;**1**: 430–442.

143. Froelicher, V.F., K.G. Lehmann, R. Thomas, et al., The electrocardiographic exercise test in a population with reduced workup bias: Diagnostic performance, computerized interpretation, and multivariable prediction. Veterans Affairs Cooperative Study in Health Services #016 (QUEXTA) Study Group. Quantitative Exercise Testing and Angiography. *Ann. Intern. Med.*, 1998;**128**: 965–974.

144. Sketch, M.H., A.N. Mooss, M.L. Butler, et al., Digoxin-induced positive exercise tests: Their clinical and prognostic significance. *Am. J. Cardiol.*, 1981;**48**: 655–659.

145. LeWinter, M.M., M.H. Crawford, R.A. O'Rourke, et al., The effects of oral propranolol, digoxin and combination therapy on the resting and exercise electrocardiogram. *Am. Heart J.*, 1977;**93**: 202–209.

146. Blackburn, H., Canadian colloquium on computer assisted interpretation of electrocardiograms, VI: importance of the electrocardiogram in populations outside the hospital. *Can. Med. Assoc. J.*, 1973;**108**: 1262–1265.

147. Cullen, K., N.S. Stenhouse, K.L. Wearne, et al., Electrocardiograms and 13-year cardiovascular mortality in Busselton study. *Br. Heart J.*, 1982;**47**: 209–212.

148. Aronow, W.S., Correlation of ischemic ST segment depression on the resting electrocardiogram with new cardiac events in 1,106 patients over 62 years of age. *Am. J. Cardiol.*, 1989;**64**: 232–233.

149. Califf, R.M., D.B. Mark, F.E. Harrell Jr, et al., Importance of clinical measures of ischemia in the prognosis of patients with documented coronary artery disease. *J. Am. Coll. Cardiol.*, 1988;**11**: 20–26.

150. Harris, P.J., F.E. Harrell Jr, K.L. Lee, et al., Survival in medically treated coronary artery disease. *Circulation*, 1979;**60**: 1259–1269.

151. Miranda, C.P., K.G. Lehmann, and V.F. Froelicher, Correlation between resting ST segment depression, exercise testing, coronary angiography, and long term prognosis. *Am. Heart J.*, 1991;**122**: 1617–1628.

152. Geleijnse, M.L., P.M. Fioretti, and J.R.T.C. Roelandt, Methodology, feasibility, safety and diagnostic accuracy of dobutamine stress echocardiography. *J. Am. Coll. Cardiol.*, 1997;**30**: 595–606.

153. Geleijnse, M.L., A. Salustri, T.H. Marwick, et al., Should the diagnosis of coronary artery disease be based on the evaluation of myocardial function or perfusion? *Eur. Heart J.*, 1997;**18**(Suppl. D): D68–D77.

154. Schinkel, A.F.L., J.J. Bax, M.L. Geleijnse, et al., Noninvasive evaluation of ischemic heart disease: Myocardial perfusion imaging or stress echocardiography? *Eur. Heart J.*, 2003;**24**: 789–800.

155. Geleijnse, M.L., A. Elhendy, and R.T. Van Domburg, Cardiac imaging for risk stratification with dobutamine–atropine stress testing in patients with chest pain. Echocardiography, perfusion scintigraphy, or both? *Circulation*, 1997;**96**: 137–147.

156. Rigo, P., I.K. Bailey, L.C. Griffith, et al., Value and limitations of segmental analysis of stress thallium myocardial imaging for localization of coronary artery disease. *Circulation*, 1980;**61**: 973–981.

157. Ritchie, J.L., T.M. Bateman, R.O. Bonow, et al., Guidelines for clinical use of cardiac radionuclide imaging: Report of the American College of Cardiology/American Heart Association Task Force on Assessment of Diagnostic and Therapeutic Cardiovascular Procedures (Committee on Radionuclide Imaging), developed in collaboration with the American Society of Nuclear Cardiology. *J. Am. Coll. Cardiol.*, 1995;**25**: 521–547.

158. Cheitlin, M.D., J.S. Alpert, W.F. Armstrong, et al., ACC/AHA guidelines for the clinical application of echocardiography: A report of the American College of Cardiology/American Heart Association Task Force on Practice Guidelines (Committee on Clinical Application of Echocardiography). Developed in collaboration with the American Society of Echocardiography. *Circulation*, 1997;**95**: 1686–1744.

159. Christian, T.F., T.D. Miller, K.R. Bailey, et al., Exercise tomographic thallium 201 imaging in patients with severe coronary artery disease and normal electrocardiograms. *Ann. Intern. Med.*, 1994;**121**: 825–832.

160. Gibbons, R.J., A.R. Zinsmeister, T.D. Miller, et al., Supine exercise electrocardiography compared with exercise radionuclide angiography in noninvasive identification of severe coronary artery disease. *Ann. Intern. Med.*, 1990;**112**: 743–749.

161. Ladenheim, M.L., T.S. Kotler, B.H. Pollock, et al., Incremental prognostic power of clinical history, exercise electrocardiography and myocardial perfusion scintigraphy in suspected coronary artery disease. *Am. J. Cardiol.*, 1987;**59**: 270–277.

162. Weiner, D.A., T.J. Ryan, C.H. McCabe, et al., Prognostic importance of a clinical profile and exercise test in medically treated patients with coronary artery disease. *J. Am. Coll. Cardiol.*, 1984;**3**: 772–779.

163. Mark, D.B., M.A. Hlatky, F.E. Harrell Jr, et al., Exercise treadmill score for predicting prognosis in coronary artery disease. *Ann. Intern. Med.*, 1987;**106**: 793–800.

164. Morrow, K., C.K. Morris, V.F. Froelicher, et al., Prediction of cardiovascular death in men undergoing noninvasive evaluation for coronary artery disease. *Ann. Intern. Med.*, 1993;**118**: 689–695.

165. Brunelli, C., R. Cristofani, and A. L'Abbate, Long term survival in medically treated patients with ischaemic heart disease and prognostic importance of clinical and electrocardiographic data (the Italian CNR Multicentre Prospective Study OD1). *Eur. Heart J.*, 1989;**10**: 292–303.

166. Luwaert, R.J., J.A. Melin, C.R. Brohet, et al., Non invasive data provide independent prognostic information in patients

with chest pain without previous myocardial infarction: Findings in male patients who have had cardiac catheterization. *Eur. Heart J.*, 1988;**9**: 418–426.

167. Gohlke, H., L. Samek, P. Betz, et al., Exercise testing provides additional prognostic information in angiographically defined subgroups of patients with coronary artery disease. *Circulation*, 1983;**68**: 979–985.

168. Hammermeister, K.E., T.A. DeRouen, and H.T. Dodge, Variables predictive of survival in patients with coronary disease: Selection by univariate and multivariate analyses from the clinical, electrocardiographic, exercise, arteriographic, and quantitative angiographic evaluations. *Circulation*, 1979;**59**: 421–430.

169. McNeer, J.F., J.R. Margolis, K.L. Lee, et al., The role of the exercise test in the evaluation of patients for ischemic heart disease. *Circulation*, 1978;**57**: 64–70.

170. Mark, D.B., L. Shaw, F.E. Harrell Jr, et al., Prognostic value of a treadmill exercise score in outpatients with suspected coronary artery disease. *N. Engl. J. Med.*, 1991;**325**: 849–853.

171. Alexander, K.P., L.J. Shaw, L.K. Shaw, et al., Value of exercise treadmill testing in women [published erratum appears in J Am Coll Cardiol 1999;33:289]. *J. Am. Coll. Cardiol.*, 1998;**32**: 1657–1664.

172. Lauer, M.S., G.S. Francis, P.M. Okin, et al., Impaired chronotropic response to exercise stress testing as a predictor of mortality. *JAMA*, 1999;**281**: 524–529.

173. Cole, C.R., E.H. Blackstone, F.J. Pashkow, et al., Heart-rate recovery immediately after exercise as a predictor of mortality. *N. Engl. J. Med.*, 1999;**341**: 1351–1357.

174. Cole, C.R., J.M. Foody, E.H. Blackstone, et al., Heart rate recovery after submaximal exercise testing as a predictor of mortality in a cardiovascularly healthy cohort. *Ann. Intern. Med.*, 2000;**132**: 552–555.

175. Diaz, L.A., R.C. Brunken, E.H. Blackstone, et al., Independent contribution of myocardial perfusion defects to exercise capacity and heart rate recovery for prediction of all-cause mortality in patients with known or suspected coronary heart disease. *J. Am. Coll. Cardiol.*, 2001;**37**: 1558–1564.

176. Watanabe, J., M. Thamilarasan, E.H. Blackstone, et al., Heart rate recovery immediately after treadmill exercise and left ventricular systolic dysfunction as predictors of mortality: The case of stress echocardiography. *Circulation*, 2001;**104**: 1911–1916.

177. Nishime, E.O., C.R. Cole, E.H. Blackstone, et al., Heart rate recovery and treadmill exercise score as predictors of mortality in patients referred for exercise ECG. *JAMA*, 2000;**284**: 1392–1398.

178. Shetler, K., R. Marcus, V.F. Froelicher, et al., Heart rate recovery: Validation and methodologic issues. *J. Am. Coll. Cardiol.*, 2001;**38**: 1980–1987.

179. McHam, S.A., T.H. Marwick, F.J. Pashkow, et al., Delayed systolic blood pressure recovery after graded exercise: An independent correlate of angiographic coronary disease. *J. Am. Coll. Cardiol.*, 1999;**34**: 754–759.

180. Bogaty, P., G.R. Dagenais, B. Cantin, et al., Prognosis in patients with a strongly positive exercise electrocardiogram. *Am. J. Cardiol.*, 1989;**64**: 1284–1288.

181. Bertrand, M.E., M.L. Simoons, K.A. Fox, et al.; Task Force on the Management of Acute Coronary Syndromes of the European Society of Cardiology, Management of acute coronary syndromes in patients presenting without persistent ST segment elevation. *Eur. Heart J.*, 2002;**23**: 1809–1840. Erratum in: *Eur. Heart J.*, 2003;**24**: 1174–1175. *Eur. Heart J.*, 2003;**24**: 485.

182. Boersma, E., K.S. Pieper, E.W. Steyerberg, et al., Predictors of outcome in patients with acute coronary syndromes without persistent ST segment elevation. Results from an international trial of 9461 patients. The PURSUIT Investigators. *Circulation*, 2000;**101**: 2557–2567.

183. Stein, R.A., B.R. Chaitman, G.J. Balady, et al., Safety and utility of exercise testing in emergency room chest pain centers: An advisory from the Committee on Exercise, Rehabilitation, and Prevention, Council on Clinical Cardiology, American Heart Association. *Circulation*, 2000;**102**: 1463–1467.

184. Gibler, W.B., J.P. Runyon, R.C. Levy, et al., A rapid diagnostic and treatment center for patients with chest pain in the emergency department. *Ann. Emerg. Med.*, 1995;**25**: 1–8.

185. Farkouh, M.E., P.A. Smars, G.S. Reeder, et al., A clinical trial of a chest-pain observation unit for patients with unstable angina. Chest Pain Evaluation in the Emergency Room (CHEER) Investigators. *N. Engl. J. Med.*, 1998;**339**: 1882–1888.

186. Froelicher, E.S., Usefulness of exercise testing shortly after acute myocardial infarction for predicting 10-year mortality. *Am. J. Cardiol.*, 1994;**74**: 318–323.

187. Mark, D.B. and V.F. Froelicher, Exercise treadmill testing and ambulatory monitoring, in *Acute Coronary Care*, R.M. Califf, D.B. Mark, and G.S. Wagner, Editors. St. Louis, Mosby-Year Book, 1995.

188. Juneau, M., P. Colles, P. Théroux, et al., Symptom limited versus low level exercise testing before hospital discharge after myocardial infarction. *J. Am. Coll. Cardiol.*, 1992;**20**: 927–933.

189. Stevenson, R., V. Umachandran, K. Ranjadayalan, et al., Reassessment of treadmill stress testing for risk stratification in patients with acute myocardial infarction treated by thrombolysis. *Br. Heart J.*, 1993;**70**: 415–420.

190. Moss, A.J., R.E. Goldstein, W.J. Hall, et al., Detection and significance of myocardial ischemia in stable patients after recovery from an acute coronary event: Multicenter Myocardial Ischemia Research Group. *JAMA*, 1993;**269**: 2379–2385.

191. Arnold, A.E., M.L. Simoons, J.M. Detry, et al., Prediction of mortality following hospital discharge after thrombolysis for acute myocardial infarction: Is there a need for coronary angiography? *Eur. Heart J.*, 1993;**14**: 306–315.

192. Hamm, L.F., R.S. Crow, G.A. Stull, et al., Safety and characteristics of exercise testing early after acute myocardial infarction. *Am. J. Cardiol.*, 1989;**63**: 1193–1197.

193. Jain, A., G.H. Myers, P.M. Sapin, et al., Comparison of symptom limited and low level exercise tolerance tests early after myocardial infarction. *J. Am. Coll. Cardiol.*, 1993;**22**: 1816–1820.

194. Krone, R.J., J.A. Gillespie, F.M. Weld, et al., Low level exercise testing after myocardial infarction: Usefulness in enhancing clinical risk stratification. *Circulation*, 1985;**71**: 80–89.

195. Nielsen, J.R., H. Mickley, E.M. Damsgaard, et al., Predischarge maximal exercise test identifies risk for cardiac death in patients with acute myocardial infarction. *Am. J. Cardiol.*, 1990;**65**: 149–153.

196. Topol, E.J., K. Burek, W.W. O'Neill, et al., A randomized controlled trial of hospital discharge three days after myocardial infarction in the era of reperfusion. *N. Engl. J. Med.*, 1988;**318**: 1083–1088.

197. Senaratne, M.P., G. Smith, and S.S. Gulamhusein, Feasibility and safety of early exercise testing using the Bruce protocol after acute myocardial infarction. *J. Am. Coll. Cardiol.*, 2000;**35**: 1212–1220.

198. Fletcher, G.F., G.J. Balady, E.A. Amsterdam, et al., Exercise standards for testing and training: A statement for healthcare professionals from the American Heart Association. *Circulation*, 2001;**104**: 1694–1740.

199. Vanhees, L., D. Schepers, and R. Fagard, Comparison of maximum versus submaximum exercise testing in providing prognostic information after acute myocardial infarction and/or coronary artery bypass grafting. *Am. J. Cardiol.*, 1997;**80**: 257–262.

200. Villella, A., A.P. Maggioni, M. Villella, et al., Prognostic significance of maximal exercise testing after myocardial infarction treated with thrombolytic agents: The GISSI 2 data base. Gruppo Italiano per lo Studio della Sopravvivenza Nell'Infarto. *Lancet*, 1995;**346**: 523–529.

201. Chaitman, B.R., R.P. McMahon, M. Terrin, et al., Impact of treatment strategy on predischarge exercise test in the Thrombolysis in Myocardial Infarction (TIMI) II Trial. *Am. J. Cardiol.*, 1993;**71**: 131–138.

202. Newby, L.K., R.M. Califf, A. Guerci, et al., Early discharge in the thrombolytic era: An analysis of criteria for uncomplicated infarction from the Global Utilization of Streptokinase and tPA for Occluded Coronary Arteries (GUSTO) trial. *J. Am. Coll. Cardiol.*, 1996;**27**: 625–632.

203. Froelicher, V.F., S. Perdue, W. Pewen, et al., Application of meta analysis using an electronic spread sheet for exercise testing in patients after myocardial infarction. *Am. J. Med.*, 1987;**83**: 1045–1054.

204. Maggioni, A.P., F.M. Turazza, and L. Tavazzi, Risk evaluation using exercise testing in elderly patients after acute myocardial infarction. *Cardiol. Elder.*, 1995;**3**: 88–93.

205. Théroux, P., D.D. Waters, C. Halphen, et al., Prognostic value of exercise testing soon after myocardial infarction. *N. Engl. J. Med.*, 1979;**301**: 341–345.

206. Shaw, L.J., E.D. Peterson, K. Kesler, et al., A meta analysis of predischarge risk stratification after acute myocardial infarction with stress electrocardiographic, myocardial perfusion, and ventricular function imaging. *Am. J. Cardiol.*, 1996;**78**: 1327–1337.

207. Volpi, A., C. de Vita, M.G. Franzosi, et al., Predictors of nonfatal reinfarction in survivors of myocardial infarction after thrombolysis: Results of the Gruppo Italiano per lo Studio della Sopravvivenza nell'Infarto Miocardico (GISSI 2) Data Base. *J. Am. Coll. Cardiol.*, 1994;**24**: 608–615.

208. Ciaroni, S., J. Delonca, and A. Righetti, Early exercise testing after acute myocardial infarction in the elderly: Clinical evaluation and prognostic significance. *Am. Heart J.*, 1993;**126**: 304–311.

209. Stone, P.H., Z.G. Turi, J.E. Muller, et al., Prognostic significance of the treadmill exercise test performance 6 months after myocardial infarction. *J. Am. Coll. Cardiol.*, 1986;**8**: 1007–1017.

210. Fioretti, P., R.W. Brower, M.L. Simoons, et al., Prediction of mortality in hospital survivors of myocardial infarction: Comparison of predischarge exercise testing and radionuclide ventriculography at rest. *Br. Heart J.*, 1984;**52**: 292–298.

211. Fioretti, P., R.W. Brower, M.L. Simoons, et al., Relative value of clinical variables, bicycle ergometry, rest radionuclide ventriculography and 24 hour ambulatory electrocardiographic monitoring at discharge to predict 1 year survival after myocardial infarction. *J. Am. Coll. Cardiol.*, 1986;**8**: 40–49.

212. Pilote, L., J. Silberberg, R. Lisbona, et al., Prognosis in patients with low left ventricular ejection fraction after myocardial infarction. *Circulation*, 1989;**80**: 1636–1641.

213. Krone, R.J., E.M. Dwyer, H. Greenberg, et al., Risk stratification in patients with first non Q wave infarction: Limited value of the early low level exercise test after uncomplicated infarcts: The Multicenter Post Infarction Research Group. *J. Am. Coll. Cardiol.*, 1989;**14**: 31–37.

214. DeBusk, R.F. and W. Haskell, Symptom limited vs heart rate limited exercise testing soon after myocardial infarction. *Circulation*, 1980;**61**: 738–743.

215. Abboud, L., J. Hir, I. Eisen, and W. Markiewicz, Angina pectoris and ST segment depression during exercise testing early following acute myocardial infarction. *Cardiology*, 1994;**84**: 268–273.

216. McConahay, D.R., M. Valdes, B.D. McCallister, et al., Accuracy of treadmill testing in assessment of direct myocardial revascularization. *Circulation*, 1977;**56**: 548–552.

217. Visser, F.C., L. van Campen, and P.J. de Feyter, Value and limitations of exercise stress testing to predict the functional results of coronary artery bypass grafting. *Int. J. Card. Imaging*, 1993;**9**(Suppl. 1): 41–47.

218. Kafka, H., A.J. Leach, and G.M. Fitzgibbon, Exercise echocardiography after coronary artery bypass surgery: Correlation with coronary angiography. *J. Am. Coll. Cardiol.*, 1995;**25**: 1019–1023.

219. Yli Mayry, S., H.V. Huikuri, K.E. Airaksinen, et al., Usefulness of a postoperative exercise test for predicting cardiac events after coronary artery bypass grafting. *Am. J. Cardiol.*, 1992;**70**: 56–59.

220. Krone, R.J., R.M. Hardison, B.R. Chaitman, et al., Risk stratification after successful coronary revascularization: The lack of a role for routine exercise testing. *J. Am. Coll. Cardiol.*, 2001;**38**: 136–142.

221. Kadel, C., T. Strecker, M. Kaltenbach, et al., Recognition of restenosis: Can patients be defined in whom the exercise ECG result makes angiographic restudy unnecessary? *Eur. Heart J.*, 1989;**10**(Suppl. G): 22–26.

222. Honan, M.B., J.R. Bengtson, D.B. Pryor, et al., Exercise treadmill testing is a poor predictor of anatomic restenosis after angioplasty for acute myocardial infarction. *Circulation*, 1989;**80**: 1585–1594.

223. Schroeder, E., B. Marchandise, P. DeCoster, et al., Detection of restenosis after coronary angioplasty for single vessel disease: How reliable are exercise echocardiography and scintigraphy in asymptomatic patients? *Eur. Heart J.*, 1989;**10**: 18–21.

224. Laarman, G., H.E. Luijten, L.G. van Zeyl, et al., Assessment of silent restenosis and long-term follow-up after successful angioplasty in single vessel coronary artery disease: The value of quantitative exercise electrocardiography and quantitative coronary angiography. *J. Am. Coll. Cardiol.*, 1990;**16**: 578–585.

225. Desmet, W., I. De Scheerder, and J. Piessens, Limited value of exercise testing in the detection of silent restenosis after successful coronary angioplasty. *Am. Heart J.*, 1995;**129**: 452–459.

226. Vlay, S.C., J. Chernilas, W.E. Lawson, et al., Restenosis after angioplasty: Don't rely on the exercise test. *Am. Heart J.*, 1989;**117**: 980–986.

227. Echt, H.S., R.E. Shaw, H.L. Chin, et al., Silent ischemia after coronary angioplasty: Evaluation of restenosis and extent of ischemia in asymptomatic patients by tomographic thallium 201 exercise imaging and comparison with symptomatic patients. *J. Am. Coll. Cardiol.*, 1991;**17**: 670–677.

228. Hecht, H.S., L. DeBord, R. Shaw, et al., Usefulness of supine bicycle stress echocardiography for detection of restenosis after percutaneous transluminal coronary angioplasty. *Am. J. Cardiol.*, 1993;**71**: 293–296.

229. Bigger, J.T., Jr, F.J. Dresdale, R.H. Heissenbuttel, et al., Ventricular arrhythmias in ischemic heart disease: Mechanism, prevalence, significance and management. *Prog. Cardiovasc. Dis.*, 1977;**19**: 255–300.

230. Faris, J.V., P.L. McHenry, J.W. Jordan, et al., Prevalence and reproducibility of exercise-induced ventricular arrhythmias during maximal exercise testing in normal men. *Am. J. Cardiol.*, 1976;**37**: 617–622.

231. Busby, M.J., E.A. Shefrin, and J.L. Fleg, Prevalence and long-term significance of exercise-induced frequent or repetitive ventricular ectopic beats in apparently healthy volunteers. *J. Am. Coll. Cardiol.*, 1989;**14**: 1659–1665.

232. Ellestad, M.H. and M.K. Wan, Predictive implications of stress testing. Follow up of 2700 subjects after maximum treadmill stress testing. *Circulation*, 1975;**51**: 363–369.

233. Ellestad, M.H., Chronotropic incompetence: The implications of heart rate response to exercise (compensatory parasympathetic hyperactivity?). *Circulation*, 1996;**93**: 1485–1487.

234. Lauer, M.S., P.M. Okin, M.G. Larson, et al., Impaired heart rate response to graded exercise: Prognostic implications of chronotropic incompetence in the Framingham Heart Study. *Circulation*, 1996;**93**: 1520–1526.

235. Corbelli, R., M. Masterson, and B.L. Wilkoff, Chronotropic response to exercise in patients with atrial fibrillation. *Pacing Clin. Electrophysiol.*, 1990;**13**: 179–187.

236. Fisher, F.D. and H.A. Tyroler, Relationship between ventricular premature contractions in routine electrocardiograms and subsequent sudden death from coronary heart disease. *Circulation*, 1973;**47**: 712–719.

237. Buckingham, T.A., The clinical significance of ventricular arrhythmias in apparently healthy subjects. *Pract. Cardiol.*, 1983;**9**: 37.

238. McHenry, P.L., S.N. Morris, M. Kavalier, et al., Comparative study of exercise-induced ventricular arrhythmias in normal subjects and patients with documented coronary artery disease. *Am. J. Cardiol.*, 1976;**37**: 609–616.

239. Froelicher, V.F., M.M. Thomas, C. Pillow, et al., Epidemiologic study of asymptomatic men screened by maximal treadmill testing for latent coronary artery disease. *Am. J. Cardiol.*, 1974;**34**: 770–776.

240. Blackburn, H., H.L. Taylor, B. Hamrell, et al., Premature ventricular complexes induced by stress testing. Their frequency and response to physical conditioning. *Am. J. Cardiol.*, 1973;**31**: 441–449.

241. McHenry, P.L., S.N. Morris, and M. Kavalier, Exercise-induced arrhythmia: Recognition, classification and clinical significance. *Cardiovasc. Clin.*, 1974;**6**: 245–254.

242. Jouven, X., M. Zureik, M. Desnos, et al., Long-term outcome in asymptomatic men with exercise-induced premature ventricular depolarizations. *N. Engl. J. Med.*, 2000;**343**: 826–833.

243. Jelinek, M.V. and B. Lown, Exercise stress testing for exposure of cardiac arrhythmia. *Prog. Cardiovasc. Dis.*, 1974;**16**: 497–522.

244. Goldschlager, N., D. Cake, and K. Cohn, Exercise-induced ventricular arrhythmias in patients with coronary artery disease: Their relationship to angiographic findings. *Am. J. Cardiol.*, 1973;**31**: 434–440.

245. Surawicz, B. and T.K. Knilans, *Chou's Electrocardiography in Clinical Practice: Adult and Pediatric*, 5th edn. Philadelphia, PA: W.B. Saunders.

246. Kotler, M.N., B. Tabatznik, M.M. Mower, et al., Prognostic significance of ventricular ectopic beats with respect to sudden death in the late postinfarction period. *Circulation*, 1973;**47**: 959–966.

247. Chiang, B.N., L.V. Perlman, L.D. Ostrander Jr, et al., Relationship of premature systoles to coronary heart disease and sudden death in the Tecumseh epidemiologic study. *Ann. Intern. Med.*, 1969;**70**: 1159–1166.

248. Coronary Drug Project Research Group, Prognostic importance of premature beats following myocardial infarction. Experience in the Coronary Drug Project. *JAMA*, 1973;**223**: 1116–1124.

249. Henry, R.L., G.T. Kennedy, and M.H. Crawford, Prognostic value of exercise-induced ventricular ectopic activity for mortality after acute myocardial infarction. *Am. J. Cardiol.*, 1987;**59**: 1251–1215.

250. Krone, R.J., J.A. Gillespie, F.M. Weld, et al., Low-level exercise testing after myocardial infarction: Usefulness in enhancing clinical risk stratification. *Circulation*, 1985;**71**: 80–89.

251. Waters, D.D., X. Bosch, A. Bouchard, et al., Comparison of clinical variables and variables derived from a limited predischarge exercise test as predictors of early and late mortality after myocardial infarction. *J. Am. Coll. Cardiol.*, 1985;**5**: 1–8.

252. Margonato, A., A. Mailhac, F. Bonetti, et al., Exercise-induced ischemic arrhythmias in patients with previous myocardial infarction: Role of perfusion and tissue viability. *J. Am. Coll. Cardiol.*, 1996;**27**: 593–598.

253. Marieb, M.A., G.A. Beller, R.S. Gibson, et al., Clinical relevance of exercise-induced ventricular arrhythmias in suspected coronary artery disease. *Am. J. Cardiol.*, 1990;**66**: 172–178.

254. Califf, R.M., R.A. McKinnis, J.F. McNeer, et al., Prognostic value of ventricular arrhythmias associated with treadmill exercise testing in patients studied with cardiac catheterization for suspected ischemic heart disease. *J. Am. Coll. Cardiol.*, 1983;**2**: 1060–1067.

255. Helfant, R.H., R. Pine, V. Kabde, et al., Exercise-related ventricular premature complexes in coronary heart disease: Correlations with ischemia and angiographic severity. *Ann. Intern. Med.*, 1974;**80**: 589–592.

256. Udall, J.A. and M.H. Ellestad, Predictive implications of ventricular premature contractions associated with treadmill stress testing. *Circulation*, 1977;**56**: 985–989.

257. Sami, M., B. Chaitman, L. Fisher, et al., Significance of exercise-induced ventricular arrhythmia in stable coronary artery disease: A Coronary Artery Surgery Study project. *Am. J. Cardiol.*, 1984;**54**: 1182–1188.

258. Schweikert, R.A., F.J. Pashkow, C.E. Snader, et al., Association of exercise-induced ventricular ectopic activity with thallium myocardial perfusion and angiographic coronary artery disease in stable, low-risk populations. *Am. J. Cardiol.*, 1999;**83**: 530–534.

259. Dimsdale, J.E., W. Ruberman, R.A. Carleton, V. DeQuattro, E. Eaker, R.S. Eliot, C.D. Furberg, C.W. Irvin Jr, A.P. Shapiro, et al., Sudden cardiac death. Stress and cardiac arrhythmias. *Circulation*, 1987;**76**(1 Pt. 2): I198–I201.

260. Pinski, S.L., The right ventricular tachycardias. *J. Electrocardiol.*, 2000;**33**: 103–114.

261. Podrid, P.J. and T.B. Graboys, Exercise stress testing in the management of cardiac rhythm disorders. *Med. Clin. North Am.*, 1984;**68**: 1139–1152.

262. Young, D.Z., S. Lampert, T.B. Graboys, et al., Safety of maximal exercise testing in patients at high risk for ventricular arrhythmia. *Circulation*, 1984;**70**: 184–191.

263. Saini, V., T.B. Graboys, V. Towne, et al., Reproducibility of exercise-induced ventricular arrhythmia in patients undergoing

evaluation for malignant ventricular arrhythmia. *Am. J. Cardiol.,* 1989;**63**: 697–701.

264. ACC/AHA guidelines for the management of patients with valvular heart disease: A report of the American College of Cardiology/American Heart Association Task Force on Practice Guidelines (Committee on Management of Patients with Valvular Heart Disease). *J. Am. Coll. Cardiol.,* 1998;**32**: 1486–1588.

265. Hochreiter, C. and J.S. Borer, Exercise testing in patients with aortic and mitral valve disease: Current applications. *Cardiovasc. Clin.,* 1983;**13**: 291–300.

266. Chandramouli, B., D.A. Ehmke, and R.M. Lauer, Exercise induced electrocardiographic changes in children with congenital aortic stenosis. *J. Pediatr.,* 1975;**87**: 725–730.

267. James, F.W., D.C. Schwartz, S. Kaplan, et al., Exercise electrocardiogram, blood pressure, and working capacity in young patients with valvular or discrete subvalvular aortic stenosis. *Am. J. Cardiol.,* 1982;**50**: 769–775.

268. Bonow, R.O., Management of chronic aortic regurgitation. *N. Engl. J. Med.,* 1994;**331**: 736–737.

5 Computer Analysis of the Electrocardiogram

Jan A. Kors · Gerard van Herpen

P. W. Macfarlane et al. (eds.), *Specialized Aspects of ECG*, DOI 10.1007/978-0-85729-880-5_5,
© Springer-Verlag London Limited 2012

This chapter deals with the use of digital computers for the handling of the resting ECG. The reader is referred to other chapters of this book for a review of computer-assisted interpretation of the exercise electrocardiogram, for ambulatory monitoring, on-line arrhythmia detection in the coronary care unit, and for surface mapping and modeling applications.

5.1   Some History

It is a deep rooted fantasy of man, told in many stories, to be able to handicraft a creature in his own image and endow it with the breath of life: a "homunculus." More often than not, the endeavor is initially successful but ends in disenchantment. The advent of the computer seemed to make it possible to equip such a creation with human intelligence. Electrocardiography appeared to be a field where the computer could be expected to deploy its intelligent capabilities to the best advantage.

The ECG was an attractive object for computerization for a number of reasons: (1) it is an electrical signal, easily recorded and easily digestible for a computer; (2) it is a rather simple, orderly and repetitive signal; (3) it carries important information about which a vast corpus of knowledge has been amassed to prime the computer program; (4) ECGs are produced in enormous quantities all over the world which makes it worthwhile to let a computer reduce human workload.

ECG diagnosis by computer would be an instance of artificial intelligence which might ultimately challenge the specific human faculty of diagnosis. When is artificial intelligence really intelligent? Turing devised a thought experiment to answer this question [1]. Suppose that a computer and a human being are sitting in separate closed chambers and that an outside investigator is questioning them. If the investigator cannot decide from the answers whether they are given by the computer or by man, then the computer has attained full human intelligence. This implies that the computer's diagnosis of the ECG must exactly copy that of man in order to satisfy this requirement. Indeed, the agreement between computer classification and man-made diagnosis of the ECG has been extensively studied. But how intelligent is man? Disagreement between computer and man might even be due to a computer's superior diagnostic power! A second approach in testing a diagnostic ECG program, therefore, had to be to gauge it against reality, the clinical diagnosis, and to compare its performance with the skills of the human reader in this respect. The outcomes of both approaches will be discussed later.

The first attempts to automate ECG analysis by computer were made as early as the late 1950s, but it took considerably more time to develop operational computer programs than had originally been anticipated. At that time, the analog electric computer dominated the field. Analog computers were being used in basic electrocardiographic research [2], but their impact on clinical electrocardiography remained insignificant and they soon disappeared from the scene [3]. To have an analog signal processed by a digital computer, it must be broken down into digital samples. However, analog-to-digital (A-D) conversion systems (see ❯ Chap. 12 of *Basic Electrocardiology: Cardiac electrophysiology, ECG Systems and Mathematical Modeling*) were not available as they are today and a special purpose A-D conversion system for ECGs had to be developed first [4].

A very crude computer program for the separation of normal from abnormal records became operational in 1959 [5]. It was based on angles and magnitude of spatial ventricular gradients, calculated from the time integrals over one PQRST cycle in the three orthogonal leads. Cycle recognition was still obtained through analog circuitry. The beginning and end of P, QRS, and T were not identified in this simple screening program. The first automatic wave-recognition program became available in 1961, opening the way for more detailed analysis of ECG records [6]. This original program, as well as its successors developed by Pipberger and coworkers [7, 8], was based on the Frank XYZ leads for the main reason that three leads laid less claim to computer capacity, still very limited both in speed and in memory space, than 12 leads. Through the pioneering work of Caceres et al. [9] the first program for conventional 12-lead ECG analysis became available in 1962. It was supported by the US Public Health Service and intended to make expert ECG analysis immediately available to all who needed it, using the telephone system. The 12 ECG leads were transmitted sequentially and, therefore, had to be analyzed individually. The loss of context between the leads, together with inherent cable noise, caused considerable waveform recognition errors and the program came to an untimely end.

User satisfaction, indeed, was not won by these early accomplishments and the initial state of excitement was to give way to one of dogged perseverance. Fresh investigators were, according to their state of awareness, attracted by the seeming easiness or the proven difficulties of the subject. Commercial suppliers started to be active in this market [10]. Gradually, a number of operational systems came into being in North America, Europe, and Japan. In the bigger hospitals, main frame computers were installed, which received the ECG signals on tape from mobile carts and could store them in databases. For the less well-equipped customers, ECG diagnosis via telephone was offered by all kinds of entrepreneurial services, which did a thriving business in the 1970s and 1980s, sometimes handling millions of ECGs a year [11, 12]. The scene changed completely with the advent of the microprocessor [13]. Microprocessor-based systems have made it possible to distribute computerized ECG analysis outside hospital and laboratory to even the smallest hospitals, to screening clinics and to practitioners of every kind. While it took minutes to process a single ECG on a main frame computer in the early years, a present-day simple PC takes a fraction of a second to do the analysis. Most of these electrocardiographs are "stand-alone," that is, have a computer and printer on board. Some manufacturers offer separate front-end equipment (amplifiers and A-D converter) that can be interfaced with the computer standing in the doctor's office.

With a widening choice of systems on the market, the consumer may wish to know how intelligent the system being considered for purchase is. But where can the consumer turn for an objective intelligence test? It is clear that objective assessment of the quality of computerized ECG systems is needed. We will return to this subject in later sections of this chapter.

5.2   ECG-Processing Computer Systems

5.2.1   Advantages

Although diagnostic accuracy and reliability are greatly desirable characteristics of an interpretation system, the program's utility in a clinical environment is also determined by other factors. Reduction of the labor spent by the cardiological and clerical staff has been a key determinant in moving toward computer-aided processing systems in hospitals [11, 14]; improvement of overall process quality has been another. Rigorous operational control, as imposed by a computer system, can substantially add to the recording quality and thus the reliability of interpretation. The quality of reporting is also improved through the use of standard terminology and formats.

Computer analysis abolishes the well-known subjective differences arising in visual interpretation, and through a quantitative approach may enhance correct classification. Pipberger and cornfield [15] have, since the early 1960s, pointed to improved accuracy of interpretation as the primary objective of computer ECG processing. Automatic storage and retrieval, with the possibility of comparing the new ECG with its predecessors (serial analysis) is another asset of computerized ECG processing.

Computerized analysis of the resting ECG has also increased the feasibility of large-scale cardiovascular screening and epidemiological studies. "Minnesota coding" of the ECG can nowadays be performed by computer, quickly and reliably (see ❷ Chap. 8).

5.2.2   ECG Management Systems

An ECG management system can come in several forms and undertake multiple functions. In its simplest form, it effectively acts as a database for storage of ECGs and offers straightforward retrieval of ECGs for display or printing. It could be in the form of a small PC, to which an ECG machine might be directly attached as might be found in a small family medical practice.

At the other extreme, a large ECG management system could be used to centrally store all ECGs recorded within a large hospital or group of hospitals. Such systems generally have the capability to store multiple ECGs for a single patient and thereby facilitate serial comparison either through visual display of several ECGs on the same monitor screen or through automated techniques (see ❷ Sect. 5.16). The large systems offer the user the ability to measure wave amplitudes, durations, and standard time intervals on an averaged ECG waveform, generally using digital calipers.

One of the major benefits of the larger systems is to allow editing, sometimes known as over-reading, of the automated interpretations. Generally, manufacturers provide facilities to assist with editing such as through acronyms to represent standard interpretative statements. In many environments, a physician will handwrite comments onto an automated report and a member of the administrative staff with appropriate knowledge can edit the changes on the ECG management system. A problem then arises if serial comparison is available on the system. In such a case, the original electronic copy of the automated interpretation also has to be edited so that any subsequent serial comparison is made with the corrected report. This is actually quite a complex issue and one which can inhibit automated serial comparison.

Clearly, the ECG management system offers the facility for the provision of statistics on throughput of ECGs, number of edits made by each cardiologist, and so on. Nowadays, there is a trend toward manufacturers providing multiple databases for ECGs, echocardiograms, x-rays, etc., on a single server, but flexibility of editing and retrieving ECGs easily on an ECG management system still remains of significant importance in many healthcare environments.

5.3   Information Content of Lead Systems; Lead Transformations

In the analysis of biological signals in general, an enormous flow of information is channeled through a limited number of transducers. The often still redundant transducer output stream is then reduced and transformed to a manageable number of parameters. These in turn are harnessed into decision machinery, which finally summarizes the input information in a few standardized "diagnostic" terms that carry significance for the user and are the basis for further action. The ECG is such a biological signal.

The electrical activity of the heart gives rise to a three-dimensional time-varying distribution of currents and potentials. To obtain a full picture of this process, it is necessary to measure the complete course of potential distributions in and on the body. Only the body surface signals are readily available for measurement and even then the amount of information generated by the heart is so large that it is necessary to curtail the information stream for practical purposes. For the recording of a body surface potential map (BSPM), grids of 64–192 electrodes are being used (see ❷ Chap. 9 of *cardiac Arrhythmias and Mapping Techniques*). In this way, in a single BSPM all ECG information of that moment may be considered to be present as to localization. However, in a sequence of BSPMs, it is not feasible to follow all these individual electrocardiograms in their time course. For practical reasons, global parameters like "isointegral maps" or "isochrone maps" have to be used, and for diagnostic purposes, "difference maps" and "departure maps" have also been used. All this manipulation of data has only become possible, thanks to the computer, but so far clinical acceptance of BSPM diagnostic systems has been poor.

The universally used standard 12-lead ECG system needs nine electrodes, the three original Einthoven electrodes and the six thoracic electrodes adapted from Wilson. With the use of nine electrodes, eight independent leads, as they are called, can be obtained. The four extra extremity leads, which complete the 12-lead system, are not independent as they are arithmetically derived from any two other extremity leads. Nine electrodes are a drastic reduction of the number of sampling sites used to create a BSPM; the diagnostic power retained in this reduced lead set is indeed amazing. The explanation lies in the large degree of redundancy present in the surface information. Even among the eight leads of the standard ECG there is much redundancy and the question arises how many leads are actually required to render all relevant information.

In the vectorcardiogram (VCG), all information is contained in only three orthogonal leads, the X, Y, and Z components of a single dipole vector that changes with time in direction and strength, but is assumed to be stationary in position. Clearly, the three leads of the VCG (composed from a set of selected primary leads by linear combination) carry less information than eight leads, but, in return, the vector depicts the temporal relation between leads, providing phase information that is largely neglected in the ECG. Vectorcardiography could properly be called "phase electrocardiography." This feature makes up for the restriction on information input so that the diagnostic performances of the ECG and VCG are comparable, as will be discussed later on. Thus, each choice of data input, whether it be BSPM, standard ECG, or VCG, incurs the sacrifice of some information aspect: time resolution, phase coherence, or localization.

Presently, all ECG computer programs which are in clinical use will handle the conventional 12-lead system. Systems processing only the VCG have been driven from the market. The advantage that the VCG offers a data reduction of 8:3 has become insignificant considering the power of present-day computers. The clinical acceptance of the VCG has been hampered by the variety of different lead systems (from which the Frank lead system [16] emerged as the most commonly embraced), by a lack of understanding by clinicians of the physical principles, by the requirement of dorsal electrodes found to be cumbersome to apply, and finally by the absence, at the time, of proper recording equipment [17].

The question remains: how many leads are actually required to render all relevant information? It is of more than anecdotal value that Dower [18] let his ECG service only take vectorcardiograms. The ECGs that were then delivered to the hospital were derived from these VCGs by means of a mathematical transformation – apparently for many years to everybody's satisfaction. The inverse transformation yields the VCG from the standard ECG [19, 20], or, for better adjustment, from the standard ECG fitted out with some extra electrodes [21]. Kornreich [22, 23] demonstrated that the ECG and VCG leave some clinically useful spaces on the surface map not covered by their electrodes. With a set of electrodes also serving these areas, nine leads were determined that yielded better diagnostic classification (using multivariate analysis) than either the VCG or ECG [24, 25]. Kors et al. [26] proposed a system containing the standard electrodes of which two chest electrodes were moved to positions higher up and lower down on the chest. From the seven not-displaced electrodes (4 chest + 3 limb) the 12 leads could be reconstructed by linear transformation in very good approximation. In fact, it was possible to compose any set of ECG leads with electrode positions chosen for local information density and ease of placement, standard or nonstandard, and from these leads derive the standard ECG by a mathematical transformation [27]. Computer analysis of such a "derived" ECG should give all but the same result as that of its directly recorded counterpart. The nonstandard extra recorded leads might then be exploited for additional information – with the difficulty that no standard diagnostic criteria are available for such leads. Even an entire BSPM can be simulated from a limited number of measured ECG leads.

The EASI lead system designed by Dower uses only four electrodes to produce the 12 standard ECG leads by linear transformation [28]. Four electrodes will yield three independent leads; four was also the number of electrodes used originally by Burger to derive the three orthogonal vector components [29]. Linear transformations were also used to reduce signal noise [30] and to identify interchanged leads [31]. The first to use a linear transformation in electrocardiography were Burger et al. [32] to transform VCGs obtained from different lead systems into those from each other.

For practical purposes, this review will be further restricted to computer analysis of the resting standard 12-lead ECG with some reference to the orthogonal 3-lead ECG. Some ECG processing systems have an option to display and print vector loops, either directly recorded from the regular (Frank) electrode positions or computed through linear transformation from the ECG leads. The reader is referred to ❷ Chap. 11 of *Basic Electrocardiology: Cardiac electrophysiology, ECG Systems and Mathematical Modeling* in this book for a review of other lead systems.

5.4   Computer Processing of the ECG

In teaching electrocardiography, and in order to start the novice reader on a career in electrocardiography, it suffices to say: "This is a QRS complex, this little wiggle in front is a P, and the hump following QRS is a T." Some more detailed descriptions are absorbed with equal ease and the final touch is added by the recommendations and guidelines for nomenclature and measurements as issued by various committees and task forces [33–36]. Reading the electrocardiogram is in the first place a matter of visual observation, if necessary, aided by calipers and magnifying glass, and relies on the amazing deftness in pattern recognition of the human brain. The subsequent electrocardiographic diagnosis is a logic built on correct pattern recognition. The computer must do without human "eye balling" skills and needs to be instructed punctiliously about every detail of measurement down to the microvolt and millisecond level. Rules and definitions for visual ECG analysis may then appear imprecise and not consistent enough for computer application, and may even show gaps in their logic. New computer-compatible prescriptions for ECG signal measurements should, however, adhere as much as possible to accepted methods of visual measurement [34]. In the sections on waveform recognition (5.12) and parameter computation (5.13) we will go further into the matter.

As in visual ECG analysis, in an ECG data-processing system, the first of the two main parts that can be distinguished is that which contains program components to perform measurements. The second part includes the program components that derive the clinical significance of these measurements. This results in a final classification, or interpretation, of the ECG in terms familiar to the physician. The words "classification" or "interpretation" are preferred by some over "diagnosis," which is then the term reserved for the human interpretative activity.

The principal components of the ECG measurement section are as follows:

1. Data acquisition
2. Preprocessing and signal conditioning
3. Detection of QRS complexes and of P waves
4. Typing of QRS complexes
5. Forming a representative (P)-QRS-T complex

6. Boundary recognition, that is, detection of points of onset and offset of waves
7. Parameter extraction

The principal components of the ECG interpretative section are:

1. Rhythm analysis
2. Diagnostic classification
3. Serial comparison

These separate program components will be discussed in detail in the following paragraphs. Many ECG processing systems implement these different tasks in separate modules, each of which has well-defined objectives [37]. The advantage of such a structured setup is its easy implementation, evaluation, and maintenance [38]. In addition, systems for clinical use will have to offer an over-reading facility, which allows manual correction of the computer output. A fixed set of codes, most commonly acronyms, takes care of producing the required text elements, thereby ensuring consistency of terminology. In addition, entries in free text are admissible.

To inform the consumer about the quality of a computerized ECG system, it is necessary to have access to reference standards for objective evaluation. A paragraph on reference databases will therefore precede the discussion of the various parts of computer processing mentioned above, since it will often be necessary to refer to these standards.

5.5   Reference Databases for Program Evaluation

"How to test the intelligence of the computer" was the question raised in the introduction of this chapter. The simple precept is to compare the computer statements with the objective "truth" embodied in the ECG readings of the human expert or the clinical findings. How to carry this out will be shown to be no simple matter.

Two qualities are to be considered separately in the operations of the computer program, namely, waveform recognition skill and diagnostic competence, with correct waveform recognition being a sine qua non for reliable interpretation. As to the first quality, large measurement differences may become apparent between programs while analyzing identical ECGs [39, 40]. As to the second aspect, where is it possible to obtain the diagnostic truth? Initially, a number of program designers compared the computer output with their own ECG interpretation [41]. Diagnostic criteria were identical for both. As could be expected, agreement between computer and human readers was excellent. It is obvious that not diagnostic accuracy but reliability of the wave-recognition and measurement parts of the programs was tested in these studies. For example, in the study by Crevasse and Ariet [42] a computer accuracy rate of 98% was reported for LVH. Both the computer and the human readers used the Romhilt-Estes point score. When this criterion was tested by the originators of this scoring system in 150 autopsy cases with LVH, they found a true accuracy of only 60% [43]. This is therefore the closest to "truth" that the computer could ever get on the strength of this criterion [8]. In other studies, computer results were compared to interpretations of human readers who used their own, individual diagnostic rules [44–47]. As had to be expected, percentages of disagreement rose sharply, reaching almost 50% in one early study [48].

Comparisons with ECG-independent clinical evidence were also carried out in due course [8, 49–53]. These investigations were mostly limited to one or two programs only. Moreover, they are difficult to compare since they utilized different databases, most of them collected within a single institute. More and more the need was felt for common, objective, impartial reference standards to test and improve different ECG computer programs [14, 54–58]. For this purpose, well-established test libraries are indispensable, together with well-defined measurement rules and evaluation procedures. On several occasions, this necessity was stressed, as at the first IFIP Working Conference on Computerized ECG Analysis [54] or in the editorial of Pipberger and Cornfield [15]. Detailed guidelines for program testing were presented at the 1977 Bethesda Conference on Optimal Electrocardiography [14].

In 1979, a concerted European action was started to develop "Common Standards for Quantitative Electrocardiography" (abbreviated: CSE). The CSE Working Party consisted of investigators from 25 institutes in Europe with the participation of investigators from six North-American and one Japanese center.

The CSE project was divided into two 5-year periods, the first dealing with measurements, the second with diagnostic interpretation [59]. The main objectives of the first part of the CSE project were, firstly, to establish standards for

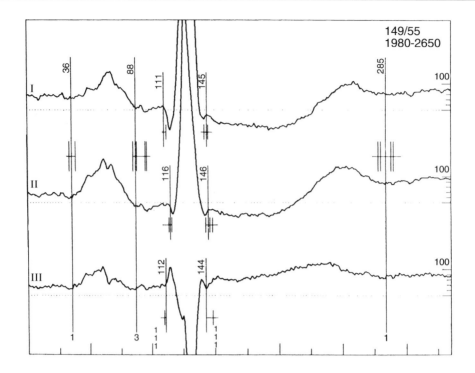

⊙ Fig. 5.1

Example of wave boundary determination by five cardiologists (from Willems et al. [62]). The *short vertical lines* depict the individual, sometimes coinciding, referee estimates, the long ones the median results. The adjacent values denote the sample point locations relative to the onset of the recording window. The figures at the *bottom* of the *vertical lines* indicate the final reviewing round in which the estimates were obtained. Note that the onset of QRS in leads I and II is at a lower level than the onset of P, due to the presence of the atrial repolarization wave. In lead III the projection of this wave is isoelectric. Also, in lead III the T wave ends in an isoelectric segment. The observers disregarded this when they established T offset over the three leads simultaneously

computer-derived ECG measurements, which implied agreement on definitions of waves and amplitude reference levels, and, secondly, to compare the results of measurements from different programs.

Thanks to this first CSE study, two reference databases came into being [60, 61]. They were composed of normal and a variety of abnormal cases. The first database [60] comprised 250 original and 310 so-called artificial ECGs. The recordings contain four lead groups of three simultaneously recorded leads each, as was common for most electrocardiographs at the time. From the original ECGs, companion artificial ECGs were constructed by concatenating one selected beat per lead group into strings of identical complexes. This artifice makes it possible to compare programs with different approaches for deriving a representative beat. To verify the effect of beat-to-beat variability, out of 30 original ECGs, two additional beats were selected to form an extra 60 artificial records. A group of five cardiologists determined the points of onset and offset of the various ECG waves (P, QRS, and T) on much enlarged tracings in an iterative, four-round, Delphi review process (⊙ Fig. 5.1).

The second database [61] comprised 250 original and 250 artificial ECGs in which all 15 leads – the 12 standard ECG leads plus the Frank XYZ leads – were recorded simultaneously. In view of the work load involved, the visual analysis strategy could not be repeated. Instead, the median wave-recognition results of 11 ECG and six VCG programs participating in the CSE study were taken as the reference. The cardiologists reviewed a random set of about 20% of the cases in a two-round process, and it was shown that the median of the program results was almost identical to the median results of the referees [61].

Both for the three-lead and multilead database, the original and corresponding artificial ECGs were divided over two sets. The waveform reference results of one set have been released [63, 64]; the results of the other set remain under lock and key at the CSE coordinating center for independent testing.

Differing mathematical algorithms may lead to similar solutions in pattern recognition [34]. For that reason, it was not seen as fitting to propose any specific algorithm as the exclusive standard for ECG wave recognition. At the same time, the CSE reference databases are strongly recommended as a bench mark for ECG measurement programs. Comparison with the standard involves two quality measures: a program should approach the reference as closely as possible, and the standard deviation of the differences of its results with respect to the reference should not exceed certain limits. These limits have been described in detail in a paper with recommendations for measurement standards in quantitative electrocardiography [34].

The second part of the CSE project aimed at the assessment of the diagnostic performance of ECG computer programs. This study commenced in 1985 and finished in 1990. A database consisting of 1,220 multilead recordings was collected, comprising seven diagnostic groups: normal (n = 382); left (n = 183), right (n = 55), and biventricular (n = 53) hypertrophy; and anterior (n = 170), inferior (n = 273), and combined (n = 73) myocardial infarction. Also some cases with both infarction and hypertrophy (n = 31) were included, but ECGs showing major intraventricular conduction defects were not. The clinical diagnosis was documented by ECG-independent evidence, such as cardiac catheterization, coronary arteriography, echocardiography, cardiac enzymes, and patient history [65]. The ECGs and VCGs were analyzed by 15 computer programs and by nine cardiologists, from seven European countries [66]. Evaluation results will be discussed later.

The CSE reference libraries have become an international standard for the evaluation and improvement of ECG and VCG computer programs. A comprehensive overview of the CSE project appeared in 1990 [59].

5.6 Data Acquisition

Before the ECG signals are transmitted to a computer system for analysis, the operator has to enter patient identification data. The patient's name, sex, and date of birth together with an identification code are essential for proper automatic handling of the ECG data. Data like weight, height, blood pressure, and medication might be useful – if they are not based on guess-work by a lackadaisical technician! The system will also store the time and date of the recording, as well as, mostly, a technician and location code. For programs that perform serial ECG analysis, the unique patient identification code is indispensable for record linking.

In order to achieve optimal performance of an ECG-processing system it is essential that the data used in the analysis are of good quality. In practice, ECG records can be disturbed by power line interference, baseline wander caused by electrode polarization, electromagnetic muscle artifacts, spikes, sudden baseline shifts due to electrode contact interruption, and amplitude saturation. Although automated systems can achieve a great deal of signal conditioning (see the following paragraphs), it devolves upon the operator to correctly apply the electrodes and to detect and remedy signal errors and disturbances before entering them in the system, according to the maxim "garbage in, garbage out." Power-line interference can be prevented or reduced by proper shielding and grounding, by appropriate skin preparation and electrode application. Muscle tremor can be reduced or removed by having the patient comfortable and relaxed, while respiratory baseline wander can be minimized by breath holding.

The front-end of an ECG processing system consists of analog amplifiers. Present-day technology even allows them to be incorporated in the electrodes and to transmit the signals by a local wireless system to the processing unit. The amplifiers must be of adequate bandwidth for a faithful rendering of the signals. For further technical details, the reader is referred to ❯ Chap. 12 of *Basic Electrocardiology: Cardiac electrophysiology, ECG Systems and Mathematical Modeling*.

A digital computer can handle data only in numerical form, and therefore, the original continuous (or analog) voltage variations of ECG signals need to be converted into a series of numbers, corresponding to the voltage levels of the leads at any moment of time. General principles concerning analog-to-digital (A-D) conversion of the ECG have been reviewed by Berson et al. [67, 68]. The time and amplitude resolution of the A-D conversion is dependent on the sampling rate, the word size of the converter and the dynamic range of the analog input.

Sampling rates for ECG data in various programs originally varied from 250 to 500 samples per second. The American Heart Association [69] and the CSE Working Party [34] have recommended for clinical application a high-frequency cutoff of the analog amplifiers of 150 Hz and a sampling rate of 500 Hz for the A-D conversion. In the pediatric ECG, the waves, especially the QRS, are of shorter duration at often elevated voltage which results in high rates of acceleration and deceleration of the signal with corresponding high frequency content. This requires an extension of the minimal high-frequency cutoff to 250 Hz [70].

The more bits per word in an A-D converter, the greater the possible resolution. In addition, the dynamic range of the amplifiers must be wide enough to accept the largest possible excursion of the signal amplitude. Modern electrocardiographs have 16 or 18 bit converters, with quantization levels of 1.22 µV–4.88 µV for the least significant bit.

Until the introduction of "stand-alone," microprocessor-equipped systems for ECG analysis, ECG records needed to be transmitted to a central computing facility. This was possible by transferring magnetic tapes on which ECGs were recorded, or by sending the signals on-line over ordinary telephone lines. This involved frequency modulation and demodulation which noticeably contributed to recorder noise. In the present digital era, the total analysis of the ECG can be done on a stand-alone electrocardiograph. The central ECG management system is required for storage and retrieval, a necessary utility for serial analysis; as well as for providing a means of editing interpretations. Interchange with the central facility may occur through a local area network, possibly by wireless transmission, or the ECGs are conveyed on some digital storage medium.

In the acquisition device, all 12 leads are acquired simultaneously so that time coherence between the signals is preserved. In practice, eight independent leads are recorded (I, II, VI-V6) and the other four are reconstructed from leads I and II using the classical relations such as lead III = II − I. In some systems, additional leads may be entered simultaneously for the VCG or for other purposes. The signals are stored in memory and can be displayed for a visual quality check. The computer may interact with the operator and warn of excessive noise in a lead or indicate electrode reversal. Reversal between right and left arm is detected by most programs. Other forms of electrode interchange require more sophisticated approaches [31, 71]. After approval by the operator, the signals are processed.

While the electrodes may have been placed in the correct order, without interchange, they still may be ill-positioned, for example, one interspace too high or too low on the chest. These errors are almost refractory to detection and correction [72, 73].

Conventionally, 12-lead ECGs were presented on multichannel writers in four lead groups of 2.5 s, often with a 10.0 s rhythm strip, on one page. Sometimes 5.0 s was taken per lead group, requiring two pages, or 6-channel writers were used. With the entire ECG present in memory and the availability of a thermal writer or laser printer, a modern device will allow considerable flexibility of output format. The signals, in addition, are preprocessed by digital techniques in such a way that mains interference and baseline drift have been reduced to a minimum to produce a neat paper output.

5.7　Signal Preprocessing and Conditioning

ECG records may be disturbed by different types of artifacts as enumerated previously, namely, power-line interference, baseline wander, muscle noise, spikes, and amplitude saturation. The aim of the preprocessing stage is to detect and correct these artifacts as far as possible. In hopeless cases, rejection of a part or the whole of the recording may be inevitable. The problems of signal improvement have been a challenge to many capable technical minds and have resulted in an abundant literature on the subject. Some of the algorithms require that the locations of the QRS complexes are known, and thus are not properly part of the preprocessing stage. This will be mentioned when the case occurs. The evaluation of the performance of these algorithms applied to real ECGs is not straightforward since the undisturbed signals are unknown. This may in particular be an issue in treating baseline wander and muscle noise. A common approach to studying the problem is to add simulated noise to a clean, "noise free," ECG signal. This approach can be carried one step further by simulating both noise and signal. As with all simulations, the validity of the evaluation results will depend on how well the simulated signals mimic those that occur in practice.

5.7.1　Power-Line Interference

Power-line interference is a common problem and is characterized by its periodicity of 50 or 60 Hz (higher harmonics may also be observed). Different digital filters have been proposed for the removal of power-line interference [74, 75]. They can be categorized in three types:

1. Notch filters, which attenuate frequencies in a narrow frequency band around the interference frequency [76, 77].
2. Global filters, which make a single estimate of the interfering noise over the total duration of the signal and then subtract this estimate from the signal. Cramer et al. [75] describe two such global approaches. One is based on a least-squares error fit of the interference. The other approach requires the sampling rate to be an integer multiple of the power-line frequency, say n, and calculates an average amplitude for each of the n phase points in one period of the interference. Both approaches only perform well if the line frequency is stable within 0.02 Hz of the nominal frequency [75], which in practice may often not be the case. Also, these methods, by definition, cannot adjust to amplitude changes of the interference. Levkov et al. [78] proposed estimating the interference from each isoelectric or slowly changing part of the ECG signal, which allows tracking of interference amplitude changes. To ensure that the sampling rate was an integer multiple of the power-line frequency, they used a hardware-synchronized A-D converter. More recently, a software solution to adjust for interference frequency variation was proposed, involving estimation of the interference period and resampling of the ECG signal [79]. An extensive review of the method is given by Levkov et al. [80].
3. Adaptive filters, which use an auxiliary reference signal containing the interference alone [74, 81–83]. This reference is adaptively filtered to match the interfering sinusoid as closely as possible, and is then subtracted from the primary signal. An interesting variant of the classical adaptive filter approach is the "incremental estimation" filter proposed by Mortara [84] and further investigated by others [74, 85–87]. The filter generates a prediction of the power-line interference $v(n)$ contained in the signal $x(n)$, based on the noise estimate $w(n)$ at the previous two samples:

$$v(n) = 2\cos(2\pi f/f_s)\, w(n-1) - w(n-2),$$

with f the nominal frequency of the interference and f_s the sampling rate. If $v(n)$ is a good prediction, then the difference $x(n) - v(n)$ should be zero apart from a possible constant offset. Assuming a slowly changing signal, the difference $x(n-1) - w(n-1)$ is taken as an estimate of this offset, and the error

$$e(n) = \big(x(n) - v(n)\big) - \big(x(n-1) - w(n-1)\big)$$

indicates how well $v(n)$ predicts the interference amplitude. A final estimate is then produced by incrementing or decrementing the value of $v(n)$ with a fixed amount δ, depending on the sign of $e(n)$:

$$w(n) = v(n) + \delta\,\mathrm{sgn}(e(n)).$$

Finally, the output $y(n)$ of the filter is

$$y(n) = x(n) - w(n).$$

The value of the increment δ is chosen heuristically. A value which is too small may cause sluggish adaptation to the interference amplitude and poor tracking of its changes. A value which is too large, on the other hand, may cause the estimate $w(n)$ to jitter around the power-line interference, introducing extra noise. Also, since the assumption of a slowly changing signal does not hold true for the QRS complex, large increments will result in ringing artifacts. An incremental value of 1.25 µV was proposed by Mortara [84]. Using a few simplifying assumptions, Talmon [85] analyzed the relationship between the amplitude of the sinusoidal disturbance, the increment, and the bandwidth of the filter. Glover [88] showed that the filter reduces to a standard notch filter if the nonlinear sign function in the update equation is replaced by a linear increment function.

A number of different filters, representative of the above filter types, were compared by McManus et al. [74]. They applied the filters both to artificial test signals simulating various forms of interference (including second and third harmonics of the nominal frequency), and to a small subset of real ECGs from one of the CSE databases. Tested against a list of 14 desiderata for an ideal interference filter, no single filter consistently performed better than the others for all requirements. Remarkably, the incremental estimation filter and the global filter were the only ones that did not produce a ringing effect at the end of the QRS as is the usual accompaniment of large-amplitude QRS complexes when filtered, as illustrated by ❷ Fig. 5.2. In another study [87], the incremental estimation filter was compared to a nonadaptive second order notch filter. The better transient behavior of the adaptive filter produced less distortion in the ST segment and removed the interference more effectively.

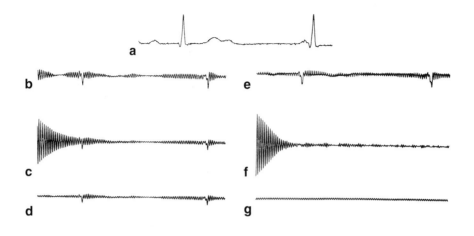

◉ Fig. 5.2
Effects of different interference removal filters on an ECG, which has no interference: **(a)** original ECG, and tenfold magnified differences between filter-input and output of two notch filter methods (**b** and **c**), three adaptive methods (**d**, **e**, and **f**; **f** is the incremental estimation filter), and a global method (**g**). Several filters can be seen to generate sizable differences during the QRS complex (From McManus et al. [74]. © Elsevier. Reproduced with permission)

5.7.2   Baseline Wander

Baseline wander is another annoyance. The source of low-frequency fluctuations of the baseline may be sought in changing electrode impedances, such as caused by respiratory movement. More abrupt changes may result from the patient being restless. The frequency content of baseline wander is typically less than 0.5 Hz. Baseline wander may severely disturb ECG beat morphology. A variety of techniques for estimating and removing baseline wander has, therefore, been developed.

In the 1975 recommendations of the American Heart Association (AHA) [89], for baseline wander removal a standard 0.05 Hz single pole high-pass filter was advised. While such a filter largely avoids the problem of phase nonlinearities, it does very little to suppress the baseline wander that can typically be observed in ECGs. In their 1990 recommendations, the AHA stipulated that a baseline removal filter should have a flat amplitude response within 0.5 dB from 1 to 30 Hz, with a −3 dB cutoff frequency of less than 0.67 Hz, and should adhere to certain test criteria based on triangular and rectangular wave impulse responses [69, 90].

A general problem in the evaluation of baseline correction methods is the difficulty in discriminating between baseline wander and the genuine ECG [85, 91]. Most studies only provide a qualitative assessment, showing ECGs before and after application of a correction algorithm. In a few studies, artificially generated baseline wander is added to "clean" ECGs constructed by concatenating identical beats [92, 93]. Since baseline correction may introduce new distortions, several algorithms try to identify periods with minimal or no baseline wander and skip these periods in the filtering [85, 93, 94].

Two main remedial approaches have been followed:

1. Interpolation.
Linear interpolation approximates the baseline by straight-line segments between isoelectric levels, usually estimated from the intervals preceding QRS onset [85, 94]. The estimated baseline is subsequently subtracted from the ECG signal. Boucheham et al. [95] proposed a piecewise linear correction based on "dominant" points as detected by a curve simplification algorithm [96]. An interesting feature of their algorithm is its capability to correct for sudden baseline shifts.

A more elaborate interpolation method estimates the baseline by a third-order polynomial, or cubic spline [97]. Each PR segment provides a "knot" through which the cubic spline must pass. Meyer [97] described an elegant and fast state-space approach for the computation of the cubic splines.

Talmon [85] compared the linear interpolation and cubic spline methods on a set of real ECGs, and concluded that both approaches performed similarly. Linear baseline correction, however, is to be favored because cubic spline correction is more difficult to apply in the presence of sudden baseline shifts.

Since all interpolation methods assume that reference points or knots can accurately be determined, they may break down if this assumption is not met, for example, in the case of a premature beat merging with the preceding T wave [98–100]. Performance may also degrade at lower heart rates as the knots become more separated.

2. High-pass filtering.

Infinite impulse response (IIR) filters are generally unacceptable due to their nonlinear phase response, which may induce distortions in particular in areas of the ECG where amplitudes change abruptly [90]. However, in off-line situations, or if some time delay between acquisition and processing of the signal is accepted, forward-backward or bidirectional filtering can be applied [100, 101], yielding overall linear-phase response [102]. Alternatively, De Pinto [103] proposed a linear-phase high-pass filter. He subtracted the output of a linear phase low-pass IIR filter from the original signal with a delay equal to the pass-band group delay of the low-pass filter. The filter was shown to adhere to the 1990 AHA recommendations.

Linear phase filtering is easily accomplished with finite impulse response (FIR) filters. However, these filters typically have very long impulse responses, resulting in many multiplications and long time delay [91, 104], which may be unacceptable for short-term resting ECG recordings. Van Alste et al. [104] proposed an FIR filter that combines removal of baseline wander with that of power line interference, and greatly saves on the number of computations. QRS complexes may heavily influence the baseline estimate. This may cause a shift of the assumed baseline with respect to the true one, resulting in measuring errors especially in diagnostically sensitive low-frequency segments such as the ST segment. Sörnmo et al. [92] described an approach in which the QRS complexes are removed prior to filtering the signal by one of a bank of linear low-pass filters with variable cut-off frequencies. The method was tested on ECGs with different types of simulated baseline wander and showed superior performance as compared to standard high-pass filtering or cubic spline interpolation (❂ Fig. 5.3), especially when the baseline wander contained frequencies >0.5 Hz. It must be noted that the method requires that beat classification is performed prior to correction, to minimize the effects of ectopic beats.

A two-step method combining interpolation and filtering techniques was proposed by Shusterman [93]. First, the magnitude of baseline wander is determined and classified as small or large. If large baseline drift is present, the signals are filtered with a bidirectional high-pass filter with a cut-off that depends on the estimated frequency content of the baseline wander. In a second step, any residual, small baseline wander is removed by simple linear interpolation between PQ and TP segments.

A two-stage cascade filter was described by Jane et al. [105]. First, a high-pass notch filter is applied with a cut-off frequency at 0.3 Hz [83]. Any remaining baseline contamination at higher frequencies is then removed with an adaptive impulse correlated filter. The reference input consists of a sequence of unit impulses correlated with the QRS complexes. This filter was shown to be equivalent to an exponentially weighted average [106] and requires a QRS detector. It also removes other disturbances not correlated with the QRS complex, such as muscle noise or line interference. When tested on a few records of the MIT-BIH database [107], the filter was shown to perform better than cubic spline correction.

Park et al. [108] described a wavelet adaptive filter. The filter consists of two parts. A wavelet transform decomposes the ECG signal into seven frequency bands. The signal of the lowest frequency band (0–1.4 Hz) is then fed into an adaptive filter. The wavelet adaptive filter was compared with a "commercial standard filter" with a cutoff of 0.5 Hz and with a general adaptive filter. Using test data from the MIT-BIH and the European ST-T [109] databases, the wavelet filter was shown to perform better than the other two filters, especially with respect to distortion of the ST segment. When tested on a triangular wave, as recommended by the AHA, the wavelet filter showed negligible distortion of the ST segment, whereas the standard filter and the adaptive filter produced severe distortions.

Finally, nonlinear filtering methods for baseline correction have been proposed [110]. Sun et al. [111], building on earlier work of Chu and Delp [112], described an approach using morphological filtering, a technique widely used in the field of image processing [113]. Testing on simulated ECG signals, they compared their approach with the wavelet adaptive filter [108] and found morphological filtering to produce better results.

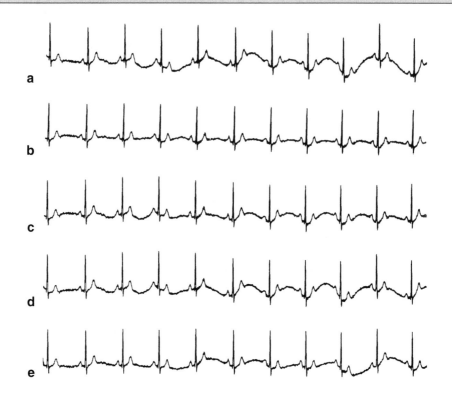

◨ Fig. 5.3

Example of baseline wander removal. **(a)** Original ECG, and resulting signal after baseline wander removal using **(b)** time-varying filter with beat subtraction, **(c)** time-varying filter without beat substraction, **(d)** time-invariant filter, and **(e)** cubic spline interpolation (From Sörnmo [92]. © Springer)

5.7.3 Muscle Noise

Muscle noise, another signal deformity, is caused by the electrical discharges of skeletal muscles. Common causes are patient restlessness, nervousness, cold shivers, and Parkinson tremor. Reduction of muscle noise is often effected by one of the other tasks in ECG signal processing as, for example, when the ECG signal is band-pass filtered for the purpose of QRS detection. Since most of the energy of the QRS complex is contained in the frequency band from 10 to 25 Hz, noise components outside the pass band can effectively be suppressed. For P-wave detection, even stronger noise reduction is possible because the frequency content of the P wave is lower. In these applications it is unnecessary to keep the original signal undistorted. For accurate amplitude and duration measurements, however, the requirement is to improve signal-to-noise ratio (SNR) without loss of signal information.

A common method to reduce muscle noise is coherent averaging. ECG complexes of one family are summed and the sum is divided by their number, giving an averaged ECG complex while uncorrelated noise averages out and disappears. Coherent averaging is one way of improving the SNR, as will be discussed later.

A number of other noise reduction techniques have been proposed. Adaptive filtering for muscle noise suppression was described by Thakor and Zhu [83]. To cancel the noise in a particular lead, they proposed employing, as a reference signal, another lead perpendicular to the first, in order to ensure that the noise in the two leads is uncorrelated.

Talmon et al. [114] describe an adaptive Gaussian filter, based on earlier work of Hodson [115]. The frequency characteristics of the filter are dependent on the estimated curvature of the signal to be filtered. A curvature estimate is obtained by fitting a polynomial function. The width of the filter is then adjusted according to the curvature, where low curvature (e.g., in the PR interval) implies a low-frequency cutoff, and a high curvature (e.g., in the QRS complex) a cutoff at higher frequencies. A related approach is proposed by De Pinto [103], who describes a low-pass filter with time-varying band-width. The bandwidth is maximal during the QRS complex, and decreases in the interval between QRS complexes. The bandwidth is varied in increments by selecting one of six sets of coefficients, controlled by an estimate of the slope of the ECG signal.

Another approach, termed noise consistency filtering, was initially proposed by Mortara [30] and later investigated by Wei et al. [116]. This filter method requires the availability of multiple, simultaneously recorded leads, and exploits the redundancy in the ECG signals. Reconstruction coefficients are determined to synthesize each of the eight independent ECG leads from the remaining seven leads. The filter output is the original lead signal multiplied by a time-varying coherence measure with a value between 0 and 1, dependent on the correspondence between the predicted and the original signal. The lower the coherence, the stronger is the filtering, and vice versa. The filter was reported to reduce noise by a factor of 10, provided the noise in the leads is uncorrelated [30].

Wei et al. [116] proposed two modifications to the filter as it was described by Mortara. Firstly, to avoid problems with baseline wander, the signal is split into a low-frequency and a high-frequency part, and only the latter is filtered according to the source consistency method. Secondly, a modified coherence measure is used, to reduce unwanted filtering effects that were observed by the authors. The modified filter performance was verified on simulated and real ECG signals, and compared with the original source consistency filter and conventional low-pass filters. Results show more effective noise suppression and less distortion of the QRS complex with the modified filter.

More elaborate filtering methods, involving the discrete cosine transform and singular-value decomposition, have been described by several investigators [117–119]. These approaches are computationally demanding and were mainly developed for the suppression of excessive muscle noise during exercise testing.

Finally, several studies used morphological filtering for muscle noise suppression [110–112]. Morphological filtering was also employed to detect muscle noise, without attempting to suppress it [120].

5.7.4   Spikes

Spikes are sudden pulses of short duration and high amplitude. They may be due to an interfering electrical source in the environment or to an implanted artificial pacemaker.

Accurate pacemaker spike detection has become increasingly important with the growing population of patients with implanted pacemakers. Because of the small spike width, in the order of 0.2–0.5 ms, many electrocardiographs use high-bandwidth front end amplifiers and analog circuitry to detect pacemaker spikes before A-D conversion. To reduce the number of false detections that this approach may induce, it has been combined with software algorithms that must confirm the presence of the spikes in the diagnostic bandwidth (0.05–150 Hz) signals. Alternatively, signals have been sampled at very high frequency, of the order of several kHz, and then software is used to detect the spikes.

Only a few algorithms have been described that attempt to detect spikes in diagnostic bandwidth signals. As these signals have been sampled at no more than 500 Hz; one may wonder how it is possible to detect pulses that have a duration well below the sampling interval. The reason is that the anti-aliasing low-pass filtering broadens the spikes. However, this filter also greatly reduces the amplitude of the spikes, which makes detection more difficult. The presence of narrow QRS complexes mimicking spikes, high-frequency noise and other artifacts further complicates the detection task.

The Louvain VCG analysis program [121] used a simple spike detector: if the spatial velocity exceeds a fixed threshold, a spike is assumed to be present [122]. In the AVA program [123] a number of tests based on slope differences between four consecutive points (8 ms) in a single lead were performed to detect spikes or discontinuities in the input signals [122]. No evaluation of these methods has been given.

Talmon [85] described a spike detector that operates in two stages. First, signals are filtered with a parabolic filter and the root-mean-square (RMS) of the residuals is computed. If the residual at a certain time instant exceeds three times the RMS value in that signal, a potential spike is assumed to be present. In a second stage, an additional number of criteria, structured in a decision tree, are tested to verify whether a spike has truly been detected. The algorithm was tested on an independent test set of 1,908 ECGs and VCGs, showing a sensitivity of 90.9% and a positive predictive value of 95.4%.

Helfenbein et al. [124] proposed another pacemaker spike detector. The algorithm detects a spike if a steep slope exceeding a threshold is followed by an opposite polarity slope within a short time window. The threshold is adaptive and computed as a function of the maximum slope in a window preceding the spike. When tested on a set of 1,108 adult ECGs containing a variety of pacemaker types and modes, excellent performance (sensitivity 99.7%, positive predictive value 99.5%) was obtained. On another set of 1,382 non-paced pediatric ECGs, only four false-positive QRS complexes were reported.

5.7.5 Amplitude Saturation and Sudden Baseline Shifts

No substantial literature is available dealing with the detection of amplitude saturation and sudden baseline shifts. In descriptions of various ECG processing systems, a statement is made that these artifacts are searched for, but the algorithms are not described.

5.8 Detection of QRS Complexes

The detection of QRS complexes is probably the most extensively studied problem in ECG signal analysis [86, 125–131]. A host of different algorithms has been proposed, most of them originating from applications in the fields of coronary care monitoring and Holter recording. Consequently, many of these QRS-detection algorithms were designed to operate on a single lead. In computerized resting ECG and VCG interpretation, three simultaneously recorded leads were used from early times. Now, multiple simultaneously recorded leads have also become increasingly common in the non-resting ECG.

Basically, a QRS detector consists of two stages [132]: a preprocessing stage, in which the signal is filtered and signal features are determined, and an identification stage, in which a decision is made about the presence and location of a QRS complex. Algorithms are commonly distinguished with respect to their preprocessing stages.

An extensive survey of single-lead QRS-detection algorithms is given by Kohler et al. [130]. The most common approaches are based on high-pass and band-pass digital filters, but many other approaches have been proposed, based on wavelet transforms [133, 134], artificial neural networks [127, 135], and genetic algorithms [136]. Some algorithms [137, 138] employ techniques from syntactic pattern recognition, but it has been difficult to demonstrate the practical utility of this approach [139].

In the multiple-lead algorithms, the simultaneous leads are transformed to a detection function. The transformation brings out the QRS complexes amongst the other parts of the signal, in order to increase the QRS detection rate. One of the most commonly used transformations is the computation of the spatial velocity of the VCG or of a similar derived function for the 12-lead ECG. The spatial velocity (SV) is defined as:

$$SV(n) = \sqrt{\sum_{k=1}^{3} (d_k(n))^2}$$

where $d_k(n)$ denotes the first derivatives of the VCG leads X, Y, and Z. Various difference equations have been proposed to approximate the derivatives [130]:

$$d(n) = x(n+1) - x(n-1);$$
$$d(n) = 2x(n+2) - x(n+1) - x(n-1) - 2x(n-2);$$
$$d(n) = x(n) - x(n-1).$$

In the case of the 12-lead ECG, the VCG leads can be reconstructed from the ECG leads by linear transformation, or approximated by a quasi-orthogonal set of ECG leads [140]. Alternatively, a pseudo-SV has been computed by combining the derivatives of all ECG leads.

The detection signal is then gauged against a threshold to detect the occurrence of a QRS complex. The threshold may be fixed, but more commonly is adaptive, changing with varying signal characteristics [140–142]. Some algorithms also require that the detected QRS complexes fulfill certain amplitude constraints. Other algorithms compute a second derivative,

$$d^2(n) = x(n+2) - 2x(n) + x(n-2),$$

and use a combination of first and second derivatives as the detection function. Balda et al. [143] used the sum of the absolute first and second derivatives over three simultaneous leads. This detection function was called the "waveform boundary indicator" as it also provided an estimate of the onset and the end of QRS complexes. A single-lead implementation of the method was given by Ahlstrom and Tompkins [86].

Once a potential QRS complex is detected, most of the algorithms apply further heuristic criteria to exclude false-positive detections, for example, by requiring a minimum time lag between adjacent QRS locations [140]. Laguna et al. [144] apply a single-lead detection algorithm to each of a set of simultaneously recorded leads, and then enter into a decision process comparing the detection positions over all leads to decide which detections are true or not.

An inventory of different methods used in seven VCG and eight ECG programs can be found in the second progress report of the CSE project [122]. However, only few developers of these ECG computer programs have published detailed evaluation results of their detection algorithms. On a set of 2,889 QRS complexes from the CSE multilead library, Kors et al. [140] found no false positive or false negative detections at all. Contrasting with the parsimonious communications on multilead QRS-detection algorithms, performance results for single-lead algorithms have been reported in fair abundance (see [130] for an overview). Many of these algorithms were evaluated on (part of) the MIT-BIH arrhythmia database, and achieved excellent results (>99% sensitivity and positive predictive value) [130]. A comparative study on noise sensitivity of nine single-lead QRS-detection algorithms for five different types of noise also indicated very good detection performance of most algorithms for all but the highest levels of noise [126]. In general, considering that the multiple leads of the standard 12-lead ECG offer redundancy of information and that noise levels in the resting situation are typically less troublesome than under monitoring conditions, it may be concluded that near-perfect QRS detection in the resting ECG is feasible.

5.9 Detection of P Waves

Detection of the P waves remains one of the most difficult tasks in automated ECG analysis. Failure of P-wave detection will jeopardize the rhythm interpretation program. Problems may arise owing to low amplitude, variable morphology and diverse timing of P waves. A P wave superimposed on a T wave, and even more so, a P wave that coincides with a QRS complex, are difficult to distinguish in surface ECGs (❷ Fig. 5.4). Their probable location can only be extricated by considering the sequence of the preceding and following P waves and by recognizing small irregularities in the expected contour of QRS or T. This requires long and continuous recordings. Even then, problems remain in deciphering morphology and polarity. While P-wave detection on surface ECG leads may already pose problems to the eye of the cardiologist,

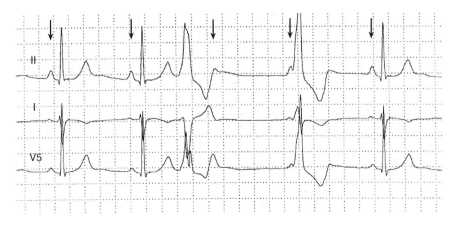

❏ Fig. 5.4
ECG showing an AV dissociation, with one P wave superimposed on a T wave and another P wave merging into a QRS complex

more problems await the computer programmer working in this field [145]. The human ability to recognize even low-voltage P waves hidden in other waves and amidst noise and artifacts is indeed still far superior to the performance of all presently available ECG wave-recognition programs.

Different approaches with respect to automatic detection of P waves have been described in the literature. Stallman and Pipberger [6] applied a threshold approach to the smoothed spatial velocity curve. McManus [146] has worked further on this method. Bonner and Schwetman [147] used a piecewise approximation of the ECG, followed by tests on level crossings and slope changes. A two-stage detection method was introduced by Hengeveld and Van Bemmel [148], and later on refined by Talmon [85]. First, QRS-linked P waves are searched for, based on histograms of local signal extrema in the intervals preceding the QRS complexes. If they are not found, non-QRS-linked P waves are sought by cross-correlation of signal amplitudes with an empirical P-wave template. Schnyders and Jordan [149] applied an energy correlation technique on the 12-lead ECG with apparently good results. Martinez et al. [131] proposed a wavelet-based P-wave detector. Once the location of the QRS complex is found, local maxima in the wavelet transform of the higher scales (i.e., in the lower frequency bands) are sought in an RR-dependent search interval. If at least two local extrema exceed a certain threshold, a P wave is considered present. Gritzali et al. [150] used as a detection function the length transformation of a signal, which essentially is the length of the signal curve within a time window. The length transformation can be defined for more than one lead by adding the curve lengths of the individual leads. Simple thresholding of the transformation is used to detect the P waves, as well as their onsets and ends.

It can be very difficult to distinguish P waves from flutter waves. In the presence of 2:1 AV block it may be hard, even for a human observer, to choose between flutter and sinus tachycardia. In various programs, separate routines are applied to determine whether atrial flutter waves are present [37, 141]. Talmon et al. [151] described a method that detects the periodic components characteristic of flutter waves (❷ Fig. 5.5). After appropriate filtering and removal of the QRS complexes, the resulting signal is autocorrelated. Flutter waves are assumed to be present if the autocorrelation function has a sufficiently large local maximum at a lag between 150 and 300 ms (corresponding with flutter rates between 200 and 400/min) and a second local maximum at twice the lag of the first maximum. A sensitivity of 86% and a specificity of 99.9% were reported. Taha et al. [152] employed a QRST subtraction technique and spectral methods to distinguish between atrial flutter, atrial fibrillation, and other rhythms. They obtained a sensitivity for flutter of 80%, at a specificity of 98.7%. Giraldo et al. [153] tried to detect the boundaries of atrial flutter and fibrillation waves, and used the coefficient of variation of the wave amplitudes to distinguish between flutter and fibrillation. They tested their approach on 40 short signal segments with flutter or fibrillation from the MIT-BIH database, but did not include segments with other heart rhythms in their analysis. Christov et al. [142] propose an atrial flutter-fibrillation parameter that is the mean value of the filtered and rectified signal, after subtraction of QRS-T complexes. On a test set, they obtained 76% sensitivity for flutter and fibrillation combined, at 97.9% specificity.

The detection rate of P waves varies according to the different algorithms that are applied. McManus [146] reported failures from 0–3%. For the 250 ECGs in the multilead CSE library [61], Kors et al. [140] obtained a sensitivity of 98.1% and a positive predictive value of 99.9%. Oversensitive methods cause difficulties in cases with atrial fibrillation. In the AVA program [123], as well as in several other programs, a P-wave search is only performed in an interval between the end of the T wave and the onset of QRS. In addition, only one P wave can be detected per QRS complex, which practically excludes the diagnosis of AV block or AV dissociation with an atrial rate higher than the ventricular rate. Programs that do attempt to detect more than one P wave per cycle have not reported detailed results [37, 141, 154], but judging from the results of arrhythmia detection (see section on rhythm interpretation), the success rate of these algorithms must be rather unsatisfying. A confounding factor is that P waves may alter their appearance in one recording, suddenly, from one beat to the other, or gradually, and that precisely this behavior is an element in rhythm diagnosis. To our knowledge, no work has been done on P-wave typing, that is, the distinction between different P-wave morphologies in one and the same recording.

5.10　QRS Typing

QRS typing is essentially a clustering task followed by a classification task, as the case requires. The clustering attempts to distinguish between different types, or families, of QRS complexes (if more than one). Within one family the complexes are similar in QRS morphology. If more than one type has been detected, the classification task is to determine which one

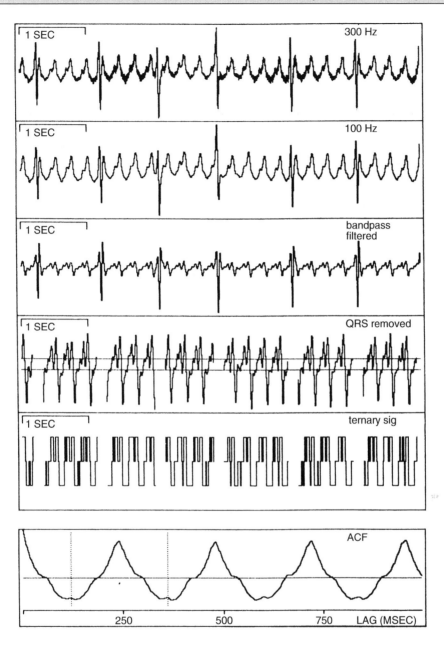

◻ Fig. 5.5
Example of the processing steps in a flutter wave detection algorithm (From Talmon et al. [151]). From *top* to *bottom*: original signal; signal after sampling rate reduction; signal after bandpass filtering; bandpass filtered signal after removal of QRS complexes; ternary signal; autocorrelation function

is the dominant type. The term "dominant" is not synonymous with "most numerous." It may well be that in a recording the "dominant" sinus complexes are outnumbered by ectopics, for example. We define the term dominant as the indication for the family of complexes to be used for the morphological (or contour) diagnosis. The nondominant complexes may be further divided into several types, such as premature ventricular or supraventricular complexes (possibly from different foci) and escape beats. This makes it clear that correct QRS typing is indispensable for a reliable rhythm interpretation. Typing, however, is a less straightforward endeavor than one would wish. Commonly, the dominant complexes are sinus beats, but they might also be of atrial or nodal, or even ventricular origin. What if the pacemaker site changes during the recording? And, quite annoyingly, complexes from the same origin may show sudden variation in QRS morphology, for example, in intermittent right bundle branch block. Which one will be labeled as the dominant morphology? Differentiating aberrantly conducted complexes from ectopic complexes is the next problem. Also, similar QRS complexes are not always followed by similar ST-T segments, a complication that inspired only a few investigators to take a closer look at ST-T typing [85, 155].

A variety of clustering methods and features for QRS typing has been proposed. All methods compute a similarity measure between a newly presenting complex and one or more of the complexes in each of the already existing clusters. The new complex is then assigned to the group with the complexes that are most similar to it, unless the similarity is below a certain threshold, in which case a new group is formed. Different similarity measures have been proposed, such as the area between the normalized spatial velocity curves of the two complexes [156], the difference in so-called arc lengths of the complexes [94], or the Mahalanobis distance using four morphological QRS features [157]. To determine whether two complexes were of similar type, Talmon [85] used a decision tree that involved two similarity measures, reflecting similarity in shape and in power. Lagerholm et al. [158] decomposed the QRS complexes into five orthogonal Hermite functions and used the resulting coefficients, together with RR-interval parameters, as features to cluster the complexes into 25 groups by means of a self-organizing map.

When more than one type of QRS complex has been found, it must be decided which is the dominant type. As mentioned above, this may not be so self-evident since the most frequent type is not necessarily the dominant one. More elaborate decision logic has been developed [85, 141], involving QRS duration, RR interval length preceding the complex, and the number of beats of each type.

Few quantitative results on QRS typing in the resting ECG have been published. Using the ECGs from the CSE multilead library, Kors et al. [140] found an error rate of 0.3% for their multilead ECG program in classifying four types of complexes. Lagerholm et al. [158], using the MIT-BIH database with 16 different beat types, report a chance of 1.5% that a beat ends up in the wrong cluster.

Several investigators have approached QRS typing primarily as a beat classification task [127, 159–162], rather than as a clustering task, possibly followed by a classification stage. They trained one or more classifiers based on a labeled set of beats of different morphology. For example, Hu et al. [127] applied artificial neural networks to distinguish between normal and abnormal beats (involving 12 different beat morphologies), using raw QRS samples from the MIT-BIH arrhythmia database as the input. They obtained a total accuracy of 90.6%, which compared favorably with the 73.0% accuracy of a simple nearest neighbor classifier, but this level of accuracy would not seem high enough for clinical application. This may not come as a surprise considering the large interindividual variability of QRS morphology. Only when the classifier was trained on patient-specific ECG data, were more acceptable results obtained [159]. Christov et al. [162] applied a nearest neighbor rule to 26 parameters derived from two ECG leads. Again, when tested on the MIT-BIH arrhythmia database, a general classifier performed poorly, but patient-specific classifiers showed good performance. However, the patient-specific approach to QRS typing requires initial human labeling of beats and, therefore, is of little value for computer programs that should analyze the short-duration resting ECG fully automatically.

5.11   Forming a Representative Complex

Most diagnostic ECG computer programs operate on a single "representative" P-QRS-T complex from the "dominant" family [37, 121, 122, 141, 163, 164]. From this representative complex, the measurements needed for the diagnostic interpretation stage are derived. Mostly, the representative complex (sometimes called a "template" complex) is obtained by the computation of an averaged beat or a median beat from as many complexes in the record as may qualify for the purpose. Such a procedure presupposes complexes of similar morphology, and thus requires that QRS typing has been performed. The following techniques are in use:

1. Coherent or ensemble averaging is a simple technique in which the average of the time-aligned complexes is calculated at each sample point. The technique has been shown to be equivalent to low-pass comb filtering and to yield optimal noise reduction for Gaussian distributed noise [165, 166]. Under this condition, the SNR improvement is equal to the

square root of the number of complexes being averaged. Since the average is vulnerable for outliers, it is imperative that complexes affected by sudden baseline shifts or other major disturbances are excluded from averaging.

2. Another approach is finding the median value for each sample point of the time-aligned complexes. The median beat is less sensitive to baseline shifts, but low-frequency baseline wander may introduce discontinuities in the median beat and result in reduced noise suppression [85, 167].

3. To reduce the effect of averaging widely differing amplitudes, Macfarlane et al. [94] compute a so-called modal beat. They assign weights to each sample of each QRS complex, with similar amplitudes across complexes having a high weight, the others having lower weights. The approach performed well [85], but was computationally expensive. In later versions of the Glasgow program, the technique was, therefore, abandoned in favor of simple averaging or, if any individual beat significantly deviated from the average, computation of a median cycle [141].

4. A hybrid approach, trying to combine the advantages of the averaging and median techniques, was proposed by Mertens and Mortara [167]. They first split the QRS complexes in three equally-sized groups and determine the averaged complex for each group. These three averaged complexes are then partitioned in their low- and high-frequency components with a simple moving average filter, and for both signals the median complex is determined. Finally, the two median complexes are added to form the representative complex.

For all these methods precise beat alignment is essential. In several programs [122, 163, 164], synchronization is performed by a cross-correlation method. In the MEANS program [37, 85], alignment is based on a reference point within the QRS complex, the position of an extremum in the band-pass filtered signal, whereas the Louvain program [121] uses the onset of individual QRS complexes. If complexes are not accurately aligned, beat-to-beat variations in the timing between peaks in the complexes may reduce the peak amplitudes [85]. To avoid this problem, some programs select only one "typical" complex for further analysis [168]. While this approach obviously does not need beat alignment, it does not help to improve the SNR.

The single complex approach is being taken a step further when wave recognition and measurements are done on each individual complex followed by computing an average or median of the measurements across the complexes [123, 143, 154, 169, 170].

There has been some discussion on the merits of signal averaging versus measurement averaging. Talmon [85] was not able to show any significant difference in QRS duration if wave recognition were performed on single complexes or on an averaged complex, after proper beat alignment [85]. The averaging method, however, offers the advantage of increasing the SNR. Based on results of extensive noise tests performed in the CSE project, a measurement strategy that uses selective averaging has been recommended for diagnostic ECG computer programs [171, 172].

5.12   Waveform Recognition

The goal of waveform or boundary recognition is to determine the inflectional points P onset, P end, QRS onset, QRS end, and T end, as much as possible in conformity with their visually determined counterparts (❷ Fig. 5.6). No attempt is made in any ECG computer program to determine the end of the U wave, the orphan wave of electrocardiology. The CSE Working Party [34] stated that the inclusion or exclusion of isoelectric segments in the initial or terminal parts of a wave may lead to differences in wave duration of more than 10 ms between leads, and, therefore, urges that "the true onsets and offsets of P and QRS as well as the end of T should be determined using at least three simultaneously recorded leads." (cf. ❷ Fig. 5.1) The end of T deserves special attention in this respect. In 1990, Campbell and his group introduced the concept of QT dispersion (QTd) [173], defined as the difference between the longest and the shortest QT in any of the 12 surface ECG leads. QTd was supposed to reflect the dispersion of repolarization within the myocardium. The idea caused a tidal wave of papers but in due course became severely criticized [174–177]. Differences in QT duration will arise from differences in the projection of the spatial T vector onto the different leads, which in some leads may result in terminal isoelectric segments of various lengths and hence in shortened QT [174]. Also in QTd measurements, the U wave was regarded as a nuisance, obscuring the end of T. If it were too prominent, the lead was simply excluded from QTd determination. The U wave, however, might deserve more attention than this. Viewed in simultaneous leads, it may be seen in some as a separate wave, detached from the T; in other leads it may encroach on the T wave, and in still other leads it may blend in with the T wave. In fact, searching for the common end of the T wave is not pertinent if T and

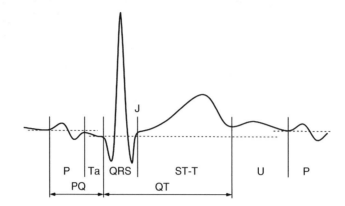

▫ **Fig. 5.6**
In the waveform recognition, onset and offset of P, QRS, and T are determined, as indicated by the *vertical bars*. QRS offset and J are identical points. A true 0-level cannot be identified: the onset of QRS is superimposed on the atrial repolarization wave (*Ta*), at the J point ventricular repolarization is already underway, and the end of T coalesces with the U wave, the end of which is hidden in the next P. As the operational 0-level for QRS and T the *horizontal line* through QRS onset is recommended, likewise for the P the horizontal through P onset. Amplitudes are measured with respect to these 0-levels

U form a continuum as has been proposed [178], in the same way as it is impossible to ask for the common end of a Q wave in the QRS. Whatever the ultimate truth, it seems best for the time being and for practical purposes, for example, for QT duration measurement in drug safety testing, to let the computer determine T offset over multiple simultaneous leads.

As pointed out above, single lead, "one-dimensional" measurements systematically produce shorter measurements of wave duration than when, "multidimensionally," the first onset and latest offset in any lead are taken. Most ECG computer programs, therefore, use the spatial velocity or a similar multidimensional function as the detection function for waveform recognition (see ❷ Sect. 5.8). For single-lead recordings, other detection functions, such as the envelope of the ECG signal [179] or wavelet transforms [131, 133], have been applied. Basically, three different approaches of boundary recognition can be distinguished [180]. Each has to be trained and tested by human observers.

1. Thresholding

The most straightforward method is to apply a simple threshold to the detection function. For the onset, usually the maximum of the detection function is localized from where it is traced backward until where it first becomes smaller than an absolute or relative threshold. This point is considered to be the wave onset. The end of a wave is determined similarly.

According to an inventory of waveform-recognition methods used in various ECG computer programs in the CSE project [122], most programs applied threshold detectors. A number of different thresholding algorithms to detect the end of the T wave in single leads were described and compared by McLaughlin et al. [181, 182]. Using a threshold detector, Vila et al. [183] attempted to determine not only the end of the T but also the end of the U wave. They mathematically modeled the TU complex and used the modeled signal for detection. Laguna et al. [144] applied a single-lead threshold detector to each of the leads of multilead ECGs and then combined the wave boundaries in the individual leads to find overall onsets and offsets of P, QRS, and T.

2. Signal matching

A second approach is to search for the point where the weighted least-square difference between a reference waveform and the detection function is minimal [184]. The reference waveform is obtained from a learning set of detection functions with known wave boundaries, as indicated by one or more human observers. Rubel and Ayad [184] compared the performance of a signal matching algorithm for different detection functions using the CSE database. They obtained the best results for QRS onset and offset detection with an unfiltered spatial area detection function.

3. Template matching

The template method takes into account information on the time-amplitude distribution of the detection function in a window around the inflectional point [185]. A template is constructed from a series of detection functions in which the wave boundaries have visually been assessed by a human observer. The boundary point in a new ECG is then located at that point where the cross-correlation between the template and the new detection function is maximal. Details of this approach and an efficient way of implementation have been described by Talmon [85].

A somewhat different approach, obviating the need for thresholding or matching, was proposed by Zhang et al. [186]. As a detection function, they took the output of a signal integrator in a window sliding over the T wave. With recourse to some simple assumptions, the maximum of the detection function was shown to coincide with the end of the T wave. A model-based approach to delineate single-lead QRS onset and offset was described by Sörnmo [187]. He statistically modeled the low-frequency segments (containing P and T waves) and high-frequency segments (QRS complex), and applied a maximum-likelihood procedure to estimate the points where a change occurred between low- and high-frequency segments.

Using the multilead CSE database, Willems et al. [61] evaluated the measurement performance of 11 ECG and 6 VCG computer programs (❷ Fig. 5.7), incorporating a variety of wave boundary detection algorithms [122]. Onset of QRS showed overall the smallest deviations from the reference, with the narrowest confidence intervals. End of T showed the largest scatter. The median of the waveform recognition results of all programs coincided best with the median results of referee cardiologists, corroborating findings of the former 3-lead CSE study [60]. However, individual program results

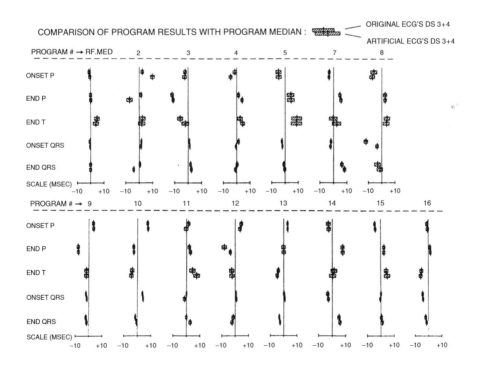

■ Fig. 5.7

Comparison of individual program results (numbered 2–16) and median referee results (RF MED) with the median of all programs in the CSE multilead library. Mean differences and 99% confidence intervals are indicated by *small vertical lines* and *horizontal bars*, respectively (From Willems et al. [61]. © American College of Cardiology. Reproduced with permission)

were widely divergent. As a consequence, P, PR, QRS, and QT interval measurements also varied widely among the various programs.

Willems et al. [171] assessed the influence of noise on wave boundary recognition of eight ECG and six VCG programs. Seven different types of high- and low-frequency noise were added to each of ten recordings. Mains interference and baseline wander had no significant effect on boundary detection for the majority of programs, but increasing levels of high-frequency noise shifted the onsets and offsets of most programs outward. Programs which apply beat averaging techniques had more stable results than programs analyzing single beats, but it was noted that these results mainly occurred at high noise levels that reflect poor operational conditions and can be avoided by proper quality control [171]. In a second related study [172], the effect of noise on amplitude measurements was examined. Programs that showed the least variability in waveform onsets and offsets also exhibited the highest stability in waveform detection and amplitude measurements.

Laguna et al. [144] compared the waveform boundary results and interval measurements obtained by their own algorithm with the median program estimates and median referee estimates of the multilead CSE database. The standard deviations of the differences were shown to be within acceptable tolerance limits [34] for most of the measurements. Martinez et al. [131] used the same data set to evaluate their wavelet transform-based approach, but they obtained less favorable results for QRS end and T end.

An interesting method to assess and compare the results of various waveform recognition algorithms was proposed by Morlet et al. [188]. They use scatter graphs that picture the standard deviation of the differences between program results and reference when the largest differences are progressively removed. This information allows us to distinguish between the reliability of an algorithm, that is, its capacity to provide wave boundary estimates without flagrant errors, and its precision, that is, the standard deviation of the differences between its estimates and the references.

5.13 Parameter Computation

Once the onsets and offsets of the various ECG waveforms have been identified, parameter or feature extraction is the next step. Time intervals and wave durations follow directly from the established time points. The ambiguities around the QT interval have been pointed out in the previous section. For the amplitudes of the various deflections, a 0-line, or baseline, must be defined. It should be understood that there is no true 0-level anywhere in the ECG (❷ Fig. 5.6). The T-P interval which has been recommended as such contains the U wave. The CSE Working Party defined baseline as "a horizontal reference line computed from a single base level" [34] and declared itself against the use of non-horizontal lines. For QRS and T combined, it recommended strongly the uniform use of a baseline through the onset of QRS in combination with a limited number of preceding sample points. For the P wave, the base level may be chosen at the onset of P. Voltage amplitudes are then simply determined with respect to the chosen baselines. A wave is defined as a discernible deviation from the baseline where at least two opposite slopes can be identified and where discernible means that both the amplitude and the duration of the deviation exceed certain minimum values [34]. Various amplitude ratios, such as Q/R and R/S, and also integrals and angles can be derived from these measurements. When simultaneously recorded orthogonal leads are available or are reconstructed from the 12-lead ECG [20, 189], spatial or planar vector magnitudes and directions, gradients and polar vectors can be obtained. The relative areas of the spatial QRS loop in each octant of the three-dimensional space are also measured in some systems [168].

Pipberger et al. [7, 8] applied the technique of time normalization of the QRS complex and the ST-T segment. Each was divided into eight equal time segments, regardless of their duration. In this way, measurements from QRS complexes with different durations can be compared one with another.

Advanced mathematical techniques, like Fourier analysis, polynomial fitting, or Karhunen–Loeve expansion, have been applied by some early investigators [190, 191]. It has been pointed out by Van Bemmel [180] that parameters derived from these techniques may allow an accurate reconstruction of the overall shape of the ECG, but are not necessarily the best discriminating features in ECG classification.

Computer processing systems frequently make 250–300 measurements per ECG. Ultimately, only a limited subset is used in the diagnostic classification stage and a still smaller number is printed out in the final computer report, which is submitted to the requesting physician. Most ECG processing systems will optionally display the averaged or median beat, if desired with markings for wave onsets and offsets as determined by the program. The ECG reader, therewith, has a check on the correctness of the measurements underlying the computer diagnosis.

5.14   Diagnostic ECG Interpretation

5.14.1   Strategies for Diagnostic Classification

After the initial waveform-detection, pattern-recognition, and measurement algorithms have been applied, the diagnostic stage is entered in which the ECG is classified into one or more of the various possible diagnostic categories. Two basically different approaches to diagnostic classification have been developed since the early days of computer assisted electrocardiography [192]. In the first, the deterministic or heuristic approach, the cardiologist's method of interpreting ECGs is simulated. The majority of existing ECG computer programs follows this approach. In the second, a statistical or probabilistic approach is adopted whereby an attempt is made by mathematical means to establish the probability that a given ECG belongs to a particular diagnostic category.

More recently, other approaches to diagnostic ECG classification have been tried. Some investigators have applied fuzzy set theory [170, 193, 194], others the "expert system" approach [195, 196] and, finally, neural-network techniques have been used [197–201]. However, clinical application of the latter techniques on a larger scale is lacking.

5.14.2   Deterministic ECG Computer Programs

The analysis follows a logical path of questions regarding the presence or absence of certain predetermined criteria for every diagnostic category, to be answered with yes or no. The questions and answers can be arranged in a decision table or in a decision tree resulting in diagnostic statements [85]. Such decision schemes, often quite elaborate, are implemented in all programs using the deterministic approach. The likelihood of the resulting diagnostic statements may be indicated by modifiers like "definite," "probable," and "possible."

Deterministic programs have the advantage that the diagnostic criteria used are familiar to the cardiologist, and that the logic is easy to follow and comprehend [192]. Much experience with conventional ECG interpretation present in the brain of the developer or published in the literature can, theoretically at least, be incorporated in these programs. Decision-tree programs are organic and flexible in structure and remain open for modification. With advancing insight and experience diagnostic pathways can be improved. Criteria selection can be guided by deductive reasoning based on knowledge of electrophysiological processes, a design that is inherently excluded in the statistical diagnostic approach. Also, new diagnostic categories can be added quite easily without the need for recruiting new statistical data.

Emulation of the human reader brings advantages but has also its limitations. The criteria selection might tend to be arbitrary and based on impressions rather than founded on solid quantitative information. In some systems, criteria selection was the work of a single expert, in others the effort of a group [154]. The appreciation of ECG criteria may vary considerably between cardiologists, as demonstrated by many studies on intra- and inter-observer variability of ECG interpretation [202–204]. The set of criteria proposed by one cardiologist may be met with another cardiologist's disapproval. This lack of agreement on criteria and the dearth of reliable quantitative data on their sensitivity and specificity have resulted in a diversity of commercial systems, even in one where each user could incorporate his own preferences, if so desired [205].

Many studies on ECG criteria have demonstrated a considerable overlap between normal and abnormal populations with respect to almost all ECG parameters, notably of Q-wave durations and voltage measurements. This necessarily gives rise to a proportion of false-positive and false-negative statements. The addition of a new, independent criterion to an existing decision tree increases sensitivity, but is almost invariably accompanied by a loss in specificity. This practice led to intolerably high false-positive rates in some of the early programs that, as a result, were dismissed as unsuitable for clinical use [45, 206]. A weighty argument of the adherents of the probabilistic approach was that conventional ECG programs can never surpass an accuracy level of 54–60%, the level reached by eminent experts in Simonson's study [203], who read the ECGs and VCGs of patients whose diagnoses were known and documented by ECG-independent means. In the CSE study, later to be discussed, the level of accuracy against the clinical "truth" was much higher, ranging between 73% and 81% [207].

Nowadays, however, decision-logic programs may also employ statistical tools. Computer programs are available that automatically generate decision-tree logic based on a given choice of features [208, 209]. Sensitivity and specificity of thresholds used in different criteria can be statistically optimized on population samples with well-defined disease entities. In a way, conventional ECG programs thereby move toward the statistical programs and, as we will see, vice versa.

5.14.3 Statistical ECG Computer Programs

The availability of the computer to perform voluminous mathematical computations for statistical purposes would seem to make the statistical approach the easy solution for diagnostic classification, but it will be shown that there are no easy solutions. For each diagnostic category, a population of ECGs has to be collected. The presence of normality or of the various types of abnormality (infarction, LVH, etc.) has preferably been established from clinical data, although ECG information does not have to be excluded. Next, the probabilities of occurrence of the various ECG measurements are determined for each diagnostic category. Having done this in a learning stage, any new ECG can be assigned to its presumed appropriate population in a test stage to evaluate the validity of the classification method. The measurements going into the statistical procedure are in principle just the amplitude values of samples in each lead of an ECG, in addition to certain duration measurements, not the values of the customary diagnostic ECG criteria, although, again in principle, there could be nothing against using them.

The main claim to preeminence of statistical over conventional programs is that diagnostic performance should be better and that mathematical objectivity takes the place of the personal idiosyncrasies of conventional program developers [192, 210]. Also, in the neighborhood of critical thresholds, minute changes in measurements may alter the interpretation in heuristic programs, but less so in statistical programs and certainly not when the probabilities for the diagnoses are above 70% [211, 212].

There are, however, distinct disadvantages [192]. First of all, large databases are needed for developing and testing. For each diagnostic category, a separate population of clinically documented records has to be collected. Case collection carries with it the problem of selection. The AVA program [123] has been developed almost exclusively on a database collected in a male and war veteran population. Statistical parameters may differ significantly in other populations that are more heterogeneous with respect to sex or to age and more homogeneous, on the other hand, with respect to race (see the Appendix on normal limits).

Furthermore, the diagnostic categories are mutually exclusive. A case may have a probability of 60% of belonging to the single category of, say, left ventricular hypertrophy (LVH), 30% of belonging to anterior myocardial infarction (AMI), and 10% of being normal. The individual probabilities add up to 100%. With this approach, it is not possible to have 100% probability of LVH and at the same time 100% probability of AMI. For this to be possible a separate collection of cases with LVH + AMI would have to be created and every other combination of diagnoses would again necessitate a different data base. In this way, the required number of cases soon increases out of control. Also, when one ECG presents an abnormality which does not belong to any of the existing categories, the probabilities will be spread over the existing categories [7]. To handle this problem, some diagnostic-tree type decisions were added in the AVA program in order to deal with some abnormalities not listed by the main AVA classification [123].

The common denominator of all the proposed statistical techniques is multivariate analysis. The first program using such methods dates back to 1961 and was described by Cady et al. [213]. They separated 23 normal tracings from 19 records with a typical pattern of LVH. Bayes' theorem was first applied to ECG diagnosis by Kimura et al. [214]. There were more early attempts to use multivariate analysis for ECG classification [215–218], but particularly Pipberger and coworkers have for many years persistently promoted the statistical method at numerous conferences and in many articles [7, 8, 41, 123, 219–222]. Following this lead, other investigators have applied statistical techniques for computer processing mainly to the VCG [163, 223]. Multivariate analysis has less frequently been applied to the standard 12-lead electrocardiogram [53, 163, 224].

The Bayes' formula is given by

$$P(i|\mathbf{x}) = \frac{f(\mathbf{x}|i) \cdot P(i)}{\sum_{j=1}^{m} f(\mathbf{x}|j) \cdot P(j)}$$

where $P(i|\mathbf{x})$ is the posterior or conditional probability that an ECG belongs to diagnostic category i (out of m possible categories) given the measurement vector $\mathbf{x}$; $f(\mathbf{x}|i)$ represents the conditional probability that the measurement vector $\mathbf{x}$ is produced in the cases belonging to category i; and $P(i)$ is the unconditional or prior probability for an ECG to belong to category i [7].

An essential feature of the classification strategy in the AVA program developed by Pipberger et al. [7, 8], as well as by some other investigators [223, 224], is the application of prior probabilities as expressed in the Bayes' formula. For this purpose, the relative frequencies of occurrence of various clinical diagnostic categories in the environment in question must be estimated. Thus, in Pipberger's approach, different prior probabilities were assigned to patients of different provenance (cardiological out-patient, general medicine, pulmonary disease) even to the extent of introducing "individual prior codes" [8]. This concept was argued to emulate the thought process of a physician who, when interpreting an ECG, weighs his diagnosis in the light of age, sex, and clinical condition of the patient, and the likelihood of occurrence of the disease in the specific population to which he happens to belong. The "proper prior code" for an individual is indicated on the ECG request form as one of several broad clinical categories, according to the tentative clinical diagnosis [8]. When entered with the patient's vital statistics, the prior probabilities are automatically set for computation of the posterior probabilities. The sensitivity and specificity for certain diagnostic categories of the AVA program can easily be adapted through manipulation of prior probabilities [8].

By including the prior probabilities of the various diagnostic categories, non-electrocardiographic information is introduced in a formalized way. In an extreme example, when a prior probability is set to zero or to one for a certain group, no case or every case will respectively be diagnosed in this disease category, no matter what the ECG appearance may be. These are the mathematical facts of this classification procedure [192]. Proponents of the use of prior probabilities argue that in a non-formalized way, prior knowledge and bias are applied by the clinician as well in routine ECG reading, in a justifiable and natural way. The opponents state that, by using clinical information, the role of the ECG is reduced to futility. They claim that evaluation of the ECG, in the larger framework of a final clinical diagnosis, should independently contribute to the diagnosis. In all these considerations, the element of "cost" cannot be neglected. The cost of missing the diagnosis of a single case of bubonic plague in a population hitherto thought to be free of the disease may be huge, as is the cost of overdiagnosing cervical cancer in a population where the disease is not uncommon. Prior probabilities should not be applied without discernment!

5.14.4   Methodology of ECG Computer Program Evaluation

The following paragraphs mainly address the topics of diagnostic accuracy and reliability of ECG computer programs. For other aspects such as utility, efficacy, and cost-benefit analysis, the reader is referred to some specific publications [12, 225–229].

It was pointed out earlier that comparison between computer and truth is a more cumbersome and problematic task than one would anticipate. To list the main complications:

1. There are ECG statements for which there is no clinical confirmation. Three types of statements can be made by human readers or computer programs [14], as follows:
    (a) Type A statements refer to an anatomic lesion or pathophysiologic state, such as myocardial infarction or hypertrophy, the presence of which can be confirmed by non-electrocardiographic evidence like cardiac catheterization, serum enzyme levels, ventriculograms, echocardiograms, scintigrams, and autopsy findings.
    (b) Type B statements apply to conditions which belong intrinsically to the realm of electrocardiography itself. They refer to electrophysiological processes such as arrhythmias and atrioventricular and intraventricular conduction disturbances. Sometimes these type B statements can be corroborated by the results of other diagnostic methods, such as scintigraphy in the case of a statement of ischemia based on a typical ST-T change. Most often, the physician's interpretation is the reference.
    (c) Type C statements refer to purely descriptive ECG features for which no substrate can be demonstrated by other means. Under this category, statements are subsumed like "nonspecific ST-T changes" or "axis deviation."

At the tenth Bethesda conference, Task force III [14] strongly recommended evaluation of type A statements by means of independent, clinical evidence. For type B and C statements, the human observer is the reference. A distinction was made between a constrained and a free observer, the constraint being a given set of measurements or criteria agreed upon before the evaluation. In fact, this again boils down to a test on the waveform recognition proficiency of the program. The free observer applies his own individual rules, or the majority opinion of a group of free observers may be obtained, but if these rules are formalized they can be put into computer logic and the observer is again constrained.

2. Collecting a type A database is a laborious and tedious task. In the early years, investigators were quite satisfied when they could single out one disease condition, say D, from a population composed of only D and normals. A simple 2×2 contingency table suffices to describe the diagnostic results, with sensitivity, specificity, positive predictive value, etc., as the indices of performance. This simple situation is already spoilt when non-D can be anything, not just normal. Non-normal conditions other than D may resemble D in some features and lead to false positive diagnoses of D and so degrade performance. In the real-life situation, the population contains all types of abnormality and the program is expected to classify each one correctly. This results in as many sensitivities and specificities as there are diagnostic conditions, and total performance cannot be expressed in a single, representative figure. The same "total accuracy" could be attained by one program scoring low on infarct recognition but high on LVH and a second one doing the reverse. Whatever the problems of assessing the agreement between computer and reference, it is mandatory that the database includes a spectrum of disease states, with different grades of severity and a representative number in each category, as well as combinations of different diseases. A database without any bias, however, is an illusion. Mostly, noisy recordings are excluded from the collection although noise is a fact of life (for testing purposes noise could be added afterward). Also, arrhythmias and conduction defects are sometimes excluded. Finally, databases differ in the populations they were drawn from, with respect to race, age, sex, social status, etc.

3. Output statements are not standardized and their meanings must be established first. What is to be understood by septal myocardial infarction? Does it mean the same thing as antero-septal myocardial infarction? What are the clinical grounds for diagnosing right ventricular hypertrophy (RVH)? Is RVH caused by pulmonary valve stenosis the same as RVH caused by an atrial septal defect? Such questions were addressed in the CSE study [65]. These considerations not only apply to type A statements, but to B and C as well. What is a nonspecific ST-T change? How will RBBB or LBBB be defined? Regarding the latter, a set of criteria for conduction disturbances and pre-excitation have previously been recommended [35].

4. Probability statements constitute another problem. A human observer may make a diagnosis of "probable inferior infarct." Does this mean "70% probability of IMI," but still a chance of 30% normal? Do the probabilities add up to 100%? In the case of "probable anterior infarct, possible LVH" does this mean 70% probability of AMI, 30% of LVH, and 0% normal, or must we understand that the case is probably abnormal (70%) with a preference for AMI (50%), a residual chance of 20% for LVH and leaving a 30% likelihood of normality? The problem is compounded by the tendency of ECG readers to cover all contingencies by statements like "posterior wall infarct not entirely excluded." It is, therefore, necessary that the reporting follows strictly prescribed rules. As an example, in the CSE study the number of categories was limited to seven. For each category, four certainty qualifiers were allowed: definite, probable, possible, and absent with numerical values of 3, 2, 1, and 0, respectively. The computer statements had to be transcribed into the same format by the program developers. As per diagnostic category, the scores were averaged over all readers or programs, and rounded. The category with highest score was taken to be the diagnosis of the "combined cardiologist" or "combined program." Additional rules were defined to handle some more complex situations [230].

5. Instability of interpretation is not restricted to man. Intra-observer variability is recognized to be sometimes considerable, but computer programs are generally viewed as robust against the diagnostically insignificant short-term variations that may occur between two successive ECGs of the same person. This is not entirely the case [231–233]. Even one and the same ECG may give rise to two different outcomes, as demonstrated by Bailey et al. [44, 45, 234, 235]. They processed two sets of digital samples, 1 ms apart, from the same recording, and, surprisingly, the separate results were by no means identical. The reproducibility of some of the older programs tested in this way proved to be unacceptably low. Spodick and Bishop [236] assessed the variability in the interpretations by an unspecified computer program of 92 unselected pairs of ECGs recorded 1 min apart. In 36 (39%) pairs, they found "grossly" different interpretations. The clinical significance of part of the differences, however, is debatable.

5.14.5   Comparison of Computer Interpretations with Physician's Interpretations

The 1,220 ECGs and VCGs from the CSE diagnostic library were read by nine cardiologists of whom four read ECGs and VCGs, four read only the ECGs and one read only the VCGs. For each recording, a combined result was derived in the above described manner. The results of nine ECG and six VCG computer programs were then compared with the "combined cardiologist." Different misclassification matrices, as well as sensitivity, specificity, predictive values of positive and negative test results, total accuracy, information content, and other measures of performance, were calculated [66, 207, 237]. The specificity of the ECG programs (median 87.7%, range 73.4–96.8%) was higher than that of the VCG program (median 75.5%, range 69.1–84.8%). Median sensitivities for LVH, RVH, AMI, and inferior myocardial infarction (IMI) were 71.6%, 58.6%, 81.0%, and 78.1%, respectively, but among the programs, sensitivities varied widely (❯ Table 5.1). Total agreement between an individual program and the combined cardiologist varied between 68.1% and 80.3% for the ECG programs and between 69.2% and 78.1% for the VCG programs. The combined program agreed with the combined cardiologist in 87.9% of the cases, which was significantly higher than for any individual program. The figure may be compared with the intra-observer variability of the cardiologists, who interpreted 125 randomly selected cases a second time without their knowing. Reproducibility was then seen to vary between a low of 73.6% and 90.8% (median 82.4%) [66].

It should be noted that the cardiologists in the CSE study were experienced, highly-motivated electrocardiographers. In a study by Jakobsson et al. [238], the interpretations of 69 physicians (only four of them being cardiologists) were compared with those of a computer-based ECG recorder in routine clinical practice. The authors took their own judgment as the reference. The study population consisted of 474 routine ECGs taken in a general practice, a medical emergency department, and an out-patient department. No single physician interpreted more than 7% of the ECGs. A written physician's interpretation was lacking in 11% of the ECGs. The diagnostic sensitivity for myocardial infarction of the doctors was significantly lower than that of the program. The overall quality of the computer interpretations was judged as being satisfactory in 82% of the ECGs, whereas this was only 64% for the physicians' written interpretations. Most computer misinterpretations could be attributed to poor signal quality, and it was suggested that the nonexpert physician should team up with the computer to approach the performance of an experienced ECG reader.

The CSE study only dealt with type A diagnostic statements. Computer–physician comparison is the usual method for assessing type B and type C interpretative statements, for which the ECG itself is the reference. Although this may seem to be less essential than diagnostic type A accuracy, such comparison is important since agreement between computer and physician is a convincing argument for the clinical acceptability of an ECG computer program [46, 52, 239]. Further, physician review is mandatory for legal and other reasons [240].

5.14.6   Comparison of Computer Results with Clinical "Truth"

The results of the nine ECG and six VCG computer programs obtained in the same 1,220 clinically validated ECGs and VCGs in the CSE diagnostic library, as well as those from the nine readers, were now compared with the "clinical truth" [66, 207]. The classification accuracies of the different programs (❯ Table 5.2), and to a lesser extent of the cardiologists

◻ Table 5.1

Percentage agreement of nine ECG and six VCG computer programs and the combined program results with the combined cardiologists' interpretations on the 1,220 cases of the CSE diagnostic library (Adapted from Willems [66], p. 183)

Program	Normal	LVH	RVH	Anterior MI	Inferior MI	Total accuracy
ECG	87.7 (73.4–96.8)[a]	73.4 (63.2–90.7)	58.3 (25.0–66.7)	83.6 (65.1–89.3)	71.1 (44.6–87.5)	76.6 (68.1–80.3)
VCG	75.5 (69.1–84.8)	71.3 (47.9–77.8)	63.3 (21.7–85.0)	72.3 (50.9–82.1)	85.1 (74.4–91.9)	71.1 (69.2–78.1)
Combined program results						
ECG	95.6	88.2	66.7	87.7	81.0	85.4
VCG	85.3	80.3	78.3	83.0	93.4	82.1
ECG+VCG	95.2	87.9	75.0	88.7	91.0	87.9

[a] Median (range)

Table 5.2

Percentage correct classifications of nine ECG and six VCG computer programs and the combined program results against the clinical "truth" on the 1,220 cases of the CSE diagnostic library (Adapted from Willems [66], p. 181)

Program	Normal	LVH	RVH	Anterior MI	Inferior MI	Total accuracy
ECG	91.3 (86.3–97.1)[a]	56.6 (50.3–76.2)	31.8 (14.5–52.8)	77.1 (58.8–81.5)	58.8 (38.7–82.8)	69.7 (62.0–77.3)
VCG	80.9 (71.4–86.6)	55.4 (47.2–76.2)	35.9 (28.2–64.5)	68.0 (54.5–74.1)	74.1 (63.6–86.5)	68.3 (64.3–76.2)
Combined program results						
ECG	96.7	67.9	40.6	79.6	68.8	76.3
VCG	87.1	67.3	53.0	77.3	82.2	77.0
ECG+VCG	95.5	69.0	45.8	80.0	76.7	78.5

[a]Median (range)

Table 5.3

Percentage correct classifications of eight ECG readers and five VCG readers and the combined cardiologist results against the clinical "truth" on the 1,220 cases of the CSE diagnostic library (Adapted from Willems [66], p. 180)

Cardiologist	Normal	LVH	RVH	Anterior MI	Inferior MI	Total accuracy
ECG	96.1 (92.7–97.6)[a]	63.9 (54.8–69.3)	46.6 (40.6–51.5)	84.9 (79.0–87.5)	71.7 (59.2–84.1)	76.3 (72.6–81.0)
VCG	80.6 (73.8–87.2)	63.4 (48.4–68.5)	50.0 (45.5–56.4)	65.2 (62.4–79.4)	75.1 (69.8–82.1)	70.3 (67.5–74.4)
Combined cardiologist results						
ECG	97.1	65.8	47.6	87.3	75.1	79.2
VCG	84.7	64.7	53.0	74.1	78.6	74.8
ECG+VCG	96.5	68.2	50.3	85.7	78.3	80.3

[a]Median (range)

(● Table 5.3), vary widely. The median specificity of the ECG programs was 91.3% (range 86.3–97.1%) against 80.9% (range 71.4–86.6%) for the VCG programs. Corresponding values for the cardiologists were 96.1% (range 92.7–97.6%) for the ECG and 80.6% (range 73.8–97.2%) for the VCG. The median sensitivities for LVH, RVH, AMI, and IMI were 55.7%, 32.7%, 74.1%, and 65.1%, respectively, for ECG and VCG computer programs together, versus 63.4%, 48.5%, 82.9%, and 73.3%, respectively, for all cardiologists. Total accuracy varied between 62.0% and 77.3% (median 69.7%) for the ECG programs, and between 64.3% and 76.2% (median 68.3%) for the VCG programs. Total accuracy of the cardiologists varied between 72.6% and 81.0% (median 76.3%) for the ECG, and between 67.5% and 74.4% (median 70.3%) for the VCG. However, the programs with the best performance reached almost equal levels as the best cardiologists.

The cardiologists obtained more accurate results for the ECG than for the VCG. The VCG readers had a lower specificity and, somewhat surprisingly, a lower sensitivity for anterior infarction, while sensitivities for RVH, inferior infarction, and combined infarction were slightly higher. These results largely corroborate those of other investigators demonstrating that the VCG is superior for most diagnostic categories as far as sensitivity is concerned, at the expense of specificity [241]. In another study [53], using 3,266 cases and the same statistical classification technique, the ECG and VCG were shown to have identical diagnostic information. One reason for the lower performance of the VCG readers in the CSE study may be, for some readers, an unusual display of the vector loops. It should be noted that the total accuracies of the combined ECG program (76.3%) and combined VCG program (77.0%) were almost identical.

Total accuracy of the four statistical programs was significantly higher (median 76.0%) than for the heuristic programs (median 67.4%). This may, at least in part, be explained by the fact that 87% of the database consisted of single-disease cases. The statistical programs were designed to classify a case into one of seven or eight disease categories, which is not the case for the open-ended heuristic programs. Thus, the composition of the database may have resulted in a bias favoring the statistical programs. Moreover, results of the AVA program may have been inflated thanks to its being fed with clinical information to adjust the prior probabilities on a case-by-case basis.

Combined results of programs and cardiologists were in almost all cases more accurate than those of the individual programs and cardiologists. This confirms previous findings on a subset of the CSE library [204].

The advantageous effect of combining programs was used in a study by Kors et al. [242] to improve the performance of their MEANS program. MEANS comprises two different classification programs, one for the ECG and one for the VCG. The interpretations of both programs in analyzing the ECGs and VCGs of the CSE diagnostic library were combined. The total accuracy of the combined program against clinical evidence was 74.2% (❷ Fig. 5.8), significantly better than the total accuracy of each program separately (69.8% for the ECG, 70.2% for the VCG). Interestingly, to avoid the necessity of recording a VCG, in addition to the ECG, the VCGs were also reconstructed from the ECGs and then interpreted by the VCG classification program. The combined ECG and reconstructed VCG results (73.6%) were almost the same as those of the combined ECG and original VCG. Thus, the performance of an ECG computer program was improved by incorporating both ECG and VCG classificatory knowledge, drawing only on the ECG itself.

Another strategy, which takes into account possible beat-to-beat variations in the ECG was proposed by the same group [243]. In the first step, all individual complexes of the dominant type are analyzed and a classification is derived for each. In a second round, the individual classifications are combined in one final interpretation. When tested on the CSE diagnostic library, the total accuracy of MEANS against the clinical evidence significantly increased from 69.8% for the interpretations of the averaged complexes to 71.2% for the combined interpretations of the individual complexes.

Rather than combining the diagnostic outputs of an ECG and a VCG program, Andresen et al. [244, 245] integrated ECG and VCG criteria for acute and prior MI in one algorithm. VCG leads were synthesized using the "inverse Dower" transformation [19]. Using a database containing normals and patients with infarctions validated by ECG-independent means, the algorithm achieved sensitivity equal to that of three cardiologists and three primary care physicians, but had

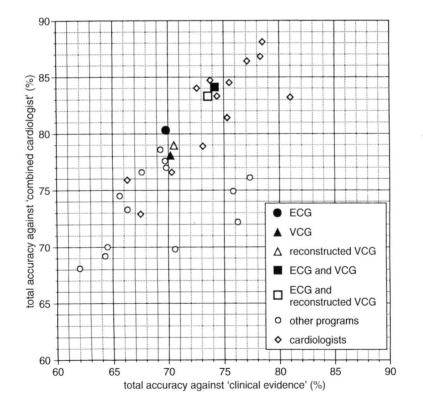

◼ Fig. 5.8

Total accuracies for the MEANS interpretation of the ECG, VCG, reconstructed VCG, and the combined interpretations. Also, the total accuracies of the other programs and of the cardiologists participating in the CSE study are shown (From Kors et al. [242]. © Elsevier. Reproduced with permission)

much higher specificity than the primary care physicians [246]. An improved version of the algorithm even outperformed the human readers [244], but these results might tend to be enhanced because the test database did not contain abnormalities other than infarctions.

The results of the CSE study showed that some ECG computer programs perform almost as well as the best cardiologists in classifying seven main diagnostic entities. However, it also became clear that some other programs were in need of considerable overhaul to meet reasonable standards.

5.14.7   Computer-Aided Physician's Interpretation of the ECG

Several studies evaluated the effect of computerized ECG interpretation on physicians' readings of ECGs. Milliken et al. [247] collected 180 ECGs from patients with various cardiac disorders known from ECG-independent data. Nine readers first read the ECG twice at an interval of several months without computer printouts. Months later, they reread the same ECGs, this time with the computer printout being available. The interpretations with several months intervening, but without computer output, resulted in an average change of 13.8% of the statements with 7.3% becoming correct and 6.5% becoming incorrect. When they reread the ECGs together with a computer output, the changes from incorrect to correct averaged 12% and from correct to incorrect 3%. From this study, it is apparent that the effect of priming the reader with computer results was in the direction of greater accuracy.

Hillson et al. [248] performed a randomized controlled trial to examine the effects of computer-assisted ECG interpretation on ECG reading time and agreement with the clinical diagnosis. Forty family physicians and general internists evaluated ten clinical vignettes accompanied by ECGs. Half of the physicians received the ECGs with computer-generated reports, the other half without. Those receiving the reports spent, on average, 25% less time in reading the ECGs. The first-listed diagnosis of those physicians who did not receive computer support agreed with the clinical diagnosis in only 15.3% of the cases, while the score rose to 30.1% in those who received support (p = 0.004). This effect could mainly be attributed to two cases with somewhat uncommon diagnoses (Wolff–Parkinson–White syndrome and pericarditis), which were correctly identified by the computer. However, in one of three cases that had erroneous computer reports, physicians who received the misleading reports were likely to adopt the diagnostic error. Another study [249] involved 22 cardiologists who each interpreted 80 ECGs, half of them with a computer report. Computer-assisted ECG interpretation gave an average reduction in reading time of 28% and significantly improved concordance of the cardiologists' interpretations with a gold standard established by a panel of five expert electrocardiographers.

In still another study, ten senior house officers were recruited in an emergency department [250]. They interpreted 50 ECGs and five of these junior doctors had access to the computer report. Their interpretations and the computer reports were compared with the consensus interpretation of two experienced clinicians. The computer made only two major errors. Access to the computer report improved the physicians' error rate (22.4% without report versus 18.4% with), but not significantly.

Tsai et al. [251] examined the effects of correct and incorrect computer advice. They performed a randomized controlled trial in which 30 internal medicine residents each interpreted 23 ECGs with a total of 54 findings. The gold standard was established by two cardiologists. Computer interpretations were correct in almost 60% of the findings. Overall, without computer report, the physicians' interpretations were correct in 48.9% of the findings. With the reports, they interpreted 55.4% correctly (p < 0.0001). For the subset in which the computer findings agreed with the gold standard, physicians without the computer report interpreted 53.1% correctly; when the computer report was included, accuracy increased to 68.1% (p < 0.0001). When computer advice that did not agree with the gold standard was not given to the physicians, accuracy was 56.7%. Accuracy dropped to 48.3% when the incorrect computer report was provided (p = 0.13). In the subset of findings in which the computer interpretation was incorrect, physicians agreed with the incorrect interpretation twice as often when they were prompted by the computer than when they were not (67.7% versus 34.6%, p < 0.0001).

Most studies have shown a clear improvement in ECG reading of physicians when they are provided with a computer-generated report. "Computerized electrocardiography – an adjunct to the physician" is the title of an editorial by Laks and Selvester [252] hailing the CSE report. Indeed, but there is a danger that nonexpert physicians let themselves be persuaded by an incorrect computer interpretation. This underlines the need for well-validated ECG computer programs that should perform at the level of expert electrocardiographers.

5.15   Rhythm Analysis Programs

Automatic identification of various arrhythmias poses major problems in the routine resting ECG. The rhythm interpretation logic in all clinically used programs follows a deterministic approach, using measurements (RR intervals and PR intervals, results of QRS wave typing, morphology of P waves, etc.) derived by the measurement program. The quality of the rhythm section rests largely on the quality of the measurement algorithms. While QRS complexes can be detected quite reliably, serious problems persist in P-wave recognition, especially in noisy recordings. For this reason, in many programs the logic has been constructed so as to allow for a degree of wave-recognition failure and measurement error [145, 253]. The record length poses another major problem. With the current multichannel recorders, usually 10 s of data are analyzed. This is too short for reliable detection of parasystole, for example, or other complicated arrhythmias. Providentially, the shortcomings of routine rhythm analysis programs are generally not too apparent, thanks to the low incidence of complex arrhythmias in the general hospital environment [254, 255].

The first extensive program for rhythm analysis was developed by Bonner and Schwetman in 1968 [256]. In a second program [257], five sets of three simultaneously recorded leads were used as input. The basic rhythm was derived from each 5 s record and a "combining" program made a decision as to the final rhythm statement. The total number of rhythm statements was forty.

These statements were also implemented in the AVA program [145]. The arrhythmia logic was divided into four main sections dealing, respectively, with regular and irregular rhythms and single and multiple aberrant beats. In the regular rhythm section, three major branchings were made depending on the ratio of P waves to the number of QRS complexes found (P:QRS). If P:QRS ≤ 0.25, entry into the AV-junctional section was made. If P:QRS ≥ 0.75, sinus rhythm was considered, as was AV-junctional rhythm depending on the polarity of the P wave. If $0.25 <$ P:QRS < 0.75, further tests were made and in the case of inconclusive results, the statement "regular rhythm" was printed. In the irregular-rhythm section, P:QRS was also used as a major branching point.

The same ratio (P:QRS) was also used in the more elaborate rhythm program developed by Plokker [253]. He considered 13 different types of arrhythmias, each represented by and programmed according to a detailed flowchart. Instead of decision trees, Wartak et al. [258] used decision tables. The whole arrhythmia logic is subdivided into a set of tables, which are linked to each other.

A comparison of results published by different investigators is difficult and sometimes delusive. For rhythm program evaluation, there are no approved databases comparable to that of CSE. The ideal case collection would contain sufficient numbers of records in every rhythm category and evaluation should provide figures for sensitivity and specificity for each category. However, arrhythmia cases tend to be in short supply. Evaluation is then often restricted to the sensitivity and specificity of sinus rhythm diagnosis, in which specificity is calculated with respect to all non-sinus cases. The results are thus heavily influenced by the diagnostic difficulty of the cases in the non-sinus category.

The results of a number of programs were evaluated by several authors. Bailey et al. [44] analyzed results of the IBM-Bonner program, and reported a sensitivity for arrhythmias of 87.2% while specificity was 98.2%. Of the 31 false-negative arrhythmias, the statement "undetermined rhythm" was made in 18 cases, all found to be atrial fibrillation. Sensitivity for atrial fibrillation was 85.5%. Of eight cases with second-degree AV block, the program correctly identified two. The prevalence of complex arrhythmias was too low to derive any meaningful conclusions.

Similar detection rates of cardiac arrhythmias have been reported for other processing systems [52, 239, 253, 259]. For example, Bernard et al. [239] reported an overall correct detection rate of 86% in 240 arrhythmias by the Telemed program. They did not specify whether the missed arrhythmias were incorrectly called sinus rhythm or any other arrhythmia.

A comparative study of five computer programs in the diagnosis of various types of AV block was undertaken by Shirataka et al. [260], using an ECG signal generator. Although all systems correctly detected normal sinus rhythm and first-degree AV block, only one system recognized second-degree AV block with classic Wenckebach periodicity, and no system was able to classify atypical Wenckebach periods. Most systems performed reasonably well for Mobitz II AV block, third-degree AV block, and ventricular bigeminy and trigeminy.

Plokker [253] tested the rhythm analysis of an early version of the MEANS program. On a set of 2,769 ECGs, he found a sensitivity for sinus rhythm of 96.6% and a specificity of 98.0%. Using the HP program, Thomson et al. [261] reported a sensitivity for sinus rhythm of 96.6% and a specificity of 97.0% on a set of 5,110 ECGs.

Several reports [255, 262, 263] were devoted to the rhythm analysis program of GE Health Technologies (formerly Marquette). Farrell et al. [263] used 70,000 physician-confirmed ECGs from four teaching hospitals. Patients with pacemakers were excluded. Primary rhythm statements of a new and a previous program version were compared with the confirmed interpretations. Overall disagreement decreased from 6.9% for the older version to 4.1% for the new version. Increased sensitivities were observed for sinus rhythm (98.2%), atrial fibrillation (89.0%), and AV-junctional rhythms (63.1%), while specificity and positive predictive value improved for all arrhythmias. However, specificity for sinus rhythm was 85.5%, which means that as much as 14.5% of abnormal rhythms were called sinus. This would disqualify such a program for arrhythmia case-finding purposes.

Using a nearly identical software version as in Farrell's study, Poon et al. [255] assessed the performance of the GE program in 4,297 consecutive ECGs recorded in a university teaching hospital. Over-reading was performed by either one of two cardiologists. Overall, 13.1% of the ECGs required revision of the computer's rhythm interpretation, but about half of these ECGs involved patients with pacemakers. In the unpaced population, sensitivity for sinus rhythm was 98.7%, but specificity was again rather low at 90.1%. For atrial fibrillation, sensitivity was 90.8% and specificity 98.9%. Sensitivity for atrial flutter was 61.0%, whereas sensitivity for atrial tachycardia was only 2.8%. It was concluded that physician over-reading remains mandatory, in particular to confirm a computer statement of normal sinus rhythm, or rhythm statements in patients with pacemakers.

In another study involving the GE 12SL program, 2,072 ECGs collected in a tertiary care hospital were processed by the computer and then over-read by two cardiologists [264]. In 9.9% of the ECGs there were significant disagreements between the computer and the cardiologists; 86% of these related to arrhythmias, conduction disorders, and electronic pacemakers. Sensitivities for atrial fibrillation and atrial flutter were 76.1% and 65.9%, respectively, at specificities of more than 99.5%.

Sinus rhythm appears uniformly well recognized, but other results depend quite heavily on the material analyzed, not only with respect to the mix of various arrhythmias, but also to the noise content of the database.

5.16　Serial Comparison Programs

Comparison with previous records is a part of normal routine in ECG reading. It must, therefore, also be seen as a necessary adjunct to computerized ECG analysis. A prerequisite is an efficient database management system for storage and retrieval of results. In the past, restricted storage capacity limited the number of records and the type of data that could be kept on line. Pryor et al. [265] developed the first serial ECG comparison program but the comparison was essentially limited to the final diagnostic statements. Others compared measurements as well [266]. In some systems, raw data from one representative cycle for up to three records were stored [267], or the entire record could potentially be regenerated in case of arrhythmias [143, 268].

Nowadays, with vastly expanded storage capacity and transmission and processing speed boosted to previously unimagined heights, technical limitations hardly seem to be a consideration. Nevertheless, an operational difficulty remains. The modern stand-alone microprocessor-based electrocardiograph is able to perform a complete ECG analysis but does not contain the information of the central management system. If one wants serial analysis, a way of communication with the management system must be chosen from several options, the most advanced being instantaneous wireless transmission of data [269, 270].

The more fundamental problem of serial comparison is that of semantics: which meaning must be attached to a difference in measurements or in diagnostic statements between successive interpretations? As is well known, there is a certain variability in recordings from 1 day to the next or from 1 year to the next [271, 272]. This variability is caused by differences in electrode placement, variations in depth of respiration, alterations in posture, changes in body fat, and by other factors [273]. Measurement changes from one tracing to the next should be given attention only if they exceed the natural variability. As mentioned earlier, in deterministic programs, it is quite possible that small, insubstantial measurement fluctuations around a threshold value cause a material difference in diagnostic statements [234]. But which of the statements in this borderline situation is the correct one? Each serial analysis program deals with this problem in its own way.

Different checks are made to ascertain whether or not changes are the result of a borderline crossover of decision criteria. As an option, a graphic display of trends in measurements and diagnostic statements has been implemented in some processing systems [274–276]. Also, serial comparison summary statements, such as "no significant change" or "descriptive differences only," have been proposed as a means of taking into account normal ECG fluctuations [277]. Alternative methods for improving the consistency of serial ECG analysis are the use of smooth decision functions rather than binary thresholds [278, 279], or VCG loop alignment (if not available as such, the VCGs may be derived from the two ECGs to be compared by mathematical transformation) [280, 281].

On the other hand, as long as the measurements are essentially identical, a good program will produce the same diagnostic result which may mean persisting in making the same error. Meanwhile, the initial statement may have been corrected by a reviewer [282]. Only if the corresponding changes are made in the central ECG management system may a serial analysis program take them into account in the comparison with a subsequent ECG from the same patient [277].

Most programs for serial ECG analysis use decision rules to arrive at their diagnostic interpretation [141, 163, 267, 283]. Two studies investigated the use of artificial neural networks. Sunemark et al. [281] described a neural network to classify serial changes indicative of newly developed infarcts, taking the consensus opinion of three interpreters as the reference. The input data consisted of measurements from the ECG and the reconstructed VCG. At 90% specificity, the use of only ECG or VCG measurements gave a sensitivity of 63% and 60%, respectively, and increased to 69% when measurements were combined. Ohlsson et al. [284] also used neural networks to detect acute MI based on either the current ECG only, or on the combination of the previous and the current ECGs. Acute MI was diagnosed according to characteristic chest pain, elevated enzyme levels, or characteristic ECG changes. There was a small but significant improvement in the neural network performance when a previous ECG was used as an additional input. On the same set of ECGs, the neural network appeared to perform better than two physicians, an experienced cardiologist and an intern.

No independent evaluation studies of different systems for serial ECG analysis have been published.

5.17   Computer Analysis of Pediatric Electrocardiograms

The ECG in children differs considerably in signal characteristics from that of the adult. Small children usually have high heart rates, and the recordings are often much noisier and show more baseline wander than in adults. There is a fast and profound evolution of electrocardiographic patterns especially in the first days and weeks after birth, but changes continue up to adolescence [285, 286]. Consequently, normal limits of ECG and VCG parameters are heavily dependent on age, and for diagnostic criteria, especially in young children, it is necessary to rely on extensive tables of values for amplitudes, durations, and angles [287–292]. Here, obviously, the computer can be of assistance. Also, congenital heart diseases can be quite complex and can produce a variety of electrocardiographic patterns. In addition, qualified readers of pediatric ECGs are rare and mostly located in university centers [293]. Inter- and intra-observer variability in reading pediatric ECGs was shown to be substantial [294]. These were the main incentives for the development of pediatric ECG programs.

In the past, the Mayo computer system routinely processed pediatric VCGs for some time [295], and in the VA Research Center for Cardiovascular Data, a large cooperative study has been undertaken in this field [296]. Other programs have been developed for pediatric VCG [163, 223] and 12-lead ECG [297–300]. The combination of ECG and synthesized VCG measurements to discriminate between mild RVH with terminal conduction delay and partial RBBB in children was described by Zhou et al. [301].

Relatively few evaluation studies of pediatric ECG programs have been performed. In a study of 248 pediatric ECGs that were diagnosed by ECG-independent means, the HP pediatric program had a 70% sensitivity and 82% specificity for RVH and a 38% sensitivity and 93% specificity for LVH [302].

Based on a test set of 642 ECGs diagnosed by two pediatric cardiologists, Rijnbeek et al. [300] assessed the performance of the pediatric version of the MEANS program (❷ Table 5.4). Sensitivities for RVH, LVH, RBBB, and LBBB were 74%, 79%, 84%, and 75%, respectively, at specificities of at least 95%. The program employs continuous age-dependent normal limits that in a separate study were shown to be considerably different from those commonly used in children [292].

In a study by Hamilton et al. [303], the diagnoses of RVH and LVH by the Glasgow program was compared with those of two pediatric cardiologists. When the cardiologists were not provided with clinical information, sensitivity of

◻ Table 5.4

Performance of the computer program PEDMEANS on a training set (n = 1,076) and test set (n = 642) of pediatric ECGs (from Rijnbeek et al. [300])

Abnormality	Training set		Test set	
	Sensitivity (%)	Specificity (%)	Sensitivity (%)	Specificity (%)
LVH	71.7	97.1	74.3	96.5
RVH	80.0	95.0	79.4	95.6
LBBB	86.4	97.9	84.0	95.3
RBBB	62.5	99.3	75.0	99.7

the program for RVH was 73% at a specificity of 97%, but sensitivity for LVH was only 25% at 96% specificity though the sensitivity for LVH increased to 44% at the same specificity when the clinical information was provided. Interestingly, if the cardiologists had disagreed initially with each other, their consensus opinion was twice as likely to be in agreement with the program.

Finally, pediatric ECG interpretations by the Marquette 12 SL program were compared with those of emergency department physicians in a 12-month prospective study, taking the interpretation by a pediatric electrophysiologist as the reference [304]. The computer proved to be more accurate than the physicians for interpretations considered to be of minimal or indeterminate clinical significance, but both performed poorly in interpreting the few cases of definite clinical significance (prolonged QTc, acute MI, supraventricular tachycardia, and atrial fibrillation).

5.18   Conclusion

In 1989, the late Jos Willems, the author of this chapter on computerized electrocardiography in the first edition of this handbook, wrote: "Nowadays computerized ECG analysis is being utilized widely in many medical institutions" and "Microprocessor-equipped electrocardiographs are proliferating and are on the verge of widespread application in smaller hospitals, general practitioners' offices and the health-screening environment." Now, in 2010, it will be hard to find a non-microprocessor-based electrocardiograph outside a museum for medical instruments, where it may stand next to an Einthoven string-galvanometer-based electrocardiograph invented in 1902. Willems also wrote: "Since 1982, definite progress has been made in the development of reference standards aimed at the evaluation of ECG measurement programs. This has largely been the result of the cooperative study "Common Standards for Quantitative Electrocardiography" (CSE project). Much work still needs to be done in the objective assessment of the diagnostic performance of ECG-analysis computer programs. Many challenges are still ahead . . .."

In almost 20 years since the closure of the CSE project, certainly much work has been done, but many challenges remain. The volume per annum of publications on computerized ECG analysis has steadily decreased. It looks as if a certain amount of saturation has set in. The providers of "intelligent" ECG equipment seem to be less keen on improving their diagnostic programs: has not the CSE study shown that programs rival the cardiologists' intelligence in diagnosis? But the time has not arrived to sit back complacently. It must be remembered that the CSE study applies to an idealized breed of ECGs. In real life, ECGs are not selected for good appearance and straightforward character. They may be of unshapely physiognomy due to combinations of abnormalities and be disfigured by noise, arrhythmias, and conduction defects. Here, the computer's painstakingly taught tricks for detecting waves and inflectional points are eclipsed by man's innate talents for pattern recognition. Especially P-wave detection and, connected with it, rhythm analysis need improvement and it would help if electrocardiographs would routinely acquire records of at least 30 s for this purpose. On the other hand, man is unreliable and, except where waveform recognition is suddenly led astray – a weakness that still should be amended – computer measurements are much more consistent. Presently, computer measurement of the QT interval is widely used for drug safety testing. In general, computer diagnosis is very specific, that is, a statement of "normal" can be relied on almost blindly and computerized ECG analysis is, therefore, an adequate screening instrument. Also, population screening by Minnesota coding through computer is much more reliable, faster, and cheaper than by hand. For clinical purposes, an abnormal computer classification still requires over-reading by an expert. The confrontation of the reader with the computer report was shown to improve quality and consistency of diagnosis. The huge advantages offered by a computerized system for automatic reporting, filing, and retrieval do not have to be emphasized. Finally, on the list-to-do in computerized electrocardiography, we should put the further development of serial analysis and perfection of the diagnosis of acute coronary syndromes. For this latter purpose, well-validated data bases are necessary.

The electrocardiograph with diagnostic facilities is often called "intelligent." Shannon once exclaimed: "Man is a machine, man can think, therefore some machines can think." The reader may speculate whether the third term of this syllogism will at some point apply to the computerized ECG machine.

References

1. Turing, A.M., Computing machinery and intelligence. *Mind*, 1950;**59**: 433–460.

2. Rijlant, P.B.L., L'analyse par un calculateur analogique des electrocardiogrammes scalaires et vectoriels. *Bull. Acad. Royal Med. Belgique*, 1962;**2**: 363.

3. Rautaharju, P.M., The impact of computers on electrocardiography. *Eur. J. Cardiol.*, 1978;**8**: 237–248.

4. Taback, L., E. Marden, H.L. Mason, and H. Pipberger, Digital recording of electrocardiographic data for analysis by means of a digital electronic computer. *IRE Trans. Med. Electron.*, 1959;**6**: 167–171.

5. Pipberger, H.V., R.J. Arms, and F.W. Stallmann, Automatic screening of normal and abnormal electrocardiograms by means of a digital electronic computer. *Proc. Soc. Exp. Biol. Med.*, 1961;**106**: 130–132.

6. Stallmann, F.W. and H.V. Pipberger, Automatic recognition of electrocardiographic waves by digital computer. *Circ. Res.*, 1961;**9**: 1138–1143.

7. Cornfield, J., R.A. Dunn, C.D. Batchlor, and H.V. Pipberger, Multigroup diagnosis of electrocardiograms. *Comput. Biomed. Res.*, 1973;**6**: 97–120.

8. Pipberger, H.V., D. McCaughan, D. Littmann, H.A. Pipberger, J. Cornfield, R.A. Dunn, et al., Clinical application of a second generation electrocardiographic computer program. *Am. J. Cardiol.*, 1975;**35**: 597–608.

9. Caceres, C.A., C.A. Steinberg, S. Abraham, J. CW, J.M. McBride, and W.E. Tolles, et al., Computer extraction of electrocardiographic parameters. *Circulation*, 1962;**25**: 356–362.

10. Rautaharju, P.M., The current state of computer ECG analysis: a critique, in *Trends in Computer-Processed Electrocardiograms*, J.H. van Bemmel and J.L. Willems, Editors. Amsterdam: North-Holland, 1976, pp. 117–124.

11. Drazen, E.L., Use of computer-assisted ECG interpretation in the United States, in *Computers in Cardiology 1979*, K.L. Ripley and H.G. Ostrow, Editors. Long Beach: IEEE Comp Soc. 1979, pp. 83–85.

12. Drazen, E.L., N. Mann, R. Borun, M. Laks, and A. Bersen, Survey of computer-assisted electrocardiography in the United States. *J. Electrocardiol.*, 1988;**21**(Suppl): S98–104.

13. Macfarlane, P.W., A brief history of computer-assisted electrocardiography. *Methods Inf. Med.*, 1990;**29**: 272–281.

14. Rautaharju, P.M., M. Ariet, T.A. Pryor, R.C. Arzbaecher, J.J. Bailey, R. Bonner, et al., The quest for optimal electrocardiography. Task force III: computers in diagnostic electrocardiography. *Am. J. Cardiol.*, 1978;**41**: 158–170.

15. Pipberger, H.V., J. Cornfield, What ECG computer program to choose for clinical application. The need for consumer protection. *Circulation*, 1973;**47**: 918–920.

16. Frank, E., An accurate, clinically practical system for spatial vectorcardiography. *Circulation*, 1956;**13**: 737–749.

17. Rautaharju, P.M., H.W. Blackburn, H.K. Wolf, and M. Horacek, Computers in clinical electrocardiology. Is vectorcardiography becoming obsolete? *Adv. Cardiol.*, 1976;**16**: 143–156.

18. Dower, G.E., H.B. Machado, and J.A. Osborne, On deriving the electrocardiogram from vectoradiographic leads. *Clin. Cardiol.*, 1980;**3**: 87–95.

19. Edenbrandt, L. and O. Pahlm, Vectorcardiogram synthesized from a 12-lead ECG: superiority of the inverse Dower matrix. *J. Electrocardiol.*, 1988;**21**: 361–367.

20. Rubel, P., I. Benhadid, and J. Fayn, Quantitative assessment of eight different methods for synthesizing Frank VCGs from simultaneously recorded standard ECG leads. *J. Electrocardiol.*, 1992;**24**(Suppl): 197–202.

21. Macfarlane, P.W., M.P. Watts, and T.D.V. Lawrie, Hybrid electrocardiography, in *Optimization of Computer ECG Processing*, H.K. Wolf and P.W. Macfarlane, Editors. Amsterdam: North-Holland, 1980, pp. 57–61.

22. Kornreich, F. and P.M. Rautaharju, The missing waveform and diagnostic information in the standard 12 lead electrocardiogram. *J. Electrocardiol.*, 1981;**14**: 341–350.

23. Kornreich, F., The missing waveform information in the orthogonal electrocardiogram (Frank leads). I. Where and how can this missing waveform information be retrieved? *Circulation*, 1973;**48**: 984–995.

24. Kornreich, F., P. Smets, and J. Kornreich, About challenging the uniqueness of a new, so-called "optimal", "total" or "maximal" 9-lead system, in *Trends in Computer-Processed Electrocardiograms*, J.H. van Bemmel and J.L. Willems, Editors. Amsterdam: North-Holland, 1977, pp. 293–301.

25. Kornreich, F., R.L. Lux, and R.S. MacLeod, Map representation and diagnostic performance of the standard 12-lead ECG. *J. Electrocardiol.*, 1995;**28**(Suppl): 121–123.

26. Kors, J.A. and G. van Herpen, How many electrodes and where? A "poldermodel" for electrocardiography. *J. Electrocardiol.*, 2002;**35**(Suppl): 7–12.

27. Nelwan, S.P., J.A. Kors, S.H. Meij, J.H. van Bemmel, and M.L. Simoons, Reconstruction of the 12-lead electrocardiogram from reduced lead sets. *J. Electrocardiol.*, 2004;**37**: 11–18.

28. Dower, G.E., A. Yakush, S.B. Nazzal, R.V. Jutzy, and C.E. Ruiz, Deriving the 12-lead electrocardiogram from four (EASI) electrodes. *J. Electrocardiol.*, 1988;**21**(Suppl): S182–S187.

29. Burger, H.C. and J.B. Van Milaan, Heart-vector and leads. *Brit. Heart J.*, 1946;**8**: 157–161.

30. Mortara, D.W., Source consistency filtering. Application to resting ECGs. *J. Electrocardiol.*, 1992;**25**(Suppl): 200–206.

31. Kors, J.A. and G. van Herpen, Accurate automatic detection of electrode interchange in the electrocardiogram. *Am. J. Cardiol.*, 2001;**88**: 396–399.

32. Burger, H.C., A. van Brummelen, and G. van Herpen, Compromise in vectorcardiography. II. Alterations of coefficients as a means of adapting one lead system to another. Subjective and mathematical comparison of four systems of VCG. *Am. Heart J.*, 1962;**64**: 666–678.

33. Surawicz, B., H. Uhley, R. Borun, M. Laks, L. Crevasse, K. Rosen, et al., The quest for optimal electrocardiography. Task force I: standardization of terminology and interpretation. *Am. J. Cardiol.*, 1978;**41**: 130–145.

34. The CSE Working Party, Recommendations for measurement standards in quantitative electrocardiography. *Eur. Heart J.*, 1985;**6**: 815–825.

35. Willems, J.L., E.O. Robles de Medina, R. Bernard, P. Coumel, C. Fisch, D. Krikler, et al., Criteria for intraventricular conduction disturbances and pre-excitation. World Health Organizational/International Society and Federation for Cardiology Task Force Ad Hoc. *J. Am. Coll. Cardiol.*, 1985;**5**: 1261–1275.

36. Kadish, A.H., A.E. Buxton, H.L. Kennedy, B.P. Knight, J.W. Mason, C.D. Schuger, et al., ACC/AHA clinical competence statement on electrocardiography and ambulatory electrocardiography: A report of the ACC/AHA/ACP-ASIM task force on clinical competence. *Circulation*, 2001;**104**: 3169–3178.

37. van Bemmel, J.H., J.A. Kors, and G. van Herpen, Methodology of the modular ECG analysis system MEANS. *Methods Inf. Med.*, 1990;**29**: 346–353.

38. Talmon, J.L. and J.H. van Bemmel, The advantage of modular software design in computerized ECG analysis. *Med. Inform.*, 1986;**11**: 117–128.

39. Willems, J.L. and J. Pardaens, Differences in measurement results obtained by four different ECG computer programs, in *Computers in Cardiology 1977*, H.G. Ostrow and K.L. Ripley, Editors. Long Beach: IEEE Comput Soc, 1977, pp. 115–121.

40. Willems, J.L., A plea for common standards in computer aided ECG analysis. *Comput. Biomed. Res.*, 1980;**13**: 120–131.

41. Pipberger, H.V., Comparative evaluation of electrocardiography computer programs, in *Computers in Cardiology 1976*, H.G. Ostrow and K.L. Ripley, Editors. Long Beach: IEEE Computer Society, 1976, pp. 85–88.

42. Crevasse, L. and M.A. Ariet, New scalar electrocardiographic computer program. Clinical evaluation. *JAMA*, 1973;**226**: 1089–1093.

43. Romhilt, D.W. and E.H. Estes, A point-score system for the ECG diagnosis of left ventricular hypertrophy. *Am. Heart J.*, 1968;**75**: 752–758.

44. Bailey, J.J., S.B. Itscoitz, J.W. Hirshfeld, L.E. Grauer, and M.R.A. Horton, Method for evaluating computer programs for electrocardiographic interpretation. I. Application to the experimental IBM program of 1971. *Circulation*, 1974;**50**: 73–79.

45. Bailey, J.J., S.B. Itscoitz, L.E. Grauer, J.W. Hirshfeld, and M.R.A. Horton, Method for evaluating computer programs for electrocardiographic interpretation. II. Application to version D of the PHS program and the Mayo clinic program of 1968. *Circulation*, 1974;**50**: 80–87.

46. Hodges, M., A clinical evaluation of the H-P ECG analysis program: program accuracy and value of adjustable criteria, in *Computers in Cardiology 1979*, K.L. Ripley and H.G. Ostrow, Editors. Long Beach: IEEE Comput Soc, 1979, pp. 167–170.

47. Garcia, R., G.M. Breneman, and S. Goldstein, Electrocardiogram computer analysis. Practical value of the IBM Bonner-2 (V2 MO) program. *J. Electrocardiol.*, 1981;**14**: 283–288.

48. Caceres, C.A. and H.M. Hochberg, Performance of the computer and physician in the analysis of the electrocardiogram. *Am. Heart J.*, 1970;**79**: 439–443.

49. Bourdillon, P.J. and D. Kilpatrick, Clinicians, the Mount Sinai program and the Veterans' Administration program evaluated against clinico-pathological data derived independently of the electrocardiogram. *Eur. J. Cardiol.*, 1978;**8**: 395–412.

50. Willems, J.L., H. Ector, J. Pardaens, J. Piessens, and H. de Geest, Computer and conventional ECG analysis: correlation with cineangiographic data. *Adv. Cardiol.*, 1978;**21**: 177–180.

51. Khadr, N.E., C.L. Bray, D.C. Beton, R.S. Croxson, M. Hughes, C. Jeffery, et al., Diagnosis of left ventricular hypertrophy and myocardial infarction by Bonner/IBM program verified by ECG-independent evidence, in *Computers in Cardiology*, K.L. Ripley and H.G. Ostrow, Editors. Long Beach: IEEE Comput Soc, 1979, pp. 93–97.

52. Macfarlane, P.W., D.I. Melville, M.R. Horton, and J.J. Bailey, Comparative evaluation of the IBM (12-lead) and Royal Infirmary (orthogonal three-lead) ECG computer programs. *Circulation*, 1981;**63**: 354–359.

53. Willems, J.L., E. Lesaffre, and J. Pardaens, Comparison of the classification ability of the electrocardiogram and vectorcardiogram. *Am. J. Cardiol.*, 1987;**59**: 119–124.

54. Zywietz, C. and B. Schneider, Editors. *Computer Application in ECG and VCG Analysis*. Amsterdam: North-Holland, 1973.

55. van Bemmel, J.H. and J.L. Willems, Editors. *Trends in Computer-Processed Electrocardiograms*. Amsterdam: North-Holland, 1977.

56. Wolf, H.K. and P.W. Macfarlane, Editors. *Optimization of Computer ECG Processing*. Amsterdam: North-Holland, 1980.

57. Willems, J.L., P. Arnaud, R. Degani, P.W. Macfarlane, J.H. van Bemmel, and C. Zywietz, Protocol for the Concerted Action Project "Common Standards for Quantitative Electrocardiography". Leuven: ACCO, 1980.

58. The CSE European Working Party, An approach to measurement standards in computer ECG analysis, in *Optimization of Computer ECG Processing*, H.K. Wolf and P.W. Macfarlane, Editors. Amsterdam: North-Holland, 1980, pp. 135–137.

59. Willems, J.L., P. Arnaud, J.H. van Bemmel, R. Degani, P.W. Macfarlane, C. Zywietz, Common standards for quantitative electrocardiography: goals and main results. CSE Working Party. *Methods Inf. Med.*, 1990;**29**: 263–271.

60. Willems, J.L., P. Arnaud, J.H. van Bemmel, P.J. Bourdillon, R. Degani, B. Denis, et al., Establishment of a reference library for evaluating computer ECG measurement programs. *Comput. Biomed. Res.*, 1985;**18**: 439–457.

61. Willems, J.L., P. Arnaud, J.H. van Bemmel, P.J. Bourdillon, R. Degani, B. Denis, et al., A reference data base for multilead electrocardiographic computer measurement programs. *J. Am. Coll. Cardiol.*, 1987;**10**: 1313–1321.

62. Willems, J.L., P. Arnaud, J.H. van Bemmel, P.J. Bourdillon, C. Brohet, S. Dalla Volta, et al., Assessment of the performance of electrocardiographic computer programs with the use of a reference data base. *Circulation*, 1985;**71**: 523–534.

63. Willems, J.L., *Common Standards for Quantitative Electrocardiography. CSE Atlas.* Referee Results First Phase Library – Data Set 1. Leuven: ACCO, 1983.

64. Willems, J.L., *Common Standards for Quantitative Electrocardiography. CSE Multilead Atlas.* Measurement Results – Data Set 3. Leuven: ACCO, 1988.

65. Willems, J.L., *Common Standards for Quantitative Electrocardiography*, 4th Progress Report. Leuven: ACCO, 1984.

66. Willems, J.L., *Common Standards for Quantitative Electrocardiography*, 10th Progress Report. Leuven: ACCO, 1990.

67. Berson, A.S., Analog-to-digital conversion, in: *Computer Application on ECG and VCG Analysis*, C. Zywietz and R. Schneider, Editors. Amsterdam: North-Holland, 1973, pp. 57–72.

68. Berson, A.S., T.A. Ferguson, C.D. Batchlor, R.A. Dunn, and H.V. Pipberger, Filtering and sampling for electrocardiographic data processing. *Comput. Biomed. Res.*, 1977;**10**: 605–616.

69. Bailey, J.J., A.S. Berson, A. Garson, L.G. Horan, P.W. Macfarlane, D.W. Mortara, et al., Recommendations for standardization and specifications in automated electrocardiography: bandwidth and digital signal processing. A report for health professionals by an ad hoc writing group of the Committee on Electrocardiography and Cardiac Electrophysiology of the Council on Clinical Cardiology, American Heart Association. *Circulation*, 1990;**81**: 730–739.

70. Rijnbeek, P.R., J.A. Kors, and M. Witsenburg, Minimum bandwidth requirements for recording of pediatric electrocardiograms. *Circulation*, 2001;**104**: 3087–3090.

71. Hedén, B., M. Ohlsson, L. Edenbrandt, R. Rittner, O. Pahlm, and C. Peterson, Artificial neural networks for recognition of electrocardiographic lead reversal. *Am. J. Cardiol.*, 1995;**75**: 929–933.

72. Schijvenaars, R.J., J.A. Kors, G. van Herpen, and J.H. van Bemmel, A method to reduce the effect of electrode position variations on automated ECG interpretation. *J. Electrocardiol.*, 1995;**28**: 350–351.

73. Brodnick, D., A method to locate electrode placement. *J. Electrocardiol.*, 2000;**33**(Suppl): 211–218.

74. McManus, C.D., K.D. Neubert, and E. Cramer, Characterization and elimination of AC noise in electrocardiograms: a comparison of digital filtering methods. *Comput. Biomed. Res.*, 1993;**26**: 48–67.

75. Cramer, E., C.D. McManus, and D. Neubert, Estimation and removal of power line interference in the electrocardiogram: a comparison of digital approaches. *Comput. Biomed. Res.*, 1987;**20**: 12–28.

76. Lynn, P.A., Online digital filters for biological signals: some fast designs for a small computer. *Med. Biol. Eng. Comput.*, 1977;**15**: 534–540.

77. Weaver, C.S., J. von der Groeben, P.E. Mantey, J.G. Toole, C.A. Cole, J.W. Fitzgerald, et al., Digital filtering with applications to electrocardiogram processing. *IEEE Trans. Audio Electroacoust.*, 1968;**16**: 350–391.

78. Levkov, C., G. Michov, R. Ivanov, and I.K. Daskalov, Subtraction of 50 Hz interference from the electrocardiogram. *Med. Biol. Eng. Comput.*, 1984;**22**: 371–373.

79. Dotsinsky, I. and T. Stoyanov, Power-line interference cancellation in ECG signals. *Biomed. Instrum. Technol.*, 2005;**39**: 155–162.

80. Levkov, C., G. Mihov, R. Ivanov, I. Daskalov, I. Christov, and I. Dotsinsky, Removal of power-line interference from the ECG: a review of the subtraction procedure. *Biomed. Eng. Online*, 2005;**4**: 50.

81. Widrow, B., J.R. Glover, M. McCool, J. Kaunitz, C.S. Williams, R.H. Hearn, et al., Adaptive noise cancelling: principles and applications. *Proc. IEEE*, 1975;**63**: 1692–1716.

82. Glover, J.R., Adaptive noise canceling applied to sinusoidal interferences. *IEEE Trans. Acoust. Speech Signal Process.*, 1977;**25**: 484–491.

83. Thakor, N.V. and Y.S. Zhu, Applications of adaptive filtering to ECG analysis: noise cancellation and arrhythmia detection. *IEEE Trans. Biomed. Eng.*, 1991;**38**: 785–794.

84. Mortara, D.W., Digital filters for ECG signals, in *Computers in Cardiology 1977*, H.G. Ostrow and K.L. Ripley, Editors. New York: IEEE Comput Soc, 1977, pp. 511–514.

85. Talmon, J.L., *Pattern recognition of the ECG. A structured analysis*, dissertation. Amsterdam: Free University, 1983.

86. Ahlstrom, M.L. and W.J. Tompkins, Digital filters for real-time ECG signal processing using microprocessors. *IEEE Trans. Biomed. Eng.*, 1985;**32**: 708–713.

87. Hamilton, P.S., A comparison of adaptive and nonadaptive filters for reduction of power line interference in the ECG. *IEEE Trans. Biomed. Eng.*, 1996;**43**: 105–109.

88. Glover, J.R., Comments on "Digital filters for real-time ECG signal processing using microprocessors". *IEEE Trans. Biomed. Eng.*, 1987;**34**: 962–963.

89. Pipberger, H.V., R.C. Arzbaecher, A.S. Berson, S.A. Briller, D.A. Brody, N.C. Flowers, et al., Recommendations for standardization of leads and of specifications for instruments in electrocardiography and vectorcardiography: report of the Committee on Electrocardiography, American Heart Association. *Circulation*, 1975;**52**: 11–31.

90. Bailey, J.J., The triangular wave test for electrocardiographic devices: a historical perspective. *J. Electrocardiol.*, 2004;**37**(Suppl): 71–73.

91. van Alste, J.A., W. van Eck, and O.E. Herrmann, ECG baseline wander reduction using linear phase filters. *Comput. Biomed. Res.*, 1986;**19**: 417–427.

92. Sörnmo, L., Time-varying digital filtering of ECG baseline wander. *Med. Biol. Eng. Comput.*, 1993;**31**: 503–508.

93. Shusterman, V., S.I. Shah, A. Beigel, and K.P. Anderson, Enhancing the precision of ECG baseline correction: selective filtering and removal of residual error. *Comput Biomed Res* 2000; **33**:144–160.

94. Macfarlane, P.W., J. Peden, G. Lennox, M.P. Watts, and T.D.V. Lawrie, The Glasgow system, in *Trends in Computer-Processed Electrocardiograms*, J.H. van Bemmel and J.L. Willems, Editors. Amsterdam: North-Holland, 1977, pp. 143–150.

95. Boucheham, B., Y. Ferdi, and M.C. Batouche, Recursive versus sequential multiple error measures reduction: a curve simplification approach to ECG data compression. *Comput. Methods Programs Biomed.*, 2005;**78**: 1–10.

96. Douglas, D.H. and T.K. Peucker, Algorithms for the reduction of the number of points required to represent a digitized line or its caricature. *Can. Cartographer*, 1973;**10**: 112–122.

97. Meyer, C.R. and H.N. Keiser, Electrocardiogram baseline noise estimation and removal using cubic splines and state-space computation techniques. *Comput. Biomed. Res.*, 1977;**10**: 459–470.

98. Gradwohl, J.R., E.W. Pottala, M.R. Horton, and J.J. Bailey, Comparison of two methods for removing baseline wander in the ECG, in *Computers in Cardiology 1988*, K.L. Ripley, Editor. Los Angeles: IEEE Comput Soc, 1988, pp. 493–496.

99. Froning, J.N., M.D. Olson, and V.F. Froelicher, Problems and limitations of ECG baseline estimation and removal using a cubic spline technique during exercise ECG testing: recommendations for proper implementation. *J. Electrocardiol.*, 1988;**21**(Suppl): S149–157.

100. Pottala, E.W., J.J. Bailey, M.R. Horton, and J.R. Gradwohl, Suppression of baseline wander in the ECG using a bilinearly transformed, null-phase filter. *J. Electrocardiol.*, 1989;**22**(Suppl): 243–247.

101. Frankel, R.A., E.W. Pottala, R.W. Bowser, and J.J. Bailey, A filter to suppress ECG baseline wander and preserve ST-segment accuracy in a real-time environment. *J. Electrocardiol.*, 1991;**24**: 315–323.

102. Longini, R.L., J.P. Giolma, C. Wall, and R.F. Quick, Filtering without phase shift. *IEEE Trans. Biomed. Eng.*, 1975;**22**: 432–433.

103. de Pinto, V., Filters for the reduction of baseline wander and muscle artifact in the ECG. *J. Electrocardiol.*, 1992;**25**(Suppl): 40–48.

104. van Alste, J.A. and T.S. Schilder, Removal of base-line wander and power-line interference from the ECG by an efficient FIR filter with a reduced number of taps. *IEEE Trans. Biomed. Eng.*, 1985;**32**: 1052–1060.

105. Jane, R., P. Laguna, N.V. Thakor, and P. Caminal, Adaptive baseline wander removal in the ECG: comparative analysis with cubic spline technique, in *Computers in Cardiology 1992*, A. Murray and R.C. Arzbaecher, Editors. Los Alamitos: IEEE Comput Soc, 1992, pp. 143–146.

106. Laguna, P., R. Jane, O. Meste, P.W. Poon, P. Caminal, H. Rix, et al., Adaptive filter for event-related bioelectric signals using an impulse correlated reference input: comparison with signal averaging techniques. *IEEE Trans. Biomed. Eng.*, 1992;**39**: 1032–1044.

107. Moody, G.B. and R.G. Mark, The impact of the MIT-BIH arrhythmia database. *IEEE Eng. Med. Biol. Mag.*, 2001;**20**: 45–50.

108. Park, K.L., K.J. Lee, and H.R. Yoon, Application of a wavelet adaptive filter to minimise distortion of the ST-segment. *Med. Biol. Eng. Comput.*, 1998;**36**: 581–586.

109. Taddei, A., G. Distante, M. Emdin, P. Pisani, G.B. Moody, C. Zeelenberg, et al., The European ST-T database: standard for evaluating systems for the analysis of ST-T changes in ambulatory electrocardiography. *Eur. Heart J.*, 1992;**13**: 1164–1172.

110. Chu, C.H. and E.J. Delp, Nonlinear methods in electrocardiogram signal processing. *J. Electrocardiol.*, 1990;**23**(Suppl): 192–197.

111. Sun, Y., K. Chan, and S.M. Krishnan, ECG signal conditioning by morphological filtering. *Comput. Biol. Med.*, 2002;**32**: 465–479.

112. Chu, C.H. and E.J. Delp, Impulsive noise suppression and background normalization of electrocardiogram signals using morphological operators. *IEEE Trans. Biomed. Eng.*, 1989;**36**: 262–273.

113. Haralick, R.M., S.R. Sternberg, and X. Zhuang, Image analysis using mathematical morphology. *IEEE Trans. Pattern Anal. Mach. Intell.*, 1987;**9**: 532–550.

114. Talmon, J.L., J.A. Kors, and J.H. van Bemmel, Adaptive Gaussian filtering in routine ECG/VCG analysis. *IEEE Trans. Acoust. Speech Signal Process.*, 1986;**34**: 527–534.

115. Hodson, E.K., D.R. Thayer, and C. Franklin, Adaptive Gaussian filtering and local frequency estimates using local curvature analysis. *IEEE Trans. Acoust. Speech Signal Process.*, 1981;**29**: 854–859.

116. Wei, D., E. Harasawa, and H. Hosaka, A low-distortion filter method to reject muscle noise in multi-lead electrocardiogram systems. *Front Med. Biol. Eng.*, 1999;**9**: 315–330.

117. Acar, B. and H. Koymen, SVD-based on-line exercise ECG signal orthogonalization. *IEEE Trans. Biomed. Eng.*, 1999;**46**: 311–321.

118. Paul, J.S., M.R. Reddy, and V.J. Kumar, A transform domain SVD filter for suppression of muscle noise artefacts in exercise ECG's. *IEEE Trans. Biomed. Eng.*, 2000;**47**: 654–663.

119. Nikolaev, N., A. Gotchev, K. Egiazarian, and Z. Nikolov, Suppression of electromyogram interference on the electrocardiogram by transform domain denoising. *Med. Biol. Eng. Comput.*, 2001;**39**: 649–655.

120. Raphisak, P., S.C. Schuckers, and A. de Jongh Curry, An algorithm for EMG noise detection in large ECG data, in *Computers in Cardiology 2004*, A. Murray, Editor. Piscataway, NJ: IEEE Comput Soc, 2004, pp. 369–372.

121. Brohet, C.R., C. Derwael, A. Robert, and R. Fesler, Methodology of ECG interpretation in the Louvain program. *Methods Inf. Med.*, 1990;**29**: 403–409.

122. Willems, J.L., *Common Standards for Quantitative Electrocardiography*, 2nd CSE Progress Report. Leuven: ACCO, 1982.

123. Pipberger, H.V., C.D. McManus, and H.A. Pipberger, Methodology of ECG interpretation in the AVA program. *Methods Inf. Med.*, 1990;**29**: 337–340.

124. Helfenbein, E.D., J.M. Lindauer, S.H. Zhou, R.E. Gregg, and E.C. Herleikson, A software-based pacemaker pulse detection and paced rhythm classification algorithm. *J. Electrocardiol.*, 2002;**35**(Suppl): 95–103.

125. Hamilton, P.S. and W.J. Tompkins, Quantitative investigation of QRS detection rules using the MIT/BIH arrhythmia database. *IEEE Trans. Biomed. Eng.*, 1986;**33**: 1157–1165.

126. Friesen, G.M., T.C. Jannett, M.A. Jadallah, S.L. Yates, S.R. Quint, and H.T. Nagle, A comparison of the noise sensitivity of nine QRS detection algorithms. *IEEE Trans. Biomed. Eng.*, 1990;**37**: 85–98.

127. Hu, Y.H., W.J. Tompkins, J.L. Urrusti, and V.X. Afonso, Applications of artificial neural networks for ECG signal detection and classification. *J. Electrocardiol.*, 1993;**26**(Suppl): 66–73.

128. Suppappola, S. and Y. Sun, Nonlinear transforms of ECG signals for digital QRS detection: a quantitative analysis. *IEEE Trans. Biomed. Eng.*, 1994;**41**: 397–400.

129. Afonso, V.X., W.J. Tompkins, T.Q. Nguyen, and S. Luo, ECG beat detection using filter banks. *IEEE Trans. Biomed. Eng.*, 1999;**46**: 192–202.

130. Kohler, B.U., C. Hennig, and R. Orglmeister, The principles of software QRS detection. *IEEE Eng. Med. Biol. Mag.*, 2002;**21**: 42–57.

131. Martinez, J.P., R. Almeida, S. Olmos, A.P. Rocha, and P. Laguna, A wavelet-based ECG delineator: evaluation on standard databases. *IEEE Trans. Biomed. Eng.*, 2004;**51**: 570–581.

132. Pahlm, O. and L. Sörnmo, Software QRS detection in ambulatory monitoring—a review. *Med. Biol. Eng. Comput.*, 1984;**22**: 289–297.

133. Li, C., C. Zheng, and C. Tai, Detection of ECG characteristic points using wavelet transforms. *IEEE Trans. Biomed. Eng.*, 1995;**42**: 21–28.

134. Kadambe, S., R. Murray, and G.F. Boudreaux-Bartels, Wavelet transform-based QRS complex detector. *IEEE Trans. Biomed. Eng.*, 1999;**46**: 838–848.

135. Vijaya, G., V. Kumar, and H.K. Verma, ANN-based QRS-complex analysis of ECG. *J. Med. Eng. Technol.*, 1998;**22**: 160–167.

136. Poli, R., S. Cagnoni, and G. Valli, Genetic design of optimum linear and nonlinear QRS detectors. *IEEE Trans. Biomed. Eng.*, 1995;**42**: 1137–1141.

137. Belforte, G., R. De Mori, and F. Ferraris, A contribution to the automatic processing of electrocardiograms using syntactic methods. *IEEE Trans. Biomed. Eng.*, 1979;26: 125–136.

138. Papakonstantinou, G., E. Skordalakis, and F. Gritzali, An attribute grammar for QRS detection. *Pattern Recog.*, 1986;**19**: 297–303.

139. Skordalakis, E., Syntactic ECG processing: a review. *Pattern Recog.*, 1986;**19**: 305–313.

140. Kors, J.A., J.L. Talmon, and J.H. van Bemmel, Multilead ECG analysis. *Comput. Biomed. Res.*, 1986;**19**: 28–46.

141. Macfarlane, P.W., B. Devine, S. Latif, S. McLaughlin, D.B. Shoat, and M.P. Watts, Methodology of ECG interpretation in the Glasgow program. *Methods Inf. Med.*, 1990;**29**: 354–361.

142. Christov, I., G. Bortolan, and I. Daskalov, Automatic detection of atrial fibrillation and flutter by wave rectification method. *J. Med. Eng. Technol.*, 2001;**25**: 217–221.

143. Balda, R.A., G. Diller, E. Deardorff, J.C. Doue, and P. Hsieh, The HP ECG analysis program, in *Trends in Computer-Processed Electrocardiograms*, J.H. van Bemmel and J.L. Willems, Editors. Amsterdam: North-Holland, 1977, pp. 197–204.

144. Laguna, P., R. Jane, and P. Caminal, Automatic detection of wave boundaries in multilead ECG signals: validation with the CSE database. *Comput. Biomed. Res.*, 1994;**27**: 45–60.

145. Willems, J.L. and H.V. Pipberger, Arrhythmia detection by digital computer. *Comput. Biomed. Res.*, 1972;**5**: 273–278.

146. McManus, C.D., A re-examination of automatic P-wave recognition methods, in *Optimization of Computer ECG Processing*, H.K. Wolf and P.W. Macfarlane, Editors. Amsterdam: North-Holland, 1980, pp. 121–127.

147. Bonner, R.E. and H.D. Schwetman, Computer diagnosis of electrocardiograms. II. A computer program for EKG measurements. *Comput. Biomed. Res.*, 1968;**1**: 366–386.

148. Hengeveld, S.J. and J.H. Bemmel, Computer detection of P-waves. *Comput. Biomed. Res.*, 1976;**9**: 125–132.

149. Schnyders, H.C. and M. Jordan, Energy correlation technique for small P-wave detection in the presence of noise, in *Computers in Cardiology 1980*, K.L. Ripley and H.G. Ostrow, Editors. Los Angeles: IEEE Comput Soc, 1980, pp. 161–164.

150. Gritzali, F., G. Frangakis, and G. Papakonstantinou, Detection of the P and T waves in an ECG. *Comput. Biomed. Res.*, 1989;**22**: 83–91.

151. Talmon, J.L., J.A. Kors, and J.H. van Bemmel, Algorithms for the detection of events in electrocardiograms. *Comput. Methods Programs Biomed.*, 1986;**22**: 149–161.

152. Taha, B., S. Reddy, Q. Xue, and S. Swiryn, Automated discrimination between atrial fibrillation and atrial flutter in the resting 12-lead electrocardiogram. *J. Electrocardiol.*, 2000;**33**(Suppl): 123–125.

153. Giraldo, B.F., P. Laguna, R. Jane, and P. Caminal, Automatic detection of atrial fibrillation and flutter using the differentiated ECG signal, in *Computers in Cardiology 1995*, A. Murray and R.C. Arzbaecher, Editors. Piscataway, NJ: IEEE Comput Soc, 1995, pp. 369–372.

154. Bonner, R.E., L. Crevasse, M.I. Ferrer, and J.C. Greenfield, A new computer program for analysis of scalar electrocardiograms. *Comput. Biomed. Res.*, 1972;**5**: 629–653.

155. van Bemmel, J.H. and S.J. Hengeveld, Clustering algorithm for QRS and ST-T waveform typing. *Comput. Biomed. Res.*, 1973;**6**: 442–456.

156. Simoons, M.L., H.B. Boom, and E. Smallenburg, On-line processing of orthogonal exercise electrocardiograms. *Comput. Biomed. Res.*, 1975;**8**: 105–117.

157. Moraes, J.C.T.B., M.O. Seixas, F.N. Vilani, and E.V. Costa, A real time QRS complex classification method using Mahalanobis distance, in *Computers in Cardiology 2002*, A. Murray, Editor. Piscataway, NJ: IEEE Comput Soc, 2002, pp. 201–204.

158. Lagerholm, M., C. Peterson, G. Braccini, L. Edenbrandt, and L. Sörnmo, Clustering ECG complexes using hermite functions and self-organizing maps. *IEEE Trans. Biomed. Eng.*, 2000;**47**: 838–848.

159. Hu, Y.H., A patient-adaptable ECG beat classifier using a mixture of experts approach. *IEEE Trans. Biomed. Eng.*, 1997;**44**: 891–900.

160. Wieben, O., V.X. Afonso, and W.J. Tompkins, Classification of premature ventricular complexes using filter bank features, induction of decision trees and a fuzzy rule-based system. *Med. Biol. Eng. Comput.*, 1999;**37**: 560–565.

161. de Chazal, P., M. O'Dwyer, and R.B. Reilly, Automatic classification of heartbeats using ECG morphology and heartbeat interval features. *IEEE Trans. Biomed. Eng.*, 2004;**51**: 1196–1206.

162. Christov, I., I. Jekova, and G. Bortolan, Premature ventricular contraction classification by the Kth nearest-neighbours rule. *Physiol. Meas.*, 2005;**26**: 123–130.

163. Zywietz, C., D. Borovsky, G. Gotsch, and G. Joseph, Methodology of ECG interpretation in the Hannover program. *Methods Inf. Med.*, 1990;**29**: 375–385.

164. Rautaharju, P.M., P.J. MacInnis, J.W. Warren, H.K. Wolf, P.M. Rykers, and H.P. Calhoun, Methodology of ECG interpretation in the Dalhousie program; NOVACODE ECG classification procedures for clinical trials and population health surveys. *Methods Inf. Med.*, 1990;**29**: 362–374.

165. Rompelman, O. and H.H. Ros, Coherent averaging technique: a tutorial review. Part 1: Noise reduction and the equivalent filter. *J. Biomed. Eng.*, 1986;**8**: 24–29.

166. Rompelman, O. and H.H. Ros, Coherent averaging technique: a tutorial review. Part 2: Trigger jitter, overlapping responses and non-periodic stimulation. *J. Biomed. Eng.*, 1986;**8**: 30–35.

167. Mertens, J. and D.W. Mortara, A new algorithm for QRS averaging, in *Computers in Cardiology 1984*, K.L. Ripley, Editor. Long Beach: IEEE Comput Soc, 1984, pp. 367–369.

168. Arnaud, P., P. Rubel, D. Morlet, J. Fayn, and M.C. Forlini, Methodology of ECG interpretation in the Lyon program. *Methods Inf. Med.*, 1990;**29**: 393–402.

169. Goetowski, C.R., The Telemed system, in *Trends in Computer-Processed Electrocardiograms*, J.H. van Bemmel and J.L. Willems, Editors. Amsterdam: North-Holland, 1977, pp. 207–210.

170. Degani, R. and G. Bortolan, Methodology of ECG interpretation in the Padova program. *Methods Inf. Med.*, 1990;**29**: 386–392.

171. Willems, J.L., C. Zywietz, P. Arnaud, J.H. van Bemmel, R. Degani, and P.W. Macfarlane, Influence of noise on wave boundary recognition by ECG measurement programs. Recommendations for preprocessing. *Comput. Biomed. Res.*, 1987;**20**: 543–562.

172. Zywietz, C., J.L. Willems, P. Arnaud, J.H. van Bemmel, R. Degani, P.W. Macfarlane, et al., Stability of computer ECG amplitude

measurements in the presence of noise. *Comput. Biomed. Res.*, 1990;**23**: 10–31.

173. Day, C.P., J.M. McComb, and R.W. Campbell, QT dispersion: an indication of arrhythmia risk in patients with long QT intervals. *Br. Heart J.*, 1990;**63**: 342–344.

174. Kors, J.A., G. van Herpen, and J.H. van Bemmel, QT dispersion as an attribute of T-loop morphology. *Circulation*, 1999;**99**: 1458–1463.

175. Rautaharju, P.M., QT and dispersion of ventricular repolarization: the greatest fallacy in electrocardiography in the 1990s. *Circulation*, 1999;**99**: 2477–2478.

176. Malik, M., B. Acar, Y. Gang, Y.G. Yap, K. Hnatkova, and A.J. Camm, QT dispersion does not represent electrocardiographic interlead heterogeneity of ventricular repolarization. *J. Cardiovasc. Electrophysiol.*, 2000;**11**: 835–843.

177. van Herpen, G., H.J. Ritsema van Eck, and J.A. Kors, The evidence against QT dispersion. *Int. J. Bioelectromagn.*, 2003;**5**: 231–233.

178. Ritsema van Eck, H.J., J.A. Kors, and G. van Herpen, The U wave in the electrocardiogram: a solution for a 100-year-old riddle. *Cardiovasc. Res.*, 2005;**67**: 256–262.

179. Nygards, M.E. and L. Sörnmo, Delineation of the QRS complex using the envelope of the e.c.g. *Med. Biol. Eng. Comput.*, 1983;**21**: 538–547.

180. van Bemmel, J.H., C. Zywietz, and J.A. Kors, Signal analysis for ECG interpretation. *Methods Inf. Med.*, 1990;**29**: 317–329.

181. McLaughlin, N.B., R.W. Campbell, and A. Murray, Comparison of automatic QT measurement techniques in the normal 12 lead electrocardiogram. *Br. Heart J.*, 1995;**74**: 84–89.

182. McLaughlin, N.B., R.W. Campbell, and A. Murray, Accuracy of four automatic QT measurement techniques in cardiac patients and healthy subjects. *Heart*, 1996;**76**: 422–426.

183. Vila, J.A., Y. Gang, J.M. Rodriguez Presedo, M. Fernandez-Delgado, S. Barro, and M. Malik, A new approach for TU complex characterization. *IEEE Trans. Biomed. Eng.*, 2000;**47**: 764–772.

184. Rubel, P. and B. Ayad, The true boundary recognition power of multidimensional detection functions. An optimal comparison, in *Computer ECG Analysis: Towards Standardization*, J.L. Willems, J.H. van Bemmel, and C. Zywietz, Editors. Amsterdam: North-Holland, 1986, pp. 97–103.

185. van Bemmel, J.H., J.L. Talmon, J.S. Duisterhout, and S.J. Hengeveld, Template waveform recognition applied to ECG-VCG analysis. *Comput. Biomed. Res.*, 1973;**6**: 430–441.

186. Zhang, Q., A. Illanes Manriquez, C. Medigue, Y. Papelier, and M. Sorine, Robust and efficient location of T-wave ends in electrocardiogram, in *Computers in Cardiology*, A. Murray, Editor. Piscataway, NJ: IEEE Comput Soc, 2005, pp. 711–714.

187. Sörnmo, L., A model-based approach to QRS delineation. *Comput. Biomed. Res.*, 1987;**20**: 526–542.

188. Morlet, D., P. Rubel, P. Arnaud, and J.L. Willems, An improved method to evaluate the precision of computer ECG measurement programs. *Int. J. Biomed. Comput.*, 1988;**22**: 199–216.

189. Kors, J.A., G. van Herpen, A.C. Sittig, and J.H. van Bemmel, Reconstruction of the Frank vectorcardiogram from standard electrocardiographic leads: diagnostic comparison of different methods. *Eur. Heart J.*, 1990;**11**: 1083–1092.

190. Young, T.Y. and W.H. Huggins, Intrinsic component theory of electrocardiograms. *IEEE Trans. Biomed. Eng.*, 1963;**9**: 214–221.

191. Horan, L.G., N.C. Flowers, and D.A. Brody, Principal factor waveforms of the thoracic QRS complex. *Circ. Res.*, 1964;**15**: 131–145.

192. Willems, J.L., Introduction to multivariate and conventional computer ECG analysis: pro's and contra's, in *Trends in Computer-Processed Electrocardiograms*, J.H. van Bemmel and J.L. Willems, Editors. Amsterdam: North-Holland, 1977, pp. 213–220.

193. Smets, P., New quantified approach for diagnostic classification, in *Optimization of Computer ECG Processing*, H.K. Wolf and P.W. Macfarlane, Editors. Amsterdam: North-Holland, 1980, pp. 229–237.

194. Degani, R. and G. Bortolan, Combining measurement precision and fuzzy diagnostic criteria, in *Computer ECG Analysis: Towards Standardization*, J.L. Willems, J.H. van Bemmel, and C. Zywietz, Editors. Amsterdam: North-Holland, 1986, pp. 177–182.

195. Doue, J.C., The role of artificial intelligence in standardizing ECG criteria, in *Computer ECG Analysis: Towards Standardization*, J.L. Willems, J.H. van Bemmel, and C. Zywietz, Editors. Amsterdam: North-Holland, 1986, pp. 53–57.

196. Matthes, T., G. Götsch, and C. Zywietz, Interactive analysis of statistical ECG diagnosis on an intelligent electrocardiograph. An expert system approach, in *Computer ECG Analysis: Towards Standardization*, J.L. Willems, J.H. van Bemmel, and C. Zywietz, Editors. Amsterdam: North-Holland, 1986, pp. 215–220.

197. Edenbrandt, L., B. Devine, and P.W. Macfarlane, Neural networks for classification of ECG ST-T segments. *J. Electrocardiol.*, 1992;**25**: 167–173.

198. Yang, T.F., B. Devine, and P.W. Macfarlane, Use of artificial neural networks within deterministic logic for the computer ECG diagnosis of inferior myocardial infarction. *J. Electrocardiol.*, 1994;**27**(Suppl): 188–193.

199. Kennedy, R.L., A.M. Burton, and R.F. Harrison, Neural networks and early diagnosis of myocardial infarction. *Lancet*, 1996;**347**: 407.

200. Hedén, B., H. Ohlin, R. Rittner, and L. Edenbrandt, Acute myocardial infarction detected in the 12-lead ECG by artificial neural networks. *Circulation*, 1997;**96**: 1798–1802.

201. Olsson, S.E., M. Ohlsson, H. Ohlin, and L. Edenbrandt, Neural networks—a diagnostic tool in acute myocardial infarction with concomitant left bundle branch block. *Clin. Physiol. Funct. Imaging*, 2002;**22**: 295–299.

202. Segall, H.N., The electrocardiogram and its interpretation: a study of reports by 20 physicians on a set of 100 electrocardiograms. *Can. Med. Assoc. J.*, 1960;**82**: 847–850.

203. Simonson, E., N. Tuna, and N. Okamoto, Diagnostic accuracy of the vectorcardiogram and electrocardiogram. A cooperative study. *Am. J. Cardiol.*, 1966;**17**: 829–878.

204. Willems, J.L., C. Abreu-Lima, P. Arnaud, J.H. van Bemmel, C. Brohet, R. Degani, et al., Effect of combining electrocardiographic interpretation results on diagnostic accuracy. *Eur. Heart J.*, 1988;**9**: 1348–1355.

205. Balda, R.A., A.G. Vallance, J.M. Luszcz, F.J. Stahlin, and G. Diller, ECL—a medically oriented ECG criteria language and other clinical research tools, in *Computers in Cardiology 1977*, H.G. Ostrow and K.L. Ripley, Editors. New York: IEEE Comput Soc, 1977, pp. 481–495.

206. Bruce, R.A. and S.R. Yarnall, Reliability and normal variations of computer analysis of Frank electrocardiogram by Smith-Hyde program (1968 version). *Am. J. Cardiol.*, 1972;**29**: 389–396.

207. Willems, J.L., C. Abreu-Lima, P. Arnaud, J.H. van Bemmel, C. Brohet, R. Degani, et al., The diagnostic performance of computer programs for the interpretation of electrocardiograms. *N. Engl. J. Med.*, 1991;**325**: 1767–1773.

208. Breiman, L., J.H. Friedman, R.A. Olshen, and C.J. Stone, *Classification and Regression Trees*. Belmont, CA: Wadsworth, 1984.

209. Kors, J.A. and A.L. Hoffmann, Induction of decision rules that fulfill user-specified performance requirements. *Pattern Recognit. Lett.*, 1997;**18**: 1187–1195.

210. Pipberger, H.V., R.A. Dunn, and J. Cornfield, First and second generation computer programs for diagnostic ECG and VCG classification, in *XIIth International Colloquium Vectorcardiographicum*, P. Rijlant, Editor. Brussels: Presses Académiques Européennes, 1972, pp. 431–439.

211. Willems, J.L. and J. Pardaens, Reproducibility of diagnostic results by a multivariate computer ECG analysis program (AVA 3.5). *Eur. J. Cardiol.*, 1977;**6**: 229–243.

212. Dunn, R.A., R. Babuska, J.M. Wojick, and H.V. Pipberger, Variation in probability levels in electrocardiographic diagnosis. *Comput. Biomed. Res.*, 1978;**11**: 41–49.

213. Cady, L.D., M.A. Woodbury, L.J. Tick, and M.M.A. Gertler, Method for electrocardiogram wave pattern estimation. Example: left ventricular hypertrophy. *Circ. Res.*, 1961;**9**: 1078–1082.

214. Kimura, E., Y. Mibukura, and A. Miura, Statistical diagnosis of electrocardiogram by theorem of Bayes. A preliminary report. *Jpn. Heart J.*, 1963;**4**: 469–488.

215. Young, T.Y. and W.H. Huggins, Computer analysis of electrocardiograms using a linear regression technique. *IEEE Trans. Biomed. Eng.*, 1964;**11**: 60–67.

216. Stark, L., J.F. Dickson, G.H. Whipple, and H. Horibe, Remote real-time diagnosis of clinical electrocardiograms by a digital computer system. *Ann. N.Y. Acad. Sci.*, 1965;**126**: 851–872.

217. Specht, D.F., Vectorcardiographic diagnosis using the polynomial discriminant method of pattern recognition. *IEEE Trans. Biomed. Eng.*, 1967;**14**: 90–95.

218. Yasui, S., M. Yokoi, Y. Watanabe, K. Nishijima, and S. Azuma, Computer diagnosis of electrocardiograms by means of the joint probability. *Jpn. Circ. J.*, 1968;**32**: 517–523.

219. Goldman, M.J. and H.V. Pipberger, Analysis of the orthogonal electrocardiogram and vectorcardiogram in ventricular conduction defects with and without myocardial infarction. *Circulation*, 1969;**39**: 243–250.

220. Kerr, A., A. Adicoff, J.D. Klingeman, and H.V. Pipberger, Computer analysis of the orthogonal electrocardiogram in pulmonary emphysema. *Am. J. Cardiol.*, 1970;**25**: 34–45.

221. Eddleman, E.E. and H.V. Pipberger, Computer analysis of the orthogonal electrocardiogram and vectorcardiogram in 1,002 patients with myocardial infarction. *Am. Heart J.*, 1971;**81**: 608–621.

222. Pipberger, H.V., ECG computer analysis: past, present and future, in *Computer ECG Analysis: Towards Standardization*, J.L. Willems, J.H. van Bemmel, and C. Zywietz, Editors. Amsterdam: North-Holland, 1986, pp. 3–10.

223. Brohet, C.R., A. Robert, C. Derwael, R. Fesler, M. Stijns, A. Vliers, et al., Computer interpretation of pediatric orthogonal electrocardiograms: statistical and deterministic classification methods. *Circulation*, 1984;**70**: 255–262.

224. Willems, J.L., E. Lesaffre, J. Pardaens, and D. de Schreye, Multivariate logistic classification of the standard 12- and 3-lead ECG, in *Computer ECG Analysis: Towards Standardization*, J.L.

Willems, J.H. van Bemmel, and C. Zywietz, Editors. Amsterdam: North-Holland, 1986, pp. 203–210.

225. Rios, J., F. Sandquist, D. Ramseth, R. Stratbucker, E. Drazen, and J. Hanmer, The quest for optimal electrocardiography. Tast force V: cost effectiveness of the electrocardiogram. *Am. J. Cardiol.*, 1978;**41**: 175–183.

226. Okajima, M., Current status and future optimization of computerized electrocardiography in Japan, in *Optimization of Computer ECG Processing*, H.K. Wolf and P.W. Macfarlane, Editors. Amsterdam: North-Holland, 1980, pp. 293–307.

227. Moorman, J.R., M.A. Hlatky, D.M. Eddy, and G.S. Wagner, The yield of the routine admission electrocardiogram. A study in a general medical service. *Ann. Intern. Med.*, 1985;**103**: 590–595.

228. Salerno, S.M., P.C. Alguire, and H.S. Waxman, Competency in interpretation of 12-lead electrocardiograms: a summary and appraisal of published evidence. *Ann. Intern. Med.*, 2003;**138**: 751–760.

229. Eisenstein, E.L., Conducting an economic analysis to assess the electrocardiogram's value. *J. Electrocardiol.*, 2006;**39**: 241–247.

230. Willems, J.L., C. Abreu-Lima, P. Arnaud, C.R. Brohet, B. Denis, J. Gehring, et al., Evaluation of ECG interpretation results obtained by computer and cardiologists. *Methods Inf. Med.*, 1990;**29**: 308–316.

231. Farb, A., R.B. Devereux, and P. Kligfield, Day-to-day variability of voltage measurements used in electrocardiographic criteria for left ventricular hypertrophy. *J. Am. Coll. Cardiol.*, 1990;**15**: 618–623.

232. van den Hoogen, J.P., W.H. Mol, A. Kowsoleea, J.W. van Ree, T. Thien, and C. van Weel, Reproducibility of electrocardiographic criteria for left ventricular hypertrophy in hypertensive patients in general practice. *Eur. Heart J.*, 1992;**13**: 1606–1610.

233. de Bruyne, M.C., J.A. Kors, S. Visentin, G. van Herpen, A.W. Hoes, D.E. Grobbee, et al., Reproducibility of computerized ECG measurements and coding in a nonhospitalized elderly population. *J. Electrocardiol.*, 1998;**31**: 189–195.

234. Bailey, J.J., M. Horton, S.B. Itscoitz, A method for evaluating computer programs for electrocardiographic interpretation. 3. Reproducibility testing and the sources of program errors. *Circulation*, 1974;**50**: 88–93.

235. Bailey, J.J., M. Horton, and S.B. Itscoitz, The importance of reproducibility testing of computer programs for electrocardiographic interpretation: application to the automatic vectorcardiographic analysis program (AVA 3.4). *Comput. Biomed. Res.*, 1976;**9**: 307–316.

236. Spodick, D.H. and R.L. Bishop, Computer treason: intraobserver variability of an electrocardiographic computer system. *Am. J. Cardiol.*, 1997;**80**: 102–103.

237. Michaelis, J., S. Wellek, and J.L. Willems, Reference standards for software evaluation. *Methods Inf. Med.*, 1990;**29**: 289–297.

238. Jakobsson, A., P. Ohlin, and O. Pahlm, Does a computer-based ECG-recorder interpret electrocardiograms more efficiently than physicians? *Clin. Physiol.*, 1985;**5**: 417–423.

239. Bernard, P., B.R. Chaitman, J.M. Scholl, P.G. Val, and M. Chabot, Comparative diagnostic performance of the Telemed computer ECG program. *J. Electrocardiol.*, 1983;**16**: 97–103.

240. Willems, J.L., Is human verification of computerized ECGs mandatory? *Adv. Cardiol.*, 1978;**21**: 193–194.

241. Chou, T.C., When is the vectorcardiogram superior to the scalar electrocardiogram? *J. Am. Coll. Cardiol.*, 1986;**8**: 791–799.

242. Kors, J.A., G. van Herpen, J.L. Willems, and J.H. van Bemmel, Improvement of automated electrocardiographic diagnosis by

combination of computer interpretations of the electrocardiogram and vectorcardiogram. *Am. J. Cardiol.*, 1992;**70**: 96–99.

243. Kors, J.A., G. van Herpen, and J.H. van Bemmel, Variability in ECG computer interpretation. Analysis of individual complexes vs analysis of a representative complex. *J. Electrocardiol.*, 1992;**25**: 263–271.

244. Andresen, A., J. Dobkin, C. Maynard, R. Myers, G.S. Wagner, R.A. Warner, et al., Validation of advanced ECG diagnostic software for the detection of prior myocardial infarction by using nuclear cardiac imaging. *J. Electrocardiol.*, 2001;**34**(Suppl): 243–248.

245. Andresen, A., M.D. Gasperina, R. Myers, G.S. Wagner, R.A. Warner, and R.H. Selvester, An improved automated ECG algorithm for detecting acute and prior myocardial infarction. *J. Electrocardiol.*, 2002;**35**(Suppl): 105–110.

246. Wagner, G.S., C. Maynard, A. Andresen, E. Anderson, R. Myers, R.A. Warner, et al., Evaluation of advanced electrocardiographic diagnostic software for detection of prior myocardial infarction. *Am. J. Cardiol.*, 2002;**89**: 75–79.

247. Milliken, J.A., H. Pipberger, H.V. Pipberger, M.A. Araoye, R. Ari, G.W. Burggraf, et al., The impact of an ECG computer analysis program on the cardiologist's interpretation. A cooperative study. *J. Electrocardiol.*, 1983;**16**: 141–149.

248. Hillson, S.D., D.P. Connelly, and Y. Liu, The effects of computer-assisted electrocardiographic interpretation on physicians' diagnostic decisions. *Med. Decis. Making*, 1995;**15**: 107–112.

249. Brailer, D.J., E. Kroch, and M.V. Pauly, The impact of computer-assisted test interpretation on physician decision making: the case of electrocardiograms. *Med. Decis. Making*, 1997;**17**: 80–86.

250. Goodacre, S., A. Webster, and F. Morris, Do computer generated ECG reports improve interpretation by accident and emergency senior house officers? *Postgrad. Med. J.*, 2001;**77**: 455–457.

251. Tsai, T.L., D.B. Fridsma, and G. Gatti, Computer decision support as a source of interpretation error: the case of electrocardiograms. *J. Am. Med. Inform. Assoc.*, 2003;**10**: 478–483.

252. Laks, M.M. and R.H. Selvester, Computerized electrocardiography – an adjunct to the physician. *N. Engl. J. Med.*, 1991;**325**: 1803–1804.

253. Plokker, H.W.M., *Cardiac Rhythm Diagnosis by Digital Computer*, dissertation. Amsterdam: Free University, 1978.

254. Reddy, S., B. Young, Q. Xue, B. Taha, D. Brodnick, and J. Steinberg, Review of methods to predict and detect atrial fibrillation in post-cardiac surgery patients. *J. Electrocardiol.*, 1999;**32**(Suppl): 23–28.

255. Poon, K., P.M. Okin, and P. Kligfield, Diagnostic performance of a computer-based ECG rhythm algorithm. *J. Electrocardiol.*, 2005;**38**: 235–238.

256. Bonner, R.E. and H.D. Schwetman, Computer diagnosis of electrocardiograms. 3. A computer program for arrhythmia diagnosis. *Comput. Biomed. Res.*, 1968;**1**: 387–407.

257. Bonner, R.E., IBM rhythm analysis program, in *Computer Application on ECG and VCG Analysis*, C. Zywietz and B. Schneider, Editors. Amsterdam: North-Holland, 1973, pp. 375–397.

258. Wartak, J., J.A. Milliken, and J. Karchmar, Computer program for diagnostic evaluation of electrocardiograms. *Comput. Biomed. Res.*, 1971;**4**: 225–238.

259. Brohet, C., C. Derwael, R. Fesler, and L.A. Brasseur, Arrhythmia analysis by the Louvain VCG program, in *Computers in Cardiology*, K.L. Ripley, Editor. Los Angeles: IEEE Comput Soc, 1982, pp. 47–51.

260. Shirataka, M., H. Miyahara, N. Ikeda, A. Domae, and T. Sato, Evaluation of five computer programs in the diagnosis of second-degree AV block. *J. Electrocardiol.*, 1992;**25**: 185–195.

261. Thomson, A., S. Mitchell, and P.J. Harris, Computerized electrocardiographic interpretation: an analysis of clinical utility in 5110 electrocardiograms. *Med. J. Aust.*, 1989;**151**: 428–430.

262. Reddy, B.R., B. Taha, S. Swiryn, R. Silberman, and R. Childers, Prospective evaluation of a microprocessor-assisted cardiac rhythm algorithm: results from one clinical center. *J. Electrocardiol.*, 1998;**30**(Suppl): 28–33.

263. Farrell, R.M., J.Q. Xue, and B.J. Young, Enhanced rhythm analysis for resting ECG using spectral and time-domain techniques, in *Computers in Cardiology*, A. Murray, Editor. Piscataway, NJ: IEEE Comput Soc, 2003, pp. 733–736.

264. Guglin, M.E. and D. Thatai, Common errors in computer electrocardiogram interpretation. *Int. J. Cardiol.*, 2006;**106**: 232–237.

265. Pryor, T.A., A.E. Lindsay, and R.W. England, Computer analysis of serial electrocardiograms. *Comput. Biomed. Res.*, 1972;**5**: 709–714.

266. Macfarlane, P.W., H.T. Cawood, and T.D. Lawrie, A basis for computer interpretation of interpretation of serial electrocardiograms. *Comput. Biomed. Res.*, 1975;**8**: 189–200.

267. Bonner, R.E., L. Crevasse, M.I. Ferrer, and J.C. Greenfield, A new computer program for comparative analysis of serial scalar electrocardiograms: description and performance of the 1976 IBM program. *Comput. Biomed. Res.*, 1978;**11**: 103–118.

268. Schnyders, H.C. and G.A. Kien, Computer-assisted serial comparison of ECGs: the Telemed version, in *Computer Application in Medical Care*, R.A. Dunn, Editor. New York: IEEE Comput Soc, 1979, pp. 652–659.

269. Rubel, P., J. Fayn, J.L. Willems, and C. Zywietz, New trends in serial ECG analysis. *J. Electrocardiol.*, 1993;**26**(Suppl): 122–128.

270. Rubel, P., J. Fayn, G. Nollo, D. Assanelli, B. Li, L. Restier, et al, Toward personal eHealth in cardiology. Results from the EPI-MEDICS telemedicine project. *J. Electrocardiol.*, 2005;**38**(Suppl): 100–106.

271. Willems, J.L., P.F. Poblete, and H.V. Pipberger, Day-to-day variation of the normal orthogonal electrocardiogram and vectorcardiogram. *Circulation*, 1972;**45**: 1057–1064.

272. de Bruyne, M.C., J.A. Kors, S. Visentin, G. van Herpen, A.W. Hoes, D.E. Grobbee, et al., Reproducibility of computerized ECG measurements and coding in a nonhospitalized elderly population. *J. Electrocardiol.*, 1998;**31**: 189–195.

273. Schijvenaars, B.J., *Intra-individual Variability of the Electrocardiogram*, dissertation. Rotterdam: Erasmus University, 2000.

274. Pipberger, H.V., R.A. Dunn, and H.A. Pipberger, Automated comparison of serial electrocardiograms. *Adv. Cardiol.*, 1976;**16**: 157–165.

275. Rubel, P., N. Saccal, J.L. Sourrouille, and M.C. Forlini, Multidimensional techniques for the optimal display of trends in sequential vectorcardiograms, in *Medinfo 1980*, D.A.B. Lindberg and S. Kaihara, Editors. Amsterdam: North-Holland, 1980, p. 274.

276. Zywietz, C., B. Widiger, and R. Fischer, A system for comprehensive comparison of serial ECG beats and serial ECG recordings, in *Computers in Cardiology*, A. Murray, Editor. Piscataway, NJ: IEEE Comput Soc, 2003, pp. 689–692.

277. Hedstrom, K. and P.W. Macfarlane, Development of a new approach to serial analysis. The manufacturer's viewpoint. *J. Electrocardiol.*, 1996;**29**(Suppl): 35–40.

278. McLaughlin, S.C., T.C. Aitchison, and P.W. Macfarlane, Methods for improving the repeatability of automated ECG analysis. *Methods Inf. Med.*, 1995;**34**: 272–282.

279. McLaughlin, S.C., P. Chishti, T.C. Aitchison, and P.W. Macfarlane, Techniques for improving overall consistency of serial ECG analysis. *J. Electrocardiol.*, 1996;**29**(Suppl): 41–45.

280. Fayn, J. and P. Rubel, CAVIAR: a serial ECG processing system for the comparative analysis of VCGs and their interpretation with auto-reference to the patient. *J. Electrocardiol.*, 1988;**21**(Suppl): S173–S176.

281. Sunemark, M., L. Edenbrandt, H. Holst, and L. Sörnmo, Serial VCG/ECG analysis using neural networks. *Comput. Biomed. Res.*, 1998;**31**: 59–69.

282. Bonner, R.E., L. Crevasse, M.I. Ferrer, and J.C. Greenfield, The influence of editing on the performance of a computer program for serial comparison of electrocardiograms. *J. Electrocardiol.*, 1983;**16**: 181–189.

283. van Haelst, A.C., D.K. Donker, F.C. Visser, C.C. de Cock, A. Hasman, and J.L. Talmon, A computer program for the analysis of serial electrocardiograms from patients who suffered a myocardial infarction. *Int. J. Biomed. Comput.*, 1985;**17**: 273–284.

284. Ohlsson, M., H. Ohlin, S.M. Wallerstedt, and L. Edenbrandt, Usefulness of serial electrocardiograms for diagnosis of acute myocardial infarction. *Am. J. Cardiol.*, 2001;**88**: 478–481.

285. Schwartz, P.J., A. Garson, T. Paul, M. Stramba-Badiale, V.L. Vetter, and C. Wren, Guidelines for the interpretation of the neonatal electrocardiogram. A task force of the European Society of Cardiology. *Eur. Heart J.*, 2002;**23**: 1329–1344.

286. Dickinson, D.F., The normal ECG in childhood and adolescence. *Heart*, 2005;**91**: 1626–1630.

287. Davignon, A., P.M. Rautaharju, E. Boisselle, F. Soumis, M. Megelas, and A. Choquette, Normal ECG standards for infants and children. *Pediatr. Cardiol.*, 1979/80;**1**: 123–131.

288. Brohet, C.R., C. Hoeven, A. Robert, C. Derwael, R. Fesler, and L.A. Brasseur, The normal pediatric Frank orthogonal electrocardiogram: variations according to age and sex. *J. Electrocardiol.*, 1986;**19**: 1–13.

289. Perry, L.W., H.V. Pipberger, H.A. Pipberger, C.D. McManus, and L.P. Scott, Scalar, planar, and spatial measurements of the Frank vectorcardiogram in normal infants and children. *Am. Heart J.*, 1986;**111**: 721–730.

290. Macfarlane, P.W., E.N. Coleman, E.O. Pomphrey, S. McLaughlin, A. Houston, and T. Aitchison, Normal limits of the high-fidelity pediatric ECG. Preliminary observations. *J. Electrocardiol.*, 1989;**22**(Suppl): 162–168.

291. Macfarlane, P.W., S.C. McLaughlin, B. Devine, and T.F. Yang, Effects of age, sex, and race on ECG interval measurements. *J. Electrocardiol.*, 1994;**27**(Suppl): 14–19.

292. Rijnbeek, P.R., M. Witsenburg, E. Schrama, J. Hess, and J.A. Kors, New normal limits for the paediatric electrocardiogram. *Eur. Heart J.*, 2001;**22**: 702–711.

293. Horton, L.A., S. Mosee, and J. Brenner, Use of the electrocardiogram in a pediatric emergency department. *Arch. Pediatr. Adolesc. Med.*, 1994;**148**: 184–188.

294. Hamilton, R.M., K. McLeod, A.B. Houston, and P.W. Macfarlane, Inter- and intraobserver variability in LVH and RVH reporting in pediatric ECGs. *Ann. Noninvasive Electrocardiol.*, 2005;**10**: 330–333.

295. Guller, B., P.C. O'Brien, R.E. Smith, W.H. Weidman, and J.W. DuShane, Computer interpretation of Frank vectorcardiograms in normal infants: longitudinal and cross-sectional observations from birth to 2 years of age. *J. Electrocardiol.*, 1975;**8**: 201–208.

296. Guller, B., F.Y. Lau, R.A. Dunn, H.A. Pipberger, and H.V. Pipberger, Computer analysis of changes in Frank vectorcardiograms of 666 normal infants in the first 72 hours of life. *J. Electrocardiol.*, 1977;**10**: 19–26.

297. Francis, D.B., B.L. Miller, and D.W. Benson, A new computer program for the analysis of pediatric scalar electrocardiograms. *Comput. Biomed. Res.*, 1981;**14**: 63–77.

298. Laks, M.M., A computer program for interpretation of infant and children electrocardiograms, in *Computer ECG Analysis: Towards Standardization*, J.L. Willems, J.H. van Bemmel, and C. Zywietz, Editors. Amsterdam: North-Holland, 1986, pp. 59–65.

299. Macfarlane, P.W., E.N. Coleman, B. Devine, A. Houston, S. McLaughlin, T.C. Aitchison, et al., A new 12-lead pediatric ECG interpretation program. *J. Electrocardiol.*, 1990;**23**(Suppl): 76–81.

300. Rijnbeek, P.R., M. Witsenburg, A. Szatmari, J. Hess, and J.A. Kors, PEDMEANS: a computer program for the interpretation of pediatric electrocardiograms. *J. Electrocardiol.*, 2001;**34**(Suppl): 85–91.

301. Zhou, S.H., J. Liebman, A.M. Dubin, P.C. Gillette, R.E. Gregg, E.D. Helfenbein, et al., Using 12-lead ECG and synthesized VCG in detection of right ventricular hypertrophy with terminal right conduction delay versus partial right bundle branch block in the pediatric population. *J. Electrocardiol.*, 2001;**34**(Suppl): 249–257.

302. Guller, B., T. Jones, J. McCloskey, and S.P. Herndon, The Hewlett-Packard pediatric ECG computer program (HP-P3) and independent clinical information. *J. Electrocardiol.*, 1990;**23**(Suppl): 204.

303. Hamilton, R.M., A.B. Houston, K. McLeod, and P.W. Macfarlane, Evaluation of pediatric electrocardiogram diagnosis of ventricular hypertrophy by computer program compared with cardiologists. *Pediatr. Cardiol.*, 2005;**26**: 373–378.

304. Snyder, C.S., A.L. Fenrich, R.A. Friedman, C. Macias, K. O'Reilly, and N.J. Kertesz, The emergency department versus the computer: which is the better electrocardiographer? *Pediatr. Cardiol.*, 2003;**24**: 364–368.

6 Pacemaker Electrocardiography

Thomas Fåhraeus

P. W. Macfarlane et al. (eds.), *Specialized Aspects of ECG*, DOI 10.1007/978-0-85729-880-5_6,
© Springer-Verlag London Limited 2012

6.1   Introduction

When artificial cardiac stimulation was introduced in 1958 as a permanent treatment for bradycardia, the interpretation of pacemaker ECGs posed little difficulty. The indication for pacemaker implantation at that time was total atrioventricular block, and the available pacemaker systems provided fixed-rate ventricular stimulation (❯ Fig. 6.1). Today multiprogrammable pacemaker devices are available with many different pacing modes, sophisticated functions, and diagnostic tools. Pacing during various arrhythmias creates ECG recordings which are sometimes rather difficult to analyze, and nowadays there are many methods for performing an evaluation of the pacemaker function other than looking at a standard surface ECG. To perform a comprehensive examination, an appropriate pacemaker programmer is sometimes necessary where the initial interrogation will allow retrieval of programmed settings and diagnostic data. The ECG (usually both surface ECG and intracardiac electrograms) monitoring capability simultaneously with telemetry event markers on the display facilitates the interpretation.

In this chapter, the basic principles of the interpretation of pacemaker ECGs will be presented, first concerning normal pacemaker function and thereafter concerning malfunction and pseudomalfunction. Most of the ECG recordings have been selected from the daily clinical work at the Skåne University Hospital, Lund, Sweden, and the intention is to provide a survey of the field of pacemaker ECG. Questions concerning the choice of the stimulation mode and clinical application have to be referred to text books dealing with pacemaker treatment.

The different pacing modes used are identified according to the recommendations of the 1987 NASPE and NASPE/BPEG codes. The original three-position letter code (since 1974) was revised to a five-position code in 1981, and has subsequently been expanded further in 2002 (❯ Table 6.1). Usually, the first three letters are used, for example, VVI, DDD, AAI, VDD, etc., but today most pulse generators have a built-in sensor for rate modulation. When this function is activated, the code will be VVIR, DDDR, AAIR, and so on. The use of the letter code facilitates rapid acquisition of information about the programmed basic mode of the pacemaker and how it is pacing and sensing the heart.

6.2   Registration of Pacemaker Impulses

Pacemaker impulses should be clearly visible in the ECG tracings and are commonly called "spikes." An ECG recording of good quality facilitates correct interpretation of pacemaker performance. The typical standard pacemaker ECGs recorded when the lead tip is in the apex area of the right ventricle show broad QRS complexes with an LBBB pattern. New modes with different pacing sites have in some cases changed the QRS morphology. The print-out with data and ECG -markers from a programmer are very useful when difficult and problematic ECG's occur (❯ Figs. 6.2 and ❯ 6.3).

The reproduction of the pacemaker spikes is influenced by many factors. One of the most important is the use of the interference filter of the ECG recorder (❯ Fig. 6.4). While the amplitude of the spikes is huge in unipolar systems, much less stimulus artifact can be seen on the recording when a bipolar lead is used with anode and cathode only about a centimeter apart (❯ Fig. 6.5). Furthermore, the spike amplitude is related to the actual pulse generator output as demonstrated by the example in ❯ Fig. 6.6, where the energy content of the pacemaker impulse is temporarily reduced to 10% for test purposes. The spike amplitude and vector orientation when dealing with unipolar systems are dependent on the choice of ECG lead and the position of the pulse generator (❯ Fig. 6.7).

Digital ECG recorders are responsible for additional variation of the spike amplitude. If the sampling interval is 4 ms, ordinary pacemaker impulses of 0.2–0.5 ms duration may not be registered consistently, resulting in the changes of their reproduction (❯ Fig. 6.8). The variation of the spike amplitude may easily be misinterpreted as a lead or stimulation problem. This can partly be circumvented by sampling the signal at a much higher rate; for example, every 0.25 ms.

6.3   Relationship Between the Stimulation Impulse and Cardiac Activity

In most transvenous ventricular pacing systems with only one electrode, the lead tip is usually positioned in the right ventricle, and during stimulation the ECG will show a left bundle branch block pattern. If the lead tip is located close to the ventricular septum or is positioned on the left ventricle with an epicardial technique, a right bundle branch block pattern will be produced (❯ Fig. 6.9).

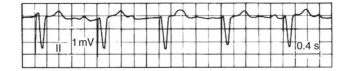

Fig. 6.1

Continual asynchronous ventricular pacing at a rate of 60 bpm in the presence of complete AV block. A left bundle block pattern with wide QRS complexes appears due to stimulation first of the right ventricle and then the left

Table 6.1

The revised NASPBE/BPEG generic code for antibradycardia, adaptive rate, and multisite pacing. Pace, 25(2), 260–264, February 2002

I What is stimulated?	II What is sensed?	III Reaction to sensing	IV Rate modulation	V Multisite pacing
0 = None	0 = None	0 = None	0 = None	0 = None
A = Atrium	A = Atrium	T = Triggered	R = Rate	A = Atrium
V = Ventricle	V = Ventricle	I = Inhibited	Modulation	V = Ventricle
D = Dual (A + V)	D = Dual (A + V)	D = Dual (T + I)		D = Dual (A + V)
S = Single	S = Single			
(A or V)	(A or V)			

The simultaneous occurrence of spontaneous cardiac activity and pacemaker impulses is not uncommon. When the endocardium close to the lead tip is already depolarized spontaneously, the pacemaker impulse will not affect the myocardium. However, the ECG will be distorted by the spike, a phenomenon referred to as a pseudofusion beat. If parts of the myocardium are depolarized by intrinsic activity while others are activated by the pacemaker impulse, fusion beats will occur. When the spontaneous heart rate and the basic stimulation rate are almost the same, fusion and pseudofusion beats are commonly seen (❷ Fig. 6.10).

In atrial pacing, intermittent ventricular extrasystoles may result in a confusing ECG when the atrial spike is followed by a QRS complex, referred to as a pseudopseudofusion beat (❷ Fig. 6.11). Tachycardia-terminating pacemakers provide additional variation to the relationship between spikes and the PQRS complexes; for example, during the termination of reentry tachycardias with rapid overdrive pacing with short sequences (bursts) of stimuli. In ❷ Sect. 6.10, there are more examples of tachycardia treatment (❷ Fig. 6.12).

6.4 The ECG Appearance of Different Pacing Modes

One of the most commonly used modes is VVI pacing, which comprises ventricular stimulation and inhibition. A VVI pacemaker operates with two timing circuitries; the basic rate counter and the technical refractory period, both of which are initiated either by stimulation or sensing events. Possible ECG combinations are demonstrated in the timing diagram shown in ❷ Fig. 6.13. The basic rate interval in a VVI pulse generator is programmable. When the pulse generator detects ventricular depolarization within the basic interval, stimulation will be inhibited and a new basic interval will start (❷ Fig. 6.14).

In the VVT mode, instead of inhibition, the pulse generator delivers an impulse triggered by the QRS complex during the refractory period, thereby leaving the spontaneous depolarization unaffected (❷ Fig. 6.15). This pacing mode is very seldom used but can be useful when sensing problems occur (inhibition is avoided).

A sensing event followed by either inhibition (VVI) or triggering (VVT) occurs when the intracardiac signal reaches a certain amplitude at the site of the electrode. Sometimes the intrinsic deflection of this signal coincides with the beginning of the QRS complex in the surface ECG. Whether or not ectopic ventricular activity causes inhibition of a VVI pulse

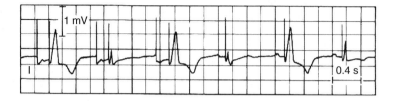

◙ Fig. 6.2
Dual-chamber pacing and sensing (DDD) during second-degree AV block. The basic rate and intrinsic atrial rate are almost the same, which explains the additional variations of the QRS-T morphology

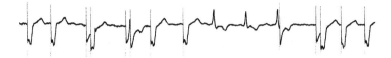

◙ Fig. 6.3
To interpret this ECG from a patient with a DDD pacemaker, a pacemaker programmer is very useful. Parameters such as rate, AV interval, and modes can be changed, diagnostic marker tools are available

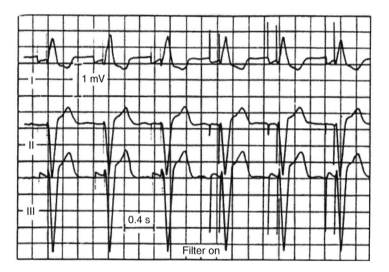

◙ Fig. 6.4
DDD pacing recorded without and with an interference filter. As the spike recording is more clearly seen with the low-pass filter switched on, it is recommended for routine use

generator depends on the duration of the refractory period (❯ Fig. 6.16). Multiprogrammable pulse generators offer a selection of different refractory periods.

Variation in the rate, because of different timing intervals, is provided in pulse generators where the hysteresis function has been activated. Without hysteresis, the automatic basic interval is equal to the escape interval. With hysteresis, the basic rate interval is constant during stimulation, but after an inhibition the escape interval is prolonged. Thus, a pulse generator with a fixed or programmable hysteresis function operates with an inhibition rate lower than the basic stimulation rate (❯ Fig. 6.17).

Atrial pacing (AAIR) is achieved in a manner quite similar to ventricular pacing. Reliable AV conduction is, however, essential for the use of atrial pacing (❯ Fig. 6.18). As the amplitude of the atrial signal is considerably lower than the corresponding QRS signal in ventricular sensing, the sensitivity of an AAI device must be high enough to allow correct sensing.

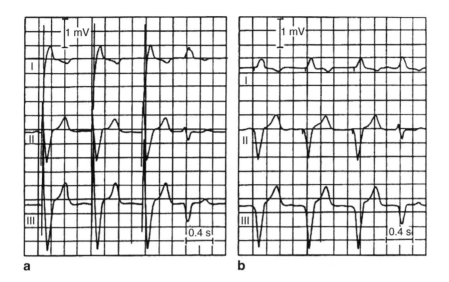

Fig. 6.5

Unipolar pacing to the left (a) compared with bipolar (b) ventricular pacing through the same electrode system, which was achieved by means of a pulse generator with programmable polarity

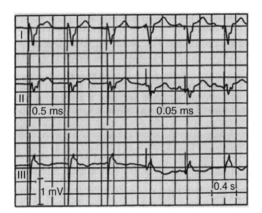

Fig. 6.6

Unipolar ventricular pacing, during an automatic stimulation threshold test with reduction of impulse duration from 0.5 to 0.05 ms. Note the change of spike configuration. The output pulse corresponds to the spike on the ECG

6.5   Dual-Chamber Pacing

The expression *dual-chamber pacing* is used to describe a pacing modality capable of delivering pacing stimuli to two chambers, usually the atrium and the ventricle (DOO, DDD, DDI, and DVI). During the last few years, the term *biventricular pacing* has been used to indicate cardiac resynchronization of the ventricles in heart failure. It is easy to be confused by the terms; resynchronization will be described later in this chapter. In the DVI mode, the stimulation of the atria is followed by ventricular pacing after a technical AV delay. As there is no sensing in the atria, a DVI pulse generator may only be inhibited by intrinsic ventricular activity. Atrial stimulation occurs at the programmed basic rate as long as the pulse generator is not inhibited by spontaneous ventricular beats (❯ Fig. 6.19).

In the VDD mode, atrial sensing is followed by synchronous ventricular stimulation, but without the possibility of stimulating the atria during sinus bradycardia (❯ Fig. 6.20). Ventricular inhibition is accomplished when spontaneous QRS complexes are sensed during the AV delay (❯ Fig. 6.21). Ectopic beats sensed after the end of the technical refractory

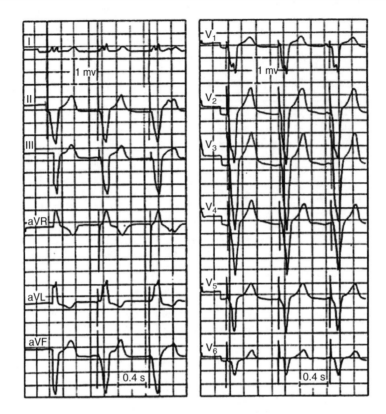

◘ Fig. 6.7
The vector orientation and amplitude of the spikes are depended on placement of the pulse generator and the ECG electrodes. The illustration is an example of unipolar right ventricular pacing with the pacemaker pocket located in the left pectoral region

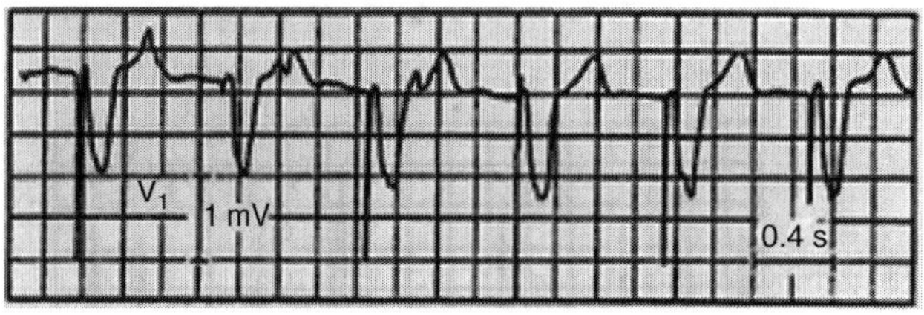

◘ Fig. 6.8
A digital ECG recording of unipolar ventricular pacing. The variation in the spike amplitude is caused by the digital sampling technique of this particular ECG recorder

period may also cause inhibition and resetting of the basic rate interval. The disadvantages of only ventricular stimulation in the absence of spontaneous atrial activity make the VDD mode less attractive from a clinical point of view. The VDD mode is still available as a programmable mode in DDD pulse generators.

In the DDD mode, the pulse generator operates with sensing and stimulation of both the atrial and the ventricular chambers depending on the presence or absence of spontaneous cardiac activity and the programmed time intervals. Thus, it presents a functional combination of AAI, VAT, and VVI principles. The coincidence between dual-chamber pacing and the occurrence of spontaneous atrial and/or ventricular activity can cause many different ECG morphologies, including atrial and ventricular fusion or pseudofusion beats.

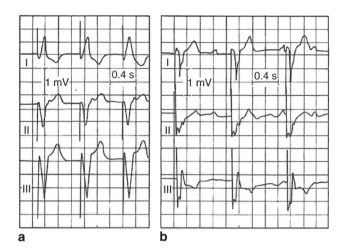

■ Fig. 6.9

(a) Unipolar pacing through a transvenous right ventricular lead resembles a left bundle branch block (LBBB) pattern. (b) Left ventricular stimulation through a myocardial screw-in electrode produces a right bundle branch block (RBBB) pattern

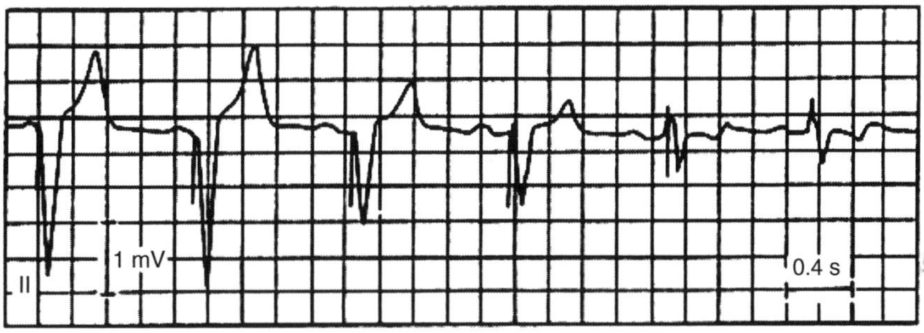

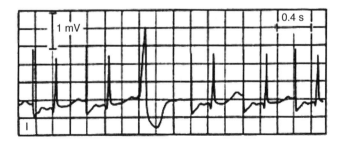

■ Fig. 6.10

Unipolar ventricular-inhibited pacing demonstrating the difference between pacemaker-induced QRS complexes (QRS complexes #1 and #2) and different degrees of fusion beats (QRS complexes #3 and #4) caused by simultaneous depolarization via stimulation and normal AV conduction. The T-wave configuration in complex #5 indicates a spontaneously induced depolarization together with an ineffective pacemaker spike – a pseudofusion beat

■ Fig. 6.11

Atrial pacing at a rate of 100 min⁻¹. A ventricular ectopic beat (complex #3) coincides with an atrial spike producing a pseudopseudofusion beat

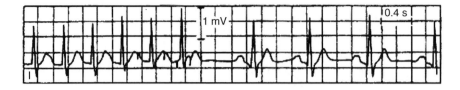

☐ Fig. 6.12

Atrial bipolar burst stimulation (300 min⁻¹) terminating a supraventricular tachycardia. The spikes in the burst sequence are clearly visible

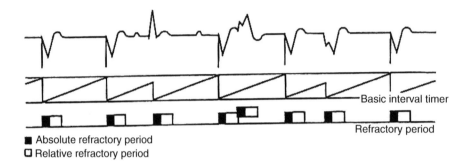

☐ **Fig. 6.13**

Schematic ECG illustration demonstrating the operation of the basic interval timer and the refractory period. In this example the refractory period is programmed to 312 ms. The absolute refractory period is 125 ms and the relative refractory period is thus 187 ms. A conducted ventricular complex which occurs during the relative refractory period (noise-sampling period) does not accomplish inhibition, that is, does not reset the basic interval timer, but restarts a new refractory period, as in the case of complex #5

☐ Fig. 6.14

Ventricular-inhibited pacing (VVI mode) at a programmed rate of 70 min⁻¹. Inhibition will occur as soon as a spontaneous QRS complex at a higher rate occurs, as in this case

The resulting ECG appearance is even more confusing when spontaneous AV conduction varies intermittently (❂ Fig. 6.22). Furthermore, the ECG appearance may be altered by different AV delay settings in the presence of AV conduction (❂ Fig. 6.23). It is of clinical interest to have a long AV delay to support possible AV conduction and a normal activation of the ventricles. There are functions in pacemakers that automatically test the AV delay looking for intrinsic conduction and prolong the technical AV delay if the AV conduction is acceptable. During the last few years, the negative effects in some patients have been documented by long-term stimulation through the apex lead with an LBBB pattern. This electrical asynchrony can result in heart failure and in some cases a biventricular (❂ Sect. 6.9) pacemaker system will be implanted.

Pathological atrial tachycardia or sensing interference may trigger DDD pulse generators to high rates. In order to avoid unacceptable fast-triggered ventricular pacing, different solutions for rate limitations have been introduced,

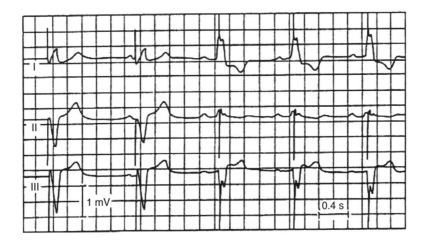

◘ Fig. 6.15

The ventricular-triggered pacing (VVT mode) at a basic rate of 50 min⁻¹ followed by sinus rhythm at a higher rate (60 min⁻¹), and triggered ventricular spikes (pseudofusion beats)

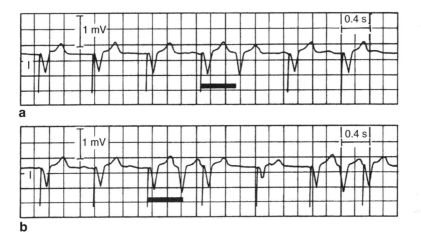

◘ Fig. 6.16

Ventricular pacing in the VVI mode at a rate of 80 min⁻¹. Ventricular ectopic beats accomplish inhibition as in (a) only if they occur after the end of the technical refractory period, denoted here by a horizontal bar. Early ectopic beats in (b) are ignored because the technical refractory period is 500 ms in this case

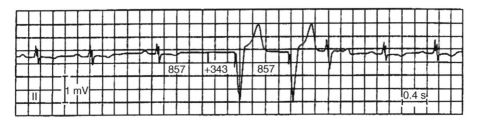

◘ Fig. 6.17

VVI pacing with a programmed basic rate of 70 min⁻¹ and an activated hysteresis function. After an inhibition, a hysteresis delay of 343 ms is added to the basic rate interval of 857 ms thus permitting a slower intrinsic rhythm by consistent inhibition of the pulse generator. Lack of spontaneous rhythm is followed by stimulation at the programmed basic rate until a new inhibition occurs

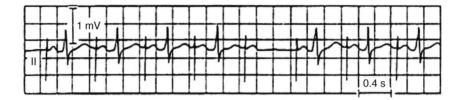

■ Fig. 6.18

Atrial pacing at a programmed rate increased to 100 min⁻¹ for test purposes. While consistent atrial capture can be seen, a blocked P wave indicates unreliable AV conduction

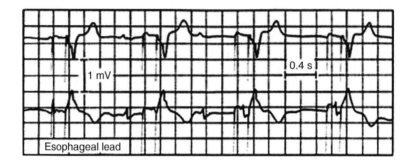

■ Fig. 6.19

Dual-chamber stimulation (DVI mode) at a rate of 50 min⁻¹ in the presence of AV block, and an intrinsic atrial rate of approximately 60 bpm. The esophageal ECG clearly indicates the asynchronous atrial stimulation owing to the lack of atrial sensing in a DVI pulse generator. Esophageal recordings are not used so often nowadays, due to availability of atrial electrograms

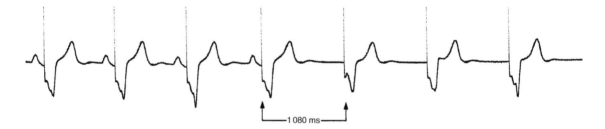

■ Fig. 6.20

The basic function of a VDD pulse generator. In the absence of triggering P waves during sinus arrest or bradycardia, compensation by basic rate stimulation is achieved (The time interval is 1 080 ms)

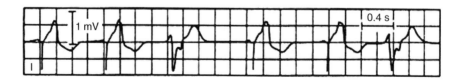

■ Fig. 6.21

Atrial-triggered ventricular stimulation combined with ventricular inhibition (VDD mode). Every P wave is followed by ventricular pacing unless an ectopic beat inhibits the system. Hence, a spontaneous or retrograde P wave within the ectopic ventricular beat cannot initiate a new triggering

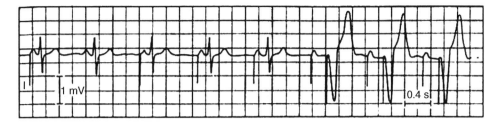

▣ Fig. 6.22
Dual-chamber pacing in the DDD mode at a basic rate of 70 min^{-1} alternating with sinus rhythm at a somewhat faster rate. As long as the AV conduction is normal, inhibition of the ventricular output is accomplished (complexes 1–5), but atrial activation is followed by ventricular pacing during impaired AV conduction (complexes 6–8)

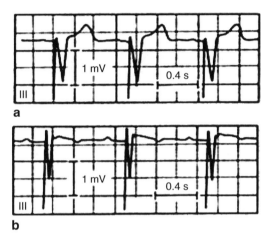

▣ Fig. 6.23
Atrial-triggered ventricular stimulation in the same patient as in ❷ Fig. 6.22, but with different technical AV delay settings. In the ECG shown in (a), the AV delay is 100 ms followed by typical pacemaker-induced ventricular complexes, while in the ECG in (b), a delay of 200 ms permits AV conduction resulting in pseudofusion beats

for example, the technical Wenckebach behavior shown in ❷ Fig. 6.24. In atrial fibrillation, the amplitude and the configuration of the intrinsic fibrillation waves may intermittently be too low to be sensed by the atrial amplifier.

If too many high-frequency signals are detected, the pulse generator converts to basic rate stimulation (interference rate stimulation) as a protective countermeasure (❷ Fig. 6.25).

It is therefore impossible to provide a complete survey of all conceivable ECG appearances regarding all different technical solutions, program settings, and changes in the intrinsic cardiac activity (❷ Fig. 6.26).

6.6   Diagnostic Tools

Earlier, standard ECG registration remained the main tool for the evaluation of the pacemaker function. However, complete information about a particular pacemaker system and its function today requires the use of a pacemaker programmer.

Measures have to be taken for assessment of possible stimulation response. Most pulse generators can be converted to fixed-rate stimulation by the application of a magnet. Different manufacturers have chosen different features of the magnet test response. The magnet test rate can be the same as the programmed basic rate (❷ Fig. 6.27a). As long as interference between the intrinsic rhythm and pacemaker stimulation is followed by pseudofusion beats, no conclusion

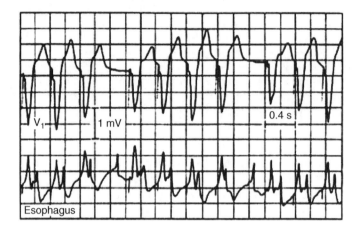

⬛ Fig. 6.24

Atrial-triggered ventricular stimulation (DDD mode) at the highest synchronous rate. Esophageal registration discloses an atrial tachycardia, which runs at a rate of 175 bpm, while ventricular stimulation is running at 160 min^{-1} (the highest synchronous rate) resulting in repetitive Wenckebach block

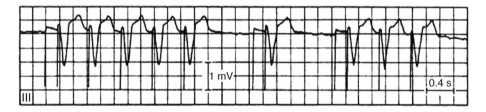

⬛ Fig. 6.25

Atrial-triggered ventricular stimulation (DDD mode) running at different rates alternating with basic rate stimulation. This is a typical example of the impact of atrial fibrillation on a DDD pacemaker system without automatic mode switch when atrial fibrillation occurs

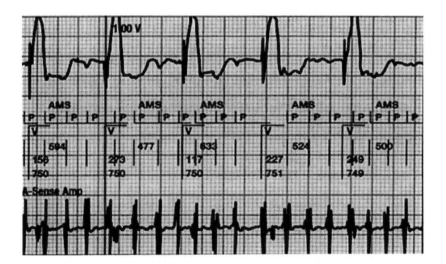

⬛ Fig. 6.26

Print out from a pacemaker programmer with markers and intracardiac recordings. The intracardiac atrial ECG at the bottom reveals atrial fibrillation during DDDR pacing, but the rate of the ventricles is normal. The adequate sensing of the fibrillation waves results in an automatic mode shift (AMS) to DDIR pacing

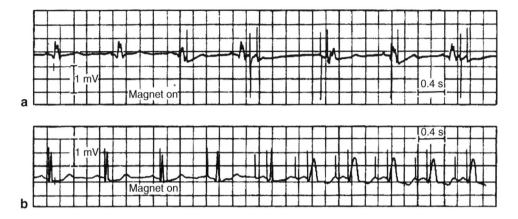

◻ Fig. 6.27

Two examples of DDD pacing in the presence of inhibiting atrial rates followed by normal AV conduction, which causes either inhibition of the ventricular output or pseudofusion beats. In (a), magnet application reverts the pulse generator to asynchronous stimulation (DOO) at the programmed basic rate. The interference between intrinsic activity and pacemaker stimulation produces pseudofusion beats without diagnostic information. In (b), the magnet test rate of 100 min^{-1} overdrives both spontaneous atrial activity and conducted ventricular beats thus providing information about atrial and ventricular capture

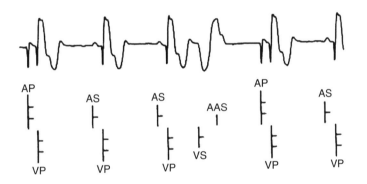

◻ Fig. 6.28

An early pacemaker example of the first markers of intracardiac ECG complexes. Dual-chamber pacing and simultaneous display of marker pulses indicating alternation between atrial pacing (*AP*), atrial sensing (*AS*), ventricular pacing (*VP*), ventricular sensing (*VS*), and abolished atrial sensing (*AAS*) after ventricular sensing of an ectopic beat

can be drawn about capture. Magnet tests running at higher rates facilitate the clinical investigation when overdrive suppression is accomplished (❷ Fig. 6.27b).

Besides the assessment of stimulation response, the magnet test rate also reflects information about the battery condition. Today, telemetric data about the condition of the battery is a more reliable method of controlling the expected lifetime of the battery. Once more, it is necessary to emphasise the individual nature of the technical behavior of different pacemaker models and the need to obtain specific, relevant information before conclusions can be drawn.

The interpretation of a pacemaker ECG is easier when pulse generators with telemetric function are used. By means of corresponding programmers, marker pulses can be recorded indicating which chamber has been involved and whether sensing or stimulation is occurring (❷ Fig. 6.28). In the new models, even the duration of the different refractory periods is displayed, together with the ongoing intracardiac ECG registration.

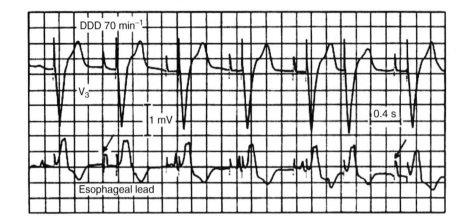

□ Fig. 6.29
Esophageal-lead registration permits atrial activity to be visualized very clearly and discloses alternation between atrial fusion beats (*arrows*), normal atrial capture, and a supraventricular ectopic beat localized within the T wave of the preceding QRS complex. Today, intracardiac recordings and markers from the atrium make esophageal ECG recordings unnecessary

Besides marker pulses, intracardiac ECG recording can also be obtained via telemetry (❷ Fig. 6.29).

The evaluation of atrial stimulation response in dual-chamber pacing is often difficult because of the distortion of the ECG registration by atrial impulses. It is not uncommon that standard ECG leads fail to permit any conclusion. Earlier, esophageal registration was therefore necessary to analyze atrial activity both concerning stimulation response and spontaneous ectopic beats if intracardiac atrial recording from the programmer is not available.

Nowadays, each patient should be equipped with a pacemaker "passport," including relevant data on the latest program setting. Pacemaker–ECG interpretation can be further facilitated when programmed parameters and information are printed out simultaneously on the ECG strip together with marker pulses.

6.7   Pacemaker Malfunction and Pseudomalfunction

When analyzing a "pathological" pacemaker ECG, it is necessary to differentiate between malfunction owing to lead or pulse generator disorders and pseudomalfunction caused by inappropriate program settings with regard to the underlying arrhythmia.

Technical disorders of pacemaker systems are mainly related to lead problems, but other factors may also disturb the pacemaker operation. A collection of possible causes is given in ❷ Fig. 6.30. Some complications are accompanied by typical ECG patterns, and their diagnosis and assessment can be undertaken through the interpretation of standard ECG recordings. However, several malfunctions may cause the same ECG pattern, thereby creating difficulties in making a correct diagnosis and in deciding adequate countermeasures. The disclosure of intermittent and sporadic disorders sometimes requires a closer look at the diagnostic memory of the pacemaker or Holter monitoring.

The most important question regarding pacemaker function is whether there is adequate response (capture) to all pacemaker stimuli. A lack of capture is called *exit block*, a descriptive ECG term, which does not provide any information about the underlying cause. Hence, it is not possible to discriminate between lead dislodgment and pathological threshold rise with an unchanged lead-tip position (❷ Fig. 6.31).

The presence of ventricular exit block is obvious in dual-chamber systems when there is AV block (❷ Fig. 6.32). Sometimes, it is difficult to see if the exit block is from the atrial or the ventricular lead. However, it can be overlooked when spontaneous AV conduction occurs and initiates ventricular depolarization resulting in pseudofusion beats (❷ Fig. 6.33).

As mentioned earlier, the assessment of atrial capture demands visualization of atrial activity (❷ Fig. 6.34). If standard ECG leads do not provide sufficient information, intracardiac recording or reprogramming procedures may help to disclose possible atrial exit block.

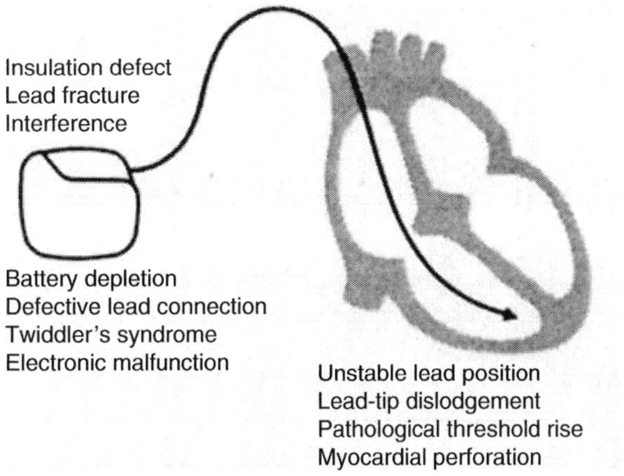
Insulation defect
Lead fracture
Interference
Battery depletion
Defective lead connection
Twiddler's syndrome
Electronic malfunction
Unstable lead position
Lead-tip dislodgement
Pathological threshold rise
Myocardial perforation

Fig. 6.30
Different pacemaker malfunctions detailed concerning cause and location

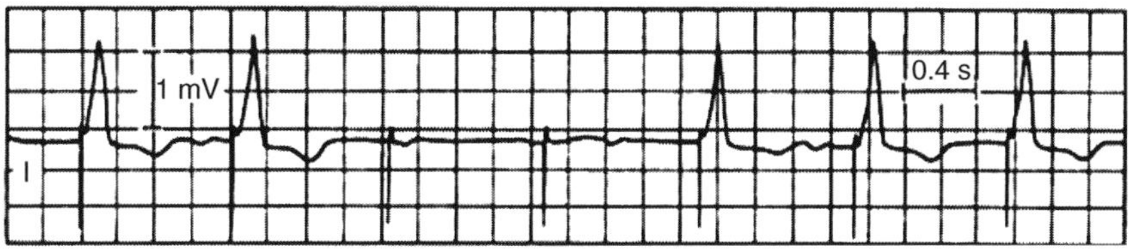
1 mV
0.4 s
I

Fig. 6.31
VVI pacing at a rate of 70 min^{-1} and intermittent exit block, but without any information about the cause of loss of capture

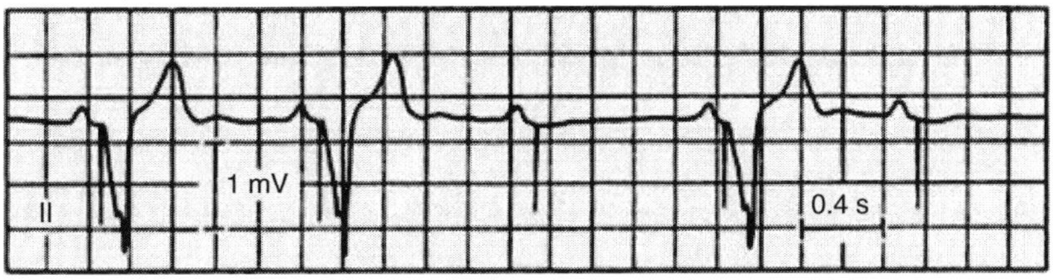
1 mV
0.4 s
II

Fig. 6.32
DDD mode. Atrial-triggered ventricular stimulation is followed by intermittent ventricular exit block

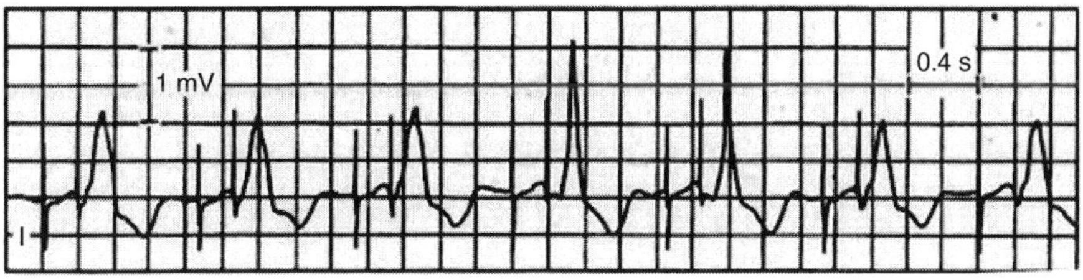
1 mV
0.4 s
I

Fig. 6.33
Dual-chamber pacing at a rate of 70 min^{-1}. Two of the ventricular complexes differ in configuration and occur approximately 80 ms after the ventricular stimulus is delivered. This indicates the presence of an intermittent ventricular exit block "somewhat concealed" by the spontaneously conducted QRS complexes

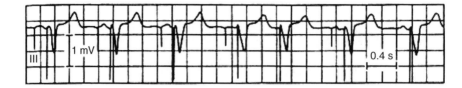

Fig. 6.34
Dual-chamber pacing at a rate of 70 min^{-1}. Atrial depolarizations are clearly visible in this recording. The loss of atrial capture in complex #4 is followed by triggered ventricular stimulation, probably because of a spontaneous P wave hidden somewhere in the T wave of the preceding QRS complex

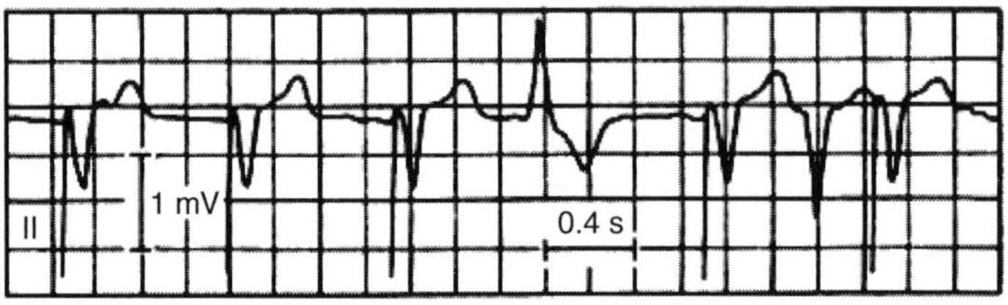

Fig. 6.35
VVI pacing at a rate of 80 min^{-1}. The first premature ectopic ventricular beat accomplishes inhibition indicated by the reset of the basic rate interval, while the second one differs in configuration and remains unsensed

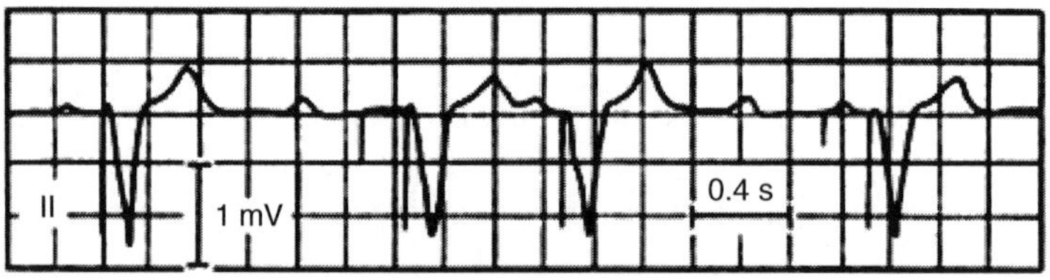

Fig. 6.36
Dual-chamber pacing. Intermittent P wave undersensing is followed by atrial stimulation at a basic rate of 50 min^{-1}. Atrial capture can be obtained when the biological refractory period of the unsensed spontaneous P wave has passed

The sensing function also has to be assessed in an ECG analysis. Ventricular ectopic activity may be sensed with different amplitudes and slew rates. The actual program setting may cover normal ventricular complexes, but not all ectopic beats (● Fig. 6.35).

In dual-chamber pacing, one of the major concerns is consistent P-wave sensing. In the presence of AV block, P-wave undersensing is easily detected (● Fig. 6.36). However, during normal AV conduction, P-wave undersensing may be overlooked when the pacemaker is correctly inhibited via the ventricular amplifier owing to sensing of spontaneous QRS complexes (● Fig. 6.37).

Unfortunately, other signals may affect the pacemaker function; for example, myopotentials. In unipolar pacemaker systems, myopotentials near the pulse generator pocket may be sensed causing inhibition or interference rate pacing, the signals being perceived as cardiac activity. Inhibition by myopotentials is supposed to be a pseudomalfunction, as the pulse generator operates correctly according to the technical specifications (● Fig. 6.38). Another example of pseudomalfunction is given in ● Fig. 6.39, which demonstrates far-field R wave oversensing in AAI pacing. In unipolar AAI pacing, sometimes rather large intra-atrial R waves can be seen resulting in sensing problems.

Rather confusing ECG patterns are obtained when a lead insulation defect appears (● Fig. 6.40). Pathological inhibition alternating with interference rate stimulation resulting in pseudoundersensing may occur as intracardiac insulation

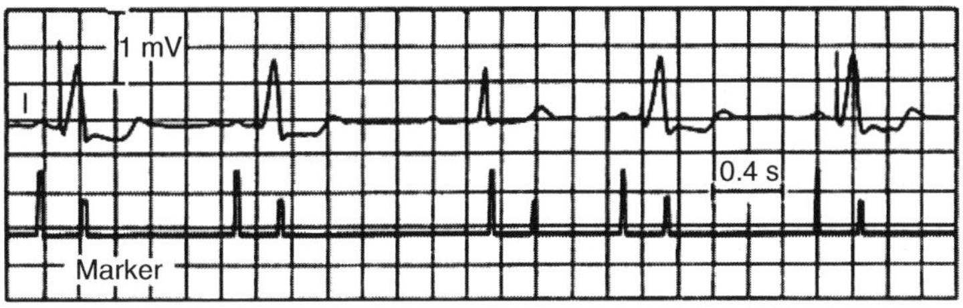

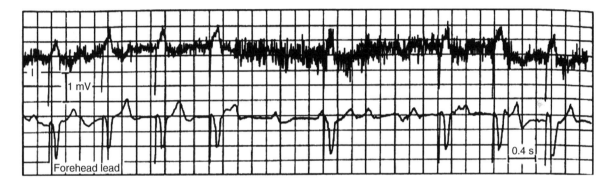

Fig. 6.37
Dual-chamber pacing. One P wave (number 3) is not detected by the atrial amplifier. The following spontaneously conducted QRS complex is sensed by the ventricular amplifier as is clearly indicated by the simultaneous marker-pulse recording

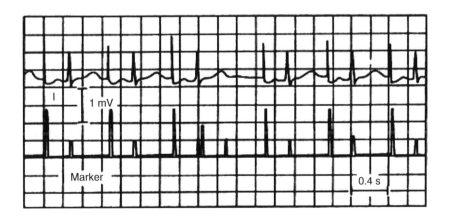

Fig. 6.38
VVI pacing at a rate of 80 min^{-1}. The occurrence of myopotentials clearly seen in standard lead I causes intermittent inhibition. The lack of interference in the lower-lead recording is a result of the temporary placement of the ECG lead on the patient's forehead

Fig. 6.39
AAI pacing at a rate of 90 min^{-1} with an intermittent pause. Marker-pulse registration indicates a reset of the technical refractory period and the basic interval timer. The reset can be related to the QRS complex and the diagnosis is intermittent far-field R-wave oversensing; that is, the actual sensing program detects the "distant" ventricular activity

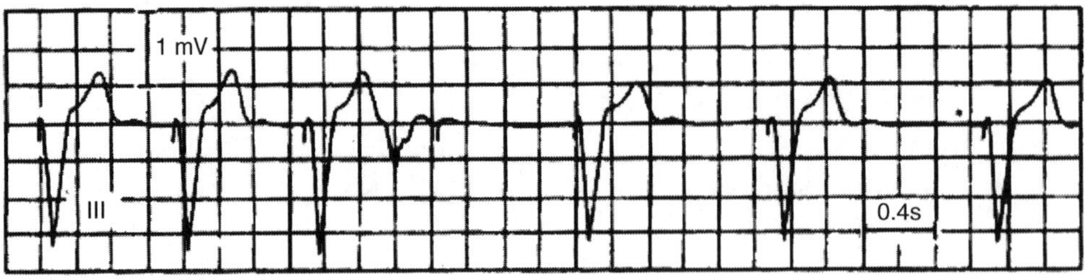

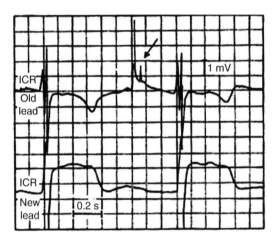

Fig. 6.40

VVI pacing system with a programmed basic rate of 80 min⁻¹. A premature ventricular ectopic beat is not followed by inhibition. Intermittent and irregular variation of pacing intervals indicates inhibition owing to oversensing. Because there are neither signs of external electrical interference nor myopotentials, signals occurring within the lead system can be assumed to cause the intermittent inhibition or conversion to interference rate stimulation thus mimicking undersensing. In this particular patient, an insulation defect of the transvenous lead at the site of the tricuspid valve was found to be the reason for the pathological ECG

Fig. 6.41

Intracardiac ECG recording (ICR) (paper speed 50 mm s⁻¹) obtained from the same patient as in ❯ Fig. 6.40 during lead replacement. Simultaneous registration discloses pathological signals with maximum amplitude of 5 mV from the old lead, but not from the newly implanted second ventricular lead

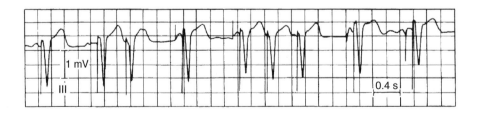

Fig. 6.42

DDD pacing system operating with irregular triggered ventricular stimulation, alternating with basic rate stimulation and occasionally P-wave undersensing. The reason for this confusion ECG turned out to be an insulation defect of the epicardial atrial lead a few centimeters from the lead tip

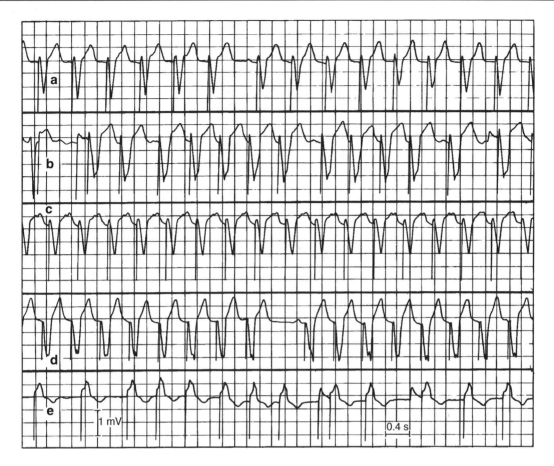

◘ Fig. 6.43

DDD-mode tachycardias. Recordings from five different patients, each with a different diagnosis. The recording taken from the patient shown in (a) illustrates sinus tachycardia at a rate slightly ahead of the programmed upper rate limit of 110 min^{-1} resulting in prolonged AV delay and a Wenckebach block type of behavior; (b) shows a patient with atrial fibrillation with irregular ventricular triggering limited by a programmed upper rate of 128 min^{-1}; (c) illustrates pacemaker-mediated reentrant tachycardia owing to sensing of retrograde P waves following ventricular stimulation; (d) shows repetitive far-field R-wave oversensing owing to inappropriate program setting with respect to the duration of the atrial refractory period and high atrial sensitivity; and (e) illustrates irregular triggered ventricular stimulation owing to "oversensing" of potentials generated by an insulation defect of the atrial lead

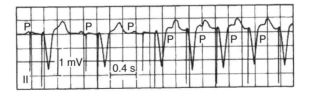

◘ Fig. 6.44

DDD pacing with good recording of atrial activity. After three unsensed P waves, ventricular stimulation is followed by a retrograde P wave, which is obviously sensed, subsequently triggering the next ventricular stimulation. Repetitive occurrence and consistent sensing of retrograde P waves maintain the running of an endless-loop reentrant tachycardia

defects giving rise to pathological potentials (❯ Fig. 6.41). Another puzzling ECG is given in ❯ Fig. 6.42, where an insulation defect in an atrial lead is responsible for pathological triggering of ventricular stimulation.

Tachyarrhythmias in dual-chamber pacing pose challenging diagnostic problems as they may look alike despite different underlying mechanisms (❯ Fig. 6.43). As mentioned earlier, a good ECG recording is necessary for the detection of P waves, which may help to disclose the cause of the arrhythmia (❯ Fig. 6.44).

6.8   Functional Tests

The days when only a magnet was available as a test instrument have more or less disappeared. In multiprogrammable pacemakers, output can be reduced either by shortening the impulse duration or decreasing the amplitude with the programmer. Some manufacturers have chosen to provide an automatic stepwise decrease or a one-step change of the pacing threshold measurement (❯ Fig. 6.45). This is a temporary programming, which necessitates access to the specific programmer and knowledge of how to handle this device. Episodes of asystole may occur during the stimulation tests (❯ Figs. 6.46 and ❯ 6.47).

In dual-chamber pacing, the evaluation of the atrial stimulation threshold by the temporary reduction of voltage or impulse duration is facilitated when the atrial depolarization is clearly visible (❯ Fig. 6.48). In some cases, it is difficult to see the P waves, but if the test is done with the programmer, markers and intracardiac ECG recordings are useful tools.

The clinical information obtained from only reading standard pacemaker ECG registration is limited. Even if the adequate pacemaker function can be assessed, it is advisable to evaluate safety margins for stimulation and sensing, as well as the battery condition during follow-up. Almost all programmers measure sensing automatically or semi-automatically (❯ Fig. 6.48).

The assessment of atrial sensing threshold always requires a reprogramming procedure. P-wave sensing is subjected to changes in the postoperative course without correlation with the variation of stimulation thresholds. Additional provocation tests with ECG recordings in different postures and during maximal inspiration can expose intermittent undersensing (❯ Fig. 6.49).

During the follow up of the AAI/R mode, special attention should be paid to the AV conduction. This can be done by reevaluation of the Wenckebach block by temporary incremental rate increase. Valsalva maneuvers and carotid massage can also provide useful information about the AV conduction properties (❯ Fig. 6.50).

When normal AV conduction is present in the DDD mode, it is possible that – in the presence of long technical AV delay – the ventricular spikes will coincide with spontaneous QRS complexes or be inhibited depending on the critical timing. Hence, no information can be obtained about ventricular stimulation response unless the technical AV delay is reprogrammed to a very short value (❯ Fig. 6.51). A possible exit block may thus be disclosed which is otherwise well-concealed by pseudofusion beats or inhibition.

In unipolar pacing, sensing of myopotentials from muscles close to the pulse generator constitutes a well-known problem. To determine the extent to which an individual patient may experience myopotential inhibition, routine testing is recommended before a final decision on program setting is made. In the DDD pulse generators, both the atrial and the

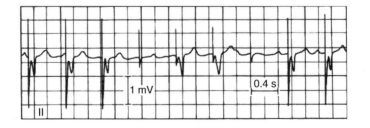

◼ **Fig. 6.45**
VVI pacing during a threshold test where the output of four stimuli is automatically reduced by a decrease in impulse duration from 0.5 to 0.07 ms. Intermittent loss of capture occurs

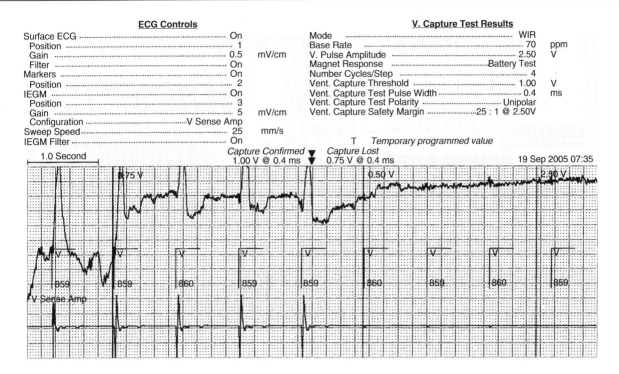

ECG Controls

Surface ECG	On	
Position	1	
Gain	0.5	mV/cm
Filter	On	
Markers	On	
Position	2	
IEGM	On	
Position	3	
Gain	5	mV/cm
Configuration	V Sense Amp	
Sweep Speed	25	mm/s
IEGM Filter	On	

V. Capture Test Results

Mode	WIR	
Base Rate	70	ppm
V. Pulse Amplitude	2.50	V
Magnet Response	Battery Test	
Number Cycles/Step	4	
Vent. Capture Threshold	1.00	V
Vent. Capture Test Pulse Width	0.4	ms
Vent. Capture Test Polarity	Unipolar	
Vent. Capture Safety Margin	25 : 1 @ 2.50V	

T   *Temporary programmed value*

Capture Confirmed ▼   Capture Lost
1.00 V @ 0.4 ms   0.75 V @ 0.4 ms

1.0 Second   19 Sep 2005 07:35

Fig. 6.46
An automatic ventricular pacing threshold test with a printout from the programmer is done with reduction of the voltage of the pacing amplitude. The surface ECG has some muscle potential disturbances but loss of capture is clearly seen at 0.75 V. The markers line in the middle has a V sign indicating a ventricular output from the pacemaker. The bottom ECG is an intrinsic recording of the sensed amplitude, which, of course, disappears when capture is lost. No ventricular escape rhythm is detected

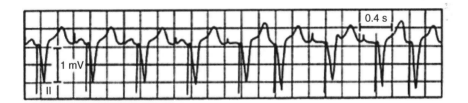

Fig. 6.47
Automatic atrial stimulation threshold test of a DDD pacemaker. As the P waves are clearly visible it is simple to estimate when loss of capture occurs

ventricular amplifier may be influenced by myopotentials depending on their amplitude and slew rate in relation to the sensitivity setting (❱ Fig. 6.52).

6.9   Biventricular Pacing, Cardiac Resynchronization

During the last few years, there has been an enormous interest in treating patients with heart failure with pacing both ventricles at the same time or almost simultaneously by implanting an extra pacing lead on the left ventricle. This is

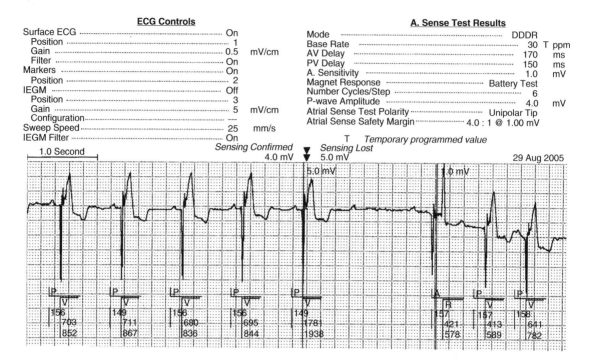

ECG Controls

Surface ECG	On
Position	1
Gain	0.5 mV/cm
Filter	On
Markers	On
Position	2
IEGM	Off
Position	3
Gain	5 mV/cm
Configuration	---
Sweep Speed	25 mm/s
IEGM Filter	On

A. Sense Test Results

Mode	DDDR
Base Rate	30 T ppm
AV Delay	170 ms
PV Delay	150 ms
A. Sensitivity	1.0 mV
Magnet Response	Battery Test
Number Cycles/Step	6
P-wave Amplitude	4.0 mV
Atrial Sense Test Polarity	Unipolar Tip
Atrial Sense Safety Margin	4.0 : 1 @ 1.00 mV

T   *Temporary programmed value*

Sensing Confirmed — 4.0 mV   *Sensing Lost* — 5.0 mV

1.0 Second   5.0 mV   5.0 mV   29 Aug 2005

P	P	P	P	P	A	P	P
V	V	V	V	V	R	V	V
156	149	156	156	149	157	157	158
703	711	680	695	781	421	413	641
852	867	836	844	938	578	589	782

⊡ **Fig. 6.48**

Here is an example of an automatic atrial-sensing test in a DDD system. Sensing of the P waves is lost at 5.0 mV, which the two arrows indicate. To simplify the test, the base rate is programmed to 30 bpm temporary.

P spontaneous P wave, *A* paced atrium, *V* paced ventricle, *R* spontaneous ventricular beat

⊡ **Fig. 6.49**

DDD pacing with obviously reliable atrial sensing. However, a test during deep inspiration discloses intermittent atrial undersensing

⊡ **Fig. 6.50**

AV conduction test in an AAI system. When carotid sinus pressure is applied, intermittent second-degree AV block is exposed

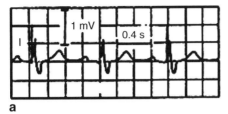

Fig. 6.51

A DDD pacemaker with a technical AV delay programmed to 200 ms is shown in (**a**). Atrial triggered ventricular stimulation coincides with spontaneous conducted beats and the ECG could be interpreted as normal pacemaker function. However, reprogramming to a shorter AV delay of 120 ms discloses an underlying ventricular exit block, which is shown in (**b**)

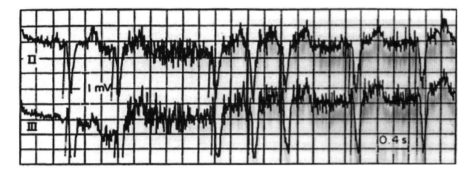

Fig. 6.52

Myopotential provocation test. In DDD pacing, myopotentials sensed by the atrial amplifier will cause triggered ventricular stimulation, while sensing by the ventricular amplifier is followed by inhibition or conversion to interference rate stimulation. The type of reaction depends on the program setting and the amplitude of the myopotentials obtained

possible by using branches of the coronary sinus vein and specially designed pacemaker leads for this purpose. It is not necessary that the patient has bradycardia; a major intraventricular electromechanical asynchrony with heart failure is the indication for CRT (cardiac resynchronization therapy). Instead of pacing only the right ventricle with bundle branch block as a result, stimulation of both ventricles at the same time is a more optimized treatment for each patient. If chronic atrial fibrillation does not exist, the patient will have three leads implanted: one in the right atrium, another in the right ventricle, and the third one in the coronary sinus (❯ Fig. 6.53). In chronic atrial fibrillation, the atrial lead is skipped.

The ECGs from biventricular pacing can be very similar to the ordinary DDD ECGs, but during different tests it is easier to see how the system works. The pacing ventricular threshold tests can be done with a short AV delay or in the VVI modes for each ventricle (❯ Fig. 6.54).

In the early stages of biventricular pacing, many different systems were available. For example, the ventricular ports were connected together to provide simultaneous pacing of both ventricles. The pacemaker senses RV and LV activity simultaneously. Today, the modern biventricular pulse generator usually has two independent ventricular ports and it is possible to program a short time delay between the LV and RV stimuli and optimize the therapy for each patient.

6.10 Tachycardia and ICD

Many patients with a life-threatening tachycardia will receive an ICD. The ICD (implantable cardioverter defibrillator) has a built-in pacemaker, and depending on the lead configuration, the pulse generator can pace and sense in single or double chamber mode or even in biventricular configuration. Many patients need pacing just after termination of a

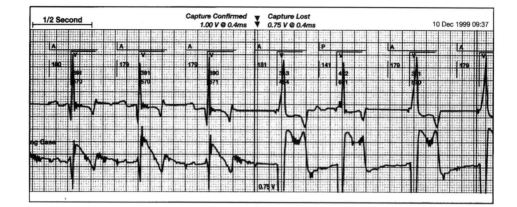

◼ Fig. 6.53

In the upper ECG lead, the three first QRS complexes are narrow due to biventricular stimulation. During an automatic thresh-old test, capture is lost at 0.75 V on one pacemaker channel resulting in a bundle branch block pattern visible both on the surface ECG and the intracardiac electrogram (EGM) in the lower part [7]

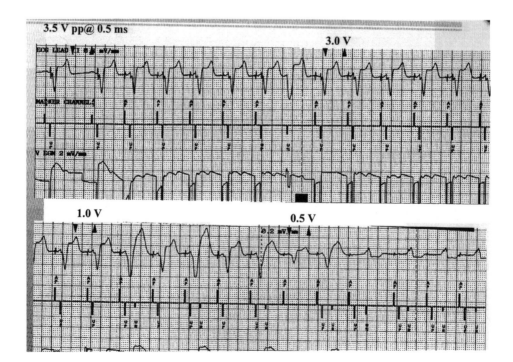

◼ Fig. 6.54

Another example of biventricular pacing. The first complexes are similar to ordinary DDD pacing. During the threshold test, bundle branch block occurs on one channel and at 0.5 V the spontaneous intrinsic QRS complex is seen

tachycardia, when a short asystole can appear. During implantation, ventricular fibrillation is initiated in order to check that the shock therapy terminates the life-threatening tachycardia (❷ Fig. 6.55).

Most implantable defibrillators have the opportunity to terminate a ventricular tachycardia by using a function called ATP (antitachycardia pacing). Instead of a painful shock therapy, a preprogrammed rapid overdrive (bursts) stimuli is automatically delivered with a low-pacing amplitude when the tachycardia starts (❷ Fig. 6.56). If VF is initiated, shocks will be delivered.

The pacemaker in the ICD device has a sensor which is very useful when antiarrhythmic drug therapy sometimes results in bradycardia.

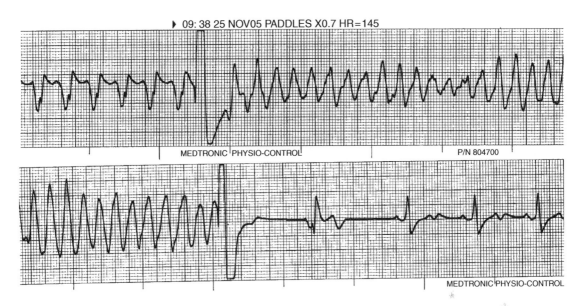

◼ Fig. 6.55
Initiation and automatic termination of VF in a test during an implantation of an ICD. The first six beats are overdrive pacing with a shock on the vulnerable phase of the T wave to start the VF. The bottom ECG has a pacemaker beat after the shock has been delivered and then sinus rhythm is established

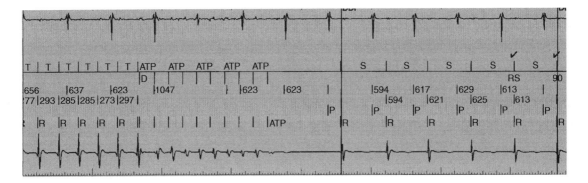

◼ Fig. 6.56
Print out from an ICD programmer with a stored ECG, EGM, and markers from an ICD device. The print out demonstrates a ventricular tachycardia and a burst of pacing stimuli is given (*ATP*) and the VT terminates to sinus rhythm (*S*). Markers of the P and R waves are also seen

The interpretation of stored ECGs in the ICD devices focuses a lot on the correct sensing of VT and VF. Unfortunately, many shocks are delivered due to false sensing (rapid atrial fibrillation, lead insulation defects, etc.). The pacing/sensing ventricular lead is tested in the same way as an ordinary pacing lead regarding thresholds.

References

1. Parsonnet, V., S. Furman, N.P.D. Smyth, and M. Bilitch, Optimal resources for implantable cardiac pacemakers. Pacemaker study group. *Circulation*, 1983;**68**: 227A–244A.
2. Barold, S.S, Editors. *Modern Cardiac Pacing*. Mount Kisco, New York: Futura, 1986.
3. Furman, S., D. Hayes, and D. Holmes, *A Practice of Cardiac Pacing*. Mount Kisco, New York: Futura, 1986.
4. Levine, P.A and R.C. Mace, *Pacing Therapy: A Guide to Cardiac Pacing for Optimum Hemodynamic Benefit*. Mount Kisco, New York: Futura, 1983.
5. Schüller, H. and T. Fåhraeus, *Pacemaker Electrocardiograms – An Introduction to Practical Analysis*. Solna, Sweden: Siemens-Elema, 1983.
6. Serge, B.X.S. Roland, and F.S. Alfons,*Cardiac Pacemakers Step by Step, an Illustrated Guide*. Futura: Blackwell, 2004.
7. Levine, P.A. *Guidelines to the Routine Evaluation, Programming and Follow-Up of the Patient with an Implanted Dual-Chamber Rate-Modulated Pacing System*. St Jude Medical, 2003.
8. Kenneth, E.A., K.G. Neal, and L.W. Bruce, *Clinical Cardiac Pacing*. W.B. Saunders, 1995.

7 The Signal-Averaged Electrocardiogram

Leif Sörnmo · Elin Trägårdh Johansson · Michael B. Simson

P. W. Macfarlane et al. (eds.), *Specialized Aspects of ECG*, DOI 10.1007/978-0-85729-880-5_7,
© Springer-Verlag London Limited 2012

7.1   Introduction

The signal averaging technique is applied to electrocardiographic recordings to reduce extraneous noise, which masks low-amplitude bioelectric signals from the heart. Although modern amplifier design and good recording techniques can minimize certain types of noise, other sources of noise, such as muscle activity, obscure low amplitude potentials. With signal averaging, the noise level can be reduced so that repetitive waveforms at the microvolt level can be reliably detected and analyzed. The noise level after averaging is, in most studies, below 1 μV, the equivalent of 1/100 of a millimeter at a standard ECG display scale.

This chapter discusses the methodology of signal averaging and its use in studying high-frequency components of the QRST complex, manifested either as ventricular late potentials (❷ Sects. 7.3 through ❷ 7.7) or within the QRS complex (❷ Sects. 7.8 and ❷ 7.9). Signal averaging is useful also in other ECG applications such as exercise testing (see ❷ Chap. 4), although the dynamic changes of the ST segment call for recursive signal averaging with a forgetting factor.

7.2   Methods of Signal Averaging

Signal averaging reduces the level of noise that contaminates a repetitive signal such as the ECG [1–3]. The most commonly used form is ensemble averaging in which multiple samples of a repetitive waveform are averaged with equal weights; random noise, which is not synchronized with the waveform of interest, is reduced. The process of averaging begins by measuring the voltage of an ECG fed through a high-gain (×1,000) amplifier with bandwidth ranging from 0.05 Hz to several 100 Hz. The analog signal is converted into digital form at a sampling rate of 1,000 Hz or more and stored. Once all beats of the ECG have been identified and aligned in time, the ensemble average is computed by first summing the samples at a particular instant within the beat and then dividing the sum by the total number of beats. This procedure is repeated for all the samples of the beat.

Several requirements must be met so that the signal averaging technique can reduce noise effectively [1, 3]. First, the waveform of interest must be repetitive so that multiple samples can be obtained to form an average waveform. Second, there must exist a unique feature in the ECG, which can be used as a reference time so that appropriate points of the repetitive signal can be averaged. The time of the maximum amplitude or maximum slope of the QRS complex may be used as reference time; however, such simplistic definitions are useful only when the noise level of the ECG is known to be low. A more robust approach is to cross-correlate each new waveform with a template waveform, determining the reference time as that point in time which corresponds to the highest cross-correlation value [4, 5]. If the algorithm for determining the reference time is inaccurate, that is, causing "trigger jitter," the averaged waveform becomes smoothed and the high-frequency components of the waveform are reduced. For example, it can be shown that a normally distributed jitter with a standard deviation of 1 ms causes the averaging operation to act as a linear, time-invariant low-pass filter with cut-off frequency at about 140 Hz [1]. Similarly, if the QRS complex is used as reference time, then the high-frequency components of an averaged P wave is smoothed because the PR interval varies slightly from beat to beat.

Third, the signal of interest must be uncorrelated with the contaminating noise. If so, the reduction of noise by signal averaging is proportional to the square root of the number of beats contained in the ensemble. For example, averaging of 100 beats will reduce the noise by a factor of 10 [1]. However, the noise must have certain properties to be reduced effectively by signal averaging: it should be random, uncorrelated with the beats, and characterized by an unchanging statistical distribution.

The noise that masks low-level electrical events of the heart has three primary origins:

1. Skeletal muscle noise, typically 5–20 μV even with a relaxed patient
2. Power line interference (50 or 60 Hz and related harmonics) and
3. Electronic and thermal noise from amplifiers and electrodes

Myoelectrical and electrode noise are the most troublesome ones in practice; modern isolation amplifiers have greatly reduced interference originating from power lines. Another noise source is the presence of ectopic beats. These complexes can be eliminated by their premature timing and through matching of a new beat against a template of the desired beat before averaging is performed [5–7].

7.3 Late Potentials and Time Domain Analysis

7.3.1 Introduction

One of the most frequent applications of signal averaging in electrocardiology has been the detection of ventricular late potentials, most often in patients with ventricular tachyarrhythmias. Late potentials are micro-volt level, high-frequency waveforms that are contiguous with the QRS complex and last a variable time into the ST segment. Such potentials are postulated to originate from small areas of delayed and fragmented ventricular depolarization, resulting primarily from myocardial infarction (MI).

7.3.2 Filtering and Time Domain Parameters

Characterization of late potentials is facilitated by linear, time-invariant high-pass filtering of the signal averaged ECG so as to reduce the influence of large-amplitude low-frequency content. Such filtering permits high-frequency components, that is, the late potentials, to pass without loss of amplitude, while low-frequency components are attenuated. High-pass filtering is used because depolarization of cells generates rapid changes in membrane voltage, fast movement of wave fronts of activation, and high frequencies on the body-surface ECG. The plateau or repolarization phases of the action potential generate more slowly changing membrane voltages and lower-frequency signals on the body surface [8]. Microvolt-level waveforms, arising from the late depolarization of small areas of myocardium, would be difficult to perceive if displayed at high gain without filtering. High-pass filters with a cut-off frequency ranging from 25 to 100 Hz have been employed in most studies.

The use of conventional linear, time-invariant high-pass filtering is, however, complicated by the fact that a transient event in the input signal, that is, the QRS complex, produces ringing in the output signal that is subsequent to the event (❱ Fig. 7.1a) [5]. This property is most unfortunate because it impedes the detection of low-amplitude potentials occurring immediately after the QRS complex. While the ringing problem is inherent to linear, time-invariant high-pass filtering, its harm can be largely reduced by employing "bidirectional" filtering–a technique which is implemented in most systems for late potential analysis. The main idea behind this technique is to delay ringing by filtering the signal in different directions so that ringing occurs within the mid-QRS. Forward filtering starts at the P wave and continues until the mid-QRS is reached, whereas backward filtering starts at the T wave and ends at the mid-QRS (❱ Fig. 7.1b) [5]. Evidently, bidirectional filtering suffers from the disadvantage of an undefined output at mid-QRS, and thus no measurements should be done from the bidirectionally filtered signal that involves the entire QRS complex.

❱ Figures 7.2 and ❱ 7.3 show examples of recordings made with signal-averaging technique in patients with and without late potentials. The tracings at the top of each figure are signal-averaged bipolar X, Y, and Z leads (as used in most studies of late potentials) from about 150 beats. Each lead is then high-pass filtered with a bidirectional filter (cut-off frequency at 25 Hz) and combined into a vector magnitude ($\sqrt{(X^2 + Y^2 + Z^2)}$), a signal that combines the high-frequency information contained in all three leads. This signal, shown on the bottom of each figure, is here termed the "filtered QRS complex." In patients without late potentials, the filtered QRS complex exhibits an abrupt onset, a peak of high-frequency voltage 40–50 ms after QRS onset, and an abrupt decline to noise level at the end of the QRS complex (❱ Fig. 7.2). There is no high-frequency signal above the noise level in the ST segment. The peak of the T wave is associated with a small amount of high-frequency content. In patients with late potentials (❱ Fig. 7.3), the initial portion of the filtered QRS complex is similar to that in patients without late potentials, except that the voltage tends to be lower [9]. At the end of the filtered QRS complex, however, there is a "tail" of low-amplitude signal which is not present in recordings from patients without late potentials. The low-level signal, a late potential, is contiguous with the QRS complex and corresponds to low-amplitude activity which can be seen at the end of the QRS complex in the unfiltered leads when displayed at high gain. The amplitude of the late potential varies from 1 to 20 µV when 25 Hz filtering is used.

The accuracy of the endpoint of the filtered QRS complex is a crucial parameter in time domain analysis as all other parameters are computed with reference to this point. Poor accuracy of the endpoint definition obviously limits the overall accuracy of the analysis. Clearly, the presence of late potentials causes the transition from signal to noise to be much less clear-cut than when late potentials are absent. The endpoint may be found by a backward search in the vector magnitude for the first samples which exceed a certain threshold; the threshold value is related to the residual noise level

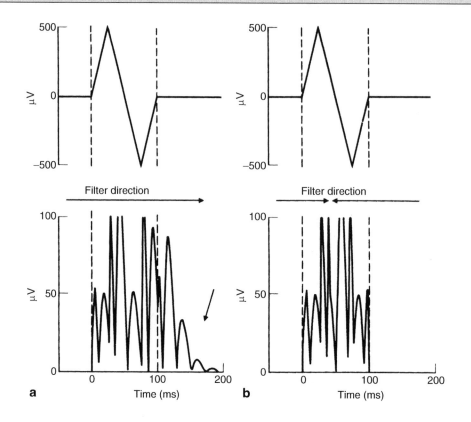

◘ Fig. 7.1

In (**a**), a test ECG signal is shown on top, while below the effect of a unidirectional filter with highpass (>25 Hz) characteristics is shown. Filtering starts at QRS onset and progresses, but it can be clearly seen that undesired signals (*ringing, arrowed*) have been introduced after the end of the QRS complex. In (**b**), however, the same filter is applied from QRS onset for 40 ms only and then applied from QRS end in the opposite direction, that is, toward QRS onset, again for 40 ms. This time no ringing outside the test ECG is apparent from the use of bidirectional filtering (After Simson [5]. American Heart Association, Dallas, Texas. Reproduced with permission)

of the averaged beat [5]; see also [10] for description of a more robust approach in individual leads. Several studies have required that the noise level of the averaged beat is reduced to a root mean square (RMS) level no more than 1 μV. However, it has been shown that the accuracy of the late potential endpoint, as well as the sensitivity and specificity of late potential analysis as such, can be further improved by extending the averaging period so that additional beats are included [11].

Time domain parameters are usually computed from the vector magnitude and include the RMS amplitude of the last 40 ms and the duration of the terminal filtered QRS amplitude <40 μV. These parameters are generally measured in commercially available equipment, as is the filtered QRS duration. The following, commonly used, diagnostic criteria for ventricular late potentials are based on filtering of the QRS complex with pass band 40–250 Hz:

1. RMS amplitude of last 40 ms of filtered QRS complex <20 μV (RMS40)
2. Duration of terminal low amplitude of filtered QRS complex below 40 μV < 38 ms (LAS40)
3. In the absence of a conduction defect, a filtered QRS duration >114 ms (FQRSd)

Using instead filtering with passband 25–250 Hz, the following criteria are commonly used: RMS40 <25 μV, LAS40 >30 ms, and fQRSd >100 ms. At least two criteria should be met for late potentials to be considered present. A signal-averaged ECG with the three measurements (RMS40, LAS40, and FQRSd) is displayed in ❷ Fig. 7.4.

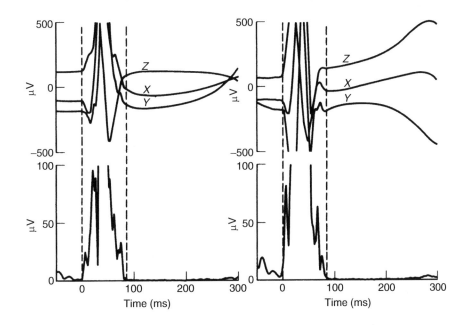

□ Fig. 7.2
Recordings in patients without late potentials. These patients had anterior (*left*) and inferior (*right*) MI respectively. Bipolar signal-averaged leads are shown in high gain (*top*). On the bottom is the filtered signal-averaged QRS complex which is less than 100 ms in duration in both patients. There is a large RMS amplitude of signal in the last 40 ms of the filtered QRS complex (80 and 129 μV, respectively). The dashed vertical lines denote QRS onset and offset

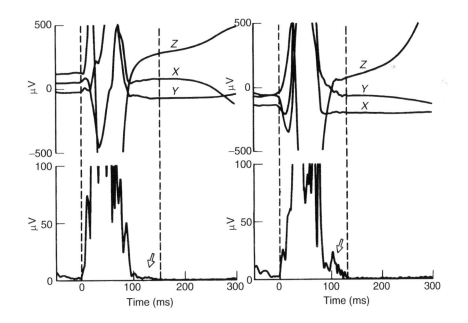

□ Fig. 7.3
Signal processing in patients with VT and late potentials. The patient on the left had an anterior MI and the patient on the right had an inferior MI. The filtered QRS complex shows a longer duration in both patients and late potentials (*arrows*). The RMS voltages in the last 40 ms of the filtered QRS complex measured 2.0 and 11.2 μV, respectively. The *dashed vertical lines* denote QRS onset and offset

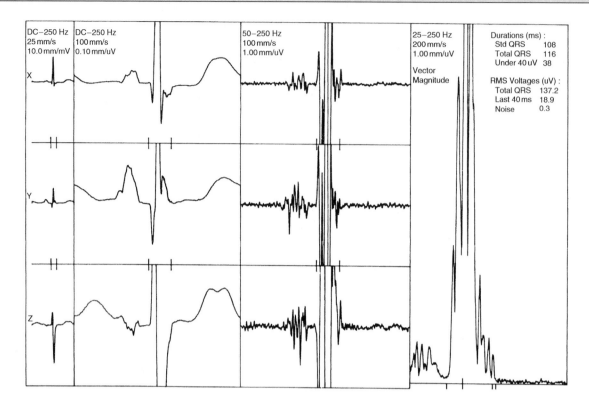

◘ Fig. 7.4

An example of the display of the signal-averaged ECG. The ECG is recorded from a 69-year old female with documented VT. The RMS voltage in the last 40 ms (RMS40) is abnormally low at 18.9 μV, the filtered QRS duration (fQRSd) is abnormally long at 116 ms, and the duration of late activity under 40 μV (LAS40) is also abnormally long at 38 ms

7.3.3 Physiological Background

Late potentials are considered to originate from small areas of delayed ventricular depolarization. Disorganized and late ventricular activation has been recorded directly from infarcted and ischemic myocardium in animals and in humans [12–18]. Studies in animals with experimental infarcts have shown that the delayed ventricular activation can span diastole and that it relates to the occurrence of ventricular arrhythmias [12, 15, 16]. Josephson et al. demonstrated with endocardial recordings in man that fragmented electrical activity can outlast the surface QRS complex, and that the onset and maintenance of ventricular tachycardia (VT) depends on continuous diastolic activity [19]. When VT ceased, the continuous diastolic activity was no longer present. These studies provide evidence that VT after infarction has a reentrant mechanism and involves areas of abnormally slow and protected ventricular activation.

Several groups have reported examples of delayed epicardial ventricular activation in patients with late potentials [20–22]. To establish the time relationship between the body surface late potential and delayed ventricular activation, Simson et al. studied eight patients with signal-averaged ECGs and ventricular mapping [17]. The patients had medically intractable and inducible VT after infarction and underwent surgery for control of the arrhythmia. Twelve to 16 left ventricular endocardial sites were mapped with a catheter and 32–54 epicardial sites were directly recorded in the operating room at normal body temperature. Studies were performed during sinus rhythm. All patients showed evidence of fragmented and low-level electrograms which were prolonged (>60 ms) in duration. These electrograms were recorded from 6.6 ± 3.3 sites per patient; 88% of the fragmented electrograms began during the QRS complex and the latest fragmented electrogram for each patient ended a mean of 161 ms after QRS onset. Six patients with VT had late potentials and the late potentials on the body surface corresponded in time to fragmented and delayed electrogram activity. During the last 40 ms of the filtered QRS complex, when the late potentials were recorded, 68% of the electrograms active showed fragmented activity. In contrast, in earlier segments of the QRS complex only 27% of the active electrograms showed fragmented activity. The mapping studies demonstrated that the late potentials correlated in time with fragmented electrogram activity, which begins during the normal QRS complex but which outlasts normal ventricular activation. The studies are in agreement with those performed in animals with experimental infarcts and late potentials [18, 23].

The mapping studies suggest that fragmented electrogram activity could be detected on the body surface as a low-level waveform only when it outlasted normal ventricular activation. Late potentials were not detected in a patient with left bundle branch block because the late epicardial activation occurred simultaneously with delayed and fragmented endocardial electrograms. When the fragmented electrograms were of brief duration and ended less than 90 ms after QRS onset, then no late potentials could be detected [17]. Because the duration of fragmented ventricular activation is prolonged with premature beats or at rapid heart rates, pacing the heart or inducing a premature beat may enhance the detection of late potentials [15, 16]. The frequency content of late potentials is similar to that of the entire QRS complex and it is unlikely that frequency analysis could detect small areas of fragmented ventricular activation occurring simultaneously with activation of a larger mass of normal myocardium.

7.4 Late Potentials and Time Domain Analysis in Clinical Applications

7.4.1 Recent Myocardial Infarction

Hundreds of articles have been published on clinical applications of analysis of late potentials. Most of these focus on patients after MI. It has been found that the prevalence of late potentials in patients with old MI varies between 71% and 90% in patients with sustained ventricular arrhythmias, compared to 26–34% in patients without ventricular arrhythmias [24–26]. The presence of late potentials after an MI has been associated with increased risk for VT in prospective studies [27, 28]. Breithardt et al. [28] studied 132 patients a mean of 22 days after acute MI. The prevalence of sustained VT on a mean follow-up of 15 months was 11.9% in patients with, and only 2.7% in patients without late potentials. The prevalence of VT increased with the duration of late potentials; VT occurred in 5% of those with late potential duration <40 ms, compared to 25% in whom the late potential lasted >40 ms.

Between 14% and 29% of the patients with late potentials have been shown to have sustained VT within the first year after MI, compared to only 0.8–4.5% of patients without late potentials [29]. The prevalence of late potentials is higher in patients with inferior MI (58%) compared to patients with anterior infarction (31%) [27], which is not surprising when considering the normal activation sequence of the ventricles, but the prognostic value for ventricular tachycardia is higher for anterior infarctions. Analysis of late potentials has higher prognostic value for ventricular tachycardia than offered by long-term ECG and left ventricular ejection fraction [27].

There is a correlation between the prevalence of late potentials and the degree of ventricular dysfunction. Breithardt et al. [25] found that in patients without a history of ventricular arrhythmia, late potentials were detected in only three of 32 patients (9%) with normal ventricular function, but were present in 32 of 69 patients (46%) who had ventricular akinesia or aneurysm. Hombach et al. [2] found a similar relation between the incidence of late potentials and increasing degrees of ventricular dysfunction. Regardless of the degree of ventricular dysfunction, however, late potentials were found more frequently and had a longer duration in patients with ventricular tachycardia or fibrillation [25]. A retrospective study compared the findings on a signal-averaged ECG, prolonged ECG monitoring and cardiac catheterization to determine which combination of findings best characterized patients with VT after MI [26]. A multivariate statistical analysis showed that the abnormalities on the signal-averaged ECG, including the late potentials, provided independent information useful in identifying patients with VT after MI. An abnormal signal-averaged ECG (presence of late potentials or a long-filtered QRS duration), a peak premature ventricular contraction rate >100 h^{-1} and the presence of a left ventricular aneurysm were the only three variables identified which provided significant information to characterize patients with VT. The study suggested that the abnormal signal-averaged ECG may be combined with other clinical information to provide a more specific identification of patients with VT.

The ACC expert consensus document from 1996 [30] concludes that a normal signal-averaged ECG indicates a low risk for developing life-threatening ventricular arrhythmias. The positive predictive accuracy of only 14–29%, however, is not high enough to justify interventions in individual patients with abnormal results.

7.4.2   Myocardial Reperfusion

Successful treatment of acute MI with thrombolytic agents has been shown to reduce the incidence of late potentials (range 5–24% in patients treated with thrombolytic agents compared to 18–43% in patients not treated) [31–40]. Maki et al. [41] investigated the relationship between the time required for reperfusion by percutaneous transluminal coronary angioplasty and the incidence of late potentials in 94 patients with acute MI. They found that the incidence of late potentials in patients undergoing primary angioplasty at ≤4, 4–6, 6–8, 8–10, and >10 h after infarction was 8%, 12%, 14%, 33%, and 43%, respectively. In the control group, consisting of 31 patients who were treated conventionally, the incidence of late potentials was 48%. The presence of late potentials has been shown to have a low positive predictive value in patients who undergo reperfusion after acute MI [42, 43]. The presence of late potentials has also been shown to be a poor predictor of sudden death after surgical revascularization [44]. Thus, signal-averaged ECG has limited value for risk stratification in an unselected postinfarction population, and is currently not recommended as a risk marker for increased mortality [45].

7.4.3   Sudden Death

The incidence of sudden death has been too infrequent in the studies to date to form a firm conclusion on the value of late potentials as a prognostic indicator for that event. Nevertheless, some prospective studies have been undertaken [46, 47] to evaluate whether the presence of late potentials is an independent risk factor for sudden death or serious ventricular arrhythmias after MI, and to establish the role of the signal-averaged ECG along with other noninvasive tests in identifying patients at high risk.

The combination of late potentials with a low left ventricular ejection fraction, as determined by radionuclide techniques, together with complex ventricular ectopy on Holter monitoring have been used to identify those patients at highest risk of sudden death or developing sustained VT from 6 months to 2 years following MI. Kuchar et al. [46] found that an abnormal signal-averaged ECG together with an ejection fraction <40% predicted arrhythmic events with 34% probability. On the other hand, if the patient had abnormal left ventricular function but a normal signal-averaged ECG, there was only 4% risk of the occurrence of an arrhythmia. The signal-averaged ECG, Holter monitoring, and ejection fraction were independently related to outcome, but a left ventricular ejection fraction <40% was the most powerful indicator.

In a similar study, Gomes et al. [47] also found that the presence of late potentials, an abnormal ejection fraction, and high-grade ectopic activity on Holter monitoring were the variables most significantly related to a future arrhythmic event. Their overall conclusion was that the combination of these abnormalities identified the group of patients at highest risk of VT, sudden death or both in the first year after MI.

7.4.4   Unexplained Syncope

The presence of late potentials in patients with unexplained syncope has been associated with high sensitivity and specificity for inducement of VT during electrophysiological studies. Kuchar et al. [48] evaluated 150 patients with syncope. Late potentials were detected in 29 patients, of whom 16 were found to have VT. In the patients with syncope due to other causes than VT, none of the patients had late potentials on signal-averaged ECG. In this study, the sensitivity was 73%, the specificity 55%, the positive predictive value 55%, and the negative predictive value 94%. Another study by Lacroix et al. [49] found that the positive predictive value of late potentials was 39% for predicting the inducibility of sustained VT. The clinical value of analysis of late potentials in patients with unexplained syncope is mainly in its negative predictive accuracy.

7.4.5   Success of Arrhythmia Surgery

Several investigators have reported that late potentials may disappear after a successful operation for VT [20, 22, 50–52]. The operation generally includes an aneurysmectomy and an additional procedure, such as endocardial excision,

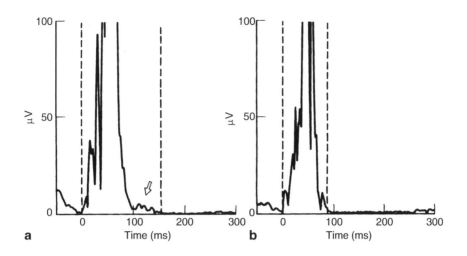

⬛ Fig. 7.5
The filtered QRS complexes from a patient with VT who underwent aneurysmectomy and endocardial excision for control of the arrhythmia. In (**a**), before the operation, a 2.8 μV level of LP is present (*arrow*). In (**b**), after the operation, VT could not be induced and the LPs were no longer present

to remove or isolate the apparent site of origin of VT. In one study, 24 patients in whom VT could not be induced after operation, the FQRSd decreased (from a mean of 137 to 121 ms) and the incidence of late potentials decreased (71–33%) [52] (❯ Fig. 7.5). Eight patients continued to have late potentials, despite surgical control of the arrhythmias. The incidence of late potentials in the filtered QRS complex was not changed in 13 patients in whom VT could be induced after operation.

Experience indicates that a successful operation for control of VT may cause the late potentials to vanish, but they may persist despite successful control of the arrhythmia. This finding suggests that the operation need not remove all areas of delayed activation in order to control VT. In patients with persistent late potentials, despite surgical control of the arrhythmias, it is hypothesized that either the delayed activation does not outlast the refractoriness of the myocardium or that the interface between the slowly conducting tissue and normal myocardium is sufficiently disrupted so that reentry cannot occur.

7.4.6 Efficacy of Anti-Arrhythmic Drugs

Analysis of late potentials has not yet been established as a method for accurately assessing anti-arrhythmic drug efficacy. Class IA, IC, and II [53–58] anti-arrhythmic drugs have been shown to elicit changes in the late potentials, where especially class IC drugs are associated with a marked increase in FQRSd [58]. Only a few studies have examined the effects of class III drugs [59, 60]. In general, time domain analysis of the signal-averaged ECG has not shown a correlation between the changes induced during drug therapy and anti-arrhythmic drug efficacy [53, 54, 58]. A few studies have shown a correlation between the prolongation of the total FQRSd induced by class I drugs and prolongation of the cycle length of ventricular tachycardia [55–57].

Simson et al. [60] investigated the effect of anti-arrhythmic drug therapy on the signal-averaged ECG in 36 patients with VT after MI. Twenty-nine patients, or 81%, had late potentials on medications. The drugs evaluated, alone and in combination, were procainamide, quinidine, disopyramide, amiodarone, phenytoin, and mexiletine. Electrophysiological stimulation was used to evaluate the control of VT. The duration of the filtered QRS complex was increased by a mean of 8–13 ms by procainamide, quinidine, and amiodarone. Procainamide decreased the voltage in the last 40 ms of the

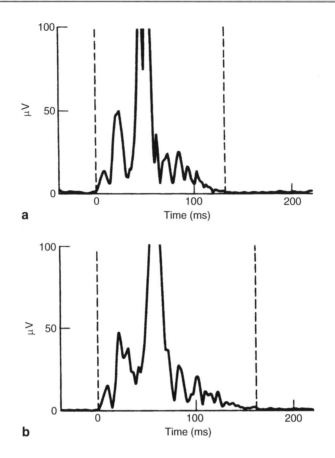

Fig. 7.6

The effects of procainamide on the LPs in a patient with VT after MI. In (**a**), during the period without medication, the patient had a FQRSd of 129 ms and a 4.6 μV level LPs present at the end of the filtered QRS complex. In (**b**), when receiving the pro-cainamide at a serum level of 16 μg/ml, the patient had a longer FQRSd (162 ms) but the LPs persisted. The VT remained inducible (After Simson, (c) Saunders, Philadelphia, Pennsylvania. Reproduced with permission)

filtered QRS complex by 4 μV; however, the incidence of late potentials with anti-arrhythmic drug therapy did not change (❯ Fig. 7.6). Ventricular tachycardia was no longer inducible after anti-arrhythmic drug therapy in ten patients; nor was the late potentials abolished by any agent in these patients. There was no pattern of change in the filtered QRS complex that would indicate a successful response to anti-arrhythmic agents.

7.4.7 Cardiac Transplant

Several studies have investigated possible noninvasive methods for detection of cardiac transplant rejection. A few of them have examined the extent to which late potentials are a measure of heart transplant rejection [61–64]. One report showed a sensitivity of 65%, positive predictive accuracy of 92%, and negative predictive accuracy of 68% for acute rejection [61]. RMS values have also been shown to provide high sensitivity and specificity for rejection [62]. Thus, the potential of signal-averaged ECG analysis to detect acute rejection is promising, but more studies need to be done before the method can be used clinically.

7.4.8 Nonischemic Cardiomyopathy

The occurrence of late potentials in patients with nonischemic congestive cardiomyopathy has been investigated in a group of 41 patients and the findings compared with 55 normal controls [65]. It was found that the FQRSd was longer in patients with sustained ventricular arrhythmia than in those without (130.2 ± 19.5 ms as opposed to 105 ± 13.1 ms); a highly significant difference. The mean control value was 95.9 ms. The RMS voltage in the last 40 ms of the filtered QRS was lower in the group with arrhythmia than in those without (11.3 ± 9.3 as opposed to 53.5 ± 28.3 µV), again a highly significant difference. The corresponding normal group values were 53.7 ± 25.2 µV. Overall, 83% of patients in the group with sustained ventricular arrhythmia had both an abnormally long FQRSd and abnormally low late-potential amplitude; 14% of patients without an arrhythmia and 2% of controls had similar findings. Findings from other [66, 67], but not all [68–70] studies of patients with dilated nonischemic cardiomyopathy have shown similar results.

Arrhythmogenic right ventricular cardiomyopathy was one of the first pathologic entities in which late potentials were identified. Analysis of late potentials can be useful for screening purposes or detection of arrhythmogenic right ventricular cardiomyopathy in family members [71, 72]. Nava et al. [73] evaluated signal-averaged ECGs in 138 patients with arrhythmogenic right ventricular cardiomyopathy and compared the results with those of 146 healthy controls. Late potentials were found in 57% of the patients, and in 4% of the controls. They also found that there is a closer correlation between late potentials and the extent of the disease than with the presence of ventricular arrhythmias. Late potentials have also been found in a significant proportion of patients with the Brugada syndrome. Research suggests that late potentials might be helpful to identify patients at a higher risk of life-threatening arrhythmic events in this population, both in a retrospective [74] and a prospective [75] study, but the results need to be confirmed in larger studies.

7.5 Late Potentials and Frequency Analysis

As described above, late potentials are composed of frequencies which are higher than those of the ST segment, that is, higher than about 25 Hz. However, no specific information is available beforehand on their particular frequency content. By employing frequency analysis based on the discrete-time Fourier transform (and typically implemented by the fast Fourier transform, FFT), it would be possible to pinpoint the range of frequencies which is characteristic of late potentials. The main advantage of the frequency domain approach is that no prior knowledge is required on signal characteristics, whereas the time domain approach requires that the cut-off frequency of the high-pass filter is predetermined. However, this advantage comes at the sacrifice of temporal information as it is not possible to pinpoint the occurrence of late potentials as being late in the QRS complex or early in the ST segment. In practice, frequency analysis is also hampered by certain undesirable properties of the Fourier power spectrum related to frequency leakage and large variance [1, 76]. While these properties can be mitigated to a certain extent by various techniques, care should still be exercised when interpreting the outcome of frequency analysis.

In time domain analysis, a crucial signal processing step is to determine the endpoint of the high-pass filtered QRS complex in order to assure that the diagnostic measurements, that is, RMS amplitude, duration of low-amplitude signals, and filtered QRS duration are accurate. In frequency analysis, the corresponding crucial step is to determine the location and length of the signal segment to be processed. Since the segment begins in the terminal part of the QRS – a part of the heartbeat with drastic changes in amplitude – a displacement of its onset by just a few milliseconds can produce quite different spectra. The segment location should preferably be determined by an algorithmic procedure so as to avoid the subjectivity of manual delineation; one approach is to choose the segment onset as the point when the vector magnitude drops below 40 µV [77].

Different lengths of the segment are associated with different spectral resolution, implying that it is important to keep the length fixed from one patient to another in order to facilitate comparison of results. In the literature, lengths have ranged from 40 ms, thus only including the terminal part of the QRS, to about 200 ms so that a large part of the ST segment is included.

Prior to frequency analysis, it should be standard procedure to subtract the mean value of the ECG samples contained in the segment, that is, the DC component. Windowing is another common time domain operation with which samples at the boundaries of the segment are multiplied with weights smaller than those applied to samples in the middle of the segment, thus reducing the influence of abrupt changes which may occur at the segment boundaries. On the other hand, windowing may have the undesirable effect of reducing the contribution of late potentials when these happen to be located at any of the segment boundaries.

Once the power spectrum has been computed, one or several parameters must be derived which condense its main features. The absolute power can be computed in frequency bands whose limits are determined by some prior knowledge. Alternatively, it may be more appropriate to compute relative power, defined as the ratio of the power in a single frequency band to either the total power or the power contained in certain bands. Relative power measurements are often preferred since the absolute power may be influenced by various nonphysiological factors.

It is sometimes convenient to display and analyze the power spectrum with a logarithmic magnitude scale since it allows detail to be displayed over a wider dynamic range. The scale is defined in units of $20 \cdot \log_{10}$, referred to as decibel (dB). With this scale, 0 dB corresponds to a magnitude equal to 1, -20 dB corresponds to a ten times smaller magnitude, -40 dB corresponds to a 100 times smaller magnitude, and so on. The magnitude function is normalized with respect to its maximum value, thus corresponding to 0 dB. It should be noted that although the power spectrum is commonly employed in the literature, that is, the squared magnitude of the FFT, the (unsquared) magnitude of the FFT is also sometimes employed.

As described earlier, the conventional time domain approach to handle multiple-lead recordings is to simply combine the filtered leads into a vector magnitude from which a set of descriptive parameters is derived. However, the vector magnitude does not lend itself to frequency analysis as this function may obscure the frequency content of the ECG. Instead, the power spectra of individual leads may be averaged into one spectrum from which a set of parameters is derived. Alternatively, parameters can be derived from each spectrum and combined with some suitable technique, for example, averaging of the resulting parameter values.

7.6   Late Potentials and Frequency Analysis in Clinical Applications

The first clinical study exploiting frequency analysis was presented by Cain et al. in 1984 for the purpose of distinguishing patients prone to sustained VT [78]. The analysis method was assessed in three groups of subjects, consisting of 16 patients with previous MI and sustained VT, 35 patients with previous MI but no sustained VT, and ten normal subjects, respectively. The ECG was recorded from the X, Y, and Z Frank leads, digitized, and subjected to signal averaging of 100 beats such that a noise level of 1.5 μV was reached.

In each lead, Fourier-based frequency analysis was performed on a manually delineated 40 ms segment at the terminal part of the QRS, windowed using the Blackman–Harris window. The power spectrum was characterized by two parameters derived from the logarithmic magnitude scale, the spectral value in decibels at 40 Hz and the area enclosed between the 0 and -60 dB level (❷ Fig. 7.7). It should be noted that these two parameters are correlated since a large spectral value, in most cases, implies a large area.

The results for the three groups of subjects suggested that the area was considerably higher in patients with VT than in the other two groups, that is, the amplitude of the high-frequency components of the ECG in patients with VT was much greater than in those without. As one may expect, the spectral value in decibels at 40 Hz was larger in patients with VT than in the other two groups. Besides the terminal part of the QRS, frequency analysis was also performed on segments defined by the QRS complex, the ST segment, and the T wave; the ST segment was associated with results similar to those of the terminal part of the QRS, whereas the other two segments did not offer any discrimination between the VT group and non-VT groups.

In a subsequent study, Cain et al. modified their original way of deriving parameters from the spectrum by instead computing a ratio between the spectral areas defined by the intervals 20–50 Hz and 0–20 Hz [79]. Based on the findings of their previous study, the processed ECG segment was extended from the 40 ms at the terminal part of the QRS to also include the remaining part of the ST segment (though the segment was still manually delineated). The spectral area ratio was tested in 16 patients with a previous MI and sustained VT, 53 patients with a previous MI but without sustained VT, and 11 normal subjects. The results presented in ❷ Fig. 7.8 show that the VT patients have considerably larger ratios than the other two groups. However, the groups could not be discriminated when the 20–50 Hz interval was replaced by 70–120 Hz, a result which is somewhat surprising since the higher frequencies are important to the outcome of time domain analysis.

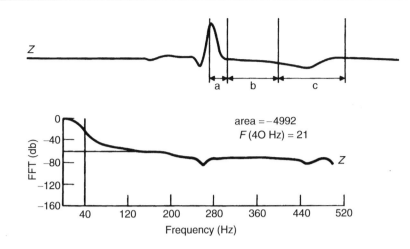

Fig. 7.7
The logarithmic power spectrum characterized by the value in dBs at 40 Hz and the area enclosed between the 0 and −60 dB level (Reprinted from Lindsay et al. [80] with permission)

It should be noted that the spectral area ratio may account for signal properties unrelated to the presence of late potentials. Since the spectral area ratio involves frequencies in the interval 0–20 Hz, it is obvious that low-frequency components originating from, for example, baseline wander or a slowly changing ST segment will also influence the area ratio. In a later study, however, the lower limit was increased to 10 Hz so as to avoid this problem [80].

The studies by Cain and coworkers were followed by several studies from other groups who also employed frequency analysis to find out if late potentials present during sinus rhythm can be used as a marker for ventricular arrhythmias. The results presented in the literature have been most variable, ranging from "inability of frequency domain parameters to distinguish VT from non-VT patients" to "improved identification with frequency domain parameters." In the remaining part of this section, a number of studies are briefly summarized with variable outcomes. It should be noted that each of these studies has a slightly different approach to the implementation of frequency analysis, for example, the definitions of analyzed signal segment and frequency interval of interest.

In a study by Kelen et al., involving ten patients with spontaneous or inducible VT and ten normal subjects, it was shown that the spectral area ratio was markedly dependent on the length of the analyzed signal segment [81]. In fact, a change of as little as 3 ms in segment length changed the results across proposed boundaries of normalcy in normal subjects and in patients with VT. In contrast, the use of time domain analysis established that the patients had late potentials, whereas the normal subjects did not, using the standard diagnostic criteria.

Similar results were also obtained in a study by Machac et al. where the purpose was to determine whether time domain or frequency domain parameters were better in distinguishing patients with and without sustained VT [82, 83]. The two methods were tested in 26 patients with sustained VT, 18 control patients with organic heart disease but without sustained VT, and 11 normal volunteers. Frequency domain analysis was performed on three different segment lengths (the terminal 40 ms of the QRS complex, either alone or with 216 or 150 ms of the ST segment), and both power and power ratios were calculated in different frequency bands. At a fixed specificity of 78%, the best time domain sensitivity was 85%, whereas the best frequency domain sensitivity was 77%. It was thus concluded that frequency domain analysis did not offer any improvement over time domain analysis in distinguishing patients with VT from those without.

The study performed by Worley et al. was also designed to compare the value of time domain and frequency domain parameters [84]. However, they investigated the spectral area ratio, defined in the same way as in [79], not only for segments related to QRS end but also to QRS onset. Six different 140 ms segments started at 0, 40, 50, and 60 ms after QRS onset, two segments started at 40 and 50 ms before QRS end, and a variable-length segment started 40 ms before QRS end and extended to the T wave. The study included 36 patients with remote MI and sustained VT, 29 asymptomatic patients with remote MI, and 23 normal subjects. The results showed that the spectral area ratios from segments starting at 0, 40, and 60 ms after QRS onset were significantly different between infarct patients with and without VT; however,

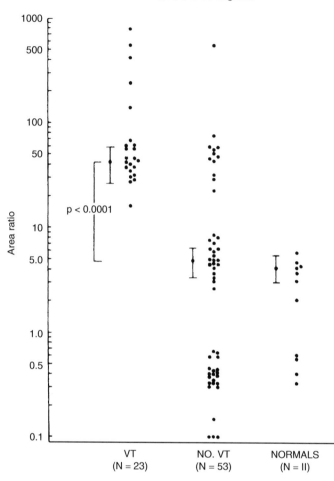

Comparison of the spectral area ratio for patients with sustained VT, without sustained VT, and normal subjects. The terminal QRS and the ST segment are analyzed (Reprinted from Cain et al. [79] with permission)

this finding did not apply to any of the segments related to QRS end. Thus, the results showed that the spectral content of the QRS complex is a marker to discriminate between the two patient groups. The time domain parameters studied were all found to be significantly different between the groups.

The idea to investigate the influence of the analyzed segment location was also pursued in a study by Buckingham et al. [85]. They used a data set consisting of 84 patients with VT and 150 patients without VT, all patients having had prior MI. All analyzed segments had a length of 140 ms and were located 0, 20, 40, 60, and 80 ms after QRS onset and 20, 40, 60, and 80 ms before QRS end. In each segment the spectral area ratio was computed using the same definition as the one given in [79]. Significant differences between the patient groups were only observed for ratios computed in segments 60 and 80 ms after QRS onset and 80 ms before QRS end.

The importance of higher-frequency components was investigated by Pierce et al. on a data set consisting of 24 patients with coronary artery disease and recurrent VT, 24 control patients with coronary artery disease, and 23 normal subjects [77]. The analyzed segment had its onset at the QRS end and a length of 120 ms. Unlike the studies by Cain et al., the frequency domain parameters involved considerably higher frequencies as contained in the interval 60–120 Hz; normalization was done with the entire interval 0–120 Hz. Quantifying performance in terms of the area under the receiver operating characteristic, the frequency domain parameters were associated with larger areas than the time domain parameters. It was therefore concluded that the higher frequencies in late potentials better identified patients with coronary artery disease being prone to VT than did the time domain parameters.

7.7 Late Potentials and Time–Frequency Analysis

7.7.1 Spectrotemporal Mapping

Frequency analysis for identification of late potentials is, as indicated above, flawed by difficulties to accurately delimit the signal segment to be processed; small changes in segment position may lead to substantial changes in frequency domain parameters. The introduction of a sliding segment, whose initial position is located well before the end of the QRS complex and final position well into the T wave, has been suggested as a means to mitigate such difficulties; "sliding" means that the analysis segment is shifted by one or a few milliseconds at a time. For each segment, the power spectrum is computed so that, when the segment has reached its endpoint, a series of successive power spectra has been produced. Similar to frequency analysis, each segment is windowed and the DC level subtracted. This time-frequency approach is widely known as the short-term Fourier transform (STFT) and represents a standard signal processing tool for characterizing the time-varying spectral properties of a nonstationary signal. In the context of ventricular LPs, the STFT is commonly referred to as spectrotemporal mapping [86–89].

❯ Figure 7.9a illustrates spectrotemporal mapping when implemented using an 80 ms segment whose position slides around the end of the QRS complex so that the presence of late potentials may be identified through spectral changes. In this particular case, the signal-averaged ECG contains low-amplitude activity at the end of the QRS complex, that is, late

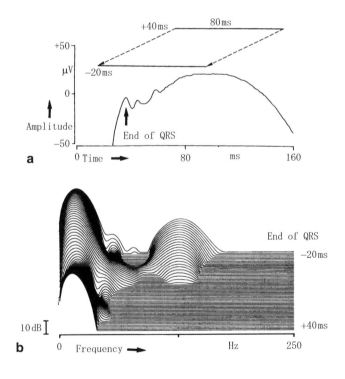

◗ Fig. 7.9

(a) Spectrotemporal mapping is created by computing successive Fourier transforms within a sliding window which, in this example, has 80-ms duration. (b) The spectrotemporal map of a patient with late potentials (Reprinted from Haberl et al. [86] with permission)

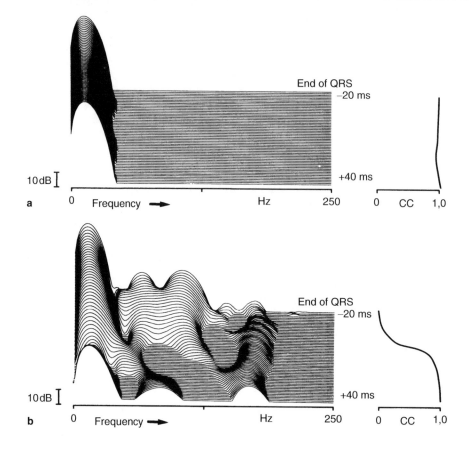

◘ Fig. 7.10
Spectrotemporal map for (a) a patient without late potentials, and (b) a patient with late potentials, manifested by a "landscape with ridges." The curve of cross-correlation coefficients is displayed to the right of each map (Reprinted from Haberl et al. [86] with permission)

potentials are considered to be present. The corresponding series of successive power spectra is displayed in ❷ Fig. 7.9b as a three-dimensional plot where the three axes of the diagram describe frequency, time, and spectral power, respectively. The plot shows that high-frequency components above 50 Hz, contained in segments at the QRS end, gradually vanish as the segment slides toward the T wave, that is, from top to bottom of the plot. The last few spectra are similar in that they do not contain any high-frequency components. In this case, the transition from late potentials to noise is clearly visible using spectrotemporal mapping since the signal-to-noise ratio of the signal-averaged ECG is high.

Although the parameters of frequency analysis can be applied to each individual power spectrum, parameters that exploit the time-dependent properties of spectrotemporal mapping can be expected to add information for identification of late potentials. An early approach to such characterization was the so-called normality factor which determines the similarity of successive spectra through the computation of a series of cross-correlation coefficients [87]; these coefficients have the property of being normalized to the interval [−1,1]. Each individual spectrum is correlated to a template spectrum being determined by averaging the last few spectra positioned at the end of the analysis interval. The curve of cross-correlation coefficients is illustrated for ECGs with and without late potentials in ❷ Fig. 7.10a and ❷ b, respectively. It is obvious from ❷ Fig. 7.10a that the correlation curve increases from almost 0 in segments where high-frequency components are present to a value well outside the QRS complex. On the other hand, ❷ Fig. 7.10b displays a correlation curve which remains close to one throughout all spectra, suggesting that late potentials are absent.

In the original work by Haberl et al. [87] an 80 ms segment was analyzed sliding in steps of 3 ms from a start time 23 ms before the QRS end until 52 ms after; the resulting 25 segments were indexed backward in time so that the last segment had index 1. The normality factor was obtained as the ratio between the mean of the cross-correlation coefficients of segments 20–25, where late potentials were expected to occur, and the mean of the cross-correlation coefficients of the segments 1–5. The factor was then multiplied by 100 and interpreted as a percentage. Late potentials were considered to be present when the normality factor dropped below 30%.

The initial results obtained with spectrotemporal mapping surpassed those obtained by conventional time domain analysis when identifying patients prone to sustained VT in the presence of coronary artery disease [87]. Furthermore, most patients with bundle branch block were correctly classified with spectrotemporal mapping, while these patients had to be excluded in time domain analysis. Despite these promising initial results, this technique is not in widespread use, probably due to its poor reproducibility. In a study comparing spectrotemporal mapping to both time domain and frequency domain analysis, the reproducibility of spectrotemporal mapping was substantially lower than that of the other two types of analysis [89].

7.7.2 Spectral Turbulence Analysis

Spectral turbulence analysis defines another approach to time-frequency characterization of the signal-averaged ECG, originally developed to detect abnormal variations in frequency content during depolarization of the diseased myocardium [90]. The word "turbulence" signifies the transient spectral changes that were hypothesized to occur in the ECG as depolarization propagates throughout the ventricles around areas of abnormal conduction, thus resulting in a high degree of spectral turbulence. While spectral turbulence analysis has the short-term Fourier transform in common with spectrotemporal mapping, the analysis embraces the entire QRS complex and the ST segment and is not limited to an interval at the QRS end. Usually, the first segment starts 25 ms before QRS onset and ends 125 ms after QRS end, incremented in 2 ms steps. The resulting power spectra from all available leads are then normalized with respect to the spectrum with the highest magnitude; this magnitude is designated as 100% while the other magnitudes are smaller. A number of parameters are derived from the normalized spectra which describe the similarity between adjacent spectra expressed in terms of the above-mentioned cross-correlation coefficient. It was claimed that spectral turbulence analysis is applicable to patients irrespective of the QRS duration and the presence or absence of bundle branch block.

In the original study by Kelen et al. [90] both spectral turbulence analysis and conventional time domain late potential analysis (40–250 Hz) were employed for identifying patients with inducible sustained monomorphic VT. The signal-averaged ECG was obtained from 144 subjects using a recording configuration of three orthogonal bipolar leads. The data set contained 71 normal control subjects, 33 with both late potentials by time domain analysis and inducible sustained monomorphic VT, 28 with time domain late potentials but no evidence of spontaneous or inducible sustained monomorphic VT, and ten with inducible sustained monomorphic VT but absence of time domain late potentials. The total predictive accuracy for all groups was 94% with spectral turbulence analysis, whereas only 73% could be achieved with time domain analysis.

Spectral turbulence analysis has been employed in several subsequent studies with results that sometimes improve upon those obtained by conventional time domain analysis. In a study by Malik et al. [91], both techniques were considered for risk prediction after acute MI, using a material of 553 survivors of acute MI (bundle branch blocks and other conduction abnormalities were excluded); the patients were followed for at least 1 year. Spectral turbulence analysis provided significantly lower positive predictive accuracy than the time domain analysis for prediction of ventricular tachycardia/fibrillation during 1 year after infarction. On the other hand, it provided significantly higher positive predictive accuracy for the prediction of 1-year all-cause mortality. The study by Copie et al. [92] also made use of both time domain and spectral turbulence analysis for the prediction of cardiac death and arrhythmic events after acute MI in 603 patients (patients with bundle branch block and other conduction abnormalities were excluded). The results showed that spectral turbulence analysis was essentially equivalent to time domain analysis for the prediction of arrhythmic events after MI, but performed significantly better than time domain analysis for the prediction of cardiac death.

Although it was initially claimed that spectral turbulence analysis is equally suitable for patients with bundle branch block, the study by Englund et al. [93] came to the opposite conclusion, that is, spectral turbulence analysis is applicable only to patients without bundle branch block. Their results were based on a material of 169 patients of whom 120 had a QRS duration $\leq$120 ms; 47 patients had inducible sustained monomorphic VT and were compared to 122 control patients.

The total predictive accuracy for predicting inducible VT was as low as 47% when the whole material was analyzed, however, it increased to 73% when only patients with QRS duration <120 ms were included.

7.7.3   Combined Time Domain and Spectral Turbulence Analysis

The idea to combine time domain and spectral turbulence analysis has been investigated in a number of studies for the purpose of increasing the power of predicting serious arrhythmic events in post-infarction patients [94–96]. The results of these studies indicated that the combined approach may lead to a higher total predictive accuracy than can be achieved using each of the analysis techniques independently. Based on a material of 262 patients with acute MI, Ahuja et al. [94] obtained a total predictive accuracy of 92% when combined analysis was employed for predicting arrhythmic events. The corresponding performance figures for time domain analysis and spectral turbulence analysis were 87% and 78%, respectively.

Improved risk stratification was also found in a study by Mäkijärvi et al. [95] though the levels of predictive accuracy were considerably lower than those reported in [94]. The study comprised a prospective material of 778 males who survived the acute phase of MI. The most powerful prediction of arrhythmic events was achieved by combining time domain and spectral turbulence analysis, reaching a total predictive accuracy of 61% when one of the two techniques showed abnormality and a total predictive accuracy of 87% when both showed abnormality. Spectral turbulence analysis was clearly inferior to time domain analysis in predicting arrhythmic events when used separately.

In yet another study, Vazquez et al. [96] investigated the value of combined analysis on a material of 602 patients after acute MI (of which 38 patients had a major arrhythmic event during the 1-year follow-up period). The total predictive accuracy of combined analysis was 89.9%, significantly higher than achieved separately by time domain analysis (75%) and spectral turbulence analysis (78%).

7.8   High-Frequency QRS Components

7.8.1   Introduction

Frequency analysis of an ECG signal shows that the signal also includes frequencies above the standard frequency range [97]. These high-frequency components are mainly found within the QRS complex, having a low amplitude compared to the components of the standard ECG (μV compared to mV) (❷ Fig. 7.11). Early attempts to visualize high-frequency ECG components employed signal amplification in combination with high paper speed. With this technique, "notches" and "slurs" could be observed within the QRS complex [98, 99]. Studies in the 1970s showed that patients with heart disease had an increased number of notches and slurs compared to healthy individuals. Later analysis of the ECG signal showed that the notches and slurs contained frequencies between 40 and 185 Hz [100].

The development of high-resolution recording techniques combined with digital filtering and signal averaging enabled better analysis of high-frequency components in the ECG signal. Several studies, both on humans and animals, have investigated whether high-frequency QRS components (HF-QRS) contain diagnostic information. Several heart diseases have been studied, such as acute myocardial ischemia [101–109], old MI [109–117] and left ventricular hypertrophy [118, 119]. It is still unknown, however, if the method is useful as a complement to standard ECG for the clinical diagnosis of different heart diseases.

The physiological mechanisms underlying HF-QRS are still not fully understood. One theory is that HF-QRS are related to the conduction velocity and the fragmentation of the depolarization wave in the myocardium. In a three-dimensional model of the ventricles with a fractal conduction system it was shown that high numbers of splitting branches are associated with HF-QRS. In this experiment, it was also shown that the changes seen in HF-QRS in patients with myocardial ischemia might be due to the slowing of the conduction velocity in the region of ischemia [120]. Further electrophysiological studies are needed, however, to better understand the underlying mechanisms of HF-QRS.

There is no standardized method for the recording and quantification of HF-QRS. Both orthogonal leads and all or some of the 12 standard leads have been used in different studies. Several frequency ranges (most commonly 150–250 Hz) and filters have been used as well. Different methods for quantification have also been used. The two most commonly used

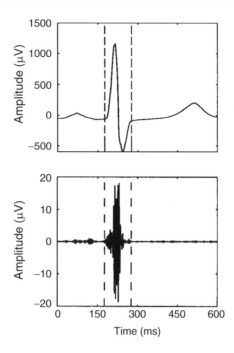

Fig. 7.11

A signal-averaged ECG in the standard frequency range (*upper panel*) and the same ECG within the 150–250 Hz frequency range (*lower panel*). *Dashed lines* indicate the QRS duration determined from the standard frequency range (Reprinted from Pettersson et al. [126] with permission)

methods for quantification are RMS values during the entire QRS duration and "reduced amplitude zones" (RAZ), a way of describing zones in the filtered QRS complex with reduced amplitudes. Due to the low amplitude of the HF-QRS, noise reduction is necessary before analysis. In order to achieve this in a clinical environment, signal averaging is necessary.

7.8.2 Signal Recording and Analysis

To be able to extract HF-QRS it is important to use recording equipment with high resolution acquisition, both in time and amplitude. The sampling rate should be 1,000 Hz or higher [1], and the amplitude resolution at least 1 μV. Since the amplitudes of HF-QRS are in the microvolt range, a low noise level is required. For example, the influence of noise due to skeletal muscle can be reduced by moving the electrodes on the legs and arms to a more proximal position according to Mason and Likar [121]. More importantly, signal averaging must be performed in order to attain an acceptable noise level, sometimes requiring a recording time of several minutes. If the ECG morphology is subject to dynamic changes, for example, observed during percutaneous transluminal coronary angioplasty, recursive averaging with a forgetting factor must be used instead as conventional ensemble averaging is unsuitable.

The HF-QRS is extracted from the signal averaged beats through band pass filtering, often by employing a Butterworth filter [122]. This filter type has a nonlinear phase response which may distort temporal relationships of the various signal components. Linear phase filtering can be obtained, however, by first filtering the entire signal in a forward direction and then filtered signal once more but backward. Different studies have used different bandwidths when extracting HF-QRS, although the frequency range 150–250 Hz is the most common choice.

Several methods have been used for quantification of HF-QRS of which calculation of RMS values during the entire QRS duration is the most common one. For a correct RMS value it is necessary to correctly identify the onset and end of the QRS complex. It has been shown that the most correct delineation of the QRS complex is obtained when determining the QRS duration in the standard frequency range.

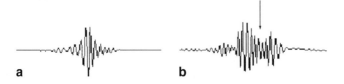

▫ Fig. 7.12

HF-QRS (150–250 Hz) from two individuals, with (**a**) and without (**b**) RAZ

Another method for quantification of HF-QRS is calculation of reduced amplitude zones (RAZ). The RAZ measure is a morphological measure and is defined as an interval between two adjacent local maxima or two adjacent local minima in the HF-QRS, where a local maximum or minimum must have an absolute value higher than the three preceding and three following envelope points (❷ Fig. 7.12). The method was first introduced by Abboud in the 1980s [103]. It was discovered that areas with lower amplitude were present in the high-frequency signal in dogs with myocardial ischemia but not in normal dogs. The method has been developed further, and a scoring system has been proposed [123, 124]. Other methods for quantification of HF-QRS include peak-to-peak amplitude and the integral of the signal.

A recent approach to HF-QRS quantification is to compute the upward and downward slopes of the QRS complex [125]. This technique was designed with the aim to reduce the leakage and smearing caused by linear band pass filtering of the QRS complex. It was shown that both slope coefficients are more sensitive to ischemic changes than is the RMS value obtained from the band pass filtered QRS complex.

The amplitude of HF-QRS differs among the 12 standard leads (❷ Fig. 7.13). The largest amplitudes are usually found in the anterior-posterior-oriented leads V2–V4 and in the inferior-superior-oriented leads II, aVF, and III. The lowest amplitudes are found in the left-right-oriented leads aVL, I, -aVR, V1, V5, and V6 [126]. In the transverse plane, the leads V1 and V6 are located furthest away from the left ventricle, which is a possible explanation for the low amplitudes recorded in these leads. In the frontal plane, however, no leads are located close to the heart, but there is still a large difference in amplitude of HF-QRS between these leads.

The correlation between HF-QRS and the QRS amplitudes in standard ECG is generally low. Thus, factors other than the QRS amplitude in standard ECG seem to influence the size of HF-QRS. There is also a large variation in HF-QRS between individuals. During consecutive registrations on the same individual, however, only small variations in HF-QRS are registered [126]. When studying healthy individuals, no significant differences in HF-QRS regarding sex and age have been found [117].

7.9 HF-QRS in Heart Disease

7.9.1 Ischemic Heart Disease

Several studies have compared HF-QRS in patients with old MI to HF-QRS in normal subjects. The vast majority of these studies show reduced amplitudes after old MI. In the frequency range 80–300 Hz HF-QRS are significantly lower in leads V2 and V5 in patients with old anterior MI [112]. In patients with old inferior infarction, HF-QRS are reduced in leads II, aVF, and III [110, 112]. When recording with Frank leads (X, Y, and Z leads), reduced HF-QRS are found in patients with old anterior and/or inferior infarction [114]. There are some studies, however, that show higher HF-QRS in patients with old MI compared to normal individuals, measured with frequencies >90 Hz using Frank leads [115].

Studies on patients with angiographically documented ischemic heart disease, with and without signs of old MI on ECG, do not show any difference in HF-QRS between the two populations [116]. When comparing a healthy population with patients with ischemic heart disease, both with and without old MI, the healthy population shows higher HF-QRS than the patient group [117]. These results indicate that ischemic heart disease, with and without old MI, causes a reduction of HF-QRS. A possible explanation is that chronic ischemic heart disease leads to structural changes in the myocardial tissue. These changes may contribute to abnormal impulse propagation in the ischemic heart. This abnormal propagation might be the reason for the reduced high-frequency content in patients with ischemic heart disease.

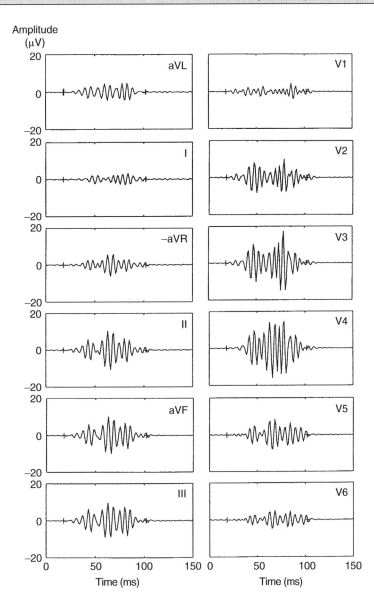

◻ Fig. 7.13
Filtered QRS complexes (150–250 Hz) in 12 standard leads from a patient with typical amplitude distribution among the leads. *Tick marks* indicate QRS onset and offset, determined from the standard frequency ECG (Reprinted from Pettersson et al. [126] with permission)

7.9.2   Acute Myocardial Ischemia

Several studies have reported lower HF-QRS during acute myocardial ischemia. In a study on dogs, ECG was recorded both from epicardial electrodes and from surface electrodes during occlusion of the left anterior descending coronary artery. HF-QRS recorded from the epicardium of the left ventricle were significantly reduced during the occlusion, while HF-QRS recorded from the nonischemic right ventricle remained unchanged. Reduced HF-QRS from the surface electrodes were also found [102]. Other animal studies have shown similar results [101, 104–106].

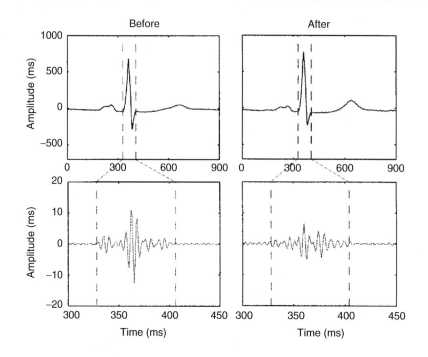

⬛ **Fig. 7.14**

Lead V5. *Upper panel*: Pre-inflation and inflation ECGs in the standard frequency range. *Lower panel*: The same ECGs within the HF range (150–250 Hz). The *dashed lines* indicate the QRS duration, determined from the standard frequency ECG (Reprinted from Pettersson et al. [109] with permission)

In humans, the ECG has been recorded during percutaneous transluminal coronary angioplasty [108, 109]. The results from these studies show that ischemia leads to changes in HF-QRS in a majority of the patients. These changes can be observed even when no ST changes in standard ECG are seen (❯ Fig. 7.14). The results indicate that acute myocardial ischemia can be detected with higher sensitivity with analysis of HF-QRS compared to conventional analysis with standard ECG. Analysis of HF-QRS might therefore serve as a complement to standard ECG in the detection of myocardial ischemia. The large inter-individual variation in HF-QRS, however, probably makes high-frequency analysis most applicable to monitoring situations when changes from baseline can be identified.

During occlusion of the left anterior descending coronary artery a reduction in HF-QRS is observed in many leads, most commonly in lead V3. During occlusion of other large coronary arteries a reduction in HF-QRS is seen in various leads. Thus, HF-QRS seem to be poorer than standard ECG in detecting the location of ischemia.

7.9.3   Reperfusion

To assess the resolution of ST segment elevation is the most commonly used method for detecting reperfusion during thrombolytic therapy for acute MI. A couple of studies have shown that successful reperfusion also results in a significant increase in HF-QRS (❯ Fig. 7.15) [127, 128]. More and larger studies are needed, however, to determine if analysis of HF-QRS could be a useful method for monitoring patients during treatment of acute MI.

7.9.4   Stress-Induced Ischemia

Analysis of HF-QRS during exercise test has been suggested as a complement to assessment of the ST segment reaction for detection of exercise-induced ischemia. It has been shown that HF-QRS increase during exercise in healthy

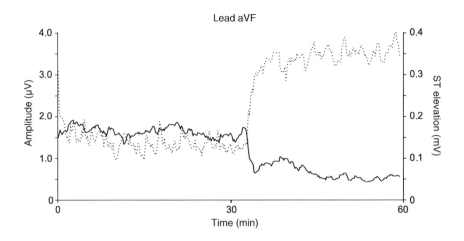

◻ Fig. 7.15

Dynamic changes in lead aVF in HF-QRS (*dashed line*) and ST segment (*solid line*) during reperfusion therapy for acute inferior MI. After 30 min of therapy, the ST elevation decreases and the HF-QRS simultaneously increases

individuals [129]. In a study comparing healthy individuals to patients with ischemic heart disease, it was found that HF-QRS are significantly higher in the healthy population, both during and after exercise [130]. Two other studies have shown that a large relative change in HF-QRS during exercise is more sensitive for detecting ischemia in myocardial perfusion imaging test compared to conventional ST analysis [131, 132]. A recent study investigated changes in HF-QRS during adenosine myocardial perfusion imaging stress tests [133]. It was found that analysis of HF-QRS is highly sensitive and specific for detecting reversible perfusion defects, and significantly more sensitive than conventional ST segment analysis. Another study trying to reproduce these findings found, however, that analysis of HF-QRS was no better than tossing a coin for detecting reversible perfusion defects [134]. A problem with analysis of HF-QRS recorded during exercise is the high noise level generated by skeletal muscle.

7.9.5 Left Ventricular Hypertrophy

Standard ECG is one of the most common methods to detect left ventricular hypertrophy. Several different ECG-based criteria are used clinically. These methods, however, have low sensitivity when a high level of specificity is required. Studies on rabbits, with and without left ventricular hypertrophy, have shown that HF-QRS correlate well with left ventricular mass [119]. In the study, the vector magnitude from orthogonal leads in different frequency ranges was studied. High-pass filtering at 44 Hz showed the best correlation between left ventricular mass and HF-QRS ($r = 0.84$). A high correlation between left ventricular mass and HF-QRS was also found among the healthy rabbits alone.

Studies on humans have shown more diverging results. A study on 15 patients, both with normal and pathologic left ventricular mass, determined by echocardiography, showed that the sum of vectors in orthogonal leads in the 2–250 Hz range had approximately the same correlation with left ventricular mass as do established electrocardiographic criteria for left ventricular hypertrophy [118]. Another study on 60 healthy individuals, using magnetic resonance imaging as gold standard, found no correlation between HF-QRS and left ventricular mass [135]. Thus, it is not certain whether HF-QRS can be of value in the electrocardiographic diagnosis of left ventricular hypertrophy.

7.9.6 Conduction Abnormalities

In dogs, HF-QRS are reduced during slow conduction velocity in the heart [136]. By infusing sodium channel blockers (lidocaine, disopyramide) in the left anterior descending coronary artery at the same time as recording ECGs from the entire ventricular surface, it has been shown that HF-QRS are significantly lower in the areas affected by the sodium channel blockers. These results indicate that HF-QRS is a potent indicator of disturbed local conduction.

7.9.7   Heart Transplantation and Heart Surgery

Allograft rejection is a major cause of morbidity and mortality in patients who have undergone heart transplant. There is no reliable method for detecting rejection except endomyocardial biopsy. Some studies have investigated whether HF-QRS could be used as a noninvasive marker for rejection [137, 138]. The results from the studies have in part showed diverging results, with both an increase and a decrease in HF-QRS at rejection.

In a study on patients after heart surgery, a reduction of HF-QRS correlating with the dysfunction of the heart has been found [139]. It is therefore suggested that HF-QRS could be used as a noninvasive marker of myocardial dysfunction after heart surgery. In children who have undergone heart surgery, the change in HF-QRS during aortic clamping has been investigated [140]. I was found that the recovery time of the HF-QRS significantly correlated with cardioplegic arrest time during surgery.

References

1. Sörnmo, L. and P. Laguna, *Bioelectrical Signal Processing in Cardiac and Neurological Applications*. Amsterdam: Elsevier (Academic Press), 2005.
2. Hombach, V., V. Braun, H.W. Hopp, et al., The applicability of the signal averaging technique in clinical cardiology. *Clin. Cardiol.*, 1982;**5**: 107–124.
3. Ros, H.H., A.S.M. Koeleman, and T.J. Akker, The technique of signal averaging and its practical application in the separation of atrial and His Purkinje activity, in *Signal Averaging Technique in Clinical Cardiology*, V. Hombach and H.H. Hilger, Editors. Stuttgart: Schattauer, 1981, p. 3.
4. Rompelman, O. and H.H. Ros, Coherent averaging technique: a tutorial review. Part 1: noise reduction and the equivalent filter. Part 2: trigger jitter, overlapping responses and nonperiodic stimulation. *J. Biomed. Eng.*, 1986;**8**: 24–35.
5. Laciar, E., R. Jané, and D.H. Brooks, Improved alignment method for noisy high-resolution ECG and Holter records using multiscale cross-correlation. *IEEE Trans. Biomed. Eng.*, 2003;**50**: 344–353.
6. Simson, M.B., Use of signals in the terminal QRS complex to identify patients with ventricular tachycardia after myocardial infarction. *Circulation*, 1981;**64**: 235–242.
7. Berbari, E.J. and P. Lander, Principles of noise reduction, in *High-Resolution Electrocardiography*, N. El-Sherif and G. Turitto, Editors. Armonk: Futura, 1992, pp. 51–66.
8. Plonsey, R., *Bioelectric Phenomena*. New York: McGraw-Hill, 1969, pp. 281–299.
9. Kienzle, M.G., R.A. Falcone, and M.B. Simson, Alterations in the initial portion of the signal averaged QRS complex in acute myocardial infarction with ventricular tachycardia. *Am. J. Cardiol.*, 1988;**61**: 91–103.
10. Atarius, R. and L. Sörnmo, Maximum likelihood analysis of cardiac late potentials. *IEEE Trans. Biomed. Eng.*, 2006;**43**: 60–68.
11. Steinberg, J.S. and J.T. Bigger, Importance of the endpoint of noise reduction in analysis of the signal-averaged electrocardiogram. *Am. J. Cardiol.*, 1989;**63**: 556–560.
12. Boineau, J.P. and J.L. Cox, Slow ventricular activation in acute myocardial infarction: A source of reentrant premature ventricular contraction. *Circulation*, 1973;**48**(4): 702–713.
13. Waldo, A.L. and G.A. Kaiser, A study of ventricular arrhythmias associated with acute myocardial infarction in the canine heart. *Circulation*, 1973;**47**(6): 1222–1228.
14. El-Sherif, N., B.J. Scherlag, and R. Lazzara, Electrode catheter recordings during malignant ventricular arrhythmias following experimental acute myocardial ischemia. *Circulation*, 1975;**51**(6): 1003–1014.
15. El-Sherif, N., B.J. Scherlag, R. Lazzara, and R.R. Hope, Reentrant ventricular arrhythmias in the late myocardial infarction period. 1. Conduction characteristics in the infarction zone. *Circulation*, 1977;**55**(5): 686–702.
16. El-Sherif, N., R.R. Hope, B.J. Scherlag, and R. Lazzara, Reentrant ventricular arrhythmias in the late myocardial infarction period. 2. Patterns of initiation and termination of re-entry. *Circulation*, 1977;**55**(5): 702–719.
17. Simson, M.B., W.J. Untereker, S.R. Spielman, L.N. Horowitz, N.H. Marcus, R.A. Falcone, et al., The relationship between late potentials on the body surface and directly recorded fragmented electrograms in patients with ventricular tachycardia. *Am. J. Cardiol.*, 1983;**51**(1): 105–112.
18. Berbari, E.J., B.J. Scherlag, R.R. Hope, and R. Lazzara, Recording from the body surface of arrhythmogenic ventricular activity during the S-T segment. *Am. J. Cardiol.*, 1978;**41**(4): 697–702.
19. Josephson, M.E., L.N. Horowitz, and A. Farshidi, Continuous local electrical activity. A mechanism of recurrent ventricular tachycardia. *Circulation*, 1978;**57**(4): 659–665.
20. Breithardt, G., R. Becker, L. Seipel, R.R. Abendroth, and J. Ostermeyer, Non-invasive detection of late potentials in man–a new marker for ventricular tachycardia. *Eur. Heart J.*, 1981;**2**(1): 1–11.
21. Fontaine, G., G. Guiraudon, R. Frank, et al., Stimulation studies and epicardial mapping in ventricular tachycardia. Study of mechanisms and selection for surgery, in *Reentrant Arrhythmias*, H. Kulbertus, Editor. Lancaster: MTP; 1977, p. 334.

22. Rozanski, J.J., D. Mortara, R.J. Myerburg, and A. Castellanos, Body surface detection of delayed depolarizations in patients with recurrent ventricular tachycardia and left ventricular aneurysm. *Circulation*, 1981;**63**(5): 1172–1178.

23. Simson, M.B., D. Euler, and E.L. Michelson, Detection of delayed ventricular activation on the body surface in dogs. *Am. J. Physiol.*, 1981;**241**(3): H363–H369.

24. Denniss, A.R., D.A. Richards, D.V. Cody, P.A. Russell, A.A. Young, D.L. Ross, et al., Correlation between signal-averaged electrocardiogram and programmed stimulation in patients with and without spontaneous ventricular tachyarrhythmias. *Am. J. Cardiol.*, 1987;**59**(6): 586–590.

25. Breithardt, G., M. Borggrefe, U. Karbenn, R.R. Abendroth, H.L. Yeh, and L. Seipel, Prevalence of late potentials in patients with and without ventricular tachycardia: correlation and angiographic findings. *Am. J. Cardiol.*, 1982;**49**(8): 1932.

26. Kanovsky, M.S., R.A. Falcone, C.A. Dresden, M.E. Josephson, and M.B. Simson, Identification of patients with ventricular tachycardia after myocardial infarction: signal-averaged electrocardiogram, Holter monitoring, and cardiac catherization. *Circulation*, 1984;**70**(2): 264–270.

27. Gomes, J.A., S.L. Winters, M. Martinson, J. Machac, D. Stewart, and A. Targonski, The prognostic significance of quantitative signal-averaged variables relative to clinical variables, site of myocardial infarction, ejection fraction and ventricular premature beats: a prospective study. *J. Am. Coll. Cardiol.*, 1989;**13**(2): 377–384.

28. Breithardt, G., M. Borggrefe, and K. Haerten, Role of programmed ventricular stimulation an noninvasive recording of ventricular late potentials for the identification of patients at risk of ventricular tachyarrhythmias after acute myocardial infarction, in *Cardiac Electrophysiology and Arrhythmias*, D.P. Zipes and J. Jalife, Editors. New York: Grune and Stratton, 1985, pp. 553–561.

29. Breithardt, G. and M. Borggrefe, Recent advances in the identification of patients at risk of ventricular tachyarrhythmias: role of ventricular late potentials. *Circulation*, 1987;**75**(6): 1091–1096.

30. Cain, M.E., J.L. Anderson, M.F. Arnsdorf, J.W. Mason, M.M. Scheinman, and A.L. Waldo, Signal-averaged electrocardiography. *J. Am. Coll. Cardiol.*, 1996;**27**(1): 238–249.

31. Gang, E.S., A.S. Lew, M. Hong, F.Z. Wang, C.A. Siebert, T. Peter, Decreased incidence of ventricular late potentials after successful thrombolytic therapy for acute myocardial infarction. *N. Engl. J. Med.*, 1989;**321**(11): 712–716.

32. Eldar, M., J. Leor, H. Hod, Z. Rotstein, S. Truman, E. Kaplinsky, et al., Effect of thrombolysis on the evolution of late potentials within 10 days of infarction. *Br. Heart J.*, 1990;**63**(5): 272–276.

33. Chew, E.W., P. Morton, J.G. Murtagh, M.E. Scott, and D.B. O'Keeffe, Intravenous streptokinase for acute myocardial infarction reduces the occurrence of ventricular late potentials. *Br. Heart J.*, 1990;**64**(1): 5–8.

34. Turitto, G., A.L. Risa, E. Zanchi, and P.L. Prati, The signal-averaged electrocardiogram and ventricular arrhythmias after thrombolysis for acute myocardial infarction. *J. Am. Coll. Cardiol.*, 1990;**15**(6): 1270–1276.

35. Tranchesi, B.J., M. Verstraete, F. van de Werf, C.P. de Albuquerque, B. Caramelli, O.C. Gebara, et al., Usefulness of high-frequency analysis of signal-averaged surface electrocardiograms in acute myocardial infarction before and after coronary thrombolysis for assessing coronary reperfusion. *Am. J. Cardiol.*, 1990;**66**(17): 1196–1198.

36. Aguirre, F.V., M.J. Kern, J. Hsia, H. Serota, D. Janosik, T. Greenwalt, et al., Importance of myocardial infarct artery patency on the prevalence of ventricular arrhythmias and late potentials after thrombolysis in acute myocardial infarction. *Am. J. Cardiol.*, 1991;**68**(15): 1410–1416.

37. Vatterott, P.J., S.C. Hammill, K.R. Bailey, C.M. Wiltgen, and B.J. Gersh, Late potentials on signal-averaged electrocardiograms and patency of the infarct-related artery in survivors of acute myocardial infarction. *J. Am. Coll. Cardiol.*, 1991;**17**(2): 330–337.

38. Santarelli, P., G.A. Lanza, F. Biscione, A. Natale, G. Corsini, C. Riccio, et al., Effects of thrombolysis and atenolol or metoprolol on the signal-averaged electrocardiogram after acute myocardial infarction. Late Potentials Italian Study (LAPIS). *Am. J. Cardiol.*, 1993;**72**(7): 525–531.

39. Moreno, F.L., L. Karagounis, H. Marshall, R.L. Menlove, S. Ipsen, and J.L. Anderson, Thrombolysis-related early patency reduces ECG late potentials after acute myocardial infarction. *Am. Heart J.*, 1992;**124**(3): 557–564.

40. de Chillou, C., N. Sadoul, S. Briancon, and E. Aliot, Factors determining the occurrence of late potentials on the signal-averaged electrocardiogram after a first myocardial infarction: a multivariate analysis. *J. Am. Coll. Cardiol.*, 1991;**18**(7): 1638–1642.

41. Maki, H., Y. Ozawa, N. Tanigawa, I. Watanabe, R. Kojima, S. Yakubo, et al., Effect of reperfusion by direct percutaneous transluminal coronary angioplasty on ventricular late potentials in cases of total coronary occlusion at initial coronary arteriography. *Jpn. Circ. J.*, 1993;**57**(3): 183–188.

42. Kawalsky, D.L., K.N. Garratt, S.C. Hammill, K.R. Bailey, and B.J. Gersh, Effects of infarct-related artery patency and late potentials on late mortality after acute myocardial infarction. *Mayo Clin. Proc.*, 1997;**72**(5): 414–421.

43. Savard, P., J.L. Rouleau, J. Ferguson, N. Poitras, P. Morel, R.F. Davies, et al., Risk stratification after myocardial infarction using signal-averaged electrocardiographic criteria adjusted for sex, age, and myocardial infarction location. *Circulation*, 1997;**96**(1): 202–213.

44. Scharf, C., H. Redecker, F. Duru, R. Candinas, H.P. Brunner-La Rocca, A. Gerb, et al., Sudden cardiac death after coronary artery bypass grafting is not predicted by signal-averaged ECG. *Ann. Thorac. Surg.*, 2001;**72**(5): 1546–1551.

45. Bauer, A., P. Guzik, P. Barthel, R. Schneider, K. Ulm, M.A. Watanabe, et al., Reduced prognostic power of ventricular late potentials in post-infarction patients of the reperfusion era. *Eur. Heart J.*, 2005;**26**(8): 755–761.

46. Kuchar, D.L., C.W. Thorburn, and N.L. Sammel, Prediction of serious arrhythmic events after myocardial infarction: Signal-averaged electrocardiogram, Holter monitoring and radionuclide ventriculography. *J. Am. Coll. Cardiol.*, 1987;**9**(3): 531–538.

47. Gomes, J.A., S.L. Winters, D. Stewart, S. Horowitz, M. Milner, and P.A. Barreca, New noninvasive index to predict sustained ventricular tachycardia and sudden death in the first year after myocardial infarction: based on signal averaged electrocardiogram, radionuclide ejection fraction and Holter monitoring. *J. Am. Coll. Cardiol.*, 1987;**10**(2): 349–357.

48. Kuchar, D.L., C.W. Thorburn, and N.L. Sammel, Signal-averaged electrocardiogram for evaluation of recurrent syncope. *Am. J. Cardiol.*, 1986;**58**(10): 949–953.

49. Lacroix, D., M. Dubuc, T. Kus, P. Savard, M. Shenasa, and R. Nadeau, Evaluation of arrhythmic causes of syncope; correlation between Holter monitoring, electrophysiologic testing,

and body surface potential mapping. *Am. Heart J.*, 1991;**122**(5): 1346–1354.

50. Uther, J.B., C.J. Dennett, and A. Tan, The detection of delayed activation signals of low amplitude in the vectorcardiogram of patients with recurrent ventricular tachycardia by signal averaging, in *Management of Ventricular Tachycardia – Role of Mexiletine*, E. Sabndoe, D.J. Julian, and J.W. Bell, Editors. Amsterdam: Excerpta Medica, 1978, p. 80.

51. Breithardt, G., L. Seipel, J. Ostermeyer, U. Karbenn, R.R. Abendorth, M. Borggrefe, et al., Effects of anti-arrhythmic surgery on late ventricular potentials recorded by precordial signal averaging in patients with ventricular tachycardia. *Am. Heart J.*, 1982;**104**(5 Pt 1): 996–1003.

52. Marcus, N.H., R.A. Falcone, A.H. Harken, M.E. Josephson, and M.B. Simson, Body surface late potentials: Effects of endocardial resection in patients with ventricular tachycardia. *Circulation*, 1984;**70**(4): 632–637.

53. Denniss, A.R., A.J. Ross, D.A. Richards, D.V. Cody, P.A. Russell, A.A. Young, et al., Effect of anti-arrhythmic therapy on delayed potentials detected by the signal-averaged electrocardiogram in patients with ventricular tachycardia after acute myocardial infarction. *Am. J. Cardiol.*, 1986;**58**(3): 261–265.

54. Simson, M.B., E. Kindwall, A.E. Buxton, and M.E. Josephson, Signal averaging of the ECG in the management of patients with ventricular tachycardia: prediction of anti-arrhythmic drug efficacy, in *Cardiac Arrhythmias: Where to Go From Here?* P. Brugada and H.J. Wellens, Editors. Armonk, NY: Futura, 1987, p. 299.

55. Hopson, J.R., M.G. Kienzle, A.M. Aschoff, and D.R. Shirkey, Noninvasive prediction of efficacy of type IA anti-arrhythmic drugs by the signal-averaged electrocardiogram in patients with coronary artery disease and sustained ventricular tachycardia. *Am. J. Cardiol.*, 1993;**72**(3): 288–293.

56. Kulakowski, P., Y. Bashir, S. Heald, V. Paul, M.H. Anderson, S. Gibson, et al., Effects of procainamide on the signal-averaged electrocardiogram in relation to the results of programmed ventricular stimulation in patients with sustained monomorphic ventricular tacycardia. *J. Am. Coll. Cardiol.*, 1993;**21**(6): 1428–1439.

57. Freedman, R.A. and J.S. Steinberg, Electrophysiologic Study Versus Electrocardiographic Monitoring Trial (ESVEM) Investigators. Selective prolongation of QRS late potentials by sodium channel blocking anti-arrhythmic drugs: relation to slowing of ventricular tachycardia. *J. Am. Coll. Cardiol.*, 1991;**17**(5): 1017–1025.

58. Greenspon, A.J., G.A. Kidwell, M. DeCaro, and S. Hessen, The effects of type I anti-arrhythmic drugs on the signal-averaged electrocardiogram in patients with malignant ventricular arrhythmias. *Pacing Clin. Electrophysiol.*, 1992;**15**(10 Pt 1): 1445–1453.

59. Goedel-Meinen, L., M. Hofmann, G. Schmidt, W. Maier-Rudolph, P. Barthel, A. Schrag, et al., Amiodarone-efficacy and late potentials during long-term therapy. *Int. J. Clin. Pharm. Ther. Toxicol.*, 1990;**28**(11): 449–454.

60. Simson, M.B., H.L. Waxman, R. Falcone, N.H. Marcus, and M.E. Josephson, Effects of anti-arrhythmic drugs on noninvasively recorded late potentials, in *New Aspects in the Medical Treatment of Tachyarrhythmias*, G. Breithardt and F. Loogen, Editors. Munich: Urban and Schwarzenberg, 1983, pp. 80–86.

61. Keren, A., A.M. Gillis, R.A. Freedman, J.C. Baldwin, M.E. Billingham, E.B. Stinson, et al., Heart transplant rejection monitored by signal-averaged electrocardiography in patients receiving cyclosporine. *Circulation*, 1984;**70**(3 Pt 2): 1124–1129.

62. Lacroix, D., S. Kacet, P. Savard, F. Molin, J. Dagano, A. Pol, et al., Signal-averaged electrocardiography and detection of heart transplant rejection: comparison of time- and frequency-domain analyses. *J. Am. Coll. Cardiol.*, 1992;**19**(3): 553–558.

63. Haberl, R., M. Weber, H. Reichenspurner, B.M. Kemkes, G. Osterholzer, M. Anthuber, et al., Frequency analysis of the surface electrocardiogram for recognition of acute rejection after orthoptic cardiac transplantation in man. *Circulation*, 1987;**76**(1): 101–108.

64. Valentino, V.A., H.O. Ventura, F.M. Abi-Samra, C. van Meter, H.L. Price, The signal-averaged electrocardiogram in cardiac transplantation. *Transplantation*, 1992;**53**(1): 124–127.

65. Poll, D.S., F.E. Marchlinski, R.A. Falcone, M.E. Josephson, and M.B. Simson, Abnormal signal averaged electrocardiograms in patients with nonischemic congestive cardiomyopathy: relationship to sustained ventricular tachyarrhythmias. *Circulation*, 1985;**72**(6): 1308–1313.

66. Mancini, D., K.L. Wong, and M.B. Simson, Prognostic value of an abnormal signal-averaged electrocardiogram in patients with nonischemic congestive cardiomyopathy. *Circulation*, 1993;**87**(4): 1083–1092.

67. Ohnishi, Y., T. Inoue, and H. Fukuzaki, Value of the signal-averaged electrocardiogram as a predictor of sudden death in myocardial infarction and dilated cardiomyopathy. *Jpn. Circ. J.*, 1990;**54**(2): 127–136.

68. Middlekauff, H.R., W.G. Stevenson, M.A. Woo, D.K. Moser, and L.W. Stenvenson, Comparison of frequency of late potentials in idiopathic dilated cardiomyopathy and ischemic cardiomyopathy with advanced congestive heart failure and their usefulness in predicting sudden death. *Am. J. Cardiol.*, 1990;**66**(15): 1113–1117.

69. Denereaz, D., M. Zimmermann, and R. Ademec, Significance of ventricular late potentials in non-ischemic dilated cardiomyopathy. *Eur. Heart J.*, 1992;**13**(7): 895–901.

70. Keeling, P.J., P. Kulakowski, G. Yi, A.K. Slade, S.E. Bent, and W.J. McKenna, Usefulness of signal-averaged electrocardiogram in idiopathic dilated cardiomyopathy for identifying patients with ventricular arrhythmias. *Am. J. Cardiol.*, 1993;**72**(1):78–84.

71. Santangeli, P., F. Infusino, G.A. Sgueglia, A. Sestito, and G.A. Lanza, Ventricular late potentials: a critical overview and current applications. *J. Electrocardiol.*, 2008;**41**: 318–324.

72. Francés, R.J., Arrhythmogenic right ventricular dysplasia/cardiomyopathy. A review and update. *Int. J. Cardiol.*, 2006;**110**: 279–287.

73. Nava, A., A.F. Folino, B. Bauce, P. Turrini, G.F. Buja, L. Daliento, and G. Thiene, Signal-averaged electrocardiogram with arrhythmogenic right ventricular cardiomyopathy and ventricular arrhythmias. *Eur. Heart J.*, 2000;**21**: 58–65.

74. Ikeda, T., H. Sakurada, K. Sakabe, T. Sakata, M. Takami, N. Tezuka, T. Nakae, M. Noro, Y. Enjoji, T. Tejima, K. Sugi, and T. Yamaguchi, Assessment of noninvasive markers in identifying patients at risk in the Brugada syndrome: insight into risk stratification. *J. Am. Coll. Cardiol.*, 2001;**37**: 1628–1634.

75. Ikeda, T., M. Takami, K. Sugi, Y. Mizusawa, H. Sakurada, and H. Yoshino, Noninvasive risk stratification of subjects with a Brugada-type electrocardiogram and no history of cardiac arrest. *Ann. Noninvasive Electrocardiol.*, 2005;**10**: 396–403.

76. Marple, S.J., *Digital Spectral Analysis with Applications*. New Jersey: Prentice-Hall, 1987.

77. Pierce, D.L., A.R. Easley, J.R. Windle, and T.R. Engel, Fast Fourier transformation of the entire low amplitude late QRS potential to predict ventricular tachycardia. *J. Am. Coll. Cardiol.*, 1989;**14**: 1741–1743.

78. Cain, M.E., H.D. Ambos, F. Witkowski, and B.E. Sobel, Fast-Fourier transform analysis of signal-averaged electrocardiograms for identification of patients prone to sustained ventricular tachycardia. *Circulation*, 1984;**69**: 711–720.

79. Cain, M.E., H.D. Ambos, J. Markham, A.E. Fischer, and B.E. Sobel, Quantification of differences in frequency content of signal-averaged electrocardiograms in patients with compared to those without sustained ventricular tachycardia. *Am. J. Cardiol.*, 1985;**55**: 1500–1505.

80. Lindsay, B.D., J. Markham, K.B. Schechtman, H.D. Ambos, and M.E. Cain, Identification of patients with sustained ventricular tachycardia by frequency analysis of signal-averaged electrocardiograms despite the presence of bundle branch block. *Circulation*, 1988;**77**: 122–130.

81. Kelen, G.J., R. Henkin, J. Fontaine, and N. El-Sherif, Effects of analysed signal duration and phase on the results of fast fourier transform analysis of the surface electrocardiogram in subjects with and without late potentials. *Am. J. Cardiol.*, 1987;**60**: 1282–1289.

82. Machac, J., A. Weiss, S.L. Winters, P. Barecca, and J.A. Gomes, A comparative study of frequency domain and time domain analysis of signal averaged electrocardiograms in patients with ventricular tachycardia. *J. Am. Coll. Cardiol.*, 1988;**11**: 284–296.

83. Machac, J. and J.A. Gomes, Frequency domain analysis, in *Signal-Averaged Electrocardiography. Concepts, Methods and Applications*, chapter 6, J.A. Gomes, Editor. Boston, MA: Kluwer, 1993, pp. 81–123.

84. Worley, S.J., D.B. Mark, W.M. Smith, P. Wolf, R.M. Califf, H.C. Strauss, M.G. Manwaring, and R.E. Ideker, Comparison of time domain and frequency domain variables from the signal-averaged electrocardiogram: a multivariable analysis. *J. Am. Coll. Cardiol.*, 1988;**11**: 1041–1051.

85. Buckingham, T.A., C.M. Thessen, D. Hertweck, D.L. Janosik, and H.L. Kennedy, Signal-averaged electrocardiography in the time and frequency domains. *Am. J. Cardiol.*, 1989;**63**: 820–825.

86. Haberl, R., G. Jilge, R. Pulter, and G. Steinbeck, Comparison of frequency and time domain analysis of the signal-averaged electrocardiogram in patients with ventricular tachycardia and coronary artery disease: methodologic validation and clinical relevance. *J. Am. Coll. Cardiol.*, 1988;**12**: 150–158.

87. Haberl, R., G. Jilge, R. Pulter, and G. Steinbeck, Spectral mapping of the electrocardiogram with Fourier transform for identification of patients with sustained ventricular tachycardia and coronary artery disease. *Eur. Heart. J.*, 1989;**10**: 316–322.

88. Lander, P., D.E. Albert, and E.J. Berbari, Spectrotemporal analysis of ventricular late potentials. *J. Electrocardiol.*, 1990;**23**: 95–108.

89. Malik, M., P. Kulakowski, J. Poloniecki, A. Staunton, O. Odemuyiwa, T. Farrell, and J. Camm, Frequency versus time domain analysis of signal-averaged electrocardiograms. I. Reproducibility of the results. *J. Am. Coll. Cardiol.*, 1992;**20**: 127–134.

90. Kelen, G.J., R. Henkin, A.M. Starr, E.B. Caref, D. Bloomfield, and N. El-Sherif, Spectral turbulence analysis of the signal-averaged electrocardiogram and its predictive accuracy for inducible sustained monomorphic ventricular tachycardia. *Am. J. Cardiol.*, 1991;**67**: 965–975.

91. Malik, M., P. Kulakowski, K. Hnatkova, A. Staunton, and A.J. Camm, Spectral turbulence analysis versus time-domain analysis of the signal-averaged ECG in survivors of acute myocardial infarction. *J. Electrocardiol.*, 1994;**27**: S227–S232.

92. Copie, X., K. Hnatkova, A. Staunton, A.J. Camm, and M. Malik, Spectral turbulence versus time-domain analysis of signal-averaged ECG used for the prediction of different arrhythmic events in survivors of acute myocardial infarction. *J. Cardiovasc. Electrophysiol.*, 1996;**7**: 583–593.

93. Englund, A., M. Andersson, and L. Bergfeldt, Spectral turbulence analysis of the signal-averaged electrocardiogram for predicting inducible sustained monomorphic ventricular tachycardia in patients with and without bundle branch block. *Eur. Heart J.*, 1995;**16**: 1936–1942.

94. Ahuja, R.K., G. Turitto, B. Ibrahim, E.B. Caref, and N. El-Sherif, Combined time-domain and spectral turbulence analysis of the signal-averaged ECG improves its predictive accuracy in postinfarction patients. *J. Electrocardiol.*, 1994;**27**: S202–S206.

95. Mäkijärvi, M., T. Fetsch, L. Reinhardt, A. Martinez-Rubio, M. Shenasa, M. Borggrefe, and G. Breithardt, Comparison and combination of late potentials and spectral turbulence analysis to predict arrhythmic events after myocardial infarction in the Post-Infarction Late Potential (PILP) study. *Eur. Heart J.* 1995; **16**: 651–659.

96. Vazquez, R., E.B. Caref, F. Torres, M. Reina, A. Espina, and N. El-Sherif, Improved diagnostic value of combined time and frequency domain analysis of the signal-averaged electrocardiogram after myocardial infarction. *J. Am. Coll. Cardiol.*, 1999;**33**: 385–394.

97. Golden, D.P. Jr., R.A. Wolthuis, and G.W. Hoffler, A spectral analysis of the normal resting electrocardiogram. *IEEE Trans. Biomed. Eng.*, 1973;**20**: 366–372.

98. Reynolds, E.W., B.F. Muller, G.J. Anderson, and B.T. Muller, High frequency components in the electrocardiogram. A comparative study of normals and patients with myocardial disease. *Circulation*, 1967;**35**: 195–206.

99. Flowers, N.C., L.G. Horan, J.R. Thomas, and W.J. Tolleson, The anatomic basis for high-frequency components in the electrocardiogram. *Circulation*, 1969;**39**: 531–539.

100. Mor-Avi, V., S. Abboud, and S. Akselrod, Frequency content of the QRS notching in high-fidelity canine ECG. *Comput. Biomed. Res.*, 1989;**22**: 18–28.

101. Abboud, S., Subtle alterations in the high-frequency QRS potentials during myocardial ischemia in dogs. *Comput. Biomed. Res.*, 1987;**20**: 384–395.

102. Mor-Avi, V., B. Shargorodsky, S. Abboud, S. Laniado, and S. Akselrod, Effects of coronary occlusion on high-frequency components of the epicardial electrogram and body surface electrocardiogram. *Circulation*, 1987;**76**: 237–243.

103. Abboud, S., R.J. Cohen, A. Selwyn, P. Ganz, D. Sadeh, and P.L. Friedman, Detection of transient myocardial ischemia by computer analysis of standard and signal-averaged high-frequency electrocardiograms in patients undergoing percutaneous transluminal coronary angioplasty. *Circulation*, 1987;**76**: 585–596.

104. Abboud, S., J.M. Smith, B. Shargorodsky, S. Laniado, D. Sadeh, and R.J. Cohen, High frequency electrocardiography of three orthogonal leads in dogs during a coronary artery occlusion. *PACE*, 1989;**12**: 574–581.

105. Abboud, S., R.J. Cohen, and D. Sadeh, A spectral analysis of the high frequency QRS potentials observed during acute myocardial ischemia in dogs. *Int. J. Cardiol.*, 1990;**26**: 285–290.

106. Mor-Avi, V. and S. Akselrod, Spectral analysis of canine epicardial electrogram; short term variations in the frequency content induced by myocardial ischemia. *Circ. Res.*, 1990;**66**: 1681–1691.

107. Abboud, S., High-frequency electrocardiogram analysis of the entire QRS in the diagnosis and assessment of coronary artery disease. *Prog. Cardiovasc. Dis.*, 1993;**35**: 311–328.

108. Pettersson, J., P. Lander, O. Pahlm, L. Sörnmo, S.G. Warren, and G.S. Wagner, Electrocardiographic changes during prolonged coronary artery occlusion in man: comparison of standard and high-frequency recordings. *Clin. Physiol.*, 1998;**18**: 179–186.

109. Pettersson, J., O. Pahlm, E. Carro, L. Edenbrandt, M. Ringborn, L. Sörnmo, S.G. Warren, and G.S. Wagner, Changes in high-frequency QRS components are more sensitive than ST segment deviation for detecting acute coronary artery occlusion. *J. Am. Coll. Cardiol.*, 2000;**36**: 1827–1834.

110. Goldberger, A.L., V. Bhargava, V. Froelicher, J. Covell, and D. Mortara, Effect of myocardial infarction on the peak amplitude of high frequency QRS potentials. *J. Electrocardiol.*, 1980;**13**: 367–372.

111. Bhargava, V. and A. Goldberger, Myocardial infarction diminishes both low and high frequency QRS potentials: power spectrum analysis of lead II. *J. Electrocardiol.*, 1981;**14**: 57–60.

112. Goldberger, A.L., V. Bhargava, V. Froelicher, and J. Covell, Effect of myocardial infarction on high-frequency QRS potentials. *Circulation*, 1981;**64**: 34–42.

113. Talwar, K.K., G.S. Rao, U. Nayar, and M.L. Bhatia, Clinical significance of high frequency QRS potentials in myocardial infarction: analysis based on power spectrum of lead III. *Cardiovasc. Res.*, 1989;**23**: 60–63.

114. Berkalp, B., E. Baykal, N. Caglar, C. Erol, G. Akgün, and T. Gürel, Analysis of high frequency QRS potentials observed during acute myocardial infarction. *Int. J. Cardiol.*, 1993;**42**: 147–153.

115. Novak, P., L. Zhixing, V. Novak, and R. Hatala, Time-frequency mapping of the QRS complex in normal subjects and in postmyocardial infarction patients. *J. Electrocardiol.*, 1994;**27**: 49–60.

116. Ringborn, M., O. Pahlm, G.S. Wagner, S.G. Warren, and J. Pettersson, The absence of high-frequency QRS changes in the presence of standard electrocardiographic QRS changes of old myocardial infarction. *Am. Heart J.*, 2001;**36**: 1827–1834.

117. Trägårdh, E., O. Pahlm, G.S. Wagner, and J. Pettersson, Reduced high-frequency QRS components in patients with ischemic heart disease compared to normal subjects. *J. Electrocardiol.*, 2004;**37**: 157–162.

118. Vacek, J.L., D.B. Wilson, G.W. Botteron, and J. Dobbins, Techniques for the determination of left ventricular mass by signal-averaged electrocardiography. *Am. Heart J.*, 1990;**120**: 958–963.

119. Okin, P.M., T.M. Donnelly, T.S. Parker, D.C. Wallerson, N.M. Magid, and P. Kligfield, High-frequency analysis of the signal-averaged ECG. Correlation with left ventricular mass in rabbits. *J. Electrocardiol.*, 1992;**25**: 111–118.

120. Abboud, S., O. Berenfeld, and D. Sadeh, Simulation of high-resolution QRS complex using a ventricular model with a fractal conduction system. Effects of ischemia on high-frequency QRS potentials. *Circ. Res.*, 1991;**68**: 1751–1760.

121. Mason, R.E. and I. Likar, A new system of multiple-lead exercise electrocardiography. *Am. Heart J.*, 1966;**71**: 196–205.

122. Proakis, J.G. and D.G. Manolakis, *Digital Signal Processing – Principles, Algorithms, and Applications.* Upper Saddle River, NJ: Prentice-Hall, 1996.

123. Schlegel, T.T., W.B. Kulecz, J.L. DePalma, A.H. Feiveson, J.S. Wilson, M.A. Rahman, and M.W. Bungo, Real-time 12-lead high-frequency QRS electrocardiography for enhanced detection of myocardial ischemia and coronary artery disease. *Mayo Clin. Proc.* 2004;**79**: 339–350.

124. Schlegel, T.T., B. Arenare, V. Starc, E.C. Greco, G. Poulin, D.R. Moser, and R. Delgado, The best identifiers of cardiomyopathy in short duration ECG recordings: high frequency QRS reduced amplitude zone score, QT interval variability, low frequency RR interval power and heart rate turbulence slope. *Folia Cardiol.*, 2005;**12**(SupplC): 1–4.

125. Pueyo, E., E. Sörnmo, and P. Laguna, QRS slopes for early ischemia detection and characterization. *IEEE Trans. Biomed. Eng.*, 2008;**55**: 468–477.

126. Pettersson, J., E. Carro, L. Edenbrandt, C. Maynard, O. Pahlm, M. Ringborn, L. Sörnmo, S.G. Warren, and G.S. Wagner, Spatial, individual, and temporal variation of the high-frequency QRS amplitude in the 12 standard electrocardiographic leads. *Am. Heart J.*, 2000;**139**: 352–358.

127. Abboud, S., J. Leor, and M. Eldar, High frequency ECG during reperfusion therapy of acute myocardial infarction. *IEEE Comput. Soc. Comput. Cardiol.*, 1990; 351–353.

128. Aversano, T., B. Rudicoff, A. Washington, S. Traill, V. Coombs, and J. Raqueno, High frequency QRS electrocardiography in the detection of reperfusion following thrombolytic therapy. *Clin. Cardiol.*, 1994;**17**: 175–182.

129. Bhargava, V. and A.L. Goldberger, Effect of exercise in healthy men on QRS power spectrum. *Am. J. Physiol.*, 1982;**243**: H964–H969.

130. Beker, A., A. Pinchas, J. Erel, and S. Abboud, Analysis of high frequency QRS potential during exercise testing in patients with coronary artery disease and in healthy subjects. *PACE*, 1996;**19**: 2040–2050.

131. Lipton, J.A., S.G. Warren, M. Broce, S. Abboud, A. Beker, L. Sörnmo, D.R. Lilly, C. Maynard, B.D. Lucas Jr, and G.S. Wagner, High-frequency QRS electrocardiogram during exercise stress testing for detecting ischemia. *Int. J. Cardiol.*, 2008;**124**: 198–203.

132. Toledo, E., J.A. Lipton, S.G. Warren, S. Abboud, M. Broce, D.R. Lilly, C. Maynard, B.D. Lucas Jr, and G.S. Wagner, Detection of stress-induced myocardial ischemia from the depolarization phase of the cardiac cycle – a preliminary study. *J. Electrocardiol.*, 2009;**42**: 240–247.

133. Rahman, M.A., A. Gedevanishvili, Y. Birnbaum, L. Sarmiento, W. Sattam, W.B. Kulecz, and T.T. Schlegel, High-frequency QRS electrocardiogram predicts perfusion defects during myocardial perfusion imaging. *J. Electrocardiol.*, 2006;**39**: 73–81.

134. Trägårdh, E., T.T. Schlegel, M. Carlsson, J. Petterson, K. Nilsson, and O. Pahlm, High-frequency electrocardiogram analysis in the ability to predict reversible reperfusion defects during adenosine myocardial perfusion imaging. *J. Electrocardiol.*, 2007;**40**: 510–514.

135. Trägårdh, E., H. Arheden, J. Pettersson, G.S. Wagner, and O. Pahlm, High-frequency QRS components vs left ventricular mass in humans. *Folia Cardiol.*, 2005;**12**(suppl C): 68.

136. Watanabe, T., M. Yamaki, H. Tachibana, I. Kubota, and H. Tomoike, Decrease in the high-frequency QRS components depending on the local conduction delay. *Jpn. Circ. J.*, 1998;**62**: 844–848.

137. Valentino, V.A., H.O. Ventura, F.M. Abi-Samra, C.H. Van Meter, and H.L. Price, The signal-averaged electrocardiogram in cardiac transplantation. A non-invasive marker of acute allograft rejection. *Transplantation*, 1992;**53**: 124–127.

138. Graceffo, M.A. and R.A. O'Rourke, Cardiac transplant rejection is associated with a decrease in the high-frequency components of the high-resolution, signal-averaged electrocardiogram. *Am. Heart J.*, 1996;**132**: 820–826.

139. Matsushita, S., Y. Sakakibara, T. Imazuru, M. Noma, Y. Hiramatsu, O. Shigeta, T. Jikuya, and T. Mitsui, High-frequency QRS potentials as a marker of myocardial dysfunction after cardiac surgery. *Ann. Thorac. Surg.*, 2004;**77**: 1293–1297.

140. Abe, M., S. Matsushita, and T. Mitsui, Recovery of high-frequency QRS potentials following cardioplegic arrest in pediatric cardiac surgery. *Pediatr. Cardiol.*, 2001;**22**: 315–320.

8 Electrocardiography in Epidemiology

Pentti M. Rautaharju

P. W. Macfarlane et al. (eds.), *Specialized Aspects of ECG*, DOI 10.1007/978-0-85729-880-5_8,
© Springer-Verlag London Limited 2012

8.1   Introduction

Like other areas of electrocardiography, epidemiological electrocardiography has grown and evolved in content since the publication of the first edition of this book. The emphasis in epidemiological electrocardiography has shifted from primarily descriptive population studies to follow-up studies with risk evaluation. Electrocardiographic (ECG) recording technology has evolved, and computer electrocardiography has matured, developments that have greatly enhanced the feasibility of high-volume ECG acquisition and analysis with substantially enhanced precision and reproducibility.

At the time of the preparation of the material for the first volume of this book, computer electrocardiography in epidemiology was still a novelty that required special consideration. This is no longer necessary. The second area of epidemiological electrocardiography that has gone through a similar period of maturation and growth is the use of electrocardiography in clinical trials. This subject area has, in fact, grown so much that it is no longer feasible to cover it any more in the context of this chapter, with a few exceptions. Exercise electrocardiography and ambulatory electrocardiography are covered in separate chapters of this book.

The subject areas covered in this chapter belong in the realm of epidemiological electrocardiography that includes the following broad topics of ECG investigation:

- Estimation of the prevalence and incidence of ECG abnormalities in cross-sectional population studies.
- Determination of the normal limits for ECG intervals, amplitudes, and waveform patterns.
- Assessment of the evolution with age, significance of ECG findings in relation to physiological and anthropometric measurements, and coronary heart disease (CHD) risk factors and natural history of disease processes.
- Assessment of the risk of future adverse events, morbidity, and mortality associated with ECG abnormalities.

Each of these major application areas has certain special requirements which may be different from the needs of the traditional electrocardiographic practice in clinical diagnostic applications. Consideration of normal limits for ECG patterns is covered elsewhere in this book.

There is a scarcity of systematic reviews of epidemiological aspects of electrocardiography. One of the few, published since the first edition of Comprehensive Electrocardiography is the review from 2000 by Ashley et al. [1].

8.1.1   ECG Coding Schemes from Historical Perspective

Modern cardiovascular epidemiological studies were initiated in the USA, several European countries, and Japan during the 1950s when little was still known about the epidemiology of CHD and hypertensive heart disease (HHD). Many of these studies were inspired by the pioneering efforts of Ancel Keys at the Laboratory of Physiological Hygiene, School of Public Health of the University of Minnesota. Dr. Keys initiated a 15-year prospective study in 1947 of business and professional men from Minnesota [2], and in the 1950s, the classic Seven Countries study [3, 4]. These studies led to intensive electrocardiographic research and developmental work in this area of epidemiology. The Framingham study was initiated around 1948–1950 [5]. That study, as well as the studies in Albany, New York [6], Los Angeles [7], and Chicago [8, 9], are other milestones among modern cardiovascular epidemiology. However, the state-of-the-art of ECG coding in the 1950s was appalling. The only common guidelines for ECG wave definitions and measurements were those proposed by the Criteria Committee of the New York Heart Association [10]. Most wave definitions and classification criteria were largely qualitative descriptions and thus were too ambiguous for epidemiological applications. It was evident that the comparability of the reported prevalence of ECG abnormalities from these studies in the 1950s was questionable.

The Minnesota code (MC) was developed between 1956 and 1960. Its primary purpose was to improve the comparability of ECG classification and thus the consistency of the assessment of the coronary heart disease prevalence rates among the cohorts of the Seven Countries study. At that time, it was a formidable task to reach an agreement within any group of cardiologists on any set of ECG criteria, for instance for myocardial infarction (MI) or ventricular hypertrophies. The authors of the Minnesota code were cautious to avoid any reference to diagnostic classification. The code was described strictly as a scheme for objective reporting of morphological ECG wave measurements without prejudice to any interpretation. However, the classification criteria were based on clinical ECG criteria commonly used at that time, many of which were developed during the late 1950s. Dr. Henry Blackburn was in charge of the Minnesota code development. One of the earliest field trials of the new code was carried out in Finland from 1956 to 1959 in epidemiological studies, which assessed the prevalence of arteriosclerotic and hypertensive heart disease among ostensibly healthy working populations [11]. The report concluded that with the aid of the Minnesota code, the ECG can be successfully used as an objective tool in the study of cardiovascular epidemiology. After the publication of the original Minnesota code in Circulation in 1960 [12], it rapidly gained widespread acceptance. The code was systematically used in the Seven Countries study and in a variety of other population studies such as the Tecumseh study of a total natural community in Michigan [13], the Tukisenta study in New Guinea [14], and the National Cooperative Pooling project including Tecumseh and four other longitudinal investigations in the USA [15].

A more recent development is the Novacode [16], which has been used in a variety of epidemiological studies sponsored by the National Institutes of Health. There are several other ECG coding schemes, which have been proposed for morphological description of ECG patterns or for diagnostic ECG classification [17–21]. However, most of these schemes are more suitable for clinical than for epidemiological applications.

8.1.2 Minnesota Code

The Minnesota code belongs to the group of classification systems called linguistic or syntactic. In general, these classifiers extract "morphs" or various feature patterns observed or measured and use a "grammar" to categorize the morphs into a given set of usually, but not necessarily, mutually exclusive diagnostic classes. In most instances, the grammar can be expressed as a branching tree of Boolean decisions. Boolean logic uses the presence or absence of various features in each decision node to determine which branch of the diagnostic decision tree to follow.

8.1.2.1 ECG Measurement Rules

The ECG measurement rules were left fairly ill defined and incomplete in the original version of the Minnesota code. These rules were defined a little more clearly in the 1968 version of the Minnesota code [22]. The Minnesota code ECG measurement rules are best described in the 1982 version of the code [23], which provides detailed illustrations of visual ECG wave measurement devices and procedures. The older hot stylus electrocardiographs, with ECGs recorded on thermosensitive paper produced a tracing that had a thick "baseline." This can considerably bias wave-duration measurements, depending on the writing characteristics of the stylus and the paper speed [24]. Proper measurement procedures can reduce but cannot eliminate these errors, which can have a significant impact on ECG coding.

It was recommended in the original version of the Minnesota code that the majority rule should be applied throughout without exception and a majority of codable complexes was required from each ECG lead coded. The measurement rules for the 1982 version of the Minnesota code specify several exceptions to the majority rule. For instance, an initial R wave exceeding 0.025 mV even in one complex in a given lead (except V_1) rules out codable Q and QS waves in that lead. For some other codes (for instance code 1.2.8), a given feature has to be present in all complexes in order to qualify as a codable item.

Three different reference or baseline points are used for amplitude measurements in the Minnesota code. All QRS-complex and ST-segment amplitude measurements are made with respect to the PR segment immediately preceding the onset of QRS. P-amplitude measurements are referred to the TP segment preceding the P-wave and T-amplitude measurements to the flattest part of the TP segment following the T wave. The amplitudes of positive deflections are measured from the upper margin of the tracing and negative deflections from the lower margin of the tracing at the baseline point.

8.1.2.2 Definition of Codable Waves

An attempt to give unambiguous definitions for codable ECG waves was one of the most important contributions of the Minnesota code. The logic for wave definitions is relatively simple as described in the following sequence:

- The first codable wave is the first deflection within the QRS complex ≥ 0.025 mV or ≤ -0.1 mV. The first codable wave is denoted as R wave if it is positive and a Q or QS wave if it is negative.
- The second codable wave is the first deflection following the first codable wave with an opposite polarity and an absolute amplitude ≥ 0.1 mV. The second wave is an R wave if it is positive and an S wave if it is negative.
- Subsequent codable waves within QRS, with alternating signs, are defined similarly with 0.1 mV amplitude thresholds. The third codable wave is an R$'$ wave if it is positive and S$'$ wave if it is negative. The fourth codable wave is an R$'$ wave if it positive and an S$'$ wave if it is negative.
- A Q wave is the first codable wave within QRS if it is negative and is followed by a codable R wave.
- A QS wave is the first codable wave if it is negative and is not followed by another codable wave within QRS.

The above definitions are adequate for describing objectively all possible combinations of QRS patterns of type R, RS, RSR$'$, RSR$'$S$'$, QR, QRS, QRSR$'$, and QS.

8.1.2.3 Coding Criteria for Serial ECG Changes

The basic problem with the initial set of the Minnesota code criteria for serial ECG changes was that trivial changes in ECG amplitudes or wave durations frequently induced artifactual new codable events in myocardial infarction (MI) classification. The coding scheme was vulnerable to considerable coding variation. A new classification scheme for coding of serial ECG changes [25] was developed for determining the incidence rate of reinfarction in the Coronary Drug Project [26], a large secondary prevention trial. This was done when it was noted that up to 27% of ECG changes, coded as significant worsening or reinfarction in the Coronary Drug project, were caused by coding variation alone. Similar problems were encountered in another large intervention study, the Multiple Risk Factor Intervention Trial (MRFIT) [27].

The serial change criteria for the Minnesota code are not based on changes in ECG measurements or simultaneous comparison of successively recorded ECGs acquired from periodic examinations. Instead, the coding scheme is based on changes in the severity level of the coding category of independently coded records. For major Q–QS changes, a jump over one severity level in code 1 is required (e.g., from 1.3 to 1.1). For minor Q–QS changes, a worsening by one severity level in code 1, plus a worsening by one severity level in code 5 (T waves) is needed (excluding code 5.4).

A significant worsening for ST changes requires a transition over one severity level (e.g., from 5.3 to 5.2). There are no serial change criteria for items related to ventricular hypertrophies.

The coding rules suitable for use in algorithms for classification of serial changes in Q–QS patterns are summarized in ❏ Table 8.1. There are additional rules for certain other items. For instance, a codable new left bundle branch block (LBBB) (7.1) requires a QRS-duration increase of 0.020 s or more from the baseline ECG.

❏ Table 8.1

Serial change comparison rules for significant worsening of Minnesota Code (MC) Q and QS waves

Follow-up ECG Minnesota Code	Qualifying conditions for a significant change
1.1.6, 1.1.7, 1.2.3, 1.2.7, 1.3.2, 1.3.6, 1.1.1, 1.1.4, 1.1.5, 1.2.1, 1.2.2, 1.2.4	Initial R amplitude decrease ≥ 0.1 mV or Q:R amplitude ratio increase $\geq 50\%$
1.1.2	Initial R-amplitude decrease ≥ 0.15 mV and Q: R ratio increase $\geq 50\%$
1.1.3	Initial R-amplitude decrease ≥ 0.10 mV or Q: R ratio increase $\geq 75\%$
1.2.6	(Initial R-amplitude decrease > 0.10 mV or Q: R ratio increase $\geq 75\%$) and appearance of a new codable Q wave in a VF
1.2.8	R-amplitude decrease in the "lead to the left" causing new code ≥ 0.10 mV

8.2   Prevalence of ECG Abnormalities

Most cardiovascular epidemiological studies have primarily focused on coronary heart disease (CHD) and hypertensive heart disease. ECG coding of Q waves and associated ST-T abnormalities has been considered as an index of old myocardial infarction (MI) in comparison with contrasting populations. Left ventricular hypertrophy (LVH) by ECG criteria (ECG-LVH), in turn, has been considered as an index of true anatomical LVH. Limited diagnostic accuracy of more moderate ECG-MI criteria and low prevalence of more strict ECG-MI criteria limits the utility of ECG-MI prevalence estimation in free-living populations. As will be shown later, similar or even more severe limitations are encountered with the application of ECG-LVH criteria. Prognostic evaluation in early epidemiological studies was done for broad categories of ECG abnormalities, in part because of limited sample size in categories considered disease specific.

8.2.1   Contrasting Prevalence and Age Trends of ECG Abnormalities in Middle-Aged Men and Women

The coronary heart disease study of the Social Insurance Institution of Finland is one of the best-documented recent prevalence surveys conducted in free-living male and female populations [28]. The study population of 5,738 men and 5,224 women consisted of whole or random samples of rural or semi-urban populations, with an overall participation rate of 90%.

❯ Table 8.2 summarizes the prevalence of selected Minnesota code (MC) abnormalities for various age-groups of men and women ranging from 30 to 59 years. In Finnish men, the prevalence of major and minor Q waves (MC 1.1 to 1.3) was nearly four times higher than in Finnish women. These prevalence rates are nine times higher than in a 1965 report from Tecumseh population in the corresponding age range (30–59 years and less) [13]. The linear gradient in increase of the prevalence of Q waves with age was not significant in Finnish men and only of borderline significance in women. The prevalence of Q waves was higher in men than in women. However, the gender difference was no longer significant for the age-group 55–59 years.

In the Finnish study group, the prevalence of left axis deviation (MC 2.1) was 4.1% in men and 2.3% in women. The prevalence increased significantly with age in a fashion similar to that in the Tecumseh population and several others. Interestingly, such left axis trend with age was not present in men in a Polynesian community of Pukapuka [29]. Blood pressure levels in Pukapuka men have low mean values and show no rise with age and the prevalence of obesity is reportedly low.

Among the most intriguing observations in the study of Finnish communities was the contrasting age trend between men and women in the prevalence of high-amplitude R waves in leads V_5, V_6, or the frontal plane limb leads (MC 3.1). The prevalence was very high (25.9%) among Finnish men and showed no significant age trend. Evidently, the decrease of R-wave amplitudes with age observed among normotensive men is offset by R-wave amplitude increase with hypertension. The prevalence of high blood pressure ($\geq$ 160 mm Hg systolic, or $\geq$95 mm Hg diastolic) among men increased from 12.9% in the age-group 30–39 years to 33.1% in the age-group 50–59 years.

The prevalence of high-amplitude QRS waves in Finnish women was substantially lower than in men, and particularly in women younger than 50 years. The gradient with age in women is significant. The striking sex differences in the prevalence indicate the inappropriateness of using identical criteria for men and women. These differences also reflect the influence on these voltage criteria of factors other than LVH associated with hypertension, such as physical activity level, age, sex, and other anthropometric extracardiac factors.

The inclusion of high-voltage criteria of Sokolow and Lyon (MC 3.1 and 3.3) causes a substantial increase in the LVH prevalence estimates. With these criteria, the prevalence was 41.9% in men and 19.5% in women. The prevalence of LVH according to the high-voltage criteria combined with ST-T changes is very low in most populations studied and these criteria are likely to be too insensitive to be used as an index for LVH in hypertension.

Abnormal ST depression in the resting ECG (MC 4.1, 4.2 or 4.3) was present significantly more often in women (4.3%) than in men (2.2%), and the prevalence increased markedly with age in both sex groups. The inclusion of the borderline abnormal ST category (J depression in excess of 0.1 mV with upsloping ST where the J point denotes the end of the QRS complex) added merely 0.8% to the prevalence in men and 1.4% in women. This reflects a deficiency in the hierarchical structure of abnormal ST codes regarding the severity of the ST abnormality, since prevalence would be expected to

Table 8.2

Prevalence (%) of Minnesota Codes among a Finnish cohort representing total or random samples of middle-aged rural or semi-urban community dwellers or factory employees by age and gender

Age and Gender	MC Category N	Q, QS Waves 1.1–1.3	Left Axis 2.1	High R Waves 3.1	Abnormal ST 4.1–4.3	Abnormal T 5.1–5.3	PR Prolonged 6.3	LBBB 7.1	RBBB 7.2	R' Wave 7.3	Atrial Fibrillation 8.3	ST Elevation 9.2
30–34												
M	1,073	6.1	2.4	26.6	0.7	2.5	1.4	0.0	0.4	0.6	0.0	22.3
F	865	3.0	0.9	3.9	1.5	7.4	0.6	0.0	0.1	0.2	0.2	0.4
35–39												
M	1,076	5.7	3.0	25.1	0.9	3.2	1.3	0.1	0.2	0.5	0.1	18.8
F	889	4.6	1.2	5.0	1.1	8.2	0.0	0.1	0.1	0.3	0.0	0.3
40–44												
M	1,099	6.6	2.8	25.8	0.9	3.1	1.8	0.5	0.0	1.0	0.1	15.2
F	997	4.0	1.8	5.3	2.7	10.7	0.2	0.1	0.1	0.3	0.0	0.5
45–49												
M	906	5.7	5.0	23.1	1.6	6.2	1.9	0.3	0.6	0.9	0.2	14.6
F	927	3.8	3.0	7.7	3.9	13.1	0.5	0.1	0.2	0.5	0.0	0.4
50–54												
M	791	8.2	6.6	25.2	3.2	9.2	1.4	0.3	0.9	1.1	0.4	9.2
F	793	5.2	3.3	11.1	7.8	18.5	0.8	0.5	0.4	0.9	0.3	0.9
55–59												
M	793	8.1	5.8	29.5	6.3	13.1	1.3	1.0	1.3	0.8	1.0	10.6
F	753	6.9	3.9	16.1	9.7	24.0	1.3	0.9	0.4	0.5	0.4	0.9
All												
M	5,738	6.6	4.1	25.9	2.2	5.8	1.5	0.4	0.5	0.8	0.3	15.6
F	5,224	4.5	2.3	7.9	4.3	13.3	0.6	0.3	0.2	0.5	0.1	0.6

M males, *F* females, *MC* Minnesota code. Data from the Finnish Social Insurance Institution's Coronary Heart Disease Study, Reunanen et al. [28], Acta Med Scand 1983;673 (suppl.):1–120

increase with decreasing severity of the code. For instance, for men, the prevalences for codes 4.1 to 4.4 were 0.9%, 0.7%, 0.6%, and 0.8%, respectively.

Abnormal T waves (MC 5.1 to 5.3) were coded in 5.8% of men and 13.3% of women. The prevalence increased with age and was significantly higher in women. In women aged 55–59 years, the prevalence of abnormal T waves at rest was as high as 24%. Over 60% of abnormal T waves were flat or biphasic (MC 5.3).

The high prevalence of T-wave abnormalities in women observed in the Finnish populations, Tecumseh, and other studies, evidently indicates that repolarization abnormalities in women are often associated with factors not related to CHD. Similar relatively high prevalence rates have been reported in nonindustrialized native female populations relatively free from CHD. For instance, about one quarter of the women aged 40–59 years had T-wave abnormalities (MC 5.1 to 5.3) in a non-urbanized population of Tukisenta, New Guinea [14].

The prevalence of other coded ECG abnormalities in men and women was low, with the exception of ST elevation in men. Prolonged PR (MC 6.3) was present in 1.5% of men and in 0.6% of women, left bundle branch block in 0.4% of men and 0.3% of women, right bundle branch block (RBBB) in 0.5% of men and 0.2% of women, incomplete right bundle branch block in 0.8% of men and 0.5% of women, and atrial fibrillation in 0.3% of men and 0.1% of women.

One striking contrast between the prevalence rates of men and women was the high prevalence of ST elevation in Finnish men (15.6%). The corresponding prevalence in women was only 0.6%. The prevalence of ST elevation in men was seen to decrease significantly with age. An opposite, less-pronounced trend was observed in women. The high prevalence of ST elevation in men is apparently associated with tall T waves in the chest leads, which is a common finding especially in younger men. For other abnormalities of interest, the prevalence of Wolff–Parkinson–White syndrome (MC 6.4) was 0.2% in men and 0.1% in women. Frequent ventricular ectopic complexes (over 10% of QRS complexes) were present in 1.0% of men and 1.4% of women. Occasional ventricular ectopic complexes were observed in 1.2% of men and 1.4% of women. The prevalence of frequent supraventricular ectopic complexes (over 10%) was 0.5% in both sex groups, and the prevalence of occasional supraventricular complexes was 0.8% in men and 1.0% in women.

The reported prevalence of abnormal ECG findings in three major coding categories of the Minnesota code in five male and female population studies [13, 28, 30–32] is summarized in ❏ Table 8.3. The data confirm the uniform trend toward higher prevalence of ST depression and lower prevalence of significant Q waves in women. The prevalence of significant Q waves varies little between male populations, as a contrast to quite dramatic variations in the prevalence of high-amplitude QRS waves.

The prevalence of high-amplitude QRS waves in Finnish men is unusually high. Comparable prevalence rates have been reported only for black Jamaican males [33], with a reported prevalence of 29.9% for MC 3.1. Prevalence rates for code 3.1 as low as 0.6% have been reported for British men aged 50–59 years employed as civil servants [34]. However, this Whitehall study of Rose et al. was based on limb-lead ECGs only. As pointed out by Reunanen et al. [28], differences in occupational distributions may partly explain these differences in prevalence that, however, remain largely unresolved discrepancy.

❏ Table 8.3

Contrasting prevalence (%) of major Q waves, high-amplitude R waves, and ST depression in five studies on male and female populations aged 50–59 years

	No. Subjects		Major Q Waves MC 1.1, 1.2		High-Amplitude R Waves MC 3.1		ST Abnormalities MC 4.1–4.3	
Study/Ref.	Male	Female	Male	Female	Male	Female	Male	Female
Tecumseh [13]	331	327	4.2	0.6	3.3	3.4	3.3	12.2
Framingham [30]	650	808	3.5	1.9	9.5	5.0	5.2	6.7
Busselton [31]	310	375	2.3	0	6.8	1.1	3.2	2.7
Copenhagen [32]	2,014	2,791	2.2	0.7	12.0	4.1	4.0	4.7
Finland's Soc. Ins. Inst. [28]	1,584	1,546	3.9	2.5	27.3	13.5	4.7	8.7

MC Minnesota code

As a contrast to the variability of the high R-wave amplitude prevalence, the ST-depression prevalence among male populations was relatively uniform.

8.2.2 Prevalence of ECG Abnormalities in Adult Male Populations

❯ Table 8.4 summarizes prevalence data for ECG findings from the classic Seven Countries study of Keys et al. [3]. Twelve of these 17 cohorts of men aged 40–59 years represent total populations of males in each geographical area. Four occupational groups included in the study consisted of rail employees from the USA and Italy. One of the European populations (Zutphen) was drawn as a random (five out of nine) subsample.

The prevalence of any codable Q, QS waves, and related items ranged from 0.6% in the Japanese fishing village of Ushibuka to 6% among US railroad executives. An even larger range of variation was found in the prevalence of high-amplitude R waves (code 3.1): 1.2% among US railroad executives and 17.9% in Karelia, Finland. However, the prevalence of MI and LVH according to more stringent criteria, which gives a higher specificity, was very low. The total prevalence of diagnostic Q waves (code 1.1), lesser Q waves plus negative T waves (code 1.2 or 1.2 with code 5.1 or 5.2) or ventricular conduction defects (7.1, 7.2, or 7.4) ranged from 0.9% in Crete to 7.1% among non-sedentary US railroad clerks. The range for the prevalence of high-amplitude R waves combined with ST changes (code 3.1 and any of the codes 4.1 to 4.4) was from 0.13% for the Italian railwaymen to 1.98% in the farming village of Tanushimaru in Japan.

Rose et al. [35] compared prevalence rates for Minnesota code ECG abnormalities in six cohorts of middle-aged male clerical workers from five European countries (Belgium, Denmark, Italy, The Netherlands, and the USSR). The prevalence of Q, QS waves (MC 1.1 to 1.3) ranged from 3.4% to 5.5%, ST abnormalities (MC 4.1 to 4.3) from 2.6% to 3.6%,

◻ Table 8.4
Prevalence (%) of Minnesota Code ECG abnormalities among 17 cohorts of adult male populations in the Seven Countries Study of Keys et al.[a]

MC Category/Cohort	N	Major Q 1.1	Any Q 1.1–1.3	Minor Q + Abn. T 1.3 + 5.1, 5.2	Major Abn. T 5.1	High R 3.1	High R + Abn. ST 3.1 + 4.1–4.4	Abn. ST, Isolated 4.1–4.4	Abn. T, Isolated 5.1–5.3	Ventricular Conduction 7.1, 7.2, 7.4
Crete, Greece	683	1 (0.2)	9 (1.3)	0 (0.0)	0 (0.0)	35 (5.1)	2 (0.3)	4 (0.6)	5 (0.7)	5 (0.7)
Corfu, Greece	529	3 (0.6)	17 (3.2)	0 (0.0)	1 (0.2)	40 (7.6)	5 (1.0)	6 (1.1)	3 (0.6)	11 (2.1)
Velikakrsna, Yugoslavia	510	5 (1.0)	14 (2.7)	0 (0.0)	0 (0.0)	62 (12.2)	6 (1.2)	1 (0.2)	0 (0.0)	6 (1.2)
Dalmatia, Yugoslavia	669	0 (0.0)	14 (2.1)	1 (0.2)	0 (0.0)	19 (2.8)	1 (0.2)	5 (0.8)	5 (0.8)	7 (1.1)
Slavonia, Yugoslavia	694	3 (0.4)	13 (1.9)	0 (0.0)	0 (0.0)	79 (11.4)	5 (0.7)	2 (0.3)	9 (1.3)	6 (0.9)
Finland, West	857	6 (0.7)	15 (1.8)	0 (0.0)	0 (0.0)	139 (16.2)	10 (1.2)	1 (0.1)	21 (2.5)	12 (1.4)
Finland, Karelia	814	7 (0.9)	18 (202)	4 (0.5)	0 (0.0)	146 (17.9)	12 (1.5)	2 (0.3)	25 (3.1)	5 (0.6)
Italy, Crevalcore	993	5 (0.5)	35 (3.5)	3 (0.3)	0 (0.0)	55 (5.5)	13 (1.3)	1 (0.1)	18 (1.8)	14 (1.4)
Italy, Montegiorgio	717	4 (0.6)	15 (2.1)	1 (0.1)	0 (0.0)	24 (3.6)	3 (0.4)	4 (0.6)	3 (0.4)	5 (0.7)
Rome, Railwaymen	766	4 (0.5)	22 (2.9)	0 (0.0)	0 (0.0)	26 (3.4)	1 (0.1)	4 (0.5)	13 (1.7)	9 (1.2)
Netherlands, Zuthen	877	8 (0.9)	33 (3.8)	0 (0.0)	0 (0.0)	38 (4.3)	8 (0.9)	2 (0.2)	5 (0.6)	21 (2.4)
Japan, Tanushimaru	504	3 (0.6)	11 (2.2)	0 (0.0)	0 (0.0)	38 (7.5)	10 (2.0)	38 (7.5)	4 (0.8)	4 (0.8)
Japan, Ushibuka,	484	2 (0.4)	3 (0.6)	0 (0.0)	0 (0.0)	71 (14.7)	7 (1.5)	32 (6.6)	2 (0.4)	6 (1.2)
USA, Switchmen	835	8 (1.0)	31 (3.7)	0 (0.0)	0 (0.0)	13 (1.6)	2 (0.2)	4 (0.5)	16 (1.9)	11 (1.3)
USA Clarks Sedentary	847	10 (1.2)	29 (3.5)	1 (0.1)	0 (0.0)	29 (3.4)	4 (0.5)	6 (0.7)	15 (1.8)	12 (1.4)
USA Clarks, Nonsedentary	155	2 (1.3)	8 (5.2)	2 (1.3)	0 (0.0)	10 (6.5)	1 (0.7)	2 (1.3)	1 (0.7)	7 (4.5)
USA, Executives	250	4 (1.6)	15 (6.0)	1 (0.4)	0 (0.0)	3 (1.2)	1 (0.4)	1 (0.4)	2 (0.8)	7 (2.8)
Totals	11184	75 (0.7)	302 (2.7)	13 (0.1)	1 (0.0)	827 (7.4)	91 (0.8)	115 (1.0)	147 (1.3)	148 (1.3)

[a] From Keys et al., Acta Medica Scand 1966; Suppl 460, pp 1–392, Tampereen Kirjapaino, Tampere, Finland

and T-wave abnormalities from 3.4% to 5.9%. No significant heterogeneity was evident between the cohorts except for T-wave abnormalities in the younger age-group (40–49 years). Rose et al. also concluded that the codable ECG abnormalities did not directly reflect national CHD mortality except the prevalence of major Q, QS waves (MC 1.1, 1.2), and even this association may have been owing to the small number of men with these changes (1.6%).

The World Health Organization (WHO) European Collaborative Group [36] reported contrasting prevalence rates for major Q, QS waves, and ST-T segment abnormalities in industrial populations (mainly factories) in five countries (Belgium, Italy, Poland, Spain, and the UK). The prevalence estimates for the intervention group of this large multi-factorial prevention trial (63,732 men aged 40–59 years, employed in 88 factories) varied significantly between centers in various countries. The prevalence of major Q, QS waves (MC 1.1 and 1.2) ranged from 0.74% in Italy to 1.34% in Poland.

There was no apparent parallelism between the prevalence of major Q, QS waves, and the mean CHD risk for each center estimated using multiple logistic coefficients derived from the Seven Countries study based on age, number of cigarettes smoked per day, systolic blood pressure, plasma or serum cholesterol, and body mass index (BMI). The prevalence of other ECG abnormalities considered to be related to suspect myocardial ischemia (ST depression, MC 4.1 to 4.3, T-wave abnormalities, MC 5.1 to 5.3 or complete bundle branch block, MC 7.1) also varied significantly between centers, with prevalence rates for the UK and Belgian centers more than double those of the Polish and Spanish centers. The authors of the report suggest that these independent variations in the prevalence of Q, QS, and ST-T changes may indicate that populations may differ in the type of CHD as well as the extent, possibly in relation to the severity, chronicity, or age at the onset of ischemia.

The determination of prevalence estimates for ECG abnormalities for clinically normal populations as well as the establishment of normal ECG standards based on unselected samples of the general population can be problematic because of difficulties in setting up criteria for "clinically normal." This is evident, for instance, by considering the problem of clinically unrecognized "silent" MI. On the other hand, results from studies in highly selected populations cannot easily be extrapolated to general populations as pointed out by Barrett et al. [37]. However, some of these studies in selected populations (e.g., aviators) have provided information regarding the significance of ECG abnormalities. This holds true particularly for the natural history studies on conduction defects and other evolutionary investigations. One key question is whether given ECG abnormalities are indicators of latent CHD in asymptomatic individuals such as healthy aviators.

The reported prevalence rates in various occupational groups vary widely, evidently dependent on the selection criteria and differences in ECG classification criteria. For instance, the prevalence of ST-segment abnormality in the resting ECG was 0.08% among 3,983 aviators with a mean age of 27 years [38]. In contrast, the prevalence of ST abnormalities (myocardial ischemia) was 11.7% in a large random sample of Israeli male permanent civil service employees aged 40 years or over [39]. It appears that in the latter study, the ischemic category included negative T waves (−0.1 mV or more negative) and incomplete left bundle branch block [40]. On the other hand, nearly 3% of the aviators in the former study had T-wave abnormalities (primary T-wave changes). Differences in classification criteria make it difficult to compare reported prevalence rates in different occupational groups.

There is increasing evidence that repolarization abnormalities in the resting ECG have significant association with latent CHD in asymptomatic men. For instance, Froelicher et al. have reported coronary angiographic findings in 58 asymptomatic aviators with repolarization abnormalities in their resting ECG [41]. Twenty six (45%) of these men had 50% or greater obstruction in one or more coronary arteries and 55% had some evidence of coronary lesions.

8.2.3   Prevalence of ECG Abnormalities in Ostensibly CHD-Free US Male Populations

The 1978 report of the Pooling Project Research group [15] provides detailed information on the prevalence of codable ECG abnormalities from three studies on samples of working male populations drawn from employment groups and from two studies based on community populations samples (❷ Table 8.5). The report is limited to white males aged 40–59 years. Excluded were all men with definite, probable, or suspect MI, definite angina pectoris by history, or Minnesota code 1.1 or 1.2 Q or QS waves.

◪ Table 8.5

Prevalence (percent) of major and minor ECG abnormalities in five adult populations of US males considered free from coronary heart disease at study baseline

Population	N	No Codable Abnormality	Minor Abnormality[a]	Major Abnormality[b]	Minor of Major Abnormality
Albany	1,765	90.4	7.1	2.5	9.6
Chicago Peoples Gas Co.	1,264	92.2	4.7	3.1	7.8
Chicago Western Electric Co.	1,981	86.4	11.1	2.5	13.6
Framingham	1,375	90.0	5.1	4.9	10.0
Tecumseh	691	73.0	20.7	6.4	27.1
Total	7,076	88.0	8.7	3.5	12.2

[a] Minnesota code 1.3; 4.3; 5.3; 6.3; 3.1; 9.1; 2.1, 2.2
[b] Minnesota code 5.5, 5.2; 6.1, 6.2; 7.1, 7.2, 7.4; 8.1; 8.3

The following Minnesota code items were coded as major abnormalities:

MC 4.1	Significant ST depression
MC 5.1 and 5.2	Negative T waves
MC 6.1 and 6.2	Complete and second-degree atrioventricular (AV) block
MC 7.1, 7.2 and 7.4	Complete left bundle branch block, complete right bundle branch block. and intraventricular (IV) block
MC 8.3	Atrial flutter or fibrillation and
MC 8.1	Frequent ventricular ectopic complexes

The prevalence of major ECG abnormalities ranged from 2.5% to 3.1% in the employee groups and 5.0% and 6.4% in the two community samples in ❷ Table 8.5. ST depression, T-wave inversion, and frequent premature ventricular complexes accounted for the majority of major abnormalities, each category having an individual prevalence of approximately 1%.

The wide prevalence difference of minor ECG abnormalities among these five male populations is of interest. The Framingham and Tecumseh study groups represent male populations of total communities. The 5.1% prevalence rate of minor ECG abnormalities in Framingham contrasts with 20.7% prevalence in Tecumseh. A closer examination of the data reported reveals that this highly significant difference in the prevalence is caused by left axis deviations and flat or biphasic T waves in Tecumseh in comparison with Framingham and other populations. The prevalence of code 5.3 (flat T waves) was 11.6% in Tecumseh and 4.2% in Framingham. The prevalence of left axis deviation (code 2.1) was 7.2% in Tecumseh and 0.9% in Framingham. The fact that the ECGs in Tecumseh were recorded during a glucose tolerance test may explain the higher prevalence of minor T-wave changes in that population. There is no obvious reason for the high prevalence of left axis deviation in Tecumseh. Perhaps systematic coding differences may at least in part be responsible.

8.3 Broad Abnormal ECG Categories and Mortality Risk

Early epidemiological studies commonly reported mortality risk for broad categories of ECG abnormalities, mainly because sample size and endpoint events were too low for a meaningful risk evaluation of disease-specific abnormalities.

8.3.1 ECG Abnormalities and Mortality Risk in General Male Populations

Blackburn et al. reported detailed analyses of the 5-year risk of incident CHD for various ECG findings by Minnesota code among men aged 40–59 years [42, 43] The groups compared for risk were matched for age, skinfold thickness, systolic blood pressure, serum cholesterol, smoking, and physical activity. Diagnostic Q waves (code 1.1), negative T waves (code 5.2), and atrial fibrillation (code 8.3) were all highly significant predictors of CHD death. The ratio of observed to expected number of deaths ranged from 10 to 15 for these three categories. Moderately large Q waves associated with T-wave inversion (1.2 and (5.1 or 5.2)) and bundle branch blocks (7.1, 7.2, 7.4) were not significant predictors of CHD death.

In prediction of all CHD events, both fatal and nonfatal, minor T-wave abnormalities (code 5.3), first-degree AV block (code 6.3), and frequent ventricular ectopic complexes (code 8.1) were significant predictors of subsequent clinical CHD in cohorts outside the USA but not in the US cohorts. Any level of ST depression (codes 4.1 to 4.3) carried a significant association with future CHD. Smaller Q waves (code 1.3) and high-amplitude R waves (code 3.1) were not significant independent predictors of CHD; nor was sinus tachycardia (heart rate >100).

Blackburn et al. also reported a more detailed breakdown of the association of ST depression with 5-year mortality from all causes in their pooled European populations (without any exclusion and irrespective of other ECG findings). The results are best summarized by expressing the risk ratio (RR), or the ratio of death rate in the subgroup with a certain ST code to the rate in the subgroup with no codable ST items. The ratios were 10.1, 4.3, 4.0 and 3.3 for codes 4.1, 4.2, 4.3 and 4.4, respectively.

Keys has subsequently reported 10-year follow-up data for a subgroup of the Seven Countries study populations [44]. This subgroup was considered CHD-free at the initial examination. However, nonspecific resting ECG abnormalities in the absence of clinical judgment of definite or possible heart disease did not qualify for exclusion, thus men with any of the following codes were included in the CHD-free subgroup: 1.2, 1.3, 4.1, 4.2, 5.1, 5.2, 6.1, 6.2, 7.1, 7.2, 7.4. and 8.3. The observed-to-expected ratio of the death rate from all causes among men with any of these nonspecific ECG abnormalities ranged from 1.0 to 2.7 in different populations, with the average value of 1.7. Adjusting for the age difference between men with and without ECG abnormalities reduced to the observed-to-expected ratio to 1.48. Thus, the all-causes 10-year death rate among men with nonspecific ECG abnormalities was 48% greater than that for the other men. High-amplitude criteria for LVH showed no predictive significance among the CHD-free cohorts of the Seven Countries study.

Risk of incident CHD for newly acquired ECG-LVH was reported by Kannel et al. in the 14-year follow-up of 5,127 men and women in the Framingham study [45]. Life-table analysis from that study showed that persons who acquired definite LVH by their ECG criteria at any time during the first seven biennial examinations, had a threefold increase in risk of clinical CHD after adjustment for coexisting hypertension. A twofold increase in risk of incident CHD was found among persons with possible LVH by ECG. However, the latter association was no longer significant after adjustment for hypertension.

Criteria for definite LVH in the above-mentioned Framingham study included primarily high voltage associated with ST-segment and T-wave changes or left axis deviation or increased left ventricular activation time. Criteria for possible LVH were based solely on QRS-amplitude criteria without ST-T changes. Thus, in both the Framingham study and the Seven Countries study, high-voltage criteria alone did not carry predictive information independently of other CHD risk factors, in contrast to criteria that included ST-T changes.

8.3.2   Major and Minor ECG Abnormalities and CHD Risk in Industrial Populations

Findings from three longitudinal studies on white, middle-aged, male populations screened from industrial companies and organizations in Chicago provide new information on the importance of major and minor ECG abnormalities for subsequent risk of death from CHD and other causes [46]. Excluded were men who had major Q waves (codes 1.1, 1.2) at the entry examination. Two of these studies, the Chicago Peoples Gas Company study and the Chicago Western Electric Company study are follow-up projects included in the Pooling project described earlier. The third major study reported is the Chicago Heart Association detection project in industry. The combined population of the three projects is 11,204 men aged 40–59 years at baseline, with 5–20 years of follow-up.

8.3.2.1   Major Abnormalities

The following Minnesota codes were included among the major abnormalities: ST depression (codes 4.1, 4.2), T-wave inversion (codes 5.1, 5.2), complete atrioventricular (AV) block (code 6.1), second-degree AV block (code 6.2), complete left bundle branch block (code 7.1), complete right bundle branch block (code 7.2), intraventricular (IV) block (code 7.4), frequent ectopic ventricular beats (code 8.1), and atrial flutter/fibrillation (code 8.3).

Major abnormalities were found in 11.2% among subgroups, which had a full 12-lead ECG recorded. The yield was significantly lower when only 5-lead or 6-lead ECGs were used. The risk ratio for CHD death for men with major ECG abnormalities relative to men with normal ECG was 1.57 for the Chicago Peoples Gas Company, 2.85 for the Western Electric Company, and 6.89 for the men in the Chicago Heart Association detection project in industry. The corresponding risk ratios for death from all causes were 1.64, 1.79, and 3.85. Thus, the death rates for men with major ECG abnormalities were considerably higher than those among men with a normal ECG. ECG abnormalities retained a significant association with death rates when baseline age, diastolic blood pressure, serum cholesterol, relative weight, and number of cigarettes smoked per day were taken into consideration in multivariate analysis.

8.3.2.2 Minor ECG Abnormalities

The following items were included among minor ECG abnormalities: Borderline Q waves (code 1.3), borderline ST depression (code 4.3), flat or biphasic T waves (code 5.3), first-degree AV block (code 6.3), low-voltage QRS (code 9.1), high-amplitude R waves (code 3.1), left axis deviation (code 2.1), and right axis deviation (code 2.2). The risk ratio for CHD death for men with minor ECG abnormalities in relation to men with normal ECG was 1.04 for the Chicago Peoples Gas Company, 1.63 for the Chicago Western Electric Company, and 3.67 for the Chicago Heart Association detection project in industry. The corresponding risk ratios for death from all causes were 1.29, 1.35, and 2.42. Minor ECG abnormalities were shown to carry significant predictive information independently from CHD risk factors in the Chicago Western Electric Company study and the Chicago Heart Association study groups. The association with excess mortality and ECG abnormalities was demonstrated for deaths, which occurred within the first 10 years of follow-up as well as for deaths that occurred more than 10 years after entry.

The overall CHD death risk ratio for men with major or minor ECG abnormalities in relation to men with a normal ECG in the Chicago studies was 1.79 and the risk ratio for death from all causes was 1.57. These risk ratios are similar to those reported by Keys from the Seven Countries study (and the follow-up data from the pooling project [44]). The Pooling Project Research group reported an average risk ratio of 1.7 for a first major or minor ECG abnormality defined as in the Chicago study report summarized above.

8.3.3 Comparative Value of the ECG in Prediction of CHD Risk in Men and Women

The coronary heart disease study of the Finnish Social Insurance Institution [28] provides well-documented information on the relative risk of CHD death and total mortality within 5 years in men and women for various severity levels of Minnesota code abnormalities. The results of the study concerning prognostic value of ECG-MI are summarized later in the ❷ Sect. 8.4.1. Gender comparison of more nonspecific categories is summarized here.

The Finnish study consisted of whole or random samples of rural or semi-urban dwellers. The reported relative risk for CHD death and total mortality within 5 years for a subgroup of 3,589 men and 3,470 women aged 40–59 years is of particular interest here. The relative risk was expressed as the age-adjusted risk ratio for subgroups with defined CHD-related abnormalities compared to those without such abnormalities. In judging the practical utility of risk ratios, it is important to consider what fraction of the total population has such abnormalities. It is possible to achieve, by strict classification criteria, very high-risk ratios in subgroups so small that they would be of limited value in screening and prevention because of an insufficient fraction of the total risk in a given population for a preventive effort with an adequate efficacy.

The combined category of other ischemic abnormalities (smaller Q, QS waves, ST changes, significant conduction defects, or atrial fibrillation) had a substantial increase in relative risk in men for CHD death (risk ratio 7.2) and death from all causes (risk ratio 3.1). Nonspecific T-wave changes (MC 5.3, flat or biphasic T) had over threefold excess risk for CHD death and nearly twofold risk ratio for death from all causes.

The results from the Finnish study illustrate the difficulties encountered in the evaluation of the prognostic significance of ECG abnormalities in female populations. Only 16 of the 3,470 women (0.46%) aged 40–59 years had ECG findings compatible with a probable old MI, and none of them died in 5 years of follow-up. The prevalence of ischemic findings in the resting ECG was quite high (12.8%) in women aged 40–59 years. Ten of these 445 women died within 5 years (risk ratio of 2.2 for death from all causes compared to women without CHD-related ECG abnormalities). There were only two CHD deaths in this group. Similarly, there was only one CHD death in the group of

509 women in this age range who had nonspecific T-wave changes. Thus, although there was some indication of a trend toward an increased risk ratio for death from all causes among women with increasing severity level of ECG abnormalities, the predictive power of such ECG changes for CHD deaths appears weak, and the low overall incidence of CHD deaths does not permit meaningful analysis of a possible association between ECG abnormalities and coronary mortality.

Similar problems were encountered in other studies in attempts to compose risk ratios for ECG abnormalities in men and women owing to the relatively low incidence of CHD death in women during the follow-up period involved. The report from the Framingham study [30] compared the risk of CHD (8-year incidence of CHD including angina pectoris, MI, and sudden death) in 2,336 men and 2,873 women with various combinations of Minnesota code ECG abnormalities. This cohort, aged 32–62 years at entry to the study, included only those persons who were considered CHD-free at the initial examination. The relative risk of CHD for a given category of ECG abnormalities was determined by calculating the ratio of the observed and expected number of cases with CHD. For both men and women without codable ECG abnormalities, the risk was 0.9. For 241 men with any Q waves (MC 1.1 to 1.3), ST or T abnormalities (MC 4.1 to 4.3, 5.1 to 5.3), the risk was 1.8, and for 375 women with any of these abnormalities, the risk was 1.1. Thus, there was a twofold risk for men with these abnormalities compared to men without codable abnormalities, and the risk ratio for women was 1.2.

The Copenhagen City heart study [32] evaluated the risk of death from all causes in a random sample of men and women for eight major categories of the Minnesota code. This prognostic evaluation was done for age-groups 50 years or older, and the association with mortality was assessed by comparing the ratio of the observed and expected number of deaths in a given coding category with the ratio in the group with a completely normal ECG. There was a total of 325 deaths among males and 135 among females during the variable follow-up period between February 1, 1976 and March 31, 1980. The log-rank test in the age-group 50–59 years indicated significant association with mortality in men for high-amplitude R waves, bundle branch blocks (MC 7.1, 7.4), and arrhythmias (MC 8.1 to 8.3). In women, aged 50–59 years the expected number of deaths in all these categories was too low to permit a meaningful evaluation of risk. In the older age-groups of women, there was a significant association with mortality for abnormal T waves in the age-group 70–79 years.

8.3.4   Contrasting Prognostic Significance of ECG Abnormalities in Symptomatic and Asymptomatic Men

Rose et al. reported on the 5-year incidence of CHD death according to the initial ECG findings in standard limb-lead ECGs among 18,403 male civil servants aged 60–64 years (❷ Table 8.6) [34]. The men were divided into subgroups according to the presence or absence of symptomatic heart disease, defined at the initial examination as either a positive response to the chest-pain questionnaire (angina or history of possible MI) or being under medical care for heart disease or high blood pressure. Age-adjusted CHD mortality incidence rates were given in the report so that the outcome in men with and without given ECG abnormalities can be compared in spite of differences in age distribution.

Of interest is the overlap between predictive information from different sources. As expected, men who were under medical care, had a history of angina or possible MI and also had an ischemic ECG had the highest mortality (20%) but the prevalence was also low (0.6%), and this category contributed only 7% of all deaths. An ischemic ECG included the following abnormalities: any Q waves, any ST abnormality, negative or flat T waves, or left bundle branch block. The prevalence of an isolated ischemic ECG was 6.5%, and this category contributed 27 of the total of 274 deaths (9.9%), a relatively small fraction. The 5-year age-adjusted CHD mortality for men with ischemic ECG only was 3.3%, slightly higher than the mortality rate for men with chest pain only (2.5%).

For asymptomatic men, only three categories of Minnesota code abnormalities were associated with excess CHD deaths at ≤5% level of statistical significance (in a two-tailed test): Q, QS waves (MC 1.1 to 1.3), T-wave abnormalities (MC 1.1 to 1.3), and left bundle branch block (MC 7.1). The 5-year CHD mortality rate was in general low for asymptomatic men. It exceeded 5% only for men with prominent Q waves (MC 1.1 to 1.2) and atrial fibrillation (MC 8.3). For the total group of asymptomatic men, the 5-year CHD mortality was 1%. It was 2% for asymptomatic men with left axis deviation (MC 2.1) and 2% for men with ventricular conduction defects (MC 7.1, 7.3, 7.4). There was no excess CHD mortality among asymptomatic men with prolonged PR interval (MC 6.3).

◘ Table 8.6

Five year coronary heart disease mortality among 18,228 men according to mutually exclusive combinations of baseline findings

Status Combinations	N (%)	Number of CHD Deaths	Age-adjusted Percentage
Chest pain[a] only	1,453 (8.0)	38	2.5
Ischemic ECG[b] only	791 (6.5)	27	3.3
Under medical care, no chest pain or ischemic ECG	313 (1.7)	16	4.5
Chest pain and under medical care, no ischemic ECG	201 (1.1)	17	6.0
Ischemic ECG and under medical care, no chest pain	98 (0.5)	11	7.6
Ischemic ECG and chest pain, not under medical care	147 (0.8)	22	10.2
Ischemic ECG and chest pain and under medical care	107 (0.6)	20	20.2
Remainder of men	15,118 (82.9)	123	0.84

[a] Positive response to questionnaire (angina or history of possible myocardial infarction

[b] Minnesota codes 1.1–1.3; 4.1–4.4; 5.1–5.3; 7.1

Recomposed from ❷ Fig. 8.2, Rose et al., Ref. [34], British Heart J 1978;40:636–643, © 1978 BMJ Publishing Group, amended with permission

The Israel ischemic heart disease project [39, 40] introduced new information on the value of nonspecific ECG abnormalities in predicting future symptomatic and asymptomatic ischemic heart disease. The results were based on a 5-year follow-up of a random sample of 10,000 Israeli male permanent civil service employees aged 40 years and over in 1963.

Two categories of resting ECG abnormalities were associated with a significant increase in the 5-year incidence of angina pectoris: nonspecific T-wave abnormalities, and probable infarct by computer criteria when two electrocardiographers disagreed with the computer interpretation! The prevalence of these nonspecific T waves by computer was close to 6% of the Israeli study population chosen for the follow-up, and the prevalence of probable MI was 3.3%.

8.3.5 Contrasting Racial Differences in Prognostic Significance of ECG Abnormalities

Substantial differences have been reported in many studies in the prevalence of ECG abnormalities between black and white populations. The increased prevalence of ST-T abnormalities in black males compared to white males has been known a long time [33, 47, 48].

The Evans County study gave a comprehensive description of the rather drastic differences in the prevalence of Minnesota code ECG abnormalities in black and white males and females, and also differences in the prognostic significance of various ECG abnormalities [49]. The Evans County study population screened between 1960 and 1962 consisted of 3,009 persons 15 years or older who were considered free of evidence of past or present CHD at the time of the initial examination. Also excluded from the CHD incidence comparisons were individuals with diagnosed hypertensive heart disease in the initial examination. The reported age-adjusted prevalence of abnormal ECGs (any specified abnormality) was considerably higher in blacks than in whites. The excess prevalence of ECG abnormalities in black men and women was largely due to high prevalence of high-amplitude R waves and T-wave abnormalities (both major and minor).

In sharp contrast to the highly significant increased prevalence of ECG abnormalities in black men, the 1971 follow-up report showed a significantly lower CHD incidence associated with an abnormal ECG in black males. Small sizes of the subgroups and small number of CHD events does not permit a meaningful comparison in specific categories of abnormalities in men and particularly in women. The comparability of the prognostic significance of ECG abnormalities from this study is also limited by the age structure of the study population. Approximately 39% of the black makes, 22.2% of the white males, and about 43% of the black and white females were from the age-group 15–45 years.

A more recent 20-year mortality follow-up report from the Evans County heart study clarified the role of the racial differences regarding the prognostic value of ECG abnormalities in this cohort. That newer report was restricted to black and white men who were aged 40–64 years of age at entry. Men with major or moderate Q waves (MC 1.1, 1.2) and men with a history of angina pectoris or myocardial infarction at the initial examination were excluded.

Baseline ECG abnormalities were categorized into major and minor abnormalities using a similar grouping of the Minnesota codes as was done in the pooling project cited above [15]. The association between baseline ECG abnormalities and time to death was examined using the Cox proportional hazards model to adjust for standard CHD risk factors. Relative risks were estimated for CHD, cardiovascular disease (CVD), and all cause mortality. They were not significantly increased for black or for white men with respect to minor ECG abnormalities, which included minor Q waves (MC 1.3) and high-amplitude R waves (MC 3.1).

For major ECG abnormalities, the unadjusted relative risk of CHD, CVD, and all-cause mortality was significantly increased in both race groups. The relative risks of CVD and all-cause mortality remained significant in both races after adjustment for age at entry, systolic blood pressure, cholesterol, current and past smoking, and body mass index (BMI). The adjusted relative risk was over twofold for CVD mortality (2.3 for black men and 2.2 for white men, with 95% CI 1.1–4.5 and 1.2–4.2, respectively) and the relative risk of CHD mortality was nearly as high although no longer significant after adjustment for standard CHD risk factors. It thus appears that the adjusted relative risks of CVD mortality for major ECG abnormalities were of the same order of magnitude in black and white men.

8.4   ECG-MI and Mortality Risk

CHD prevalence is known to differ drastically in populations from different geographic locations, as was initially demonstrated by the Seven Countries study. The massive WHO MONICA project used carefully standardized procedures for data entered into population registers by MONICA centers selected for the study for documenting death rates in men and women aged 35–64 years [50]. The survey was conducted during the 1985–1987 period in 38 selected communities from 21 countries. The data revealed a 12-fold range in age-standardized annual event rates (coronary deaths and definite MI) in men and an 8.5-fold range in women. Event rates for men were highest in North Karelia, Finland (907/100,000) and lowest in Beijing, China (73/100,000). In women, event rates were highest in Glasgow, UK (241/100,000) and the rates were lowest in Toulouse, France (24/100,000) and Catalonia, Spain (25/100,000).

8.4.1   Mortality Risk in Q Wave Myocardial Infarction

Data from three well-documented studies reporting mortality risk for Q wave MI are listed in ❷ Table 8.7. In a CHD-free cohort of the Seven Countries study, there was a drastic, over 15-fold increase in short-term mortality risk (up to 5 years) for diagnostic Q waves (large Q waves or major Q waves with ST-T abnormalities) and an over fourfold increased risk for the combined category of any Q waves with or without ST-T abnormalities [51, 52]. The long-term (6–25 years) mortality risk was increased over threefold for diagnostic Q waves but was not significant for the combined category of any Q waves.

In Finland's Social Insurance Institute's study [28], the mortality risk was increased in men for diagnostic Q wave MI (defined similarly as in the Seven Countries study) for all mortality endpoints: RR was 19.5 for CHD mortality, 13.3 for CVD mortality, and 5.6 for all-cause mortality. There were too few events in women for risk evaluation in this ECG category. The risk for Minnesota code 1.1 large Q waves in men was 13.4, and for smaller Q waves in codes 1.2, 1.3 approximately threefold compared to men without significant Q waves. The prevalence of diagnostic Q wave myocardial infarction was quite low. The prevalence of the category labeled as "other ischemic abnormalities" was considerably higher, and also the risk of CHD, CVD, and all-cause mortality was markedly increased in all men, in men with an apparent silent MI, and also in women for CVD and all-cause mortality.

The Italian RIFLE Pooling project [53] reported mortality risk for large group of CHD-free men (n = 12,180) and women (n = 10,373) aged 30–69 years. CHD mortality risk for combined category of any Minnesota code Q waves was not significant in men or in women. There was a profound, over 17-fold increased risk of CHD mortality in men with major Q waves combined with major T waves. Again, there were too few events in women for risk evaluation.

As seen from ❷ Table 8.7, the low prevalence of diagnostic Q wave codes in all three of the populations is too low for population screening for preventive efforts, in spite of the extremely high mortality risk associated with them. However, when identified in any other connection, they warrant consideration for intensified secondary prevention. The Italian study suggests that the prevalence and the mortality risk for the combined category of ischemic abnormalities is at least potentially high enough for identification of subgroups for intervention.

● Table 8.7

Three population studies with evaluation of the risk for ECG manifestations of an old myocardial infarction (MI)

Study/Ref.	Seven Countries Study [15, 16]	Finland's Social Insurance Institution's CHD study [17]	Italian Rifle Pooling Project [18]
Geographic Location	Finland, Greece, Italy, the Netherlands, former Yugoslavia, Japan, the USA	South-western, western, central, and eastern districts of the country	Eight regions in Italy.
Source population	12,763 men (11 cohorts from rural areas of Finland, Greece, Japan, and Yugoslavia; three other more diverse cohorts from Yugoslavia; the town of Zutphen, the Netherlands; and cohorts of railroad employees from the USA and Italy.	Men and women of the districts. Participation rate 90% (5,738 men and 5,224 women).	Reported four out of nine studies, 23 cohorts total. Participation rate 65–70%.
Baseline	1958–1964	1966–1972	1978–1987
Exclusions	Sampling goal: total male population from selected geographic areas. Participation rate ≥60%. For CHD-free sample, excluded 854 with prevalent CHD at baseline; no ECG exclusions.	All participants included; risk evaluated separately for subjects with ischemic ECG free from symptoms typical of MI.	History of angina pectoris by Rose questionnaire, hospitalization with discharge diagnosis of MI, history of other heart disease.
CHD-free sample	11,860		12,180 men, 10,373 women.
Age range	40–59 years	30–59 years	30–69 years.
Follow-up	Initial 5-years and subsequent 6–25 years	5 years	6 years
Q wave MI-related ECG findings evaluated for risk	1. Any Q wave codes, with or without other ECG abnormalities (MC 1.1–1.3) 2. Diagnostic Q wave MI (MC 1.1 OR (MC 1.2 and MC 5.1–5.2)).	1. Diagnostic Q wave MI (MC 1.1 OR (MC 1.2 and MC 5.1–5.2). 2. Other "ischemic" categories (MC 1.2–1.3, 4.1–4.3, 5.1–5.3, 6.1–6.2, 7.1, 7.2, 7.4, 8.3))	Any Q wave codes (MC 1.1–1.3) Any Q wave codes with any T wave codes (5.1–5.3) 3. Q codes 1.1–1.2 with T codes 5.1, 5.2

▣ **Table 8.7**   (Continued)

Study/Ref.	Seven Countries Study [15, 16]	Finland's Social Insurance Institution's CHD study [17]	Italian Rifle Pooling Project [18]
Baseline prevalence	MC 1.1–1.3 (all men combined): 2.7% CHD-free men: 2.1%	1. Diagnostic Q wave MI Men 40–59 years: 1.3% Women 40–59 years: 0.5% Other "ischemic" ECG Men 40–59 years: 10.4% Women 40–59 years: 12.8%	Men Any Q codes 30–49 years: 0.6% 50–69 years: 1.1% Women Any Q codes 30–49 years: 0.5%; 50–59 years: 1.2%
Follow-up (Years)	25	5	6
Associated risk (hazard ratio HR)	Short-term (Years 0–5), Risk for CHD death (CHD-free men) Any Q: HR 4.1 (2.20, 7.61) Large Q or major Q with ST-T: HR 15.6 (7.2, 34.1) (not significant if large Q category excluded) Long-term (Years 6–25), Risk for CHD Death 1. Any Q: HR 1.2 (0.84, 1.58) 2. Large Q or major Q with ST-T: HR 3.4 (1.9, 6.2)	1. Diagnostic Q wave MI (5-year, age-standardized risk for age-group 40–49) Men: CHD mortality RR = 19.5 CVD mortality RR = 13.3 All-cause mortality RR = 5.6 Women: too few events for risk evaluation 2. "Other ischemic" ECG Men: CHD mortality RR = 7.2 CVD mortality RR = 6.4 All-cause mortality RR = 3.1 Women: CVD mortality RR = 3.0; All-cause mortality 2.2 Symptom-free men with "other ischemic" ECG CHD mortality, RR = 4.4 CVD mortality, RR = 3.9	CHD mortality Any Q waves: not significant in men or in women Any Q waves with any T waves: not significant for men or for women Major Q waves with major T waves: Men: RR 17.2 (1.54, 1.92) Women: Too few events for RR calculations

8.4.2   Other Studies with Mortality Risk Assessed for Major and Minor Q Waves

Mortality risk for various categories of Q waves has been evaluated in many other diverse populations. The Whitehall study on 18,403 male civil servants in the age-group 40–60 years conducted in early 1970s evaluated the 5-year CHD mortality risk for Q waves coded from limb-lead ECGs [34]. The study population contained a subgroup of 15,974 non-symptomatic men with no history of angina pectoris or MI and who were not under medical care for heart disease or hypertension. The prevalence of codes 1.1–1.3 was 2.0% in the whole group and 1.6% in the non-symptomatic group. Approximately two thirds of the Q waves were minor, Minnesota code 1.3. The age-adjusted CHD mortality ratio for men with any Q waves was 6.1 with all men in the study as the reference. In the non-symptomatic group, the mortality ratio was 4.0.

The Busselton study on 2,119 unselected subjects reported that the 13-year standardized CVD mortality rate was significantly higher in the pooled group of men and women with Minnesota code 1.1–1.3 Q waves than among those with a normal ECG [54].

The cross-sectional data from the Copenhagen City Heart Study involved a random sample of 9,384 men and 10,314 women aged 20 years and older [32]. In the age-group 60–69 years, 92 men (5.9%) and 38 women (2.4%) had Minnesota code 1.1–1.3 Q waves. Among 25 men who died, 21 had major Q waves (Minnesota code 1.1, 1.2), a highly significant difference between the observed and expected number of deaths compared to men without Q waves. There was only one death among women with Q waves.

8.4.3   Unrecognized Compared to Recognized Myocardial Infarction

Three studies listed in ❷ Table 8.8 evaluated mortality risk for recognized versus unrecognized MI: the Reykjavik study, the Framingham study, and the Honolulu study. Unrecognized MI was defined in these studies as either totally asymptomatic or associated with symptoms atypical for acute MI.

8.4.3.1   The Reykjavik Study

This study in a large male cohort ($N = 9,141$) was performed in five stages, 3–5 years apart, with the last stage conducted in 1983–1987 [55]. The overall prevalence of unrecognized MI at the first (0.5%) stage of the study increased sharply with age, from 0.5% at age 50 years to over 5% at age 75 years. The prevalence also increased at the later phases of the study, to 2.8% in 1987. About 30% of all MIs in the pooled data from all phases of the study were unrecognized. In logistic regression analysis, angina, age, smoking, serum cholesterol level, cardiomegaly, and diuretic therapy were associated with both types of MI. Impaired glucose tolerance and digoxin therapy were significantly associated only with recognized MI. Factors with predictive power for future unrecognized and recognized MI from Poisson regression included age, diastolic blood pressure, and hypertension medication. Digoxin therapy was significantly predictive for future unrecognized MI. Current smoking had a more consistent association with future recognized MI than with unrecognized MI.

Relative risk of CHD mortality for MI without angina pectoris was 4.6 (2.4, 8.6) for unrecognized MI and 6.3 (3.7, 10.6) for recognized MI. For all-cause mortality, the corresponding relative risks were 2.7 (1.5, 4.8) for unrecognized MI and 2.9 (1.8, 4.6) for recognized MI. The survival probabilities for both types of MI from life table analysis were relatively similar for subjects with and without MI in the first four stages of the study. Ten-year survival probabilities for unrecognized and recognized MI were 49% and 45%, respectively, and 15-year survival probabilities 62% and 48%, respectively.

8.4.3.2   Framingham Study

In a 1984 report from the Framingham study population, subjects with unrecognized MI were as likely as those with recognized MI to be at increased risk of death, heart failure, or strokes [56]. In subjects initially free from CHD, three successive 10-year periods since the start of the Framingham study in 1948 were used as the baseline for comparing the risk for the two types of MI. Of all baseline MIs in 5,127 subjects at the initial examination, 130 of 469 (27.7%) among men

■ Table 8.8

Mortality risk for recognized versus unrecognized myocardial infarction

Study/Ref.	The Reykjavik Study [21]	Framingham [22]	Hawaii Heart Program [24]
Geographic Location	Reykjavik area, Iceland	Framingham, Massachusetts	Oahu Island, Hawaii
Source population	Male residents born between 1907 and 1934. Response rate 64–75%.	Town's representative adult population, 2,336 men, 2,873 women	Men of Japanese ancestry born between 1900 and 1919. Participation rate 73%.
Baseline	1967–1968	Onset of each of the three successive 10-year periods starting 1948	1965–1968
Selection criteria	Whole cohort included	Free from overt CHD at baseline, excluding from next follow-up subjects with MI during the preceding period	CHD-free at baseline, with at least one follow-up examination
Sample size	9,141	5,127 men and women	7,331
Age range	33–80 years	35–62 years	45–68 years
Follow-up period	4–24 years (in four stages, at 3–5 year intervals)	30 years	10 years from the examination where incident MI was detected
Definition of MI	1. Recognized MI: MONICA criteria (Patients with MC 1.1,1.2 Q waves, or with MI by enzymes, chest pain, borderline Q waves) 2. Unrecognized MI: MC 1.1, 1.2 with no history of MI	Appearance of pathologic (≥40 ms) Q waves or loss of initial R waves Unrecognized MI: Incident MI when neither the patient nor the attending physician had considered heart attack.	1. Serial ECG changes at follow-up considered diagnostic for old or age-undetermined MI; 2. Hospitalization with acute chest pain with evolving ECG changes and/or elevated enzymes 3. Serial ECG changes at hospital surveillance considered as old or age-undetermined MI
Prevalence/incidence of MI	Prevalence of unrecognized MI 0.5% at first stage, increased at later stages to 2.8% in 1980. Prevalence increased sharply with age, from 0.5% at age of 50 years to over 5% at age of 75 years. About 30% of all MI unrecognized (in pooled data from all phases).	Incidence of all MIs (during three 10-year periods): Increased in men from 7.1%, in women from 1.3% at age 45–54 years to 12.8% at age 75–84 years. Over one quarter of all MIs in men and over one third in women were unrecognized.	Average annual rate/1,000 of recognized MI (in category 1 above) 1.46, unrecognized MI 0.71, with significant age trend in both. Unrecognized MIs 32.6%.

Associated Risk	CHD death, MI without angina: RR = 4.6 (2.4, 8.6) for unrecognized MI, RR = 6.3 (3.7, 10.6) for recognized MI CHD death, MI with angina: RR = 16.9 (9.4, 30.3) for unrecognized MI, RR = 8.5 (5.8, 12.6) for recognized MI	Ten-year age-adjusted mortality risk ratio (unrecognized MI versus recognized MI) from proportional hazards model Men CHD death 1.0 CVD death 1.2 Sudden coronary death 0.6 All deaths 1.2 Women CHD death 0.6 CVD death 0.5 Sudden coronary death 0.8 All deaths 0.7	Ten-year CHD mortality 35% versus 25% (p = 0.107), CVD mortality 39% versus 28% (p = 0.045), total mortality 45% versus 35% (p = 0.045), for unrecognized versus recognized MI, respectively.
Multivariate adjustment	Not clearly stated. Age, cholesterol level, antihypertensive medication, diastolic pressure, and smoking were associated with risk of unrecognized MI	Age-adjusted, controlling also for the effect of the loss of subjects to follow-up because of death from unrelated causes.	Unadjusted (age distribution similar in both groups).
Comments	Ten-year survival probabilities for CHD death: 49% for unrecognized MI, 62% for recognized MI; 15 years: 45% for unrecognized MI, 48% for symptomatic MI.	p < 0.05; not significant difference for other recognized versus non-recognized MI	

and 83 of 239 (34.7%) among women were unrecognized, almost half without any symptoms. A similar proportion as mentioned above was unrecognized among incident MI during the three 10-year follow-up periods. ❷ Table 8.8 shows that the cause-specific mortality and all-cause mortality in men was similar for unrecognized and recognized MI. In women, the mortality was lower for unrecognized compared to recognized MI, and the difference was significant (p < 0.05) for CVD mortality.

A 1986 report from the Framingham study compared the relative 10-year risk of clinical CHD for unrecognized, asymptomatic ECG-MI and ECG-LVH [57]. The evaluation group was CHD-free at the baseline and new asymptomatic ECG-MI and ECG-LVH was detected as a 2-year incidence before the start of the follow-up. There was a profound two- to fourfold increase in CHD mortality, particularly sudden death, for both ECG abnormalities, with similar rates for both. Of interest was also the finding that ECG-LVH carried a significantly greater risk than ECG-MI for CHD death in women.

8.4.3.3   Honolulu Heart Program

The prognosis of recognized and unrecognized MI was also evaluated in the Honolulu Heart Program in a 10-year follow-up among 7,331 men who were CHD-free at baseline examination and who had serial ECG changes classified as incident Q-wave MI at the second or third examinations (2 and 6 years following the baseline) [58]. There was a total of 89 Q-wave MIs classified from serial ECG changes, 33% of them asymptomatic. Among men who were classified as MI from hospital surveillance of the study, the proportion of silent MIs among all nonfatal MIs was 22%. (The average annual incidence rate (per 1,000) for all nonfatal MIs was 3.29). The unrecognized MI group had a consistently higher (60–70%) total CVD and CHD mortality than the group with recognized MI. The number of events in groups compared in the Honolulu study was small and the difference in risk was not significant. However, consistent with the other studies mentioned above, the results suggest that the mortality risk for silent MI is at least as high as for recognized, symptomatic MI.

8.4.3.4   Other Studies Comparing Recognized Versus Unrecognized MI

A Finnish cohort of 697 men aged 65–84 years of the Seven Countries study, who had survived at the time of the 23-year follow-up examination, was followed up for the next 5-year period [59]. At the time of the beginning of the follow-up, 98 of the men (14.1%) had Minnesota code 1.1–1.3 Q waves. Q waves combined with ST depression (codes 4.1–4.3) or negative T waves (codes 5.1 or 5.2) were significantly associated with excess risk of fatal and nonfatal MI and total mortality. Isolated Q waves were not associated with independent risk with any of the endpoints.

The Bronx Aging Study assessed the prognosis of recognized and unrecognized MI in 390 elderly (75–85 years) community-based men and women in an 8-year prospective evaluation [60]. In this older group, baseline prevalence of MI was 18.5%, over one third (34.7%) of them unrecognized (completely silent MI and MI with atypical symptoms were included in this category). During the follow-up, the proportion of unrecognized MIs among all incident or recurrent MIs was 44%. The total mortality rate in subjects with recognized or unrecognized MI was 5.9/100 person–years compared with 3.9/100 person–years in the group without MI (p = 0.059). The sample size is small and the event rates in study subgroups are low, but the mortality rates were similar among those with recognized and unrecognized MI. The report reviewed other studies on unrecognized MI and noted that in newer reports (often from prospective studies) the average proportion of unrecognized MI was 30%.

In the older Israel ischemic heart disease project [61], the mortality follow-up was conducted 5 years from the initial examination in 1963. The second clinical examination took place in 1965 and the third in 1968. The occurrence of the MI was assumed to have taken place halfway between the two closest examinations before and after the abnormality developed. The average annual mortality rate in the group of men without any signs of MI during the follow-up period was 4.6/1,000.

There was a total of 170 men with clinically unrecognized MI during the follow-up and the annual mortality rate in this group of men was 17.3/1,000, or 3.8 times the mortality rate in men without any sign of MI. One half of all unrecognized MIs were silent and classified strictly on the basis of ECG findings in the 1965 or 1968 reexamination. The other half of clinically unrecognized MIs was not asymptomatic but their complaints were considered atypical for MI. The annual mortality rate of 17.3/1,000 for men with unrecognized MI can be compared with the rate of 36.3/1,000 for the group of 120 men with clinically recognized MI.

The incident (or recurrent) MI rate, particularly that of unrecognized MI, was high among men with possible or probable MI at baseline according to computer criteria but who were considered as non-MI by electrocardiographers reviewing the computer interpretation. A sizable fraction of these men may have had latent CHD already at the onset of the study.

No serial ECG change classification criteria were evidently used in the study and it is possible that relatively minor changes from the baseline ECG were more likely to cause a classification as a new unrecognized MI in this subgroup. In any case, ECG signs of unrecognized MI seemed to be associated with excess mortality, with a prognosis perhaps half as serious as that for clinically recognized MI. It is noted that in the Israel study, 62% of the unrecognized MIs were categorized as possible old anterior MI, defined by the presence of a Q wave in V_2 or V_3 or R wave ≤ 100 mV in any two of the leads V_2–V_5. Multivariate analyses also indicated that the increased incidence of unrecognized MIs was associated with age, cigarette smoking, blood pressure (systolic and diastolic), left axis deviation, and LVH on the ECG. Poor progression of R waves in anterior chest leads is often seen in hypertensives with LVH, and it is possible that a significant proportion of these unrecognized MIs were false positives because of the limited specificity of the criteria used.

8.4.4 ECG Risk Predictors in Heart Attack Survivors

The Coronary Drug project was the first large-scale clinical trial that reported on systematic analyses of the prognostic value of ECG abnormalities among survivors from a first heart attack during a 3-year period of a longer follow-up [62]. Baseline ECGs, including the placebo group, were recorded at least 3 months after the acute phase.

ST depression had the strongest association of any ECG items with excess mortality. The risk ratio for major ST depression (>0.1 mV J depression with horizontal or downsloping ST segment) relative to normal ST was 4.0, and any degree of ST depression, except J-point depression with upsloping ST had a significant association with excess mortality. Actually, any degree of ST depression, except J-point depression with upsloping ST, was associated with a significant excess mortality. T waves more negative than −0.1 mV were also associated with over twofold excess mortality, and there was also a significant excess among men with minor T-wave abnormalities (flat or biphasic T waves).

Of particular importance was the observation that resting ECG ST depression was related to excess mortality also among men with no history of heart failure and among men not taking digitalis.

Extensive multivariate analyses were performed using Coronary Drug project data to elucidate possible independent prognostic value of ECG findings after simultaneous adjustment for all major known CHD risk factors and clinical risk indicators. Minnesota code items that contain independent prognostic information included the following categories: Q, QS waves (any code 1), ST depression (codes 4.1 to 4.4), ventricular conduction defects (e.g. codes 7.1 and 7.4) except complete right bundle branch block (code 7.2), atrial flutter/fibrillation (code 8.3), and any ventricular premature beats (code 8.2).

ST depression in the resting ECG turned out to be the strongest single ECG predictor of mortality and as strong an independent risk predictor as cardiac enlargement and functional class. This is clinically important because codable ST changes are common among survivors of a first heart attack (25% of men in the Coronary Drug project had codable ST changes) and a considerable proportion of all deaths occur among this subgroup.

8.4.5 Heart Attack Prevention Programs and Prognostic Value of Rest and Exercise ECG Abnormalities

Numerous studies cited in previous sections have demonstrated the adverse prognostic value of several resting ECG abnormalities. Relatively little is known, however, on how the presence of these abnormalities may influence heart attack prevention efforts, for instance, whether persons with defined ECG abnormalities might respond particularly favorably to intervention. The MRFIT project was designed to test the effect of a multifactor intervention program on mortality from CHD in 12,866 high-risk men aged 35–57 years. The two a priori ECG-based subgroup hypotheses were formulated with the expectation that intervention would be especially beneficial in men with a normal resting ECG and a normal exercise

ECG, respectively. No significant difference in CHD mortality was found between the special intervention and usual care (UC) groups of the trial [63]. The findings from the MRFIT study even brought up the possibility that hypertensive high-risk men with resting ECG abnormalities may have experienced increased CHD mortality in the special intervention group of the trial, an observation that created a great deal of interest because of its potential implications on diuretic therapy [64]. Similar adverse trends in coronary events were reported from the Oslo study trial on mild hypertension although the number of events involved was too low to reach nominal statistical significance [65].

The Hypertension Detection and Follow-up Program (HDFP) [66] compared CHD and total mortality in a subgroup of mild hypertensives (diastolic pressure 90–104 mm Hg) with resting ECG abnormalities similar to the MRFIT study population. CHD mortality for persons receiving systematic antihypertensive therapy in special program centers (stepped care group) was compared to that for persons referred to existing community medical care (referred care group.) The CHD mortality rate was slightly but not significantly higher in the stepped care group than in the referred care group in white men and black women, but not in black men. However, the rates for all-cause mortality were consistently lower in the stepped care group than in the referred care group. This 24% difference in favor of the stepped care group did not reach a nominal level of statistical significance because the subgroups with ECG abnormalities of HDFP cohort were small, again demonstrating problems in reaching adequate statistical power even in very large clinical trials.

In primary prevention trials, the emphasis is in demonstrating the effectiveness of risk-factor intervention in subgroups without ECG abnormalities. This is based on the assumption that intervention should be most beneficial in an early, asymptomatic phase of the disease process before end-organ damage develops.

As a contrast to the unexpected negative overall outcome of the intervention among men with a normal ECG response to exercise in MRFIT, men with an abnormal exercise ECG seemed to benefit substantially from risk-factor reduction [67]. There was a 57% lower rate of CHD deaths among men in the special intervention group with an abnormal ECG response to exercise compared with men in the usual care group (22.2 versus 51.8/1,000). Abnormal ECG response to exercise was defined as an ST-depression integral measured by a computer as 16 μVs or more in peak exercise or immediate recovery records in any of leads CS5, aVL, aVF, or V$_5$, with the ST-depression integral being less than 6 μVs in the above leads in the pre-exercise sitting record. These abnormal responses to a submaximal heart-rate-limited treadmill exercise test represented mainly early repolarization abnormalities with upsloping ST in lead CS5 during peak exercise. At the baseline of the study, 12.2% of the usual care men of the study had an abnormal exercise ECG. There was a nearly fourfold increase in 7-year coronary mortality among men with an abnormal response to exercise compared with men with a normal response [68].

Changing trends in CHD mortality can cause formidable problems for primary prevention trials. Unexpectedly, low CHD and total mortality particularly among subgroups or high-risk men selected on the basis of normal resting and exercise ECG can become problematic. In MRFIT, the CHD mortality rate was only about 2 per 1,000 per year in the large subgroup (61%) of these high-risk men with a normal resting and exercise ECG. It is difficult to demonstrate a significant reduction of CHD deaths below this level because a very large sample size is required for attaining adequate statistical power.

MRFIT mortality follow-up data were later extended to cover a 10.5-year follow-up period [69]. Ischemic response to exercise remained the only abnormality in the UC men with a significant association with CHD mortality, confirming the results from the initial 7-year mortality data. In the SI group, ST-T abnormalities at rest, absent or low-amplitude U waves and an abnormal cardiac infarction injury score (CIIS) [20] were all significantly associated with 10.5-year CHD mortality. However, absent or low-amplitude U waves were the only ECG abnormalities with a significant difference between the special intervention and usual care men in the relative risk estimates ($p = 0.004$).

In the Belgian heart disease prevention project [70], there was no significant difference in CHD incidence between intervention and control groups among men with a normal resting ECG. However, reduction of CHD risk factors among men with ischemic changes in their resting ECG by the Minnesota code criteria was associated with a significant reduction in 6-year CHD incidence and total mortality.

8.4.6   Time Trends: Are Risk Evaluation Data from Older Studies Still Valid?

To what extent are risk evaluation results from the older studies still valid in view of the reported decline in-hospital MI mortality rate? For instance, a survey of patients hospitalized for acute Q-wave MI in Worcester, Massachusetts, metropolitan area hospitals, compared two periods 1 decade apart (1995–1997 versus 1986–1988) [71]. The in-hospital case fatality rate had declined from 19% to 14%. Controlled clinical trials have demonstrated reduced mortality with more common use of primary angioplasty and improved treatment of acute MI with more widespread use of coronary reperfusion and antiplatelet therapy.

It is apparent that the short-term risk of acute MI patients has improved at least in industrialized countries that have benefited from improved acute care. The question remains to what extent the long-term prognosis has improved. Already before the introduction of the major improvements in the care of CHD patients, factors other than ECG evidence of old MI seemed to determine the long-term outcome. Unrecognized MI may be less likely to benefit from improved care until a later phase of the evolution of the disease. The proportion of unrecognized MI has been approximately one third of all MIs in the studies cited above, including the Western Collaborative Group Study [72].

It takes a prolonged period of time and a large sample size to produce results from long-term studies, and by the time the results come in, the question of obsolescence often arises. The popularity of the traditional observational population studies has declined, in part because of funding problems and because clinical drug trials have taken a higher priority for funding as well as for the acceptance of manuscripts for publication in high-impact medical journals.

8.5   ECG-LVH: A Spectrum of Connotations

8.5.1   Age Trends and Ethnic Differences in ECG-LVH

The Copenhagen City Heart Study [32] conducted from 1976 to 1978, reported in 1981, combined Minnesota code 3.1, 3.3 prevalence data of 6,505 men and 7,713 women. The data showed the well-known drop in LVH prevalence in young adult men until age 40–49 years. There was little subsequent variation with age in men but in women, there is a steady increase in ECG-LVH prevalence by these criteria after age 40–49 years.

In US populations, there are rather striking differences in age trends of ECG-LVH by Cornell voltage and Sokolow–Lyon voltage criteria [73]. The Cornell voltage increases by age in men and in women (❷ Figs. 8.1 and ❷ 8.2). Cornell voltage patterns are relatively similar in Hispanic and white men and women, and the amplitudes are drastically higher in African–American men and women. In contrast to Cornell voltage, Sokolow–Lyon voltage decreases with age in all three ethnic groups except African–American women (❷ Figs. 8.3 and ❷ 8.4).

Many studies have reported a higher ECG-LVH prevalence in blacks compared to whites. In the Evans County study, LVH prevalence by Sokolow–Lyon criteria was threefold in blacks compared to whites, and also the ECG estimate of LV mass was significantly higher [49, 74, 75]. By Sokolow–Lyon criteria, LVH prevalence was over fourfold in the Charleston study [76]. In the Chicago Heart Study, LVH was defined by Minnesota code 3.1 criteria combined with repolarization abnormalities (MC 4.1–4.3 or MC 5.1–5.3) [77]. Although the overall LVH prevalence by this combination was substantially lower, the black and white differences were still pronounced in all age-groups from 20 to 64 years. ECG-LVH prevalence in Nigerian civil servants by Minnesota code 3.1–3.3 criteria was reported as 36.3% in men and 16.9% in women [78].

8.5.2   Time Trends in ECG-LVH Prevalence

A notable decline was found in ECG-LVH prevalence from 1950 to 1989 in the predominantly white combined original and offspring cohorts of the Framingham study [79]. ECG-LVH by combined high R and abnormal ST criteria had decreased from 4.5% to 2.5% in men and from 3.6 to 1.1% in women. The mean age-adjusted Cornell voltage amplitude had declined 80 μV per decade in men (p = 0.03) and 60 μV per decade in women (p = 0.06). Similar, profound decline has been observed in other US populations, including data from the National Health and Nutrition Surveys [80]. Although increasing use and improved effectiveness of antihypertensive medications parallel this decrease in ECG-LVH prevalence, questions remain about the reliability of ECG-LVH criteria in general and possible confounding factors.

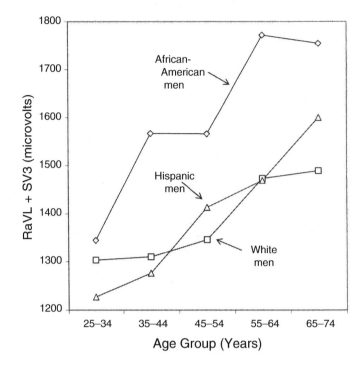

⬛ Fig. 8.1

Cornell voltage (RaVL + SV3) by age in white (*squares*), Hispanic (*triangles*), and African–American men (*diamonds*). Note consistent increasing trend with age in all three ethnic groups and the substantially higher mean values in African–American compared to white and Hispanic men (Data modified from ref. [73], Rautaharju et al., J Electrocardiol 1994; 27(suppl): [20–30]. © 1994 Churchill Livingstone, reproduced with permission)

8.5.3   Echo-LVH Versus ECG-LVH: Gender and Racial Differences

In the Treatment of Mild Hypertension Study (TOMHS) [81], Echo-LVH (LV mass index $\geq 134 \, g/m^2$ for men and $\geq 110 \, g/m^2$ for women) was present in 13% of men and in 20% of women. ECG-LVH was reported to be "virtually absent" by Minnesota code 3.1 criteria combined with abnormal repolarization (Minnesota code 4.1–4.3 or 5.1–5.3).

Okin et al. concluded that gender differences in body size and LV mass do not completely account for gender differences in voltage measurements and QRS duration [82].

Although available echocardiographic data are limited, it has become evident that standard electrocardiographic criteria overestimate racial differences in LVH prevalence [83]. There was no notable difference in the echocardiographic LV mass between white and African–American men or women in CHD-free subgroups of the CHS population of men and women 65 years old and older [84]. In that report, relatively strict selection criteria were used to establish upper normal limits for LV mass ($116 \, g/m^2$ for men and $104 \, g/m^2$ for women). LVH prevalence was 18.1% in white men, 15.5% in African–American men, 14.7% in white women, and 12.8% in African–American women. Thus, racial differences in Echo-LVH were relatively small. These relative differences are not overly dependent on the LV mass cut points chosen.

8.5.4   LVH and Overweight

The role of overweight and obesity in relation to ECG-LVH and Echo-LVH is a relatively complex issue, and space limitations do not permit presentation of any data here. Classification accuracy of ECG-LVH by Sokolow–Lyon criteria is limited in general, and in particular in the presence of obesity. Revaluation of the CHS data indicated that there is a

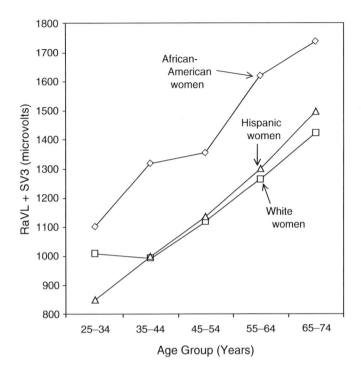

◨ **Fig. 8.2**
Cornell voltage (RaVL + SV3) by age in white (*squares*), Hispanic (*triangles*), and African–American women (*diamonds*). Note
consistent increasing trend with age in all three ethnic groups and the substantially higher mean values in African–American
compared to white and Hispanic men (Data modified from ref. [73], Rautaharju et al., J Electrocardiol 1994;27(suppl):20–30.
© 1994 Churchill Livingstone, reproduced with permission)

substantial underestimate in ECG-LVH by the Cornell voltage criteria particularly in white men. In white and in African–American women, being overweight is associated with a notably higher Echo-LVH [85]. The overall LVH prevalence estimates by both methods may not differ substantially but the fraction of cases where both methods agree with the classification is relatively small.

Various studies have produced differing results about the role of overweight and LVH. The results differ depending on the method of indexing of LV mass to body size [82–86]. The availability of lean body weight data may be necessary to resolve the role of overweight in LVH.

8.5.5 ECG-LVH Prevalence in Hypertensive Cohorts

Higher ECG-LVH prevalence in blacks than in whites has also been reported in hypertensive cohorts. The Hypertension Detection and Follow-up Program (HDFP) evaluated ECGs of 10,940 hypertensive men and women with diastolic blood pressure (fifth phase) at the second screening visit of 90 mm Hg or above [54]. By Minnesota code 3.1, 3.3 plus 4.1–4.3, 5.1–5.3 criteria, the prevalences were 2.7% and 8.6% for white and black men, and 1.7% and 7.7% for white and black women, respectively. With high QRS amplitudes combined with ST-T abnormalities, the specificity of the criteria is very high, but the sensitivity is very low. The question of the need for improved LVH criteria arises again.

The Italian PIUMA study [87] reported Cornell voltage sensitivity as 16% and specificity as 97%. The authors reported that for the Perugia score for LVH [88], the sensitivity was 34% and specificity 93%. The operating points for various criteria can be expected to be quite different in hypertensive hospital populations compared to community-dwelling populations.

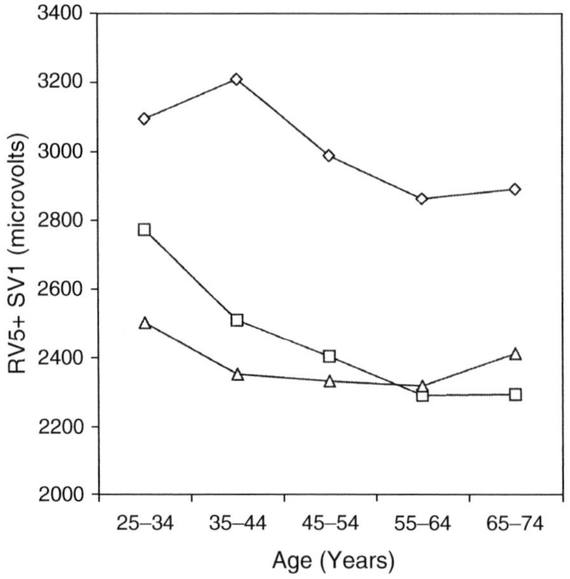

Fig. 8.3
Sokolow–Lyon voltage (RV5 + SV1) by age in white (*squares*), Hispanic (*triangles*), and African-American men (*diamonds*). Note the opposite age trend in Sokolow–Lyon voltage in all three ethnic groups in comparison to the systematic increase in Cornell voltage with age in Fig. 8.1. The mean values of the Sokolow–Lyon voltage in African-American men are substantially higher compared to white and Hispanic men. Rautaharju, PM, unpublished data

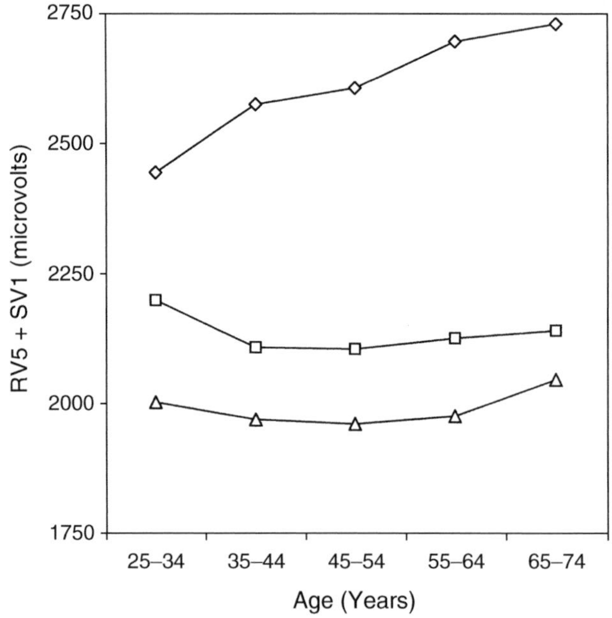

Fig. 8.4
Sokolow–Lyon voltage (RV5 + SV1) by age in white (*squares*), Hispanic (*triangles*), and African-American women (*diamonds*). Increasing age trend in Sokolow–Lyon voltage is present only in African-American women and their mean values are substantially higher compared to white and Hispanic women (From NHANES 3 and HHANES ECG data, ref. [73], Rautaharju, PM, unpublished)

In summary, there are profound problems in using ECG-LVH criteria for estimating LVH prevalence in contrasting populations. LVH prevalence estimates by echocardiographic criteria will face similar, although not quite as severe, problems when some more accurate evaluation method will become available as an independent standard.

8.5.6 Visual Coding Errors as Source for Limited Sensitivity

The primary reason for visual coding errors is the complexity of the Minnesota code coding rules, particularly for serial comparison. All significant findings, particularly in code 1 category, are usually verified by an experienced supervisor in case there are any coding disagreements after duplicate reading by two coders (the procedure usually followed). Thus, false coding of significant abnormalities is actually rare. From experience in large clinical trials such as the Multiple Risk Factor Intervention Trial, the major problem in visual coding is the relatively frequent miss rate of truly codable items in spite of duplicate or even triplicate coding of each record. This miss rate can be 20% or even 30% when high volumes of records have to be coded. These error rates were found when visually coded items were verified with a computer program and all disagreements were again arbitrated.

Rautaharju et al. used a statistical model in an attempt to elucidate the reasons for the high miss rate with visual coding [89]. The authors concluded that a high miss rate in certain difficult categories of Code 1 will explain the high overall miss rate, and they also suggested that an initial screening by a computer and possible visual verification of selected items may substantially improve the accuracy and efficiency of ECG coding.

8.5.7 Prognostic Value of ECG-LVH in General Populations

Population characteristics and ECG-LVH criteria used differ from study to study, and the reported CVD mortality risk data differ considerably as seen from data derived from five diverse populations in ❷ Table 8.9. In the Framingham cohort, ECG-LVH by high QRS amplitude with LV strain was associated with a substantial excess of CVD, CHD, and all-cause mortality [51], and the mortality rates for ECG-LVH were similar as for MI by ECG, and in women they were always higher for ECG-LVH. Two-year age-adjusted incidence of ECG-LVH increased sharply both in men and in women with hypertensive status classified as mild and definite, compared with non-hypertensive groups.

LVH by Cornell voltage criteria was associated with an over threefold increased risk in black men and with an over twofold increased risk in white women in the NHANES one survey from the early 1970s. The risk was not significantly increased in any of the subgroups for Sokolow–Lyon criteria (PM Rautaharju, unpublished observations).

The Belgian Inter-University Research on Nutrition and Health (BIRNH) found a significantly increased age-adjusted and multivariately adjusted relative risk for ECG-LVH by high QRS amplitude criteria of the Minnesota code in men for CVD mortality but not for CHD mortality or total mortality [70]. The risk model included an adjustment for other major ECG abnormalities. The multivariately adjusted risk ratio for ECG-LVH was 3.14 (1.36–7.26). The risk was not significantly increased in women for any of the three major endpoints.

Data in ❷ Table 8.9 includes data from two elderly cohorts, namely an older Finnish cohort of men aged 65–84 years of the Seven Countries study [59] and the Bronx Longitudinal Aging Study that included men and women aged 75–85 years [90]. In the Finnish study with a 5-year follow-up of 697 survivors aged 65–85 years subsequent to the 25-year examination of the initial Finnish cohort of the Seven Countries study, the mortality risk for high-amplitude QRS waves and other Minnesota code items was evaluated, first separately for each abnormality and then according to a clearly defined hierarchic scheme. In the latter scenario, high QRS codes (MC 3.1, 3.3) without significant Q, ST, and T codes were entered into logistic regression models also adjusted for major CHD risk factors. High QRS amplitude codes entered without considering other coexisting codes were associated with a significant excess risk of all-cause mortality, and also with risk of fatal and nonfatal MI. The risk for isolated high R waves alone in the absence of ST-T abnormalities was not significant for any of the study endpoints. This finding again suggests that the inclusion of repolarization abnormalities with high-amplitude QRS variables is essential, not only for diagnostic applications but in particular for improved risk identification.

Table 8.9

ECG-LVH and CVD Mortality risk in general adult populations, including two old cohorts

Study/Baseline years	Age (years)	Follow-Up	Criteria	Endpoint	Gender/Race	RR (95% CI)	Comments
Framingham 1948	> 28	18 biennials	High QRS, ST Strain	CVD mortality	Men Women	3.4 (p < 0.05) 3.4 (p < 0.05)	RR = age-adjusted mortality rate versus general Framingham sample.
BIRNH 1981–1984	25–74	≥ 10 years	High R MC	CVD mortality	Men Women	3.14 (1.36–7.26) 2.20 (0.53–9.16)	CHD-free at baseline;
NHANES 1 1971–1975	35–74	7–13 years	High QRS + ST-T MC		White Men Black Men White Women Black Women	3.26 (1.91, 5.56) 4.29 (2.00, 9.18) 2.59 (1.29, 5.19) 1.90 (0.64, 5.65)	RR multivariately adjusted RR age-adjusted
RIFLE Pooling Project 1978–1987	30–69	6 years	High R MC High QRS + ST-T MC	CVD mortality CVD mortality	Men Women Men Women	1.86 (1.13, 3.07) 3.66 (0.96, 14.0) 6.33 (3.02, 13.3) 5.91 (0.70, 49.9)	Reference group free from LVH; multivariately adjusted, also for other ECG abnormalities
Bronx Longitudinal Aging Study 1980	75–85	10 years	High QRS, ST-T MC	CVD mortality All-cause mortality	Men and women Men and women	2.72 (0.53, 2.09) 2.18 (1.06, 4.45)	
Finnish cohort of the Seven Countries Study 1984	65–84	5 years	High QRS MC With or without Q, ST-T codes High QRS alone MC	All-cause mortality All-cause mortality	Men Men	1.27 (p = 0.034) 0.68 (0.22, 1.45)	p value from chi-square test adjusted for age and geographic area Reference group men with no major ECG abnormalities

In the Bronx Longitudinal Aging Study, ECG-LVH (MC 3.1, 3.3 with 4.1–4.3 or 5.1–5.3) had a significantly higher risk of CVD mortality than no ECG-LVH, with risk ratio 2.65 (1.58–4.41). In a multivariate model adjusting for common risk factors, CVD mortality risk was increased but not statistically significant.

One of the most informative reports from evaluation of the risk of LVH with various combinations of the relevant Minnesota codes comes from the Copenhagen City Heart Study [91]. In that report, ECG abnormalities for risk evaluation were classified as normal (reference group) together with five hierarchic, mutually exclusive abnormal categories: high-voltage QRS alone, negative T wave, ST depression with negative T wave, high-voltage QRS with negative T, and high-voltage QRS with ST depression and negative T. Each abnormality was an isolated finding, with no other abnormalities. Short-term (7-year) risk and long-term (21-year) risk were estimated for three endpoints: fatal and nonfatal MI, ischemic heart disease (ICD 8:410–414), and CVD mortality. The short-term risks for ischemic heart disease and CVD mortality are listed in ❯ Table 8.10, reproduced from ❯ Tables 4 and ❯ 5 of the Copenhagen study report. The study found no evidence of significant interaction between gender and ECG abnormalities in the Cox risk models when evaluated as individual categories or as a combined group.

The results confirm the findings from other studies that high QRS voltage alone is of little importance for risk identification, particularly when adjusted for blood pressure. Negative T waves and ST depression as isolated findings and not associated with high-voltage QRS were important predictors. The highest relative risk was found for high QRS voltage combined with negative T waves and high QRS voltage with ST depression was the strongest risk predictor of all five abnormal combinations. The report did not try to identify dominant predictors by entering all ECG abnormal categories simultaneously into the multivariately adjusted risk model. It is most likely, however, that such a model would have identified high-voltage QRS with ST depression and possibly also with negative T wave as dominant predictors among the abnormal categories.

Using ECG predictors as continuous variables will, in principle, improve the risk prediction power. An older ECG model for estimation of LV mass indexed to body surface area was used in an older study to evaluate mortality risk using NHANES1 data [92]. Comparing relative risk for an increment from 20th to 80th percentile, age-adjusted risks for CVD mortality were 1.39 (1.21, 1.60) for white men, 1.67 (1.21, 2.29) for black men, 1.62 (1.17, 2.24) for white women, and 2.08 (1.27, 3.42) for black women. With an additional adjustment for systolic blood pressure and history of heart attack, CVD mortality risk remained significant in white men (RR = 1.21 (1.03, 1.43)), white women (RR = 1.36 (1.08, 1.70)), and in black women (RR = 1.95 (1.44, 2.66)) but not for black men (RR = 1.26 (0.81, 1.96)). These data suggest that the risk is graded across a wide range of estimated LV mass values.

8.5.8 Incident ECG-LVH

The Framingham study is among the very few with adequate documentation of CHD risk in persons developing new ECG evidence of LVH during a long follow-up period [93]. It is of practical importance that the incidence of ECG-LVH is higher than anticipated from the cross-sectional prevalence data. In the Framingham population, one in ten people developed some evidence of ECG-LVH in the first 12 years of follow-up. In about 3% of the cohort, ECG findings were categorized as definitive new LVH (mostly high-amplitude R waves combined with repolarization abnormalities).

There was a pronounced increase in the risk of every manifestation of CHD in men and women with definite LVH, including stroke and heart failure. The incidence of angina, MI, and sudden death in this group was about as high as in persons surviving a first MI. Data from 20-year follow-up of the Framingham study indicate a risk ratio for the age-adjusted overall mortality of about five for both males and females with definitive LVH compared to those without ECG evidence of LVH. For men, this risk ratio was nearly six for CHD death and sudden death. For women, the risk ratio for total cardiovascular mortality was nearly ten. The excess mortality associated with definite LVH on ECG carried a greater risk of cardiovascular events than cardiac enlargement. The risk was three times the risk associated with hypertension alone. As a contrast, electrocardiographic LVH based on high-amplitude R-wave criteria alone carried a risk for CHD mortality, which was about half of the risk for definite LVH. Furthermore, this excess risk was no longer manifest when adjustment was made for the coexisting hypertension.

◻ Table 8.10

Age-standardized incidence and relative risk of ischemic heart disease events and of cardiovascular disease mortality during 7 years of follow-up in relation to ECG findings among those without ischemic heart disease at baseline, for the age range 35–74 years in Copenhagen City Heart Study

	Ischemic Heart Disease Events			Cardiovascular Disease Mortality		
	N (Inc.)	Age-adjusted RR	Multivariately adjusted RR^a (95% CI)	N (Inc.)	Age-adjusted RR	RR^a (95% CI)
Normal ECG (n = 8,460)	345 (6.7)	1	1	223 (4.5)	1	1
Voltage-only LVH (n = 1,197)	66 (10.2)	1.16 (0.89–1.52)	1.15 (0.88–1.51)	45 (6.6)	1.23 (0.89–1.69)	1.28 (0.92–1.77)
T, n = 799	73 (11.6)	1.69 (1.31–2.18)*	1.56 (1.21–2.03)[†]	55 (8.5)	1.82 (1.35–2.45)*	1.61 (1.19–2.18)[†]
ST/T, n = 257	27 (14.1)	2.25 (1.52–3.34)*	2.07 (1.39–3.08)*	17 (9.1)	1.98(1.21–3.26)[†]	1.68 (1.02–2.77)[†]
LVH with neg. T (n = 137)	17 (16.2)	1.95 (1.20–3.19)[†]	1.89 (1.15–3.09)[††]	14 (13.4)	2.28 (1.32–3.92)[†]	2.16 (1.25–3.74)[†]
LVH with ST/T (n = 132)	32 (30.5)	4.27 (2.95–6.16)*	3.62 (2.47–5.30)*	22 (17.8)	3.75 (2.41–5.85)*	2.96 (1.87–4.68)*

CI confidence interval RR relative risk, ECG electrocardiographic, LVH left ventricular hypertrophy, ST/T LVH with ST depression and negative T wave, Inc. age-standardized number of endpoint events per 1,000 years of follow-up.

^{a}Adjusted for age, systolic and diastolic blood pressure, heart rate, body mass index, cholesterol, smoking, diabetes, alcohol, physical exercise, and family history of ischemic heart disease.

* P < 0.001

[†] P <0.01

[††] P < 0.05

8.6   Incident Bundle Branch Blocks: Prognostic Value

The Framingham study cited above has also reported on the prognostic significance of newly acquired left and right bundle branch block [93]. There were 55 individuals in the Framingham population who acquired a left bundle branch block and 70 who acquired a right bundle branch block during 18 years of follow-up. The CVD mortality in these two subgroups of men and women was compared to the mortality in a group of age-matched members of the Framingham population who were presumed free from bundle branch block. Within 10 years after the onset of the block, the cumulative cardiovascular disease mortality was more than four times greater in those with left bundle branch block and more than three times greater in those with right bundle branch block than in the age-matched group of the study population. The proportion of sudden deaths was similar in those with left and right bundle branch block. In women, there was no indication of a different trend in cardiovascular disease mortality rates for left and right bundle branch block.

The acquired bundle branch blocks were all associated with prospective cardiovascular abnormalities during the 18-year follow-up. In men with right bundle branch block and in women with either kind of block, the presence of a block did not contribute to the increased risk of death from cardiovascular disease independently from associated cardiovascular abnormalities, whereas the appearance of a new left bundle branch block in men contributed important independent predictive information.

The University of Manitoba follow-up study report on a 29-year follow-up of 3,983 young pilots included observations on 28 men who developed complete left bundle branch block [94]. Excluded were blocks associated with ischemic or valvular heart disease at the time of the occurrence of the conduction defect. The 5-year incidence of sudden death as the first manifestation of heart disease was at least ten times higher among men with acquired left bundle branch block than among the remainder of the men without left bundle branch block (and apparently also free from ischemic heart disease). However, this marked excess risk of sudden death was not manifest for men who were less than 45 years old at the occurrence of the left bundle branch block.

It is uncertain to what extent observations from these highly selected special occupational groups can be extrapolated to general populations. The low incidence of these incident abnormalities makes risk assessment for them difficult.

8.7   ADDENDUM

8.7.1   New Reports on Repolarization Abnormalities as Mortality Predictors from Large Population-Based Cohorts

Several new reports have been published since the preparation of the manuscript for this chapter five years ago. Some of these reports on large population-based cohorts have brought new information about the risk associated with repolarization abnormalities as mortality predictors. Summary tables describing most salient results from these studies can be found in a 2007 monograph Investigative Electrocardiography in Epidemiological Studies and Clinical Trials by Rautaharju and Rautaharju [80].

Of particular interest are the results from the Women's Health Initiative (WHI) involving nearly 40,000 women aged 50 years and older. One of the WHI reports evaluated the risk of CHD and all-cause mortality for ECG abnormalities and a second report the risk of incident CVD and congestive heart failure (CHF) [95, 96]. With all significant individual risk predictors entered simultaneously into a multivariably-adjusted CHD mortality risk model, QRS-T angle was associated with an over two-fold increase in risk, and the rate-adjusted QT interval also remained a significant predictor [95]. QRS nondipolar voltage, possibly reflecting fragmented excitation, was a dominant predictor in these women, together with an old ECG-MI. Wide QRS-T angle, ST V5 depression, high T V1 amplitude and prolonged QT were dominant predictors of incident CHF [96]. The investigators concluded that ventricular repolarization abnormalities are as important as an old ECG-MI as predictors of incident CHD, CHF and mortality.

CHF is one of the leading causes of mortality and morbidity in the USA, and the prevalence of diastolic dysfunction has been reported to be higher in women than in men [97, 98]. In the Cardiovascular Health Study (CHS), the prevalence of CHF was 8.8% and was associated with increased age, particularly for women [99]. In women with CHF, systolic ventricular function was normal significantly more often than in men (67% vs. 42%). Diagnosis of diastolic dysfunction is presently done by clinical exclusion of other cardiac conditions. Potential importance of repolarization abnormalities as markers of CHS and for monitoring its evolution is obvious..

A report from CHS compared the relative risk of CHD and all-cause mortality during a 9-year follow-up in 4,912 men and in women aged 65 years old and older [100]. In men and in women, the relative risk of CHD mortality was increased 60% for wide QRS-T angle and there was a two-fold increase in risk of CHD mortality for ST depression. These risk levels were as high as for an old ECG-MI. Relative risk for left ventricular mass (LVM) from an ECG model with Cornell voltage and body weight as model covariates was significant in women only, as was QRS nondipolar voltage. These investigators concluded that the association of ECG abnormalities with mortality risk in women was consistently as strong as in men.

Acknowledgement

Dr. Farida Rautaharju has contributed to the contents and the preparation of this chapter.

References

1. Ashley, E.A., V.K. Raxwal, and V.F. Froelicher, The prevalence and prognostic significance of electrocardiographic abnormalities. *Curr. Probl. Cardiol.*, 2000;**25**: 1–72.

2. Keys, A., H.L. Taylor, H. Blackurn, J. Brozek, J.T. Anderson, and E. Simonson, Coronary heart disease among the Minnesota business and professional men followed fifteen years. *Circulation*, 1965;**28**: 381–395.

3. Keys, A., C. Aravanis, H.W. Blackburn, et al., Epidemiological studies related to coronary heart disease: characteristics of men aged 40–59 in seven countries. *Acta Med. Scand.*, 1967;**460**(Suppl): 1–392.

4. Keys, A., Editor. *Coronary Heart Disease in Seven Countries.* Heart Association Monograph Number 29. New York: American Heart Association, Inc., 1970.

5. Dawber, T.R., F.E. Moore, and G.V. Mann, Coronary heart disease in the Framingham study. *Am. J. Public Health*, 1957;**47**(Suppl. 1): 4–24.

6. Doyle, J.T., A.S. Heslin, H.E. Hilleboe, P.F. Formel, and R.F.A. Korns, prospective study of degenerative cardiovascular disease in Albany. Report of three years' experience –I. Ischemic heart disease. *Am. J. Public Health*, 1957;**47**(Suppl. I): 25–32.

7. Chapman, J.M., L.S. Goerke, W. Dixon, D.B. Loveland, and E. Phillips, The clinical status of a population group in Los Angeles under observation for two to three years. *Am. J. Public Health*, 1957;**47**(Suppl. 1): 33–42.

8. Stamler, J., H.A. Lindberg, D.M. Berkson, A. Shaffer, W. Miller, and A. Poindexter, Prevalence and incidence of coronary heart disease in strata of the labor force of a Chicago industrial corporation. *J. Chronic Dis.*, 1960;**11**: 405–420.

9. Paul, O., M.H. Lepper, W.H. Phelan, et al., A longitudinal study of coronary heart disease. *Circulation*, 1963;**28**: 20–31.

10. New York Heart Association, Subcommittee on Electrocardiographic Criteria. *Nomenclature and Criteria for Diagnosis of Diseases of the Heart and Blood Vessels*, 5th edn. New York: New York Heart Association, 1953.

11. Rautaharju, P.M., M.J. Karvonen, and A. Keys, The frequency of arteriosclerotic and hypertensive heart disease among ostensibly health working populations in Finland. *J. Chronic Dis.*, 1961;**13**: 426–438.

12. Blackburn, H., A. Keys, E. Simonson, P. Rautaharju, and S. Punsar, The electrocardiogram in population studies. A classification system. *Circulation*, 1960;**21**: 1160–1175.

13. Ostrander, L.D. Jr, R.L. Brandt, M.O. Kjelsberg, and F.H. Epstein, Electrocardiographic findings among the adult population of a total natural community, Tecumseh, Michigan. *Circulation*, 1965;**31**: 888–898.

14. Sinnett, P.F. and H.M. Whyte, Epidemiological studies in a total highland population. Tukisenta, New Guinea, Cardiovascular disease and relevant clinical, electrocardiographic, radiological and biochemical findings. *J. Chronic Dis.*, 1973;**26**: 265–290.

15. The Pooling Project research Group, Relationship of blood pressure, serum cholesterol, smoking habit, relative weight and ECG abnormalities to incidence of major coronary events: Final report of the Pooling Project. *J. Chronic Dis.*, 1978;**31**: 201–306.

16. Rautaharju, P.M., H.P. Calhoun, and B.R. Chaitman, Novacode serial ECG classification system for clinical trials and epidemiological studies. *J. Electrocardiol.*, 1992;**24**: 179–187.

17. Burch, G.E. and T. Winsor, *A Primer of Electrocardiography*, 5th edn. Philadelphia, PA: Lea and Febiger, 1966.

18. Robles de Medina, E.O., *A New Coding System for Electrocardiography*. Assen: Royal van Gorcum, 1966.

19. Schamroth, L. and H.D. Friedberg, A coding system for cardiac arrhythmias. *J. Electrocardiol.*, 1970;**3**: 169–172.

20. Rautaharju, P.M., J.W. Warren, U. Jain, H.K. Wolf, and C.L. Nielsen, Cardiac infarction injury score: an electrocardiographic coding scheme for ischemic heart disease. *Circulation*, 1981;**64**: 249–256.

21. Pipberger, H.V., E. Simonson, E.A. Lopez Jr, A. Araoye, and H.A. Pipberger, The electrocardiogram in epidemiologic investigations. A new classification system. *Circulation*, 1982;**65**: 1456–1464.

22. Rose, G.A. and H. Blackburn, *Cardiovascular Survey Methods*. Geneva: World Health Organization, 1968. Monograph Series, no. 56

23. Prineas, R.J., R.S. Crow, and H. Blackburn, *The Minnesota Code Manual of Electrocardiographic Findings. Standards and Procedures for Measurement and Classification*. Boston, MA/Bristol/London: John Wright PSG Inc, 1982.

24. Rautaharju, P.M., D. Seale, R. Prineas, H. Wolf, R. Crow, and J. Warren, Changing electrocardiographic recording technology and diagnostic accuracy of myocardial infarction criteria. Improved standards for evaluation of ECG measurement precision. *J. Electrocardiol.*, 1978;**11**: 321–230.

25. Crow, R., R.J. Prineas, D.R. Jacobs, and H. Blackburn, A new epidemiological classification system for interim myocardial infarction from serial electrocardiographic changes. *Am. J. Cardiol.*, 1989;**64**: 454–461.

26. The Coronary Drug Project Research group, The coronary drug project: design, methods, and baseline results. *Circulation*, 1973;**47**(Suppl. 1): 11–50.

27. Rautaharju, P.M., S.K. Broste, R.J. Prineas, W.J. Eifler, R.S. Crow, and C.D. Furberg, Quality control procedures for the resting electrocardiogram in the multiple risk factor intervention trial. *Controlled Clin. Trials*, 1986;**7**(Suppl. 3): 46S–65S.

28. Reunanen, A., A. Aromaa, K. Pyörälä, S. Punsar, J. Maatela, and P. Knekt, The Social Insurance Institution's Coronary Heart Disease Study. Baseline data and 5 year mortality experience. *Acta Med. Scand.*, 1983;**673**(Suppl): 1–120.

29. Evans, J.G., I.A.M. Prior, and W.M.G. Turnbridge, Age-associated change in QRS axis: intrinsic or extrinsic aging? *Gerontology*, 1982;**28**: 132–137.

30. Higgins, I.T.T., W.B. Kannel, and T.R. Dawber, The electrocardiogram in epidemiological studies: reproducibility, validity and international comparison. *Br. J. Prev. Soc. Med.*, 1965;**19**: 53–68.

31. Cullen, K.J., B.P. Murphy, and G.N. Cumpston, Electrocardiograms in the Busselton population. *Aust. N.Z. J. Med.*, 1974;**4**: 325–330.

32. Ostor, E., P. Schnohr, G. Jensen, J. Nybe, and A.T. Hansen, Electrocardiographic findings and their association with mortality in the Copenhagen city heart study. *Eur. Heart J.*, 1981;**2**: 317–328.

33. Miall, W.E., E. Campo, J. Fodor, et al., Longitudinal study of heart disease in a Jamaican rural population. 1. Prevalence, with special reference to ECG findings. *Bull. W.H.O.*, 1972;**46**: 429–441.

34. Rose, G., P.J. Baxter, D.D. Reid, and P. McCartney, Prevalence and prognosis of electrocardiographic findings in middle aged men. *Br. Heart J.*, 1989;**1**: 73–80.

35. Rose, G.A., M. Ahmeteli, L. Checcacci, et al., Ischemic heart disease in middle-aged men: Prevalence comparisons in Europe. *Bull. W.H.O.*, 1968;**38**: 885–895.

36. World Health Organization European Collaborative Group, Multifunctional trial in the prevention of coronary heart disease: 1. Recruitment and initial findings. *Eur. Heart J.*, 1980;**1**: 73–80.

37. Barrett, P.A., C.T. Peter, H.J.C. Swan, B.N. Singh, and W.J. Mandel, The frequency and prognostic significance of electrocardiographic abnormalities in clinically normal individuals. *Prog. Cardivasc. Dis.*, 1981;**23**: 299–319.

38. Mathewson, F.A.L. and G.S. Varnam, Abnormal electrocardiograms in apparently healthy people. I. Long term follow-up study. *Circulation*, 1960;**21**: 196–203.

39. Medalie, J.H., M. Snyder, J.J. Croen, H.N. Neufeld, U. Goldbourt, and E. Riss, Angina pectoris among 10,000 men: 5 year incidence and univariate analysis. *Am. J. Med.*, 1973;**55**: 583–594.

40. Medalie, J.H., H.A. Khan, H.N. Neufeld, et al., Myocardial infarction over a five-year period. I. Prevalence, incidence and mortality experience. *J. Chronic Dis.*, 1973;**26**: 63–84.

41. Froelicher, V.F. Jr, F.G. Yanowitz, A.J. Thomson, and M.C. Lancaster, The correlation of coronary arteriography and the electrocardiographic response to maximal treadmill testing in 76 asymptomatic men. *Circulation*, 1973;**48**: 597–604.

42. Blackburn, H., H.I. Taylor, and A. Keys, The electrocardiogram in prediction of five-year coronary heart disease incidence among men aged forty through fifty-nine. *Circulation*, 1979;41(Suppl. 1): 154–161.

43. Blackburn, H., The importance of electrocardiograms in populations outside the hospital. *Can. Med. Assoc. J.*, 1973;**108**: 1262–1265.

44. Keys, A., *Seven Countries. A Multivariate Analysis of Death and Coronary Heart Disease*. Cambridge, MA: Harvard University Press, 1960.

45. Kannel, W.B., T. Gordon, W.P. Castelli, and J.R. Margolis, Electrocardiographic left ventricular hypertrophy and risk of coronary heart disease. The Framingham study. *Ann. Int. Med.*, 1970;**72**: 813–822.

46. Cedres, B.L., K. Liu, J. Stamler, et al., Independent contribution of electrocardiographic abnormalities to risk of death from coronary heart disease, cardiovascular diseases and all causes. Findings of three Chicago epidemiological studies. *Circulation*, 1982;**65**: 146–153.

47. Walker, A.R.P. and B.F. Walker, The bearing of race, sex, age, and nutritional state on the precordial electrocardiograms of young South African Bantu and Caucasian subjects. *Am. Heart J.*, 1969;**77**: 441–459.

48. Gottschalk, C.W. and E. Craige, A comparison of the precordial S-T and T waves in the electrocardiograms of 600 healthy young negro and white adults. *South. Med. J.*, 1956;**49**: 453–457.

49. Beaglehole, R., H.A. Tyroler, J.C. Cassel, D.C. Deubner, A.G. Bartel, and C.G. Hames, An epidemiological study of left ventricular hypertrophy in the biracial population of Evans County, Georgia. *J. Chron. Dis.*, 1975;**28**: 549–559.

50. WHI MONICA Project, Myocardial infarction and coronary deaths in the World Health Organization MONICA Project. Registration procedures, event rates, and case-fatality rates in 38 populations from 21 countries in four continents. *Circulation*, 1994;**90**: 583–612.

51. Menotti, A. and H. Blackburn, Electrocardiographic predictors of coronary heart disease in the seven countries study, in *Prevention of Coronary Heart Disease. Diet, Lifestyle and Risk Factors in the Seven Countries Study*, D. Kromhout, A. Menotti, and H. Blackburn, Editors. Norwell, MA: Kluwer, 2002, pp. 199–211.

52. Menotti, A., H. Blackburn, D.R. Jacobs, et al., *The predictive value of resting electrocardiographic findings in cardiovascular disease-free men. Twenty-five-year follow-up in the Seven Countries Study*. Internal document, Division of Epidemiology, School of Public Health, University of Minnesota, 2001.

53. Menotti, A., F. Seccaraccia, and the RIFLE Research Group, Electrocardiographic Minnesota Code findings predicting short-term mortality in asymptomatic subjects. The Italian RIFLE Pooling Project (Risk Factors and Life Expectancy). *G. Ital. Cardiol.*, 1997;**27**: 40–49.

54. Cullen, K., N.S. Stenhouse, K.L. Wearne, and G.N. Cumpston, Electrocardiograms and 13 year cardiovascular mortality in Busselton study. *Br. Heart J.*, 1982;**47**: 209–212.

55. Sigurdson, E., M. Sigfusson, H. Sigvaldason, and G. Thorgeirsson, Silent ST-T changes in an epidemiologic cohort study – A marker of hypertension or coronary artery disease, or both: The Reykjavik study. *J. Am. Coll. Cardiol.*, 1996;**27**: 1140–1147.

56. Kannel, B.W. and R. Abbott, Incidence and prognosis of unrecognized myocardial infarction. An update on the Framingham study. *N. Engl. J. Med.*, 1984;**311**: 1144–1147.

57. Kannel, W.B. and R.A. Abbott, Prognostic comparison of asymptomatic left ventricular hypertrophy and unrecognized myocardial infarction: The Framingham Study. *Am. Heart J.*, 1986;**111**: 391–397.

58. Yano, K. and C.J. MacLean, The incidence and prognosis of unrecognized myocardial infarction in the Honolulu, Hawaii, Heart Program. *Arch. Intern. Med.*, 1989;**149**: 1526–1532.

59. Tervahauta, M., J. Pekkanen, S. Punsar, and A. Nissinen, Resting electrocardiographic abnormalities as predictors of coronary events and total mortality among elderly men. *Am. J. Med.*, 1996;**100**: 641–645.

60. Nadelmann, J., W.H. Frishman, W.L. Ooi, et al., Prevalence, incidence and prognosis of recognized and unrecognized myocardial infarction in persons aged 75 years or older: The Bronx Aging Study. *Am. J. Cardiol.*, 1990;**6**: 533–537.

61. Medalie, J.H. and U. Goldbourt, Unrecognized myocardial infarction: five-year incidence, mortality, and risk factors. *Ann. Intern. Med.*, 1976;**84**: 526–531.

62. The Coronary Drug Project Research Group, The prognostic importance of the electrocardiogram after myocardial infarction. Experience from the Coronary Drug Project. *Ann. Intern. Med.*, 1972;**77**: 677–679.

63. The MRFIT Research Group, Relationship between baseline risk factors and coronary heart disease and total mortality in the Multiple Risk Factor Intervention Trial. *Prev. Med.*, 1986;**15**: 254–273.

64. The Multiple Risk Factor Intervention Trial Research Group, Baseline rest electrocardiographic abnormalities, antihypertensive treatment and mortality in the Multiple Risk Factor Intervention Trial. *Am. J. Cardiol.*, 1985;**55**: 1–15.

65. Holme, I., A. Helgeland, I. Hjermann, P. Leren, and P.G. Lund-Larsen, Treatment of mild hypertensives with diuretics: the importance of ECG abnormalities in the Oslo Study and in MRFIT. *J. Am. Med. Assoc.*, 1984;**251**: 1298–1299.

66. The Hypertension Detection and Follow-up Program Cooperative Research Group, The effect of antihypertensive drug treatment on mortality in the presence of resting electrocardiographic abnormalities at baseline: the HDFP experience. *Circulation*, 1984;**70**: 996–1003.

67. The Multiple Risk Factor Intervention Trial Research Group, Exercise electrocardiogram and coronary heart disease mortality in the Multiple Risk Factor Intervention Trial. *Am. J. Cardiol.*, 1985;**55**: 16–24.

68. Rautaharju, P.M., R.J. Prineas, W.J. Eifler, C.D. Furberg, J.D. Neaton, R.S. Crow, J. Stamler, and J.A. Cutler for the Multiple Risk Factor Intervention Trial Research Group, Prognostic value of exercise ECG in men at high risk of future coronary heart disease. *J. Am. Coll. Cardiol.*, 1986;**8**(1): 1–10.

69. Rautaharju, P.M. and J.D. Neaton for, the MRFIT Research Group, Electrocardiographic abnormalities and coronary heart disease mortality among hypertensive men in the Multiple Risk Factor Intervention Trial. *Clin. Invest. Med.*, 1987;**10**: 606–615.

70. De Bacquer, D., G. De Backer, M. Kornitzer, and H. Blackburn, Prognostic value of ECG findings for total, cardiovascular disease, and coronary heart disease death in men and women. *Heart*, 1998;**80**: 570–577.

71. Dauerman, H.L., D. Lessard, J. Yarzebski, M.I. Furman, J.M. Gore, and R.J. Goldberg, Ten-year trends in the incidence, treatment, and outcome of Q-wave myocardial infarction. *Am. J. Cardiol.*, 2000;**86**: 730–735.

72. Rosenman, R.H., M. Friedman, C.D. Jenkins, R. Straus, M. Wurm, and R. Kosichek, Clinically unrecognized myocardial infarction in the Western Collaborative Group Study. *Am. J. Cardiol.*, 1967;**19**: 776–782.

73. Rautaharju, P.M., S.H. Zhou, and H.P. Calhoun, Ethnic differences in electrocardiographic amplitudes in North American white, black and hispanic men and women: effect of obesity and age. *J. Electrocardiol.*, 1994;**27**(Suppl): 20–30.

74. Strogatz, D.S., H.A. Tyroler, L.O. Watkins, and C.G. Hames, Electrocardiographic abnormalities and mortality among middle-aged black men and white men of Evans County, Georgia. *J. Chron. Dis.*, 1987;**40**: 149–155.

75. Arnett, D.K., D.S. Strogatz, S.A. Ephross, C.G. Hames, and H.A. Tyroler, Greater incidence of electrocardiographic left ventricular hypertrophy in black men than in white men in Evans County, Georgia. *Ethn. Dis.*, 1992;**2**: 10–17.

76. Arnett, D.K., P. Rautaharju, S. Sutherland, B. Usher, and J. Keil, Validity of electrocardiographic estimates of left ventricular hypertrophy and mass in African Americans (The Charlston Heart Study). *Am. J. Cardiol.*, 1997;**79**: 1289–1292.

77. Xie, X., K. Liu, J. Stamler, and R. Stamler, Ethnic differences in electrocardiographic left ventricular hypertrophy in young and middle-aged employed American men. *Am. J. Cardiol.*, 1994;**73**: 564–567.

78. Huston, S.L., C.H. Bunker, F.A.M. Ukoli, P.M. Rautaharju, and H.K. Lewis, Electrocardiographic left ventricular hypertrophy by five criteria among civil servants in Benin City, Nigeria: prevalence and correlates. *Int. J. Cardiol.*, 1999; **70**: 1–14.

79. Mosterd, A., R.B. D'Agostino, H. Silbershatz, P.A. Sytkowski, W.B. Kannel, D.E. Grobbee, and D. Levy, Trends in the prevalence of hypertension, antihypertensive therapy, and left ventricular hypertrophy from 1950 to 1989. *N. Engl. J. Med.*, 1999;**340**: 1221–1227.

80. Rautaharju P, Rautaharju F. *Investigative Electrocardiography in Epidemiological Studies and Clinical Trials.* Springer-Verlag London Limited, London, 2007, pp 1:289.

81. Liebson, P.R., G. Grandits, R. Prineas, S. Dianzumba, J.M. Flack, J.A. Cutler, R. Grimm, and J. Stamler, Echocardiographic correlates of left ventricular structure among 844 mildly hypertensive men and women in the Treatment of Mild Hypertension Study (TOMHS). *Circulation*, 1993;**87**: 476–486.

82. Okin, P.M., J. Sverker, R.B. Devereux, S.E. Kjeldsen, and B. Dahlof, Effect of obesity on electrocardiographic left ventricular hypertrophy in hypertensive patients: the Losartan Intervention for Endpoint (LIFE) Reduction in Hypertension Study. *Hypertension*, 2000;**35**: 13–18.

83. Lee, D.K., P.R. Marantz, R.B. Devereux, P. Kligfield, and M.H. Alderman, Left ventricular hypertrophy in black and white hypertensives. Standard electrocardiographic criteria overestimate racial differences in prevalence. *J.A.M.A.*, 1992;**267**: 3294–3299.

84. Rautaharju, P.M., L.P. Park, J.S. Gottdiener, D. Siscovick, R. Boineau, V. Smith, and N.R. Powe, Race-and sex-specific ECG models for left ventricular mass in older populations. Factors influencing overestimation of left ventricular hypertrophy prevalence by ECG criteria in African-Americans. *J. Electrocardiol.*, 2000;**33**: 205–218.

85. Rautaharju, P.M., T.A. Manolio, D. Siscovick, S.H. Zhou, J.M. Gardin, R. Kronmal, C.D. Furberg, N.O. Borhani, and A. Newman, for the Cardiovascular Health Study Collaborative Research Group. Utility of new electrocardiographic models for left ventricular mass in older adults. *Hypertension*, 1996;**28**: 8–15.

86. Levy, D., K.M. Anderson, D.D. Savage, W.B. Kannel, J.C. Christiansen, and W.P. Castelli, Echocardiographically detected left ventricular hypertrophy: prevalence and risk factors. The Framingham study. *Ann. Intern. Med.*, 1988;**108**: 7–13.

87. Verdecchia, P., G. Schillaci, C. Borgioni, A. Ciucci, R. Gattobigio, I. Zampi, G. Reboldi, and C. Porcellati, Prognostic significance of serial changes in left ventricular mass in essential hypertension. *Circulation*, 1998;**97**: 48–54.

88. Schillaci, G., P. Verdecchia, Borgioni, A. Ciucci, M. Guerrieri, I. Zampi, M. Battistelli, C. Bartoccini, and C. Porcellati, Improved electrocardiographic diagnosis of left ventricular hypertrophy. *Am. J. Cardiol.*, 1994;**74**: 714–719.

89. Rautaharju, P.M., J. Warren, R.J. Prineas, and P.h. Smets, Optimal coding of electrocardiograms for epidemiological studies. The performance of human coders – a statistical model. *J. Electrocardiol.*, 1979;**13**: 55–59.

90. Kahn, S., W.H. Frishman, S. Weissman, W.L. Ooi, and M. Aronson, Left ventricular hypertrophy on electrocardiogram: prognostic implications from a 10-year cohort study of older subjects: a report from the Bronx longitudinal aging study. *J. Am. Geriatr. Soc.*, 1996;**44**: 524–529.

91. Larsen, C.T., J. Dahlin, H. Blackburn, H. Scharling, M. Appleyard, B. Sigurd, and P. Schnohr, Prevalence and prognosis of electrocardiographic left ventricular hypertrophy, ST segment depression and negative T-wave. *Eur. Heart J.*, 2002;**23**: 315–324.

92. Rautaharju, P.M., A.Z. LaCroix, D.D. Savage, S. Haynes, J.H. Madans, H.K. Wolf, W. Hadden, J. Keller, and J. Cornoni-Huntly, Electrocardiographic estimate of left ventricular mass vs. Radiographic cardiac size and the risk of cardiovascular disease mortality in the epidemiologic follow-up study of the First National Health and Nutrition Examination Survey. *Am. J. Cardiol.*, 1988;**62**: 59–66.

93. Levy, D., M. Salomon, R.B. D'Agostino, A.J. Belanger, and W.B. Kannel, Prognostic implications of baseline electrocardiographic features and their serial changes in subjects with left ventricular hypertrophy. *Circulation*, 1994;**90**: 1786–1793.

94. Mathewson, F.A.L., J. Manfreda, R.B. Tate, and T. Cuddy, The University of Manitoba Follow-up Study-an investigation of cardiovascular disease with 35 years of follow-up (1948–1983). *Can. J. Cardiol.*, 1987;**3**: 378–382.

95. Rautaharju, P.M., C. Kooperberg, J.C. Larson, and A. LaCroix, Electrocardiographic abnormalities that predict coronary heart disease events and Mortality in Postmenopausal Women. The Women's Health Initiative. *Circulation*, 2006;**113**: 473–480.

96. Rautaharju, P.M., C. Kooperberg, J.C. Larson, and A. LaCroix, Electrocardiographic Predictors of Incident Congestive Heart Failure and All-cause Mortality in Postmenopausal Women. The Women's Health Initiative. *Circulation*, 2006;**113**: 481–489.

97. Zile, M.R. and D.L. Brutsaert, New concepts in diastolic dysfunction and diastolic heart failure: Part I: diagnosis, prognosis, and measurements of diastolic function. *Circulation*, 2002;**105**: 1387–1393.

98. Zile, M.R. and D.L. Brutsaert, New concepts in diastolic dysfunction and diastolic heart failure: Part II: causal mechanisms and treatment. *Circulation*, 2002;**105**: 1503–1508.

99. Kitzman, D.W., J.M. Gardin, J.S. Gottdiener, A. Arnold, R. Boineau, G. Aurigemma, E.K. Marino, M. Lyles, M. Cushman, and P.L. Enright, Importance of heart failure with preserved systolic function in patients ≥65 years of age. CHS Research Group. Cardiovascular Health Study. *Am. J. Cardiol.*, 2001;**87**: 413–419.

100. Rautaharju, P.M., S.G. Ge, J. Clark Nelson, E.K. Marino Larsen, B.M. Psaty, C.D. Furberg, Z.M. Zhang, J.A. Robbins, MD, MHS, J.S. Gottdiener, MD, and P. Chaves, Comparison of Mortality risk for Electrocardiographic Abnormalities in Men and Women With and Without Coronary Heart Disease (From the Cardiovascular Health Study). *Am. J. Cardiol.*, 2006;**97**: 309–315.

9 The Dog Electrocardiogram: A Critical Review

David K. Detweiler[†]

[†]For this 2nd Edition of "Comprehensive Electrocardiology," Dr. Sydney Moise has updated this 1st Edition chapter, which was originally written by the late Dr. Detweiler.

P. W. Macfarlane et al. (eds.), *Specialized Aspects of ECG*, DOI 10.1007/978-0-85729-880-5_9,
© Springer-Verlag London Limited 2012

9.1 History and Literature

Electrocardiographic studies in dogs date back to the pioneering investigations of Augustus Waller [1] with the capillary electrometer and Willem Einthoven's development of the string galvanometer electrocardiograph [2–4]. As late as 1914 [5], Waller considered electrocardiography (ECG) as an experimental method, useful to physiologists rather than as a clinical tool for physicians. However, clinical application in man had already started and advanced rapidly (Lewis, 1909–1925 [6]; Rothberger, 1912–1930 [7]; Winterberg, 1912–1930 [9]; Scherf, 1921–present [8]; Wenckebach, 1899–1930 [9]; and Wilson, 1919–1945 [10]). Clinical use in canine medicine was modest in those early days (Nörr, 1913–1931 [11]; Roos, 1925 [12]; Haupt, 1929 [13]; Ludwig, 1924 [14]; and Gyarmati, 1939 [15]) and subsequently, until Nils Lannek's systematic study and statistical analysis of clinical records from healthy and diseased dogs [16]. Lannek also introduced a precordial-lead system that is still in use. Scherf and Schott's encyclopedic monograph, *Extrasystoles and Allied Arrhythmias* [8], reviews much of the electrocardiographic literature on experimental cardiac arrhythmias and drug effects in dogs. Burch and DePasquale's *A History of Electrocardiography* [17], Sir Thomas Lewis's classical *The Mechanism and Graphic Registration of the Heart Beat* [6], and Wilson's collected works (edited by Johnston and Lepeschkin [10]) are rich sources of information on earlier canine studies.

Modern imaging of the heart with echocardiography, angiography, magnetic resonance imaging (MRI), endocardial mapping, computer-assisted tomography (CT) and other modalities potentially provides more valuable information of the structure, function, and electrical competency than the routine surface electrocardiogram. However, the ECG is the mainstay for the diagnosis of arrhythmias in all animals. In the complete diagnosis of disease, the ECG must be supplemented with other technologies. The ECG remains a cornerstone for the initial screening and recognition of disease. Moreover, in pharmacological studies, the dog remains a key animal of study for which the review of ECG changes for the treatment effect or toxicity involves routine examinations.

Besides the routine analysis of the ECG in the dog, more thorough approaches to the clues of the disease, drug effect, or toxicity that the ECG offers are in use today. These include 24-h ambulatory ECG monitoring (Holter monitoring), telemetry recordings via implantable recording devices, loop-recording devices to capture arrhythmias, and heart rate variability.

9.1.1 Canine Electrocardiography

An enormous amount of literature has been published on experimental electrocardiographic studies in dogs. Historical and useful reviews are found in textbooks and monographs on arrhythmias and conduction disorders such as Bellet [18, 19], Scherf and Schott [8], and Schamroth [20]. Normal values for dog ECGs have been summarized in several textbooks (Ettinger and Suter [21], Detweiler et al. [22], Bolton [23], and Tilley [24]). In early papers and textbooks, generalized statements were frequently made with regard to the interpretation of ECG measurements to heart size based on the amplitude and duration of a specific waveform. Today, we recognize that some of these conclusions were too specific because of breed, age, and body conformation. Some examples will be addressed in the following discussions on the ECG waveforms.

9.1.2 Beagle Electrocardiogram

The ECG of the beagle is of special interest because of its widespread use as a research animal [25]. The published normal values for the ECG waveforms with regard to time and amplitude serve as a guideline to the evaluation of the ECG for the beagle. ❯ Table 9.1 lists findings that are commonly found when evaluating the electrocardiogram of the research beagle.

◘ **Table 9.1**

Electrocardiographic findings of the research beagle that are not within the usual normal range for dogs and that are not likely pathologic[a]

Number	Electrocardiographic finding	Comments	Level of concern for use of dog in cardiovascular studies
1	Deep (not wide) S waves in lead III (1.0 mV > S wave > 0.7 mV)	Common singular finding without known association to structural or electrical abnormality	Low
2	Deep (not wide) S waves in lead III (S wave ⩾ 1 mV) only	Less common than #1. May be an insignificant finding	Low-medium
3	Deep (not wide) S waves in leads II, III, and aVF (0.5 mV > S wave > 0.3 mV in lead II, 1 mV > S wave > 0.5 mV in lead III, and 1 mV ⩾ S wave > 0.5 mV in lead III)	Common cluster finding without known association to structural or electrical abnormality or may be associated with right ventricular enlargement, incomplete right bundle branch block, or left anterior fascicular block	Medium
4	Very deep (not wide) S waves in II, III, and aVF (S wave > 0.5 mV in lead II, S wave > 1 mV in lead III, and S wave > 1 mV in lead III)	Much less common cluster finding without known association to structural or electrical abnormality but more likely than #3 to be associated with right ventricular enlargement, incomplete right bundle branch block, or left anterior fascicular block	High
5	T_a wave (Tsub "a" wave)	Occasionally seen. A negative deflection immediately following the P wave. Indicates the T wave of the P wave (repolarization of the atria)	None unless associated with large P wave
6	Tall (not wide) R wave (3.5 mV > R wave > 3.0 mV)	Common. Mild elevation in the amplitude of the R wave is usually not associated with structural or functional abnormality, but could indicate left ventricular hypertrophy	Low
7	Very tall (not wide) R waves (R wave > 3.5 mV)	Less common than #6. Moderate elevation in the amplitude may still not be associated with structural or functional abnormality, but more likely to be associated with left ventricular hypertrophy than #6	Medium
8	Splintered or notched QRS complex	Occasionally seen. The appearance of this finding can be affected by the filter settings of the ECG recording device. Splintered R waves are associated with tricuspid dysplasia in the dog, but this congenital anomaly has not been reported in the beagle	Low, but if marked could affect ease of interpretation
9	Low amplitude QRS complex (QRS complex < 0.7 mV)	Occasionally seen. Although low R waves are reported for a variety of conditions (e.g., pericardial effusion, ascites, pleural effusion, obesity, hypothyroidism, pulmonary embolism) in the beagle this is seen with a normal heart	Low
10	Deep Q waves (Q wave > 1.2 mV)	Common. May be a singular finding or with a tall or very tall R wave. Can be a normal variation or indicative of septal hypertrophy or right ventricular hypertrophy	Low as a singular finding
11	Large T wave (>25% of the R wave)	Occasionally seen as a singular finding. May be present with tall and very tall R wave. In the latter situations the T wave is large as a negative deflection	Low as a singular finding

■ Table 9.1 (Continued)

Number	Electrocardiographic finding	Comments	Level of concern for use of dog in cardiovascular studies
12	Second-degree heart block (low grade with only single P waves not associated with QRS complex)	Occasionally seen in dogs more than 4 months of age. Common in dogs less than 2 months of age. In these situations usually not associated with disease, but with high vagal tone	Low as a singular finding, but most investigators do not want dogs with this finding[b]
13	Sinus bradycardia or long sinus pauses (heart rate < 60 bpm, PP interval > 1.5 s)	Occasionally seen. Dogs bred for calm personality tend to have slower heart rates due to higher vagal tone and less sympathetic tone. Many of these dogs have heart rates that approach the lower limit of 60 bpm	Low to medium depending on the degree of the bradycardia and the length of the sinus pause. Extreme bradycardia or pauses would have a high concern
14	Presence of a J wave. The J wave is a positive deflection at the very terminal point of the downstroke of the R wave. It may be a complete secondary positive deflection with amplitudes of 0.2 mV or just a widening of the R wave usually beginning at the amplitude of 0.1–0.2 mV	Common finding and is due to the current density of I_{to}. Seen in other breeds too	None, but in some cases can make the determination of the QRS duration problematic because the end of the QRS is difficult to determine Some include this wave in the duration of the QRS

[a]This table is not a listing of electrocardiographic abnormalities per se, but is a listing of findings often found in the beagles that usually are not associated with pathology. However, as described, the findings may be associated with an abnormality although frequently they are not
[b]In 2,232 beagles on which two 1-min recordings were taken was about 1% [26], while that in 11 resting dogs monitored for about 6 h by radiotelemetry was about 64%. This figure increased to 100% in 12 puppies, 8–11 weeks old [47]

9.2 Recording Techniques

9.2.1 Lead Systems

A variety of lead systems has been used for decades in the dog. Most commonly used is the six-lead limb system which includes leads I, II, III, aVR, aVL, and aVF. However, the addition of other leads may be beneficial for some studies.

Historically, Waller [1] initiated the limb-lead system of recording from dogs when he taught his pet bulldog "Jimmie" to stand in beakers filled with a conducting solution into each of which an electrode was fixed (❷ Fig. 9.1). In Waller's earliest experiments, wires connected these electrodes to the capillary manometer (❷ Fig. 9.2). This method of recording was also used with other species including humans and anticipated the technique that Einthoven adopted for his string galvanometer.

Because of the offset potentials generated at the metal–skin surface interface, nonpolarizable electrode systems were required with the capillary electrometer and the early string galvanometers of the Einthoven type. This was accomplished by immersing the limb in a bath containing a salt of the metal used in the electrode; for example, silver chloride solution with silver electrodes or zinc chloride with zinc or nickel silver (German silver, a silver white alloy of copper, zinc, and nickel) electrodes. Soon, the bath was replaced by cloth strips that were saturated with the solution and wrapped about the limb to form contact between the electrode and the skin. Later, the material was replaced by conducting electrolyte pastes and gels placed between the skin and the electrodes. In animals, a variety of needle and clip electrodes was used to fix the leads firmly in place despite inadvertent movement of the subjects.

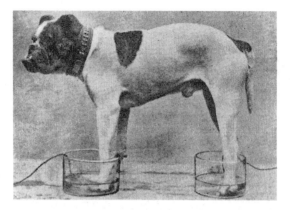

☐ **Fig. 9.1**

Waller's pet dog "Jimmie" patiently standing with his left foreleg and connected by wires to an electrometer (A. Waller. *Physiology, the Servant.* London Press/Hodder & Stoughton, London, 1888. Reproduced with permission)

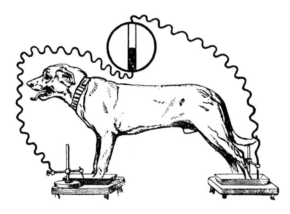

☐ **Fig. 9.2**

Probably the first picture of an ECG being recorded from a dog. The instrument is a capillary electrometer. The line drawing depicts a dog standing with the left foreleg and hindleg in pans of saline solution and wires leading from electrodes immersed in the solution to a schema of the electrometer (Waller [1]. © British Medical Association, London. Reproduced with permission)

The idea prevailed for some years [13, 26] that a bipolar lead along the imaginary anatomical longitudinal axis of the heart would be best for animals. A single lead with one electrode attached to the left precordium over the cardiac apex and the other electrode attached over the base of the heart at the junction of the neck and thorax, the scapular spine, or anterodorsal edge of the scapula on the right side, became popular. It was not realized that this was essentially a precordial lead with a neck or scapular electrode acting more or less as the indifferent electrode. A later modification of this was a three-lead triangular system similar to that of Nehb [27] with the three limb electrodes placed at the cardiac apex (left leg [LF] electrode), the base of the neck (anterodorsal edge of the scapula) on the right side (right arm [RA] electrode), and the sacral region (left arm [LA] electrode). The leads thus obtained are termed dorsal (RA to LA), axial (RA to LF), and inferior (LA to LF) [28]. This system never gained popularity in the dog, but has been used more often in large farm animals and the laboratory rat [29].

Lannek [16] developed a precordial-lead system that has been used in the dog. This system utilized anatomical criteria to position one electrode over the right ventricle and two electrodes over the left ventricle. In taking these precordial leads, he paired the exploring electrode with the right foreleg electrode and used the symbol CR for these chest leads. Wilson's central terminal soon replaced the right leg as the indifferent electrode and by early 1960, Hamlin [30] initiated the use of a lead corresponding to V_{10} in man to the chest leads for the dog. V_{10} is uncommonly used today.

The original lead symbols introduced by Lannek were CR_5RL, CR_6LL, and CR_6LU. With the introduction of Wilson's central terminal, these symbols were changed to CV_5RL, CV_6LL, and CV_6LU. In 1977, the Committee of the American Academy of Veterinary Cardiology introduced new lead symbols [31] similar to those used for man. Although these electrode positions in the dog roughly approximate, they do not correspond, accurately, to the identically named lead positions in man. Both nomenclatures are given here. The electrode positions for each lead are as follows:

(a) V_2 (CV_6LL): sixth left intercostal space near the edge of the sternum at the most curved part of the costal cartilage
(b) V_4 (CV_6LU): sixth left intercostal space at the costochondral junction
(c) V_{10}: over the dorsal spinous process of the seventh thoracic vertebra (on the dorsal midline vertically above the V_4 position)
(d) rV_2 (CV_5RL): fifth right intercostal space near the edge of the sternum at the most rounded part of the costal cartilage

The abbreviations in the parentheses are the terms originally used by Lannek [16] to designate these electrode positions. The terminology and corresponding equivalent in humans has been questioned [32]. The conformation of the thorax of the dog is dissimilar to humans. Thus, the positioning of the leads at the same points on the thorax does not correspond exactly to that of the humans. Also, the location and effect of the diaphragm on cardiac position is different between the two species. Importantly, the morphology of the thorax varies greatly amongst different somatotypic breeds of dogs, such that even within the canine species, variability must be expected when trying to make anatomical comparisons to the location and direction of the electrical depolarization. Moreover, consistent positioning of these leads and additional precordial leads (V_1, V_2, V_3, V_4, V_5, and V_6) is critical for an acceptable amount of variability between recordings.

Three-lead (X, Y, and Z)-corrected orthogonal systems such as those of McFee and Parungao [33] ($\bullet$ Fig. 9.3) and Frank [34, 35] ($\bullet$ Fig. 9.4) have been used historically for vectorcardiography. Vectorcardiography has been replaced by more sophisticated means of electrical mapping of the heart. Such systems are beyond the scope of this review. The X-, Y-, and Z-lead system has been used extensively in the Holter Laboratory of Cornell University, College of Veterinary Medicine. Such a system typically provides excellent recordings for analysis in the dog.

A more complex lead system is used in Japan [37]. Takahashi [38], on the basis of experimental studies in the dog, introduced an elaborate 12-lead precordial system with 6 leads on each side of the thorax as follows ($\bullet$ Fig. 9.5): C_1, C_2, and C_3 at the left costochondral junction anterior to rib one and at the second and fifth intercostal space, respectively; C_4, C_5, and C_6 at the right costochondral junctions in the seventh, fifth, and third intercostal spaces, respectively; M_1, M_2 at the widest portion of the thorax in the third and sixth left intercostal spaces, respectively; M3 at the left of the xiphoid process; M_4 at the right of the xiphoid process; and M_5, M_6 at the widest portion of the thorax in the right seventh and third intercostal spaces, respectively.

In 1966, the Japanese Association of Animal Electrocardiography recommended a bipolar base-apex (termed A-B) lead similar to that recommended in 1929 by Haupt [13], one of Nörr's [11] pupils, for use in dogs. The positive electrode (A) is placed at the costochondral junction of the left sixth rib and the negative electrode at the right scapular spine (Japanese Association of Animal Electrocardiography, 1975) [36]. In addition, they recommend the use of the Takahashi precordial leads $C_1 - C_6$, M_1, and M_6.

In summary, although multiple lead systems have been proposed, the most common one used for the evaluation of the electrical activity of the dog is the six-lead limb system. Importantly, in modern times, a critical evaluation demanded in pharmacological studies is the evaluation of the QT interval. Most of time and amplitude measurements are done in lead II; however, in approximately 10–20% of the canine recordings, the clarity of the T wave and particularly the offset point is not clear in lead II or other limb leads. In such situations, other leads may be better suited to more definitively make the QT interval measurement (see below).

9.2.2 Position and Restraint

In quadrupeds, the magnitude and direction of electrocardiographic vectors determined from limb leads can be vastly altered by changes in the position of the muscular attachments of the shoulder girdle to the thorax ($\bullet$ Fig. 9.6).

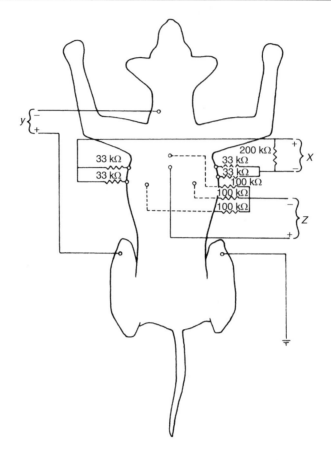

◘ Fig. 9.3
The corrected orthogonal-lead system designed for the canine thorax by McFee and Parungao [33]. Electrode placement for transverse (*X*), longitudinal (*Y*), and sagittal (*Z*) axis leads. Viewed from the dorsal aspect of the dog. Note that the Z+ electrode is on the back of the dog (After Chastain et al. [83]. ©American Veterinary Medical Association, Schaumburg, Illinois. Reproduced with permission)

Thus consistent positioning of the forelimbs, and especially the scapulae, is crucial to obtaining reproducible vectors in serial ECGs. This was not known until the early 1950s, while Lannek [16] reported that in dogs, the mean manifest QRS vector in the frontal plane could be highly variable. This finding was later confirmed independently by Cagan et al. [39, 40], Hulin and Rippa [41], and was studied systematically by Hill [42, 43]. The following technique is recommended: The dog is placed in right lateral recumbency. The head and neck are held flat on the table in line with the long axis of the trunk. The forelegs are positioned parallel to one another and perpendicular to the long axis of the body so that the point of the left shoulder (anterior aspect of the scapulohumeral joint) is vertically above the point of the right shoulder. The complexes in lead aVL are often those most sensitive to changes in foreleg position. Therefore, in serial records, complexes in lead aVL can be compared to verify the consistency in foreleg positioning.

To restrain the dogs on a table, the handler should face the right side of the standing animal with its head to his right side, reach over the animal's back, grasp the forelegs in his right hand and the hind legs in his left hand. The dog is then laid on its right side, the head and neck pressed flat against the table with the right forearm, and its back restrained against the handler's body. The technician operating the electrocardiograph then attaches the electrodes and arranges the forelimbs and head and neck as described. The handlers must avoid touching moist surfaces or electrodes in case AC interference is introduced.

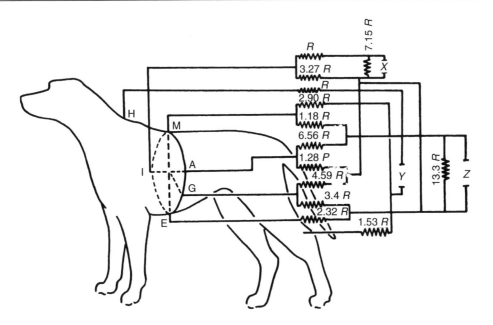

◻ Fig. 9.4
Frank's orthogonal-lead system applied to the dog. $R = 100,000Q$ (After Bojrab et al. [35]. © American Veterinary Medical Association, Schaumburg, Illinois. Reproduced with permission)

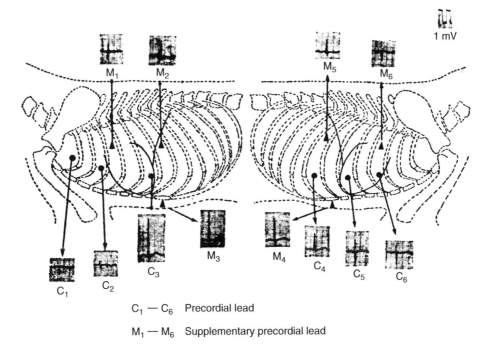

$C_1 - C_6$ Precordial lead

$M_1 - M_6$ Supplementary precordial lead

◻ Fig. 9.5
The precordial-lead system proposed by Takahashi for clinical use (After Takahashi [38]. Society of Veterinary Science, Tokyo. Reproduced with permission)

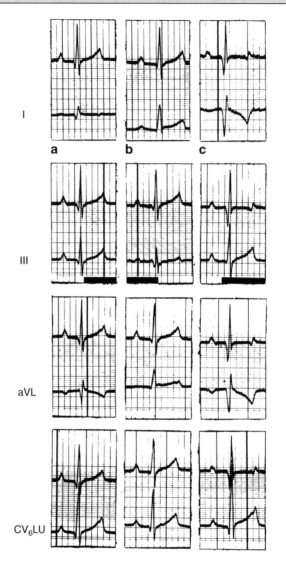

◘ Fig. 9.6
The effect of foreleg position on the ECG. The upper tracing in each recording is lead II. The dog was positioned in right lateral recumbency. In column (a) the forelegs are parallel and at right angles to the long axis of the body. In column (b) the right foreleg is pulled forward and the left foreleg pulled backward. In column (c) the right foreleg is pulled backward and the left forward. Note the dramatic alterations in the QRS complexes and T waves in leads I, III, and aVL that falsely suggest changes in ventricular excitation and recovery pathways. See also ◗ Table 9.5

9.2.3   Electrodes

From the standpoint of their electrical characteristics, plate electrodes are superior to electronic alligator clips, while needle electrodes are unacceptable for use in conscious dogs [44]. Electronic alligator clips are recommended, however, because their somewhat inferior electrical characteristics compared to those of plate electrodes are offset by their convenience in application and their tendency to remain in place when dogs struggle. They must all be of the same metal (copper is preferred) to avoid offset voltages that can cause baseline instability. The serrations on the jaws should be flattened to reduce discomfort and maximize the area of contact with the skin. The contact area (including both jaws of the clip) should be approximately $1.0\,cm^2$. The skin and hair under the electrodes are saturated with a conductive gel or solution. The site of foreleg attachment must be well below the ventral thoracic surface (e.g., halfway between the olecranon and carpus) to avoid the influence of precordial potentials.

9.2.4 Duration of Recording

It is generally possible to restrain untrained and unsedated dogs in the recommended recording position (right lateral recumbency) for about 1 min before struggling becomes excessive. Electronic ECG systems are available now that have enhanced the ability to keep recording until the dog is relaxed. Such systems also allow the electronic storage of the ECG. Because arrhythmias are sporadic events, if it is required to compare arrhythmia prevalence rates in groups such as in the chronic toxicity testing, the duration of recording should be the same in each individual dog and a standard recording time of 1 min has been proposed for such studies [26]. However, it must be emphasized that such a duration actually evaluates less than 0.1% of the QRS complexes that a dog has in 24 h. Most normal beagles have approximately 150,000–175,000 beats in 24 h, and realizing that a 1-min recording only documents approximately 75–100 of these beats gives a perspective for conclusions.

As is well known, for the comparison of the incidence of cardiac arrhythmias, 24-h monitoring of the ECG (Holter monitoring) is optimal [45–47]. In veterinary practice, Holter monitoring is commonly performed. Despite its common use clinically, an appreciation of the need for validation of the accuracy is lacking. When arrhythmias are infrequent, the accuracy of modern analyzing systems is acceptable. However, when complex, frequent, and rapid arrhythmias are present, the accuracy of the analysis suffers. Importantly, quality control and validation of the accuracy of the reports is required, yet few labs have such oversight for canine recordings. Consequently, if Holter monitoring is required for studies, confirmation of high standards in the evaluation of the recordings should be sought.

9.2.5 Artifacts

Since the occurrence of artifacts (see reference [26] for a description of common artifacts) is nearly universal in dog ECGs, they must be identified as such in screening for abnormalities. The most common artifacts that cause problems in diagnosis are:

(a) Skeletal muscle movements
(b) Baseline drift (including oscillations associated with normal breathing and with panting)
(c) Fifty- or 60-Hz electrical inference (❯ Fig. 9.7)

Somatic muscle artifacts appear in most ECGs taken from unanesthetized dogs. Three general types may be recognized:

(a) *Somatic muscle tremor*. The frequency of skeletal muscle tremor artifact is irregular, ranging from about 15 to 35 Hz. Often a constant baseline "jiggle" is caused in long stretches of the record. Typically, such trembling intensifies on inspiration and diminishes on expiration so that it may wax and wane, or appear and disappear periodically.
(b) *Intermediate frequency somatic muscle artifacts*. These are caused by more sporadic muscle twitching that are discontinuous and occur at a frequency of about 1–15 Hz in tense subjects. Their amplitude is generally from 0.1 to 0.5 mV. These artifacts are likely to distort electrocardiographic complexes and may mimic the morphology of P waves.
(c) *Gross muscle movement artifact*. High-amplitude deflections with rapid voltage change (high Vmax) may resemble bizarre QRS complexes and mimic ventricular ectopic beats, or when rapid, paroxysmal ventricular tachycardia. Their amplitudes are often from 1.0 to 5.0 mV or greater and may exceed the excursion limit of the electrocardiographic stylus. Rhythmic tail wagging sometimes transmits movement to electrode–skin–surface interfaces, mimicking a run of ventricular tachycardia (VT), while panting can cause baseline oscillations with the frequency and amplitude of those seen in atrial flutter or atrial fibrillation.

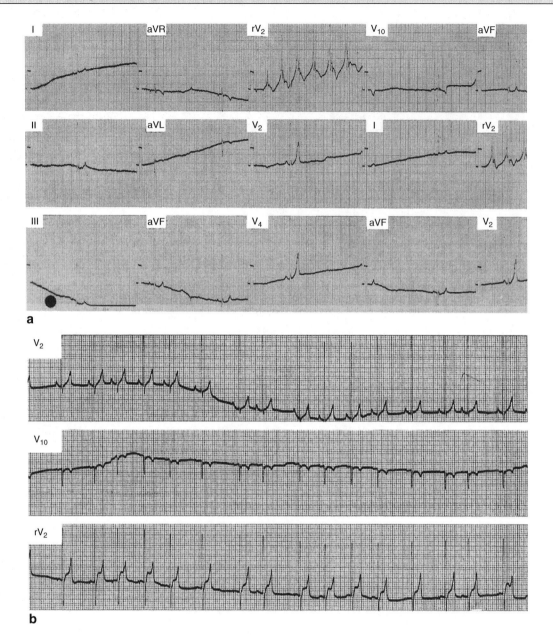

⬛ Fig. 9.7

The ECG in (**a**) illustrates several artifacts caused by skeletal muscle movement in dogs. Five sets of three leads, each are recorded automatically in each of four 2.6-s panels. Baseline drift is present in all panels. Muscle tremor artifact at 30–35 Hz and intermediate frequency muscle movement artifact at a frequency of about 15 Hz are present in the limb leads. "Tail-wag" artifact simulates paroxysmal ventricular rhythm in lead rV_2; this is caused by the movement of the rV_2 electrode (which is situated between the right thorax wall and the table surface) as the chest is moved synchronously with the wagging tail. The R wave in lead V_2 in the third panel from the left is clipped. In (**b**), the rV_2 lead illustrates simulated ST-segment elevation caused by the apex beat artifact in which the thrust of the heart against the chest wall at the fifth right intercostal space moves the electrode. Note the variability in the ST-segment elevation and contour

Artifacts present should be identified and the records examined more closely if they:

(a) Resemble electrocardiographic abnormalities
(b) Interfere with interval measurement
(c) Distort many complexes

9.3 The Normal Electrocardiogram

9.3.1 Values

The chief sources summarizing normal values are Lannek [16], Grauwiler [48], Hill [42, 43], Ettinger and Suter [21], Bolton [23], Hahn et al. [31], Tilley [24], and Detweiler [25]. A representative normal ECG is shown in ❯ Fig. 9.8. It should be emphasized that there is breed variability in the normal values for the dog. Most dogs "fit" within the "established normals"; however, some breeds have their own particular standard. For example, giant large-boned dogs with a somatotype similar to a Saint Bernard will have R waves of lower amplitude than dogs of similar weight such as a Great Dane. Also, dogs such as the Saint Bernard can have P waves with a duration that exceeds the "usual" standard in most breeds. Most research dogs are beagles; however, in recent years, pharmaceutical and device companies have requested larger mongrels. Obviously, this stresses the importance of pretrial electrocardiographic recordings for comparisons to be made.

Importantly, it should be stated that although most of the differences in the ECG discussed are the result of the conformation of the dog, there are likely differences in the current density of certain ion channels amongst breeds, particularly those of repolarization.

9.3.1.1 Amplitude

Because foreleg position affects limb-lead potentials, the limb-lead data from Hill [42], who standardized foreleg position, are given in ❯ Tables 9.2 and ❯ 9.3.

9.3.1.2 Intervals

Representative lead II time intervals are 0.03–0.06 s for P, 0.06–0.14 s for PR, 0.03–0.07 s for QRS, and 0.15–0.23 s for QT, all at heart rate 60–180 bpm [23, 26, 33]. In ❯ Table 9.4, the available regression formulae are given, and ❯ Table 9.5 relates PR and QT intervals and heart rate in beagles. The values represented by these three sources do not agree, probably because the authors used different criteria to determine where the time intervals begin and end.

Today the ECG measurement that garnishes the greatest attention is the QT interval. This duration measured from the first depolarization deflection to the end of the T wave must be considered in the context of heart rate. Thus, the QT interval is often corrected using formulas. The Bazett formula [49] has historically been the one most commonly used across species, although a variety of others have also been proposed [50–57]. However, the limitations and inaccuracies of this formula should be stressed. The Bazett formula was specifically developed by Bazett to correct for the influence of heart rate under specific conditions. Unfortunately, for decades, his original work was applied widely across species and conditions that were not in the original intent for heart rate correction of the QT interval. The majority of formulas either over or under correct the QT interval depending on the rate. This problem has been addressed with a proposal to specifically adjust the QT to the HR [50–57]. The latter is the only one of many proposals for the evaluation of the QT interval. Because the accurate interpretation of the QT interval is imperative to the evaluation of drugs, international conferences have been held to address the proper approach in the pharmacological evaluations of drugs.

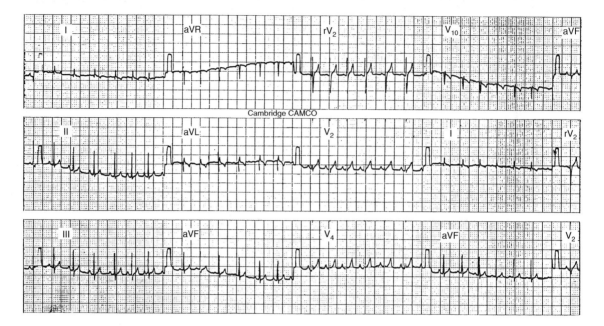

◘ Fig. 9.8
A ten-lead ECG from an 8-month-old male beagle recorded with the dog in right lateral recumbency with the forelegs held parallel and at a right angle to the long axis of the body. The recording format for each 2.8-s panel separated by 1.0 mV = 10 divisions sensitivity standardization signal is shown. Panel 5 is the beginning of a rhythm strip of 48-s duration to complete a standard (approximately) 1-min recording interval, which is the duration recommended for routine ECGs taken on groups of dogs in toxicological studies. Note that the R waves in leads V2 and V4 are clipped (by 0.2 mV for lead V2), because the true amplitude determined when the baseline was adjusted exceeds the maximum positive excursion of the stylus. Because such clipping often goes unnoticed, the true amplitude of R waves in these leads frequently present in young dogs (sometimes exceeding 6.0 mV) has been underestimated in the literature except by Lannek [16], who recorded at half sensitivity (10 divisions = 2.0 mV). The T-wave polarity in the dog changes with body position and age in addition to physiologic, pharmacologic, and pathaologic alterations. See also ❷ Fig. 3.7

9.3.2　P-Wave Amplitude and Configuration

The form and amplitude of P waves are more variable in canines than in most other animals. The variability is generally far more pronounced in limb leads than in the conventional thoracic leads (rV_2, V_2, V_4, and V_{10}), where it may be minimal or absent. When the P wave varies in association with respiration (RR interval), it is referred to as a "wandering pacemaker." The P wave also may vary within a dog during serial recordings. The P-wave amplitude can change quickly with changes in heart rate. The faster the heart rate, the taller the P wave. The T wave also changes with heart rate. Both are related to the changes in parasympathetic/sympathetic tone.

9.3.2.1　Wandering Pacemaker

As the heart rate speeds and slows with respiratory sinus arrhythmia, there are cyclic P-wave changes, both in form and amplitude. These are most pronounced in the limb leads in which the P waves are usually of greatest amplitude (e.g., II, III, and aVF). Ordinarily, there is no change in the PR interval, except when the initial part of the P wave becomes isoelectric, or having been isoelectric, becomes positive or negative.

◘ Table 9.2

The amplitude of positive and negative P and T waves (in millivolts) from 70 normal dogs with standardized body and limb positions [43]

	I	aVF	V_{10}	V_4	rV_2
Positive P waves					
Relative frequency	97.1	100.0	47.1	100.0	72.9
Range	0.05–0.15	0.05–0.25	0.05–0.10	0.05–0.25	0.05–0.15
Median	0.05	0.15	0.05	0.10	0.05
Mean	0.063	0.133	0.055	0.126	0.065
Variance	0.00084	0.0037	0.00023	0.0029	0.00073
Negative P waves					
Relative frequency			38.6		10.0
Range			0.05–0.10		0.05–0.10
Median			0.05		0.05
Mean			0.059		0.066
Variance			0.0004		
Positive T waves					
Relative frequency	44.3	45.7	8.6	65.7	98.5
Range	0.05–0.25	0.05–0.45	0.05–0.20	0.05–0.90	0.05–0.80
Median	0.05	0.20	0.05	0.25	0.30
Mean	0.071	0.186	0.075	0.320	0.346
Variance	0.002	0.012		0.048	0.037
Negative T waves					
Relative frequency	51.4	45.7	87.1	15.7	1.5
Range	0.05–0.25	0.05–0.60	0.05–0.40	0.05–0.35	0.15
Median	0.05	0.25	0.20	0.25	
Mean	0.095	0.236	0.211	0.236	
Variance	0.003	0.019	0.006		

The cause of these changes is currently attributed to shifting of the pacemaker within the sinoatrial node, induced by variations of vagal tone (wandering pacemaker within the sinoatrial node). As is well known, experimental vagal stimulation can move the apparent pacemaker site from the upper to the lower end of the sinoatrial node [58–60]. The effect of such vagally induced shifts in pacemaker location in experimental dogs has been confirmed and related to P-wave configurational changes in leads I, aVF, and V_{10} [61]. The pacemaker location was established by plotting wave-front vectors from two sets of bipolar electrodes located close to the sinoatrial node. The inspiration was accompanied by an increase in the heart rate and a shift in the pacemaker location toward the head of the sinoatrial node and the expiration (or electrical stimulation of the right vagus or carotid sinus pressure) by slowing of the heart rate and movement of the pacemaker location toward the tail of the sinoatrial node. The shift of the plotted pacemaker location amounted to about 1.4 cm. With slowing of the heart rate, P waves increase slightly in amplitude in leads I and V_{10} and decrease (often markedly) in lead aVF, frequently becoming notched or bifid in lead aVF. Rarely, P-wave polarity may reverse in leads III (becoming negative) and aVL (becoming positive) during expiration. When pacemaker locations were determined [61], the P-wave in lead aVF was:

(a) Peaked when the pacemaker was located in the head of the sinoatrial node
(b) Of lower amplitude and bifid when the pacemaker was located in the middle area of the sinoatrial node and a low amplitude
(c) Flat when the pacemaker was low in the tail of the sinoatrial node

◻ Table 9.3

Amplitudes of the QRS complex (in millivolts) from 70 normal dogs with standardized body and limb positions

	I	II	III	aVR	aVL	aVF	V2	V4	V10	rV2
Q wave										
Relative frequency	90.0	98.6	87.1	1.5	37.1	97.1	40.0	81.5	100.0	None
Range	0.05–0.60	0.05–1.20	0.05–1.00	0.30	0.05–0.65	0.05–1.05	0.05–0.35	0.05–0.55	0.15–1.20	
Median	0.15	0.30	0.25		0.30	0.25	0.05	0.15	0.65	
Mean	0.22	0.38	0.27		0.30	0.31	0.09	0.17	0.65	
Variance[a]	0.022	0.075	0.046		0.0324	0.052	0.004	0.013	0.057	
R wave										
Relative frequency	100.0	100.0	100.0	100.0	100.0	100.0	100.0	100.0	98.6	100.0
Range	0.10–1.50	0.45–3.00	0.25–2.35	0.05–0.70	0.05–0.90	0.20–2.40	0.50–4.00	0.25–5.40	0.05–0.80	0.15–3.60
Median	0.60	1.60	1.10	0.25	0.15	1.35	1.90	1.90	0.30	1.00
Mean	0.64	1.61	1.12	0.27	0.23	1.37	1.96	1.97	0.31	1.11
Variance[a]	0.117	0.334	0.247	0.032	0.042	0.366	0.593	0.828	0.0286	0.449
S wave										
Relative frequency	8.6	32.9	34.3	100.0	64.3	35.7	80.0	54.3	None	100.0
Range	0.05	0.05–0.35	0.05–0.70	0.15–2.30	0.10–1.10	0.05–0.55	0.05–1.60	0.05–1.30		0.05–1.60
Median		0.15	0.20	1.10	0.40	0.10	0.30	0.20		0.60
Mean		0.16	0.22	1.09	0.42	0.16	0.39	0.28		0.67
Variance[a]		0.009	0.029	0.223	0.054	0.014	0.093	0.067		0.156

[a]Standard deviations are not listed because of the number of asymmetrical distributions found in this series

◻ Table 9.4

Linear regression formulae for time intervals (R-R in milliseconds)

	Grauwiler [48]	Lannek [16]
PQ (ms)	82 + 0.023 (R-R) ± 30 (3SD)	
QT (ms)	136 + 0.084 (R-R) ± 10 (5SD)	160 + 0.03 (R-R) ± 38 (2SE)

It appeared that in each dog there were several specific locations in the sinoatrial node for pacemaker activity, and that a change in vagal tone caused a sudden shift in the location of pacemaker activity from one of these preferred sites to another. This is in accordance with the view that major changes in sinoatrial node discharge rate result from, say, suppression of a faster pacemaking cell and shift of pacemaking dominance to a slower discharging cell, rather than from a slowing in rate of the original pacemaker cell. Stellate ganglion stimulation or norepinephrine injection can also cause shifts in pacemaker site and alterations in P-wave morphology [62]. Mapping studies [63] have demonstrated three regions of origin of atrial depolarization located at anterior, middle, and posterior regions of the anterior vena cava-right atrial junction. The middle position was near the sinoatrial node. The anterior and posterior positions were 1–2 cm away from the sinoatrial node area. Changes in P-wave morphology resulted from abrupt shifts in the region of earliest activation among these three points, two of which were outside the sinoatrial node. The multiple points of origin of atrial activation might represent a trifocal, distributed pacemaker or the epicardial exits of three specialized pathways that rapidly conduct the impulse from a single focus. Higher heart rates and taller P waves in lead II were associated with the higher centers of early activation, while lower rates and lower-amplitude notched P waves were linked with the lower centers of early activation. Others have demonstrated that in the dog, the sinus node is long (4 cm in length), providing multiple areas for discharge that are influenced by autonomic tone and the affected spontaneous discharge rate. In summary, when ECGs are monitored in the dog, the autonomic tone will alter the P wave, and thus, this parameter is not one which is likely to be reliable in detecting differences between recordings that have impact on a study.

Table 9.5

Variation of PR and QT intervals with heart rate in the beagle ECG [165]

Group number	Heart rate (bpm)	Sex	Number of ECGs	Interval (s) PR	QT
1	61–80	Male	16	0.105 ± 0.029	0.214 ± 0.037
		Female	16	0.100 ± 0.027	0.213 ± 0.041
2	80–100	Male	96	0.102 ± 0.028	0.206 ± 0.031
		Female	86	0.104 ± 0.032	0.203 ± 0.028
3	101–120	Male	210	0.096 ± 0.025	0.195 ± 0.030
		Female	219	0.101 ± 0.028	0.192 ± 0.027
4	121–140	Male	353	0.095 ± 0.020	0.183 ± 0.031
		Female	324	0.097 ± 0.028	0.182 ± 0.029
5	141–160	Male	295	0.092 ± 0.026	0.173 ± 0.028
		Female	326	0.095 ± 0.026	0.174 ± 0.028
6	161–180	Male	172	0.088 ± 0.020	0.167 ± 0.026
		Female	187	0.078 ± 0.020	0.165 ± 0.028
7	181–200	Male	51	0.086 ± 0.020	0.160 ± 0.020
		Female	47	0.083 ± 0.021	0.160 ± 0.023
Student's t for groups 1 vs 7		Male		3.366*	5.036**
		Female		3.198*	4.942*

Values for PR and QT intervals are the means and 95% range for the numbers of ECGs shown. The asterisks indicate the degree of significance associated with the differences between the values for the lowest and highest heart-rate groups

$^*p < 0.001$; $^{**}p < 0.01$

Table 9.6

QRS patterns in various leads. For each lead the patterns are given in the order of frequency of occurrence. Patterns that are encountered less often or rarely are placed in parentheses. Refer to ❷ Fig. 9.6 and note how these patterns are altered by changing forelimb position

Lead	Pattern	Lead	Pattern	Lead	Pattern
I	QR, qR, (qRS)	aVR	rS, rSr', (qrS)	rV_2	RS, (Rs)
II	qR, zRs, Rs, (QrS)	aVL	Qr, QR, (qRs)	V_2	Rs, qRs, (qR)
III	qR, qR, Rs, (rS)	aVF	qR, Rs, (QrS)	V_4	Rs, qRs, (qR)
				V_{10}	Qr, rS, (qR, QR)

Given the above discussion, if the P wave is measured, it has not to our knowledge been stated which P wave to measure on an ECG recording (e.g., tallest, shortest, average). This in itself is problematic. We have arbitrarily decided to always measure the tallest P wave. It should also be emphasized that in an evaluation, if the heart rate changes, the P-wave values are likely to change as a consequence of rate, and not because of pathology of the atria.

9.3.3 QRS Complex

Typical QRS patterns in the various leads are given symbolically in ❷ Table 9.6. The QR pattern in lead I corresponds to the high incidence of counterclockwise rotation of the QRS vector loops in dogs (see ❷ Sect. 9.5).

9.3.4　ST-T Wave

In dogs, the ST segment is seldom horizontal and often the onset of T is imperceptible. Except for leads rV_2 and V_{10}, the polarity of the T waves may be positive or negative. In ❷ Fig. 9.9, a series of ST-T patterns observed in lead II are depicted. ST segment or ST junction (STj) deviations, especially in leads II, aVF, V_2, and V_4 are common. These ST deviations seldom remain consistent in serial records, but vary or disappear entirely from record to record. Also, the degree of ST deviation often varies cyclically with the changing R ~ R intervals of respiratory sinus arrhythmia. In this case, the degree of deviation increases with shorter preceding R-R intervals. Recent work in serial recordings of beagles and mongrels studied at Cornell University has demonstrated further that the polarity of the T wave is dependent on the age of the dog. The younger the dog, the more likely the T wave is to be positive. The T wave does not "stabilize" in the dog until approximately 12 months of age. This is an important notation for long-term studies in the dog in which the evaluation of repolarization as assessed by the ECG is important. The T wave is changing during the first year of life, so if a study is begun when the dog is 3–6 months of age, changes at 12 months of age must be assessed in conjunction with the expected changes seen developmentally with a more negative T wave at the older age. Again, the importance of control dogs is obvious for all studies.

9.3.5　U Wave

When present, U waves are generally most prominent in leads rV2, V_2, and V_4. They may vary in amplitude or disappear in consecutive beats and are usually less than 0.05 mV in amplitude and concordant with positive T waves. The TU interval approximates 0.04 s and U-wave duration approximates 0.07–0.09 s. The electrophysiological genesis of U waves is controversial [64]. They have been attributed to:

(a)　Purkinje cell repolarization potentials
(b)　An afterpotential gradient from endocardium to epicardium created during ventricular relaxation [65]

Tall U waves appear in hypokalemia, and in humans, have been described in hypomagnesemia, and in patients receiving digoxin, phenothiazines or tricyclic antidepressants [64]. U-wave inversion in humans has been described in hypertension, valvular, pulmonary, congenital, and ischemic heart disease [64]. In dogs, U-wave amplitude exceeding 0.05 mV has been associated with hypertension and anemic heart disease, but this finding is not consistent and is therefore diagnostically unreliable. U-wave values of 0.08 ~ 0.15 mV may occur in otherwise normal dogs.

9.3.6　Evolution During the First 3 Months of Life

Consistent with the functional and morphological cardiovascular changes during the first few weeks after birth [66–68], the mean (sometimes termed modal) QRS vector moves from a rightward, cranial and ventral orientation to the leftward, caudal and ventral direction [69–71]. The principal cause of this change is that the two ventricles are of about equal mass at birth, and this 1:1 ratio of right to left ventricular mass changes to a ratio of 1:2 or 1:3 [67] depending on how the ventricles are separated.

The mean QRS axis (derived from leads I and aVF) in the frontal plane is directed toward the right and either cranially or caudally at birth. By the 12th week, the mean QRS axis is directed to the left and usually resides in the left caudal quadrant of the frontal plane. In the transverse plane (leads I and V_{10}), the mean QRS axis changes from the right ventral quadrant at birth to the left ventral quadrant at week 12. The shift in the sagittal plane is from a more cranial ventral direction to a more caudal ventral orientation.

The R/S ratio in the left precordial leads increases primarily between the first and second week. It is less than 1.0 at birth and exceeds 1.0 at the sixth week. Later, this ratio becomes larger and may reach infinity because the S wave disappears. There is little change in the R/S ratio in lead rV2. In the frontal plane, the mean QRS vector shift may be from the right cranial through the left cranial to the left caudal quadrant (i.e., clockwise), or from the right cranial through the right caudal to the left caudal quadrant (i.e., counterclockwise).

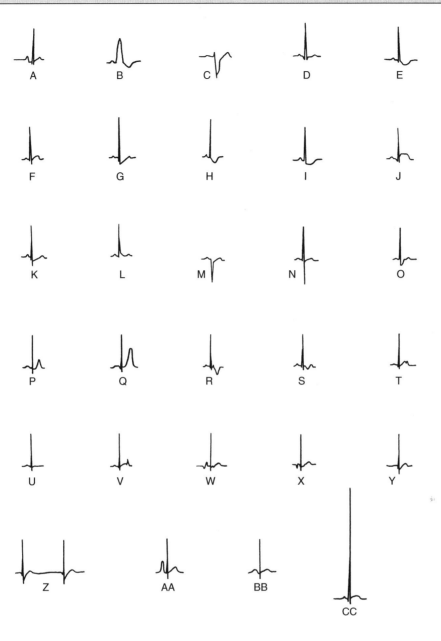

◘ Fig. 9.9

Pattern code: *A* increased Ta amplitude, *B* left bundle branch block like pattern (LBBB-like), *C* right bundle branch block like pattern (RBBB-like), *D* flat ST segment, *E* coved ST segment, *F* arched ST segment, *G* ascending ST segment, *H* descending ST segment, *I* depressed ST segment, *J* elevated ST segment, *K* STj depressed, *L* STj elevated, *M* QS complex, *N* deep S wave, *O* broad S wave, *P* symmetrical T wave, *Q* tall T wave, *R* deep negative T wave, *S* diphasic T wave: −/+ or +/−, *T* notched T wave: − or −t, *U* flat T wave, *V* dome-dart ST-T complex, *W* diphasic P wave: −/+ or +1/−, *X* negative P wave, *Y* flat P wave, *Z* absent P waves, *AA* tall P waves: >0.4 mV, *BB* broad P waves: >60 ms, and *CC* tall RV$_2$, V$_4$: >5.0 mV

9.3.7   Classification

All canine ECGs fall into one of the following three general categories: normal, normal variant, or abnormal.

(a) *Normal ECGs.* These are ECGs in which all variables (heart rate, time intervals, amplitude and polarity of waves in all leads, and rhythm) fall within the specified ranges given in ❯ Tables 9.2–9.6.
(b) *Normal variant ECGs.* These ECGs have characteristics as described in ❯ Table 9.1 without pathology of the heart.
(c) *Abnormal ECGs.* These include any electrocardiographic feature that is outside normal limits and is definitely more prevalent in the presence of heart disease or cardiotoxicity.

9.3.8   Normal/Abnormal ECG Screening

Screening becomes necessary when records of large numbers of experimental dog ECGs are examined to eliminate any dogs with abnormal or questionable ECGs. Since the beagle is the breed normally used in such studies (e.g., chronic toxicity trials in preclinical drug testing), the criteria listed apply primarily to this breed, although they would apply equally well to most mongrels and other breeds of similar size and conformation.

Since over 95% of experimental beagle ECGs will ordinarily be within normal limits, the initial goal in examining pretest records is to identify the few abnormal records rapidly. This is done by quickly scanning the records for a series of features that establish normality. The criteria should be conservative so that borderline records will be scrutinized more closely.

9.3.8.1   Normal Criteria

The following criteria are customized from our experiences in the interpretation of the ECG recorded from the beagle. These criteria are not exactly the same as the normal published values for dogs in general.

(a) Intervals and rhythm
    (i) Heart rate: 60–190 bpm (R-R interval 316–1,000 ms)
    (ii) P interval: less than 50 ms
    (iii) PR interval: greater than 70 ms, less than 130 ms
    (iv) QRS interval: less than 60 ms
    (v) QT interval: less than 220 ms
    (vi) Sinus arrhythmia present
    (vii) No abnormal arrhythmias
(b) Wave amplitudes and patterns
    (i) T wave amplitude: 0.05–1.0 mV in any lead
       (Flat T waves are not necessarily abnormal especially in leads I, aVR, aVL, and V_{10})
    (ii) ST deviation: less than 0.20 mV in limb leads and less than 0.25 mV in chest leads
    (iii) ST-T complex: no dome-dart complexes
    (iv) R wave:
- Less than 3.0 mV in limb leads rV_2 and V_{10}
- Less than 5.0 mV in leads V_2 and V_4
- More than 0.5 mV in II, III, and aVF

    (v) QRS axis in frontal plane: $-20°$ to $+110°$
    (vi) P wave: less than 0.4 mV
    (vii) R/S amplitude ratio:
- Greater than 0.5 in rV_2; and
- Greater than 0.9 in V_2 and V_4

(viii) QRS: no rs, rS, Rs or RS patterns

(ix) S/QRS duration ratio: less than 50%

Records that do not meet these normal criteria require closer examination to determine if they are abnormal or normal variants.

9.3.9 Normal Variants

A large number of electrocardiographic characteristics are sufficiently rare or puzzling to attract attention in records from dogs not known to have cardiac disease. These are grouped together here as normal variants. They are based primarily on findings in young dogs (5–18 months old) of a single breed, the beagle [26].

9.3.9.1 QRS Complex

(a) *Variant frontal plane QRS vector loop.* This is also known as the "butterfly" QRS vector loop and requires a special mention. In a small number of beagles and in some other breeds as well, the mean QRS frontal plane axis is negative, ranging from $-30°$ to $-110°$ (❷ Figs. 9.11 and ❷ 9.12). The QRS complexes in thoracic leads are within normal limits. In leads II, III, and aVF, the QRS pattern is characterized by having a small r wave (e.g., qrS or QrS pattern) or a W-shaped pattern in which the "r" wave fails to reach the isoelectric line. In lead I, there is usually a deep Q and pronounced R wave, the descending limb of which is slurred or notched as it approaches the isoelectric level. The QRS in lead aVL is usually markedly positive. If a frontal plane vector diagram is constructed from leads I and aVF, the early forces are directed counterclockwise to the right and craniad, then return close to their starting point before passing counterclockwise to the left and craniad. Thus, two connected vector loops are formed vaguely resembling butterfly wings, hence the name "butterfly" QRS vector loop (❷ Figs. 9.10 and ❷ 9.11).

This variant has neither been studied systematically nor investigated electrophysiologically. Since the thoracic lead complexes are essentially normal with tall R waves in leads V_2 and V_4 and typical configuration in leads rV2 and V_{10}, there does not appear to be an electrophysiological abnormality. It is obvious, however, that the vector forces producing tall R waves in leads V_2 and V_4 do not do so in the limb leads. This pattern, when seen in 5–7-month-old dogs, may persist into adulthood, or within a few months or a year, tall R waves may appear in leads II, III, and aVF, while the chest lead complexes remain the same. The hearts are normal at necropsy.

The conclusion that can be drawn from the information at hand is that these low-amplitude R waves in leads II, III, and aVF and the "butterfly" QRS frontal plane vector loop result from the position of the heart in the thorax relative to the limbs, such that the major vector forces during the inscription of QRS are directed largely craniad and ventrad. As shown in ❷ Figs. 9.10 and ❷ 9.11, the two components of the QRS frontal plane-constructed vector loops may be more or less symmetrically disposed, with the initial part of the loop being directed toward the right arm and the final part of the loop directed toward the left arm.

(b) Other QRS complex variants (see ❷ Table 9.1 for most common variants):

 (i) Circular frontal plane QRS vector loop

 (ii) QRS slurring and notching

 (iii) Delayed terminal forces causing broad SII, III, and aVF and broader RaVL; patterns variously (and often erroneously) described as incomplete RBBB, left anterior fascicular block

 (iv) Rr' pattern in II, III, aVF, and rV$_2$ unaccompanied by broad S waves (see also (v))

 (v) "Foot" or slur terminating QRS

 (vi) Variable SrV$_2$ and V$_2$ amplitude

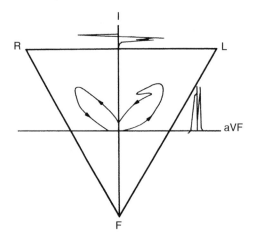

◘ Fig. 9.10

Butterfly QRS complex. A vector diagram constructed from QRS complexes of leads I and aVF. The QRS complexes are each traced on their respective zero potential lines, which intersect at zero potential in the center. The winged appearance of the vector diagrams of the variant QRS complexes gave rise to the term "butterfly" QRS complex. Note that the QRS complexes from leads I and aVF are drawn on their respective zero or isopotential lines which intersect at the middle of the triangle. To view lead aVF in its conventional orientation as recorded, the diagram must be rotated 90° counterclockwise. To view lead aVF in its conventional orientation, the diagram must be rotated 180° (i.e., lead aVF appears upside down here). The positive pole for lead I is toward L from its zero potential line and that for lead aVF is toward F, in the diagram

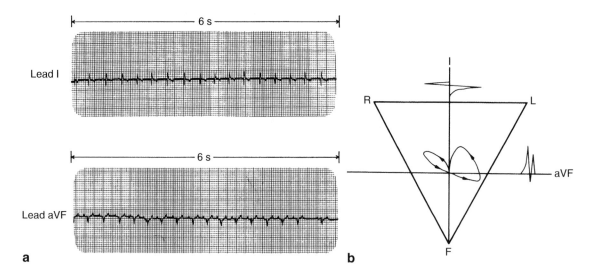

◘ Fig. 9.11

Butterfly QRS complex: (a) leads I and aVF and (b) vector diagram constructed from the QRS complex as in leads I and aVF. Note that the QRS complexes from leads I and aVF are drawn on their respective zero or isoelectric lines which intersect at the middle of the triangle. To view lead I in its conventional orientation as recorded, the diagram must be rotated 90° counterclockwise. To view lead aVF in its conventional orientation, the diagram must be rotated 180° (i.e., lead aVF appears upside down here). The positive pole for lead I is toward L from its zero potential line and that for lead aVF is toward F

9.3.9.2   T wave and ST-T Complex: U Wave

(a) T wave in V_{10} flat, diphasic $-/+$ or positive
(b) T wave in rV_2 negative terminally or diphasic $+/-$
(c) Biphasic T waves in other leads
(d) T wave variable in amplitude and form (including polarity reversal) related to varying R-R intervals
(e) Tall-peaked T waves
(f) Dome-dart ST-T complex without QT prolongation
(g) Prominent U wave (>0.5 mV)
(h) TU fusion

9.3.9.3   P Wave and T_a Wave

(a) P-wave reversal in limb leads except lead I (wandering pacemaker within the sinoatrial node)
(b) Notched P waves
(c) High-amplitude (negative deflection) T_a waves (>0.05 mV; up to 0.15 mV in lead II)

9.3.9.4   Amplitude

(a) ST deviation (with accompanying ST-segment deviation or followed by rapid return of ST segment to baseline level) up to 0.20 mV in limb leads and 0.25 mV in chest leads. Variable deviation related to R-R-interval duration
(b) Amplitude variation of QRS and T waves with breathing cycle and R-R-interval duration
(c) Tall P wave in leads II and aVF (greater than 0.4 mV). Tall R wave in leads V_2 and V_4 (> 5.5 mV)

9.3.9.5   Rhythm and Rate

(a) Bradycardia (40–55 bpm)
(b) Tachycardia (rate > 200 bpm)
(c) First-degree AV block (PR > 0.14 s)
(d) Second-degree AV block

9.4   Normal Rhythm

9.4.1   Sinus Rhythm and Rate

In the denervated heart of the dog, the sinoatrial node discharges regularly at an intrinsic rate of about 90–120 bpm (see reference [72] for literature). Parasympathectomy alone results in a persistently rapid rate of 140–160 bpm. In intact, resting, and adult dogs, heart rates of 70–120 bpm are representative; with exercise, rates of 220–325 bpm are recorded; and in newborn and young puppies, the range is 140–275 bpm. In ECGs, the heart rates tend to be more rapid than in the resting dog owing to the effect of restraint. The ranges given in ❯ Sect. 9.3.1 and ❯ Table 9.5 are characteristic of those obtained from ECGs and show that the usual range in ECGs from beagles is 100–180 bpm. At the more rapid frequencies, respiratory sinus arrhythmia is decreased or abolished.

9.4.2   Respiratory Sinus Arrhythmia

In resting dogs, the heart rate decreases and increases with the breathing cycle, owing to a waxing and waning of vagal activity with respiration, although the primary reason is a central effect on the heart rate with variation in autonomic tone. The usual pattern is acceleration with inspiration and deceleration with expiration, but this relationship is not absolute [73].

The control systems that interact to cause sinus arrhythmia include the radiation of respiratory center activity to medullary cardiovascular centers, the cardiac component of the Hering–Breuer reflex, the Bainbridge reflex (reflex cardioacceleration caused by increased stretch of the right atrium and great veins during inspiration), and the baroreceptor reflex (reflex cardiac slowing when the blood pressure rises during the accelerating phase of sinus arrhythmia). The degree of respiratory sinus arrhythmia decreases as vagal tone is decreased with exercise or excitement. The degree of sinus arrhythmia can be expressed as an index I [74]:

$$I = (\text{standard deviation of R-R} \times 100)/\text{mean R-R}.$$

This index is variable in serial records. For accuracy, 100 R-R intervals should be averaged for the calculation. Certain drugs can decrease this index or abolish sinus arrhythmia altogether at heart rates where it is ordinarily present. Other methods to evaluate heart rate variability have been studied extensively. These include time and frequency domains to assess the balance of autonomic tone [75].

In resting dogs, the rapid beats in respiratory sinus arrhythmias often occur in sets of two (bigeminy), three (trigeminy), or sets of three beats with a fourth beat during expiration [76]. Sets of four or five beats are rare. These cyclic changes in the R-R-interval duration are often accompanied by cyclic alterations in the amplitude of electrocardiographic complexes and, sometimes, in the form (and occasionally, polarity) of T waves. In puppies, Lange [77] found that respiratory sinus arrhythmia does not appear before 4 weeks of age.

Usually, the respiratory sinus arrhythmia tends to become more pronounced (i.e., the disparity between R-R intervals increases) as the heart rate slows. Rarely, this fails to occur and a slow heart rate with a relatively regular rhythm may be present. Certain drugs appear to depress the brain stem and ameliorate or abolish respiratory arrhythmia in dogs (see ❯ Sect. 9.10.1.3).

Over the years, the breeding of beagles for research purposes has led to some dogs being particularly calm with slow rates and more pronounced sinus arrhythmias.

9.5   Normal Vectorcardiogram

Starting in 1957 with the study of Horan et al. [78], vectorcardiography became a useful investigation tool in canine cardiology. Various lead systems have been employed: for example, the Wilson equilateral tetrahedral reference system [31, 78–82], the Frank corrected lead system [35, 37] (❯ Fig. 9.4), and the orthogonal-lead system of McFee and Parungao [23, 34, 43, 82–84] (❯ Fig. 9.3). Of these, the only lead system specifically corrected for the dog is that of McFee and Parungao [33]. Rarely is vectorcardiography performed today in clinical veterinary patients, in screening research dogs, or as a part of the evaluation of treatment. We continue a discussion of this method here because, although not performed, it is a valuable concept to grasp in the often two-dimensional representation of the frontal limb leads to which we are limited. In electrophysiology laboratories, extensive mapping has replaced the vectorcardiogram.

9.5.1   Normal Values

Vectorcardiographic data from 50 mongrel dogs using the axial-lead system of McFee and Parungao are given in ❯ Tables 9.7–9.9 [84]. In these tables, the term prevalent direction or θ expressed in degrees is used (see ❯ Chap. 1 of *Electrocardiology: Comprehensive Clinical ECG*) rather than the mean of observed angular directions. This variable is an estimate of the average angle of the prevalent direction, and the range of distribution of the individual points is given in the tables for 5–95% of the grouping.

■ Table 9.7

Angles and magnitudes of P, QRS, and T maximal vectors [84]

	Maximal P vector	Maximal QRS vector	Maximal T vector
Frontal plane			
Amplitude (mV)[a]	0.42 ± 0.12	2.17 ± .0.44	0.28 ± 0.12
Prevalent direction $\hat{\theta}$ (°)	71	69	84
5–95% directional range (°)	44–85	38–95	−55 to −124
Horizontal plane			
Amplitude (mV)[a]	0.21 ± 0.11	1.72 ± 0.36	0.36 ± 0.19
Prevalent direction $\hat{\theta}$ (°)	9	71	87
5–95% directional range (°)	−55 to 72	−66 to 137	30 to −163
Left sagittal plane			
Amplitude (mV)[a]	0.41 ± 0.11	2.27 ± 0.43	0.42 ± 0.22
Prevalent direction $\hat{\theta}$ (°)	95	117	161
5–95% directional range (°)	70–125	47–153	119 to −104

[a]Mean ± standard deviation

■ Table 9.8

Maximal projections of QRS vectors on W, Y, and Z [84]

	Mean ± SD (mV)	5–95% range (mV)
X axis		
Initial right	−0.21 ± 0.30	0.0 to −0.60
Left	0.91 ± 0.43	0.20–0.160
Terminal right	−0.18 ± 0.28	0.00 to −0.80
Y axis		
Initial cranial	−0.04 ± 0.08	0.00 to −0.20
Caudad	1.9 ± 0.63	1.00–2.75
Terminal cranial	−0.21 ± 0.16	0.00 to −0.50
Z axis		
Sternal	−1.50 ± 0.54	−0.50 to −2.25
Vertebral	0.98 ± 0.44	0.20–1.80

■ Table 9.9

Spatial angles and magnitudes of instantaneous QRS vectors [84]

Time after onset of QRS (ms)	$\hat{\alpha}$[a] (°)	$\hat{\beta}$[b] (°)	Magnitude[c] (mV) Mean ± SD	5–95% range
5	97	86	0.29 ± 0.17	0.12–0.46
15	81	128	1.81 ± .0.45	0.63–2.59
25	29	154	2.11 ± 0.53	1.03–2.89
35	292	128	1.28 ± 0.63	0.39–2.31
45	262	84	0.60 ± 0.48	0.08–1.62
55	257	97	0.27 ± 0.22	0.08–0.98

[a] $\hat{\alpha}$, longitude or angular deviation from the left in the horizontal plane (0°–360°) for the spatial prevalent direction
[b] $\hat{\beta}$, colatitude or angular deviation from the cranial (0°–180°) for the spatial prevalent direction
[c]Magnitude = $(X^2 + Y^2 + Z^2)^{1/2}$

9.5.2 P and T Vector Loops

With the lead system of McFee and Parungao, the P loop is a thin ellipse pointing sternally and to the left. The mean P-wave axis is within ±90° of the maximal QRS vector in 100% of the cases in the frontal plane, 82% in the horizontal plane, and 98% in the left sagittal plane [84]. With the McFee and Parungao lead system, the T loop is a moderately open ellipse with the mean axis within ±90° of the maximal QRS axis in 80% of the cases in the frontal plane, 77% in the horizontal plane, and 82% in the left sagittal plane. With the Frank system, the T vector loop is usually concordant with the QRS vector loop in the frontal (86%), transverse (90%), and sagittal (97%) planes [34]. Thus, the major T vector axis points either cranially or caudally in the frontal plane, ventrally in the horizontal plane, and sternocranially or sternocaudally in the left sagittal plane.

9.5.3 QRS Vector Loops

The incidence of counterclockwise rotation of QRS vector loops in frontal, left sagittal, and transverse ("horizontal") planes is very high with the three (Wilson tetrahedral, Frank, and McFee) lead systems. For example, with the McFee system, counterclockwise rotation of QRS in the frontal, transverse, and sagittal planes, respectively, was 52–60%, 80–98%, and 98–100% [43, 83, 84]. These percentages are similar to those reported for the frontal and left sagittal planes (85% and 100%) with the Wilson tetrahedron reference system and in all three planes with the Frank system (66%, 97%, and 100%, respectively) [35]. This predominance of counterclockwise QRS rotation in the dog frontal plane is in sharp contrast to the clockwise rotation more commonly found (65%) in the human VCG, which has a similar mean frontal axis. Since the spread of excitation through the heart in both species is similar, the difference must relate to the differing orientation of the heart within the thoracic cavity of man and dog.

Chest conformation has a distinct effect on the electrical axis of the heart such that narrow-chested breeds (e.g., Doberman pinschers, German shepherds) have more ventrally oriented QRS axes in the transverse plane and more caudally oriented QRS axes in the frontal plane than do broad-chested breeds (e.g., cocker spaniels and boxers) [83].

Vectorcardiographic appearances have been reported in dogs with a variety of spontaneous and experimental abnormal cardiac conditions such as right ventricular hypertrophy [23, 82, 85, 86], imperforate ventricular septal defect [87], congenital peritoneopericardial diaphragmatic hernia [88], patent ductus arteriosus [23, 89], idiopathic cardiomyopathy [23], coronary occlusion and other localized myocardial destruction [72, 73], ventricular ectopic beats [90], and bundle branch block patterns [23, 91–94].

9.5.4 The Vector Diagram

Despite the knowledge gained from these various investigations, vectorcardiography has been little used in the routine diagnostic cardiology in dogs. The vector diagram, however, derived from the limb-lead scalar ECG has a special usefulness in evaluating the QRS vector changes in the canine ECG [85] (❯ Fig. 9.12). This is because the normal range of mean QRS axis values is broad and the normal limits for the various breeds have not been established statistically. For example, in right ventricular hypertrophy, the usual counterclockwise rotation of the constructed QRS vector loops in the frontal, transverse, and sagittal planes is reversed. In the frontal plane, early forces are usually directed cephalically or caudally toward the left and late forces toward the right and cranially. In left ventricular hypertrophy, in contrast, the QRS axis and loop are not usually altered in form or in direction of inscription.

9.5.5 Evolution During the First 3 Months of Life

With the Wilson tetrahedron system, the QRS loops shortly after birth are directed chiefly toward the right (frontal and transverse planes) and cranially (frontal and sagittal planes); at week 12, the major orientation is toward the left and caudally. The inscription of the QRS vector loops in all three planes changes from clockwise just after birth to a counterclockwise rotation at week 12 [69, 70].

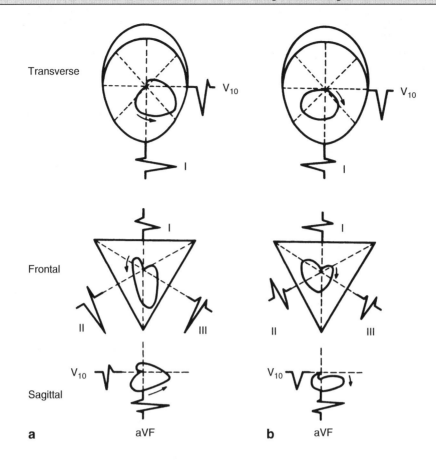

◘ Fig. 9.12
Vector diagrams in three planes constructed from limb-lead scalar ECGs (leads I, II, III, aVF, and V_{10}): (a) normal pattern and (b) right ventricular hypertrophy pattern. Note that the direction of rotation is counterclockwise in the normal record (a) and clockwise in right ventricular hypertrophy (b) in all three planes (After Detweiler et al. [78]. © New York Academy of Sciences, New York. Reproduced with permission)

The direction of the T-wave vector loop at birth in some dogs produces negative T waves in rV_2 and positive T waves in V_{10}. This changes with aging, so that by the fourth to the eighth week, the adult pattern (positive T wave in rV_2 and negative T wave in V_{10}) is present in most dogs. Positive T waves in V_{10} may persist in some dogs beyond the third month and become negative only between months 5 and 7. This T-wave polarity change from negative to positive in the right precordial lead (rV_2) is opposite to that observed in human infants, where the right precordial T waves are generally positive at birth and become negative after the first week after birth.

9.6 ECG Descriptors and Pattern Code

A number of electrocardiographic features that change spontaneously or are altered by drugs and disease are often described rather than quantified. Thus, wave contour, polarity, and amplitude characteristics require descriptive terms that are sufficiently specific to convey the intended meaning. Many terms in use are part of the jargon of electrocardiography, and few have found their way into medical dictionaries. Consequently, changes in meaning, elimination from use, or modification of terminology are continuing processes. The terms offered here have been found useful as descriptors for various recognizable characteristics of the dog ECG. Some are self explanatory while others require definition or examples. They are compiled here as an approach toward standardizing descriptive terms.

9.6.1 Descriptors Applicable to All Leads

(a) *Amplitude variable.* Amplitude variation of any of the electrocardiographic waves (P, Q, R, S, and T) from beat to beat. Example of use: P-wave amplitude variable from beat to beat in all limb leads.

   (i) Related to previous R-R interval. The form and amplitude of P and T waves and the degree of deviation of the STj or ST segment may vary predictably with changes in the R-R interval during respiratory sinus arrhythmia. The P-wave changes have been discussed in previous sections. The changes in T waves and STj or segment deviations occur because the degree of recovery of conductivity in the heart is time dependent and less complete with shorter R-R intervals. When the R-R intervals are short enough, the conduction and recovery processes are somewhat aberrant and the form of the ST-T complex changes.

   (ii) Electrical alternation. While this may occur in diseased hearts, minor variations (e.g., of the S wave in one of the chest leads) occurring in alternate beats are found in occasional records from the same dog and are not associated with any other abnormality.

(b) *Low amplitude.* Although all wave amplitudes vary in serial records, this term is used when the recorded potential is far below the average for a particular wave in a given lead. When cardiomyopathy is extensive, the entire QRST complex may be of reduced amplitude. The term is relative and the amplitudes may not be below the normal range when this term is applied. It is used primarily to describe P waves and R, R+S, or T waves. In the case of P and T waves, their polarity must be indicated as positive ($+$) or negative ($-$).

(c) *High amplitude.* The reverse of (b)

(d) *Polarity reversal.* The term is used when P and T waves change their polarity from beat to beat or from record to record in serial ECGs.

(e) *STj deviation.* The J (or junction) point is the sharp inflection marking the end of the QRS complex and the beginning of the ST segment. It deviates to some extent from the baseline in normal records. Increased STj deviation may accompany cardiac hypoxia, necrosis and epicardial inflammation. Depending on the polarity of the deviation, it is described as elevation or depression of the STj.

(f) *ST-segment deviation.* This term is used when the entire ST segment is elevated or depressed above or below the isoelectric line. The ST segments are seldom horizontal in dogs. They either ascend or descend from the STj to the T wave and a clear inflection point separating the ST segment from the beginning of T is often not present. Accordingly, it is necessary to measure the degree of ST deviation at some defined point in the ventricular complex. It is recommended that this point be located 0.04 ms after the J point.

(i) Variable ST-segment deviation (see (a) (i) above)

(g) *Coved ST segment.* Concave upward

(h) *Arched ST segment.* Convex upward

(i) *Ascending ST segment*

(j) *Descending ST segment*

(k) *Flat ST segment*

   The terms (g)–(k) are used alone or together with items (e) and (f).

(l) *Dome-dart ST-T complex.* A relatively stereotyped drug effect (rarely also seen in control records) consists of ST-T complexes in which the ST segment and first limb of the T wave form a rounded arch. This terminates in a spike that peaks and is followed by the terminal limb of the T wave. These dome-dart T waves are positive in leads rV_2 and V_2, and negative in lead V_{10} (see ❷ Fig. 9.13).

(m) *Symmetrical T waves.* Ordinarily, the first limb of the T wave has a more gradual slope than the final limb. T waves that increase in amplitude may also become symmetrical (e.g., with excitement or during hyperkalemia).

(n) *Concordant T waves.* These have the same polarity as the predominant direction of the QRS complex and discordant T waves have the opposite polarity.

(o) *Prolonged terminal QRS forces.* Delays in intraventricular conduction or heritable patterns of ventricular excitation produce broad S waves.

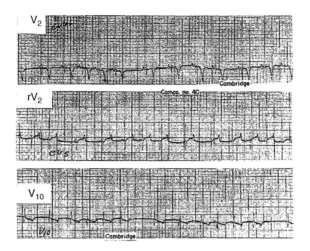

⊙ Fig. 9.13

Dome-dart T waves in leads rV$_2$ and V$_{10}$ accompanied by deep negative T waves in lead V$_2$ and QT prolongation (0.28 s). This beagle dog was receiving toxic doses of a tricyclic antidepressant neuroleptic drug with antihistaminic and local anesthetic properties (After Detweiler [25]. © CRC Press. With permission)

(p) *Prominent U wave.* U waves are ordinarily absent or less than 0.05 mV in amplitude. They are regarded as prominent when their amplitude exceeds 0.05 mV.

(q) *R/S ratio.* This amplitude ratio is usually greater than 0.5 in rV2 and greater than 0.9 in V2 and V4. In disease (e.g., cardiomyopathy, focal cardiac hypertrophy), the ratio changes ordinarily by a reciprocal decrease in R and increase in S amplitudes.

(r) *High-amplitude Ta wave.* The Ta waves are usually absent or of low amplitude. A distinct increase may be apparent after certain drugs.

(s) *Afterpotential.* This is a distinct positive or negative potential change following the T wave that is of far greater amplitude and duration than the U wave.

9.6.2 Pattern Code for Various Types of PQRST Complexes

Various influences including autonomic and electrolyte changes, drugs, and disease affect the contour of the ECG. For descriptive purposes, frequently occurring patterns may be coded by capital letters as shown in ⊙ Fig. 9.3.

9.7 Electrocardiographic Abnormalities: Diagnostic Criteria

The diagnostic criteria for specific cardiac lesions in dogs are far less reliable than those for humans for several reasons:

(a) The database for normal ranges is small.

(b) The great variation in body size and chest conformation among the various breeds of dogs increases the morphological extremes of electrocardiographic complexes in chest leads.

(c) The T waves are labile, change morphology spontaneously, and may reverse polarity in all conventional leads except rV$_2$ and V$_{10}$.

(d) ST-segment and STj-point deviation from isopotential is variable and in some normal dogs is large.

(e) Changes in the forelimb position produce marked swings in frontal plane vectors.

(f) Limb-lead P-wave morphology is normally extremely variable.

9.7.1 Hypertrophy

The electrocardiographic criteria for chamber enlargement are rather reliable for right ventricular hypertrophy (RVH), but unreliable for left ventricular hypertrophy (LVH) and for atrial enlargement.

9.7.1.1 Right Ventricular Hypertrophy

The 12 electrocardiographic criteria for the diagnosis of RVH are given in ❷ Table 9.10 [86]. Three or more of these criteria were present in 93% of dogs with RVH, the corresponding false-positive rate being about 1% [86]. An example is given in ❷ Fig. 9.14.

◻ Table 9.10

Electrocardiographic criteria in order of relative frequency in which they occurred in 70 dogs with right ventricular hypertrophy and in 70 normal dogs matched by breed, age, and sex [85]. The first column lists the rank order of 12 diagnostic electrocardiographic criteria for right ventricular hypertrophy. Two of the 12 criteria have the same rank order of 1, since their relative frequencies (given in the fourth column) are the same. The numbers listed in the sixth column are totals representing the number of abnormal dogs out of 70 which had three or more of the electrocardiographic criteria listed by rank order *above* and row in which the number appears. Thus, for example, 57 dogs out of 70 had three or more of the six criteria listed under rank orders 1–5

Rank	Criteria	Lead	Relative frequency in dogs with right ventricular enlargement	Relative frequency in normal dogs [a]	Number of abnormal dogs with three or more ECG abnormalities	Relative frequency
1	S > 0.80 mV	V2	79.4	7.1		
1	Frontal plane QRS mean electric axis from +103° clockwise to 0°	I and aVF	79.4	0		
2	S > 0.70 mV	V4	78.8	2.9		
3	S > 0.05 mV	I	77.1	0		
4	R/S ratio < 0.87	V4	62.1	0		
5	Transverse plane QRS mean electric axis from +105° clockwise to −31°	I and V10	60.7	1.4		
6	QRS algebraic sum > −0.20 mV	I	55.7	0	57	81.4
7	S > 0.35 mV	II	50.0	0	60	85.7
8	Sagittal plane QRS mean electric axis from +91° clockwise to −12°	aVF and V10	32.8	0	61	87.1
9	A > 0.30 mV	aVR	29.4	0	62	88.6
10	Positive T > 0.25 mV	I	12.9	0	63	90.0
11	R'	II	11.4	0	64	91.5
					65	92.9

[a] None of the normal dogs had ECG abnormalities

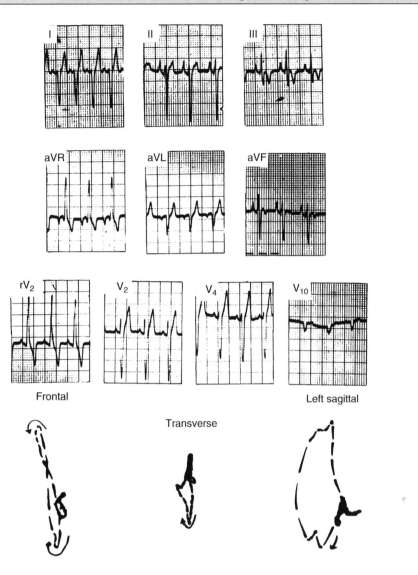

◘ Fig. 9.14
Right ventricular hypertrophy electrocardiographic patterns and VCGs from a 6-month-old Dalmatian with congenital pulmonic stenosis. The mean QRS axis is shifted far to the right (about −145 degrees), TrV_2 is negative, TV_{10} is positive and the vector loops rotate in a clockwise direction except for the final part of the figure-of-eight loop in the frontal plane (Wilson equilateral tetrahedron lead system) (Courtesy of D. F. Patterson)

9.7.1.2   Left Ventricular Hypertrophy

Reliable criteria for the electrocardiographic diagnosis of LVH in dogs are not available. This is unfortunate since LVH secondary to mitral insufficiency is the most common form of chamber enlargement seen clinically in dogs [24].

The electrocardiographic findings compatible with LVH are tall R waves, wide QRS complexes, deep negative T waves in leads II, III, aVF, and V_{10} and a mean QRS axis in the frontal plane directed toward the left. The reason these findings are not diagnostic is that they may be present in normal dogs and absent in dogs with marked LVH [24]. The QRS axis and loop are usually not altered in dogs with confirmed LVH. Young dogs between 6 and 24 months of age are especially likely to have tall R waves, exceeding 3 mV in leads II, III, and aVF, and exceeding 4 mV in leads V_2 and V4. On the other hand, such tall R waves in older dogs in the presence of QRS intervals greater than 0.07 s, a frontal mean QRS axis of less than 45°, deep negative T waves in leads I, II, III, and aVF, and the notching or slurring of the QRS complex are findings that indicate the possibility of LVH. In some cases of LVH, enormous R waves are present (e.g., 7.7 mV in lead III) [95]. On the other hand, in a series of 41 Newfoundlands with congenital subaortic stenosis, 31 had normal ECGs and the electrocardiographic features found in 10 cases with the most severe stenoses (atrial fibrillation in 4, ventricular extrasystoles in 3, RII greater than 2.5 mV in 3, and notching of QRS in 1) were not diagnostic of LVH [96].

9.7.1.3   Atrial Enlargement

Commonly in textbooks, a tall P wave is described as indicating right atrial enlargement and a wide P wave as indicating left atrial enlargement. However, these criteria are too often incorrect. It is likely better to just assume that if the P wave is either too tall or too wide that one of the atria is enlarged. Also, with atrial enlargement, the large P wave is sometimes accompanied by exaggerated T_a waves [23, 97]. Tall P waves are common in certain breeds (e.g., greyhounds) and P waves exceeding 0.4 mV are seen occasionally in young beagles as well as other breeds. Also, remember that a high sympathetic tone with fast rates results in tall P waves. This is also true if adrenergic drugs or parasympatholytic drugs are given.

9.7.2   Bundle Branch Block

The QRS interval is 0.08 s or longer in both right and left bundle branch block. In the right bundle branch block (RBBB) (❯ Fig. 9.15), the widest part of the QRS complex is directed downward in leads I, II, III, aVF, the left precordial leads V_2 and V_4, and V_{10}, while it is upright in lead aVL, the right precordial lead rV_2, and in aVR. In the left bundle branch block (LBBB) this pattern is reversed. The widest part of the QRS complex is upright in the standard limb leads and aVF, as well as the left precordial leads V_2, V_4, and V_{10}. It is negative in the leads aVR, aVL, and rV_2.

The electrocardiographic pattern of RBBB can occur in the absence of organic heart disease in dogs [78, 95]. Complete RBBB (QRS complex > 0.08 s) or incomplete RBBB (same distribution of S waves but the QRS complex < 0.08 s) can exist (❯ Fig. 9.15). When an S wave is identified in the anterior leads and left precordial leads, the following are potential reasons:

(a) Right bundle branch block (clinical and experimental)
(b) Left anterior hemiblock (experimental section of the left anterior fascicle of the left bundle branch [96])
(c) Localized hypertrophy of the free right ventricular wall at the outflow tract [94, 95]

Although the ECG criteria for bundle branch blocks are generally accepted amongst veterinary cardiologists, there is some descent as to their validity. Rosenbaum et al. [98] found that in experimental dogs, a section of the left anterior or the left posterior fascicles of the His bundle failed to produce characteristic changes in the limb-lead ECG when the heart was in the normal position, although this could be achieved by placing the heart in a more "horizontal" position by constructing a sling from the pericardium. Similarly, in a study by Okuma [99], the changes in the limb-lead and leads V_1 and V_5 of dogs caused by sectioning these fascicles were minor.

9.7.3   Bypass Conduction

(a) *Preexcitation.* Preexcitation occurs when the more distal heart is prematurely activated because supraventricular impulses travel via an accessory pathway to the distal AV node or the ventricles. This additional path of conduction is in addition to the normal conduction pathway. The accessory pathways are indeed anatomical structures [100]. In the dog, preexcitation is usually associated with a short PR interval. If this preexcitation has episodes of supraventricular tachycardia, the Wolff–Parkinson–White (WPW) syndrome is the most common diagnosis (❯ Fig. 9.16). This conduction disorder is rare in dogs, occurring in approximately 1 in 2,000 experimental beagles [25] and in 1 in 3,000 clinic patients [101]. Bypass tachycardias can be concealed such that during normal heart rates, the premature activation is not identified by a short PR interval.

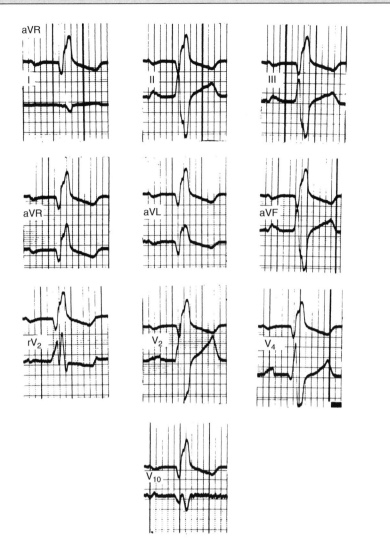

⬛ Fig. 9.15
Right bundle branch block pattern from a 12-year-old male poodle with chronic mitral insufficiency, myocardial disease, and congestive heart failure. The upper trace is lead aVR in each record. Note the RR′ complex in lead rV_2; the wide part of the QRS complex is negative in leads I, II, III, aVR, V_2, V_4, and V_{10}, while it is positive in leads aVR and aVL. Paper speed is 75 mm s^{-1}

9.8 Rhythm Abnormalities

9.8.1 Supraventricular Arrhythmias

9.8.1.1 Sinus Rhythms

The normal heart rate for dogs under clinical conditions is about 60–120 bpm. The heart rates given in data from dog ECGs [25] vary from 34 to 238 bpm. Such extremes would be abnormal if sustained, but when observed in a short ECG strip, are frequently not representative of the unperturbed heart rate. Heart rates determined from the ECG represent values obtained under some degree of duress. They must be interpreted with care.

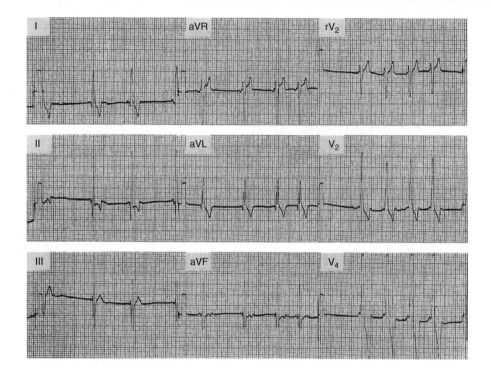

☐ **Fig. 9.16**
Wolff-Parkinson-White syndrome in a research beagle control record. The time intervals are: PR, 0.04; QRS, 0.08; and PJ, 0.12 s. The delta wave is positive in all three precordial leads

Sinus bradycardia and tachycardia. Heart rates in individual ECGs below 60 and above 180 bpm may be arbitrarily designated bradycardia and tachycardia, respectively.

(a) *Sinus bradycardia. Sinus bradycardia* can be found occasionally in otherwise normal dogs. Long and associates [102, 103] demonstrated a substantial reduction in the average heart rate of groups of dogs (e.g., from a mean of 86 bpm upon first examination to 66 bpm for a group of 60 dogs) with restraint for 2 h in a quiet, isolated environment. Under these circumstances heart rates as low as 48 bpm were observed. Sick sinus syndrome is a disorder that is characterized by sinus bradycardia that often has long sinus pauses that can extend for more than 8 s and result in syncope. Moreover, some dogs are afflicted with episodes of supraventricular tachycardias in addition to the bradycardia and pauses. Sick sinus syndrome is most common in miniature schnauzers, cocker spaniels, dachshunds, and West Highland white terriers.

(b) *Sinus tachycardia.* It can be physiologic, in response to a pathologic condition or actually pathologic in and of itself. During the recording of an ECG in some dogs, the heart rate can be as high as 180 bpm, but rates exceeding 190–200 bpm are suspect. Based on Holter recordings, normal healthy dogs can obtain heart rates as high as 300 bpm for very brief times (<10 s) associated with excitement, fear, or acute pain. Kennel activities such as feeding time and the presence of strangers are likely to induce rapid heart rates in groups of dogs, even though the ECGs are taken at a distant location. Sinus tachycardia is expected in certain disease states; for example, anemia, fever, hemorrhage, shock, and congestive heart failure. As mentioned before, it has been found in toxicological studies that sustained (e.g., several hours daily over several days) sinus tachycardia exceeding 190–200 bpm results in myocardial damage with lesions (hemorrhage and necrosis, followed by fibrosis) in left ventricular subendocardium and papillary muscles.

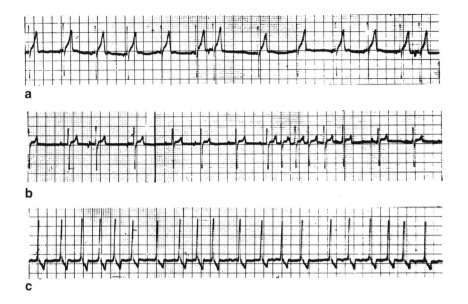

☉ Fig. 9.17
Atrial arrhythmias: (a) atrial premature beats. Two premature atrial beats with deeply inverted P waves are present, one in the middle and one at the end of the record (lead rV$_2$ of an eleven-year-old male cocker spaniel with mitral insufficiency). Part (b), a run of atrial tachycardia occurs after the seventh complex The P waves vary in shape from beat to beat, the PR interval is prolonged (0.16 s, first-degree AV block) and P waves are partially buried in the preceding T waves during the tachycardia (lead rV$_2$ of a nine-year-old male boxer with aortic body tumor infiltrating the right atrium). Part (c), atrial fibrillation. The ventricular rate has been slowed to 140 bpm with digoxin therapy (lead V$_2$ of a thirteen-year-old male Doberman pinscher with mitral insufficiency and congestive heart failure)

9.8.1.2 Atrial Rhythms

(a) *Atrial extrasystole* (see ☉ Fig. 9.17a). Premature atrial complexes are also known as atrial extrasystoles. They can originate from any location above the AV node. They may be singles, couplets, or triplets. If excessively premature, atrial extrasystoles can arrive at the AV node during the refractory period and not result in ventricular activation. In such cases, only a nonconducted P wave is identified.(b) *Atrial tachycardia* (see ☉ Fig. 9.17b). As with other atrial arrhythmias, the normally variable P waves complicate this diagnosis. Paroxysmal atrial tachycardia (PAT) with (AV) block occurs in digitalis intoxication in dogs especially when complicated by hypokalemia [98]. Such arrhythmias secondary to digitalis intoxication are far less common today because dosing (including the total dose used) is more cautious than in the past.

(c) *Atrial flutter*. It occurs at an atrial rate of usually 340–440 bpm in dogs. Although mechanistically the atrial flutter may vary from atrial tachycardia, difficulty can exist in clearly separating the two rhythms. Atrial flutter classically is characterized by undulating waves (F wave) that result in no baseline. There may be 2:1 AV block which results in a constant RR interval, although more commonly the conduction is varied and an irregular RR pattern prevails.

(d) *Atrial fibrillation*. It occurs at an atrial rate of 500–750 bpm in the dog. See ☉ Fig. 9.17c. The atrial rhythm results in fine undulations of the baseline identified as "f waves." Classically atrial fibrillation is a tachyarrhythmia in which the RR interval is very irregular.

9.8.1.3 Atrioventricular Junctional (Nodal) Rhythms

While studies in the rabbit [103] indicate that there are no pacemaker cells in the AV node, pacemaker cells have been found in the AV node of dogs [104]. Because of earlier findings in the rabbit, the term atrioventricular nodal rhythms was changed to AV junctional rhythms or His-bundle rhythms since pacemaker cells are found in the region of the AV node, especially in the His bundle [105]. Because the precise origin of these ectopic beats cannot be determined in the ECG, the more general term, AV junction, is preferable. The AV junctional escape beats occur as a subsidiary pacemaker when the sinus rate falls below 60 bpm. The inherent escape rhythm rate of the AV junctional region is 40–60 bpm. Single escape complexes can occur after long sinus pauses or after AV nodal block. The AV junctional escaperhythms occur as a sustained rhythm to "rescue" the heart when the sinus node fails to fire sufficiently or the AV node is blocked.

9.8.2   Ventricular Rhythms

9.8.2.1   Ventricular Escape Rhythm

When the sinus node and AV junctional subsidiary pacemakers fail to fire, the heart is rescued by a ventricular escape beat or, if sustained for more than three complexes in a row, a ventricular escape rhythm. For most dogs, the rate of the secondary pacemakers from the Purkinje system in the ventricle is between 20 and 30 bpm. These can be seen on occasion during Holter recordings of normal dogs that are sleeping.

9.8.2.2   Ventricular Extrasystoles

Ectopic premature complexes originating from the ventricle are termed as: (1) ventricular extrasystoles, (2) ventricular premature complexes, or (3) premature ventricular complexes. Their prevalence in control records from beagles varies from 0.6% to 1.0% [25], which approximates to that reported in human ECGs [21]. Accordingly, the occurrence of ventricular extrasystoles in an occasional animal may not be related to drugs or disease. When ventricular extrasystoles alternate with normal complexes, the term to describe the pattern is ventricular bigeminy. See ❷ Fig. 9.18.

9.8.2.3   Ventricular Parasystole

For this and more complex arrhythmias, long recording times of the cardiac rhythm are required. Of the electrocardiographic criteria for parasystole, the most controversial is the mathematical relation of the interectopic intervals. As this type of ventricular rhythm has been studied, the initial "rules" to make this diagnosis have been altered as the complexity has been more fully understood. In the simplified understanding of ventricular parasystole, the ventricular ectopic pacemaker discharges with complete regularity, and the interectopic intervals (the intervals between two consecutive ectopic beats that are separated by intervening sinus beats) are nearly an exact multiple of the ectopic cycle length (the time interval between two consecutive ectopic beats without any intervening sinus beats). This is the case in humans with this arrhythmia [8], but is more difficult to identify in dogs. The ectopic cycle length can vary for a variety of reasons including:

(a) Changes in the fundamental discharge rate
(b) Delay in conduction from the ectopic focus to responsive myocardium

In dogs, the most likely cause of alterations in the ectopic cycle length is the presence of sinus arrhythmia associated with the parasystole. It has been demonstrated experimentally [106–108] that a parasystolic focus is protected, but not insulated by a surrounding area of depressed excitability, and can be modulated by electrical events in surrounding tissues; the ectopic cycle length can be lengthened or shortened by electrotonic influences [109]. In man, the parasystolic focus is seldom completely regular and can be altered by vagal reflexes (e.g., carotid sinus pressure), while the timing of normotopic beats during interectopic intervals [110] and the ectopic cycle length can change abruptly without intervention [111]. Also, in the intact heart, neurogenic, endocrine, and hemodynamic factors can change the discharge rate of parasystolic foci

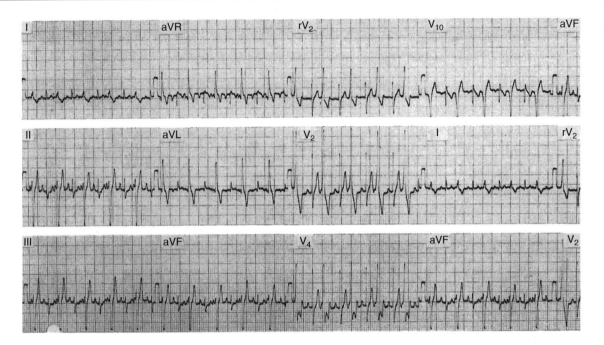

☐ Fig. 9.18
Ventricular bigeminy. This arrhythmia appeared in a control group beagle bitch in a routine ECG taken on day 1813 of a chronic drug trial. A record taken 16 days later was normal and no cardiac lesions were observed at necropsy 14 days later

[110]. Further, the human heart can give rise to coupled ventricular extrasystoles and ventricular parasystole at different times from the same focus [111].

9.8.2.4 Ventricular Tachycardia

Ventricular tachycardia (VT) is a rapid succession of impulses originating from below the AV node. The rate of VT is one which is greater than the inherent rate of the Purkinje fibers in the ventricle which is approximately 30 bpm. In the dog, the usual rate of VT can be one that approximates a normal sinus rhythm (named idioventricular tachycardia) or be as rapid as 500 bpm. The latter rate usually can be maintained for less than a second.

The causes of VT in the dog are varied and include noncardiac and cardiac diseases. Noncardiac diseases include trauma both directly to the heart and indirectly such as to the cranium, gastric torsion, neoplasia, and varied causes of hemodynamic compromise. Several breeds have inherited ventricular arrhythmias that can cause sudden death [112–138]. Boxers are afflicted with arrhythmogenic right ventricular cardiomyopathy [112–118]. This disease results in a distinctive VT that is characterized by a positive QRS complex VT in the anterior (leads II, III, and aVF) leads since the arrhythmia originates from the right ventricle. Rate of the VT in the boxer is very high (frequently 250–300 bpm) and often results in syncope when it is sustained. Some boxers die suddenly while others do not, either due to treatment or chance, but do develop congestive heart failure as the disease progresses. German shepherds are afflicted with inherited ventricular arrhythmias that primarily are manifested in young dogs between the ages of 13 and 70 weeks. Sudden death can occur without prodromes that give evidence of the disease [119? –138]. Most commonly, the VT in the German shepherd is usually characterized as a nonsustained polymorphic rapid ventricular tachycardia. Ventricular tachycardia also is documented in Dobermans with dilated cardiomyopathy and other dogs with myocardial failure.

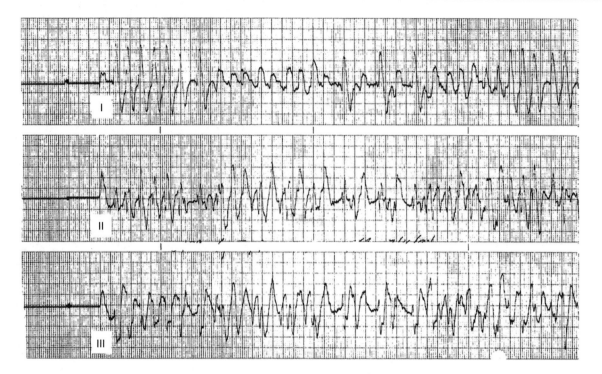

◻ Fig. 9.19

Multiform ventricular flutter (torsades de pointes). This arrhythmia was induced during a subchronic toxicity study with an experimental class I antiarrhythmic agent in an experimental beagle. The ventricular rate varies from 240 to 260 bpm

Drugs can induce VT in dogs with structurally normal hearts, but more commonly when ischemia or other disorders are present. When drugs are screened, the development of VT is considered a marked adverse response to a drug.

(a) *Torsades des pointes.* Torsades des pointes is a specific type of VT that is characterized by a rapid polymorphic VT that shows the complexes changing polarity and morphology as though around a line similar to the twisting of a fence (thus the name). This particular arrhythmia has been the reason for extensive studies of many drugs, both cardiac and noncardiac to assure that the investigated drug does not induce torsades des pointes. This rhythm is induced most likely because of the drug's effects on repolarization currents that result in prolongation of the QT interval. Many drugs have been identified to induce prolongation of the QT and torsades des pointes, and an international registry exists for the logging of cases of prolonged QT (see www.qtdrugs.org). Examples of drugs known to prolong the QT interval include quinidine, disopyramide, lidocaine, procainamide, prenylamine, phenothiazines, and tricyclic antidepressants [139]. It can be induced experimentally by burst pacing hearts with coronary occlusion in dogs, given 30 mg kg^{-1} of quinidine [140] (❯ Fig. 9.19).

9.8.2.5 Atrioventricular Dissociation

The term AV dissociation often should not be considered an "arrhythmia," but only the result of an arrhythmia [19]. AV dissociation occurs when the atria and ventricles are depolarizing independently. This general category includes arrhythmias such as the third-degree heart block and ventricular tachycardia. Isorhythmic dissociation (same rhythm rate but not associated) occurs when the rates of the sinus and ventricular discharge are almost exact (❯ Fig. 9.20).

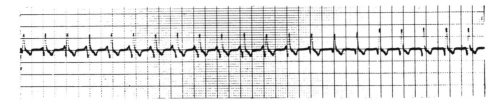

◼ Fig. 9.20

Isorhythmic atrioventricular dissociation: starting with the second complex, the p waves are seen to separate sequentially from the Q wave then move forward to fuse with the Q wave again, decreasing its amplitude for three beats, after which it moves further forward to fuse with the R wave, increasing its amplitude in the final five complexes (accrochage). Lead V_2 of a six-year-old male Labrador retriever with cor pulmonale caused by heartworm infestation and congestive heart failure is shown. The arrhythmia was caused by digoxin intoxication

9.8.3 Atrial and Atrioventricular Conduction Disorders

9.8.3.1 Intra-atrial Conduction Disorders

(a) *Sinoatrial block.* Although this arrhythmia occurs spontaneously in dogs [23], the diagnosis of SA block usually cannot be made with certainty at resting heart rates because of the ubiquitous presence of sinus arrhythmia.

(b) *Sinus arrest, sinus standstill.* This electrocardiographic diagnosis indicates that the sinus P waves are absent for an interval that should have included several heartbeats. Such periods of pacemaker arrest are occasionally caused by reflex vagal effects (carotid sinus reflex, vasovagal reflex from the esophagus as induced by passing a stomach tube, etc.) or drug effects that increase baroreceptor sensitivity, and cause central vagal nucleus stimulation (e.g., digitalis, morphine, tranquilizers). In the clinic, it is observed sometimes in the presence of intracranial tumors, atrial disease, and as a hereditary abnormality in certain breeds [25].

(c) *Intra-atrial block.* This term is applied when there is evidence of a conduction delay in the atria causing widening and deformation of the P waves beyond normal limits of variation. As discussed before, the almost universal respiratory sinus arrhythmia is accompanied by marked P-wave variation in amplitude in certain limb leads. The duration of P waves, however, varies little. The notched P waves, in the absence of increased P-wave duration beyond 0.06 s, are not abnormal per se. Conduction defects are indicated when the P-wave duration increases beyond 0.06 s in limb leads. Drugs that slow myocardial conduction, such as type I antiarrhythmic agents, are likely to delay atrial depolarization. Hyperkalemia above 7.5 mEq 1^{-1} will widen P waves and, at higher levels, abolish the P waves entirely. Widening of P waves sometimes accompanies atrial enlargement.

9.8.3.2 Atrioventricular Block

(a) *First-degree AV block.* In this case, the PR interval is prolonged beyond 0.13 s and rarely exceeds 0.20 s. The normal PR interval shortens with increasing heart rate (❯ Table 9.5). When sinus tachycardia is present (i.e., at rates exceeding 150 bpm), the PR interval ordinarily is shortened to less than 0.12 s, so that PR intervals greater than this may be considered first-degree AV block at more rapid heart rates. Not infrequently, the PR interval varies in first-degree AV block, so that only some of the intervals exceed these upper limits.

(b) *Second-degree AV block.* The block may be sporadic or frequent, regular or irregular. It may be preceded by progressively increasing PR intervals, fixed PR intervals, or PR intervals that lengthen and then shorten. The ratio of blocked to conducted beats is only rarely constant in dogs, probably because of the superimposed respiratory sinus arrhythmia that is usually also present: Type I second-degree AV block (Wenckebach phenomenon or Mobitz type I) is more common in dogs than type II. Type II second-degree AV block (Mobitz type II) occurs in otherwise normal dogs only sporadically and often at fairly rapid heart rates. Although this conduction disorder (see ❯ Chap. 6 of *Cardiac Arrhythmias and Mapping Techniques*) is reputed to occur in man only in the presence of organic heart disease [21], this is not true in dogs. Most likely, it occurs in dogs as a more-or-less physiological phenomenon when, for some reason, there is a sudden, transient increase in vagal tone that blocks AV conduction for just a single cardiac cycle. When encountered, however, the presence of organic heart disease should be ruled out by further cardiac examination. In some dogs, type I second-degree AV block develops at slower sinus rates, when type II has occurred as an isolated event at a more rapid rate.

Except for type II (Mobitz) second-degree AV block in dogs, first-degree and second-degree AV blocks are generally simply normal physiological variants.

(c) *Third-degree AV block*. Third-degree AV block is a common bradyarrhythmia in the dog that demands the implantation of a permanent pacemaker. Although underlying myocardial disease that will eventually affect hemodynamic function exists, most dogs respond well to this treatment. Usually, the atrial rate is rapid (e.g., 105–145 bpm) and the ventricular rate is slow (e.g., 25–30 bpm). Syncope or weakness is a common clinical sign. If not treated, heart failure or sudden death will result in spontaneous cases [23].

In experimental AV block, following the crushing of the His bundle, ventricular rates were 49 ± 2 bpm after surgery and reached a plateau by day 31 at 44 ± 2 bpm [141]. This rate continued to the end of the 3-year observation period. One to 4 weeks after creating the AV block, other authors have reported similar rates, for example, Hurwitz [142] found an atrial rate of 120–200 bpm and a ventricular rate of 26–54 bpm; Reynolds and DiSalvo [143] found a ventricular rate of 55 ± 13 bpm; and Robinson et al. [144] gave an atrial rate of 125 ± 10 bpm and a ventricular rate of 37 ± 3 bpm.

9.8.4　Frequency of Arrhythmias in the Human and the Dog

The ideal way to evaluate the frequency of arrhythmias in any species is with a 24-h Holter. However, with a large number of subjects, an appreciation of the number of arrhythmias in a population can be gleaned. It must be understood that if the arrhythmia number is restricted to ECG recordings for a brief period, also in the situation whereby an animal is stressed by the procedure, the amount of arrhythmias will be different than in circumstances that do not provoke the autonomic nervous system as much. These latter conditions would include the 24-h Holter and telemetry recordings. Consequently, comparisons must be made with the same techniques. Also, the age of the animal has a bearing on the arrhythmia number.

Comparable electrocardiographic series in the dog and the human are not available. The most relevant data from the human that might be compared with data from young experimental beagles of both sexes are the findings among 67,375 asymptomatic young adult male air force officers from whom 12-lead records were taken [145]. The dog ECGs are from pretest records on 5,513 young (usually 5–7 months old) experimental beagles from which pretest records were taken before being used in toxicity trials. In about 90% of the beagles, two ten-lead ECGs taken several days apart were available. The overall arrhythmia prevalence rates in the two groups were similar (27.9 per thousand for the human against 25.6 per thousand for the dog). The prevalence of ventricular ectopic beats for the human (6.2 per thousand) was about the same as for the dog (8.0 per thousand). Note that the first-degree AV block is more common in the human than in the dog, while the reverse is true for the second-degree AV block. Ventricular parasystole may be more prevalent in beagles than in humans, as may be ventricular escape rhythms, and electrical alternans. Wolff–Parkinson–White syndrome and the bundle branch block may be more common in humans. However, because of the disparities between the data and their collection and analysis, comparison is, although interesting, of questionable validity.

9.9　Comparing Serial Electrocardiogram Records

Either in clinical heart disease or in experimental cardiotoxicity, serial ECGs may permit the recognition of electrophysiological changes that presage definite electrocardiographic abnormalities. This requires that the latest record from each dog should be compared with the previous records to detect subtle changes that are not necessarily outside normal limits. Ideally, adequate numbers of dogs are included in control and treated groups such that a statistical evaluation can be made; however, often studies are undertaken with very low numbers of animals (particularly pilot investigations), and this necessitates comparisons among dogs for treatment effects. Because of the variability in recording the ECG, however, enough of a difference must be documented in order to say that the change is less likely to be due to chance. The following is a list of changes that, if exceeded, require further examination. Note that the following are suggested from experience and not based on the variability analysis. In toxicity trials, their significance is increased if several individuals in a dose group are similarly affected. It should be emphasized that these differences are based on testimonial experience of the author. Ideally, studies to document repeatability and variability between recordings for each study group are needed for precision. However, these can serve as a beginning for comparisons.

(a) Increases in time intervals
   P wave + 20 ms
   PR interval + 30 ms (when not rate related, see ❯ Table 9.5)
   Second-degree AV block
   QRS interval + 15 ms
   QT + 40 ms (when not rate related, see ❯ Table 9.5)
(b) QRS frontal plane axis: change of 30°
(c) Increases in amplitude
   R-wave amplitude increased by 0.7 mV
   T-wave amplitude increased by 50%
   ST-segment deviation greater than 0.15 mV
(d) Sinus arrhythmia index ($I = 100$ [R-R standard deviation/mean R-R]):
   substantial decrease in the absence of a commensurate increase in heart rate
(e) Contour and polarity
   P reversal in any limb lead
   ST-segment slurring

Reversal of T-wave polarity (caution is advised when the evaluation involves a very young dog and also when a dog is close to 1 year of age)

9.10 Cardiotoxic and Drug Effects on the Electrocardiogram

An important sphere of canine electrocardiography is the detection of myocardial injury and of altered regulation of cardiac activity in drug trials, nutritional studies, immunopathological responses, and in the veterinary clinic. Although the injurious agents are legion, the types of electrophysiological changes possible are limited, so that the diagnosis of specific chemical or biological agent effects is not possible through electrocardiography. Certain classes of drugs and chemicals, however, produce characteristic constellations of electrophysiological changes, so that when the test agent is known or suspected, its presence may often be predicted from the electrocardiographic findings.

Reviews of cardiotoxicity and myocardial injury include those of Böhle [146], Wenzel [147], Selye [148], Chung and Dean [149], Davies and Gold [150], Bristow [151], Balazs [152], Van Stee [153], and Spitzer [154]. Reviews dealing principally with electrocardiological drug effects include those of Scherf and Schott [8], Bellet [18, 19], Surawicz and Lasseter [155], Surawicz [156, 157], Vaughan Williams [158], Singh et al. [159], Schamroth [20], Detweiler [25], Harrison [160], and Lazdunski and Renaud [161].

9.10.1 Drug Effects on Transmembrane Action Potentials and ECG Changes

The relationship between transmembrane action potential changes and electrocardiographic changes is known for a number of drugs and electrolytes. From simultaneous records of ventricular transmembrane potentials and ECGs, the influence of transmembrane potential (TMP) effects on the ECG can be shown [161].

(a) When the slope of phase 0 of the TMP is decreased, conduction velocity is slowed, and in the ECG the QRS increases in duration (e.g., quinidine and other type I antiarrhythmics).

(b) The duration of the TMP approaches that of the QT interval, so that shortening or lengthening of TMP duration has a directly corresponding effect on the QT interval (e.g., digitalis glycosides shorten and hypocalcemia lengthens the TMP).

(c) Lengthening of phase 2 of the TMP lengthens the ST segment of the ECG and shortening phase 2 has the opposite effect (e.g., hypocalcemia prolongs and digitalis shortens the ST segment).

(d) Increased velocity of repolarization during phase 2 of the TMP reduces or abolishes this plateau and the ST segment of the ECG is abbreviated (e.g., digitalis glycosides).

(e) A more acute transition from the slope of phase 2 to that of phase 3 of the TMP, together with increased slope of phase 3, produces symmetrical peaking of the T waves in the ECG (e.g., hyperkalemia).

(f) A less acute transition from the slope of phase 2 of the TMP to that of phase 3 such that the repolarization configuration approaches a straight line and causes reduction of the T-wave amplitude in the ECG (e.g., barbiturates).

(g) Prolongation and decreased slope of phase 3 of the TMP exaggerates the U wave of the ECG (e.g., hypokalemia).

9.10.1.1   Drug Effects on the ECG

There are some electrocardiographic alterations that are somewhat less well known [26, 162]. This consists of a characteristic configurational change in the form of the ST-T segments in lead rV_2 especially and sometimes also in leads V_2, V_4, and V_{10}. In the precordial leads (rV_2, V_2, and V_4), the ST segment and first portion of the T wave form a convex upward curve and the terminal portion of the T wave forms a positive spike, hence the descriptive term "dome-dart T waves." In lead V_{10}, the ST curve is concave upward and the terminal spike is negative; that is, more or less the reciprocal of the configuration in lead rV_2. This morphological change is usually accompanied by QT-interval prolongation. The duration of QT may vary, depending on the length of the preceding R-R interval in sinus arrhythmia (e.g., from 0.30 to 0.34 s, with the longer QT intervals following the shorter R-R intervals).

This combination of electrocardiographic effects has been observed in toxicological studies with tricyclic antidepressants, phenothiazine derivative and butyrophenone derivative antipsychotic agents, and certain antihistaminic compounds. When the various pharmacological properties of these test agents were known, they combined the central nervous system, antihistaminic, and local anesthetic actions. Often, however, only their central nervous system or antihistaminic effects had been identified at the time of the toxicity trial.

One of these experimental drugs, a butyrophenone derivative neuroleptic, in addition to dome-dart T waves and QT interval prolongation, produced cardiac slowing, first-degree and second-degree AV block, left and right bundle branch block (LBBB and RBBB), and ventricular ectopic beats. Marked sinus arrhythmia was present and the LBBB and RBBB appeared sporadically following short R-R intervals. Frequently, the PR intervals preceding these bizarre complexes were not prolonged beyond normal limits. Ventricular reentrant beats with RBBB configuration followed occasional RBBB beats, and LBBB reentrant beats followed occasional LBBB complexes. Since BBB occurred in the absence of prolonged PR intervals, sometimes it appears that the depression of conduction was relatively greater on the bundle branch Purkinje fibers than on the atrioventricular junctional tissues.

9.10.1.2   The QT Interval

The important thing about QT prolongation is not its possible relation to negative inotropy, but rather its relation to arrhythmia vulnerability. It is one manifestation of increased inhomogeneity of ventricular refractory periods. The long QT syndrome has been an extensive study and the measurement of the QT interval, the subject of thousands of papers. Moreover, the correct evaluation of the QT interval in the dog for toxicological studies is one for continued discussion [51–54], and drugs that prolong the QT interval are associated with sudden death [163]. Evaluation of the QT interval is a mainstay for drug studies; however, adjusting for the QT interval relative to heart rate remains problematic for studies that involve small numbers of animals with brief recordings. The formulas derived for use in humans are not suitable for the dog [50, 51]. Full conferences have been held with this as the focus of attention. As this is a changing field of standards, it is advised to search via the Internet for the latest information at the time of design for studies in the dog for which the QT interval is an integral part of the examination.

9.10.1.3 ST-T and T-Wave Changes

The T waves in dog ECGs are markedly labile. They may be either positive or negative in most leads, and their polarity may change from record to record taken sequentially. The exceptions are lead rV_2 in which the T waves are almost always positive and lead V_{10} in which they are almost always negative. This characteristic of lead V_{10} applies only if the records are taken with the dogs in right lateral recumbency since, for example, V_{10} is frequently positive in beagles placed in the supine position.

The contour, slope, and deviation from the isopotential line of the ST segment in dog ECGs are also quite variable and change spontaneously from record to record taken at different times. Serum electrolyte alterations and cardioactive drugs often reveal their presence by changing the relative durations and contours of the ST segment and T wave. Depending on the magnitude of the change induced, such drug effects may merely alter the form of ST-T complexes in a characteristic way, but not produce a distinctly abnormal record. Thus, the complexes may be judged to be within normal limits of form and duration for the dog ECG, but because similar changes occur in several animals in a given dose group they can be attributed to drug action. For example, some drugs cause the ST-T complexes in several leads to assume a similar contour and polarity. Reversal of T waves in rV_2 and V_{10} is a reliable sign of left ventricular subendocardial and papillary muscle damage (e.g., ischemia, hemorrhage, necrosis) in the dog and, when present in toxicity trials, is accompanied by demonstrable histological lesions in myocardial tissue or small intramural coronary arteries in these regions in about 80% of the cases [164].

9.11 Interpretative Statements

When evaluating ECGs for drug studies, the interpretation is important not only to point out any relevant changes, but also to stress when the changes are unclear because of the vulnerability of the ECG. This is important when a small number of dogs are being studied. The interpretation should include an electrocardiographic diagnosis and relate this to possible electrophysiological mechanisms. It should not go beyond the scope of electrocardiography into possible cardiodynamic or hemodynamic consequences or effects on other organs and tissues. This correlative step can be made only after all the clinical or toxicological information has been assembled.

The interpretative statements should cover the following three areas:

(a) Electrophysiological characteristics detected by the ECG. This will include changes in conductivity and rhythmicity and speculations about the anatomical sites and possible effects on the transmembrane action potentials of the cardiac cell.
(b) Description of electrocardiographic features that may or may not be related to heart disease, cardiotoxicity, or physiological state. These may have a low order of significance in themselves, but may relate to other clinical or toxicological findings. Examples are nonspecific contour changes in ST segments and T waves in various leads.
(c) The likelihood that heart disease or a cardiotoxic effect is present because the physiological state of the heart has been sufficiently altered or because pathological myocardial lesions may be present.

Acknowledgement

Dr. Sydney Moise at Cornell University contributed updates to this chapter.

References

1. Waller, A., Introductory address on the electromotive properties of the human heart. *Br. Med. J.*, 1888;**2**: 751–754.

2. Einthoven, W., Enregistrement galvanométrique de l'électrocardiogramme humain et contrôle des résultats obtenus par l'emploi de l'électromètre capillaire en physiologie. *Arch. Néerland. Sci. Not.*, 1904;**11**(9): 202–209.

3. Einthoven, W., Weiteres über das Elektrokardiogramm. *Pfluegers Arch.*, 1908;**122**: 517–584.

4. Einthoven, W, G. Fahr, and A. de Waart, Über die Richtung und die manifeste Grösse **der** Potentialschwankungen immenschlichen Herzen und über den Einfluss der Herzlage auf die Form des Elektrokardiogramms. *Pfluegers Arch.*, 1913;**150**: 275–315.

5. Waller, A.D., *A Short Account of the Origin and Scope of Electrocardiography. The Harvey Lectures, 1913/14*. Philadelphia, PA: Lippincott, 1915, pp. 17–33.

6. Lewis, T., *The Mechanism and Graphic Registration of the Heart Beat*, 3rd edn. London: Shaw, 1925.

7. Rothberger, C.J., Normale und pathologische Physiologie der Rhythmik unct Koordination des Herzens. *Erg. Physiol.*, 1931;**32**: 472–820.

8. Scherf, D. and A. Schott, *Extrasysto/es and Allied Arrhythmias*, 2nd edn. Chicago, IL: Year Book Medical, 1973.

9. Wenckebach, K.F. and H. Winterberg, *Die unregelmässige-Herztätigket*. Leipzig: Engelman, 1927.

10. Wilson, F.N., F.D. Johnston, and E. Lepeschkin, Editors. *Selected Papers*. Ann Arbor, MI: Heart Station, University Hospital, 1954.

11. Nörr, J., Über Herzstromkurvenaufnahmen an Haustieren. Zur Einführung der Elektrokardiographie in die Veterinärmedizin. *Arch. Wiss. Prakt. Tierheilkd.*, 1922;**48**: 85–111.

12. Roos, J., Vorhofflimmern bei den Haustieren. *Arch. Wiss. Prakt. Tierheilkd.*, 1924;**51**: 280–293.

13. Haupt, K., *Die Aufnahmetechnik des Hundeelektrokardiogramms in der Veterinärklinik und ihre Ergebnisse*, dissertation. Giessen: University of Giessen, 1929.

14. Ludwig, K-H., *Die Elektrokardiographie beim gesunden Hund unter besonderer Berücksichtigung ihrer Anwendung in der Klinik*, dissertation. Leipzig: University of Leipzig, 1924.

15. Gyarmati, E., *Klinische elektrokardiographische Untersuchungen beim Hunde*, dissertation. Budapest: University of Budapest, 1939.

16. Lannek, N.A., *Clinical and Experimental Study on the Electrocardiogram in Dogs*, dissertation. Stockholm: Royal Veterinary College, 1949.

17. Burch, G.E. and N.P. DePasquale, *A History of Electrocardiography*. Chicago, IL: Year Book Medical, 1964.

18. Bellet, S., *Clinical Disorders of the Heart Beat*, 2nd edn. Philadelphia, PA: Lea & Febiger, 1963.

19. Bellet, S., *Essentials of Cardiac Arrhythmias: Diagnosis and Management*. Philadelphia, PA: Saunders, 1972.

20. Schamroth, L., *The Disorders of Cardiac Rhythm*, vols. 1, 2, 2nd edn. London: Blackwell Scientific, 1980.

21. Ettinger, S.J. and P.F. Suter, *Canine Cardiology*. Philadelphia, PA: Saunders, 1970.

22. Detweiler, D.K., D.F. Patterson, J.W. Buchanan, and D.N. Knight, The cardiovascular system, in *Canine Medicine*, vol. 2, 4th edn., E.J. Catcott, Editor. Santa Barbara, CA: American Veterinary, 1979, pp. 813–949.

23. Bolton, G.R., *Handbook of Canine Electrocardiography*. Philadelphia, PA: Saunders, 1975.

24. Tilley, L.P., *Essentials of Canine and Feline Electrocardiography*, 2nd edn. Philadelphia, PA: Lea & Febiger, 1985.

25. Detweiler, D.K., The use of electrocardiography in toxicological studies with Beagle dogs, in *Cardiac Toxicology*, vol. 3, T. Balazs, Editor. Boca Raton, FL: CRC Press, 1981, pp. 33–82.

26. Lautenschlager, O., *Grundlagen der Aufnahmetechnik des Elektrokardiogrammes von Pferd und Rind und ihre Ergebnisse*, dissertation. Giessen: University of Giessen, 1928.

27. Nehb, W., Zur Standardisierung der Brustwandableitungen des Elektrokardiogramms. *Klin. Wchnschr.*, 1938;**17**: 1807–1811. Cited by Lepeschkin, E., *Modern Electrocardiography*, vol. 1. Baltimore, MD: Williams & Wilkins, 1951.

28. Spörri, H., Der Einfluss der Tuberkulose auf das Elektrokardiogramm. (Untersuchungen an Meerschweinchen und Rindern.) *Arch. Wiss. Prakt. Tierheilkd.*, 1944;**79**: 1–57.

29. Detweiler, D.K., The use of electrocardiography in toxicological studies with rats, in *The Rat Electrocardiogram in Pharmacology and Toxicology*, R. Budden, D.K. Detweiler, and G. Zbinden, Editors. Oxford: Pergamon, 1981, pp. 83–115.

30. Hellerstein, H.K. and R. Hamlin, QRS component of the spatial vectorcardiogram and of the spatial magnitude and velocity electrocardiograms of the normal dog. *Am. J. Cardiol.*, 1960;**6**: 1049–1061.

31. Hahn, A.W., R.L. Hamlin, and D.F. Patterson, Standards for canine electrocardiography. *Academy of Veterinary Cardiology Committee Report*, 1977.

32. Kraus, M.S., N.S. Moise, M. Rishniw, et al. Morphology of ventricular arrhythmias in the boxer as measured by 12-lead electrocardiography with pace-mapping comparison. *J. Vet. Intern. Med.*, 2002;**16**(2): 153–158.

33. McFee, R. and A. Parungao, An orthogonal lead system for clinical electrocardiography. *Am. Heart J.*, 1961;**62**: 93–100.

34. Bloch, W.N. Jr., K.A. Busch, and T.R. Lewis, The Frank vectorcardiogram of the Beagle dog. *J. Electrocardiol.*, 1972;**5**: 119–125.

35. Bojrab, M.J., J.E. Breazile, and R.D. Morrison, Vectorcardiography in normal dogs using; the Frank lead system. *Am. J. Vet. Res.*, 1971;**32**: 925–934.

36. Morita, H., Electrocardiograms of conscious Beagle dogs by apex-base bipolar lead. *Adv. Anim. Cardiol.*, 1984;**17**: 19–23.

37. Sugano, S., Electrocardiographic studies in the beagle as an experimental dog. *Adv. Anim. Electrocardiography*, 1977;**10**: 45–50.

38. Takahashi, M., Experimental studies on the electrocardiogram of the dog. *Jpn. J. Vet. Sci.*, 1964;**24**: 191–210.

39. Cagan, S., Prespevok k elektrokardiogramu, psa. *Bratisl. Lek. Listy.*, 1959;**39**: 540–545.

40. Cagan, S. and E. Barta, Die Bedingungen des konstanten Elektrokardiogrammes beim Hund. *Z. Kreislaufforsch.*, 1959;**48**: 1101–1105.

41. Hulin, I. and S. Rippa, Why does the electrocardiogram of the dog change with a change in the foreleg position? *Am. Heart J.*, 1970;**79**: 143.

42. Hill, J.D., The significance of foreleg positions in the interpretation of electrocardiograms and vectorcardiograms from research animals. *Am. Heart J.*, 1968;**75**(4): 518–527.

43. Hill, J.D., The electrocardiogram in dogs with standardized body and limb positions. *J. Electrocardiol.*, 1968;**1**: 175–182.

44. Almasi, J.J., O.H. Schmitt, and E.F. Jankus,. Electrical characteristics of commonly used canine ECG electrodes. *Proc. Annu. Conf. Eng. Med. Biol.*, 1970;**12**: 190.

45. Rydén, L., A. Waldenström, and S. Holmberg, The reliability of intermittent ECG sampling in arrhythmia detection. *Circulation*, 1975;**52**: 540–545.

46. Morganroth, J., Ambulatory monitoring: the impact of spontaneous variability of simple and complex ventricular ectopy, in *Cardiac Arrhythmias*, D.G. Harrison, Editor. Boston, MA: Hall, 1981, pp. 479–492.

47. Moïse, N.S., Diagnosis and management of canine arrhythmias, in *Canine and Feline Cardiology*, 2nd edn., P.R. Fox, D.D. Sisson, N.S. Moïse, Editors. Philadelphia, PA: W. B. Saunders, 1999, pp. 331–385.

48. Grauwiler, J., *Herz und Kreislauf der Säugetiere: Vergleichend-Funktionelle Daten*. Batiel: Birkhäuser,1965.

49. Bazett, H.C., An analysis of the time relations of electrocardiograms. *Heart*, 1920;**7**: 353–370.

50. Chiang, A.Y., D.L. Holdsworth, and D.J. Leishman, A one-step approach to the analysis of the QT interval in conscious telemetrized dogs. *J. Pharmacol. Toxicol. Methods*, 2006 Mar 6; E-print.

51. Miyazaki, H., H. Watanabe, T. Kitayama, M. Nishida, Y. Nishi, K. Sekiya, H. Suganami, and K. Yamamoto, QT PRODACT: sensitivity and specificity of the canine telemetry assay for detecting drug-induced QT interval prolongation. *J. Pharmacol. Sci.*, 2005;**99**(5): 523–529.

52. Gauvin, D.V., L.P. Tilley, F.W. Smith Jr,, and T.J. Baird, Electrocardiogram, hemodynamics, and core body temperatures of the normal freely moving laboratory beagle dog by remote radiotelemetry. *J. Pharmacol. Toxicol. Methods*, 2006;**53**(2): 128–139.

53. Watanabe, H. and H. Miyazaki, A new approach to correct the QT interval for changes in heart rate using a nonparametric regression model in beagle dogs. *J. Pharmacol. Toxicol. Methods*, 2006;**53**(3): 234–241.

54. Camm, A.J., Clinical trial design to evaluate the effects of drugs on cardiac repolarization: current state of the art. *Heart Rhythm*, 2005;**2**(2 Suppl): S23–29. Review.

55. Harada, T., J. Abe, M. Shiotani, Y. Hamada, and I. Horii, Effect of autonomic nervous function on QT interval in dogs. *J. Toxicol. Sci.*, 2005;**30**(3): 229–237.

56. Batchivarov, V.N. and M. Makik, There is little sense in "common" QT correction methods. *J. Cardiovasc. Electrophysiol.*, 2005;**16**(7): 809.

57. Tattersall, M.L., M. Dymond, T. Hammond, and J.P. Valentin, Correction of QT values to allow for increases in heart rate in conscious Beagle dogs in toxicology assessment. *J. Pharmacol. Toxicol. Methods*, 2006;**53**: 11–19.

58. Lewis, T., J. Meakins, P.D. White, The excitatory process in the dog's heart. Part I. The auricles. *Philos. Trans. R. Soc. Lond. Ser. B*, 1914;**205**: 375–420.

59. Meek, W.J. and J.A.E. Eyster, Experiments on the origin and propagation of the impulse in the heart. IV. The effect of vagal stimulation and of cooling on the location of the pacemaker within the sino-auricular node. *Am. J. Physiol.*, 1914;**34**: 368–383.

60. Hinds, M.H., D.R. Clark, J.D. McCrady, and L.A. Geddes, The relationship among pacemaker location, heart rate, and

P-wave configuration in the dog. *J. Electrocardiol.*, 1972;**5**: 56–64.

61. Goldberg, J.M. and M.H. Lynn-Johnson, Changes in canine P wave morphology observed with shifts in intra-SA nodal pacemaker localization. *J. Electrocardiol.*, 1980;**13**: 209–217.

62. Boineau, J.P., R.B. Schuessler, and C.R. Mooney, et al., Multicentric origin of the atrial depolarization wave: the pacemaker complex. *Circulation*, 1978;**58**: 1036–1048.

63. Anonymous (editorial). U waves: unimportant undulations? *Lancet*, 1983;**2**: 776–777.

64. Watanabe, Y. and H. Toda, The U wave and aberrant intraventricular conduction. Further evidence for the Purkinje repolarization theory on genesis of the U wave. *Am. J. Cardiol.*, 1978;**41**: 23–31.

65. Kishida, H., J.S. Cole, and B. Surawicz, Negative U wave: A highly specific but poorly understood sign of heart disease. *Am. J. Cardiol.*, 1982;**49**: 2030–2036.

66. Rudolph, A.M., P.A.M. Auld, R.J. Golinko, and M.H. Paul, Pulmonary vascular adjustments in the neonatal period. *Pediatrics*, 1961;**28**: 28–34.

67. Averill, K.H., W.W. Wagner Jr., and J.H.K. Vogel, Correlation of right ventricular pressure with right ventricular weight. *Am. Heart J.*, 1963;**66**: 632–635.

68. Kirk, G.R., D.M. Smith, D.P. Hutcheson, and R. Kirby, Postnatal growth of the dog heart. *J. Anat.*, 1975;**119**: 461–469.

69. Trautvetter, E., *Untersuchungen zur EKG-Entwicklung an gesunden Welpen und Welpen mitangeborenen Pulmonalstenosen, Habilitationsschrift*. Berlin: Freie Universität Berlin, 1972.

70. Trautvetter, E., D.K. Detweiler, and D.F. Patterson, Evolution of the electrocardiogram in young dogs during the first 12 weeks of life. *J. Electrocardiol.*, 1981;**14**: 267–273.

71. Trautvetter, E., D.K. Detweiler, F.K. Bohn, and D.F. Patterson, Evolution of the electrocardiogram in young dogs with congenital heart disease leading to right ventricular hypertrophy. *J. Electrocardiol.*, 1981;**14**: 275–282.

72. Detweiler, D.K., The cardiovascular system, in *Duke's Physiology of Domestic Animals*, chaps. 5–12, 10th edn., M.J. Swenson, Editor Ithaca, NY: Cornell University Press, 1984, pp. 68–225.

73. Amend, J.F. and H.E. Hoff, Analysis of patterns and parameters of the respiratory heart rate response in the unanesthetized dog. *Southwest. Vet.*, 1970;**22**: 301–311.

74. Fuller, J.L., Genetic variability in some physiological constants of dogs. *Am. J. Physiol.*, 1951;**166**: 20–24.

75. Kleiger, R.E., P.K. Stein, and J.T. Bigger Jr., Heart rate variability: measurement and clinical utility. *Ann. Noninvasive Electrocardiol.*, 2005;**10**(1): 88–101. Review.

76. Werner, J., A. von Recum, E. Trautvetter, and H. Sklaschus, Über den Ruherhythmus des Herzens beim Hund. *Z. Kreislaufforsch.*, 1969;**58**: 593–600.

77. Lange, H., *Ober den Eintritt der Atmungsarrhythmie in der ersten Lebenszeit des Hundes*, dissertation. Munich: University of Munich, 1937.

78. Horan, L., G.E. Burch, and J.A. Cronvich, Spatial vectorcardiograms in normal dogs. *Circ. Res.*, 1957;**5**: 133–136.

79. Horan, L.G., G.E. Burch, and J.A. Cronvich, A study of the influence upon the spatial vectorcardiogram of localized destruction of the myocardium of dog. *Am. Heart J.*, 1957;**53**: 74–90.

80. Horan, L.G., G.E. Burch, and J.A. Cronvich, Spatial vectorcardiogram in dogs with chronic localized myocardial lesions. *J. Appl. Physiol.*, 1960;**15**: 624–628.

81. Hamlin, R.L., F.S. Pipers, and C.R. Smith, Computer methods for analysis of dipolar characteristics of the electrocardiogram. *Am. J. Vet. Res.*, 1968;**29**: 1867–1881.

82. Boineau, J.P., J.D. Hill, M.S. Spach, and E.N. Moore, Basis of the electrocardiogram in right ventricular hypertrophy: relationship between ventricular depolarization and body surface potentials in dogs with spontaneous RVH-contrasted with normal dogs. *Am. Heart J.*, 1968;**76**: 605–627.

83. Chastain, C.B., D.H. Riedesel, and P.T. Pearson, McFee and Parungao. Orthogonal lead vectorcardiography in normal dogs. *Am. J. Vet. Res.*, 1974;**35**: 275–280.

84. Bruninx, P. and H.E. Kulbertus, The McFee-Parungao vectorcardiogram in normal dogs. *J. Electrocardiol.*, 1974;7: 227–236.

85. Detweiler, D.K. and D.F. Patterson, The prevalence and types of cardiovascular disease in dogs. *Ann. N. Y. Acad. Sci.*, 1965;**127**: 481–516.

86. Hill, J.D., Electrocardiographic diagnosis of right ventricular enlargement in dogs. *J. Electrocardiol.*, 1971;**4**: 347–357.

87. Clark, D.R., J.G. Anderson, and C. Paterson, Imperforate cardiac septal defect in a dog. *J. Am. Vet. Med. Assoc.*, 1970;**156**: 1020–1025.

88. Bolton, G.R., S. Ettinger, and J.C. Roush II, Congenital peritoneopericardial diaphragmatic hernia in a dog. *J. Am. Vet. Med. Assoc.*, 1969;**155**: 723–730.

89. Patterson, D.F., Animal models of congenital heart disease (with special reference to patent ductus arteriosus in the dog), in *Animal Models for Biomedical Research.* Washington, DC: National Academy of Sciences Publication 1594, 1968, pp. 131–156.

90. Boineau, J.P., M.S. Spach, and J.S. Harris, Study of premature systoles of the canine heart by means of the spatial vectorcardiogram. *Am. Heart J.*, 1960;**60**: 924–935.

91. Bolton, G.R. and S.J. Ettinger, Right bundle branch block in the dog. *J. Am. Vet. Med. Assoc.*, 1972;**160**: 1104–1119.

92. Blake, D.F. and P. Kezdi, Vectorcardiography in uncomplicated canine bundle branch block. *Circulation*, 1961;**24**: 888–889.

93. De Micheli, A., G.A. Medrano, and D. Sodi-Pallares, Etude électro-vectocardiographique des blocs de branche chez le chien àla lumière du processus d'activation ventriculaire. *Acta Cardiol.*, 1963;**18**: 483–514.

94. Moore, E.N., J.P. Boineau, and D.F. Patterson, Incomplete right bundle-branch block. An electrocardiographic enigma and possible misnomer. *Circulation*, 1971;**44**: 678–687.

95. Littlewort, M.C.G., Canine electrocardiography; some potentialities and limitations of thetechnique. *J. Small Anim. Pract.*, 1967;**8**: 437–458.

96. Pyle, R.L., *A Study of Certain Clinical, Genetical, and Pathological Aspects of Congenital Fibrous Subaortic Stenosis in the Dog*, thesis. Philadelphia, PA: University of Pennsylvania, 1971.

97. Tilley, L.P., *Essentials of Canine and Feline Electrocardiography: Interpretation and Treatment*, 2nd edn. Philadelphia, PA: Lea & Febiger, 1985.

98. Rosenbaum, M.B., M.V. Elizari, and J.O. Lazzari, *The Hemiblocks.* Oldsmar, FL: Tampa Tracings, 1970.

99. Okuma, K., ECG and VCG changes in experimental hemiblock and bifascicular block. *Am. Heart J.*, 1976;**92**: 473–480.

100. Glomset, D.J. and A.T.A. Glomset, A morphologic study of the cardiac conduction system in ungulates, dog, and man. I and II. *Am. Heart J.*, 1940;**20**: 389–98, 677–701.

101. Patterson, D.F., D.K. Detweiler, K. Hubben, and R.P. Botts, Spontaneous abnormal cardiac arrhythmias and conduction disturbances in the dog. A clinical and pathologic study of 3,000 dogs. *Am. J. Vet. Res.*, 1961;**22**: 355–369.

102. Long, D.M., R.C. Truex, K.R. Friedmann, A.K. Olsen, and S.J. Phillips, Heart rate of the dog following autonomic denervation. *Anat. Rec.*, 1958;**130**: 73–89.

103. Hoffman, B.F. and P.F. Cranefield, The physiological basis of cardiac arrhythmias. *Am. J. Med.*, 1964;**37**: 670–684.

104. Tse, W.W., Evidence of presence of automatic fibers in the canine atrioventricular node. *Am. J. Physiol.*, 1973;**225**: 716–723.

105. Damato, A.N. S.H. Lau, His bundle rhythm. *Circulation*, 1969;**40**: 527–534.

106. Jalife, J. and G.K. Moe, Effect of electrotonic potentials on pacemaker activity of canine Purkinje fibers in relation to parasystole. *Circ. Res.*, 1976;**39**: 801–818.

107. Jalife, J. and G.K. Moe, A biologic model of parasystole. *Am. J. Cardiol.*, 1979;**43**: 761–712.

108. Moe, G.K., J. Jalife, W.J. Mueller, and B. Moe, A mathematical model of parasystole and its application to clinical arrhythmias. *Circulation*, 1977;**56**: 968–979.

109. Furuse, A., G. Shindo, H. Makuuchi, et al. Apparent suppression of ventricular parasystole by cardiac pacing. *Jpn. Heart J.*, 1979;**20**: 843–851.

110. Castellanos, A., E. Melgarejo, R. Dubois, and R.M. Luceri, Modulation of ventricular parasystole by extraneous depolarizations. *J. Electrocardiol.*, 1984;**17**: 195–198.

111. Soloff, L.A., Parasystole, in *Cardiac Arrhythmias*, L.S. Dreifus and W. Likoff, Editors. New York: Grune & Stratton, 1973, pp. 409–415.

112. Meurs, K.M., Boxer dog cardiomyopathy: an update. *Vet. Clin. North Am. Small Anim. Pract.*, 2004;**34**(5): 1235–1244.

113. Baumwart, R.D., K.M. Meurs, C.E. Atkins, et al., Clinical, echocardiographic, and electrocardiographic abnormalities in Boxers with cardiomyopathy and left ventricular systolic dysfunction: 48 cases (1985–2003). *J. Am. Vet. Med. Assoc.*, 2005;**226**(7): 1102–1104.

114. Basso, C., P.R. Fox, K.M. Meurs, et al., Arrhythmogenic right ventricular cardiomyopathy causing sudden cardiac death in boxer dogs: a new animal model of human disease. *Circulation*, 2004;**109**(9): 1180–1185.

115. Kraus, M.S., N.S. Moise, M. Rishniw, et al., Morphology of ventricular arrhythmias in the boxer as measured by 12-lead electrocardiography with pace-mapping comparison. *J. Vet. Intern. Med.*, 2002;**16**(2): 153–158.

116. Meurs, K.M., A.W. Spier, N.A. Wright, et al., Comparison of the effects of four antiarrhythmic treatments for familial ventricular arrhythmias in Boxers. *J. Am. Vet. Med. Assoc.*, 2002;**221**(4): 522–527.

117. Moise, N.S., From cell to cageside: autonomic influences on cardiac rhythms in the dog. *J. Small Anim. Pract.*, 1998;**39**(10): 460–468.

118. Harpster, N.K., Boxer cardiomyopathy. A review of the long-term benefits of antiarrhythmic therapy. *Vet. Clin. North Am. Small Anim. Pract.*, 1991;**21**(5): 989–1004.

119. Moïse, N.S., V. Meyers-Wallen, W.J. Flahive, et al., Inherited ventricular arrhythmias and sudden death in German shepherd dogs. *J. Am. Coll. Cardiol.*, 1994;**24**: 233–243.

120. Moïse, N.S., P.F. Moon, W.J. Flahive, et al., Phenylephrine induced ventricular arrhythmias in dogs with inherited sudden death. *J. Cardiovasc. Electrophysiol.*, 1996;7: 217–230.

121. Gilmour, R.F. Jr. and N.S. Moïse, Triggered activity as a mechanism for inherited ventricular arrhythmias in German shepherd dogs. *J. Am. Coll. Cardiol.*, 1996;**27**: 1526–1533.

122. Moïse, N.S. and R.F. Gilmour Jr., and M.L. Riccio, An animal model of sudden arrhythmic death. *J. Cardiovasc. Electrophysiol.*, 1997;**8**: 98–103.

123. Moïse, N.S., D.A. Dugger, D. Brittain, et al., Relationship of ventricular tachycardia to sleep/wakefulness in a model of sudden cardiac death. *Ped. Res.*, 1996;**40**: 344–350.

124. Moïse, N.S., R.F. Gilmour Jr., M.L. Riccio, et al., Diagnosis of inherited ventricular tachycardia in German shepherd dogs. *Am. J. Vet. Med. Assoc.*, 1997;**210**: 403–410.

125. Freeman, L.C., L.M. Pacioretty, and N.S. Moïse, et al., Decreased density of I_{to} in left ventricular myocytes from German shepherd dogs with inherited arrhythmias. *J. Cardiovasc. Electrophysiol.*, 1997;**8**: 872–883.

126. Dae, M., P. Ursell, R. Lee, C. Stilson, M. Chin, and N.S. Moïse, Heterogeneous sympathetic innervation in German shepherd dogs with inherited ventricular arrhythmias and sudden death. *Circulation*, 1997;**96**: 1337–1342.

127. Moïse, N.S., M.J. Riccio, W.J. Flahive, et al., Age dependent development of ventricular arrhythmias in a spontaneous animal model of sudden cardiac death. *Cardiovasc. Res.*, 1997;**34**: 483–492.

128. Riccio, M.L., N.S. Moïse, N.F. Otani, et al., Vector quantization of T wave abnormalities associated with a predisposition to ventricular arrhythmias and sudden death. *Ann. Noninvasive Electrocardiol.*, Jan 1998;**3**(1): 46–53.

129. Moïse, N.S., From cell to cageside cardiac rhythms in the dog: autonomic influence. *J. Small Anim. Pract.*, 1998;**39**: 460–468.

130. Sosunov, E.A., E.P. Anyukhovsky, A. Shvilkin, M. Hara, S.F. Steinberg, P. Danilo Jr., M.R. Rosen, N.S. Moïse, et al., Abnormal cardiac repolarization and impulse initialization in German shepherd dogs with inherited ventricular analysis and sudden death. *Cardiovasc. Res.*, 1999;**42**: 65–79.

131. Moïse, N.S., Inherited arrhythmias in the dog: potential experimental models of cardiac disease. *Cardiovasc. Res.*, 1999;**44**: 37–46.

132. Merot, J., V. Probst, M. Debailleul, U. Gerlacin, N.S. Moïse, et al., Electropharmacological characterization of cardiac repolarization in German shepherd dogs with an inherited syndrome of sudden death. *J. Am. Coll. Cardiol.*, 2000;**36**: 939–947.

133. Sosunov, E.A., R.Z. Gainullin, N.S. Moïse, et al., β_1 and β_2–Adrenergic receptor subtype effects in German shepherd dogs with inherited lethal ventricular arrhythmias. *Cardiovasc. Res.*, 2000;**48**: 211–219.

134. Steinberg, S.F., S.A. Alcott, E. Pak, D.H. Hu, L. Protas, N.S. Moïse, et al., Beta-receptors increase in cAMP and include abnormal CAI cycling in the German shepherd sudden death model. *Am. J. Physiol. Heart Circ. Physiol.*, 2002;**282**: H1181–H1188.

135. Obreztchikova, M.N., E.A. Sosunov, E.P. Anyukhovsky, N.S. Moïse, et al., Heterogeneous ventricular repolarization provides a substrate for arrhythmias in German shepherd model of spontaneous arrhythmic death. *Circulation*, 2003;**108**: 1389–1394.

136. Sosunov, E.A., M.N. Obreztchikova, E.P. Anyukhovsky, N.S. Moïse, et al., Mechanisms of alph adrenergic potentiation of ventricular arrhythmias in German shepherd dogs with inherited arrhythmic sudden death. *Cardiovasc. Res.*, 2004;**61**: 715–723.

137. Protas, L., E.A. Sosunov, E.P. Anyukhovsky, N.S. Moïse, et al., Regional dispersion of L-type calcium current in ventricular myocytes of German shepherd dogs with lethal cardiac arrhythmias. *Heart Rhythm*, 2005;**2**: 172–176.

138. Gelzer, A.R.M., N.S. Mo¿se, and M.L. Koller, Defibrillation of German shepherds with inherited ventricular arrhythmias and sudden death. *J. Vet. Cardiol.*, 2005;**7**(2): 97–107.

139. Wald, R.W., M.B. Waxman, and J.M. Colman, Torsade de pointes ventricular tachycardia: a complication of disopyramide shared with quinidine. *J. Electrocardiol.*, 1981;**14**: 301–307.

140. Bardy, G.H., R.M. Ungerleider, W.M. Smith, and R.E. Ideker, A mechanism of Torsades de Pointes as observed in a dog model. *Circulation*, 1981;**64**(Suppl. 4): 218.

141. Boucher, M., C. Dubray, and P. Duchene-Marullaz, Long-term observation of atri, fl and ventricular rates in the unanesthetized dog with complete atrioventricular block. *Pfluegers Arch.*, 1982;**395**: 341–343.

142. Hurwitz, R.A., Effect of glucagon on dogs with acute and chronic heart block. *Am. Heart J.*, 1971;**81**: 644–649.

143. Reynolds, R.D. and J. Di Salvo, Effects of dl-propranolol on atrial and ventricular rates in unaesthetized atrioventricular blocked dogs. *J. Pharmacol. Exp. Ther.*, 1978;**205**: 374–381.

144. Robinson, J.L., W.C. Farr, and G. Grupp, Atrial rate response to ventricular pacing in the unanesthetized A-V blocked dog. *Am. J. Physiol.*, 1973;**224**: 40–45.

145. Averill, K.H. and L.E. Lamb, Electrocardiographic findings in 67,375 asymptomatic subjects. I. Incidence of abnormalities. *Am. J. Cardiol.*, 1960;**6**: 76–83.

146. Böhle, E., Blutgefässe, in *Erkrankungen durch Arzneimittel*, R. Heinz, Editor. Stuttgart: Thieme, 1966, pp. 170–187.

147. Wenzel, D.G., Drug induced cardiomyopathies. *J. Pharm. Sci.*, 1967;**56**: 1209–1224.

148. Selye, H., *Experimental Cardiovascular Diseases*, vols. 1, 2. Berlin: Springer, 1970.

149. Chung, E.K. and H.M. Dean, Diseases of the heart and vascular system due to drugs, in *Drug-Induced Diseases*, vol. 4, L. Meyler and H.M. Peck, Editors. Amsterdam: Excerpta Medica, 1972, pp. 345–381.

150. Davies, D.M. and R.G. Gold, Cardiac disorders, in *Textbook of Adverse Drug Reactions*, D.M. Davies, Editor. Oxford: Oxford University Press, 1977, pp. 81–102.

151. Bristow, M.R., Editor, *Drug-Induced Heart Disease*. Amsterdam: Elsevier, 1980.

152. Balazs, T., Editor, *Cardiac Toxicology*, vols. 1, 2, 3. Boca Raton, FL: CRC Press, 1981.

153. Van Stee, E.W., Editor, *Cardiovascular Toxicology*. New York: Raven, 1982.

154. Spitzer, J. J., Editor, Myocardial injury. *Adv. Exp. Med. Biol; Ser.*, New York: Plenum, 1983;**161**: 421–443.

155. Surawicz, B. and K.C. Lasseter, Effect of drugs on the electrocardiogram. *Prog. Cardiovasc. Dis.*, 1970;**13**: 26–55.

156. Surawicz, B., Relationship between electrocardiogram and electrolytes. *Am. Heart J.*, 1967;**73**: 814–834.

157. Surawicz, B., The pathogenesis and clinical significance of primary T-wave abnormalities, in *Advances in Electrocardiography*, R.C. Schlant and J. Hurst, Editors. New York: Grune & Stratton, 1972, pp. 377–421.

158. Vaughan Williams, E.M., Classification of anti-arrhythmic drugs, in *Symposium of Cardiac Arrhythmias*, E. Sandøe, E. Flensted-Jensen, and K.H. Olesen, Editors. Södertälje, Sweden: Astra, 1970, pp. 449–468.

159. Singh, B.N., J.T. Collett, and C.Y. Chew, New perspectives in the pharmacologic therapy of cardiac arrhythmias. *Prog. Cardiovasc. Dis.*, 1980;**22**: 243–301.

160. Harrison, D.G., Editor, *Cardiac Arrhythmias: A Decade of Progress*. Boston, MA: Hall, 1981.

161. Lazdunski, M. and J.F. Renaud, The action of cardiotoxins on cardiac plasma membranes. *Annu. Rev. Physiol.*, 1982;**44**: 463–473.

162. Detweiler, D.K., Electrocardiographic monitoring in toxicological studies: principles and interpretations, in *Myocardial Injury*, J.J. Spitzer, Editor, *Adv. Exp. Med. Biol.*, 1983;**161**: 579–607.

163. Reynolds, E.W. and C.R. Vander Ark, Quinidine syncope and the delayed repolarization syndromes. *Mod. Concepts Cardiovasc. Dis.*, 1976;**45**: 117–122.

164. Detweiler, D.K., *Reversal of T Waves in Leads rV$_2$ and V$_{10}$ in Toxicity Trials Indicates Left Ventricular Subendocardial and Papillary Muscle Ischemia or Damage*, Personal Observation. Philadelphia, PA: University of Pennsylvania, 1985.

165. Osborne, B.E. and B.D.H. Leach, The Beagle Electrocardiogram. *Food Cosmet. Toxicol.*, 1971;**9**: 857–864.

10 The Mammalian Electrocardiogram: Comparative Features

D.K. Detweiler[†]

[†]For this 2nd Edition of "Comprehensive Electrocardiology," Dr. Sydney Moise has updated this 1st Edition chapter, which was originally written by the late Dr. Detweiler.

P. W. Macfarlane et al. (eds.), *Specialized Aspects of ECG*, DOI 10.1007/978-0-85729-880-5_10,
© Springer-Verlag London Limited 2012

10.1 Introduction

The purpose of this chapter is to summarize the characteristics that distinguish electrocardiograms recorded from different mammalian species rather than reviewing the contributions of experimental animal research to cardiac electrophysiology.

In 1888, using the capillary electrometer, Waller [1] was the first to obtain electrocardiograms from mammals (human, horse, dog, cat, and rabbit). Since that time, aside from the enormous literature on animal experimentation, a modest literature has accumulated on applied mammalian electrocardiography, written by investigators interested in the comparative aspects of electrocardiography, the use of electrocardiography to record cardiac activity in various types of laboratory animal experiments, and the application of electrocardiography in veterinary medicine. While these investigations were generally not designed to add to the mainstream of basic electrocardiographic thought and concept, they have been useful in providing a database for the interpretation of animal electrocardiograms in veterinary medicine and in a large variety of animal research applications in which electrocardiograms are monitored to detect the effects of various experimental interventions on the heart. In more recent years, the mouse has emerged as a vital animal for investigation. Although the surface electrocardiogram is frequently assessed, more detailed electrophysiologic studies have been at the forefront.

Among prominent physician cardiologists, whose interests and work have given impetus to study in this field, are Tawara (anatomy of the conduction system [2]), Paul Dudley White (elephant [3] and whale [4] electrocardiograms), Rudolph Zuckermann (atlas of animal electrocardiograms [5]), Bruno Kisch (electrocardiographic and electrographic studies in animals [6]), Eugene Lepeschkin (literature survey and analysis [7, 8]), Pierre Rijlant (pacemaker function [9]), Thomas Lewis (atrial fibrillation in horses [10, 11]), Luisada (electrocardiograms and phonocardiograms of domestic animals [12]), and Jane Sands Robb (comparative anatomy, histology, embryology, and electrophysiology [13]).

Veterinary electrocardiography had its beginnings with studies in the horse. As a prelude to this, the first normal equine electrocardiogram published (1910) was a record, which von Tschermak obtained from Einthoven [14]. Shortly thereafter, Lewis (1911) published three abnormal records from a horse with atrial fibrillation [10]. In 1911, Kahn [15] published 26 records taken from six horses and in the same year, Waller [16, 17], in two short notes, briefly discussed the cardiac electrical axis of the horse and the relationship between the duration of mechanical systole and the electrocardiogram. Also in 1913, Norr published his inaugural dissertation on the electrocardiogram of the horse and a companion article in the *Zeitschrift fur Biologie* [18]. Norr was to become the leading figure in veterinary electrocardiography for the next 25 years [19–21], contributing by himself or through his students to the literature on animal electrocardiography and comparative pathophysiology of the circulation.

Following these beginnings, until the early 1940s, in addition to Norr and Kahn, only about 20 authors contributed articles on the electrocardiogram of the horse, recommending some five different lead systems [22]. During this period, only a handful of veterinary authors published articles on the canine electrocardiogram [23] and that of other domestic species [24].

During the 1940s, owing to World War II and its aftermath, scientific publication of all kinds diminished. Notable among the few publications that appeared were those of Sporri (ox, guinea pig [25, 26]) in Switzerland; Alfredson and Sykes (cattle [27]) in the United States; Charton, Minot, and Bressou (horse [28–30]) in France; Kelso (lamb [31]) in Australia; Krzywanek and Ruud (swine [32, 33]) in Germany; and Voskanyan and Filatov (horses, cattle [34, 35]) in Russia. Roshchevsky [36] credited Voskanyan with having developed the clinical use of electrocardiography in cattle in the Soviet Union in 1938–1939. This decade was followed by a 30-year period of ever increasing publications on applied electrocardiography in veterinary medicine, toxicological studies, and records from nondomesticated mammals. Modern day electrocardiography is becoming more "paper-free" with the advent of electronic electrocardiograph systems. These systems can store continuous recordings and post-process the leads shown, with adjustable filtering, speed, and gain on the display. Storage of recordings can be facilitated with electronic retrieval, and data bases are searchable by identification and diagnosis.

10.2 Literature Reviews

Today, internet searching for electrocardiographic data on numerous species is the standard. Wide searches can result in hits not only from published papers but also from other sources of information indexed on the web. Although such means are the standard, some references may be missed from the past. From a historical perspective, the leading sources of references, listed chronologically, in comparative mammalian electrocardiography are the reviews written by Lepeschkin [7, 8], Grauwiler [37], and Roshchevsky [24, 38]. The following summarizes some of these early and important works.

Lepeschkin, in his book published in 1951 [8], covered publications on invertebrates, fish, amphibia, birds, and mammals, citing over 200 references published from 1934 to 1950 as well as publications prior to 1934 cited in his previous book [7]. Grauwiler [37] cites some 125 publications on mammalian electrocardiograms covering the period 1913–1962. Fourteen classes of mammals are represented from monotremes to primates with many illustrations of electrocardiograms and tables of electrocardiographic data for each of the 70 species.

Comparative electrocardiography was reviewed in the publications of Roshchevsky [24, 38]. His earliest effort [38] covers the entire animal kingdom and cites over 970 references. Electrocardiographic, anatomical, heart rate/body weight, and related data are reported. Roshchevsky's monograph [24] emphasizes the spread of ventricular excitation through analysis of intracardiac (endocardial), intramural, and epicardial electrograms, body-surface mapping, vectorcardiography, and the study of various electrocardiographic lead systems. This publication extended an earlier monograph published in 1958 [36]. Monographs on comparative electrocardiology edited by Roshchevsky include the *Physiological Basis of Animal Electrocardiography* (1965) [39] and proceedings of the first (1979) [40] and second (1985) [41] International Symposia on Comparative Electrocardiology held in Syktyvkar, Komi Republic, USSR.

In 1952, Kisch and his coworkers [6] summarized their studies of electrograms recorded from vertebrate hearts, including those of the rabbit, cat, dog, calf, and human. Data are given on electrocardiographic time intervals, heart rate, and pattern of ventricular excitation from unipolar epicardial and endocardial ventricular electrocardiograms recorded from five mammalian species.

In 1959, Zuckermann, as part of the third edition of his textbook on electrocardiography [5], published an extensive atlas of animal electrocardiograms from arthropods, fish, amphibians, reptiles, birds, and mammals.

Other more recent review publications that contain extensive bibliographies and illustrations, which are not listed in the bibliographies of the works already cited, are on the following animals: horse [42], dog [43–45], monkey [46], and rat [47]. ❧ Table 10.1 lists some influential publications on mammalian electrocardiography that appeared between 1888 and 1970. Today, the internet serves as a means to identify electrocardiographic data for many species. Still, compared to the data for other commercial studies on animals, not much data are available to the public on animals used in nonacademic research.

10.3   Classification of Mammalian Electrocardiograms

10.3.1   Bases for Classification

Mammalian ECGs from different species can be classified in accordance with the following general characteristics:

1. Relative duration of QT interval and ST segment
2. QRS-vector direction and sense
3. Constancy of T-wave polarity (T-wave lability) [49, 50]

These differences, in turn, are determined by three electrophysiological properties that are genetically governed: the relative duration of the ventricular cell action potential as determined by the presence or absence of phase 2 (plateau); the pattern of spread of excitation throughout the ventricles; and constancy of the pattern of repolarization, that is, the constancy of the ventricular gradient.

10.3.2   QT Duration and ST Segment

Many species (rodents, insectivores, bats, and kangaroos) have short QT intervals relative to the duration of mechanical systole [51]. The ST segment is essentially absent. The QRST complex consists of rapid QRS deflections that merge with the slower T wave, and its duration is about half that of mechanical systole. The transmembrane action potentials of these

◻ Table 10.1

Contributions important to the development of comparative mammalian electrocardiography

Year	Subject	Author	Reference
1988/9	First horse ECG (capillary electrometer).	Waller	[66]
1910	Einthoven provided horse ECG for veterinary textbook.	von Tschermak	[14]
1911	Visual proof that fibrillating atria produce f waves in ECG (from horses with atrial fibrillation)	Lewis	[10, 11]
1913	Veterinary clinical electrocardiography initiated.	Nörr	[18]
1921	Fetal electrocardiograms obtained from mares.	Nörr	[95]
1921	First elephant ECG	Forbes et al.	[216]
1924	Cardiac arrythmias in horses.	Nörr	[218]
1924	Atrial fibrillation in dogs and horses.	Roos	[219, 220]
1930	Electrocardiographic monitoring in chronic rat (nutritional) studies.	Agduhr, Drury et al.	[221, 222]
1935	Respiratory sinus arrhythmia in *canidae* (dog, fox).	Nörr	[223]
1942	Electrocardiography in dairy cattle.	Alfredson, Sykes	[27]
1949	Clinical chest leads for dogs (rV_2, V_2, V_4).	Lannek	[23]
1951	Survey of animal electrocardiography.	Lepeschkin	[8]
1952	Comparative electrocardiography in mammals.	Kisch et al.	[6]
1953	First whale ECG	King et al.	[4]
1953	First WPW in lower animals (cow).	Spörri	[161]
1953	His-bundle potentials recorded (dog).	Scher	[224]
1953	No ST segment and QT shorter than mechanical systole in adult mouse.	Richards et al.	[185]
1955	Ventricular activation pattern in the dog.	Scher	[225]
1956	QT shorter than mechanical systole and ST segment absent in adult Bennett Kangaroo but not in young in pouch.	Spörri	[186]
1957	Clinical electrocardiography in horse and cattle.	Brooijmans	[67]
1958	Right ventricular hypertrophy pattern in dog.	Detweiler	[226]
1958	Electrocardiography in cattle.	Roschchevsky	[36]
1959	Atlas of animal ECGs.	Zuckerman	[5]
1960	ECG finback whale.	Senft, Kanwischer	[181]
1960	Lead V_{10} introduced in dog.	Hamlin, Hellerstein	[84]
1965	Large atrial mass favors atrial fibrillation.	Moore et al.	[160]
1965	Survey of mammalian ECGs.	Grauwiler	[37]
1966	Monkey ECG.	Malinow	[80]
1967	Definitive criteria for right ventricular hypertrophy in the dog.	Hill	[228, 229]
1968	First journal of animal electrocardiography published (Japan).		[48]
1970	Accessory AV (Kent) bundle conduction identified in WPW syndrome (monkey, dog).	Boineau, Moore	[233]
1970	First monograph on canine cardiology.	Ettinger, Suter	[227]

species do not have a distinct plateau, which explains the absence of the ST segment (❷ Fig. 10.1). This is in contrast to the QRST complex of the remainder of mammals that have an ST segment, a QT interval equivalent to mechanical systole, and an action potential with a distinct plateau. The reason for the differences in the QT interval, ST segment, and the T wave rests in the differences in the specific ion channels that are responsible for repolarization in these varied species. The differences in the ion channels are important not only to understand from the point of recognizing the different ECG

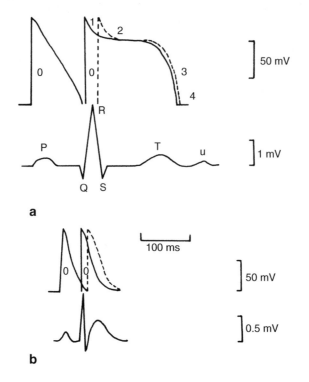

⊙ Fig. 10.1

Schema of atrial and ventricular transmembrane action potentials (TMAP) and the ECG, drawn on the same time scale. In (a), the five phases of the dog TMAP are shown; *0* initial rapid depolarization or spike, *1* initial rapid repolarization, *2* slow repolarization or plateau, *3* final rapid repolarization, *4* resting or diastolic transmembrane potential. The rat TMAP is shown in (b). Note that the rat and dog atrial and the rat ventricular TMAPs have no plateaux. The TMAPs drawn with the *solid line* represent excitation of ventricular cells early during the QRS interval; those drawn with a *dashed line* represent excitation of ventricular cells later during the QRS. Note that in the dog the plateaux of the TMAPs overlap so that there is little difference in charge between groups of cells. This period of overlap coincides with the isopotential ST segment of the ECG. The T wave of the dog ECG is generated during the final rapid repolarization, phase 3, when at any given instant in time the charges of different masses of cells are not the same. In the rat, the ventricular TMAPs do not have a plateau and there is no period during repolarization when most cells are isopotential. Thus, no ST segment appears in the ECG.

patterns, but also for comparative medicine and the effects of drugs. The latter is vital in understanding the impact that ion channel type has on the response to a pharmacologic intervention that may have little or no effect in one species, yet have a profound consequence in another. This point is of particular importance with regard to the screening for QT prolongation [52].

10.3.3 Ventricular Activation Patterns

The ventricular activation patterns of various species fall into two general classes of QRS-vector direction and sense [24, 53] as follows:

1. Class A includes those animals with QRS vectors which, generally, are directed along the long axis of the body, caudally and ventrally, and produce a largely negative deflection in lead V_{10} and a positive deflection in lead aVF; for example, dogs, humans, monkeys, cats, and rats.

2. Class B includes those animals with QRS vectors which, generally, are directed from sternum toward the spine and which produce largely positive deflections in lead V_{10} and negative deflections in lead aVF; hoofed mammals and dolphins, for example.

These differences are associated with the distributive characteristics of the Purkinje network. In animals belonging to class A, it is primarily a subendocardial network. In class B animals, the Purkinje network is more elaborate and penetrates deeply into the ventricular myocardium.

10.3.4 T-Wave Lability

In humans, primates, and many hoofed mammals, T wave amplitude and polarity tend to be fairly constant in serial records. In dogs and especially in horses, T wave vectors are quite labile. The T waves vary in polarity and amplitude in limb leads and some thoracic leads in serial records, and sometimes change during the course of recording of a given lead. In the dog, there are two conventional thoracic leads in which the T wave polarity is remarkably consistent: the T wave is normally positive in lead rV_2 (this lead approximates that of V_1 in humans and negative in V_{10} in about 90% of individuals [54–56]).

10.3.5 Effect of ECG Characteristics on Choice of Lead Systems and Terminology

For animals having QRS vector and sense of class A in ❷ Sect. 10.3.3, the conventional limb leads are oriented favorably for recording QRS potentials in the frontal plane projection. In animals with class B QRS vectors, on the other hand, the major QRS-vector forces are directed more-or-less perpendicular to the frontal plane and limb leads are not favorably disposed for recording these potentials. Hamlin and Smith's [53] use of lead V_{10} to compare species made this amply clear, but not until there had been a great deal of experimentation to find favorable lead systems, especially in large domestic animals (reviewed by Roshchevsky [24, 36]). Today the base-apex lead is the most common lead used in horses and cattle.

The discovery that another group of mammals has virtually no ST segment in the electrocardiogram caused another terminological dilemma, since ST-segment deviation is an important diagnostic term in classical electrocardiography. Actually, a flat or isopotential ST segment is abbreviated in limb leads in many mammals with the ST segment of class A (e.g., the dog) and is virtually absent in precordial leads of all species. The presence of a stable isoelectric ST segment depends on two factors: first, the occurrence of a distinct plateau and consequent long duration of the transmembrane action potential and second, in large hearts, the presence of a rapid conduction system that spreads the excitation quickly so that the plateaus of many ventricular cells overlap in time. Ventricular ectopic beats, for example, result in slowing of the depolarization throughout the ventricle such that synchrony of the plateau period in various parts of the heart is reduced and the ST segment is consequently abbreviated.

The terminological dilemma arises because the same perturbations that produce ST segment deviations in species with a distinct ST segment (for example, regional ischemia or hypoxia, "injury current") produce a similar shift of the slow-wave portion of the QRST complex in species with no ST segment (e.g., the rat). The phrase ST deviation is so ingrained in diagnostic electrocardiographic parlance as a term with definite diagnostic significance that it represents a concept. Therefore, it has been suggested that the term should be placed in quotation marks (e.g., "ST" segment elevation or depression) when used to indicate the effect of an injury potential on the immediate post-QRS portion of the ventricular complex in species lacking an ST segment [50].

Finally, for species with labile T waves in normal electrocardiograms (e.g., dog and horse), the significance of T-wave reversal in most leads in disease or cardiotoxicity cannot be evaluated. Fortunately, in the dog the T waves in leads rV_2 (V_1) and V_{10} are consistent in polarity and these leads can be used to detect T wave reversal associated with myocardial damage. No such leads have been established for the horse. Additionally, in dogs, rV_2 (V_1) may be a more reliable lead than lead II for the measurement of the QT interval because of the more consistent T wave morphology.

10.4   Technique

10.4.1   Electrocardiographs, Lead Lines, and Electrodes

Since the time of Einthoven, electrocardiographs have been designed primarily to record the cardiac potentials of humans. As the electrocardiograms of smaller mammals have frequency components that are higher than those of humans, electrocardiographs of an earlier era were found to have an inadequate frequency response for these small species [57, 58]. In the rat electrocardiogram, frequency components up to 400 Hz have been reported [59] but little distortion occurs when recording with equipment having a frequency response of 200 Hz [60]. Most modern electrocardiographs are reputed to approach an upper frequency response limit of 200 Hz. Electronic electrocardiographs now permit a longer recording time, as well as post-processing of rate, amplitude, filtering, and speed. The advantage for data storage and review is far superior performance compared to the use of paper recordings. However, these machines are often equipped with optional electronic filters that reduce response to well below that needed to record electrocardiograms of small mammals with fidelity [50]. Thus, to avoid distortion, an understanding of the filtering methods must be appreciated by the operator.

Lead lines connecting the animals to the electrocardiograph must be flexible, made of shielded cable and long enough to accommodate the size of the subject. Fine-wire extensions that are not shielded are satisfactory when dealing with very small species. The major problem to avoid is any tugging on the electrodes by swinging lead lines since this will shift the electrodes at the skin interface and cause baseline artifacts in the electrocardiogram at frequencies or harmonics of the lead-line motion that can vary from slow drift to rapid waves that mimic atrial flutter or fibrillation.

There has been considerable experimentation with electrodes in animal electrocardiography over the years but few studies of the electrical conductive properties of the various types recommended. One exception is the study of Almasi et al. [61]. Clip electrodes, such as electronic crocodile clips, are satisfactory if the total area of contact is ~1 cm^2. Clipping the fur and applying patches similar to the method used in humans is better for intermediate length recordings. The conductive properties of copper are superior to those of stainless steel. Importantly, the medal used for the different leads should not be mixed but uniform.

10.4.2   Restraint

10.4.2.1   Physical Restraint

For farm animals, the usual methods of tethering or use of stanchions are satisfactory. The main requirement is adequate control of foreleg position. For monkeys, flat restraint boards, V-boards or cradles (supine position), and monkey "chairs" (sitting position) are commonly used. Dogs and cats can generally be handled. The use of slings or support in a "begging position" [62] is not recommended. For small laboratory animals (rat, guinea pig, etc.) a variety of restraint devices have been used including the usual commercially available laboratory animal holders. Some investigators have constructed special holders for rats and guinea pigs, which confine the animal so that each limb dangles in separate beakers of saline [63] or each foot rests on electrodes covered with conducting paste [64]. A simple method is to attach the electrodes, cover the animal with a cloth to exclude light and visual stimuli, and hold by hand. For example, satisfactory records were obtained from moles by restraining by hand in a cloth, or by allowing freedom in a box containing earth under which they burrowed and became quiet [65]. For extended studies, implantable recorders are now possible for long-term recording of quality data in very small mammals.

10.4.2.2   Chemical Restraint

Whenever possible, anesthetics, narcotics, or tranquilizers should be avoided because all such agents affect heart rate, rhythm, and electrocardiographic time intervals while some are arrhythmogenic. On the other hand sedation may be required in order to obtain a quality recording. The final decision depends on the question to be answered.

10.4.3 Positioning

In all quadrupeds, it is necessary to control foreleg position to obtain consistent direction and magnitude of cardiac vectors from limb-lead scalar electrocardiograms. It must be emphasized that this precaution applies to large domestic animals as well as small laboratory species [50].

10.4.4 Leads and Lead Systems

10.4.4.1 Limb Leads

Since the time of Waller [1, 66] limb leads have been recorded in animals for scalar electrocardiograms and calculation of vector forces. They were used in Einthoven's laboratory for horses and dogs [67]. For years, some investigators rejected limb leads, considering them unsuitable for various quadrupeds. This was on the spurious ground that the heart is not in the center of an equilateral triangle as in man, not realizing that Einthoven's triangle concept relating the potentials of the three bipolar limb leads depends on Kirchhoff's second law of circuits rather than the geometry of the thorax or the location of limb attachment to the thorax.

Nörr [18] and Kahn [15], on the other hand, favored chest leads over limb leads for sounder reasons. Both investigators considered limb leads unsuitable for horses because the electrocardiographic waves were small and variable compared to those of man. For species belonging to the QRS vector and sense class A (primates, carnivores, certain rodents, etc.), the limb leads have always been considered satisfactory.

10.4.4.2 Chest Leads

In accordance with the aforementioned, Nörr [18] and Kahn [15] devised two similar bipolar electrode positions for the horse. Both placed one electrode on the ventral thoracic surface near the region of the ventricular apex. Nörr located the other electrode on the right anterior breast at the level of the scapulohumeral joint (point of the shoulder) while Kahn placed the other electrode on the right side of the base of the neck at the level of the middle of the anterior border of the scapula. The direction of the deflection was positive when the electrical vector was directed toward the anterior breast or neck electrode and vice versa. Nörr [19] later chose for cattle a location for the neck electrode similar to that used by Kahn for horses because of the more vertical anatomical axis of the ox heart.

Later, in 1928, Lautenschlager [69] investigated thoracic bipolar lead combinations systematically in horses and cattle by mapping a grid over the entire trunk, dividing the surface (right and left sides) into 106 squares measuring 15 × 15 cm. His essential conclusion was that electrode positions like those used by Kahn for horses and by Nörr for cattle were most suitable; that is, one electrode at the cardiac apex region on the left side of the chest at the level of the olecranon, and the other electrode on the right side at the base of the neck in the region of the right scapula. This bipolar thoracic lead, often referred to as a base-apex (or apex-base) lead because the electrodes are placed on the body surface where an extension of the anatomic longitudinal axis of the heart would meet the skin, has been used as a monitoring lead in hoofed mammals and is recommended by the Japanese Association of Animal Electrocardiography for use in dogs [70].

Since 1928, a large number of lead systems have been devised for domestic hoofed mammals in which the three limb-lead electrodes have been placed in some triangular configuration on the torso. These have all been detailed in Roshchevsky's book on hoofed mammal electrocardiography [24]. Spörri's [26] modification of these systems has had wide use in many species, including small animals such as the rat [50], since his 1944 publication. In this system, the Lautenschlager base-apex lead, that is, right arm electrode at the base of the neck (cervical) on the right side paired with the left leg electrode placed in the region of the cardiac apex (apical) on the left ventral chest wall at the level of the olecranon, is recorded when conventional electrocardiographs are switched to the lead II recording position. The left arm electrode is placed on the back over the last thoracic vertebra. When lead I is recorded a longitudinal lead is recorded between the neck and the last thoracic vertebral electrodes and when lead III is recorded, the recording is between the cardiac apical and last thoracic vertebral electrodes. Sporri's designation for these leads is as follows:

1. Lead D for dorsal (neck to thoracic vertebral electrode, lead I electrodes)
2. Lead A for axial (neck to cardiac apical electrode, lead II electrodes) and
3. Lead J (or I) for inferior (sacral to cardiac apical electrode, lead III electrodes)

This D, A, J lead system, therefore, is equivalent to lead II (dorsal (0) lead) and two precordial leads with the different or "exploring" electrode at the cardiac apex region and the distant electrode at the base of the neck (axial (A) lead) or posterior thoracic region (inferior (1) lead). A variant of this system is to place the left arm electrode at the cardiac apex and the left leg electrode at the last thoracic vertebra (Sander [71]).

In 1954, Brooijmans [67, 72] proposed a thoracic unipolar lead system (employing Wilson's central terminal) in which nine (horse) or seven (cattle) equidistant chest leads encircle the chest vertically at the sixth (horse) or fifth (cattle) intercostal space and five (horse) or four (cattle) electrodes encircle the anterior chest in the horizontal plane. A more complicated thoracic lead system with 28 lead positions was studied by Sellers et al. [73] for dairy cattle. None of the more elaborate chest-lead systems has come into use.

Other triangular thoracic lead systems for large hoofed mammals have been proposed to represent the electrical forces of the cardiac cycle as projected on the frontal (F), transverse (T), and sagittal (S) planes. Roshchevsky [24, 36, 39] devised such a system for hoofed animals (cattle, reindeer, etc.) in which the frontal plane is defined by placing the right arm electrode at the right scapulohumeral (shoulder) joint, the left arm electrode at the left shoulder joint (lead IF), and the left leg electrode on the ventral abdominal midline at the level of the 13th (last thoracic) vertebra (leads I IF and IIIF). The sagittal plane is defined by placing the right arm electrode at the cranial end of the manubrium sterni, the left arm electrode on the withers at the fourth vertebra (lead IS), and the left electrode on the ventral abdomen at the same site as for the frontal plane (leads IIS and IIIS). The electrocardiograph is then switched to obtain six leads in each plane (that is, IF, IIF, IIIF, aVR_F, aVL_F, aVF_F, for the frontal plane and IS; IIS; IIIS, aVR_S, aVL_S, aVF_S, for the sagittal plane). Roshchevsky, from his detailed studies of the cardiac potential over the torso surface of ungulates, considered the sagittal lead system most suitable and it was adopted by [74], for clinical studies with cattle. Sugeno et al. [75] also adopted a three-lead triangular recording system with one lead at the cardiac apex for their earlier studies. Too et al. [76] investigated a three-bipolar-lead sagittal system in cattle (placing the right arm electrode at the cardiac apex, the left arm electrode at the scapulohumeral joint, and the left leg electrode at the withers) and a bipolar transverse three-lead system (placing the right arm electrode on the right olecranon, the left arm electrode on the left olecranon, and the left leg electrode at the withers). Kusachi and Sato [77] experimented with four bipolar systems in horses, finally recommending one in which three electrodes were placed on the right foreleg, left foreleg, and withers, respectively.

In horses, Lannek and Rutqvist [78] introduced a unipolar thoracic read system (employing Wilson's central terminal) patterned after the system Lannek had used in the dog [23]. This system, with the addition of leads V_{10} and CV_6RU, has been used in horses and cattle[42, 79]. These chest leads are as follows:

1. Lead CT_1 in which the exploring electrode was placed on the right side of the thorax 3–5 cm above a horizontal line through the highest point of the olecranon and behind the posterior edge of the triceps brachii muscle
2. Lead CT_2, where the exploring electrode was placed on the left side of the thorax at the same height as a horizontal line through the highest point of the olecranon and behind the triceps brachii muscle
3. Lead CT_3, where the exploring electrode was placed on the left side of the thorax about 8 cm above the CV_6LL (or CT_2) electrode

From this system the following thoracic unipolar leads evolved [79]:

1. Lead CV_6RU, with the electrode on the right side of the thorax at the sixth rib at the level of a horizontal line drawn through the point (scapulohumeral joint) of the shoulder
2. Lead CV_6RL, with the electrode on the right side of the thorax, just above the highest point of the olecranon, behind the triceps brachii muscle at the sixth rib

3. Lead CV_6LL, where the electrode is on the left side of the thorax at the same height as a horizontal line drawn through the highest point of the olecranon, behind the triceps brachii at the sixth rib

4. Lead CV_6LU, with the electrode on the left side of the thorax directly above CV_6LL at the level of a horizontal line drawn through the point of the shoulder

5. Lead V_{10}, where the electrode is placed over the vertebral column vertically above CV_6LL (at about the dorsal spinous process of the seventh thoracic vertebra)

In primates, two systems of thoracic leads have emerged. The most common practice is to use counterparts of the six precordial leads employed in humans [46, 80, 81]. Atta and Vanace [82] introduced a precordial three-lead system for the rhesus monkey (*Macaca mulatta*) with electrodes placed as follows: MV_1 fourth right intercostal space at the midclavicular line; MV_2, fourth left intercostal space at the midclavicular line; and MV_3, fifth left intercostal space at the left, midaxillary line. These leads correspond roughly to leads V_1, V_3, and V_5 in humans [80]. A thoracic lead system found satisfactory for squirrel monkeys (*Saimiri sciurcus*) was devised by Wolf et al. [83]. The precordial electrodes were placed as follows: V_6 over the third rib 1 cm to the right of the midline; V_4, over the ninth rib 1 cm to the left of the midline; and V_6 over the eighth rib at the midaxillary line.

In drug studies, lead V_{10} is often added to these precordial leads [49]. For cynomolgus monkeys (*Macaca fascicularis*) used in drug studies, the Atta and Vanace [82] system is often used [49]. Often however, for primates the system used for humans is used.

10.4.4.3 Orthogonal Leads and Cardiac Vectors

Hamlin and associates [53, 84] used leads I, aVF, and V_{10} as X, Y, and Z leads, respectively, to define three recording planes that could be considered somewhat orthogonal to one another: frontal, leads I and aVF (or Z and Y); sagittal, leads V_{10} and aVF (or Y and Z); and transverse, leads I and V_{10} (or X and Z). While arguably a nonorthogonal system in the true sense, this approach was useful and led to the current classification of mammalian electrocardiograms on the basis of QRS direction and sense [53].

Hamlin et al. later modified the orthogonal lead system of McFee and Parungao for dogs for use in studies with the horse [85] and miniature pig [86]. Roshchevsky [24] similarly employed an uncorrected lead system to obtain approximate orthogonality in cattle. The lead pairs for each axis were: X, right scapulohumeral joint to left scapulohumeral joint; Y, cranial end of the manubrium sterni to the ventral abdominal midline a handsbreadth in front of the navel; and Z, between the withers and the left foreleg.

Holmes et al. [87, 88] developed an orthogonal system as did Grauerholz [89] for vectorial evaluation of the horse electrocardiogram.

Grauerholz adopted the lead system of Baron [89]. The lead pairs for each axis were: X, right scapulohumeral joint to left scapulohumeral joint; Z, middle of the back, halfway between the forelimbs and hindlimbs to a point vertically under this on the abdominal midline; Y, determined trigonometrically from the Z-axis lead and a lead between the dorsal back electrode of lead Z and the right shoulder electrode of lead X on the right scapulohumeral joint.

10.4.4.4 Cardiac Electric Fields and Generation of Cardiac Potentials in Hoofed Mammals

In hoofed mammals (horses, cattle, sheep, swine) that are categorized by the QRS direction and sense into class A, reliable electrocardiographic criteria for the diagnosis of left and right ventricular hypertrophy and bundle branch block have not been established. It seems that the most likely reason for this is that the elaborate Purkinje conduction system is capable of maintaining an orderly spread of excitation despite considerable disruption of the ventricular myocardium by disease in these species.

10.4.4.5   Vectorcardiography

Vectorcardiography is not commonly used today. Mapping systems that evaluate the endocardial, epicardial, and even the transmural patterns of initiation and propagation of depolarization and repolarization are used in electrophysiological studies. Historically, the vectorcardiographic approach in mammalian electrocardiology was used primarily to determine the direction of electrical forces responsible for the form of the electrocardiogram in various species and for the study of appropriate lead systems [24, 85–93]. In the horse, for example, such vectorcardiographic investigations have used a Duchosal or similar cube system [79, 96], a form of tetrahedron [53], a triangulation of leads in the horizontal (frontal) and transverse planes [90], or some similar arrangement. Holmes et al. [87, 88] first experimented with an XYZ system in which the X lead consisted of five electrodes on the left and five on the right side of the chest, distributed over the shoulders and forelimbs so as to cover the heart area anatomically [87]. In a second study, these multiple electrodes were replaced with two malleable tin plates (0.6 mm thick) that could be molded to the body surface, covering an equivalent area [88]. The Y lead consisted of an electrode at the xyphoid and one at a point on the anterior chest on the midline between and on the level of the points of the shoulders (scapulohumeral joints). The Z lead consisted of two electrodes, one just to the left of the withers and the other on the upper left foreleg [90]. The resultant vector loops were displayed using an XY plotter [94].

10.4.4.6   Fetal Electrocardiography

Fetal electrocardiography has been practised in mares since 1921 [95]. In this species, the fetal QRS complexes may appear in limb leads II and III in advanced pregnancy (for instance, about 1 month before birth) and P and QRS complexes identified in abdominal leads [96]. In middle gestational stages (for example, 150 days or so), in both cows and mares, the fetal QRS complexes may be detected with appropriate abdominal and rectal leads [97].

In the mare the most favorable bipolar electrode positions are on the back at the midline in the midlumbar position and 6 in. (~15 cm) anterior to the udder on the midline of the ventral abdominal wall [96]. In the cow, favorable bipolar electrode positions are the right side of the lower abdomen or flank paired with an electrode located on the right side of the anterior abdomen or right paralumbar fossa region, or paired with a rectal or vaginal electrode [97, 98]. The superiority of right-sided abdominal leads in cows has also been confirmed by other investigators (for example, Golikov and Vershinina [99]).

In pregnant ewes, fetal electrocardiograms from abdominal lead positions as used in cattle were obtained in only one of five animals tested [99].

As in other species, the heart rate of fetuses in cows and mares tends to decrease as pregnancy advances (for instance, in cows, fetal heart rate varies from about 140 beats per minute [bpm] at 160–191 days of pregnancy to about 120 bpm at days 251–281 of pregnancy and in mares, fetal heart rate varies from about 120 bpm in midstages of pregnancy to about 80 or 90 bpm toward the end of term) [96, 97, 99]. The fetal heart rate, however, is not stable and may vary from moment to moment independent of the maternal heart rate, possibly on account of fetal movement.

There has not been a great deal of clinical application of fetal electrocardiography in veterinary medicine although it is useful in cows and mares for monitoring fetal well-being, for making the diagnosis of fetal death after the midstage of gestation and, by identifying three spike rhythms (maternal and two fetal QRS complexes), for the diagnosis of twin pregnancies [96, 97]. In the case of twin pregnancy in cows, different bipolar lead positions were found best at different stages of pregnancy: at 5 months, vertical right-sided or longitudinal right-sided bipolar abdominal leads; at seven months bipolar leads between rectum or flank and midabdominal line on each side of lower abdomen; and at 9 months, bipolar leads from the right side to the left side of the lower abdomen [100].

Fetal electrocardiography has found another interesting application in teratological studies of toxins with rats [50, 101]. In this case, pregnant rats from the group used in a teratological study are selected and anesthetized. The fetuses are delivered surgically, and three-bipolar-lead electrocardiograms are recorded with intramuscular electrodes attached to both shoulders and one thigh of the fetus (leads I, II, III) while placental attachment is maintained. Since fetal and maternal rat electrocardiograms have different electrophysiological properties and sensitivity to such drugs as cardiac glycosides, simultaneous recording of maternal as well as fetal electrocardiograms should have other applications in toxicology and pharmacology [50].

10.4.5 Types and Duration of Recording

10.4.5.1 Clinical Records

Electrocardiography for the diagnosis of disease in clinical medicine is commonly used in veterinary practice. Here, the selection of leads and duration of records will depend on the purpose being served. In the veterinary clinic the leads selected will depend on their usefulness in diagnosis for the species being examined; in dogs, for instance, the six- or 12-lead system can be used. If the detection or diagnosis of an arrhythmia is needed, the records may be quite long, depending on the tractability of the subject, the patience of the investigator, and the pertinence of the findings, such as for clinical diagnosis in a veterinary clinic. In an epidemiological study of 4,831 dogs from a clinic population, cardiac rate and rhythm were monitored over 5 min by auscultation, palpation of the precordium, palpation of the femoral pulse, and a short casual single-lead electrocardiogram [102]. This standardized examination procedure permitted an analysis of the incidence of abnormal arrhythmias in a clinical population of dogs under these circumstances [103]. It should be stressed that today 24-h ambulatory electrocardiographic monitoring is vital in the detection of arrhythmias and the management of treatment in these animals.

10.4.5.2 Serial Records

Repeated electrocardiograms taken at predetermined intervals are useful in following clinical cases and in monitoring experimental investigations such as chronic or subchronic toxicity studies [45, 49]. In the case of toxicological studies, one important question is whether the test animal has arrhythmogenic properties. Since arrhythmias are typically episodic or sporadic events, it is important that the duration of heart rhythm monitoring be standardized for groups and individuals within groups in such studies. Ideally, this would require continuous monitoring over 24 h.

10.4.6 Telemetry and Holter Monitoring

Electrocardiographic telemetry is almost as old as the electrocardiograph itself. Einthoven, in 1903, reported using the wires of the Leiden telephone system to transmit electrocardiographic signals from a hospital patient to his laboratory, a distance of about 1.6 km [104, 105]. From these early beginnings, remote recording of the electrocardiogram developed along two general lines: telemetry by telephone and radiotelemetry [106] and then, the early Holter monitors (24 h electrocardiographic monitoring) [107].

Extensive use of radiotelemetry for measuring biological variables began with the availability of transistors in 1954 [108] and a strong stimulus for work in this area was the telemetering of biological data from a dog in Sputnik II by the USSR in 1957 [109].

Radiotelemetry was soon applied to unrestrained domestic [110–117], wild [118] and laboratory [108, 119, 120] animals and veterinary patients [121]. With miniaturization and other technological advances, totally implantable biotelemetry systems are now available that record seven channels of physiological data and are small enough (for example, 2.5 × 2.5 ×1.0 cm) to insert into animals the size of infant bonnet monkeys [122–124].

Holter monitoring is commonly used in the clinical care of veterinary patients in order to diagnose arrhythmias, determine their frequency, and verify a successful treatment. In some studies, continuous 24 h ECG monitoring may be of value in determining whether arrhythmias develop as a result of a drug. It is not realistic to think that the brief rhythm strips of a routine ECG, whether it is a casual or serial ECG, could identify accurately the frequency of arrhythmias in response to a drug. Conversely, in the evaluation of the response to therapy for arrhythmias, it is essential that a 24-h Holter be used to most fully determine the benefits or proarrhythmic effects.

10.5 Interspecies Correlations

Electrocardiography is a routine examination undertaken as part of many investigations that seek to evaluate drugs for safety. Moreover, selected species are used in research of all types, including those specific to the cardiovascular system. The most common biomedical research animals today include the mouse [125], rabbit [126], dog [127], minipig [128], and nonhuman primates [129, 130].

10.5.1 Body Size, Heart Rate, and Time Intervals

Many biological variables are related to the size of animals and such allometric relations have been described for various measures of cardiac function including the electrocardiogram [131]. The resting heart rate is related to body size, which is in turn related to metabolic rate, while both heart rate and metabolic rate are regulated by autonomic balance and humoral agents. Broadly considered, the heart weight of mammals is nearly proportional to body mass (approximately 0.6% of body mass) and heart rate per minute is inversely related to both [130–133]. The relationship between heart rate and body weight can be expressed by equations, in which HR is heart rate per minute and W (in kg) is body weight. Two such equations proposed (see [133] and [131], respectively) are in essential agreement:

$$HR = 241 \times W^{-0.25}$$
$$HR = 360 \times W^{-0.26}$$

Individual species or strains may, however, differ substantially from such generalized relationships because of special physiological adaptations. For example, the resting heart rate of the horse ranges from 28 to 48 min^{-1} while that of dairy cattle is 48–84 min^{-1}; the heart rate of the domestic rabbit is 180–350 min^{-1} while that of the hare is 70–80 min^{-1} [132]. Likewise heart weight/body weight ratios may differ in species or strains of the same general size; the wild hare heart weight/body weight ratio is four times that of the Texas jackrabbit and 1.5 times that of the domestic rabbit [135, 136]; that of wild rats is twice the value of laboratory rats [135]; the adult greyhound heart weight/body weight ratio is about 1.3 times that of the mongrel [137]; and thoroughbred race horses have larger hearts than other breeds [135]. With these exceptions to allometric generalizations in mind, it is useful to examine such electrocardiographic relationships [130].

The nearly universal positive correlation between the R-R interval (heart rate) and PR, QRS, and QT durations observed with changes in heart rate in an individual is seen to be preserved in the intraspecies correlation, that is, as heart rates increase and heart sizes decrease, PQ, QRS, and QT intervals decrease linearly, although there are some species that do not fit the regression lines, for example, dolphin and draft horse for QT and draft horse for QRS. The ratio of QRS/QT duration is seen to be about the same among the different species at about 0.20–0.25 while that of PQ/QT is approximately 0.6.

10.5.2 Heart Rate Variability and Acceleration

Different species vary enormously in their respective degree of sinus arrhythmia and some species have a remarkable ability to increase heart rate over resting levels [130, 131].

There has been considerable recent interest in using changes in the degree of heart rate variability (HRV, sometimes termed HPV for heart period variability) as a measure of psychological stress in man and animals [137–139]. In man, HRV is suppressed during sustained attention and in certain psychiatric conditions. In drug testing, agents depressing the brain stem or the sinoatrial node (for instance, calcium-channel blockers) can decrease the degree of respiratory sinus arrhythmia [45] and this variable has been incorporated into a computer-assisted electrocardiographic analysis program for drug studies [140]. Among domestic and laboratory mammals, respiratory sinus arrhythmia is most pronounced in the dog. In this species the R-R intervals may vary as much as eightfold in a given record (that is, from 250 to 2,000 ms).

While sinus arrhythmia is known to be extreme in certain exotic animals, for example, the European mole [65] and the California ground squirrel [118], there is insufficient information on occurrence of this characteristic among the various mammalian species to make valid comparisons between species.

◻ Table 10.2

Prevalence rates per thousand of common spontaneous arrhythmias and conduction disorders in pretest electrocardiograms for unanesthetized beagles (sample population N = 8,977), cynomolgus monkeys (N = 1,165) and albino rats (N = 442)

Arrhythmias or conduction disorders	Beagle	Cynomolgus monkey	Albino rat
Ventricular extrasystoles.	8.0	14.6	67.9
Second-degree AV block.	10.0	0.0	88.2
First-degree AV block.	1.9	0.0	2.3
Right bundle branch block.	0.0	42.1	0.1
Left bundle branch block.	0.0	1.7	2.3
Wolff–Parkinson–White Syndrome.	0.2	0.0	0.0
Any of the above.	20.1	38.6	160.6

With respect to cardiac acceleration, of the animals for which data are available, the horse has the greatest capacity to increase heart rate with exercise [137], for example, from 30 min^{-1} at rest to 240 min^{-1} with strenuous exercise, that is, about an eightfold increase. In man and dog the usual increase in heart rate with strenuous exercise is only about threefold although exceptional racing greyhounds may rival the horses' six to eightfold increase. There is both theoretical and experimental evidence (dog) that even at these high heart rates, continued increase in cardiac output with increase in rate prevails and that this positive relationship between increased heart rate and cardiac output is favored in thoroughbred horses and greyhounds because of their relatively larger hearts and stroke volumes [141, 142].

10.5.3 Arrhythmias and Conduction Disorders

❯ Table 10.2 compares the prevalence of cardiac arrhythmias in pretest (control) electrocardiograms from experimental beagles, cynomolgus monkeys, and albino rats. Respiratory sinus arrhythmia is not included in this table because it is ubiquitous in normal dogs at rest, although it is less frequent in restrained monkeys and rats. Except for Wolff–Parkinson–White (WPW) syndrome, the conduction disturbances are generally considered normal (see below).

In monkeys and rats (❯ Table 10.2), and in pigs as well, ventricular extrasystoles appear to be induced by the excitement and struggling caused by restraint, because their prevalence decreases with training and because their appearance will occur in a few additional subjects during a study in which serial records are taken over a sustained period.

In minipigs, premature sinus beats with aberrant ventricular conduction may be fairly common in untrained groups of animals. In cats under halothane anesthesia, atrioventricular dissociation occurs frequently and may appear occasionally merely as the result of excitement [49].

10.5.4 Heart-Rate Dependence of Electrocardiographic Time Intervals PR, QRS, and QT

The change in PR, QRS, and QT intervals with change in R-R (that is, cycle length or heart rate) makes it necessary to correct these values when comparisons of time intervals are made at different heart rates. If this is not done, the effects of disease, drugs, or toxins, for example, on the QT interval (or on PR or QRS) may be masked by changes in the interval that are dependent on heart rate.

Various linear, cubic or square root, and logarithmic or exponential equations have been proposed to describe these relations [8, 144, 145]. Most of the adjustment formulae are flawed.

Probably the most useful approach at present is for each clinic or laboratory to develop its own database, as has been done for experimental beagles [146, 147]. Either a new formula that adequately describes the relations between the heart rates and time intervals over the entire data range, or a frequency distribution table of these values may be used (see ❯ Table 9.4). The practice of correcting the observed QT interval for heart rate by dividing it by the square root of the length of R-R interval serves very little purpose. With this formula, $QT_c = QT/(RR)^{1/2}$, the observed value of QT at a given heart rate over 60 is increased and, for a rate under 60 it is decreased, but the resultant QT_c does not necessarily remain constant over the heart-rate range for the same animal. Hence, it does not increase the comparability of interval durations at different heart rates.

Since QRS is the shortest of these intervals, its absolute variation with heart-rate change is least and ordinarily is not considered, although the relationship is definitely present [8].

Determination of PR interval and QT interval change with R-R duration poses special problems with rapid heart rates in smaller species such as the rat [50]. There appear to be three reasons for this:

1. At high heart rates (475–$600 \, min^{-1}$) and paper speed of $50 \, mm \, s^{-1}$ or less, any changes in PR-interval and QT-interval duration with rate are small (that is, a few milliseconds) and therefore, difficult to measure accurately. This problem can be resolved with high-frequency sampling and electronic digital recordings that permit measurements at high speeds.
2. Also, at rapid rates (e.g., $>450 \, min^{-1}$) the succeeding P waves are superimposed on the descending limb of the previous T wave and the true QT interval cannot be determined accurately.
3. At lower heart rates (~250–$350 \, min^{-1}$) which occur frequently with anesthesia, these interval changes with rate are greater and easily measurable, but it is uncertain whether this is a rate effect or the result of anesthetic action on the myocardium.

The QT versus R-R relationship exhibits hysteresis; that is, with sudden changes in heart rate, the QT interval changes its duration gradually, requiring several heart beats at the same heart rate to attain a new steady state. Thus, with moderate variations in R-R intervals, as in respiratory sinus arrhythmia of the dog, the associated QT intervals do not undulate. This is also true with second-degree AV block in the dog in which the post-block PR interval is ordinarily shortened but the QT interval is little changed. Horses behave differently, however, because in this species both the PR and QT intervals are shortened in the post-block complex [148].

In premature ventricular extrasystoles, although the preceding R-R interval is shortened, the extrasystolic QT interval is usually longer because of the increase in QRS duration. Exceptionally, in premature ventricular extrasystoles, the QT interval may be shortened, perhaps because of the effect of the shortened R-R interval on conduction velocity and action-potential duration. This latter circumstance appears to be more common in standard swine and minipigs than in other species studied.

10.6 Normal Values

For each species, the lead II time intervals and amplitudes are presented. In these tables, only representative values (mean [above] and range [below]) for time intervals and amplitudes will be given for lead II. Unless otherwise stated, heart-rate and time-interval data are from unanesthetized and unsedated animals. Vectors (frontal plane unless otherwise designated), configuration, normal variants, and special features will be outlined in text.

Normal variants are electrocardiographic rhythm or conduction disturbances and uncharacteristic wave configurations, occurring with a sufficiently high incidence in otherwise healthy individuals of a given species that they cannot be considered abnormal [143]. Some examples are (❯ Table 10.2): first-degree and second-degree atrioventricular block in dogs, horses, and rats; RBBB and (more rarely) LBBB in monkeys; rate-dependent LBBB in rats; premature sinus beats with aberrant ventricular conduction in minipigs; QRS complexes in limb leads only, with broad S waves and low-amplitude R waves, dome-dart ST-T complexes, exaggerated U waves, tall P waves ($>0.4 \, mV$), tall R waves (RV4 up to $6 \, mV$), and P reversal in leads II, III, and a VF in dogs.

Special features mentioned include maximal heart rates with exercise, degree of sinus arrhythmia, and fetal or newborn versus adult electrocardiographic patterns when these facts are known.

10.6.1 Primates

The ECG classification and lead II time intervals and amplitudes for the primates discussed here, namely, the rhesus (❯ Fig. 10.2), cynomolgus and squirrel monkeys (❯ Fig. 10.3), the baboon, and the chimpanzee, are listed in ❯ Table 10.3.

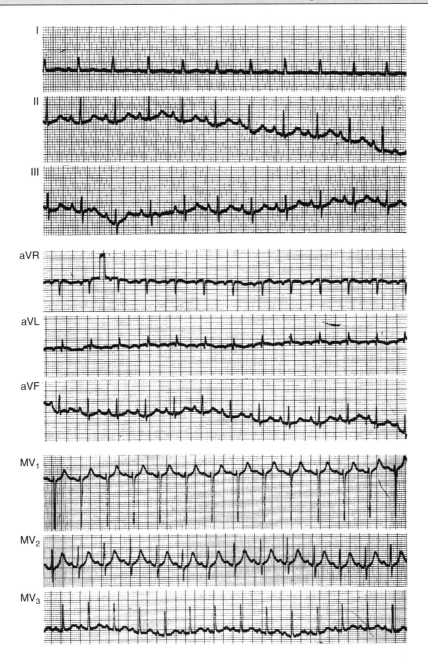

◻ Fig. 10.2

Electrocardiogram from an adult rhesus monkey (*Macaca mulatta*) restrained in a monkey chair: paper speed 50 div s^{-1}. The leads labeled MV$_1$, MV$_2$, and MV$_3$ are the thoracic leads recommended by Atta and Vanace [82]. *MV*$_1$ is located in the fourth right intercostals space, 4 cm from the midsternal line, *MV*$_2$ is on the left side symmetrical with MV$_1$; and *MV*$_3$ is registered at the left midaxillary line in the fifth intercostals space, approximately 1 cm below the level of MV$_2$. MV$_1$ is located over the right ventricle, MV$_2$ often records "transitional" type QRS potentials like those registered over the intraventricular septum and MV$_3$ is located over the left ventricle

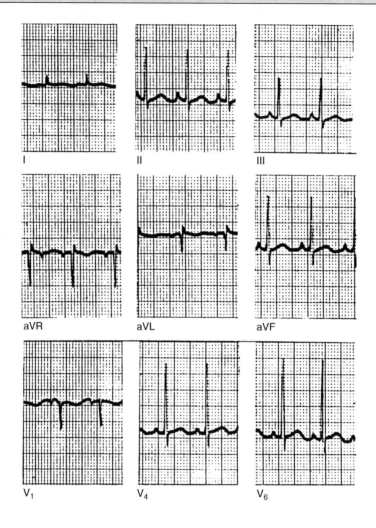

⬛ **Fig. 10.3**
Electrocardiogram from a squirrel monkey (*Saimiri sciureus*) taken under sodium thiopental anesthesia in the supine position. Paper speed 50 div s^{-1}, standardization 0.1 mV div^{-1}. The lead positions are: V_1 third right rib 1 cm to the right of the midline, V_4 ninth left rib 1 cm to the left of the midline, V_6 eighth left rib at the midaxillary line (After Wolf et al. [83]. @ American Physiological Society, Bethesda, Maryland. Reproduced with permission)

The ECG configuration of the rhesus monkey commonly has peaked P waves in II, III, and aVF, and notchings in V_1 and V_3. The QRS complex is usually positive in standard limb leads and the ST segment is generally isoelectric in limb leads. The T wave is usually positive in standard and precordial leads.

Normal variants in the rhesus monkey include RBBB, which is present in about 1.4% and LBBB, which is present in about 0.8% [80]. QRS vectors suggesting incomplete RBBB occur in about 5% [80]. Negative T waves occur in bipolar limb leads in about 6% [80]. Negative T waves in thoracic leads are less common and, in serial electrocardiograms, reversal of T wave polarity may occur occasionally in limb or thoracic leads. Coupled ventricular extrasystoles may be expected in about 1.4%.

A special feature of the rhesus monkey is that the heart rates found in electrocardiograms are far more rapid than basal rates obtained by telemetry. In telemetered electrocardiograms from rhesus monkeys resting and isolated from man, the heart rates are 80–100 min^{-1} and sinus arrhythmia is pronounced. Electrocardiograms of the cynomolgus monkey (*Macaca fascicularis*) have an ECG configuration that is the same as that of the rhesus monkey. Normal variants

◘ Table 10.3

ECG classification and normal parameters in primates

Common English name (species name)	ECG classification			Heart rate (bpm)	Lead II time interval (s)				Lead II amplitude (mV)				
	QRS[a]	QT[b]	T[c]		P	PR	QRS	QT	P	Q	R	S	T
Rhesus monkey (Macaca Mulatta) [37, 38, 46, 78, 80]	A	A	A	257 160–350	0.05 0.03–0.06	0.07 0.05–0.10	0.03 0.02–0.05	0.14 0.11–0.19	0.25 0.12–0.37	0.10 0.00–0.50	0.90 0.00–2.04	0.15 0.00–0.40	0.10 −0.10–0.20
Cynomolgus monkey (Macaca fascicularis) [82, 130, 149]	A	A	A	180 120–220	0.03 0.02–0.05	0.08 0.06–0.11	0.03 0.03–0.05	0.19 0.16–0.25	0.07 0.04–0.26	0.06 0.00–0.30	0.30 0.10–0.95	0.09 0.00–0.46	0.07 0.00–0.50
Squirrel monkey (Saimiri Sciureus) [83]	A	A	A	248 160–340	0.03 0.025–0.035	0.05 0.042–0.058	0.03 0.023–0.037	0.15 0.11–0.20	0.18 0.05–0.30	0.05 0.0–0.1	0.90 0.10–1.70	0.20 0.00–0.50	0.05 −0.10–0.20
Baboon (Papio spp) [37, 81]	A	A	A	127 80–190	0.05 0.04–0.07	0.12 0.05–0.15	0.06 0.04–0.07	0.27 0.20–0.31	0.19 0.09–0.30	0.03 0.00–0.15	1.10 0.80–1.30	0.11 0.00–0.25	0.08 −0.10–0.25
Chimpanzee (Pan Troglodytes) [37]	A	A	A	159 100–249	0.071 0.04–0.10	0.11 0.07–0.15	0.045 0.03–0.07	0.233 0.18–0.32	0.17 0.05–0.40	0.06 0.20–1.70	0.82 0.20–1.70	0.25 0.05–0.90	0.04 −0.10–0.20

a QRS-vector and sense: A along the long axis of the body, caudally and ventrally, B from sternum toward spine

b Relative QT-interval, ST-segment and action-potential duration: A long, B short

c T-wave liability: A constant, B labile

again include RBBB, which is present in about 4% of cases, and LBBB, which is present in about 0.2%. Coupled ventricular extrasystoles also occur with an incidence of 1.5%. Negative T waves may be present in bipolar limb leads and thoracic leads and reversal of previously positive T waves may occur spontaneously in serial records. An electrocardiogram (taken under sodium thiopental anesthesia in the supine position) of the squirrel monkey (Saimiri sciureus) as shown in ❷ Fig. 10.3 has a mean A QRS direction of 62° and A QRS range −60°–115°. The P wave of this species is usually positive in bipolar limb leads, occasionally tall and narrow (0.35 mV) in lead II, and sometimes its amplitude is variable in limb leads. The QRS is occasionally of low amplitude in limb leads. The ST segment is usually isoelectric but deviations of 0.1 mV are sometimes present. T is usually concordant and positive or diphasic in bipolar limb leads.

As in other monkeys, RBBB is not uncommon in its occurrence and is therefore considered a normal variant. A special feature concerning the squirrel monkey is that coupled ventricular extrasystoles occur occasionally in otherwise healthy subjects. Also, since two individuals with WPW syndrome have been found among a relatively small number of squirrel monkeys, a higher prevalence of Wolff–Parkinson–White syndrome may occur in this species than in others.

Electrocardiographic data have been obtained from several monkey species sedated with ketamine [149] including the three discussed above.

Two special features of the baboon should be mentioned. First, WPW syndrome was described among one group of 170 baboons and second, with telemetry the heart rate is 80–100 min^{-1} at rest.

ECGs from chimpanzees (Pan troglodytes) have a P wave that is usually positive in standard limb leads, but occasionally may be isoelectric in either lead I or III. The QRS complex is both of lower amplitude and lower duration than in humans and the T wave is usually concordant and positive in standard limb leads but may be isoelectric in about 30% and occasionally is discordant and negative.

Characteristics particular to the chimpanzee include sinus arrhythmia, which is frequent at heart rates below 125 min^{-1}. Also, wandering pacemaker from the SA node to the AV junction and premature atrial beats occur rarely.

10.6.2   Perissodactyla

The domestic horse (*Equus caballus*) (❷ Fig. 10.4) is the only member of the Perissodactyla discussed here. ❷ Table 10.4 lists the ECG classifications and lead II time intervals and amplitudes. In the domestic horse, the area vector A QRS in the frontal plane lies between −64° and 102°. The range of its direction in the transverse plane is −32°–100° and in the left sagittal plane is −34°–173°. The P wave in bipolar leads is usually bifid, is most often positive, is sometimes diphasic and may change its form spontaneously (for instance, from bifid to single peak) for a series of beats. Such changes in form occur in about 30% of horses. Group B ventricular activation pattern results in major QRS vector forces being directed from the sternum toward the spine. Thus, maximal QRS deflections are rarely recorded in the frontal plane limb leads but rather in the thoracic leads, especially CV$_6$LL, V$_{10}$, Z, or the base apex bipolar lead. The ST segment is usually isoelectric in limb leads and is often arched or coved in chest leads. With regard to the T lability, amplitude may change and polarity reverses with changes in heart rate. In the post-block beat in second-degree AV block, the QT interval shortens, and there is reduction in T wave amplitude or change in form, for instance, from diphasic to positive.

Normal variants in the domestic horse include periodic changes in P-wave configuration (considered as wandering pacemaker in the sinoatrial node), sinoatrial block, first-degree and second-degree atrioventricular block, and nonrespiratory sinus arrhythmia, which all occur commonly in otherwise healthy horses. All these changes are considered to be largely the result of increases in vagal tone in this "vagotonic" species.

Atrial fibrillation is more common in horses and occurs with less-severe underlying heart disease (or with no evidence of heart disease) than in other domestic species. This arrhythmia is treated with quinidine sulfate. Electrical cardioversion is another successful means of treatment. This apparent increased susceptibility to atrial fibrillation in horses is considered to be related to two predisposing factors: large atrial mass and high vagal tone.

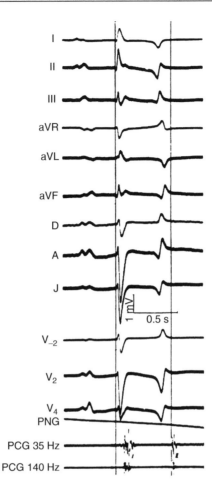

☉ Fig. 10.4

Electrocardiogram of a horse. Conventional bipolar and unipolar limb leads. D, A, and J leads after Sporri [26] as described in ❯ Sect. 10.4.4.2. The V leads are after Brooijmans [67, 72]: V_{-2} right sixth intercostal space at the junction of the lower and middle thirds of the vertical distance between the sternum and the level of the scapulohumeral joint; V_2, symmetrical with V_{-2} in the left sixth intercostal space; V_4 left sixth intercostal space at the level of the scapulohumeral joint. A pneumogram (PNG) and phonocardiograms (PCG) with cutoff filters set at two frequencies, 35 and 140 Hz, are shown at the bottom. The vertical lines are placed at the beginning of QRS and at the beginning of the second heart sound (From Grauwiler [37]. © Birkhäuser, Basel. Reproduced with permission)

10.6.3 Artiodactyla

The members of the Artiodactyla family discussed below are domestic cattle, sheep, goats, and pigs, giraffes, and camels. The ECG classifications, lead II time intervals and amplitudes, and references for further discussion are given in ❯ Table 10.4.

In domestic cattle (*Bos Taurus*), the mean *A* QRS is 70° with a range 30–90°. The P wave is usually positive in standard limb leads and may be bifid in left chest leads. QRS complexes are generally of low amplitude in the standard limb leads. T waves may be concordant or discordant in standard limb leads and are sometimes diphasic negative/positive.

P waves in the domestic pig (*Sus domesticus*) are usually upright in standard limb leads and may be bifid in V_{10} and the chest leads. The ST segment is isoelectric. T waves are often discordant in lead I and usually positive and sometimes diphasic in leads II and III.

◼ Table 10.4

ECG classification and normal parameters in Perissodactyla and Artiodactyla

Common English name (species name)	ECG classification QRS[a]	ECG classification QT[b]	ECG classification T[c]	Heart rate (bpm)	Lead II time interval (s) P	Lead II time interval (s) PR	Lead II time interval (s) QRS	Lead II time interval (s) QT	Lead II amplitude (mV) P	Lead II amplitude (mV) Q	Lead II amplitude (mV) R	Lead II amplitude (mV) S	Lead II amplitude (mV) T
Perissodactyla Domestic horse (*Equus Caballus*) [37, 42, 65, 72, 75, 76, 83, 86–89, 159, 160]	B	A	B	35 26–50	0.14 0.08–0.20	0.33 0.22–0.56	0.13 0.08–0.17	0.51 0.32–0.64	0.28 0.1–0.5	0.12 0.025–0.35	1.13 0.2–2.5	0.15 0.025–0.45	0.20 −0.20–0.90
Artiodactyla Domestic cattle (*Bos Taurus*) [19, 24, 26, 27, 35–37, 53, 67–69, 71–76, 92, 93, 100, 161]	B	A	A	70 48–98	0.06 0.03–0.08	0.19 0.1–0.3	0.095 0.065–0.120	0.40 0.29–0.47	0.10 0.03–0.18	0.16 0.03–1.00	0.37 0.03–2.60	0.07 0.03–0.10	0.31 0.03–1.10
Domestic sheep (*Ovis aries*) [37, 162–168]	B	A	A	107 60–197	0.05 0.04–0.07	0.10 0.06–0.14	0.046 0.025–0.080	0.26 0.17–0.34	0.20 0.1–0.5	0.17 0.1–0.3	0.17 0.08–0.40	0.10 0.10	0.44 0.10–1.60
Domestic goat (*Capra hircus*) [37, 169–171]	B	A	A	96 70–120	0.04 0.02–0.06	0.12 0.08–0.16	0.045 0.03–0.06	0.30 0.24–0.36	0.08 0.02–0.15	0.48 0.07–0.95	0.19 0.02–0.50	0.08 0.02–0.25	0.20 0.05–0.50
Domestic pig (*Sus domesticus*) [37, 172–176]	B	A	A	135 100–180	0.04 0.03–0.05	0.09 0.08–0.12	0.04 0.03–0.06	0.24 0.21–0.26	0.13 0.05–0.30	0.09 0.00–0.14	0.61 0.40–0.78	0.39 0.14–0.50	0.38 −0.20–0.70
Giraffe (*Giraffa camelopardalis reticulate*) [177, 178]	B	A	A	70, 83	0.10, 0.08	0.18, 0.15	0.08, 0.10	0.45, 0.33	0.10, 0.08	0.00, 0.11	0.15, 0.70	0.00, 0.00	−0.30, −0.25
Camel (*Camelus dromedarius*) [179, 180]	B	A	A	30 24–49	0.10 0.08–0.10	0.25 0.24–0.26	0.09 0.04–0.09	0.50 0.48–0.52	0.10 0.06–0.20	0.00	0.40 0.20–1.20	0.45 0.40–0.50	−0.20 −0.40–0.10

[a] QRS-vector direction and sense; A along the long axis of the body, caudally and ventrally, B from sternum toward spine
[b] Relative QT-interval, ST-segment and action-potential duration: A long, B short
[c] T-wave lability: A constant, B labile
[d] Two animals under etorphine (M99)

Ventricular extrasystoles are fairly frequent in excited pigs. In swine, the influence of body weight on electrocardiographic time intervals is separable from the influence of heart rate, as shown by holding the latter constant. When this is done, all electrocardiographic intervals can be shown to increase relatively with increasing body weight [150] (the effect of aging is not separable from that of increased body weight). When the influence of heart rate (R-R interval) alone on the electrocardiographic intervals was examined by holding the body weight constant, the R-R interval was found to have no effect on P-wave duration and a weak effect on PR and QRS intervals, but a strong effect on the QT interval [150]. Thus, both RR interval, that is, heart rate, as well as body weight W (in kg) serve to determine the expected QT interval. The following equations show these relations as calculated from data on 71 swine weighing 11–300 kg [150]:

$$P = 61 + 0.11W$$
$$PR = 107 + 0.17W$$
$$7QRS = 58.8 + 0.14W$$

and

$$QT = 159 + 0.15\,(R - R) + 0.26W$$

where P, PR, QRS, and QT are given in milliseconds.

In the ECGs of two giraffes, taken under etorphine, the QRS vectors were $-25°$ and $95°$ (an example is shown in ❯ Fig. 10.5). The R wave was either positive or negative in leads I, II, and III. The QRS was positive in leads I and II in both animals and negative in lead III in one subject. The ST segment was isoelectric and the T waves were usually discordant (see also [155]).

❯ Figure 10.6 shows the ECG of a dromedary camel (*Camelus droinedarius*) taken in the standing position and under no drugs. The mean A QRS is $+250°$ (with a range between $90°$ and $280°$). In standard limb leads, the P waves are positive, QRS complexes may be chiefly positive or negative and the ST segment is isoelectric. T waves are usually discordant. A special attribute of the camel is that sinus arrhythmia is present.

10.6.4 Cetacea

❯ Table 10.5 lists the ECG classifications, lead II time intervals and amplitudes, and references of the finback, beluga and killer whales, and the dolphin. ECGs from bottle-nosed dolphins are shown in ❯ Fig. 10.7

The ECG of a finback whale (*Balaenoptera physalus*), beached 23 h before the recordings were made, has a broad P wave with low amplitude, a QRS complex which is chiefly negative in leads II and III and an ST segment which is isoelectric. T waves are discordant in most leads. In the beluga whale (*Delphinapterus leucas*), the bipolar lead between an electrode on the back at the pectoral girdle and one about the midportion of the back did not record the P wave distinctly. The QRS pattern was qR and the T wave was negative (discordant). In the killer whale (*Orcinus orca*), no P wave was recorded, the QRS had a qR configuration, and T was discordant.

10.6.5 Marsupialia

❯ Table 10.5 lists the ECG classifications, lead II time intervals and amplitudes, and references of the Bennett's kangaroo and the opossum.

Electrocardiograms from the Bennett's kangaroo (*Macropus bennetti*) have P waves that are positive and sometimes bifid in standard limb and chest leads. In leads II, III, and in chest leads over the left ventricle, QRS complexes are somewhat similar with an RS configuration. The ST segment is absent in adults. T waves are positive, concordant in limb and chest leads, beginning immediately after QRS with no intervening ST segment.

Bennett's kangaroo was the first larger species in which it was shown that when the ST segment is absent and the QT, therefore, short, there is marked dissociation between the end of the T wave and the end of mechanical systole.

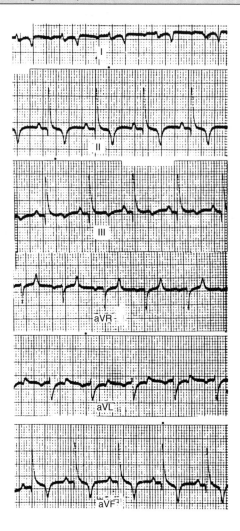

◘ Fig. 10.5

Electrocardiogram of a reticulated giraffe taken under etorphine HCl (M99) sedation in the right lateral recumbent position: paper speed 25 div s⁻¹; standardization 0.05 mV div⁻¹ (After Jefferson [154]. © American Veterinary Medical Association, Schaumburg, Illinois. Reproduced with permission)

Correct interpretation of such fusion of QRS and T and mechanical and electrical dissociation in the mouse had been made a few years earlier in 1953 [151], The single record available from a wallaby (*Macropus walabatus*) had a short ST segment in limb leads and QT intervals of 0.16–0.18 s at a heart rate of 160 bpm. In another single record labeled "kangaroo" with no species designation, a short ST segment in limb leads was present and the QT interval was 0.23 s [5]. In 14 adult Australian rock kangaroos (*Macropus robustus*) under ketamine and pentobarbital anesthesia, the mean QT intervals of 0.214 s were far shorter than the mean mechanical systole of 0.393 s [152].

In the young Bennett's kangaroos still in the maternal pouch, the ST segment is present, as is true in the fetal or newborn rat [50] and mouse [151], and the duration of QT and mechanical systole are also similar. The adult conformation appears at the time the young kangaroos leave the pouch.

In the opossum (*Didelphis marsupialis*), the P waves are small and positive in standard limb leads. QRS complexes are chiefly positive in standard limb leads. Unlike the case of the adult Bennett's kangaroo, the ST segment is present. T waves are positive and concordant in standard limb leads.

Table 10.5

ECG classification and normal parameters in the Cetacea and Marsupialia

Common English name (species name)	ECG classification			Heart rate (bpm)	Lead II time interval (s)				Lead II amplitude (mV)				
	QRS[a]	QT[b]	T[c]		P	PR	QRS	QT	P	Q	R	S	T
Cetacea Finback whale[d] (*Balaenoptera physalus*) [181]	B	A	A	27–32	0.40	0.68–0.73	0.32–0.34	0.96–1.08	0.10	0.30	0.00	0.00	0.50
Beluga whale (*Delphinapterus leucas*) [4]	B	A	A	16 12–24	not measurable	0.32	0.09–0.12	0.36–0.40	0.03	0.10	0.3–0.4	0.00	0.10–0.15
Killer whale (*Orcinus orca*) [182]	B	A	A	20–60	not visible P waves	not visible P waves	0.12	0.36	0.00	0.05	0.60	0.00	−0.30 0.10–0.25
Dolphin [183, 184]	B	A	A	100 60–137	0.82 0.06–0.10	0.178 0.120–0.210	0.065 0.05–0.08	0.257 0.05–0.320	0.03 0.03–0.20	0.03 0.00–0.15	0.30 0.20–0.40	0.20 0.03–0.40	0.15 0.10–0.25
Marsupialia Bennett's kangaroo (*Macropus bennetti*) [37, 186–231]	A	B	A	119 108–152	0.04 0.03–0.05	0.107 0.090–0.118	0.045 0.040–0.050	0.142 0.120–0.165	0.15	0.00	2.30	1.40	1.20
Opossum[e] (*Didelphis marsupialis*) [189]	A	A	A	200	not given	0.08	0.02–0.03	0.14	0.01	0.02	1.5	0.00	0.10

[a] QRS-vector direction and sense; *A* along the long axis of the body, caudally and ventrally, *B* from sternum toward spine

[b] Relative QT-interval, ST-segment and action-potential duration: *A* long, *B* short

[c] T-wave lability: *A* constant, *B* labile

[d] Beached 23 h before recordings were made

[e] Under pentobarbital sodium anesthesia

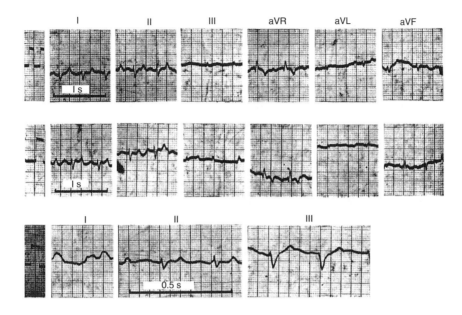

◘ Fig. 10.7

Electrocardiograms from a bottle-nosed dolphin: (a) ECG recorded immediately after loading on a truck at the port of Arari Bay: heart rate (HR) = 136.3 min⁻¹, interval times are R-R = 0.44 s, PQ = 0.16 s, QRS = 0.14 s, OT = 0.26 s, and T = 0.1 s. (**b**) ECG recorded after 4 h on the truck at Mishima: HR = 120 min⁻¹, interval times are R-R = 0.5 s, PQ = 0.2 s, QRS = 0.08 s, QT = 0.28 s, T = 0.14 s. (**c**) ECG recorded after 8 h on the truck at Enoshima: HR = 125 min⁻¹, R-R interval is 0.48 s. Needle electrodes or plate electrodes were placed at sites corresponding to the attachment of limbs in man. The pulses shown on the left of each panel indicate the scale of 1 mV (After Tokita et al. [156]. © Geirui Kenkyosho, Tokyo, Japan. Reproduces with permission)

10.6.6 Lagomorpha

The ECG classifications, lead II time intervals and amplitudes, and references of the rabbit (*Orytolagus cuniculus*) are given in ❷ Table 10.6.

The mean *A* QRS in the rabbit is 64° with a range of 0–180°. The P waves in rabbits are positive in standard limb leads and may be rather pointed in some strains. QRS complexes are generally positive, ST segments are usually isoelectric, and T waves are usually positive in standard limb leads. While a number of investigators have noted changes in T-wave polarity, especially in lead III and in chest leads, the amount of variability is only about the same as seen in nonhuman primates and is insufficient to classify this species as T labile or class B.

10.6.7 Rodentia

In recent years mice have been used extensively in genetic research. The expansion of this area of research, in addition to advances in the field of electrophysiology and the use of the mouse to match cardiac phenotype to genotype, has expanded the role of the mouse as a model. Despite this increase, criticism continues about the conclusions from the murine cardiac responses to that of other mammals and, importantly, humans [52]. The mouse has been evaluated by cardiac electrophysiological mapping studies, induction of particular arrhythmias, conduction abnormalities, infarction changes, and infectious responses by methods beyond the ECG.

The ECG classifications, lead II amplitudes and time intervals of the white laboratory rat and mouse and the guinea pig are listed in ❷ Table 10.6.

In the electrocardiograms of a white laboratory rat (*Rattus norvegicus*) for various foreleg positions the mean *A* QRS is 50° (with a range from −22° to 120°). There is some evidence that the *A* QRS shifts to the left with aging, but this has not

Table 10.6

ECG classification and normal parameters in Lagomorpha and Rodentia

Common English name (species name)	ECG classification			Heart rate (bpm)	Lead II time interval (s)				Lead II amplitude (mV)				
	QRS[a]	QT[b]	T[c]		P	PR	QRS	QT	P	Q	R	S	T
Lagomorpha Rabbit (*Orytolagus cuniculus*) [37, 190–195]	A	A	A	240 190–300	0.30 0.25–0.40	0.70 0.5–0.8	0.35 0.10–0.15		0.10 0.05–0.20	0.00	0.40 0.30–0.80	0.15 0.05–0.30	0.15 0.05–0.30
Rodentia White laboratory rat (*Ratus norvegicus*) [37, 47, 50, 196–200]	A	B	A	460 228–600	0.013 0.010–0.016	0.040 0.033–0.050	0.017 0.012–0.026	0.066 0.038–0.080	0.11 0.02–0.20	0.00	1.06 0.22–1.50	0.20 0.00–0.05	0.15 0.05–0.30
White laboratory mouse (*Mus musculus*) [37, 185, 201–204]	A	B	A	632 500–750	0.010	0.038 0.028–0.50	0.010 0.006–0.020	0.035 −0.030–0.050	0.05	0.00	0.30	0.15	0.20
Guinea pig (*Cavia porcellus*) [26, 37]	A	A	A	226 200–300	0.036 0.022–0.048	0.061 0.046–0.077	0.023 0.020–0.030	0.146 0.110–0.185	0.17 0.10–0.22	0.02 0.00–0.11	1.65 0.82–2.63	0.19 0.00–0.58	0.21 0.08–0.38

a QRS-vector direction and sense: A along the long axis of the body, caudally and ventrally, B from sternum toward spine

b Relative QT-interval, ST-segment and action-potential duration: A along, B short

c T-wave lability: A constant, B labile

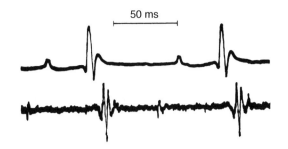

■ Fig. 10.8

Electrocardiogram (*top*) and phonocardiogram (*bottom*) from a white laboratory mouse (*Mus musculus*), lead A (right arm electrode right side at base of neck, left leg electrode at cardiac apex). The second heart sound occurs 40 ms after the end of the T wave and no ST segment is present (After Grauwiler [37]. © Birkhauser, Basel. Reproduced with permission)

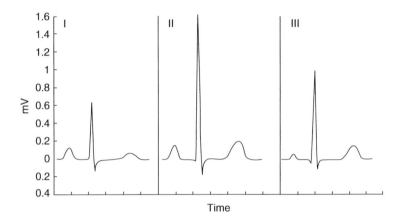

■ Fig. 10.9

Limb leads I. II, III from a guinea pig (*Cavia parcellus*) (After Sporri H. *Habilitatiansschrift*. Zurich: University of Zurich, 1944 [26]. Reproduced with permission)

been studied. In the white laboratory rat, the P wave is normally positive in leads I, II, III, and aVF, negative in aVR and flat or negative in aVL. Negative P waves are common in lead III. The Ta wave is usually discordant and appears to terminate or become isoelectric prior to the onset of the QRS complex. The Q of the QRS complex is usually absent in standard bipolar limb leads while R is prominent and S may be either prominent or absent. The ST segment is absent and the S-wave termination in bipolar leads is often difficult to separate from the onset of T. There is often no distinct isoelectric line during the electrocardiographic complex; that is, the points at which P, Ta, QRS, and T waves originate are often on different levels. This is especially true at more rapid heart rates when the P wave originates on the descending limb of the preceding T wave. The T wave is usually positive and concordant with QRS in leads II and III, but may be negative and discordant in lead I. Its ascending limb is typically steeper than its descending limb. The latter usually approaches the isoelectric line gradually, such that its termination is difficult to identify. At more rapid heart rates (450 bpm), the P wave interrupts the descent of the T wave. QT intervals are difficult to measure accurately on account of the gradual descent of T and because the succeeding P wave may interrupt the descent of T before it reaches the baseline. This has led to measuring the interval from the beginning of QRS to the apex of T (the QTa interval) instead of QT. Since the T apex can shift within the QT interval if the shape of T changes, this measurement is not a satisfactory determinant of the true QT interval.

□ Table 10.7

ECG classification and normal parameters in Carnivora and Proboscidea

Common English name (species name)	ECG classification			Heart rate rate (bpm)	Lead II time interval (s)				Lead II amplitude (mV)				
	QRS[a]	QT[b]	T[c]		P	PR	QRS	QT	P	Q	R	S	T
Carnivora Domestic cat (*Felis catus*) [37, 205–212, 232]	A	A	A	190 110–300	0.03 0.02–0.05	0.07 0.05–0.10	0.03 0.015–0.04	0.15 0.1–0.2	0.16 0.00–0.20	0.15 0.00–0.30	0.50 0.00–1.05	0.27 0.00–0.70	0.18 −0.05–0.40
Proboscidea Indian elephant (*Elephas maximus*) [3, 37, 213–216]	B	A	A	38 30–46	0.16 0.12–0.30	0.44 0.36–0.48	0.16 0.12–0.18	0.64 0.60–0.70	0.05 0.03–0.10	0.05 0.03–0.10	0.70 0.60–0.80	0.15 0.10–0.20	0.10 0.05–0.20
African elephant (*Loxodonto Africana*) [37, 216, 217]	B	A	A	46 42–53	0.11 0.10–0.12	0.28 0.20–0.32	0.13 0.12–0.19	0.55 0.48–0.60	0.10	0.05	0.30	0.35	0.20

[a] QRS-vector direction and sense; *A* along the long axis of the body, caudally and ventrally, *B* from sternum toward spine

[b] Relative QT-interval, ST-segment and action-potential duration: *A* along, *B* short

[c] T-wave lability: *A* constant, *B* labile

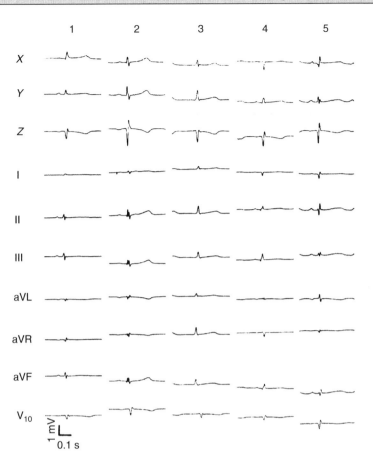

As shown in ❯ Table 10.2, ventricular extrasystoles (about 7%) and second-degree atrioventricular block (about 8%) are sufficiently frequent in control electrocardiograms from rats to be considered normal variants. This is also true for sinus arrhythmia since in some series this has been present in over half the subjects.

A shift of *A* QRS in the frontal plane has been noted by some observers during the first 4 or 5 months of life. Others have found that the percentage of rats with a leftward QRS axis increased in older and postpartum groups of rats.

The maximum heart rate found in rat electrocardiograms is usually no higher than 600 bpm. In some individuals when rates exceed 600 bpm by a few beats (e.g., 620–635 bpm) an LBBB pattern appears in the electrocardiogram. Also, in a group of 75 rats entered in a drug study, LBBB appeared spontaneously in 32% after 1 year of age (week 65) unrelated to the test agent (that is, the distribution of the bundle branch block was the same in control and treated animals). This has not been seen in other studies and probably represents an inherited characteristic of this rat strain. As mentioned previously, the ST segment is present in newborn rats but disappears during the first three to four weeks of life.

An ECG and phonocardiogram of a white laboratory mouse (*Mus musculus*) is shown in ❯ Fig. 10.8. This species of rodent has a mean *A* QRS of 31° (with a range from −10° to 70°). P waves are usually positive in the standard limb leads. QRS complexes are chiefly positive in the standard limb leads with no Q wave and the S wave is absent or, if present, is usually small. The ST segment is absent and the T waves are concordant.

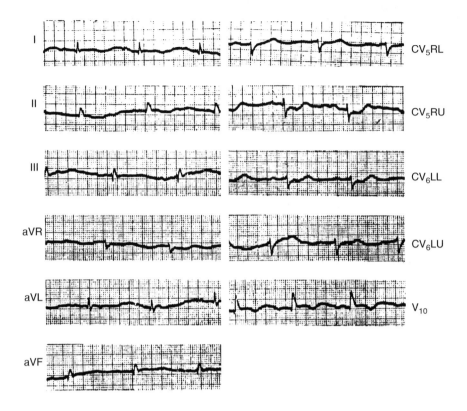

◘ Fig. 10.11

Electrocardiogram from the Indian elephant (*Elephas maximus*). The lead system is as described in ❷ Sect. 10.4.4.2 (After Jayasinghe et al. [158]. Bailliere Tindall, London. Reproduced with permission)

In the ECG of the guinea pig (*Cavia porcellus*) (❷ Fig. 10.9), the mean *A* QRS is 6° (range −20° to 60°). The ECG configuration has, in the standard limb leads, P waves which are positive and QRS complexes which generally have small q, large R and small S waves. The ST segment is present and usually isoelectric in limb leads. T waves are chiefly positive and concordant in the standard limb leads.

10.6.8   Carnivora

The domestic cat is the only member of the Carnivora discussed here. ❷ Table 10.7 lists the ECG classification lead II time intervals and amplitudes of the cat.

The ECG of the domestic cat (*Felis catus*) (❷ Fig. 10.10) has a mean *A* QRS of 70° (the range is −20°–170°). P waves are usually positive in standard limb leads. When P waves are absent in limb leads, the recording should be inspected closely for signs of AV dissociation when P waves periodically become buried in the QRS. QRS complexes are dominated by R waves in standard limb leads. The ST segment is usually isoelectric and T waves are usually concordant and stable in limb leads.

Cardiomyopathy is a common disease seen in the cat. Such afflicted cats can have a normal ECG or evidence of left anterior fascicular block or left ventricular enlargement. The ECG in the kitten has also been studied from birth to 30 days [153].

10.6.9 Proboscidea

An example of the ECG of the Indian elephant (*Elephas maximus*) is shown in ❯ Fig. 10.11. ❯ Table 10.7 gives the ECG classification and lead II time intervals and amplitudes for the Indian elephant and the African elephant (*Loxodonto africana*).

Acknowledgements

This work was supported in part by the US National Institutes of Health Grant Number LM 01660 and by Smith, Kline and French Laboratories, Philadelphia, Pennsylvania. Dr. Sydney Moise at Cornell University contributed updates to this chapter.

References

1. Waller, A.D., Introductory address on the electromotive properties of the human heart. *Br. Med. J.*, 1888;**2**: 751–754.
2. Tawara, S., *Das Reizleitungssystem des Säugetierherzens*. Jena: Fischer, 1906.
3. White, P.D., J.L. Jenks Jr, and F.G. Benedict, The electrocardiogram of the elephant. *Am. Heart J.*, 1938;**16**: 744–750.
4. King, R.L., J.L. Jenks Jr, and P.D. White, The electrocardiogram of a Beluga whale. *Circulation*, 1953;**8**: 387–393.
5. Zuckermann, R., *Grundriss und Atlas der Elektrokardiographie*, 3rd edn. Leipzig: Thieme, 1959.
6. Kisch, B., F.M. Groedel, and P.R. Borchardt, *Comparative Direct Electrography of the Heart of Vertebrates*. New York: Fordham University Press, 1952.
7. Lepeschkin, E., *Das Elektrokardiogramm. Ein Handbuchfiir Theorie und Praxis*, 2nd edn. Dresden: Steinkopff, 1947.
8. Lepeschkin, E., *Modern Electrocardiography*. Baltimore, MD: Williams and Wilkins, 1951.
9. Rijlant, P.B., Origin of the heart beat in the mammalian heart (in Russian), in *Comparative Electrocardiology International Symposium* (in Russian), M.P. Roshchevsky, Editor. Leningrad: Akademiia Nauk SSSR, 1981, pp. 20–23.
10. Lewis, T., Irregularity of the heart's action in horses and its relationship to fibrillation of the auricles in experiment and to complete irregularity of the human heart. *Heart*, 1912;**3**: 161–171.
11. Lewis, T., *The Mechanism and Graphic Registration of the Heart Beat*, 3rd edn. London: Shaw, 1925.
12. Luisada, A. L. Weisz, and H.W. Hartman, A comparative study of electrocardiogram and heart sounds in common and domestic animals. *Cardiologia*, 1944;**8**: 63–84.
13. Robb, J.S., *Comparative Basic Cardiology*. New York: Grune and Stratton, 1965.
14. von Tschermak, A., Lehre von den bioelektrischen Strömen (Elektrophysiologie), in *Lehrbuch der Vergleichenden Physiologie der Haussäugetiere*, W. Ellenberger and A. Scheunert, Editors. Berlin: Parey, 1910, p. 520.
15. Kahn, R.H., Das Pferde-Ekg. *Pfluegers Arch. Gesamle Physiol. Menschen Tiere*, 1913;**154**: 1–15.
16. Waller, A.D., Electrocardiogram of horse. *J. Physiol.*, 1913;**47**(Proc. Physiol. Soc. London): xxxii–xxxiv.
17. Waller, A.D., A short account of the origin and scope of electrocardiography. *Harvey Lect.*, 1913–1914;**9**: 17–33. (*N. Y. Med. J.* 1914;97: 719).
18. Nörr, J., Das Elektrocardiogramm des Pferdes; seine Aufnahme und Form. *Z. Biol.*, 1913;**61**: 197–229.
19. Nörr, J., Elektrokardiogrammstudien am Rind. *Z. Biol.*, 1921;**73**: 129–140.
20. Nörr, J., Über Herzstromkurvenaufnahmen an Haustieren. Zur Einfiihrung der Elektrokardiographie in die Veteriniirmedizin. *Arch. Wiss. Prakl. Tierheilkd.*, 1922;**48**: 85–111.
21. GylstorffI. Prof. Dr. Nörr 85 Jahre. Berlin u. München. *Tieraerztl. Wochenschr.*, 1971;**4**: 240.
22. Lannek, N. and L. Rutqvist, Electrocardiography in horses. A historical review. *Nord. Veterinaermed*, 1951;**3**: 435–447.
23. Lannek, N., *A Clinical and Experimental Study on the Electrocardiogram in dogs*, Thesis. Stockholm, Sweden: Royal Veterinary College, 1949.
24. Roshchevsky, M.P., *Electrocardiology of Hoofed Animals* (in Russian). Leningrad: Nauka, 1978.
25. Spörri, H., Veränderungen der Systolendauer im Elektrokardiogramm von Rind und Meerschweinchen. *Arch. Wiss. Prakl. Tierheilkd.*, 1941;**76**: 236–247.
26. Spörri, H., Der Einfluss der Tuberkulose auf das Elektrokardiogramm. (Untersuchungen an Meerschweinchen und Rindern.) *Arch. Wiss. Prakl. Tierheilkd.*, 1944;**79**: 1–57.
27. Alfredson, B.V. and J.F. Sykes, Electrocardiographic studies in normal dairy cattle. *J. Agric.Res. (Washington D.C.)*, 1942;**65**: 61–87.
28. Charton, A. and G. Minot, Electrocardiogramme normal du cheval. *C. R. Seances Soc. Biol. Ses Fil.*, 1943;**137**: 150–152.
29. Charton, A., G. Minot, and M. Bressou, Electrocardiogramme normal du cheval. *Bull. Acad Vet. Fr.*, 1943;**16**: 141–148.
30. Bressou, M., *L 'Electrocardiogramme et le Phonocardiogramme du Cheval Normal*. Paris: Foulon, 1944.
31. Kelso, W.T., Electrocardiograms of young lambs. *Queensl. J. Agric. Sci.*, 1947;**4**: 60–71.
32. Krzywanek, F.W. and G. Ruud, Die Veränderungen des Elektrokardiogramms beim sogenannten Herztod des Schweines. *Tieraerztl. Umsch.*, 1944;**2**: 23–25.

33. Ruud, G., *Das Elektrokardiogramm des Schweines und die Veränderungen desselben beim sogenannten Herztod des Schweines*, Veterinary dissertation. Berlin, 1945.

34. Voskanyan, P.M., Electrocardiography of horses (in Russian). *Trudi XV Plenum Vet. Sektsii Vses. Akad. Moskva, Nauka* 1941; 250–256.

35. Filatov, P.B., Electrocardiography of cattle, in *Non-infectious Internal Diseases of Animals* (in Russian). *Sb. Rab. Voenno-Vel. Fakulteta Mosk. Vet. Akad. Moskva. Nauka* 1949;6: 207–222.

36. Roshchevsky, M.P., *Electrical Activity of the Heart and Methods of Recording Electrocardiograms from Large Livestock(Cattle)* (in Russian). Sverdlovsk: Uralskii Gosudarstvennyi Universitet, 1958.

37. Grauwiler, J., *Herz und Kreislauf der Säugetiere; Vergleichend-Funktionelle Daten*. Basel: Birkhäuser, 1965.

38. Roshchevsky, M.P., *Evolutional Electrocardiology* (in Russian). Leningrad: Nauka, 1972.

39. Roshchevsky, M.P., Editor. *Physiological Basis of Animal Electrocardiography*. Moscow: Nauka, 1965.

40. Roshchevsky, M.P., Editor. *Comparative Electrocardiology. Proceedings of the 1st International Symposium* (in Russian). Leningrad: Nauka, 1981.

41. Roshchevsky, M.P., Editor. *Comparative Electrocardiology. Proceedings of the 2nd International Symposium* (in Russian).

42. G.F. Fregin, The cardiovascular system, in *Equine Medicine and Surgery*, vol. 1, 3rd edn, RA Mansmann, ES McAllister, and PW Pratt, Editors. Santa Barbara: American Veterinary Publishing, 1982, pp. 645–704.

43. Edwards, N.J., *Bolton's Handbook of Canine and Feline Electrocardiography*, 2nd edn. Philadelphia, PA: Saunders, 1987.

44. Tilley, L.P., *Essentials of Canine and Feline Electrocardiography*, 2nd edn. Philadelphia, PA: Lea and Febiger, 1985.

45. Detweiler, D.K., The use of electrocardiography in toxicological studies with Beagle dogs, in *Cardiac Toxicology*, vol. 3, T. Balazs, Editor. Boca Raton, FL: CRC Press, 1981, pp. 33–82.

46. Malinow, M.R., The electrocardiogram (ECG) and vectorcardiogram (VCG) of the rhesus monkey, in *Anatomy and Physiology*, G.H. Bourne, Editor. New York: Academic Press, 1975, pp. 77–105. (*The Rhesus Monkey*; vol. 1.)

47. Budden, R., D.K. Detweiler, and G. Zbinden, Editors. *The Rat Electrocardiogram in Pharmacology and Toxicology*. Oxford: Pergamon, 1981.

48. Kachiku No Shindenzu (*Advances in Animal Electrocardiography*). Tokyo: Japanese Association of Veterinary Cardiology. (Japanese language journals in existence since 1968. English translations of titles, legends, and summaries often included.)

49. Detweiler, D.K., Electrocardiographic monitoring in toxicological studies: Principles and interpretations, in *Myocardial Injury, Advances in Experimental Medicine and Biology*, vol. 161, J.J Spitzer, Editor. New York: Plenum, 1983, pp. 579–607.

50. Detweiler, D.K., The use of electrocardiography in toxicological studies with rats, in *The Rat Electrocardiogram in Pharmacology and Toxicology*, R. Budden, D.K. Detweiler, and G. Zbinden, Editors. Oxford: Pergamon, 1981, pp. 83–115.

51. Grauwiler, J. and H. Spörri, Fehlen der ST-Strecke im Elektrokardiogramm von verschiedenen Saugetierarten. *Helv. Physiol. Pharmacol. Acta.*, 1960;**C18**: 77–78.

52. Nerbonne, J.M., Studying cardiac arrhythmias in the mouse-a reasonable model for probing mechanisms? *Trends Cardiovasc. Med.*, 2004;**14**: 83–93.

53. Hamlin, R.L. and C.R. Smith, Categorization of common domestic mammals based upon their ventricular activation process. *Ann. N. Y. Acad. Sci.*, 1965;**127**: 195–203. (See also Hamlin, R.L., D.L. Smetzer, and C.R. Smith, Analysis of QRS complex recorded through a semiorthogonal lead system in the horse. *Am. J. Physiol.*, 1964;**207**: 325–333.)

54. Hill, J.D., The electrocardiogram in dogs with standardized body and limb positions. *J. Electrocardiol.*, 1968;**1**: 175–182.

55. Hill, J.D., The significance of foreleg positions in the interpretation of electrocardiograms and vectorcardiograms from research animals. *Am. Heart J.*, 1968;**75**: 518–527.

56. Detweiler, D.K., Electrophysiology of the heart, in *Dukes' Physiology of Domestic Animals*, 10th edn, M.J. Swenson, Editor. Ithaca, NY: Cornell University Press, 1984, pp. 103–130.

57. Rappaport, M.B. and I. Rappaport, Electrocardiographic considerations in small animal investigations. *Am. Heart J.*, 1943;**26**: 662–680.

58. Werth, G. and S. Wink, Das Elektrokardiogramm der normalen Ratte. *Arch. Kreislaufforsch.*, 1967;**54**: 272–308.

59. Angelakos, E.T. and P. Bernardini, Frequency components and positional changes in electrocardiogram of the adult rat. *J. Appl. Physiol.*, 1963;**18**: 261–263.

60. Godwin, K.O. and F.J. Fraser, Simultaneous recording of ECGs from disease-free rats, using a cathode ray oscilloscope and a direct writing instrument. *Q. J. Exp. Physiol.*, 1965;**50**: 277–281.

61. Almasi, J.J., O.H. Schmitt, and E.F. Jankus, Electrical characteristics of commonly used canine ECG electrodes. *Proc. Annu. Conf. Eng. Med. Biol.*, 1970;**12**: 190.

62. Osborne, B.E., A restraining device facilitating electrocardiogram recording in dogs. *Lab. Anim. Care*, 1970;**20**: 1142–1143.

63. Beinfield, W.H. and D. Lehr, Advantages of ventral position in recording electrocardiogram of rat. *J. Appl. Physiol.*, 1956;**9**: 153–156.

64. Richtarik, A., T.A. Woolsey, and E. Valdivia, Method for recording ECG's in unanesthetized guinea pigs. *J. Appl. Physiol.*, 1965;**20**: 1091–1093.

65. Detweiler, D.K. and H. Spörri, A note on the absence of auricular fibrillation in the European mole (Talpa europaea). *Cardiologia*, 1957;**30**: 372–375.

66. Waller, A.D., Ueber die den Pulsbegleitende elektrische Schwankung des Herzens (Ausserordentliche) Sitzung am 27. Dec. 1889. *Arch. Physiol. Physiologische Abtheilung des Arch. Anat. Physiol.*, 1890; 186–190.

67. Brooijmans, A.W.M., *Electrocardiography in Horses and Cattle: Theoretical and Clinical Aspects, Vet. Proefschrift Rijksuniversiteit*. Utrecht: Cantecleer, 1957.

68. Balbo, T. and U. Dotta, Gli effetti dell'eta sull'elettrocardiogramma del bovino. 1 and 2. *La Nuova Vet.*, 1966;**62**: 307–355 and Suppl. 6.

69. Lautenschlager, O., *Grundlagen der Aufnahmetechnik des Elektrokardiogrammes von Pferd und Rind und ihre Ergebnisse*, Veterinary dissertation. Giessen, 1928.

70. Morita, H., Electrocardiograms of conscious Beagle dogs by apex-base bipolar lead. *Adv. Anim. Cardiol.*, 1984;**17**: 19–23.

71. Sander, W., Das Elektrokardiogramm des Rindes. *Zentralbl. Veterinaermed.*, 1968;**15**: 587–634.

72. Brooijmans, A.W.M., Standardization of leads in veterinary clinical electrocardiography. *Tijdschr. Diergeneeskd.*, 1954;**79**: 801–811.

73. Sellers, A.F., A. Hemingway, E. Simonson, and W.E. Petersen, Unipolar and bipolar electrocardiographic studies in dairy cattle. *Am. J. Vet. Res.*, 1958;**19**: 620–624.

74. Junge, G., Über die Elektrokardiographie in der Veterinärmedizin unter besonderer Berücksichtigung der allgemeinen Elektrophysiologie und der Ableitung des Rinderelektrokardiogramms. *Arch. Exper. Veterinaermedizin*, 1967;**21**: 835–866.

75. Sugeno, H., Y. Yasuda, H. Nishikawa, and T. Takeya, Studies of the electrocardiogram of normal healthy cows. *J. Fac. Agr. Iwate Univ.*, 1956;**3**: 114–125.

76. Too, K., R. Nakamura, and K. Hirao, Studies on the applications of electrocardiogram in cattle. *Jpn. J. Vet. Res.*, 1958;**6**: 230–244.

77. Kusachi, R. and H. Sato, Fundamental studies on electrocardiograms of the horse. II. Bipolar lead. *Jpn. J. Vet. Res.*, 1955;**3**: 195–208.

78. Lannek, N. and L. Rutqvist, Normal area variation for the electrocardiogram of horses. *Nord. Veterinaermed.*, 1951;**3**: 1094–1117.

79. Detweiler, D.K. and D.F. Patterson, The cardiovascular system, in *Equine Medicine and Surgery*, 2nd edn, E.J. Catcott and J.F. Smithcors, Editors. Wheaton, IL: American Veterinary Publishing, 1972, pp. 277–347.

80. Malinow, M.R., An electrocardiographic study of *Macaca mulatta. Folia Primarol*, 1966;**4**: 51–65.

81. Herrmann, G.R. and A.H.W. Herrmann, The electrocardiographic patterns in 170 baboons in the domestic and African colonies at the primate center of the Southwest Foundation for Research and Education, in *The Baboon in Medical Research*, vol. I, H. Vagtborg, Editor. Austin, TX: University of Texas Press, 1965, pp. 251–264.

82. Atta, A.G. and P.W. Vanace, Electrocardiographic studies in the *Macaca mulatta* monkey. *Ann. N.Y. Acad. Sci.*, 1960;**85**: 811–818.

83. Wolf, R.H., N.D.M. Lehner, E.C. Miller, and T.B. Clarkson, Electrocardiogram of the squirrel monkey *(Saimiri sciureus). J. Appl. Physiol.*, 1969;**26**: 346–351.

84. Hellerstein, H.K. and R. Hamlin, QRS component of the spatial vectorcardiogram and of the spatial magnitude and velocity electrocardiograms of the normal dog. *Am. J. Cardiol.*, 1960;**6**: 1049–1061.

85. Hamlin, R.L., J.A. Himes, H. Guttridge, and W. Kirkham, P wave in the electrocardiogram of the horse. *Am. J. Vet. Res.*, 1970;**31**: 1027–1031.

86. Harolin, R.L., R.R. Burton, S.D. Leverett, and J.W. Burns, The electrocardiogram from miniature swine recorded with the McFee-axial reference program. *J. Electrocardiol.*, 1974;**7**: 155–162.

87. Holmes, J.R. and P.G.G. Darke, Studies on the development of a new lead system for equine electrocardiography. *Equine Vet. J.*, 1970;**2**: 12–21.

88. Holmes, J.R. and R.W. Else, Further studies on a new lead system for equine electrocardiography. *Equine Vet J*, 1972;**4**: 81–87.

89. Grauerholz, G., Eine Methode zur vektoriellen Auswertung des Elektrokardiogramms beim Pferd. *Zentralbl. Veterinaermed. A*, 1974;**21**: 188–197. (This article cites: Baron M. Contribution a l'etude du vectorcardiogramme du cheval de sport. Applications dans l'examen preoperative, veterinary dissertation. Paris, 1970.)

90. Holmes, J.R. and B.J. Alps, Studies into equine electrocardiography and vectorcardiography. I. Cardiac electric forces and the dipole vector theory: II. Cardiac vector distribution in apparently healthy horses. III. Vector distribution in some cardiovascular disorders. IV. Vector distributions in some arrhythmias.

Can. J. Comp. Med. Vet. Sci., 1967;**31**: 92–102; 150–155; 207–212; 219–225.

91. Darke, P.G.G. and J.R. Holmes, Studies on the equine cardiac electric field. I. Body surface potentials. II. The integration of body surface potentials to derive resultant cardiac dipole moments. *J. Electrocardiol*, 1969;**2**: 229–234; 235–244.

92. Van Arsdel, W.C., III, *Lead Selection, Cardiac Axes, and the Interpretation of Electrocardiograms in Beef Cattle*. Corvallis, OR: Oregon State College, 1959.

93. Sugeno, H., Analytical study on bovine electrocardiogram. *Jpn. Circ. J.*, 1959;**23**: 1193–1203.

94. Holmes, J.R.A., Method of vectorcardiogram: loop portrayal. *Equine Vet. J.*, 1970;**2**: 27–34.

95. Nörr, J., Fötale Elektrokardiogramme von Pferd. *Z. Biol.*, 1921;**73**: 123–128.

96. Holmes, J.R. and P.G.G. Darke, Fetal electrocardiography in the mare. *Vet. Rec.*, 1968;**82**: 651–655.

97. Too, K., H. Kanagawa, and K. Kawata, Fetal electrocardiogram in dairy cattle. I. Fundamental Studies. III. Variations in fetal QRS pattern. *Jpn. J. Vet. Res.*, 1965;**13**: 71–83; 1966;**14**: 103–113.

98. Too, K., H. Kanagawa, K. Kawata, and H. Ono, Fetal electrocardiogram in dairy cattle. II. Diagnosis for twin pregnancies. *Jpn. J. Vet. Res.*, 1965;**13**: 111–119. Too, K., H. Kanagawa, K. Kawata, T. Inoue, T.F. Odajima, et al., Electrocardiogram in cattle. V. Findings at parturition. *Jpn. J. Vet. Res.* 1967;**15**: 21–30.

99. Golikov, A.N. and R.S. Vershinina, Electrocardiographic control of the stage of pregnancy in the cow (in Russian). *Veterinariya*, 1973;**2**: 87–88.

100. Larks, S.D., L.W. Holm, and H.R. Parker, A new technic for the demonstration of the fetal electrocardiogram in the large domestic animal (cattle, sheep, horse). *Cornell Vet*, 1960;**50**: 459–468.

101. Grabowski, C.T. and D.B. Payne, An electrocardiographic study of cardiovascular problems in Mirex-fed rat fetuses. *Teratology*, 1980;**22**: 167–177.

102. Detweiler, D.K. and D.F. Patterson, The prevalence and types of cardiovascular disease in dogs. *Ann. N.Y. Acad. Sci.*, 1965;**127**: 481–516.

103. Patterson, D.F., D.K. Detweiler, K. Hubben, and R.P. Botts, Spontaneous abnormal cardiac arrhythmias and conduction disturbances in the dog. A clinical and pathologic study of 3,000 dogs. *Am. J. Vet. Res.*, 1961;**22**: 355–369.

104. Einthoven, W., Die galvanometrische Registrierung des menschlichen Elektrokardiogramms. *Pfluegers Arch. Gesamte Physiol. Menschen Tiere.*, 1903;**99**: 472–480.

105. Einthoven, W., Le Télécardiogramme. *Arch. Int. Physiol.*, 1906;**4**: 132–164.

106. Caceres, C.A., Editor. *Biomedical Telemetry*. New York: Academic Press, 1965.

107. Holter, N.J., New method for heart studies. *Science*, 1961;**134**: 1214–1220.

108. Sandler, H., H.L. Stone, T.B. Fryer, and R.M. Westbrook, Use of implantable telemetry systems for study of cardiovascular phenomena. *Circ. Res.*, 1972;**31**(Suppl. II): 85–100.

109. Denton, D., Recording of physiological functions of a suitable experimental animal during protracted space flight. *Ausl. J. Sci.*, 1958;**20**: 202–207.

110. Benazet, P., R. Bordet, A. Brion, M. Fontaine, and J. Sevestre, Étude télémétrique de l'électrocardiogramme du cheval de sport. *Rect. Med. Vel.*, 1964;**140**: 449–459.

111. Nomura, S., Adaptation of radiotelemetry to equestrian games and horse racing. *Jpn. J. Vel. Sci.*, 1966;**28**: 191–203.

112. Fregin, G.F., Radioelectrocardiography in horses. *Pennsylvania Vel*, 1967;**9**: 6–10.

113. Banister, E.W. and A.D. Purvis, Exercise electrocardiography in the horse by radiotelemetry. *J. Am. Vet. Med. Assoc.*, 1968;**152**: 1004–1008.

114. Senta, T., D.L. Smetzer, and C.R. Smith, Effects of exercise on certain electrocardiographic parameters and cardiac arrhythmias in the horse. A radiotelemetric study. *Cornell Vet*, 1970;**60**: 552–569.

115. Börnert, D., H. Seidel, R. Maiwald, and G. Börnert, Drahtlos übertragene EKG-Ableitungen vom freibeweglichen Rind. *Arch. Exp. Velerinaermed.*, 1964;**18**: 701–712.

116. Dracy, A.E. and J.R. Jahn, Use of electrocardiographic radiotelemetry to determine heart rate in ruminants. *J. Dairy Sci.*, 1964;**47**: 561–563.

117. Fregin, G.F. and D.P. Thomas, Cardiovascular response to exercise in the horse: a review, in *Equine Exercise Physiology*, D.H. Snow, S.G.B. Persson, and R.J. Rose, Editors. Cambridge: Granta, 1983, pp. 76–90.

118. Adams, L., R.E. Wetmore, R.L. Limes, and H.J. Hauer, Automated analysis of heart rate in ground squirrels using radiotelemetry and computers. *BioScience*, 1971;**21**: 1040–1042.

119. Essler, W.O. and G.E. Folk Jr, Determination of physiological rhythms of unrestrained animals by radiotelemetry. *Nature*, 1961;**190**: 90–91.

120. Essler, W.O., *Radiolelemetry of Electrocardiograms and Body Temperatures from Surgically Implanled Transmitters*, State University of Iowa Studies in Natural History; vol. 20, no. 4. Iowa City, IA: State University of Iowa, 1961.

121. Branch, C.E., S.D. Beckett, and B.T. Robertson, Spontaneous syncopal attacks in dogs. A method of documentation. *I. Am. Anim. Hosp. Assoc.*, 1972;**13**: 673–679.

122. Reite, M., Implantable biotelemetry and social separation in monkeys, in *Animal Stress*, G.P. Moberg, Editor. Bethesda, MD: American Physiological Society, 1985, pp. 141–160.

123. Patiley, J.D. and M. Reite, A microminiature hybrid multichannel implantable biotelemetry system. *Biolelem. Patient Monit.*, 1981;**8**: 163–172.

124. Kimmich, H.P. and J.W. Knutti, Editors. Implantable telemetry systems based on integrated circuits. *Bioelem. Patient Monit.*, 1979;**6**: 91–170.

125. Mohler, P.J., I. Splawski, C. Napolitano, G. Bottelli, L. Sharpe, K. Timothy, S.G. Priori, M.T. Keating, and V. Bennett, A cardiac arrhythmia syndrome caused by loss of ankyrin-B function. *Proc. Natl. Acad. Sci. USA*, Jun 15; 2004;**101**(24): 9137–9142.

126. Farkas, A., A.J. Batey, and S.J. Coker, How to measure electrocardiographic QT interval in the anaesthetized rabbit. *J. Pharmacol. Toxicol. Methods*, 2004 Nov–Dec;**50**(3): 175–185.

127. Ryu, K., S.C. Shroff, J. Sahadevan, N.L. Martovitz, C.M. Khrestian, and B.S. Stambler, Mapping of atrial activation during sustained atrial fibrillation in dogs with rapid ventricular pacing induced heart failure: evidence for a role of driver regions. *J. Cardiovasc. Electrophysiol.*, Dec 2005;**16**(12): 1348–1361.

128. Kano, M., T. Toyoshi, S. Iwasaki, M. Kato, M. Shimizu, and T. Ota, QT PRODACT: usability of miniature pigs in safety pharmacology studies: assessment for drug-induced QT interval prolongation. *J. Pharmacol. Sci.*, 2005;**99**(5): 501–511.

129. Spach, M.S., R.C. Barr, C.F. Lanning, and P.C. Tucek, Origin of body surface QRS and T wave potentials form epicardial potential distributions in the intact chimpanzee. *Circulation*, Feb 1977;**55**(2): 268–278.

130. Gauvin, D.V., L.P. Tilley, F.W. Smith Jr, and T.J. Baird, Electrocardiogram, hemodynamics, and core body temperatures of the normal freely moving cynomolgus monkey by remote radiotelemetry. *J. Pharmacol. Toxicol. Methods*, Mar–Apr 2006;**53**(2): 140–151.

131. Sawazaki, H. and H. Hirose, Comparative electrocardiographical studies on the conduction time of heart in vertebrates. *Jpn. J. Vel. Sci.*, 1974;**36**: 421–426.

132. Detweiler, D.K., Regulation of the heart, in *Dukes' Physiology of Domestic Animals*, 10th edn, M.J. Swenson, Editor. Ithaca, NY: Cornell University Press, 1984, pp. 150–162.

133. Schmidt-Nielsen, K., *Animal Physiology: Adaptation and Environment*. London: Cambridge University Press, 1975.

134. Stahl, W.R., Scaling of respiratory variables in mammals. *J. Appl. Physiol.*, 1967;**22**: 453–460.

135. Schaible, T.F. and J. Scheuer, Response of the heart to exercise training, in *Growth of the Heart in Health and Disease*, R. Zak, Editor. New York: Raven, 1984, pp. 381–419.

136. Hermann, G.R., T.E. Vice, A.R. Rodriguez, and A.W. Herrmann, Heart weight to body weight, left to right ventricular weights, and ratios of baboon hearts, in *The Baboon in Medical Research*, vol. I, H. Vagtborg, Editor. Austin, TX: University of Texas Press, 1965, pp. 269–274.

137. Detweiler, D.K., Normal and pathological circulatory stresses, in *Dukes' Physiology of Domestic Animals*, 10th edn, M.J. Swenson, Editor. Ithaca, NY: Cornell University Press, 1984, pp. 207–225.

138. Porges, S.W., P.M. McCabe, and B.G. Yongue, Respiratory-heart-rate interactions: psychophysiological implications for pathophysiology and behavior, in *Perspectives in Cardiovascular Psychophysiology*, J. Cacioppo and R. Petty, Editors. New York: Guilford, 1982, pp. 223–264.

139. Porges, S.W., Spontaneous oscillations in heart rate; potential index of stress, in *Animal Stress*, G.P. Moberg, Editor. Bethesda, MD: American Physiological Society, 1985, pp. 97–111.

140. Kitney, R.I. and E. Rompelman, Editors. *The Study of Heart-Rate Variability*. Oxford: Clarendon Press, 1980.

141. Kwatny, E., D. Peltzman, and D.K. Detweiler, Automated analysis of Beagle electrocardiograms, in *Proceedingsof the 13th North England Bioengineering Conference*, K.R. Foster, Editor. New York: IEEE, 1987.

142. Melbin, J., D.K. Detweiler, R.A. Riffle, and A. Noordergraaf, Coherence of cardiac output with rate changes. *Am. J. Physiol.*, 1982;**243**: H499–H504.

143. Detweiler, D.K., Electrocardiographic detection of cardiotoxicity in preclinical studies, in *Safely Evaluation and Regulation of Chemicals*, vol. 3, F. Homburger, Editor. Basel: Karger, 1986, pp. 76–86.

144. Bauer, K. and O. Nehring, Betrachtungen zu den mathematischen Formuliertingen der Abhängigkeit der QT-Zeit von der Frequenz und die Deutung derselben. *Z. Kreislaufforsch*, 1968;**57**: 430–436.

145. Schoenwald, R.D. and V.E.Q.T. Isaacs, Corrected for heart rate: a new approach and its application. *Arch. Int. Pharmacodyn. Ther.*, 1974;**211**: 34–48.

146. Grauwiler, J., Das normale Elektrokardiogramm des Beagle-Hundes. *Naunyn-Schmiedebergs Arch. Pharmakol.*, 1970;**266**: 337.

147. Osborne, B.E. and G.D.H. Leach, The Beagle electrocardiogram. *Food Cosmet. Toxicol.*, 1971;**9**: 857–864.

148. Patterson, D.F., D.K. Detweiler, and S.A. Glendenning, Heart sounds and murmurs of the normal horse. *Ann. N.Y. Acad. Sci.*, 1965;**127**: 242–305.

149. Gonder, J.C., E.A. Gard, and N.E.I.I.I. Lott, Electrocardiograms of nine species of nonhuman primates. *Am. J. Vel. Res.*, 1980;**41**: 972–975.

150. von Mickwitz, G., *Herz- und Kreislaufuntersuchungen beim Schwein mit Berücksichtigung des Elektrokardiogramms und des Phonokardiogramms.* Hannover: Habilitationsschrift, 1967, pp. 1–246.

151. Richards, A.G., E. Simonson, and M.B. Visscher, Electrocardiogram and phonogram of adult and newborn mice in normal conditions and under the effect of cooling, hypoxia and potassium. *Am. J. Physiol.*, 1953;**174**: 293–298.

152. O'Rourke, M.F., A.P. Avolio, and W.W. Nichols, The kangaroo as a model for the study of hypertrophic cardiomyopathy in man. *Cardiovasc. Res.*, 1986;**20**: 398–402.

153. Lourenco, M.L. and H. Ferreira, Electrocardiographic evolution in cats from birth to 30 days of age. *Can. Vet. J.*, 2003 Nov;**44**(11): 914–917.

154. Jefferson, J.W., Electrocardiographic and phonocardiographic findings in a reticulated giraffe. *J. Am. Vet. Med. Assoc.*, 1971;**159**: 602–604.

155. Rossof, A.H., An electrocardiographic study of the giraffe. *Am. Heart J.*, 1972;**83**: 142–143.

156. Tokita, K., Electrocardiographical studies on bottle-nosed dolphin (Tursiops truncatus). *Sci. Rep. Whales Res. Inst.*, 1960;**15**: 159–165.

157. Rogers, W.A. and S.P. Bishop, Electrocardiographic parameters of the normal domestic cat: A comparison of standard limb leads and an orthogonal system. *I. Electrocardiol.*, 1971;**4**: 315–321.

158. Jayasinghe, J.B., S.D.A. Fernando, and L.A.P. Brito-Babapulle, The electrocardiographic patterns of *Elephas maxim us* – the elephant of Ceylon. *Br. Vel. I.*, 1963;**119**: 559–564.

159. Stewart, J.H., R.J. Rose, P.E. Davis, and K. Hoffman, A comparison of electrocardiographic findings in racehorses presented either for routine examination or poor racing performance, in *Equine Exercise Physiology* D.H. Snow, S.G.B. Persson, and R.J. Rose, Editors. Cambridge: Granta, 1983, pp. 135–143.

160. Moore, E.N., G. Fisher, D.K. Detweiler, and G.K. Moe, The importance of atrial mass in the maintenance of atrial fibrillation, in *International Symposium on Comparative Medicine*, R.J. Tashjian, Editor. Norwich, CT: Eaton Laboratory, 1965, pp. 229–238.

161. Spörri, H., Die ersten Fälle von sog. Wolff-Parkinson-White Syndrom, einer eigenartigen Herzanomalie, bei Tieren. *Schweiz Arch. Tierheilkd.*, 1953;**95**: 13–22.

162. Giuliano, G., G. Angrisani, P.P. Campa, M. Condorelli, and V. Pennetti, L'elettrocardiogram: na nella pecora. *Boll. Soc. Ital. Biol. Sper.*, 1958;**34**: 1785–1787.

163. Mullick, D.N., B.V. Alfredson, and E.P. Reineke, Influence of thyroid status on the electrocardiogram and certain blood constituents of the sheep. *Am. J. Physiol.*, 1948;**152**: 100–105.

164. Walper, F., *Elektrokardiographische und andere kardiographische Studien am Schaf*, Dissertation. Munich, 1932.

165. Unshelm, J., H.H. Thielscher, F. Haring, H. Hohns, U.E. Pfleiderer, and W. von Schutzbar, Elektrokardiographische Untersuchungen bei Schafen unter Berücksichtigung der Rasse, des Lebensalters und anderer Einflussfaktoren. *Zentralbl. Veterinaermed. A.*, 1974;**21**: 479–491.

166. Schultz, R.A., P.J. Pretorius, and M. Terblanche, An electrocardiographic study of normal sheep using a modified technique. *Onderstepoort J. Vet. Res.*, 1972;**39**: 97–106.

167. Rozanova, T.V., Electrocardiographic indicators of sheep of various constitutional types (in Russian). *Dokl. Skh. Akad. Sofia*, 1958;**32**: 369–377.

168. Roshchevsky, M.P., Vector- i elektrokardograficheskie iccledovaniya cerdechnoi deyatel'nosti ovetz. *Skh. Biol.*, 1969;**4**: 594–600.

169. Szabuniewicz, M. and D.R. Clark, Analysis of the electrocardiograms of 100 normal goats. *Am. J. Vet. Res.*, 1967;**28**: 511–516.

170. Upadhyay, R.C. and S.C. Sud, Electrocardiogram of the goat. *Indian J. Exp. Biol.*, 1977;**15**: 359–362.

171. Senta, T., Experimental investigation of electrocardiogram in the goat. *Exp. Rep. Equme Health Lab.*, 1967;**4**: 37–72.

172. Dukes, T.W. and M. Szabuniewicz, The electrocardiogram of conventional and miniature swine (Sus scrofa). *Can. J. Comp. Med.*, 1969;**33**: 118–127.

173. Thielscher, H.H., Elektrokardiographische Untersuchungen an Deutschen veredelten Landschweinen der Landeszucht und der Herdbuchzucht. *Zentralbl. Veterinaermed. A.*, 1969;**16**: 370–383.

174. von Mickwitz, G., *Herz- und Kreislaufuntersuchungen beim Schwein mit Berücksichtigung des Elektrokardiogramms und des Phonokardiogramms.* Hannover: Habilitationsschrift, 1967, pp. 1–246.

175. Hausmann, W.O., *Das Elektrokardiogramm des Hausschweines*, Dissertation. München, 1934, pp. 1–28.

176. Cox, J.L., D.E. Becker, and A.H. Jensen, Electrocardiographic evaluation of potassium deficiency in young swine. *J. Anim. Sci.*, 1966;**25**: 203–206.

177. Jefferson, J.W., Electrocardiographic and phonocardiographic findings in a reticulated giraffe. *J. Am. Vet. Med. Assoc.*, 1971;**159**: 602–604.

178. Rossof, A.H., An electrocardiographic study of the giraffe. *Am. Heart J.*, 1972;**83**: 142–143.

179. Jayasinghe, J.B., D.A. Fernando, and L.A.P. Brito-Babapulle, The electrocardiogram of the camel. *Am. J. Vet. Res.*, 1963;**24**: 883–885.

180. Geddes, L.A., W.A. Tacker, J. Rosborough, A.G. Moore, and P. Cabler, The electrocardiogram of a dromedary camel. *J. Electrocardiol.*, 1973;**6**: 211–214.

181. Senft, A.W. and J.K. Kanwisher, Cardiographic observations on a fin-back whale. *Circ. Res.*, 1960;**8**: 961–964.

182. Spencer, M.P., T.A. Gornall III, and T.C. Poulter, Respiratory and cardiac activity of killer whales. *J. Appl. Physiol.*, 1967;**22**: 974–981.

183. Tokita, K., Electrocardiographical studies on bottle-nosed dolphin (Tursiops truncatus). *Sci. Rep. Whales Res. Inst.*, 1960;**15**: 159–165.

184. Hamlin, R.L., R.F. Jackson, J.A. Himes, F.S. Pipers, and A.C. Townsend, Electrocardiogram of bottle-nosed dolphin (*Tursiops truncatus*). *Am. J. Vet. Res.*, 1970;**31**: 501–505.

185. Richards, A.G., E. Simonson, and M.B. Visscher, Electrocardiogram and phonogram of adult and newborn mice in normal conditions and under the effect of cooling, hypoxia and potassium. *Am. J. Physiol.*, 1953;**174**: 293–298.

186. Spörri, H., Starke Dissoziation zwischen dem Ende der elektrischen und mechanischen Systolendauer bei Känguruhs. *Cardiologia*, 1956;**28**: 278–284.

187. Siegfried, J.P., *Elektrokardiographische Untersuchungen an ZOO-Tieren*, Dissertation. Zürich: University of Zurich, 1956, pp. 1–57.

188. Jayasinghe, J.B. and S.D.A. Fernando, Electrocardiograms of zoo animals, II. Leopard and Wallaby. *Ceylon Vet. J.*, 1964;**12**: 21–22.

189. Wilbur, C.G., Electrocardiographic studies on the opossum. *J. Mammal.*, 1955;**36**: 284–286.

190. Szabuniewicz, M., D. Hightower, and J.R. Kyzar, The electrocardiogram, vectorcardiogram, and spatiocardiogram in the rabbit. *Can. J. Comp. Med.*, 1971;**35**: 107–114.

191. Levine, H.D., Spontaneous changes in the normal rabbit electrocardiogram. *Am. Heart J.*, 1942;**24**: 209–214.

192. Massmann, W. and H. Opitz, Das normale Kaninchen-EKG. *Z. Gesamte Exp. Med.*, 1954;**124**: 35–43.

193. Slapak, L. and P. Hermanek, Beobachtungen über das Elektrokardiogramm des Kaninchens. I: Das normale Extremitäten-Elektrokardiogramm des Kaninchens. *Z. Kreislaufforsch.*, 1957;**46**: 136–142.

194. Slapak, L. and P. Hermanek, Beobachtungen uber des Elektrokardiogramm des Kaninchens. II: Das normale Brustwand-Elektrokardiogramm des Kaninchens. *Z. Kreislaufforsch.*, 1957;**46**: 143–166.

195. Jacotot, B., L'electrocardiogramme du lapin. Analyse des tracés de 75 animaux sains. *Recl. Med. Vet.*, 1965;**141**: 1095–1107.

196. Angelakos, E.T. and P. Bernardini, Frequency components and positional changes in electrocardiogram of the adult rat. *J. Appl. Physiol.*, 1963;**18**: 261–263.

197. Beinfeld, W.H. and D. Lehr, QRS-T variations in the rat electrocardiogram. *Am. J. Physiol.*, 1968;**214**: 197–204.

198. Beinfeld, W.H. and D. Lehr, P-R interval of the rat electrocardiogram. *Am. J. Physiol.*, 1968;**214**: 205–211.

199. Werth, G. and S. Wink, Das Elektrokardiogramm der normalen Ratte. *Arch. Kreislaufforsch.*, 1967;**54**: 272–308.

200. Langer, G.A., Interspecies variation in myocardial physiology: the anomalous rat. *Environ. Health Perspect.*, 1978;**26**: 175–179.

201. O'Bryant, J.W., A. Packchanian, G.W. Reimer, and R.H. Vadheim, An apparatus for studying electrocardiographic changes in small animals. *Tex. Rep. Bioi. Med.*, 1949;7: 661–670.

202. Lombard, E.A., Electrocardiograms of small mammals. *Am. J. Physiol.*, 1952;**171**: 189–193.

203. Giordano, G. and G. Nigro, Caratteristiche dell' elettrocardiogramma normale del Mus musculus albus. *Sperimentale*, 1957;**107**: 63–68.

204. Goldbarg, A.N., H.K. Hellerstein, J.H. Bruell, and A.F. Daroczy, Electrocardiogram of the normal mouse, *Mus musculus*: general considerations and genetic aspects. *Cardiovasc. Res.*, 1968;**2**: 93–99.

205. Callsen, A.D., *Elektrokardiographische Untersuchungen an wachen und anästhesierten Katzen mit einem System von zehn Standardableitungen*, Dissertation. Berlin: Freie University, 1983, Journal No.1130, pp. 1–105.

206. Tilley, L.P. and R.E. Gompf, Feline electrocardiography. *Vet. Clin. North Am.*, 1977;7: 257–272.

207. Rogers, W.A. and S.P. Bishop, Electrocardiographic parameters of the normal domestic cat: a comparison of standard limb leads and an orthogonal system. *I. Electrocardiol.*, 1971;4: 315–321.

208. Blok, J. and J.Th.F. Boeles, The electrocardiogram of the normal cat. *Acta Physiol. Pharmacol. Neerl.*, 1957;**6**: 95–102, 209.

209. Massmann, W. and H. Opitz, Das Katzen-Ekg. *Cardiologia*, 1954;**24**: 54–64.

210. Rothlin, E. and E. Suter, Glykosidwirkung auf Elektrokardiogramm und Myokard. I Vergleichende elektrokardiographische Untersuchungen verschiedener herzwirksamer Glykoside an der Katze bei intravenöser Infusion. *Helv. Physiol. Pharmacol. Acta*, 1947;**5**: 298–321.

211. Purchase, I.F.H., The effect of halothane on the isolated cat heart. *Br. J. Anaesth.*, 1966;**38**: 80–91.

212. Purchase, I.F.H., Cardiac arrhythmias occurring during halothane anaesthesia in cats. *Br. I. Anaeslh.*, 1966;**38**: 13–22, 213.

213. Jayasinghe, J.B., S.D.A. Fernando, and L.A.P. Brito-Babapulle, The electrocardiograpic patterns of *Elephas maxim us* - the elephant of Ceylon. *Br. Vel. I.*, 1963;**119**: 559–564.

214. Jayasinghe, J.B. and L.A.P. Brito-Babapulle, A report on an electrocardiogram of the Ceylon elephant. *Ceylon Vel. J.*, 1961;**9**: 69–70.

215. Grauweiler, J., Beobachtungen am Elektrokardiogramm von nicht-domestizierten Säugetieren. *Schweiz. Arch. Tierheilkd.*, 1961;**103**: 397–417.

216. Forbes, A. and S. Cobb, Cattell McK. An electrocardiogram and an electromyogram in an elephant. *Am. I. Physiol.*, 1921;**55**: 385–389.

217. Siegfried, J.P., *Elektrokardiographische Untersuchungen an Zoo-Tieren*, Dissertation. Zürich: University of Zürich, 1956.

218. Nörr, J., Hundert klinische Fälle von Herz und Pulsarrhythmien beim Pferde. *Mh. Prakt. Tierheilkd. Slullgarl*, 1924;**34**: 177–232.

219. Roos, J., Vorhoffiimmern bei den Haustieren. *Arch. Wiss. Prakt. Tierheilkd.*, 1924;**51**: 280–293.

220. Roos, J., Auricular fibrillation in the domestic animals. *Heart*, 1924;**11**: 1–7.

221. Agduhr, E. and N. Stenström, The appearance of the electrocardiogram in the heart lesions produced by cod liver oil treatment: electrocardiogram in rats treated with cod liver oil. *Acla Paediatr. (Uppsala)*, 1930;**9**: 280–306.

222. Drury, A.N., L.J. Harris, C. Maudsley, and B. Vitamin, deficiency in the rat. Bradycardia as a distinctive feature. *Biochem. J.*, 1930;**24**: 1632–1649.

223. Nörr, J., Über Atmungsarrhythmie bei Caniden. *Verh. Dtsch. Ges. Kreislaufforsch.*, 1935;7: 144–148.

224. Scher, A.M., Direct recording from the A-V conducting system in the dog and monkey. *Science*, 1955;**121**: 398–399.

225. Scher, A.M. and A.C. Young, The pathway of ventricular depolarization in the dog. *Circ. Res.*, 1956;**4**: 461–469.

226. Detweiler, D.K., Perspectives in canine cardiology. *Univ. Pennsylvania Bull. Vet. Ext. Q.*, 1958;**149**: 27–48.

227. Ettinger, S.J. and P.F. Suter, *Canine Cardiology*. Philadelphia, PA: Saunders, 1970.

228. Hill, J.D.A., *Correlative Study of Right Ventricular Conduction Disturbances in the Dog*, Veterinary thesis. Philadelphia, PA: University of Pennsylvania, 1967.

229. Hill, J.D., Electrocardiographic diagnosis of right ventricular enlargement in dogs. *J. Electrocardiol.*, 1971;**4**: 347–357.

230. Pruitt, R.D., Electrocardiogram of bundle-branch block in the bovine heart. *Circ. Res.*, 1962;**10**: 593–597.

231. O'Rourke, M.F., A.P. Avolio, and W.W. Nichols, The kangaroo as a model for the study of hypertrophic cardiomyopathy in man. *Cardiovasc. Res.*, 1986;**20**: 398–402.

232. Gompf, R.E. and L.P. Tilley, Comparison of lateral and sternal recumbent positions for electrocardiography of the cat. *Am. J. Vet. Res.*, 1979;**40**: 1483–1486.

233. Boineau, J.P., E.N. Moore, J.F. Spear, and W.C. Sealy, Basis of static and dynamic electrocardiographic variations in Wolff-Parkinson-White syndrome. *Am. J. Cardiol*, 1973;**32**: 32–45.

11 12 Lead Vectorcardiography

Peter W. Macfarlane · Olle Pahlm

P. W. Macfarlane et al. (eds.), *Specialized Aspects of ECG*, DOI 10.1007/978-0-85729-880-5_11,
© Springer-Verlag London Limited 2012

11.1 Vectorcardiography

11.1.1 What Is a Vector?

The term vector can have different meanings, but for the purposes of the study of vectorcardiography, the relevant definition states that a vector is an entity possessing a magnitude and a direction. For example, if a wind blows in an easterly direction at 10 km/h, it could be represented by the vector in ❷ Fig. 11.1a. On the other hand, if a light breeze blows at 5 km/h in a northeasterly direction, it would be represented using the same scheme by the vector of ❷ Fig. 11.1b. It can be seen that the length of the vector is proportional to the strength of the wind and the direction of the vector is that of the wind.

Of course, there can be many different forces that are represented by a vector. Within the context of electrocardiography (ECG), it is the cardiac electromotive force that is desired to be represented by a vector. It was Einthoven et al. [1] in their classic paper of 1913 who suggested that the electrical forces of heart could be summed and represented by a single vector.

11.1.2 Concept of Resultant Force

While a vector can be used to represent an individual force as shown in ❷ Fig. 11.1, a series of vectors can be used simultaneously to represent a variety of forces acting together or in opposition. It is possible to use some simple mathematical techniques to calculate the resultant effect of the different forces, and it is instructive to consider an example.

Imagine that a rower sets out to cross a river. He is able to row constantly at 4 km/h directly across the water but has to contend with a current that is flowing at a rate of 3 km/h. This is depicted in ❷ Fig. 11.2. It should be clear that if the rower consistently pulls directly across the river he will not reach the bank at a point directly opposite his starting point but will be carried some way downstream by the current. In fact, the distance can be calculated by what is known as the "Triangle of Forces," which shows that he would travel at a net speed of 5 km/h. The exact point at which the rower reaches the opposite bank, of course, depends on the width of the river but this can be calculated from the triangle. For example, if the river is 200 m wide, the boat should reach the opposite side 150 m downstream on the opposite side.

The combined velocity of the boat and the current produces a resultant velocity of 5 km/h depicted by the hypotenuse on the triangle. Conversely, it can be said that if there is a resultant velocity of 5 km/h, it has components of 3 and 4 km/h at right angles to each other in keeping with ❷ Fig. 11.2. Thus, there exists the concept that a resultant velocity has a component in a particular direction. The size of each component can be obtained by drawing a perpendicular from the tip of the resultant vector to a line indicating the direction in which it is desired to measure the component.

A similar concept applies in electrocardiography. Consider that in the frontal plane of the body, there is a resultant cardiac electromotive force of 2 mV acting at 45° to the horizontal, that is, approximately similar to the path of the rowing boat in ❷ Fig. 11.2. ❷ Figure 11.3 shows that there is a component of 1.41 mV in the direction of lead I. Similarly, it can be shown that there is a component of approximately 1.93 mV in the direction of lead II. This estimate assumes that the equilateral Einthoven triangle is a valid model, which in reality is not the case. However, the potential measured by lead I can be considered as the component of the resultant cardiac electromotive force acting in that direction in the frontal plane. It follows from Einthoven's Law (see ❷ Chap. 11 of *Basic Electrocardiology: Cardiac Electrophysiology, ECG Systems and Mathematical Modeling*) that the potential in lead III would be 0.52 mV at the same instant in the cardiac cycle.

11.1.3 Spatial Vector

❷ Sections 11.1.1 and ❷ 11.1.2 have dealt with the two-dimensional situation of a vector or vectors acting effectively in a plane. A more realistic situation is a force or a vector having the ability to be directed at any point in space. ❷ Figure 11.4 illustrates the concept of a spatial vector drawn within a three-dimensional coordinate reference system with axes denoted

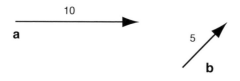

● Fig. 11.1

The direction and speed of the wind represented as a vector when the **(a)** wind blows in an easterly direction at 10 km/h **(b)** wind blows in a northeasterly direction at 5 km/h

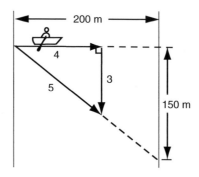

● Fig. 11.2

A rower crossing a river 200 m wide. For explanation, see text

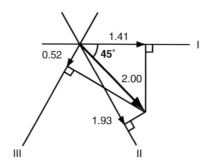

● Fig. 11.3

The cardiac electromotive force and its components in the direction of leads I, II, and III

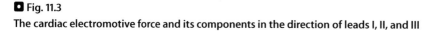

X, *Y*, and *Z*. It can be seen from the illustration that the magnitude of the vector can be calculated by using triangle OMA if the length of sides OA and AM can be determined.

However, from the Figure, it follows that:

$$OA^2 = x^2 + z^2$$

From right angled triangle OMA,

$$OM^2 = OA^2 + AM^2 = x^2 + y^2 + z^2$$

Thus, for a point M with coordinates *x*, *y*, *z* in three-dimensional space, the length of the vector OM is given by the above expression. By analogy with the two-dimensional situation, where it was shown that a vector lying in a plane could have

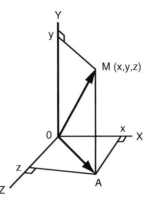

◘ Fig. 11.4

A spatial vector OM and its components *x, y, z* in a three-dimensional coordinate system

components calculated in any particular direction by drawing a perpendicular to that line, it can also be shown that in the spatial situation, a vector, for example, OM, can have components in the three mutually perpendicular directions X, Y, Z. In the forward situation, if the components *x, y, z* can be measured at a particular instant in the cardiac cycle, then a resultant OM can be calculated. This is the basis of an orthogonal lead system.

11.1.4 Orthogonal Lead Systems

11.1.4.1 Theoretical Considerations

❯ Section 11.1.3 suggests that if three leads can be designed to record components of a resultant cardiac electromotive force in three mutually perpendicular directions, then the problem of deriving the resultant cardiac electromotive force is solved. A considerable amount of research went into designing such lead systems over the past 50 years. The theory is detailed but a few simple concepts are worthy of discussion at this point. Further aspects are considered in ❯ Chap. 11 of *Basic Electrocardiology: Cardiac Electrophysiology, ECG Systems and Mathematical Modeling,* ❯ Sect. 11.5.

Assume that the potential measured by any electrocardiographic lead is represented by V. Then, assume that the resultant cardiac electromotive force is denoted by **H** or, as it is sometimes known, "The heart vector." Then from mathematical considerations, it can be shown that V = **H·L** where **L** is the vector representing the strength of the lead being used to measure the potential. In fact, it is one of the basic rules of vector mathematics that the dot product of two vectors is a scalar, that is, the potential or voltage does not have an associated direction but only a magnitude whereas the heart vector **H** and the lead vector **L** each has its own direction. This basic rule of vector mathematics can also be expanded to the following:

$$V = H_X L_X + H_Y L_Y + H_Z L_Z$$

where H_X, H_Y, H_Z are the three components of the heart vector and L_x, L_y, L_z are the three components of the lead vector. From this observation, it follows that if it is desired to measure the component of the heart vector in the X direction, then a lead should be designed that has components $(L_X, 0, 0)$. In that case,

$$V_X = H_X L_X$$

If the strength L_X of the lead is known, then when the potential V_X is measured, H_X can be calculated.

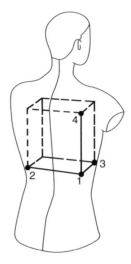

11.1.4.2 Uncorrected Lead Systems

For historical reasons, it is worth noting that the earliest attempts at designing orthogonal lead systems were made on the basis of constructing leads such that lines joining the electrodes were essentially mutually perpendicular. This is most easily understood by considering the cube system introduced by Grishman [2] (❷ Fig. 11.5). However, as experience was gained and mathematical modeling advanced, it was found that these lead systems did not accurately measure the required components.

11.1.4.3 Corrected Orthogonal Lead Systems

As a result of considerable modeling, both mathematical and physical, such as using model torsos filled with conducting solution, corrected orthogonal lead systems were gradually introduced.

The most notable and the one that is generally used wherever vectorcardiography is currently studied using an orthogonal lead system, is that of Frank [3]. This lead system is shown in ❷ Fig. 11.6. As can be seen, the lead positions are different from those of the 12-lead system, although the C and A electrodes are indeed close to the V_4 and V_6 positions, respectively.

Mathematical modeling showed that the following equations represent the derivation of the three potentials V_X, V_Y, V_Z:

$$V_X = 0.610V_A + 0.171V_C - 0.781V_I$$
$$V_Y = 0.655V_F + 0.345V_M - 1.0V_H$$
$$V_Z = 0.133V_A + 0.736V_M - 0.264V_I - 0.374V_E - 0.231V_C$$

These contributions to the individual leads from the different electrodes correspond to the resistor network also seen in ❷ Fig. 11.6. The major disadvantage of using this type of orthogonal lead system is the need to apply a completely different set of electrodes to the patient compared to that required for recording the conventional 12-lead ECG. There have been attempts to minimize the differences by doubling the C and A electrodes as V_4 and V_6, for example, and using a common left leg electrode but this still leaves four additional electrodes to be positioned on the thorax and neck.

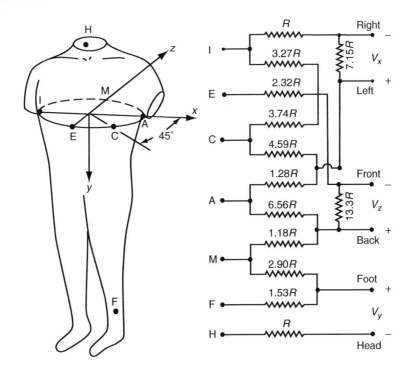

 Fig. 11.6

The Frank lead system (After Frank [3]). © American Heart Association, Dallas, Texas. Reproduced with permission

11.1.5 Cardiac Activation

11.1.5.1 Vectorial Spread of Cardiac Activation

The concept of resultant cardiac electromotive force by now should be gaining hold. It is possible to consider the various resultant forces acting throughout ventricular depolarization, for example. ❯ Figure 11.7a shows a series of individual vectors each of which represents the resultant cardiac electromotive force at one particular instant during the process of ventricular depolarization. For example, the first small vector shows the initial septal activation from left to right. Note that all of these vectors are depicted in the two-dimensional situation, which in this case is the frontal plane of the body. ❯ Figure 11.7b indicates how each of these resultant vectors can be translated to a common origin and a loop drawn to connect the tips of the vectors. This loop is a form of vectorcardiogram. Indeed, the first form of planar vectorcardiogram was introduced by Mann in 1920 [4].

11.1.5.2 Spatial Vector Loop

The previous ❯ Sect. 11.1.5.1 showed a planar loop. However, the concept of spatial vector has been introduced in ❯ Sect. 11.1.3 and it follows that if a resultant vector varies in magnitude and direction throughout the cardiac cycle, then it can be imagined that the tip of this vector will trace out a three-dimensional path. This observation is illustrated in ❯ Fig. 11.8 for the case of ventricular depolarization, that is, a spatial QRS loop is shown. In addition, the projection of this loop onto three mutually perpendicular planes is also illustrated. The collection of three planar loop projections is known as the vectorcardiogram. While only the QRS loop is depicted here for clarity, it follows that P and T loops can also be derived.

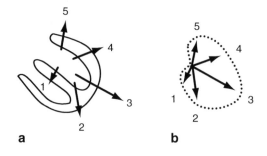

Fig. 11.7

(a) Ventricular depolarization illustrated as a sequence of vectors, *1–5*. (b) After translation of vectors to a common origin, a vectorcardiographic loop can be constructed

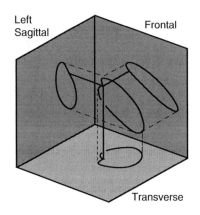

◧ Fig. 11.8

A vectorcardiographic loop in space projected onto the three orthogonal planes

11.1.6 Vector Loop Presentation

11.1.6.1 Nomenclature

The American Heart Association committee on electrocardiography (1975) [5] published a set of recommendations for vectorcardiographic terminology. The committee recommended that the lead Z be directed positively to the posterior thorax, although this does mean that the scalar presentation of lead Z is essentially opposite to that of lead V_2. This recommendation certainly causes much confusion when describing scalar lead appearances and for this reason, in this chapter, lead Z is directed positively to the anterior to be similar to V_2. Thus, R_Z can be thought of in the same way as R_{V_2}. Of more contention is the choice of whether to view the left or right sagittal planes, that is, the sagittal plane as viewed from the left or right. ❷ Figure 11.9 shows the left sagittal projection. The Committee did not make a particular recommendation, but for the purposes of illustrations in this book, the left sagittal view has been chosen in keeping with ❷ Fig. 11.9 so as to have a uniform collection of reference axes.

11.1.6.2 Display Techniques

About 20 years ago, the most common method of displaying the vectorcardiogram was via an oscilloscope. Pairs of leads such as X and Y were used to deflect the electron beam horizontally and vertically, respectively, and in this case, the

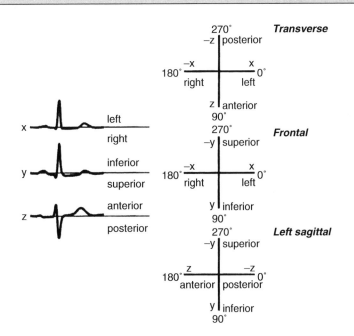

Fig. 11.9

Polarity of leads X, Y, and Z and angular reference frame of the frontal, transverse, and left sagittal planes

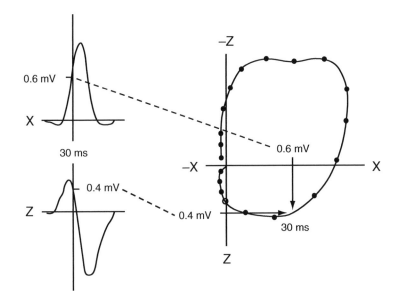

Fig. 11.10

Derivation of transverse plane loop from leads X and Z. Dots are at 4 ms intervals and the 20 ms vector is indicated with an open circle

frontal plane loop would be generated. Consider that leads X and Y are recorded simultaneously. At any instant in time, an amplitude for each lead is known, that is, an (x, y) coordinate pair of values is available. These values could be plotted simply on XY axes. If this is repeated throughout the cardiac cycle, then a complete frontal plane set of P, QRS, and T loops can be generated. ❷ Figure 11.10 shows the derivation of a QRS loop in the transverse plane.

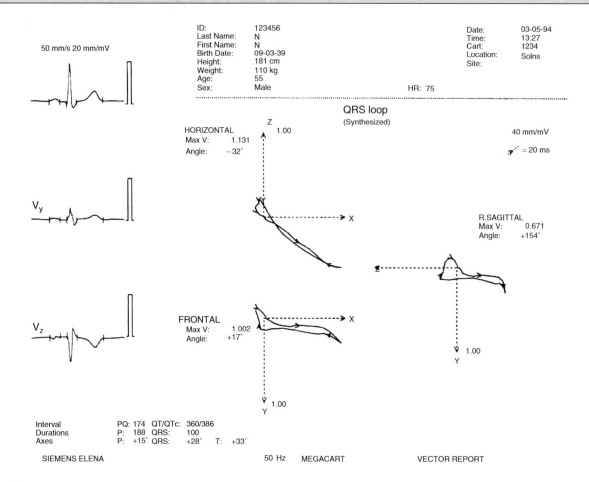

50 mm/s 20 mm/mV

ID:	123456	
Last Name:	N	
First Name:	N	
Birth Date:	09-03-39	
Height:	181 cm	
Weight:	110 kg	
Age:	55	
Sex:	Male	HR: 75

Date:	03-05-94	
Time:	13:27	
Cart:	1234	
Location:	Solns	
Site:		

QRS loop
(Synthesized)

HORIZONTAL
Max V: 1.131
Angle: −32°

40 mm/mV

⤵ ⋰ = 20 ms

R.SAGITTAL
Max V: 0.671
Angle: +154°

FRONTAL
Max V: 1.002
Angle: +17°

V_y

V_z

Interval	PQ: 174	QT/QTc: 360/386	
Durations	P: 188	QRS: 100	
Axes	P: +15°	QRS: +28°	T: +33°

SIEMENS ELENA   50 Hz   MEGACART   VECTOR REPORT

● Fig. 11.11

Vectorcardiogram printout from a commercially available electrocardiograph. Note that lead Z is inverted in comparison with other illustrations in this book

If the leads X, Y, Z are considered in pairs, then by plotting leads XY, the frontal plane vectorcardiographic loop can be obtained. Similarly, XZ plots produce the transverse plane loop and ZY plots produce the sagittal plane vectorcardiographic loop. Nowadays, with the widespread availability of computer technology, these plots can be produced in a straightforward fashion. It is somewhat more complex to program a thermal writer to produce an XY display but nevertheless this is readily attainable. Thus, vectorcardiographic loops can now be produced even on small 4″ paper displays or on the larger A4 writers such as are common at the bedside. An illustration of a typical vectorcardiographic display from a computer-based electrocardiograph is shown in ❷ Fig. 11.11.

It is important that vectorcardiographic loops have some indication of the speed of inscription as this can contain diagnostic information. A number of methods have been used. Conventionally, the vectorcardiographic loop has been interrupted so that time intervals can actually be measured by counting the number of dots between two points. Generally, 2 or 4 ms intervals have been used. An alternative is to produce a continuous loop and mark a number such as 1, 2 indicating 10, 20 ms from the onset of the QRS complex. This is helpful but creates difficulties around the onset and termination of the QRS loop, which is often the most interesting part in terms of looking for conduction problems. Either way, the direction of inscription of the loop is also of vital clinical significance. Thus, if a numbering system is not used, some indication must be given to make it quite clear to the viewer in which direction the different planar loops are inscribed. With a knowledge of the theory of vectorcardiography, the experienced cardiologist can always determine the direction of inscription but it is certainly easier if this is made obvious in a good display.

In this book, loops are presented with an arrow indicating the direction of inscription. Further, black dots indicate 4 ms intervals and the 20 ms vector is indicated with an open circle.

11.2 Normal Ranges

11.2.1 Introduction

The aim of good diagnostic criteria is to separate normal from abnormal with the highest possible sensitivity and specificity. It may be superfluous to repeat well-known definitions but for the avoidance of doubt, the following apply:

$$Specificity = A/B$$
$$Sensitivity = C/D$$

where

A = number of normals correctly reported as normal
B = total number of normals
C = number of abnormals correctly reported as abnormal
D = total number of abnormals.

❯ Figure 11.12 shows the distribution of Q wave duration in lead Y for normals and for a group of patients with inferior myocardial infarction. If a value of 20 ms is chosen as the upper limit of normal, it can be seen that the specificity of the

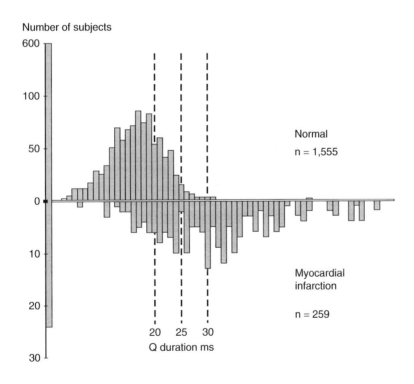

◻ Fig. 11.12

Shows distribution of Q duration in lead Y in a group of 1,555 normal subjects and in a group of 259 patients with inferior myocardial infarction. For explanation, see text

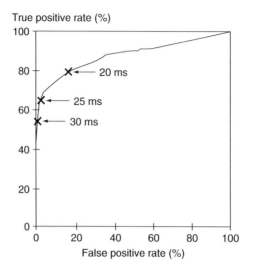

○ **Fig. 11.13**
Receiver operating characteristic (ROC) curve showing the relationship between true positive rate (sensitivity) and false positive rate (100 – specificity) for different limits of Q duration in lead 1′: The curve is based on the data in ○ Fig. 11.12

criteria would be approximately 83%. The sensitivity for inferior infarction would be the order of 79%. However, some would argue that 83% specificity, that is, close to one in five normals reported as abnormal, is not high enough and might adjust the borderline value to 25 ms. In this case, the specificity would increase to 97% and the sensitivity for infarction would decrease to 65%. This process can be continued. For example, with a borderline of 30 ms, specificity is over 99% but sensitivity decreases to 54%.

It is possible to plot the relationship between sensitivity and specificity on what is known as a receiver operating characteristic (ROC) curve. This is shown in ○ Fig. 11.13. The point on the curve, which approaches closest to 100% sensitivity and specificity, that is, the top left-hand corner, is often regarded as being optimum. In the case of electrocardiography, it is often preferable to choose a point on the curve with higher specificity (e.g., 25 ms point in ○ Fig. 11.13).

While it is clear that ROC curves are dependent on the knowledge of measurements from a normal population and patients with a particular abnormality, it should also be noted that if a user decides that 95% specificity is the desired level, then the knowledge of the abnormal data are not required. This is perhaps an extreme view but it emphasizes the value of having well-defined normal data.

In Glasgow, every effort has been made over the past 25 years to gather a population of controls from birth upward, and of different ethnic origin, in order to meet the objectives outlined above. The remainder of this chapter will deal with the techniques involved and present the results obtained from the Caucasian cohort.

11.2.2 Data Acquisition

11.2.2.1 Techniques

Data have been gathered using two separate types of electrocardiographs each with a common factor of sampling electrocardiographic waveforms at 500 samples/s. All of the recordings made outside Glasgow Royal Infirmary, for example, on infants and children, were gathered using a Mingorec 4 from Siemens-Elema AB, Solna, Sweden. This acquires eight leads simultaneously, converts from analog to digital form at a rate of 500 samples/s for further analysis. More recent work has involved the use of the Burdick Atria 6100 electrocardiograph.

For ECGs recorded within Glasgow Royal Infirmary, an electrocardiograph designed and constructed within the Department of Medical Cardiology was used ([6], 1987). This device was connected by a broadband network from wards and clinics to the central computing facility within the Department.

The methods for analyzing the ECGs have been described in detail elsewhere [7] but are summarized very briefly here.

Up to 8 s of ECG with all leads sampled simultaneously, are processed initially to remove baseline wander, if present, and also any AC interference. Thereafter, QRS detection is undertaken. The same methods apply whether the ECG is recorded from a neonate or an adult. The QRS complexes so detected are then typed into different morphologies and logic selects one particular morphology for analysis. All PQRST cycles of that morphology are then averaged to form a single synthesized beat (with all 12 leads effectively recorded simultaneously). The derived leads X, Y, Z are then obtained using the methods outlined in detail in ❷ Chap. 11 of *Basic Electrocardiology: Cardiac Electrophysiology, ECG Systems and Mathematical Modeling*. In particular, the adult X, Y, Z leads were calculated using equation and the pediatric x, y, z leads were derived using equation. The wave measurement program then locates the onsets and terminations of the various P, QRS, and T components in order to measure amplitudes and durations.

Rhythm analysis is then undertaken. This uses some measurements from the average beat matrix but also three complete leads from the initial recording. Generally, these would be II, III, and V_1. When rhythm has been determined, diagnostic logic is then entered to interpret the measurements from the average beats. The program can output several hundred diagnostic statements. The same program can now be used for adults as well as for children [8]. In other words, the ability to interpret ECGs from children is not an optional add-on to the logic but is integral to the diagnostic criteria. Some details are presented elsewhere [9].

11.2.2.2 Sampling Methods

Different approaches to the selection of an apparently healthy population can be adopted. For example, age and sex registers can be used [10], but the technique adopted for adults in the Glasgow data was essentially to seek volunteers from the different departments of local government, for example, teaching, administration, and building. All individuals admitted to the normal group were seen by a physician who obtained a complete history and undertook a physical examination. The usual blood tests were performed and in the initial part of the study, chest x-rays were obtained. It was found that a positive yield from chest x-rays was essentially nil and latterly they were discontinued as part of the screening procedure.

For sampling from children, the procedure was different. Recordings were obtained from a maternity hospital with the full consent of parents. In preschool children, it was necessary to visit postnatal clinics, health centers, and play groups in order to obtain recordings from children, again with the permission of parents. Recordings were obtained from schoolchildren by installing the Siemens electrocardiograph for periods in different schools with the permission of the local health and education authority. Volunteers were sought subject to parental permission.

11.2.2.3 Population Data

A total number of 1,555 adults were entered into the normal database. The age and sex distribution is shown in ❷ Fig. 11.14. There tends to be a preponderance of males over 30 years of age, probably because of the predominance of male workers of that age group.

❷ Figure 11.15 shows similar data for 1,782 healthy neonates, infants, and children whose ECGs were recorded. It should be pointed out that in this age group, lead V_{4R} was used in preference to lead V_3 as is the custom in many countries.

Actual numbers of males and females in the total group of 3,337 are given in ❷ Table 11.1.

In Taiwan, in collaboration with the Veterans' General Hospital in Taipei, it was possible to obtain 12-lead ECGs from 503 apparently healthy Chinese individuals [11]. From these, the 12-lead vectorcardiogram was obtained [12]. Essentially, methods used were similar to those for the collection of adult data in Caucasians although a higher percentage of individuals were in hospital with noncardiac problems.

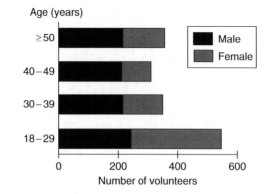
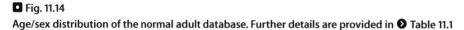

○ Fig. 11.14
Age/sex distribution of the normal adult database. Further details are provided in **❷** Table 11.1

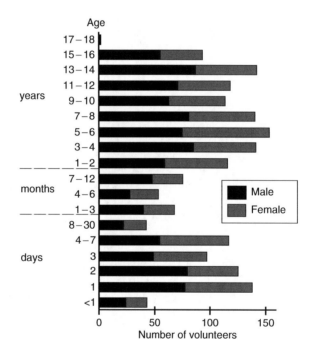

○ Fig. 11.15
Age/sex distribution of the normal children's database. Further details are provided in **❷** Table 11.1

11.2.2.4 Methods of Analysis

All measurements from each recording were stored on a computer file and added to a database. The adult and pediatric data were kept separate.

The BMDP suite of statistical programs was available for obtaining the basic data such as mean and standard deviation. The programs mainly used were P2D and P6D.

Table 11.1

Numbers of males and females in the total population group

Age	Male	Female	Total
⩽24 h	23	19	
1 day	77	61	
2 days	79	46	
3 days	48	49	
4–7 days	54	63	
⩽1 month	21	21	
⩽3 months	39	29	
⩽6 months	27	26	
⩽1 year	47	29	
1–2 years	59	57	
3–4 years	85	57	
5–6 years	75	79	
7–8 years	81	60	
9–10 years	63	51	
11–12 years	71	48	
13–14 years	87	56	
15–16 years	55	39	
17–18 years	0	1	
Children Σ	*991*	*791*	*1,782*
18–29 years	242	304	
30–39 years	217	131	
40–49 years	210	97	
⩽50 years	215	139	
Adult Σ	*884*	*671*	*1,555*
Total Σ	*1,875*	*1,462*	*3,337*

11.2.2.5 Statistical Considerations

It has been known for many years that in general terms, ECG data are not normally distributed but tend to be skewed. An illustration is shown in ❯ Fig. 11.16. For this reason, normal ranges are best described not by using the mean ± twice the standard deviation but by 96 percentile ranges, that is, by excluding 2% of measurements at the top and bottom end of a particular set of measurements. Wherever possible this has been done in analyzing the data. Only in the case of small numbers such as, for example, healthy males with a Q wave in V_1, was it necessary to include the complete range because total numbers were too small. One other point that should be noted is that the calculation of the mean is based only on measurements that were present. In other words, if there were 100 patients in a particular group but only 40 had an S wave in a selected lead, then the mean amplitude was derived using only the 40 measurements and the 60 values of 0 mV for the remaining patients were excluded from the calculation of the mean.

With respect to angular data, care was taken to ensure that all measurements were in a meaningful range. In other words, the recommendations for measuring angles would suggest that the direction in the frontal plane of the X-axis would be labeled as $0°$. If a vector measurement inferior to that was perhaps $20°$ and one superior to the X-axis was $340°$, the mean value would certainly not be $180°$ but $0°$. In other words, $340°$ would be converted to $-20°$ before calculating the mean value. Alternative methods for dealing with angular data were elaborated many years ago by Downs et al. [13].

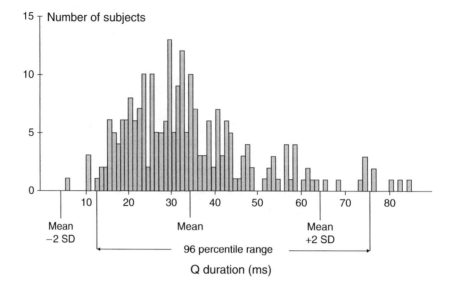

◘ Fig. 11.16

An example of a skewed distribution where there is a long tail of measurements at the upper end of the distribution. The figure shows a histogram of Q wave duration in lead Y in a group of 259 patients with proven inferior myocardial infarction. A total number of 24 patients with no Q waves in lead Y are excluded from the calculation of the mean

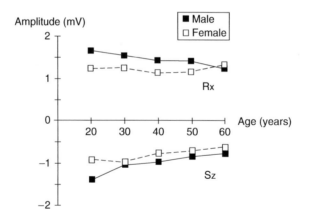

◘ Fig. 11.17

Effect of age and sex on mean R wave amplitude in lead X and mean S wave amplitude in lead Z

11.2.3   Results: Scalar Data

11.2.3.1   Wave Amplitudes and Durations

The relevant tables of normal limits of PQRST amplitudes and durations in the derived leads X, Y, and Z are presented in Appendix 5A. Again, it can be confirmed that the effects of age and sex on the amplitudes of waveforms are significant. This can be seen in ◗ Fig. 11.17 where the mean S wave amplitude in lead Z is presented.

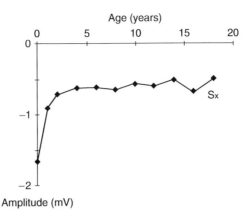

■ Fig. 11.18

The upper limit of normal S_X amplitude in children from birth to adolescence

Here the amplitude in young males is significantly higher than in young females, although the difference diminishes as age increases. These findings are similar to measurements of the S wave in V_2. The effect is not so marked for the mean R wave in lead X, which is also shown in the same figure.

In contrast, durations tended to show little difference between different age and sex groups with the exception of the QRS duration, which, as is well known, is approximately 7 ms longer in males than in females although strangely almost no cognizance is taken of this in any diagnostic criteria. This point is discussed in ❷ Chap. 1 of *Electrocardiology: Comprehensive Clinical ECG* (see ❷ Sect. 1.7.8).

11.2.3.2 Pediatric Data

It goes without saying that dramatic changes in pediatric measurements can be seen from birth onward. Again, appropriate tables are presented in Appendix 5B. As an example, the upper limit of normal S wave amplitude in lead X is shown in ❷ Fig. 11.18. There is a rapid decrease in S_X amplitude in the first year of life corresponding to a counterclockwise shift of the maximum frontal plane QRS vector.

11.2.3.3 Comparative Vectorcardiography

Yang and Macfarlane [14] reported on a comparison of the 12-lead vectorcardiogram in apparently healthy Caucasians and Chinese. To the database of 1,555 Caucasians, 503 Chinese were added giving a total of 2,058 individuals whose vectorcardiograms were derived from the conventional 12-lead ECG.

The trend of the influence of age and sex on the magnitude and direction of the derived QRS and T vectors was found to be similar in both cases. In the younger age groups, the magnitude of the maximal spatial vector was essentially greater in Caucasians than in Chinese while in the older age groups over 40, the reverse was the case. This was a somewhat surprising finding for which there is no clear explanation. ❷ Figures 11.19 and ❷ 11.20 show a comparison between the QRS and T vector magnitude in both races. It can be seen that it is essential to include the effect of age, sex, and race when interpreting 12-lead vectorcardiographic appearances.

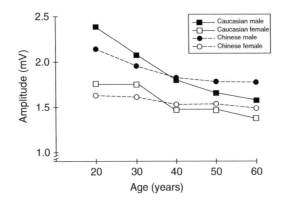

◨ Fig. 11.19

Mean magnitude of the maximal QRS vector amplitude in Caucasians and Chinese

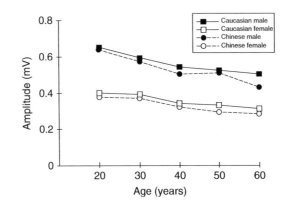

◨ Fig. 11.20

Mean magnitude of the maximal T vector amplitude in Caucasians and Chinese

11.2.4   Results: Vector Data

11.2.4.1   P Loops

In the infant, the P loop tends to be directed vertically at birth but it soon rotates superiorly in the frontal plane and remains around 55°. In the transverse plane, the P loop in children at birth is approximately 20–25° and subsequently shifts a little toward the adult value of around 0°. Sex differences between the mean P wave vector in the transverse plane are significant with the mean direction for males being 349° and for females 14° (Draper et al. [15], Nemati et al. [16]). It should be noted that the results obtained by these authors were derived using the Frank system.

11.2.4.2   QRS Loops

There is, of course, a considerable change from birth to adulthood in the QRS loop in the 12-lead vectorcardiogram. ❷ Figure 11.21 shows a 12-lead QRS loop from a neonate where the maximum QRS vector is oriented around 150° in the frontal plane. On the other hand, in the normal adult QRS in the frontal plane, ❷ Fig. 11.22, the QRS loop is oriented at around 50°. In general terms, in the frontal plane, the QRS loop is in the vast majority of cases inscribed in a

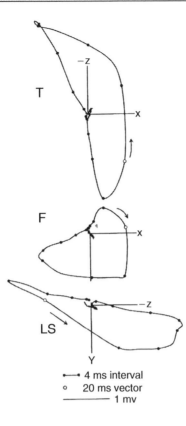

● **Fig. 11.21**
12-lead QRS and T loops from a healthy neonate

clockwise direction in the infant. In the adult, the frontal plane loop can be inscribed either in a clockwise or counter-clockwise direction, although the clockwise loop tends to predominate again. In the transverse plane, in the neonate, the inscription around birth is 43% clockwise and 45% counterclockwise but soon changes to being almost totally counterclockwise as it is in the normal adult. A figure-of-eight loop can be found in 20–40% of children up to 8 months of age using the Frank system [17] although our own 12-lead data suggest a lower incidence. ❯ Table 11.2 shows the results derived from the Glasgow data in respect of direction of inscription of the QRS loops in the frontal and transverse planes.

11.2.4.3 Left Axis Deviation

It may seem superfluous to consider a discussion on left axis deviation but the normal range of the maximum QRS vector in the frontal plane is, indeed, quite different in the 12-lead vectorcardiogram from that in the standard 12-lead ECG. A full list of ranges is given in Appendix 5.

It can be seen that in healthy females, for example, the maximum QRS vector is never superior to $0°$. In males, this seems to occur in a few individuals in the 30–59 years age group but, by and large, the vast majority of individuals have a maximum QRS vector inferior to $0°$. This observation suggests the following criteria:

Borderline/left axis deviation: $0° \rightarrow -15°$ ($360° \rightarrow 345°$)
Left axis deviation: $-15° \rightarrow -90°$ ($345° \rightarrow 270°$)

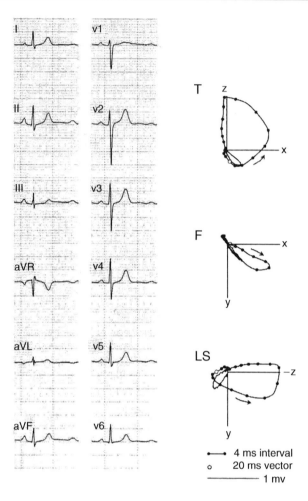

● Fig. 11.22

12-lead QRS and T loops from a healthy adult

● Table 11.2

Direction of inscription of the QRS vector loop in transverse and frontal planes expressed as a percentage from 1,555 adult Caucasian normals (CCW; Counterclockwise Rotation, CW; Clockwise Rotation)

Planes		CCW	Figure of 8	CW
Transverse	Male	98.1	0.9	1.0
	Female	97.9	1.2	0.9
Frontal	Male	22.9	19.1	58.0
	Female	21.8	25.3	52.9

11.2.4.4   Right Axis Deviation

The tables in Appendix 5 indicate that with the exception of young males <30 years of age, the normal maximum QRS vector in the frontal plane is always <65°. This indication is considerably different from the normal frontal plane vector calculated from the 12-lead ECG. It does suggest the use of the following criteria:

Borderline right axis deviation:
Females and (males > 30 years) $65° \rightarrow 75°$
Males < 30 years $90° \rightarrow 100°$

Right axis deviation:
Females and (males > 30 years) > 75°
Males < 30 years > 100°

11.2.4.5   T Loops

From ❷ Figs. 11.21 and ❷ 11.22 discussed above, the direction of the maximum T vector in the frontal and transverse planes can be seen for the average newborn and the average adult. It follows that there is a gradual change of T vector orientation from one position to another with increasing age. Details of some T vector measurements can be found in the Appendices.

11.3   Hypertrophy

11.3.1   Introduction

11.3.1.1   What is Hypertrophy?

Electrocardiographers tend to report the pattern of increased voltage in the lateral leads together with accompanying ST-T changes as left ventricular hypertrophy (LVH). The advent of echocardiography as well as cardiac catheterization has meant that the variety of pathologies, which constitute the generic term "hypertrophy" is now better known. In general terms, hypertrophy can be taken to mean an increase in mass. All four chambers of the heart can demonstrate hypertrophy or enlargement either in isolation or in combination. Enlargement is a term that is perhaps more associated with an increase in volume whereas hypertrophy strictly may relate to an increase in muscle mass.

The subdivision of different types of hypertrophy is essentially based around left ventricular geometry. Where there is an overall increase in mass with a dominant increase in muscle thickness without an increase in cavity volume, the term concentric hypertrophy is used. Where there is an increase in mass predominantly due to an increase in volume, the term eccentric hypertrophy is used.

Huwez, Pringle, and Macfarlane [18] have introduced a new classification for hypertrophy on the basis of mass and volume. The different types and the criteria are given in ❷ Table 11.3. A salutary lesson from that study was that a patient with apparently normal mass and volume could demonstrate the ECG changes of LVH described above. In addition, both concentric and eccentric hypertrophy could produce similar ECG changes or none at all.

Notwithstanding the above, the remainder of this chapter is generally concerned with the classical description of vectorcardiographic changes accompanying hypertrophy.

11.3.1.2   Effects of Age, Sex and Race

It will be apparent from the previous ❷ Sect. 11.2 on normal ranges, that QRS voltage in some leads such as X and Z increases with age until early adulthood and then decreases again. Likewise, it has also been shown that, in many cases,

■ Table 11.3

Left ventricular geometry classification

Left ventricular		Type
Mass	Volume	
Normal	Normal	Normal
Normal	Increased	Isolated left ventricular volume overload
Increased	Normal	Concentric LVH
Increased	Increased	Eccentric LVH

sex differences particularly with respect to voltage can be demonstrated in vectorcardiographic parameters. Similar effects can be seen within different races.

All these observations suggest that the criteria for ventricular hypertrophy have to be based on a knowledge of all of these three variables.

11.3.1.3 Value of Vectorcardiography

It goes without saying that the echocardiogram gives a detailed picture of left ventricular geometry. On the other hand, it is the ECG that may demonstrate secondary ST-T changes, which are well known to be associated with a poor prognosis [19, 20]. If a reasonable specificity of 95% is desired, then the best ECG criteria should have a sensitivity around 50%. Data such as these vary from one study to another depending on the gold standard, which may be postmortem weights, on the one hand, or echocardiographic measurements, on the other. The reader should therefore be aware, from the outset, that the vectorcardiographic diagnosis of LVH is somewhat insensitive.

11.3.2 Atrial Enlargement

In the normal 12-lead vectorcardiogram, the P wave may exhibit two distinct components, which probably result from asynchronous depolarization of the left and right atrium. In this event, the bifid nature of the P wave is best seen in the inferior lead Y. In view of the fact that normal atrial depolarization commences in the right atrium before spreading to the left atrium, it follows that the first component is due to right atrial excitation and the second due to left atrial excitation.

11.3.2.1 Right Atrial Enlargement

One of the manifestations of right atrial enlargement is a P wave in the inferior lead Y with an amplitude > 0.3 mV. As this abnormality not infrequently occurs in respiratory disorders, it is sometimes called P pulmonale (❷ Fig. 11.23). Occasionally, P_Y may be of normal amplitude but there may be a prominent P_Z > 0.15 mV on account of right atrial enlargement.

Chou and Helm [21] have pointed out that the P-wave changes in the inferior lead Y occasionally resemble P pulmonale when there are no clinical findings to support such a diagnosis. The cause of the abnormal P wave may be left atrial hypertrophy and the term "pseudo P pulmonale" is used to describe such a phenomenon. Clearly, this diagnosis should be made on the basis of the clinical findings taken in conjunction with the ECG appearances. The normal ranges

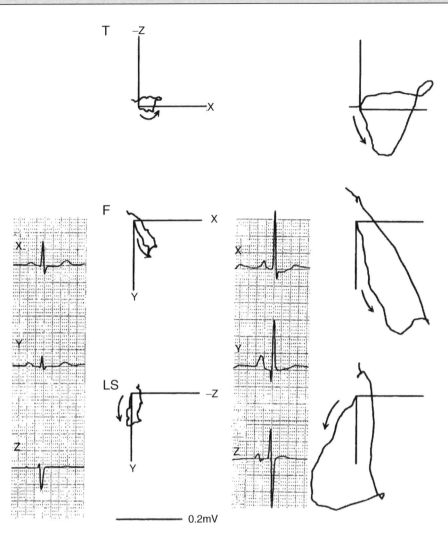

◻ Fig. 11.23
Normal P loops (*left*) and an example of combined atrial enlargement (*right*)

of the projections of the maximum P vector on to the three planes are so wide that little diagnostic advantage can be gained from a study of these parameters in respect of right atrial enlargement.

11.3.2.2 Left Atrial Enlargement

When left atrial enlargement occurs, several abnormalities may result. First, the P-wave duration may be increased beyond 120 ms. Second, bifid or M-shaped P waves of greater than normal duration may be found in the inferior lead Y and this pattern is often referred to as P mitrale because of its common association with mitral stenosis. From the vectorcardiographic point of view, enlargement of the left atrium may also cause an increase in the left atrial vectors, which in turn produce a rotation of the terminal portion of the P-wave vector posteriorly and to the left (◉ Fig. 11.23). Thus, the terminal component of the scalar P wave in lead Z can be increased in negativity and in duration.

The maximum P vector amplitude may be increased but the normal range of P-vector orientation is so wide as to be of little value. On occasions, the maximum P-vector magnitude may exceed 0.3 mV when the individual scalar components are within normal. In this case, left atrial enlargement is the most likely cause.

11.3.2.3   Combined Atrial Enlargement

In general terms, a combination of the individual criteria for left and right atrial enlargement when present would be suggestive of combined atrial enlargement (❷ Fig. 11.23).

11.3.3   Left Ventricular Hypertrophy

11.3.3.1   Diagnostic Criteria

When LVH or left ventricular enlargement produces alterations in QRS morphology, these relate generally to an increase in QRS vector amplitude. On occasions, the maximum QRS vector will be rotated posteriorly and this is seen best in the transverse plane where the resultant effect is to produce an increase in the amplitude of S_Z. Consideration of the basic principles of vectorcardiography indicates that if a vectorcardiographic loop rotates posteriorly increasing S_Z, then R_X would decrease simultaneously. Thus, one of the commonly used vectorcardiographic criteria is based on $R_X + S_Z$. The data from the 1,555 patients in the Glasgow database suggest that the upper limit of $R_X + S_Z = 3.95$ mV for males over 40 years of age. It is, however, possible to express the upper limit of normal for males as a continuous age dependent equation as follows:

$$R_X + S_Z = [72 : 81 - 0.02074 \, \text{age (months)}]^2 \, \mu V$$

Similar equations apply for women and for other races.

The typical vectorcardiographic appearances in LVH are shown in ❷ Fig. 11.24. In this case, there is increased magnitude of the QRS vector, which is more posteriorly oriented than the mean maximum QRS vector in normals in the transverse plane while the T loop is oppositely directed to the QRS loop. This is equivalent to the secondary ST-T pattern in the lateral leads.

It should be noted that the individual component amplitudes of the scalar leads may be normal while the resultant vector amplitude can be abnormal. For example, if the amplitude of R_X is 2.4 mV and, at the same instant, R_Y is 1.5 mV (although corresponding peak amplitudes might be a little higher), it follows that the amplitude of the maximum QRS vector would be

$$3.2 \, \text{mV} = \sqrt{(2.4^2 + 1.5^2 + 1.5^2)} \, \text{mV}$$

Each of the scalar amplitudes is within the normal range for a 45-year-old male, but the vector magnitude is outside normal (see Appendix 5A).

Various types of QRS loop may be seen in the vectorcardiogram. These are best differentiated by appearances in the transverse plane. Type I may simply resemble a normal QRS loop but be of increased magnitude. In Type II, there is a rotation of the projection of the maximum QRS vector posteriorly beyond 310° in the transverse plane (❷ Fig. 11.25), possibly with a normal QRS voltage.

It is not common, however, to find an abnormal orientation of the QRS vector loop in LVH without voltage evidence in addition. In Type III, where LVH is very marked, there may be a figure-of-eight loop in the transverse plane with the distal part of the loop inscribed in a clockwise direction (❷ Fig. 11.26). In Type IV, there may be slightly increased QRS

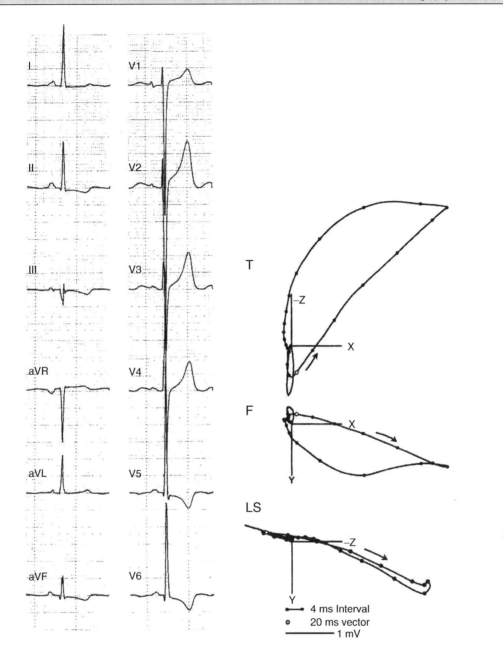

◻ Fig. 11.24

An example of left ventricular hypertrophy (LVH) Type I. Note the increased magnitude of the QRS loops best seen in the transverse plane where the T loop is essentially oppositely directed to the QRS loop

duration, and an abnormally large QRS maximum vector, but the rate of inscription of the loop is slower than normal as manifested by the closeness of the dots. This pattern is sometimes called "incomplete left bundle branch block (LBBB)" that often accompanies LVH.

Reference has already been made to secondary STT changes (❯ Fig. 11.24) sometimes called left ventricular strain or overload pattern. In a series of patients [22], it was found that this pattern of ST depression with asymmetric T wave

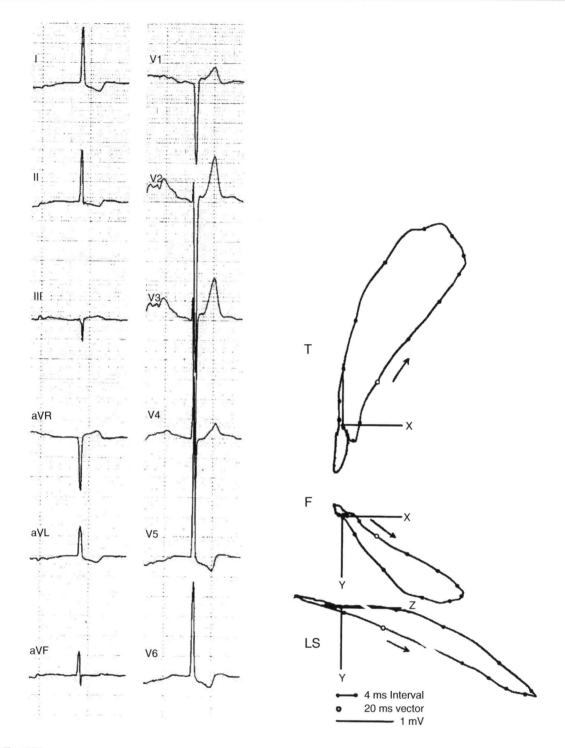

Fig. 11.25

An example of LVH Type II. Note that the maximum QRS vector in the transverse plane is posterior to 310°

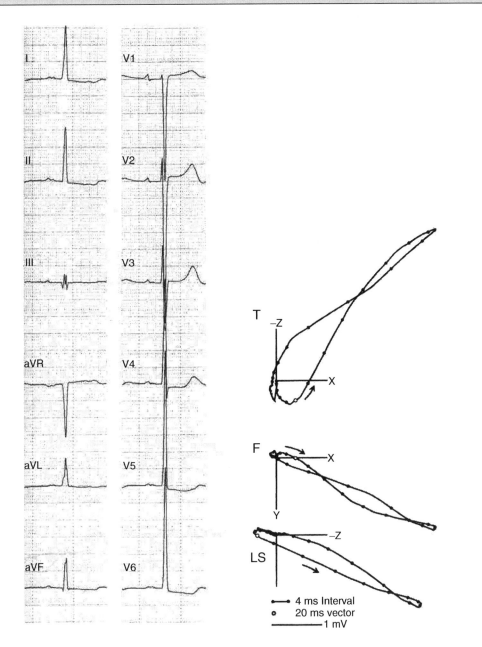

☉ Fig. 11.26

An example of LVH Type III. In this case, a figure-of-eight loop can be seen clearly in the transverse plane while the maximum QRS vector exceeds 4 mV

inversion was 94% sensitive for LVH. Thus, even in the absence of high voltage, this ECG finding in the scalar lead X should be regarded as a pointer toward the diagnosis of LVH.

One further point can be made concerning the vectorcardiographic appearances in severe LVH. It can happen that the initial QRS vectors are directed posteriorly, that is, there is a Q wave in the anteroseptal lead Z or V_2. This makes the differential diagnosis of anteroseptal infarction from LVH difficult unless the clinical picture is relatively clear-cut. For example, ☉ Fig. 11.27 shows such a pattern in a 73-year-old male with hypertension and aortic stenosis and insufficiency.

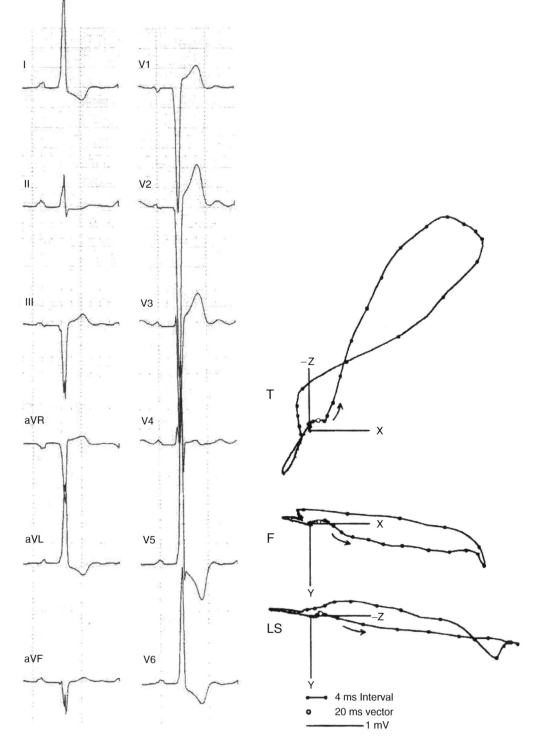

Fig. 11.27

A 12-lead ECG and vectorcardiogram recorded from a 73-year-old male with hypertension and aortic stenosis and insufficiency. Note that the initial QRS vectors are directed posteriorly, that is, there is a Q wave in lead Z. Other typical features of LVH can also be seen

The reasons for the presence of the Q wave are not fully understood although many hypotheses have been put forward. Possibly on account of there being three areas of initial activation in the left ventricle, the concept of the genesis of the Q wave may be revised. It could be postulated that the electrical activation of the area of the left ventricle adjacent to the posterior wall, which is among the first to be depolarized, predominates on account of left ventricular wall thickness, thereby leading to initial QRS forces oriented posteriorly producing a Q wave in the anteroseptal lead.

The other criteria that point to LVH include left axis deviation, which, in the vectorcardiogram, is a QRS axis superior to $0°$ in the frontal plane. Indeed, apart from the specific criteria of increased vector magnitude and posteriorly rotated maximum QRS vector orientation, other criteria mirror those for the conventional 12-lead ECG, for example, a delayed intrinsicoid deflection in lead X and increased P terminal force in lead Z.

11.3.3.2 Bundle Branch Block and LVH

The diagnosis of LVH from an ECG that shows bundle branch block is controversial. Some authors have claimed it is possible to make such a diagnosis while others have noted in various series that in the presence of LBBB, LVH is always found. Thus, no specific criteria for the diagnosis of LVH and LBBB are presented here. However, one or two points can be made.

As will be seen in ❷ Sect. 11.5, the vectorcardiographic appearances in LBBB are characteristic in having a narrow QRS loop in the transverse plane. If the scalar lead appears to have the LBBB pattern with a tall R_X but does not have the narrow bundle branch block loop, then LVH could be considered as a possible cause (incomplete LBBB/LVH pattern).

11.3.4 Right Ventricular Hypertrophy

Increased right ventricular excitation forces or increased right ventricular volume can produce varying ECG patterns depending on the time of the occurrence of the abnormal electrical activity compared to that of the left ventricle. Hypertrophy of the free wall of the right ventricle will produce abnormal anterior forces in early ventricular depolarization whereas basal hypertrophy will produce abnormal posterior forces late in ventricular depolarization. In the vectorcardiogram, there are essentially two presentations of right ventricular hypertrophy (RVH), namely, a prominent R wave in lead Z and a deep S wave in lead X. The presence of these abnormalities either singly or together produces four patterns of RVH or enlargement. These are as follows.

11.3.4.1 RVH: Type A

Type A RVH is manifested as an increase in the ratio of anterior/posterior forces in the transverse plane with counter-clockwise inscription of the QRS loop (❷ Fig. 11.28). Often the abnormal QRS loop may have a T loop directed posteriorly corresponding to the secondary ST–T abnormalities sometimes seen in V_1 and V_2.

One criterion of value in Type A is the projection of the maximum QRS vector onto the transverse plane $>30°$. Occasionally, this may be present when voltage and ratio measurements in the anteroseptal leads are normal.

11.3.4.2 RVH: Type B

One of the major advantages of the vectorcardiogram is preservation of the timing relationships between the different scalar leads. Thus, while two different scalar patterns may have similar appearances, the vectorcardiogram can be normal in one and abnormal in another. This is often apparent in Type B RVH. In this case, the QRS loop in the transverse plane

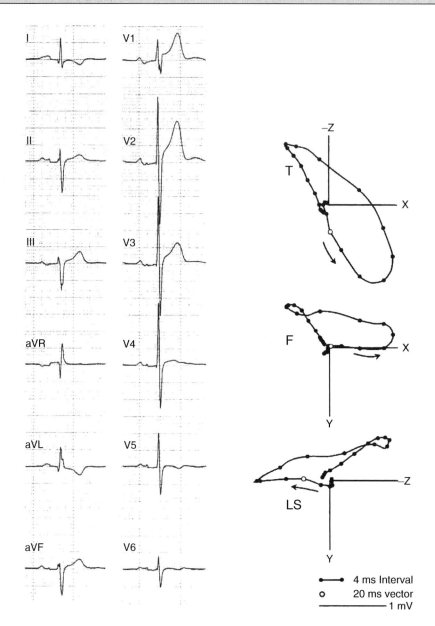

An example of right ventricular hypertrophy (RVH) Type A where there is a marked increase in anteriorly directed forces as seen in the transverse plane

initially has normal counterclockwise inscription, but the second part of the loop is deviated anteriorly so that the net effect is to have a loop with clockwise or figure-of-eight inscription in the transverse plane (● Fig. 11.29).

11.3.4.3   RVH: Type C

The third type of RVH is manifested as an abnormal transverse plane vectorcardiographic loop that is normally counterclockwise inscribed with the maximum QRS vector being oriented posteriorly and to the right (● Fig. 11.30).

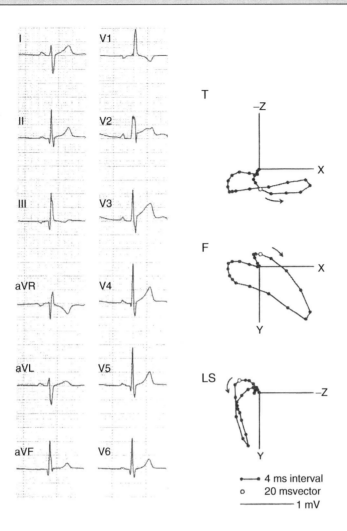

◘ Fig. 11.29
An example of RVH Type B where there is a figure-of-eight loop in the transverse plane in which all forces are seen to be anteriorly oriented. Note the late rightward-directed forces corresponding to the deep S wave in lead I

This pattern is most often found in patients with chronic respiratory disease and therefore may be accompanied by P pulmonale. However, some patients with mitral stenosis also exhibit such findings. It is thought that the posterior rightward displacement of the QRS vector is due to hypertrophy of the basal portion of the right ventricle. Secondary ST-T changes can also be found in this pattern. The abnormal rightward forces also translate into right axis deviation in the frontal plane.

11.3.4.4 RVH: Type D

In the more severe forms of RVH, as may occur in certain forms of congenital heart disease the main QRS vector may be directed abnormally not only to the anterior but also to the right with clockwise inscription of QRS in the transverse plane (❯ Fig. 11.31).

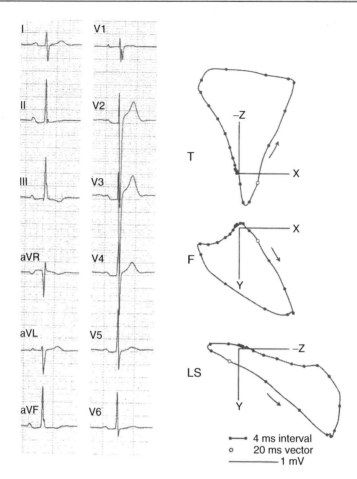

⬛ Fig. 11.30

An example of RVH Type C. In this case, there is a large posterior and rightward-directed force in the later part of QRS

11.3.5   Combined Ventricular Hypertrophy

It has been claimed that in most cases of LVH there is an accompanying RVH [23]. The vectorcardiographic diagnosis of biventricular hypertrophy is mainly based on finding features of both LVH and RVH separately. For example, if the transverse QRS loop is directed posteriorly and has an increased magnitude with the T loop oppositely directed, as in secondary changes of LVH, and the frontal QRS vector is oriented around 90°, then combined ventricular hypertrophy should be considered.

11.3.6   Pediatric Vectorcardiography

The various forms of congenital heart disease can produce a variety of vectorcardiographic patterns that can be extremely difficult to interpret. A few patterns are pathognomonic of rare forms of congenital heart disease but in any event, the report must remain an ECG interpretation. In other words, no attempt should be made to infer the anatomy of the congenital lesion in the majority of cases. Brohet [24] has reviewed the advantages of vectorcardiography in congenital heart disease.

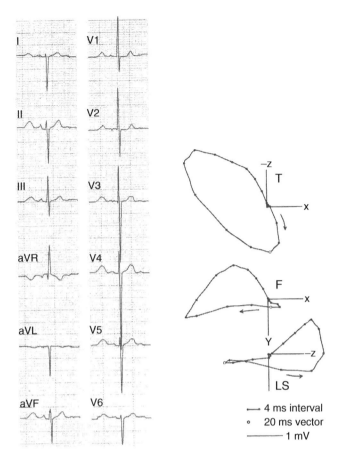

⊡ Fig. 11.31
An example of RVH Type D where the QRS loop in the transverse plane is clearly abnormal, being inscribed in a clockwise direction and lying almost entirely to the right. Marked right axis deviation can also be seen in the frontal plane loop

11.4 Myocardial Infarction

11.4.1 Introduction

11.4.1.1 Theoretical Considerations

A myocardial infarction is death of myocardial tissue as a result of insufficient blood supply, that is, due to a stenosis or occlusion of a coronary artery. An infarcted area is electrically inert and distorts the normal spread of excitation. The net effect is that the electrical forces, which are influenced by the "dead zone" or infarct vector, are directed away from the area of myocardial infarction. This is in contrast with hypertrophy that produces electrical forces directed toward the area of increased ventricular mass.

11.4.1.2 Anatomical Definitions

There is a lack of unanimity in describing myocardial infarction. In 1978, the American College of Cardiology Conference on Optimal Electrocardiography described myocardial infarction in terms of Q waves seen in the various leads of the

12-lead ECG [25]. This has resulted in terms such as septal, anteroseptal, and anterior infarction being used. However, there is still no consensus regarding the localization of an infarction among electrocardiographers.

Radiological or echocardiographic techniques can also be used to detect and localize a myocardial infarction. In coronary angiography, it is not the infarcted area per se that is detected but the stenosis or occlusion of the coronary artery that caused the myocardial infarction. An infarcted area causes abnormalities in the ventricular contraction pattern, which can usually be detected in a left ventriculogram or in an echocardiogram. The techniques described above show different aspects of the same disease. Differences in the position and orientation of the heart and a variation in the anatomy of the coronary arteries have varying influence on these techniques. Therefore, the correlations between electrocardiographic changes, abnormalities of ventricular contraction, and the degree of stenosis in relevant coronary arteries are not excellent. This should be borne in mind when comparing different techniques for the diagnosis of myocardial infarction.

Notwithstanding any of the above, in very general terms, occlusion of a left anterior descending coronary artery or a left main stem artery is likely to produce an infarct predominantly in the anterior (anteroseptal/anterosuperior) wall of the heart. An occlusion in the right coronary artery will generally produce an inferior myocardial infarction while occlusion of the left circumflex produces a lateral or posterolateral/inferior myocardial infarction.

11.4.2   The 12-Lead Vectorcardiogram in Myocardial Infarction

11.4.2.1   Anterior Infarction

In keeping with the concept of the dead zone or infarct vector, an anterior myocardial infarction will result in slightly increased posteriorly directed electromotive forces and a reduction, if not an absence, of anteriorly directed forces in the early part of ventricular depolarization. In 12-lead ECG terminology, this corresponds to a QS complex in V_2. The corresponding vectorcardiographic appearances are shown in ❯ Fig. 11.32. Here it can be seen that there is no electrical activity in the left anterior quadrant of the transverse plane vectorcardiogram. This type of clear-cut myocardial infarction, from an electrocardiographic point of view, is generally well delineated on the 12-lead ECG. Of more interest is the situation where the 12-lead ECG may be somewhat equivocal with low R waves in the anterior leads but the vectorcardiogram shows other features that are suggestive of myocardial infarction. In the transverse plane, common vectorcardiographic criteria for anterior myocardial infarction are listed in ❯ Table 11.4.

❯ Figure 11.33 gives an example of a QRS loop where there are initial anteriorly directed forces but the 30 ms QRS vector is posterior to 300°. ❯ Figure 11.34 shows a different form of vectorcardiographic change where there is an initial counterclockwise inscription leading to a bite in the vectorcardiographic loop (see ❯ Sect. 11.4.2.8). ❯ Figure 11.35 illustrates a case of anterior myocardial infarction where the area of the QRS loop in the left anterior quadrant <1%.

11.4.2.2   Anterior Myocardial Infarction Versus LVH

In cases of severe LVH, the vectorcardiographic loop may also resemble anterior myocardial infarction. In many cases, the difference between the two can clearly be separated on non-electrocardiographic considerations, clearly including the clinical history. If the QRS loop and T loop are oppositely directed in the transverse plane with lack of QRS electrical activity anteriorly, the higher probability is that appearances are due to LVH (❯ Fig. 11.27).

Of course, both abnormalities can be present simultaneously in an individual and this is more likely to be the case if the QRS–T angle is approximately 90°. A T vector directed posteriorly to the right suggests an ischemic component to the abnormality as isolated LVH would rarely produce a T vector so oriented.

11.4.2.3   Inferior Myocardial Infarction

The dead zone or infarct vector concept suggests that in inferior myocardial infarction there is an increase of electrical force superiorly. In turn, this produces a loss of inferiorly directed forces resulting in an initial superiorly directed vectorcardiographic loop in the frontal plane. However, as this is not altogether uncommon in normal individuals, the point

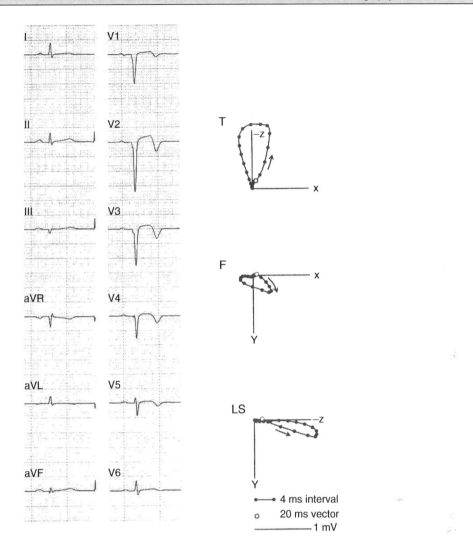

⬛ Fig. 11.32

The classical features of anterior myocardial infarction with a complete absence of anteriorly directed QRS vectors. Note that the 30 ms vector is also posterior to 300° in the transverse plane

⬛ Table 11.4

Criteria for anterior myocardial infarction

Any of the following in the transverse QRS loop
Direction of 30 ms vector 225–300°
Loop area in left anterior quadrant <1% of the total loop area
An early bite, that is, a clockwise inscription of the loop, with an amplitude >0.05 mV (see ❷ Sect. 11.4.2.8)

of importance is the length of time for which the loop persists in the superior quadrants and the ratio of superiorly to inferiorly directed forces. Common vectorcardiographic criteria for inferior myocardial infarction are presented in ❷ Table 11.5.

In addition to the superiorly directed forces having a duration >20 ms, the concept of X-intercept needs to be introduced. This is illustrated in ❷ Fig. 11.36. The X-intercept is the point at which a clockwise-inscribed frontal plane loop

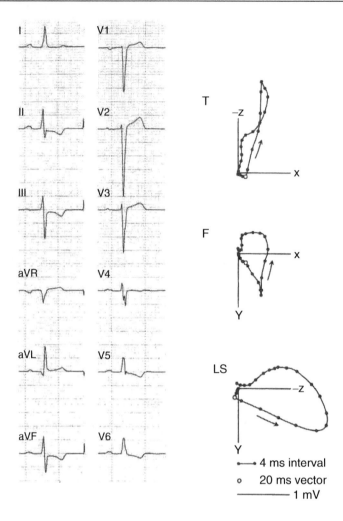

● Fig. 11.33

An example of anterior myocardial infarction where the initial QRS forces are anteriorly directed for a little over 20 ms but where the 30 ms vector is just posterior to 300°

first crosses the *X*-axis. In a sense, it is clear that the longer the QRS loop remains superior to the *X*-axis, the greater the probability that the *X*-intercept will exceed 0.3 mV. Thus, in some ways, there is a correlation between this parameter and a superior duration >20 ms. ❷ Figure 11.37 gives an example of a vectorcardiographic frontal plane loop where all the criteria are met.

Analogous to the situation of low R waves in anterior leads consistent with myocardial infarction, it is possible that there can be very low amplitude R waves in the inferior lead Y in the presence of inferior infarction, that is, there is a very short inferiorly directed initial activation in the frontal plane. If the initial vector of activation is directed inferiorly and rightward followed by clockwise inscription, then the criteria of *X*-intercept >0.3 mV and a superior/inferior amplitude ratio >0.15 can often be met.

11.4.2.4 Inferior Myocardial Infarction Versus Left Anterior Fascicular Block

Often a common feature of the inferior myocardial infarction and left anterior fascicular block is the superior orientation of the frontal plane QRS vector loop. However, the left anterior fascicular block is always accompanied by a

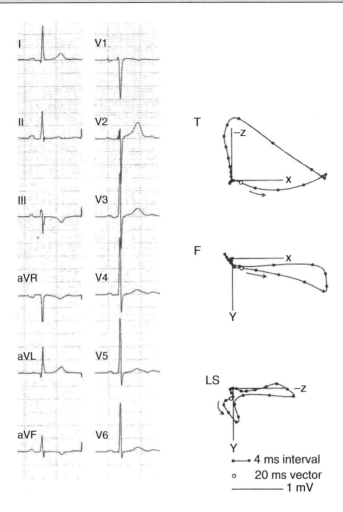

■ Fig. 11.34

Anterior myocardial infarction proven by diagnostic cardiac catheterization in a 62-year-old male. Note the early bite in the QRS loop in the transverse plane

counterclockwise inscription of the QRS loop whereas the inferior myocardial infarction invariably has a clockwise inscription of the QRS loop. A comparative example is shown in ❷ Fig. 11.38. It is also the case that in left anterior fascicular block, the QRS axis is generally more superiorly directed than in inferior myocardial infarction.

11.4.2.5   Posterior Myocardial Infarction

The theory of the dead zone or infarct vector applied to an infarction of the posterior wall of the heart indicates that there will be an increase in anteriorly directed electrical forces. The diagnosis of posterior myocardial infarction is again difficult, purely from an electrocardiographic standpoint. There may, of course, be other clinical factors that suggest a myocardial infarction which, taken together with the relevant vectorcardiographic changes, could point to infarction of the posterior wall.

The increase in anterior forces is reflected in an increased duration of the anteriorly directed forces in the transverse plane. In addition, the amplitude ratio of the anteriorly/posteriorly directed forces exceeds 1. Finally, the area

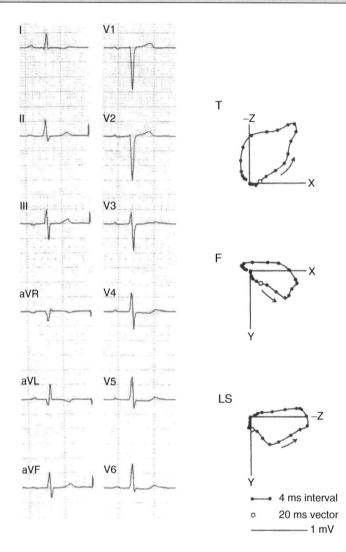

● Fig. 11.35

Anterior myocardial infarction proven by diagnostic cardiac catheterization in a 58-year-old male. Note the QRS loop area in the left anterior quadrant is almost 0% of the total QRS loop area

● Table 11.5

Criteria for inferior myocardial infarction

All of the following in the frontal QRS loop
An initial superior inscription >20 ms
A superior amplitude >0.1 mV
A superior/inferior amplitude ratio >0.15
An X-axis intercept >0.3 mV

in the left anterior quadrant of the transverse plane exceeds 50% of the total QRS loop area (● Fig. 11.39). Common vectorcardiographic criteria for posterior myocardial infarction are presented in ● Table 11.6.

The other typical feature of posterior myocardial infarction is an increase in T vector amplitude. This may well correspond to a T vector oriented in the direction of 70–80° in the transverse plane.

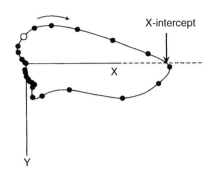

Fig. 11.36
Frontal plane QRS loop showing the X-intercept

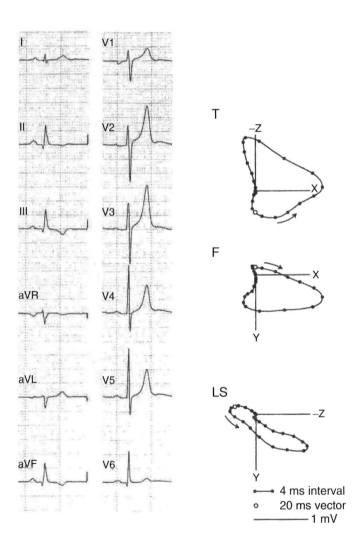

Fig. 11.37
Vectorcardiogram of inferior myocardial infarction meeting the criteria of ❷ Table 11.5

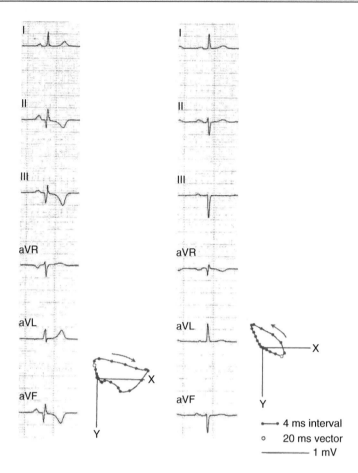

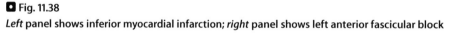

◻ Fig. 11.38

Left panel shows inferior myocardial infarction; *right* panel shows left anterior fascicular block

11.4.2.6 Posterior Myocardial Infarction Versus RVH

The features of RVH have been discussed in ❷ Sect. 11.3. The Type A vectorcardiographic loop is not too dissimilar from that of posterior myocardial infarction and therefore the differentiation between the two is difficult. However, the criteria of anteriorly directed forces exceeding 50 ms is more likely to be met in a case of posterior myocardial infarction than in RVH. Also, the T vector loop is more likely to be anteriorly directed in posterior infarction than in RVH.

Another factor that influences the situation is that an inferior or even lateral myocardial infarction, which extends toward the posterior wall of the heart, may produce, in addition, an increase in anteriorly directed forces. In that situation, a report of "increased anterior forces probably reflecting inferior/posterior myocardial infarction" is more likely to be correct than one which suggests that there is RVH in addition to inferior infarction, for example.

11.4.2.7 Anterolateral Myocardial Infarction

The effect of a lateral wall myocardial infarction is to produce an initial electrical force which is directed in the range 90–270° in the transverse plane. This is the principal requirement for the diagnosis of anterolateral myocardial infarction, an example of which is shown in ❷ Fig. 11.40. Isolated anterolateral infarction is uncommon and more often than not, the changes are associated with an anterior rather than a purely anterolateral myocardial infarction.

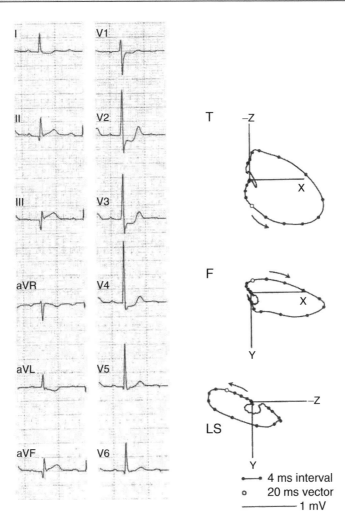

Fig. 11.39

Inferior myocardial infarction with posterior wall involvement. Note that the area of the QRS loop in the left anterior quadrant exceeds 50% of the total QRS loop area. The X-intercept also greatly exceeds 0.3 mV

Table 11.6

Criteria for posterior myocardial infarction

The QRS loop in the transverse plane shows:
an initial anteriorly directed loop >50 ms
an anterior/posterior amplitude ratio >1
a loop area in left anterior quadrant >50% of the total loop area

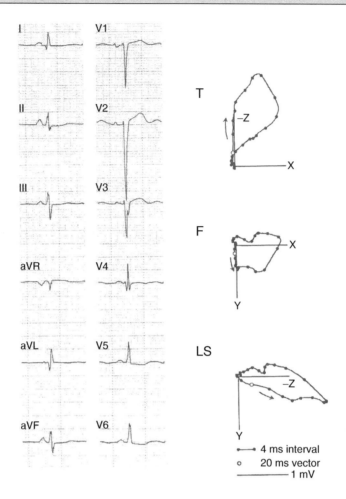

Vectorcardiographic example of anterolateral myocardial infarction. Note that in the transverse plane, the initial electrical forces are directed posteriorly to the right and that the inscription of the main body of this loop is clockwise. It should also be noted that there are no Q waves in the precordial leads of the 12-lead ECG

11.4.2.8   Bites

The concept of a vectorcardiographic bite was mentioned earlier in this chapter. This is best explained by reference to ❯ Fig. 11.41, where a comparison is made between a normal transverse plane vectorcardiogram and one exhibiting a bite, that is, an indentation of the QRS loop, which often amounts to a reversal of the direction of inscription of the loop. For example, the normal QRS loop in the transverse plane has a constant counterclockwise inscription whereas the loop with a bite has an inscription that is initially counterclockwise, then changes to clockwise before returning to counterclockwise inscription. It is suggested that the amount of deviation of the bite from the normal loop gives an indication of the size of infarcted area. Considerable work was done in this area by Selvester and Sanmarco [26] with modeling studies and, indeed, a nomogram was produced, which linked the duration of the bite with the magnitude of the difference between the normal vectorcardiographic loop and the abnormal vectorcardiographic loop (❯ Fig. 11.42). The nomogram allows calculation of an estimate of the percentage of myocardium that is damaged and in turn, an estimate of the ejection fraction of the left ventricle. Selvester et al. [27] also provided data on the occurrence of bites in diabetic patients. Edenbrandt et al. recently [28] developed a computer-assisted method for measuring the size of vectorcardiographic bites.

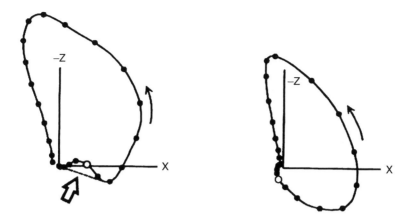

□ Fig. 11.41

Vectorcardiographic loops in the transverse plane. The left loop shows an early bite whereas the right loop has a normal inscription

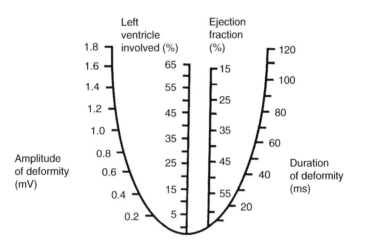

□ Fig. 11.42

Nomogram for predicting infarct size from deformities in the Frank vectorcardiogram. The amplitude and duration of the deformity are transferred to the left side and right side of the nomogram, respectively. A line is then constructed through these two points and the points where it crosses the lines in the center are used to determine the angiographic percentage of left ventricle involved and the ejection fraction

11.5 Conduction Defects

11.5.1 Introduction

It is certainly the case that conduction defects may be thought rather straightforward to diagnose from the 12-lead ECG. On the other hand, there are borderline situations where there can be doubt as to whether a QRS duration is prolonged. Indeed, it has gone almost unrecognized for many years that the normal mean QRS duration for males is almost 8 ms longer than for females in the 18–29 year age group (96.4 versus 87.7 ms) although as age increases the difference tends to decrease (92.7 versus 87.1 ms at 50 years and over) [29]. Notwithstanding, there are few if any diagnostic criteria that take cognizance of this fact.

One of the advantages of vectorcardiography is that conduction defects can be seen on the vectorcardiographic loop display as a slowing of the inscription of the loop, that is, the loop markers appear closer together. There are other features sometimes pathognomonic of particular defects, as will be seen later in this chapter.

11.5.1.1 Conduction System

The heart muscle consists of three types of tissue – automatic, specialized conducting, and contractile tissue. The process of depolarization is common to all three tissues but only the automatic and specialized conducting tissues have the ability to depolarize spontaneously.

In the human heart (❷ Fig. 11.43), the automatic tissue is concentrated mainly at the sinoatrial (SA) node. In the normal sequence of electrical events, an electrical impulse arising in the SA node, travels through the right atrium to the atrioventricular (AV) node and thereafter spreads into the ventricles via the specialized conducting tissue in the bundle of His.

Invasive recording of the signals in the atria and in particular in the area of the AV node has led to a much greater understanding of certain types of conduction defects but in particular, this approach has been of most value in the assessment of cardiac arrhythmias. On the other hand, this chapter is concerned more with abnormalities of conduction in the bundle of His and its various branches.

As seen in ❷ Fig. 11.43, the bundle of His divides at the base of the septum into the right bundle branch and the left bundle branch. The latter has been shown to divide into a variety of different forms, common to all of which are the left anterior and left posterior fascicles. Demoulin and Kulbertus [30] showed many years ago that there was often a third fascicle, which they called "the centroseptal fascicle."

Under normal circumstances, ventricular depolarization occurs first in the left ventricle, particularly on the left side of the septum, and then spreads to the free wall of the left ventricle. At the same time, shortly after left ventricular activation commences, the right ventricular excitation also starts. However, it is important to appreciate that the normal sequence of depolarization in the ventricles is from the left to the right side of the septum.

For completeness, it should be said that excitation in general terms spreads from the endocardium to the epicardium and from the apex to the base. In addition, ventricular repolarization takes place from the epicardium to the endocardium, giving rise to a normal upright T wave in the majority of precordial leads as well as most frontal plane leads with the exception of aVR. In the 12-lead vectorcardiogram, the T wave is normally upright in leads X, Y, and Z.

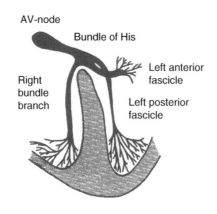

❏ Fig. 11.43
Conduction system of the human heart

11.5.2 Bundle Branch Block

11.5.2.1 Left Bundle Branch Block

When the normal conduction to the left ventricle is prevented by a block in the left bundle branch, the excitation wavefront has to find an alternative pathway via normal cardiac muscle. A major consequence of this is naturally an increase in the time taken to depolarize the ventricles and hence, there is an increase in the QRS duration.

Because of the block in the left bundle branch above its division into the various fascicles, septal activation begins on the right side and progresses from the right to left. Thus, in the 12-lead vectorcardiogram in left bundle branch block (LBBB), there is frequently no primary R wave in lead Z and almost always, an absence of a Q wave in the anterolateral lead X. Right ventricular depolarization is virtually complete before the excitation waves later spread unopposed round both anterior and posterior walls of the left ventricle to meet at the lateral wall [31].

From a vectorcardiographic point of view, the initial QRS forces are therefore directed posteriorly and to the left. Commonly, the maximum QRS vector is also similarly directed posteriorly to the left and inferiorly. The vectorcardio-graphic appearances of LBBB are as shown in ❷ Fig. 11.44. These are quite distinctive with generally a long narrow QRS

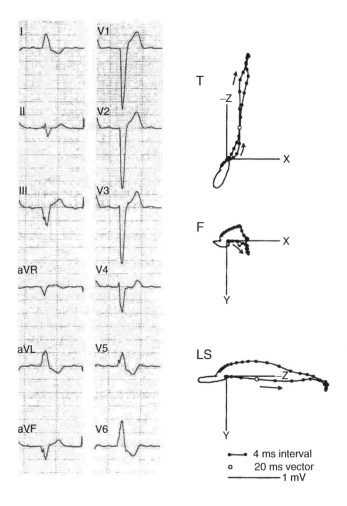

❏ Fig. 11.44
An example of left bundle branch block (LBBB). Note the closely spaced time-markers and the narrowness of the QRS loop particularly in the transverse plane. Also, it should be noted that the maximum QRS and T vectors are oppositely directed

⬛ Table 11.7

Vectorcardiographic criteria for left bundle branch block (LBBB)

A maximum QRS vector directed oppositely to the T vector
An elongated or occasionally figure-of-eight loop in the transverse plane with minimal breadth
The main body of the loop is usually inscribed in a clockwise direction in the transverse plane
The timing markers are much closer together than in the normal vectorcardiographic loop

loop in the transverse plane with the T loop being oppositely directed. This corresponds to T wave inversion in lead X. It does also suggest that ventricular repolarization takes place in a sequence parallel to that of depolarization in view of the abnormally slow spread of the ventricular activation wave fronts. The characteristic vectorcardiographic features of LBBB are shown in ❷ Table 11.7.

11.5.2.2   Incomplete Left Bundle Branch Block

The concept of incomplete LBBB is perhaps more difficult to explain. It has been suggested that the progression of excitation via the left bundle branch is slower than normal although there is not a complete block. Initial septal activation will, therefore, be on the right side of the septum. From the vectorcardiographic point of view, the QRS loop is again elongated and narrow as in complete LBBB but the overall QRS duration is of the order of 120–140 ms. The remaining markers may also be a little closer than normal. An illustration is given in ❷ Fig. 11.45.

Often this pattern is associated with a slightly increased voltage and T wave abnormalities in the lateral leads, that is, a T vector loop almost oppositely directed to the QRS loop. This has given rise to the expression "incomplete LBBB/LVH pattern." It is possible that patients with hypertensive heart disease, for example, and LVH, exhibit fibrosis, which progresses to the extent that the conduction system becomes impaired resulting in the above described abnormalities.

11.5.2.3   Right Bundle Branch Block

In complete right bundle branch block (RBBB), there is a block in the conduction system in the right bundle branch below its junction with the bundle of His. Thus, left ventricular activation commences normally so that RBBB always manifests itself as an abnormality in the terminal part of the QRS complex. This allows other abnormalities such as myocardial infarction to be reported with reasonable confidence in the presence of RBBB.

Because of the normal left ventricular activation, appearances in RBBB show normal initial depolarization. After the greater part of the left ventricle has been depolarized, the delayed excitation wave has spread to the free wall of the right ventricle so that there is an electrically unopposed (but delayed) right ventricular depolarization. This action results in the terminal portion of the QRS complex exhibiting electrical forces oriented to the right, anteriorly. In addition, the QRS duration is abnormally prolonged beyond 120 ms. In the scalar presentation of lead Z there is a broad R′ wave.

The vectorcardiographic loop is shown in ❷ Fig. 11.46. It can be seen that the terminal portion of the QRS loop shows a marked slowing of the rate of inscription as evidenced by the closeness of the timing markers. The terminal loop is directed anteriorly, rightward, with quite characteristic features being demonstrated. The major part of the loop is inscribed in a counterclockwise direction.

11.5.2.4   Incomplete Right Bundle Branch Block

There can often be dispute as to whether on a scalar presentation there is, indeed, incomplete RBBB evidenced by the secondary r′ wave in V_1, V_2, or lead Z. It has been suggested that this late QRS activity is due to hypertrophy of the basal

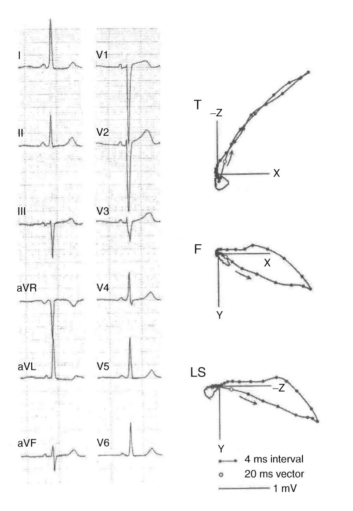

⊡ Fig. 11.45

An example of incomplete LBBB where the QRS loop in the transverse plane is extremely narrow. The time-markers are also more closely spaced than normal

portion of the right ventricle although, as it is often seen in younger individuals, it could indeed on occasions be considered a normal variant.

From the vectorcardiographic point of view, an incomplete RBBB is manifested as some slowing in the terminal inscription of the QRS loop seen best in the transverse plane. This portion of the loop will also be oriented anteriorly, rightward. In this situation, the presentation of a vectorcardiogram has an advantage over the scalar presentation in that terminal slowing can be seen.

It could be argued, since the normal QRS duration ranges from 60 to 110 ms, that an incomplete bundle branch block occurring in a patient who previously had a QRS duration of the order of 80 ms could well result in a relative prolongation of the QRS duration to 110 ms. Therefore, it should not be essential for conduction defects involving the right bundle branch in particular to be dependent on criteria which provide discrete time thresholds such as 110 ms for incomplete RBBB. On the other hand, it is unlikely in the adult that a QRS duration <90 ms would be consistent with even an incomplete RBBB. An illustration of the vectorcardiogram in incomplete RBBB is given in

❯ Fig. 11.47.

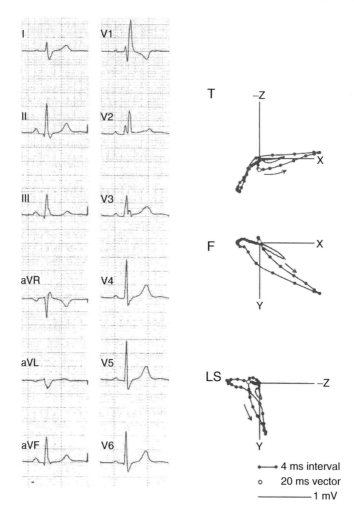

● **Fig. 11.46**

An example of right bundle branch block (RBBB) where the late QRS vectors are directed anteriorly to the right with very closely spaced time-markers in the loops corresponding to the slowed conduction. Note the terminal slowing of inscription of the QRS loop

11.5.3 Fascicular Block

In 1966, Pryor and Blount [32] suggested that the pure left axis deviation might be due to a block in the superior division of the left bundle. They termed this abnormality the "Left Superior Intraventricular Block." They also suggested that right axis deviation could be caused by a block in the inferior division of the left bundle. It was surmised that the direction of the initial excitation depended on the nature of the lesion that produced the block, for example, fibrosis or necrosis. Subsequently, Rosenbaum [33] set out criteria for conduction defects arising from different parts of the conducting system. He postulated that localized abnormalities may occur in isolation, intermittently or in association with defects in other branches of the specialized conducting system. He also introduced the term "hemiblock" to replace "superior" and "inferior" intraventricular block but since there are often more than two specialized conducting fascicles in the left ventricle, the term is perhaps a misnomer. For this reason, it has been suggested [34] that the term "fascicular block" be used. This terminology will be used in the present discussion.

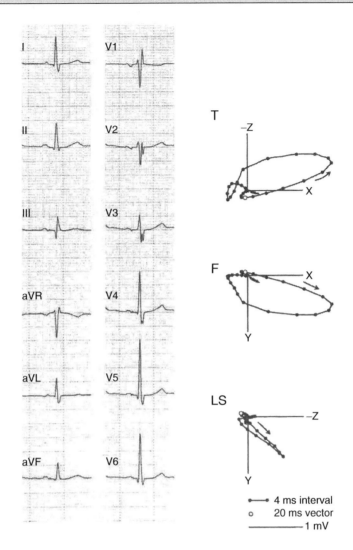

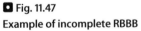

Fig. 11.47
Example of incomplete RBBB

11.5.3.1 Left Anterior Fascicular Block

In left anterior fascicular block, it is postulated that a block of the conduction of excitation arises in the anterior fascicle of the left bundle branch. In this case, ventricular depolarization probably takes place via the other intact fascicles. Excitation initially spreads inferiorly from the left posterior fascicle and it is feasible that there may also be some septal activation from another left-sided conducting fascicle such as the centroseptal fascicle. The net result is an initial, inferiorly directed and sometimes rightward spread of activation. Thereafter, the leftward upward spread of activation from the region of the left posterior fascicle becomes dominant, causing the ventricular resultant electrical force to be orientated posteriorly and superiorly producing a prominent S wave in lead Y.

The frontal plane vectorcardiographic loop shows left axis deviation in most cases, that is, the projection of the maximum QRS vector is superior to $0°$ and always has counterclockwise inscription [35]. This enables left anterior fascicular block to be differentiated from other forms of conduction abnormality such as due to inferior myocardial infarction.

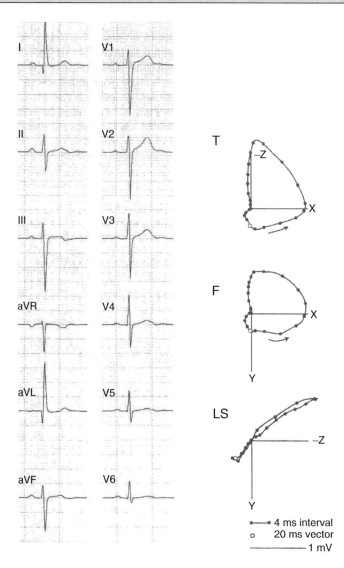

Fig. 11.48

An example of left anterior fascicular block with counterclockwise inscription of the QRS loop in the frontal plane

Table 11.8

Vectorcardiographic criteria for left anterior fascicular block

Initial QRS vectors directed inferiorly and rightward
Counterclockwise inscription in the frontal plane
QRS axis in the frontal plane superior to −30°

Figure 11.48 gives an example of left anterior fascicular block while Fig. 11.38 shows how inferior myocardial infarction can be separated from left anterior fascicular block by the fact that there is clockwise inscription in the frontal plane in the former. Lopes [36] has proposed that the vectorcardiographic criteria for left anterior fascicular block should include, those listed in Table 11.8.

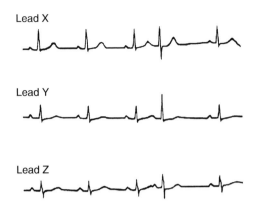

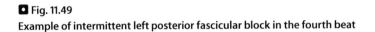

◘ Fig. 11.49

Example of intermittent left posterior fascicular block in the fourth beat

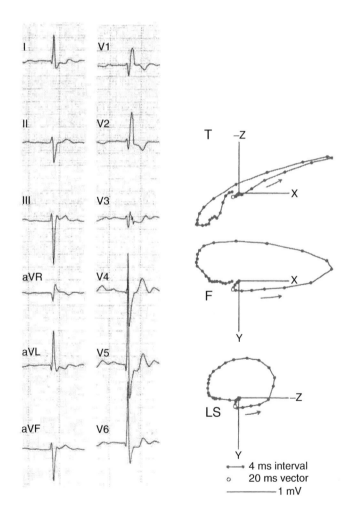

◘ Fig. 11.50

Example of RBBB + left anterior fascicular block

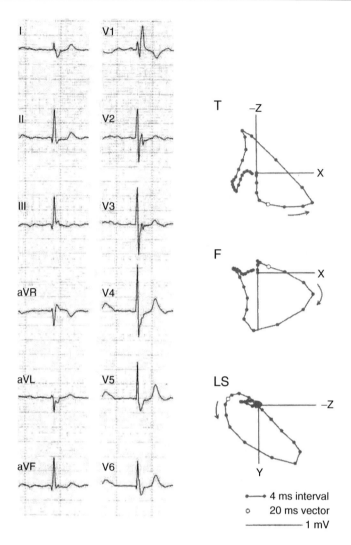

4 ms interval
○   20 ms vector
────── 1 mV

▣ Fig. 11.51

An example of RBBB plus left posterior fascicular block. Note that the QRS vector in the frontal plane exceeds 75° in this 39-year-old male

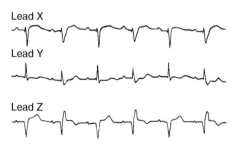

Lead X

Lead Y

Lead Z

▣ Fig. 11.52

Example of alternans where every second beat shows RBBB plus left posterior fascicular block

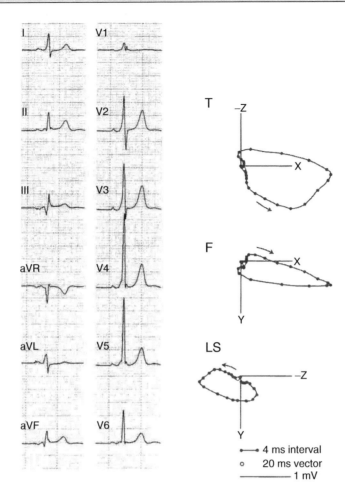

■ Fig. 11.53

An example of Wolff–Parkinson–White (WPW) Type A with initial slowing of the inscription of the QRS loop and early QRS vectors directed anteriorly

He also suggested that if the major axis of the QRS loop is not directed superiorly, but the late part of the loop lies in the left superior quadrant, possible left anterior fascicular block may be diagnosed.

11.5.3.2 Left Posterior Fascicular Block

It is postulated that if there is a block in the posterior fascicle of the left bundle branch, ventricular activation will proceed from the anterior wall of the left ventricle, spreading inferiorly. Right ventricular, and possibly septal activation are normal. However, the posterior wall of the left ventricle will be depolarized somewhat later than usual so that the excitation waves spreading anteriorly and inferiorly assume an increased importance in the development of ECG appearances. The QRS axis, therefore, shifts to the right, producing appearances suggestive of RVH. Often these appearances are best seen in an intermittent conduction defect in a rhythm strip, for example (❷ Fig. 11.49). In this example, there is an atrial extrasystole that shows a change in QRS configuration compared to the dominant complex, namely, an increase in the amplitude of the R wave in the anteroseptal and inferior leads and a deepening of the S wave in the lateral lead. These appearances are in keeping with the concept of left posterior fascicular block, which, in this case, is intermittent, presumably being produced by a refractory left posterior fascicle at the time of the occurrence of the supraventricular extrasystole.

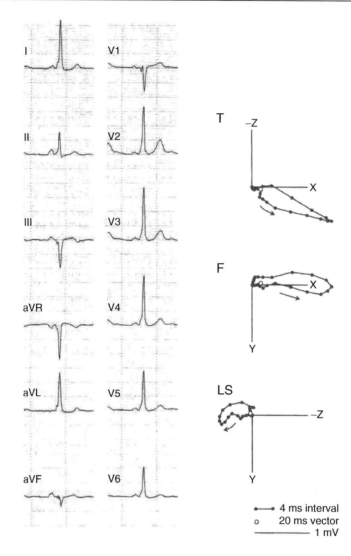

Fig. 11.54

An example of WPW Type B where there is initial slowing of the early QRS vectors that are directed leftward for the first 20 ms

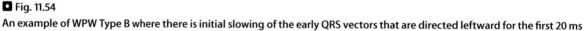

The differentiation of pure left posterior fascicular block from RVH can be difficult. The former is best diagnosed only if there is a lack of clinical evidence to support RVH. It should be clear from ❷ Fig. 11.49 that the diagnosis of pure left posterior fascicular block from a single cardiac cycle is virtually impossible.

11.5.4   Bifascicular Block

Combinations of conduction abnormalities in the right bundle branch and different fascicles of the left bundle branch lead to bifascicular block. An example of bifascicular block is RBBB in association with left anterior fascicular block (❷ Fig. 11.50). In this case, there is a marked superior displacement of the vectorcardiographic loop in the frontal plane while the terminal slowing of conduction is again apparent in the transverse plane where the terminal forces are directed anteriorly and to the right.

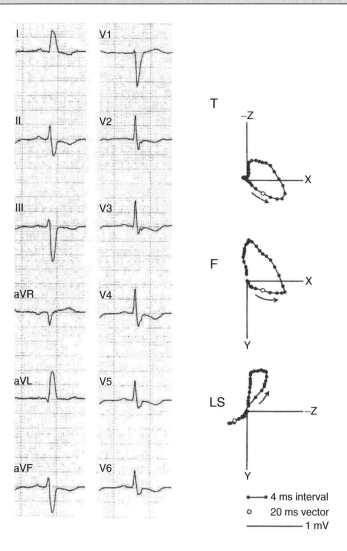

◆ Fig. 11.55

An intraventricular conduction defect exemplified by the closely spaced time-markers in all the QRS loops. The transverse loop is also open as opposed to being narrow in LBBB and does not have the late QRS vectors directed to the right as in RBBB

On the other hand, RBBB with a left posterior fascicular block may be suspected when there is right axis deviation with other typical features of RBBB (◆ Fig. 11.51). Again, the typical RBBB feature of terminal slowing of the QRS loop is apparent but the right axis deviation is abnormal. This feature can perhaps be seen more clearly in another rare example (◆ Fig. 11.52) where there is electrical alternans. The narrow QRS complex suggests myocardial infarction with possible left posterior fascicular block while the alternate beats indicate RBBB in addition.

11.5.5 Wolff–Parkinson–White Pattern

The classical features of the Wolff–Parkinson–White (WPW) [37] pattern are those of an initial slurring of the QRS complex due to the spread of activation from atria to ventricles via an accessory pathway. Note that these features describe the WPW pattern, which, if associated with episodes of paroxysmal tachycardia, gives rise to the WPW syndrome. From the vectorcardiographic point of view, the main distinguishing feature is obviously the slowing of inscription in the initial

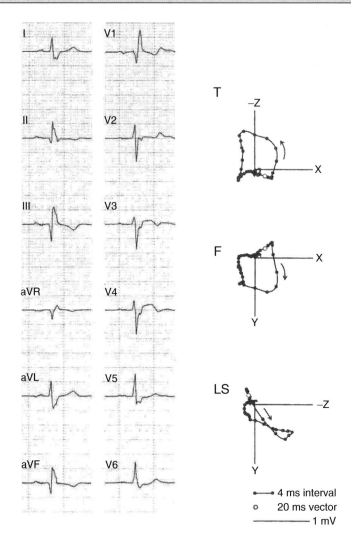

● **Fig. 11.56**

Example of RBBB and inferior myocardial infarction

part of the vectorcardiographic loop. This may facilitate the diagnosis of WPW pattern in borderline cases where the initial slurring in the scalar presentation may be questioned as being technical in origin. There is a variety of accessory pathways such that there is no typical feature of the WPW pattern on the vectorcardiogram other than the initial slowing of inscription. In other words, initial vectors may be orientated in a whole spectrum of different directions depending on the location of the accessory pathway.

In broad terms, using the older classification of Type A and Type B, the initial vector orientation will be anterior in Type A and posterior/to the left in Type B. ❷ Figures 11.53 and ❷ 11.54 give examples of the vectorcardiographic loops in the WPW pattern.

11.5.6   Intraventricular Conduction Defects

There remains a class of conduction defects that does not fit any of the categories mentioned so far. In general terms, the QRS duration is prolonged in excess of 120 ms but the features of RBBB or LBBB are not apparent. On occasions, such defects manifest themselves as an open loop in the transverse plane, which permits the diagnosis of intraventricular conduction defect as opposed to LBBB, for example, even when the QRS duration is the order of 140–160 ms (❯ Fig. 11.55). This is another area where the vectorcardiographic loop can be of considerable diagnostic value.

11.5.7 Combined Conduction Defects and Myocardial Infarction

The diagnosis of myocardial infarction in the presence of RBBB is relatively straightforward. Because RBBB affects the terminal portion of the QRS complex and classical criteria for myocardial infarction affect the initial portion of the QRS complex, it is possible for myocardial infarction to be reported in the presence of RBBB. ❯ Figure 11.56 shows an example of inferior myocardial infarction and RBBB.

On the other hand, there is still controversy over the diagnosis of myocardial infarction in the presence of LBBB. In 1982, Havelda et al. suggested that inferior myocardial infarction could be diagnosed with 100% specificity in the presence of LBBB when there were QS complexes in the inferior leads [38]. Others have subsequently suggested that anterior infarction can be diagnosed in the presence of LBBB when, for example, there is a reversed R wave progression from V_3 to V_5 or there are Q waves in the lateral leads. On the other hand, left anterior fascicular block may mask or mimic inferior infarction [39].

11.5.8 ECG Versus 12-Lead Vectorcardiogram in Conduction Defects

This chapter has shown how there are certain situations where the vectorcardiographic display can exhibit the presence of conduction defects that may be less obvious on the scalar ECG. In particular, the slowing of timing marks on the vectorcardiogram is invariably an illustration of a conduction defect, whether it is at the beginning of the QRS complex as in the WPW pattern or at the end as in RBBB. If the slowing is throughout the QRS, then most likely the diagnosis is LBBB. It has also been shown how left anterior fascicular block and inferior infarction can be separated by the direction of inscription of the frontal plane vectorcardiographic loop. All of these points lend further weight to the conclusion that the vectorcardiogram has an important role to play in the diagnosis of ventricular conduction defects.

References

1. Einthoven, W., G. Fahr, and A. de Waart, Über die Richtung und die manifeste Grosse der Potentialschwankungen im menschlichen Herzen und über den Einfluss der Herzlage auf die Form des Elektrokardiogramms. *Pflügers Arch.*, 1913;**150**: 175–315. (Translation: Hoff, H.E. and P. Sekelj, *Am. Heart J.*, 1957;**40**: 163–194.)
2. Grishman, A. and L. Scherlis, *Spatial Vectorcardiography*, Philadelphia, PA: Saunders, 1952.
3. Frank, E., An accurate, clinically practical system for spatial vectorcardiography. *Circulation*, 1956;**13**: 737–749.
4. Mann, H., A method for analyzing the electrocardiogram. *Arch. Int. Med.*, 1920;**25**: 283–294.
5. American Heart Association Committee on Electrocardiography (Pipberger, H.V., R.C. Arzbaecher, and A.S. Berson, et al.), Recommendations for standardization of leads and of specifications for instruments in electrocardiography and vectorcardiography. *Circulation*, 1975;**52**(Suppl.): 11–31.
6. Watts, M.P. and D.B. Shoat, Trends in electrocardiograph design. *J. Inst. Electron. Radio Eng.*, 1987;**57**: 140–150.
7. Macfarlane, P.W., B. Devine, S. Latif, S. McLaughlin, and M.P. Watts, Methodology of ECG interpretation in the Glasgow Program. *Meth. Inform. Med.*, 1990;**29**: 354–361.
8. Macfarlane, P.W., E.N. Coleman, B. Devine, et al., A new 12-lead pediatric ECG interpretation program. *J. Electrocardiol.*, 1990;**23**(Suppl.): 76–81.
9. Macfarlane, P.W., E.N. Coleman, E.O. Pomphrey, S. McLaughlin, and A. Houston, Normal limits of the high-fidelity pediatric ECG. *J. Electrocardiol.*, 1989;**22**(Suppl.): 162–168.
10. Lundh, B., On the normal scalar ECG. A new classification system considering age, sex and heart position. *Acta Med. Scand.*, 1984;691(Suppl.).
11. Chen, C.Y., B.N. Chiang, and P.W. Macfarlane, Normal limits of the electrocardiogram in a Chinese population. *J. Electrocardiol.*, 1989;**22**: 1–15.
12. Yang, T.F., C.Y. Chen, B.N. Chiang, and P.W. Macfarlane, Normal limits of derived vectorcardiogram in Chinese. *J. Electrocardiol.*, 1993;**26**: 97–106.
13. Downs, T.D., J. Liebman, R. Agusti, and H.C. Romberg, The statistical treatment of angular data in vectorcardiography, in

Proceedings of Long Island Jewish Hospital Symposium on Vectorcardiography, 1965, I. Hoffman and R.C. Traymore, Editors. Amsterdam: North Holland, 1966, pp. 272–278.

14. Yang, T.F. and P.W. Macfarlane, Comparison of the derived vectorcardiogram in apparently healthy Caucasians and Chinese. *Chest,* 1994;**106**: 1014–1020.

15. Draper, H.W., C.J. Peffer, F.W. Stallmann, D. Littmann, and H.V. Pipberger, The corrected orthogonal electrocardiogram and vectorcardiogram in 510 normal men (Frank lead system). *Circulation,* 1964;**30**: 853–864.

16. Nemati, M., J.T. Doyle, D. McCaughan, R.A. Dunn, and H.V. Pipberger, The orthogonal electrocardiogram in normal women. Implications of sex differences in diagnostic electrocardiography. *Am. Heart J.,* 1978;**95**: 12–21.

17. Namin, E.P., R.A. Arcilla, I.A. D'Cruz, and B.M. Gasul, Evaluation of the Frank vectorcardiogram in normal infants. *Am. J. Cardiol.,* 1964;**13**: 757.

18. Huwez, F.U., S.D. Pringle, and P.W. Macfarlane, A new classification of left ventricular geometry in patients with cardiac disease based on M-mode echocardiography. *Am. J. Cardiol.,* 1992;**70**: 681–688.

19. Kannel, W.B., Prevalence and natural history of electrocardiographic left ventricular hypertrophy. *Am. J. Med.,* 1983;**75**(Suppl. 3A): 4–11.

20. Macfarlane, P.W., British Regional Heart Study: The electrocardiogram and risk of myocardial infarction on follow-up. *J. Electrocardiol.,* 1987;**20**(Suppl.): 53–56.

21. Chou, T. and R.A. Helm, The pseudo P pulmonale. *Circulation,* 1965;**32**: 96–105.

22. Huwez, F.U., *Electrocardiography of the Left Ventricle in Coronary Artery Disease and Hypertrophy,* Ph.D. thesis. University of Glasgow, 1990.

23. Gottdiener, J.S., J.A. Gay, B.J. Maron, and R.D. Fletcher, Increased right ventricular wall thickness in left ventricular pressure overload: Echocardiographic determination of hypertrophic response of the 'non-stressed' ventricle. *J. Am. Coll. Cardiol.,* 1985;**6**: 550–555.

24. Brohet, C.R., Special value of the vectorcardiogram in pediatric cardiology. *J. Electrocardiol.,* 1990;**23**(Suppl.): 58–62.

25. American College of Cardiology, Tenth Bethesda conference report on optimal electrocardiology. *Am. J. Cardiol.,* 1978;**41**: 111–191.

26. Selvester, R.H. and M.E. Sanmarco, Infarct size in hi-gain hi-fidelity VCG's and serial ventriculograms in patients with proven coronary artery disease, in *Modern Electrocardiology,* Z Antoloczy, Editor. Amsterdam: Excerpta Medica, 1978, pp. 523–528.

27. Selvester, R.H., H.B. Rubin, J.A. Hamlin, and W.W. Pote, New quantitative vectorcardiographic criteria for the detection of unsuspected myocardial infarction in diabetics. *Am. Heart J.,* 1968;**75**: 335–348.

28. Edenbrandt, L., A. Ek, B. Lundh, and O. Pahlm, Vectorcardiographic bites. A method for detection and quantification applied on a normal material. *J. Electrocardiol.,* 1989;**22**: 325–331.

29. Macfarlane, P.W. and T.D.V. Lawrie, The normal electrocardiogram and vectorcardiogram, in *Comprehensive Electrocardiology,* Vol. 1, P.W. Macfarlane and T.D.V. Lawrie, Editors. Oxford: Pergamon Press, 1989, pp. 407–457.

30. Demoulin, J.C. and H.E. Kulbertus, Histopathological examination of the concept of left hemiblock. *Br. Heart J.,* 1972;**34**: 807–814.

31. van Dam, R.Th., Ventricular activation in human and canine bundle branch block, in *The Conduction System of the Heart,* H.J.J. Wellens, K.I. Lie, and M.J. Janse, Editors. Leiden: Stenfert Kroese, 1976, pp. 377–392.

32. Pryor, R. and S.G. Blount, The clinical significance of true left axis deviation. *Am. Heart J.,* 1966;**72**: 391–413.

33. Rosenbaum, B.M., The hemiblocks: Diagnostic criteria and clinical significance. *Mod. Concepts Cardiovasc. Dis.,* 1970;**39**: 141–146.

34. Pryor, R., Fascicular blocks and the bilateral bundle branch block syndrome. *Am. Heart J.,* 1972;**83**: 441.

35. Kulbertus, H.E., P. Collignon, and L. Humblet, Vectorcardiographic study of the QRS loop in patients with left anterior focal block. *Am. Heart J.,* 1970;**79**: 293–304.

36. Lopes, M.G., *Seminar in Vectorcardiography,* Stanford, CA: Stanford University Press, 1974.

37. Wolff, L., J. Parkinson, P.D. White, Bundle-branch block with short P–R interval in healthy young people prone to paroxysmal tachycardia. *Am. Heart J.,* 1930;**5**: 685–704.

38. Havelda, C.L.J., G.S. Sohi, N.C. Flowers, and L.G. Horan, The pathologic correlates of the electrocardiogram: Complete left bundle branch block. *Circulation,* 1982;**65**: 445–451.

39. Milliken, J.A., Isolated and complicated left anterior fascicular block: A review of suggested electrocardiographic criteria. *J. Electrocardiol.,* 1983;**16**: 199–211.

12 Magnetocardiography

Markku Mäkijärvi · Petri Korhonen · Raija Jurkko · Heikki Väänänen ·
Pentti Siltanen · Helena Hänninen

P. W. Macfarlane et al. (eds.), *Specialized Aspects of ECG*, DOI 10.1007/978-0-85729-880-5_12,

12.1 Introduction

Although magnetocardiography (MCG) was first introduced in the early 1960s, it mainly remained as an experimental method practiced by engineers in research laboratories until the 1990s [1]. Today, it has developed into one of the new technologies in cardiology employed by medical doctors in several clinical laboratories. MCG still poses technical challenges, such as the instrumentation based on the use of liquid helium and the need for magnetically shielded rooms (MSR), but the clinical application of the method has significantly benefited from the availability of modern multichannel instrumentation in hospitals at the patient's bedside. In addition, the signal-to-noise ratio in routine MCG recordings is comparable to the best of electrical measurements. MCG studies provide online results quickly, and many groups are collecting libraries of reference data. Profound efforts in the direction of standardization and data comparability are also on the way.

There are several applications in which MCG has already provided clinically useful results. For example, an MCG can diagnose and localize acute myocardial infarction, separate myocardial infarction patients with and without susceptibility to malignant ventricular arrhythmias, detect ventricular hypertrophy and rejection after heart transplantation, localize the site of ventricular preexcitation and many types of cardiac arrhythmia, and can also reveal fetal arrhythmias and conduction disturbances [2].

In addition, several other clinical applications of MCG have recently been studied: detection and risk stratification of cardiomyopathies (dilated, hypertrophic, arrhythmogenic, and diabetic), risk stratification after idiopathic ventricular fibrillation, detection and localization of myocardial viability, and the follow-up of fetal growth and neural integrity. Some studies have clearly indicated that MCG is very sensitive to the changes of repolarization, for example, after myocardial infarction or in a hereditary long-QT syndrome [3].

In this review, we briefly overview the development in instrumentation, measurement techniques, data analysis, and the clinical aspects of MCG during the last few years and present a perspective for the near future.

12.2 Sources of MCG

12.2.1 Origin of Measured Magnetic Field

The biomagnetic fields are generated by the same bioelectric activity that generates electric potentials as discussed in Vol. 1. The ion pumps on the cell membrane and the diffusion gradients impress the flow of the charged ions (such as Na^+, K^+, and Ca^{2+}) in the myocardium. These ionic currents inside and in the vicinity of excited cells are called primary current density J_p [4]. The primary current causes changes of the electric potential ϕ, which in turn creates ohmic volume currents $J_V = -\sigma \nabla \phi$, where σ is the electric conductivity. The magnetic field of total current $J_T = J_p + J_V$ can then be solved by Maxwell's equations or in quasistatic approximation from the Biot–Savart law $dB = \frac{\mu_0}{4\pi} \frac{dJ \times r}{r^3}$, where the dB is the magnetic field from the differential current dJ in relative position r. By integrating the overall current density, we obtain the magnetic field B. The resulting magnetic field from all the cardiac activity is in the range of pT, below one millionth of the earth's magnetic field (30–60 μT).

12.2.2 Forward Problem

The calculation of the external magnetic field from the known cardiac currents, the *forward problem*, has similar properties to those of the forward problem in ECG. Analytically, the forward problem in a homogeneous volume conductor can be solved with only some simple geometry. Therefore, numerical methods are used in the calculations. In the boundary-element method (BEM), an analytical equation is discretized to linear matrix equations [5, 6], which can be extended to the torso models. In the finite element model (FEM), the anisotropic properties of the material can also be included in the calculations. As with the electric forward problem, realistic torso models are needed for accurate results. However, the magnetic field is not as sensitive for material properties of the torso as the electric potential, so the requirement for the model is not quite as strict. Interestingly, preliminary results for estimating the heart outline based only on MCG mapping have also been presented [7].

12.2.3 Inverse Problem

The biomagnetic inverse problem is ill-posed and has no unique solution even if the body surface potential mapping is combined with magnetic measurements. Therefore, different equivalent source models have to be used. The equivalent current dipole (ECD) is the most elementary source of magnetic fields and can be defined as $q = \int_V J_p(r) dV$. Higher order equivalent generators, such as quadrupoles and octupoles, have also been presented by using multipole expansions [8]. Accuracies of 5–25 mm have been reported for best-fitting ECDs [9].

12.2.4 Inverse Problem with Distributed Source Model

To solve the inverse problem with a distributed source model like equivalent current density or uniform double-layer, a number of individual current dipoles are usually derived with the help of the lead field theory. The ill-posed problem of the lead field matrices requires the use of different regularization techniques for stabilizing the result. In addition to single-layer as well as double-layer sources, lead fields from each point on both the endocardial and epicardial surfaces, together with bidomain models for estimating the propagating wave front, are used [10, 11].

12.2.5 MCG vs ECG

Since the magnetocardiogram is generated by the same activity that generates the ECG, the signal waveforms corresponding to the P-, QRS-, and T-waves of the ECG are also seen in the magnetocardiogram. However, the differences in the information content between the MCG and ECG are still quite controversial; it can be shown that in an infinite and homogeneous volume conductor, J_V does not contribute to the magnetic field or electric potential which are independent of each other. In a homogeneous, semi-infinite volume conductor, all the magnetic field outside the conductor arises from the tangential current sources, while the ECG in general is more sensitive to the radial currents. In practice, due to torso inhomogeneities, conductivity differences, and anisotropy, the difference between the MCG and ECG is not that apparent. However, the sensitivity of MCG to the vortex currents seems also in practice to be remarkably different; an ideal vortex current does not produce any electric field outside the body [12]. The MCG has also been reported to be more sensitive to repolarization currents since it is not disturbed by electrode-skin potential, for example, distinguishing a real ST shift from an artifactual ST shift is possible [13]. As already discussed, the MCG is less affected by the torso inhomogeneities than the ECG, which is an advance, especially in inverse modeling. The measurement instrumentation where all the sensor localizations are always in the same relative positions to each other is also an advance, especially if the combination of measurement and torso coordinate systems is done correctly.

12.3 Measurement Technique and Instrumentation

12.3.1 History of MCG

The cardiac magnetic field was first measured by Baule and McFee [14] using a coil magnetometer. In 1970, D. Cohen et al. [15] introduced the superconducting quantum interference device (SQUID) for MCG, and 1 year after that, Zimmerman and Frederic [16] introduced a gradiometer that made MCG recording in an unshielded environment possible. In 1973 came the first modeling study [5]. Multichannel whole-thorax systems were introduced in the early 1990s, and high-Tc (high-temperature) superconductors appeared a few years later.

12.3.2 General

The DC-SQUID sensors offer the best sensitivity for MCG measurements. The strong environmental magnetic noise, unavoidable at urban hospitals and laboratories, makes the detection of biomagnetic signals impossible without special techniques for environmental interference suppression: The environmental magnetic noise is reduced by MSRs, which typically consist of a combination of μ-metal and eddy current shields. In addition, gradiometer coils are used to diminish residual magnetic noise within the shields. Alternatively, high-order gradiometers can be utilized if no magnetic shielding is employed.

12.3.3 Measurement System – Torso Position

The position of the subject's thorax with respect to the sensor array can be determined, for example, by using special marker coils attached to the skin. The positions of these coils are determined by a 3D digitizer before the measurement (in torso coordinates), and from the MCG recordings (in device coordinates) when electric current is fed to the coils. A typical measurement setup is seen in ❷ Fig. 12.1.

12.3.4 Low-Temperature and High-Temperature Sensors

The SQUID sensors are commonly classified as low-temperature SQUID sensors (LTS), which operate at the temperature of liquid helium or as high-temperature SQUID sensors (HTS) operating at liquid nitrogen temperatures. LTS are more commonly used. They are easier to manufacture and have less noise. On the other hand, cooling with liquid nitrogen is much less expensive than with liquid helium, and the cryogenic dewars for HTS are easier to manufacture.

12.3.5 Different Systems: Sensors

Most of the MCG systems have planar sensor loops, which detect the Z-component of the magnetic field, that is, the component directed toward the measurement system. Instead of measuring the magnitude of the magnetic field, the axial and planar field gradients are measured in some systems. Magnetometer sensors have the highest sensitivity for nearby and far-field sources. Thus, selecting a gradiometer with proper distance between the SQUID sensors reduces the amount of unwanted external noise components. The gradients are realized with wire-wound or bonded two or three gradiometers or by electronically combining several reference coils to one measurement coil. Therefore, it should be noted

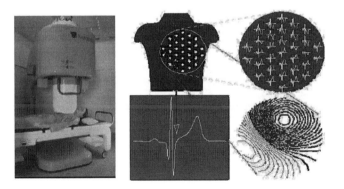

❏ Fig. 12.1

Left: MCG recording with 99-channel magnetocardiometer at 33- location (BioMag Laboratory, Helsinki, Finland). *Right*: The sensor arrangement in the cardiomagnetometer and an example of signal measured during 1 s and magnetic isofield integral map over atrial complex

that even one channel system may well contain nine SQUID sensors, and the 304-SQUID system may sample only at 57 sites. Hence, the measured number of channels does not necessarily tell everything about the effective dimension of the mapping. In some systems, gradients are also implemented with software from the separate magnetometer signals, and for multi-lead mappings also, many complex software noise cancellations are used (see below).

In addition to systems measuring only the Z-component of the field, there are also systems sensing only tangential fields or all three orthogonal vector component magnetometers. In quasistatic approximation ($\nabla \times B = 0$), it is directly seen that $\partial B_z / \partial x = \partial B_x / \partial z$, and so the tangential field gradients can be derived from the tangential gradients of the B_z.

12.3.6 Different Systems: Two Trends

Nowadays, the development of new MCG systems can be divided into two main trends: The "high-end," multichannel and high sensitivity systems mainly for research work and the "budget-priced" systems without MSRs for clinical use [17]. The lower cost systems bring MCG closer to the everyday clinical work. With efficient signal processing techniques, they can be used for single channel studies, but for mapping studies with these single or "quasi single" channel systems (seven or nine channel systems) several different measurements over certain sampling points are needed. Problems include the fact that scanning of the grid is very time-consuming, and the resulting measurement is not truly simultaneous although after averaging, signals should be time invariant. In high-end systems, more than 300 sensors are read simultaneously with a very high signal-to-noise ratio. ❷ Table 12.1 shows examples of different MCG systems with and without an MSR.

12.3.7 Different Systems: Need for Standardization

One of the problems with MCG studies is related to the number of systems with different sensor geometries, different sensor types, and different signal-to-noise ratios, which make multicenter studies difficult. In addition, the digital preprocessing of the measured signals varies. There are also problems with comparing the results obtained with different systems. Some standardization has been proposed several times including a proposal that was presented in the previous version of this book [1], but due to the huge variation of the systems in use, standardization has not been fully implemented.

❏ Table 12.1

Examples of different MCG systems

Name	Type	Number of channels	Dewar diameter (cm)
Siemens Krenikon	Shielded, multichannel	37 axial gradiometers	19
Philips	Shielded, multichannel	2*31 axial gradiometers	13.5 + 13.5
PTB Berlin	Shielded, multichannel	63 electronical gradiometers + 20 reference	21
4-D Neuroimaging (Bti) Magnes	Shielded, multichannel	61 magnetometers	32.4
(Neuromag) VectorView	Shielded, multichannel	33 magnetometers, 66 planar gradiometers	30
AtB Argos	Shielded, multichannel	Vector-magnetometers	23
Hitachi	Shielded, multichannel	64 planar gradiometers	20
Cardiomag Imaging	Unshielded	9 + second-order axial gradiometers + three vectorial reference channels	
SQUID AG	Unshielded	4 + second-order axial gradiometers + 3 reference	
Jena (FSU)	HTS, unshielded	Two planar gradiometers	
Hitachi	HTS, open-ended shielding	16	

12.4 Digital Signal Processing

12.4.1 Preprocessing

12.4.1.1 Mapping Versus Multi-Lead Analysis

All signal processing meant for improving the signal quality, removing noise, and artifacts is hereinafter called "preprocessing." The preprocessing part, just as in the actual signal analysis and the calculation of the different measures, is further divided into mapping and multichannel methods. Mapping includes methods that utilize the spatial information on measurement channels, as the multichannel methods process one channel at a time and utilize the temporal information.

12.4.1.2 Order of Signal Processing

First, noise suppression preprocessing, can be divided into different phases. Selected map analysis may utilize methods like signal-space projection (SSP), signal-space separation (SSS), independent component analysis (ICA), filtering, baseline removal, and perhaps averaging. Sometimes filtering can be undertaken before the map-operator. The data conversion is usually made on the corrected signal. Then after possible conversion, the measures (markers) are calculated.

12.4.1.3 Signal-Space Projection

There are several different methods for noise suppression: The signal-space projection (SSP) method is based on defining a noise subspace from an empty room measurement and projecting the measured multichannel signal to the signal space orthogonal to the noise subspace [18]. A similar principle is also utilized in the "eigenvector-based spatial filtering of fetal biomagnetic signals," for example [19], where the fetal signal is extracted on the basis of projecting the data to the space that maximizes the fetal and maternal eigenvector ratio.

12.4.1.4 Signal-Space Separation

Signal-space separation (SSS) is based on mathematical separation of the signal sources to the cardiac sources that are inside a predefined subspace in normal space (a ball around the heart) and outside sources. After separating sources, the signal consisting only of cardiac activity can be formed. This method can also be used together with signal conversion to the different measurement geometry or for interpolating the poor quality channels [20].

12.4.1.5 Independent Component Analysis

Independent component analysis (ICA) is a method for the blind separation of linearly mixed signals. The assumptions in the method are that the number of mixed signals is, at a maximum, the number of measured signals. Mixed signals are non-Gaussian and linearly mixed, which in practice means that their sources are spatially separable. The most commonly used algorithm was presented by Hyvärinen [21]. The actual ICA algorithm is only a part of the solution as the algorithm separates the signals blindly, which means that the wanted and the unwanted signal components have to be somehow selected. The algorithm also loses the amplitude scaling of the signal, which has to be corrected afterwards. An automatic use of ICA for separating the fetal signal from the maternal signal was presented by Comani et al. [22].

12.4.1.6   One-Channel Digital Noise Suppression

In addition to signal processing in the mapping methods described above, preprocessing methods for individual MCG channels are used. The algorithms are similar to those used with ECG channels, where signals are band-pass filtered with finite (FIR) and infinite response filters (IIR). The 50 or 60 Hz powerline interference is filtered with different adaptive notch filters. Wavelet transforms are also used [23]. Low-frequency noise, such as baseline wander, is corrected with polynomial fits to the isofield (isopotential in ECG) intervals and signals are averaged. In fetal MCG, the maternal signal average is also used for separating the fetal and maternal signals.

12.4.1.7   Conversion Between Sensor Arrays

A separate part of preprocessing is the conversion between sensor arrays. There are several different MCG systems. Sensor locations and types vary. However, since there are many different systems, the comparison of the results is difficult. For that reason, different signal conversions based on multipole and minimum normal estimates have been proposed [24, 25]. In one of these studies [24], where the conversion from measurements was done with one multichannel MCG system to another, the reconstruction succeeded with 93–95% agreement. However, the overall accepted standard system for conversion is still missing.

12.5   Signal Analysis

12.5.1   MCG Morphology Analysis

Signal processing of individual MCG channels resembles that of an ECG lead. Often only scaling constants in algorithms for waveform detection are different. Markers derived from the MCG signal morphology are also very similar to those from the ECG, namely signal amplitudes (e.g., ST level), filtered signal amplitudes (e.g., late field/potential analysis), time intervals (e.g., QT interval), spectral characteristics (e.g., fragmentation index), etc.

12.5.2   MCG Mapping Analysis

The MCG mapping markers include mapping orientations (min-max, +−, centers of gravity, and maximum field gradient) of different time instants or time intervals of the signal (QT orientation, T-wave orientation, and ST orientation) and different markers representing spatial heterogeneity (nondipolar content of QRS, STT, QRST, QT-dispersion). Also, different spatiotemporal measures (ST, T-wave orientation, and heart rate dependency) and different source modeling parameterizations have been used.

12.5.3   Visualizations

Typically, the MCG data is visualized either as temporal time traces, like an ECG trace, from one or all the measurement channels, or with different isovalue maps from one time instant or from some defined marker (e.g., integral) from each channel (see ❷ Fig. 12.1). In these maps, the signal amplitude is displayed with color coding or with isocontours.

Another commonly used way for displaying the mapping information is the current arrow map, where pseudo current at each measurement location, derived from $dB_Z/dyx + dB_Z/dxy$ (**x** and **y** being unit vectors) is represented by a vector showing the amplitude (length of the arrow) and direction of the current at that location (❷ Fig. 12.1). This current arrow map can also be projected onto a 3D model of the heart surface.

12.5.4 Experimental MCG

Experimental work utilizing MCG techniques began more than 30 years ago [26]. As a fully contactless method, MCG is ideal for noninvasive cardiac mapping of small experimental animals, for example.

MCG has also been used to detect reentry currents in cardiac flutter and fibrillation. The magnetic field produced by induced atrial flutter has been measured in isolated rabbit hearts. A moving dipole model was proposed to analyze the experimental data and to locate the reentry path [27].

In another newer study, acute myocardial infarction was induced by ligation of the left anterior descending coronary artery in a dog model. Magnetic field maps of early reperfused myocardium showed spatio-temporal field distributions consistent with anterior myocardial infarction. The use of super-paramagnetic contrast agents increased the sensitivity of standard MCG and may have an important implication for MCG in the assessment of regional myocardial ischemia, infarction, and perfusion [28].

A recent study was able to show that MCG mapping can detect age-related changes in cardiac intervals and in maps having significantly longer QTe, JTe, and T peak-Te intervals (Te = T end) in older Wistar rats. As compared to ECG recordings, MCG methodology simplified reproducible multisite noninvasive cardiac mapping of ventricular repolarization in an experimental setting [29].

12.6 Localization of Preexcitation and Cardiac Arrhythmias by Magnetocardiographic Mapping

The clinical accuracy of the MCG method has been tested by localizing the site of earliest ventricular activation during preexcitation in Wolff–Parkinson–White syndrome patients. The clinical reference has been obtained either during endocardial catheter mapping, or from successful catheter or surgical ablation of the accessory pathway. The results of the earlier studies showed that the MCG method was accurate enough for localization of cardiac electric sources for clinical purposes [30, 31]. The methodological localization accuracy of the MCG mapping has also been confirmed to be quite good [32].

In a newer study, 28 patients with Wolff–Parkinson–White syndrome were examined by MCG mapping and imaging techniques and with the five most recent accessory pathway localization ECG algorithms. ECD, effective magnetic dipole, and distributed-current imaging models were used for the inverse solution. MCG classification of preexcitation was found to be more accurate than that of ECG algorithms, and also provided additional information for the identification of paraseptal pathways and the existence of multiple accessory pathways [33].

By applying the completely noninvasive techniques of MCG and magnetic resonance imaging (MRI), it has been shown to be possible to define different origins of right ventricular ectopic beats in a complex heart model of nonischemic cardiomyopathy of 84 patients with surgically repaired Tetralogy of Fallot [34].

Postmyocardial infarction patients were investigated with cardiac MRI and signal-averaged 62-lead MCG. Three of six patients were suffering from sustained ventricular tachycardia (VT). A close matching of the low current density areas based on the QRS complexes and the high current density areas based on the late field signals were found. In three patients, the premature ventricular complexes morphologically resembling the clinical VT were localized close to the exit sites of these arrhythmias. The authors concluded that the MCG was useful in steering catheter ablation and coronary revascularization therapies [35].

An MCG was recorded pre- and post interventional therapy in three patients with atrial flutter and four patients with atrial fibrillation (AF), and in 20 healthy volunteers. The serial conduction pathway of the QRS segment was superimposed on a 3D heart outline generated by a magnetic field and verified by the silhouette on the magnetic resonance (MR) images. The MCG revealed a counterclockwise rotation of the atrial conduction in patients with atrial flutter, and random micro-reentry in the cases of AF [7]. An example of MCG localization in a patient suffering from continuous atrial tachycardia is presented in ❷ Fig. 12.2.

In conclusion, MCG has been used for localization of other sources of cardiac arrhythmias, such as the site of origin of tachycardias and extrasystoles, as well as for localization of a cardiac pacing catheter. The localization accuracies for a pacing catheter have been reported to be <1.0 cm, for extrasystoles 0.5–2.0 cm, and for tachycardias accuracy is more variable at 1.6–4.0 cm. In particular, the results in localizing a pacing catheter and the accessory pathway in preexcitation

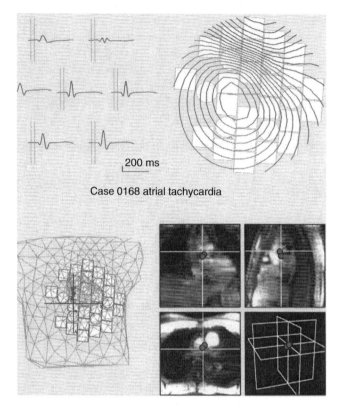

⬛ **Fig. 12.2**

An example of MCG localization in a patient suffering from incessant atrial tachycardia. The integration of the MCG and MRI results was performed using electromagnetically localized MR positive fish-oil capsules. Invasive electrophysiologic study and successful catheter ablation confirmed the localization of the tachycardia focus in the intra-atrial septum. *Upper left panel*: time interval during the P-wave used for analysis. *Upper right panel*: magnetic field morphology relative to the sensors. *Lower left panel*: location of the tachycardia (*red dots*) relative to torso and sensors. *Lower right panel*: MCG localization of the tachycardia focus (*blue dots*) integrated to MR images

confirm the good localization capability of the MCG method. The main obstacles in clinical cardiac source localization by MCG are the inherent problems concerning the clinical and imaging reference data integration.

12.7 Fetal Magnetocardiography

The fetal magnetocardiogram (FMCG) can be reliably recorded from approximately the 15th week of gestation onwards. The FMCG has the ability to accurately record cardiac time intervals, and to provide a real-time recording that reflects cardiac electrical activity. The FMCG has been demonstrated to be able to diagnose different types of atrioventricular conduction defects, paroxysmal supraventricular tachycardia, and repolarization abnormalities especially after 20 weeks of gestation. Standardization of the recording, signal processing, and measurement techniques has resulted in data that is reproducible, and when combined with normal values for different gestational ages, they can be of clinical value [36, 37].

In a study of 102 low-risk pregnant women, at the 20th to 42th gestational week, the fetal MCG provided a significant advantage via the technology available for recording the antenatal fetal heart. In the unaveraged recordings, the QRS complex was successfully detected in 68 cases (67%). Of those 68 traces, a P-wave was detected in 51 (77%) and a T-wave in 49 (72%) of the traces, using off-line signal-averaging techniques. Although good quality traces were obtained throughout the range of gestational ages, in general it was more difficult below 28 weeks. The QRS duration was found to increase significantly with increasing gestation [38]. In another study, various parameters concerning the electrical excitation of the heart, such as AV conduction, repolarization period, and morphology of the QRS complex, could be determined, leading to a more profound analysis of fetal arrhythmias [39].

Distinct patterns of initiation and termination of paroxysmal SVT have been detected using the MCG [40] as well such phenomena as Wolff–Parkinson–White syndrome, QRS aberrancy, and multiple reentrant pathways. A strong association between fetal trunk movement and the initiation and termination of SVT, suggesting autonomic influences, was also found.

The ability of the FMCG to reveal conduction system disease was evaluated in 702 fetuses initially referred on account of an arrhythmia. Altogether 306 had an irregular rhythm confirmed using either FMCG or postnatal 12-lead ECG. Eight (2.6%) had intermittent first- or second-degree AV block confirmed by FMCG and/or postnatal 12-lead ECG. Cases with conduction block may benefit from transplacental therapy with dexamethasone [41]. This method provides additional information concerning the effect of congenital heart disease (CHD) on the cardiac conduction system. As in the neonate, the FMCG changes do not reflect the severity of CHD. Indeed, the FMCG cannot serve as a primary diagnostic tool in the case of CHD for which echocardiography is more helpful.

Repolarization abnormalities in fetal heart can also be detected with the MCG during gestation. In one study, two patients were evaluated because of sustained fetal bradycardia, the diagnosis of QT-prolongation was made at the 29th and at the 35th gestational week. In both newborns, the QT-prolongation was confirmed by the postpartal ECG [42].

In general, good agreement of the magnetocardiograms and cardiac findings in newborns has been documented in a study investigating 189 fetal MCGs in 63 pregnant women between the 13th and the 42th week of pregnancy. In 16 recordings before the 20th gestational week, the signal strength was too weak to permit evaluation. Brief episodes of bradycardia, isolated supraventricular and ventricular premature beats, bigeminy and trigeminy, sinoatrial block, and atrioventricular conduction delays were found [43].

It has been suggested that the MCG can be used for noninvasive evaluation of hypertrophy of the fetal heart. In uncomplicated pregnancies, the magnitude of the MCG current dipole correlates with the gestational age, whereas in fetuses with cardiomegaly, the magnitude of the current dipole has been higher, reflecting the increased myocardial mass confirmed by ultrasound [44].

FMCG has shown that fetal P-wave and QRS complex durations increase with gestational age, reflecting a change in the cardiac muscle mass. A total of 230 FMCGs were obtained in 47 healthy fetuses between the 15th and 42nd week of gestation. The authors concluded that, from approximately the 18th week to term, fetal cardiac time intervals, which quantify depolarization times, can be reliably determined using MCG. The P-wave and QRS complex duration show a high dependence on age which to a large part reflects fetal growth. Gender instead, plays a role in QRS complex duration in the third trimester. ECD strength reflected gestational age slightly more reliably ($r^2 = 0.93$) than signal amplitude values (mean, median, maximum: $r^2 = 089, 0.88, 0.85$, respectively). The overall correlation of the amplitude to gestational age compared favorably with that of QRS complex duration. Fetal development is thus in part reflected in the fetal MCG and may be useful in the identification of intrauterine growth retardation [45, 46].

In conclusion, FMCG allows an insight into the electrophysiological aspects of the fetal heart, is accurate in the classification of fetal arrhythmias, and shows potential as a tool in defining a population at risk of congenital heart defects. FMCG offers unique capabilities for assessment of fetal heart rate (FHR) and fetal behavior, which are fundamental aspects of neurodevelopment. FMCG actograms are specific for fetal trunk movements, which are thought to be more important than isolated extremity movements and other small fetal movements. The ability to assess FHR, FHRV, and fetal trunk movement simultaneously makes fMCG a valuable tool for neurodevelopment research. In clinical reality, fMCG devices are still rare and a fetal arrhythmia or a congenital heart defect is in general discovered during prenatal evaluation by ultrasonography.

12.8 Arrhythmia Risk Assessment

MCG is sensitive to cardiac electrical activity of a very small amplitude and has therefore made it an interesting tool in the assessment of the risk of serious ventricular arrhythmias. The rapid development in instrumentation from single to multichannel devices capable of mapping large precordial areas has made clinical risk assessment studies possible.

In almost any structural heart disease, abnormalities in both depolarization and repolarization periods may lead to ventricular arrhythmias and sudden cardiac death. MCG studies considering ventricular arrhythmia risk assessment are still relatively few in number, with most of the data coming from postinfarction populations.

Postmortem studies in patients with postinfarction VT have revealed thin layers of surviving myocardial tissue, which might show mostly tangential currents and thus be detectable more readily by MCG than by ECG [47]. Late potentials in ECGs have been shown to be markers of delayed conduction serving as a substrate for reentrant ventricular arrhythmias. Late fields in MCG comparable to late potentials in ECGs have also been described [48]. Subsequently, late fields have shown a capability similar to that of late potentials in the discrimination of patients with and without ventricular arrhythmias after myocardial infarction [49, 50]. A few studies have applied magnetic source imaging in localization of the sources of late fields, which might be of value prior to catheter ablation or arrhythmia surgery [35].

In addition to late fields that may be detected at the end of the QRS, the abnormal delayed depolarization displays increased fragmentation of the whole magnetocardiographic QRS. The intra-QRS fragmentation method is based on finding the number of signal extrema during filtered QRS (❷ Fig. 12.3) and by computing the sum of the amplitude differences between neighboring extrema, thus yielding the intra-QRS fragmentation score (FRA) [51]. Recently, increased intra-QRS fragmentation in the MCG registered soon after acute MI has shown promise in the identification of patients at high risk of arrhythmic events in a prognostic study of 158 patients with acute MI and left ventricular ejection fraction (LVEF) < 50%. During follow-up of 50 +/− 15 months, 32 (20%) patients died and 18 (11%) had an arrhythmic event. Increased FRA in the MCG and LVEF < 30% yielded positive and negative predictive accuracies of 50 and 91% for arrhythmic events. The ECG predicted all-cause mortality (P < 0.05) but not arrhythmic events [52].

The dispersion of repolarization is increasingly recognized as a major factor in the genesis of malignant ventricular arrhythmias. Preliminary data from patients with hypertension and ischemic heart disease suggest that MCG might be especially sensitive to subtle changes in the repolarization period [53, 54]. Transmural repolarization in MCG, displayed as the terminal part of the T-wave, has been the subject of arrhythmia risk assessment studies in patients with ischemic

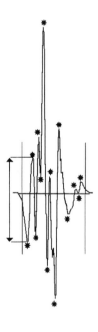

❐ Fig. 12.3

The principle of the intra-QRS fragmentation score analysis in MCG. After binomial filtering, the number of polarity changes or extrema () is computed. Next, the differences of each adjacent extrema are computed, and the differences are summed. As an example, the difference between the first and second extrema is shown with a thin arrow. Finally, the difference between the first and the last extrema is added to this sum, yielding the intra-QRS fragmentation score. The horizontal bars indicate the onset and offset of the filtered QRS

heart disease and dilated cardiomyopathy. Patients with sustained ventricular arrhythmias showed prolonged T-wave peak to T-wave end interval as a sign of dispersion of transmural repolarization [55, 56]. In another study, nondipolar isointegral maps during the repolarization phase in postinfarction patients prone to ventricular arrhythmias were found [57]. It was suggested that the non-dipolarity might serve as a marker of increased repolarization heterogeneity.

Repolarization disparities related to idiopathic long-QT syndrome also seem to be detectable with MCG. Children with long-QT syndrome, both with and without symptoms were investigated [58]. All patients showed beat-to-beat variability in T-wave morphology. When the isofield maps during the T-wave were analyzed with eigenvectors for data reduction, the symptomatic patients displayed more disparity in their maps, suggesting more heterogeneous repolarization.

Modern multichannel devices seem to allow quick MCG registrations in the hospital environment thereby rendering it a potential tool in arrhythmia risk assessment. However, a few issues need more elucidation before the role of MCG in clinical decision making can be fully assessed. First, is there really essential information in MCG not available from the ECG? In order to evaluate this, we need risk assessment studies comparing MCG not to 12-lead ECGs but to signal-averaged ECGs (SAECGs) and body surface potential mapping equally covering large precordial areas. In addition, the MCG methodology needs to be subjected to well-designed large-scale prospective studies. Until this has been done, the role of the MCG in the assessment of the risk of ventricular arrhythmias and sudden cardiac death remains to be established.

12.8.1 AF

AF is the most prevalent clinically important rhythm disturbance. The initiating and perpetuating factors of AF may vary, and prolonged AF may lead to atrial electrical and mechanical remodeling [59–61]. The effective application of new treatments for AF calls for improved diagnostics and has also led to growing interest in noninvasive methods capable of detecting and characterizing abnormalities in atrial signals.

Subtle abnormalities in atrial electric and magnetic signals could serve as markers of foci or substrates for AF. The SAECG detects abnormalities in atrial signals in patients prone to AF. These include prolongation of atrial depolarization, abnormal frequency content, and increased spatial dispersion of atrial signal duration [62–64]. Recently, magnetocardiographic techniques have also been applied to the investigation of atrial electrophysiology and pathogenesis in AF.

12.8.1.1 Magnetocardiographic P-Wave in Patients with AF, Analyses of Non-Filter Signal and Application of High-Pass Filtering Techniques

Specific changes of the P-wave in MCG were found in a study in a total of 35 subjects, including 15 AF patients (50–70 years) with persistent AF converted to sinus rhythm and 20 healthy young men. The multichannel MCG over the anterior and posterior chest and 12-lead ECG were recorded simultaneously. Sum channels from all MCG channels and separately sums from anterior and posterior channels as well as ECG channels were created. The P-wave duration was manually measured in each sum channel. Also the homogeneity and fragmentation of MCG maps were evaluated. The P-wave was divided into four segments and the correlation between maps was calculated. All segments were compared with the first segment, and the average of these three correlations, the p-score, was used as the homogeneity factor. The fragmentation index of the P-wave was calculated as the sum of amplitude differences between two amplitude peaks multiplied by the total number of amplitude peaks in each sum channel. By MCG, the P-wave duration was longer and both correlation factor and fragmentation index were lower in patients compared to normals. Similar differences were not seen in the ECG. Differences were clearest in the sum channel of all MCG channels, for example, P-wave duration was 133 ms on average in patients versus 100 ms in controls [65].

High-pass filtering techniques have also been applied to the analysis of the atrial MCG signal. Multichannel MCG over the anterior chest and orthogonal three-lead ECGs were recorded in nine patients who had paroxysmal lone AF and in ten healthy subjects in duplicate at least 1 week apart. Data were averaged using an atrial wave template and high-pass filtered at 25, 40, and 60 Hz. Atrial signal duration with automatic detection of onset and offset and root mean square amplitudes

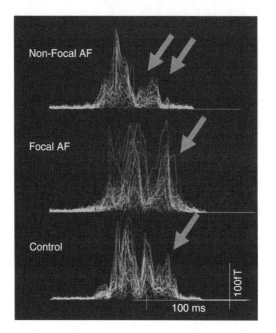

■ Fig. 12.4

Examples of typical 40 Hz high-pass filtered atrial complex in a patient with non-focal AF, in a patient with focal AF and in a healthy subject. In the patients with focal AF, the atrial signal strength was normal also during late phase of atrial complex where the left atrium is depolarized, but in a patients not defined focal triggers late phase amplitudes were reduced. Data is expressed as superimposed display of 33 magnetometer channels

(RMS) of the last portion of the atrial signal were determined. Reproducibility was best using a 40 Hz filter, somewhat better in MCG than in ECG and similar in patients and controls. For example, the difference between two measurements of atrial signal duration was 3.5 ms on average (coefficient of variation 3.3%) by MCG and 6.9 ms (coefficient of variation 6.1%) by ECG [66].

The atrial signal durations in MCG and SAECG were correlated, with $r = 0.64$ ($p < 0.01$). In addition, there was a correlation between RMS amplitudes of the first portion of the atrial complex in the MCG and the SAECG ($r = 0.49$, $p < 0.01$) but not in the last atrial portion ($r = 0.25$–0.30, $p = $ NS).

In this small population comprising patients with lone paroxysmal AF, the atrial wave duration was not longer but RMS amplitudes of the last 40 ms of the atrial complex were lower in patients.

Lately, the methods have been applied in a study of 81 patients with paroxysmal lone AF and 81 matched controls. In this study, the atrial depolarization complex was slightly prolonged in patients, namely, 109 ms on average versus 106 ms. The late RMS amplitudes were reduced in a subgroup of patients with non-focal AF but were otherwise normal (❷ Fig. 12.4). The findings are consistent with invasive measurements in focally triggered AF patients, in which only a minority of patients have shown conduction delay between or within the atria, or reduction in left atrial amplitude [67–69].

12.8.1.2   Spatial MCG Maps, Field Polarity, and Orientation during Atrial Activation and Application of Surface Gradient Methods

In another study, spatial MCG maps of 26 WPW patients were investigated [30]. Patients with AF attacks were found to have more dispersed atrial depolarization distributions compared to patients without AF. Altogether, 11/20 (55%) of the patients with AF problems were found to have more than two extrema in the atrial depolarization maps. On the other hand, 4/6 (67%) patients without AF had bipolar MCG maps. In an earlier study, multipolar MCG fields during the late phase of atrial activation have related to left atrial overloading [70]. In a study comprising patients with lone paroxysmal AF, for example, with normal left atria, multipolarity in MCG maps (integral maps over last 20 and 50 ms) was related to lone AF [71].

Magnetic field patterns can be visualized and parameterized using pseudo-current (90 degrees rotated field gradient) amplitude and direction distributions. This method is applied in some ongoing studies focused on evaluating atrial signal propagation during sinus rhythm in patients with focally triggered paroxysmal AF and in healthy subjects [71, 72]. In a study comprising 28 patients with focally triggered paroxysmal AF and 23 controls, the magnetic field orientation during the early part of atrial depolarization was mainly to the left and downward, and was similar in patients and controls. On the other hand, during the late phase of depolarization, field orientation was more variable in both groups and differed between groups as illustrated in ❷ Fig. 12.5. The degree of maximum gradient rotation over the atrial wave was larger, and the upward orientation was more common in patients. Results showed diversity and inhomogeneity in the propagation of atrial signals especially at the late phase of activation when the left atrium was depolarizing. Findings were more pronounced in patients but some seemed to occur also in healthy atria. It was concluded that the altered depolarization front may represent a conduction defect in the left atrium, and that this may be a normal variant facilitating the manifestation of AF in the presence of focal triggers.

In another study, MCG field patterns derived by the pseudo-current method were compared to invasive electro-anatomic activation maps (EAM) obtained from patients undergoing catheter ablation treatment with prior AF. The orientation of the magnetic fields during the first 30 ms of atrial depolarization representing RA activation, and during early (40-70 ms from P onset) and later part (last 50%) of LA depolarization was determined. The mean of the angles of the top 30% of the strongest pseudocurrents was used, zero angle direction pointing from subject's right to left and positive clockwise. Breakthrough of electrical activation to LA occurred through Bachmann bundle (BB) in 14, margin of fossa ovalis (FO) in 3, coronary sinus ostial region (CS) in 2, and their combinations in 10 cases by invasive reference in total of 29 different P-waves. The pseudocurrent direction in MCG maps over the first 30 ms of atrial complex was mostly leftward down, with a mean angle of 43° (CSD 28°). Over the time interval of 40–70 ms from the onset of the atrial complex, the mean angle was 39° (CSD 30°). Over the time interval of last 50% of atrial complex, the mean angle was 3° (CSD 51°).

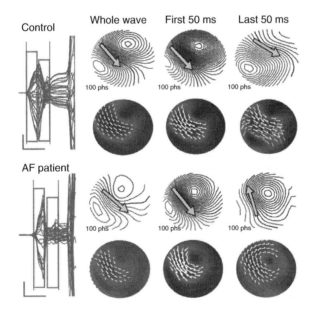

❑ Fig. 12.5

An example of orientation of magnetic fields during atrial depolarization from one healthy control (*upper rows*) and one patient with focally triggered lone AF (*lower rows*) performed as isofield integral maps (*rows 1 and 3*) and as pseudo-current maps (*rows 2 and 4*)

In the applied time interval the MCG pseudo-current angle corresponded the direction of propagation in EAM. When both the early and late LA MCG maps were viewed together, three types of combinations emerged: Type 1 with both maps showing pseudocurrent orientation leftward down, Type 2 with the map over the 40–70 ms orienting leftward down and the map over last 50% of atrial signal orienting leftward up, and Type 3 with both maps orienting leftward up. The three MCG atrial wave types correctly identified the LA breakthrough sites to BB, CS, FO, or their combinations in 27 of 29 (93%) cases [73].

Later on the method was applied in a population comprising 107 patients with lone paroxysmal AF (age 45 ± 12 years) and 94 controls. The Pd was longer in AF patients than in controls (112 ± 13 vs. 104 ± 13; p < 0.001), which was most obvious in Type 1 wave (109 ± 12 vs. 102 ± 11 ms, p = 0.003). The distribution of the atrial wave types differed between AF patients and controls: Type 1 occurred in 67% and Type 2 in 20% of controls whereas Type 1 occurred in 54% and Type 2 in 42% of AF patients, p < 0.01 for difference. Accordingly susceptibility to paroxysmal lone AF is associated with propagation of atrial signal to LA via margin of fossa ovalis or multiple pathways. When conduction occurs via Bachmann bundle, it is related with prolonged atrial activation. Thus altered and alternative conduction pathways may contribute to pathogenesis of lone AF [74].

12.8.1.3   Analyses of Atrial Signals during AF

The adaptation of QRS subtraction techniques and time frequency analysis has revealed the diagnosis of partial atrial standstill in an adult [75] and diagnosis of atrial flutter and AF in fetuses [76]. Now there are also ongoing studies designed to test the diagnostic performance of MCG mapping to separate clinical subgroups of AF, such as focal AF, by analyzing the atrial signal and its time domain as well as its spatial distribution during AF.

In conclusion, the effective application of new treatments for AF calls for improved diagnostics and has also led to a growing interest in noninvasive methods capable of detecting and characterizing abnormalities in atrial signals. The first applications of magnetocardiographic techniques to investigate atrial electrophysiology and pathogenesis in AF have presented extra dipoles in magnetic field maps during the last portion of the atrial depolarization signal in WPW patients with paroxysmal AF and in lone paroxysmal AF. Other abnormal features are altered field orientation during the late phase of atrial activation particularly in focally triggered lone AF, and reduced atrial signal amplitudes in AF patients without demonstrable focal triggers. In patients with persistent AF converted to sinus rhythm, prolongation and increased fragmentation of the atrial signal have been detected. Overall, abnormalities seem to be more pronounced in the late phase of the atrial complex corresponding to the depolarization of the left atrium. The diversity and inhomogeneity of propagation throughout the atrial signal seem to vary in different AF cohorts.

Currently, the patient series are still small, and further investigation is warranted before the real value of MCG in the clinical assessment of AF can be evaluated. However, MCG mapping techniques seem to be capable of noninvasively detecting abnormalities in the atrial activation sequences common in AF, even when the standard ECG is normal. It also seems that the MCG method may be applied to the study of pathophysiologic processes in AF and may identify subsets of patients with different underlying mechanisms for AF. Improved diagnostics could guide the selection of new treatment modalities, for example, catheter ablation or pharmacological treatment of AF.

12.9   Myocardial Ischemia and viability

One of the most interesting areas in clinical MCG is the detection and characterization of myocardial ischemia and viability. So far, few studies have been reported in this field, but the results are very encouraging. A new and accurate noninvasive method for recognition of acute and chronic ischemia could have important clinical applications, especially because therapeutic interventions for rapid and effective revascularization, such as percutaneous coronary interventions, are widely available.

It has been stated that some changes of the ST-segment could be explained by the ability of the MCG to detect DC currents, thus being more sensitive to ST changes than ECG or body surface mapping [53, 77–79]. In addition, the results of the equivalent dipole calculation during cardiac depolarization and repolarization has enabled the separation of patients with coronary artery disease from healthy controls [80].

The magnetic field orientation at rest has been proposed to separate coronary artery disease patients from healthy controls, with more prominent changes in the field orientation in severe disease. The magnetic field orientation is the angle between the line joining the field extrema and the right-left line of the torso [81]. In some studies, a semiautomatic surface gradient method helped to define the magnetic field orientation as the orientation of the maximum spatial field gradient, and this has been shown to separate both single-vessel and triple-vessel coronary artery disease patients from healthy controls during exercise-induced ischemia [82, 83]. Later, a method for heart rate adjustment of the magnetic field orientation during the recovery phase of exercise stress testing, which further improved ischemia detection, was developed [84].

The ST-segment depression and ST-segment slope, used in 12-lead ECG as ischemia parameters, can also detect ischemia in MCG. The ischemia-induced ST-depression takes place over the lower middle anterior thorax, and the reciprocal ST-elevation over the left anterior shoulder, locations orthogonal to those found in body surface potential mapping. The most prominent T-wave changes were found in patients with inferior ischemia and in patients with a history of myocardial infarction (❯ Fig. 12.6) [83, 85]. The ratio of the ST-T and QRS isointegral maxima has been reported to be reduced in coronary artery disease patients compared to healthy controls [86].

A few smaller studies have been designed to test the diagnostic performance of MCG mapping in detecting and localizing areas of hibernating myocardium. The viability of the myocardium has been first confirmed by a full set of other diagnostic tests: exercise ECG, thallium stress test, dobutamine MRI, and positron emission tomography (PET). Preliminary results look promising, but there are still some problems concerning the modeling of chronic ischemia. Both the MCG and the ECG showed a significant elevation or depression of the ST-segment during exercise-induced ischemia when they were investigated using a nonmagnetic bicycle ergometer in a MSR. The injury currents were in most cases directed from the ischemic area to the nonischemic area. For example, anterior ischemia caused an injury current directed from the apex to the base of the heart. The injury currents induced by transient ischemia and infarction of the same anatomical region were found to flow in the opposite direction. This change of direction was reflected as either ST-depression or ST-elevation in morphological signals. The anatomical location of the injury currents was in topographical agreement with the results of the reference methods (coronary angiography and myocardial scintigraphy) [87].

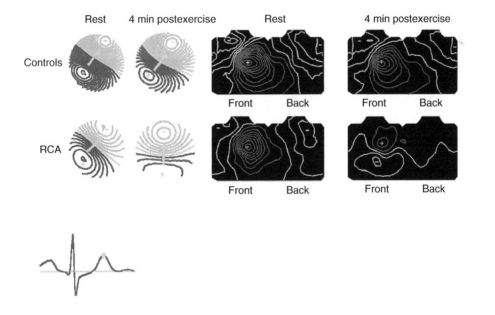

❏ Fig. 12.6

Exercise MCG in a coronary artery disease patient with a significant stenosis of the right coronary artery (*RCA*). The patient had the most extensive map rotation of the T-wave 4 min postexercise. Compared to the control group, the map rotation was more extensive ($45 \pm 39°$ vs $9 \pm 8°$, $p < 0.005$). Sensitivity for RCA was 75% at the specificity of 82% (Hänninen et al. 2000)

Corresponding to the absence of electrically active myocardial tissue, reduced current magnitudes were observed for the regions of infarcted myocardium (less than $1 \, \mu A/mm^2$) in a series of 40 subjects, including normals and patients with a history of myocardial infarction. The current density distributions correlated well with other cardiological investigations (e.g., left ventricle catheterization, scintigraphy, echocardiography) [88]. Ischemia localization was attempted in a small study of four patients with single-vessel coronary artery disease with no previous myocardial infarction. Current density estimation (CDE) was focused on in the ischemic regions confirmed by positron emission tomography in all four patients and injury currents were restricted to the region of the stenosed coronary artery [89]. A recent large clinical study included 417 subjects: 177 patients with angiographically documented CAD (stenoses $\geq 50\%$), 123 symptomatic patients without hemodynamically relevant stenosis, and 117 healthy subjects [90]. Contrary to the ECG, unshielded MCG revealed significant differences between normals and symptomatic patients with and without relevant stenoses using current density reconstruction during repolarization at rest. The discrimination between normals and CAD patients was achieved with a sensitivity of 73.3%, and specificity of 70.1%. In another series of 50 patients with CAD ($62 +/- 10$ years; EF = $76 +/- 11\%$; registration: before, 24 h, and 1 month ($n = 25$) after PCI) and 57 normals ($51 +/- 9$ years), current density vector (CDV) maps were reconstructed within the ST-T interval and classified from category 0 (normal) to category 4 (grossly abnormal) [91]. Twenty-four hours after PCI, more maps were classified as category 2 ($P < 0.05$) and less as category 4 ($P < 0.005$). One month after PCI, the MCG results further improved: more maps were classified as category 1 ($P < 0.05$) and 2 ($P < 0.005$) and fewer maps as category 4 ($P < 0.0001$). The ECG remained unchanged in the course of PCI.

A few clinically interesting studies on acute myocardial ischemia in the emergency room setting have been published. A 6-min resting MCG scan has been shown to have sensitivity, specificity, positive and negative predictive values of 76.4, 74.3, 70.0, and 80.0%, respectively, for the detection of ischemia ($p < 0.0001$) in 125 patients with presumed ischemic chest pain [92]. In another new series of 264 acute chest pain patients without ST-elevation, T vector changes in the MCG were found to have a specificity and positive predictive value > 90% for angiographically confirmed diagnosis of significant coronary artery disease. It is noteworthy that 25% patients had to be excluded from the study for poor signal quality [93].

In conclusion, magnetocardiographic mapping seems to be an accurate method for ischemia and viability detection. Moreover, it is able to localize ischemic regions in the heart in a comparable fashion to other methods. Recent larger clinical series stress the potential of this noninvasive method for current clinical decision making. However, it is the task of future large-scale clinical studies to establish a clear mandate for the MCG method in every day patient work.

12.10   Discussion

The clinical application of any method means that it has to contribute at least in one of the following fields of clinical medicine: diagnosis, therapy, or prognosis. In particular, noninvasive methods improving the accuracy of diagnosis of a cardiac disease are valuable. However, most important new methods are able to deliver current palliative or curative therapy, either by improving the results of existing therapies or by providing new modes of therapy. Methods helping to assess better the prognosis of certain heart diseases in individual patients are also desired.

MCG has many advantages, and it may become a clinically accepted method. First of all, it is totally noninvasive. It is not necessary to attach electrodes or other sensors requiring direct contact to the patient to record an MCG. Currently operating multichannel magnetometers are feasible to use and enable fast MCG recordings. A full measurement can be carried out in few minutes. Such advantages of MCG recordings also mean high patient comfort. In addition, multiple temporal and spatial parameters can be extracted from a single heartbeat for complete electromagnetic characterization of the function of the patient's heart. The spatiotemporal resolution of MCG mapping is much higher than that of conventional ECG methods. Moreover, the MCG methods still have unexplored potential for extracting new physiological and pathophysiological information about the electrical activation in the myocardium.

However, the MCG has some disadvantages. The equipment is currently expensive, and requires the use of liquid helium and an MSR. Such technical demands so far exclude the wider applicability of MCG as a quick bedside test and during catheter interventions. The development of new supra-conducting materials, operating in higher temperatures achieved using liquid nitrogen, has not yet been able to solve this problem. Low-cost multichannel devices operating in an unshielded environment have recently been introduced with promising clinical results. This way of development might be one of the ways to bring this method closer to clinicians. One profound obstacle still remains: MCG systems are generally sensitive to moving magnetic objects, which excludes some patients from the studies.

12.11 Conclusions

From all magnetocardiographic studies published so far, it can be concluded that the diagnostic performance of the MCG is superior in several applications when compared to the conventional ECG or even body surface mapping. However, this advantage has not yet encouraged clinicians to widely accept and utilize the method, mostly because of the high cost, low availability, and lack of standardization. Nevertheless, clinical applications of MCG in the fields of therapy and prognosis are currently of growing interest. The localization of arrhythmias and the detection of arrhythmia risk are already established therapy-related applications. Non-pharmacologic antiarrhythmic and antirejection medical therapies guided by MCG have been proposed, but such suggestions need more comprehensive studies. The detection and localization of acute and chronic ischemia and assessment of myocardial viability would be applicable to a large number of cardiac patients, if the MCG method proves to be successful in larger patient series. Studies on the prognostic value of MCG after myocardial infarction, in long-QT syndrome, congenital heart disease, and cardiomyopathy, may offer new applications, taking into account the promising results of recent studies on the prophylactic use of implantable defibrillators in high-risk patient groups. The increasing availability of high-performance multichannel MCG systems in the clinical environment will strongly contribute to these efforts.

References

1. Siltanen, P.P., Magnetography, in *Comprehensive Eletrocardiology, Theory and Practice in Health and Disease*, vol. 2, M.W. Lawrie and T.D. Veitch, Editors. New York: Pergamon, 1989, pp. 1405–1438.

2. Stroink, G., W. Moshage, and S. Achenbach, Cardiomagnetism, in *Magnetism in* Medicine, W. Andrä and H. Nowak, Editors. Berlin: Wiley, 1998, pp. 136–189.

3. Mäkijärvi, M., K. Brockmeier, and U. Leder, et al.,, New trends in clinical magnetocardiography, in C. Aine*Biomag96: Proceedings of the 10th International Conference on Biomagnetism*, C. Aine, et al., Editors. New York: Springer, 2000, pp. 410–417.

4. Trip, J.H., Physical concepts and mathematical models, in *Biomagnetism: An Interdisciplinary Approach*, S.J. Williamson, Editor. New York: Plenum, 1982, pp. 101–149.

5. Horacek, B. M., Digital model for studies in magnetocardiography. *IEEE Trans. Magn.*, 1973;**9**: 440–444.

6. Nenonen, J., C. Purcell, B.M. Horacek, G. Stroink, et al.,, Magnetocardiographic functional localization using a current dipole in a realistic torso. *IEEE Trans. Biomed. Eng.*, 1991;**38**: 658–664.

7. Nakai, K., K. Kawazoe, H. Izumoto, J. Tsuboi, Y. Oshima, T. Oka, K. Yoshioka, M. Shozushima, A. Suwabe, M. Itoh, K. Kobayashi, T. Shimizu, and M. Yoshizawa, Construction of a three-dimensional outline of the heart and conduction pathway by means of a 64-channel magnetocardiogram in patients with atrial flutter and fibrillation. *Int. J. Cardiovasc. Imag.*, 2005;**21**: 555–561; discussion 563–564.

8. Katila, T. and P. Karp, Magnetocardiography: morphology and multipole presentations, in *Biomagnetism, An Interdisciplinary Approach*, S.J. Williamson, G.L. Romani, L. Kaufmann, and I. Modena, Editors. New York: Plenum, 1983, pp. 237–263.

9. Nenonen, J., Magnetocardiography, in *SQUID Handbook*, Vol. 2, Sect. 9.3, J. Clarke, and A. Braginski, Editors. Berlin: Wiley, 2005.

10. van Oosterom, A., T.F. Oostendorp, G.J. Huiskamp, and M. ter Brake, The magnetocardiogram as derived from electrocardiographic data. *Circ. Res.*, 1990;**67**: 1503–1509.

11. Sepulveda, N.G., B.J. Roth, and J. Wikswo Jr., Current injection into a two-dimensional anistropic bidomain. *Biophysical. J.*, 1989;**55**: 987–999.

12. Liehr, M., J. Haueisen, M. Goernig, P. Seidel, J. Nenonen, and T. Katila, Vortex shaped current sources in a physical torso phantom. *Ann. Biomed. Eng.*, 2005;**33**: 240–247.

13. Cohen, D. and L.A. Kaufman, Magnetic determination of the relationship between the S-T segment shift and the injury current produced by coronary artery occlusion. *Circ. Res.*, 1975;**36**: 414–424.

14. Baule, G. and R. McFee, Detection of the Magnetic Field of the Heart. *Am. Heart. J.*, 1963;**66**: 95–96.

15. Cohen, D. and E. Edelsack, J. Zimmerman, Magnetocardiograms taken inside a shielded room with a superconducting point-contact magnetometer *Appl. Phys. Lett.*, 1970;**16**: 278–280.

16. Zimmerman, J.E. and N.V. Frederick, Miniature ultrasensitive superconducting magnetic gradiometer and its use in cardiography and other applications. *Appl. Phys. Lett.*, 1971;**19**: 16–19.

17. Koch, H., Recent advances in magnetocardiography. *J. Electrocardiol.*, 2004;**37**: 117–122.

18. Uusitalo, M.A. and R.J. Ilmoniemi, Signal-space projection method for separating MEG or EEG into components. *Med. Biol. Eng. Comput.*, 1997;**35**: 135–140.

19. Chen, M. and R.T. Wakai, and B. Van Veen, Eigenvector based spatial filtering of fetal biomagnetic signals. *J. Perinat. Med.*, 2001;**29**(6): 486–496.

20. Taulu, S., M. Kajola, and J. Simola, Suppression of interference and artifacts by the signal space separation method. *Brain Topogr.*, 2004;**16**: 269–275.

21. Hyvärinen, A., Fast and robust fixed-point algorithms for independent component analysis. *IEEE Trans. Neural Networks*, 1999;**10**(3): 626–634.

22. Comani, S., D. Mantini, G. Alleva, S. Di Luzio, G.L.F. Romani, et al., Magnetocardiographic mapping using independent component analysis. *Physiol. Meas.*, 2004;**25**: 1459–1472.

23. Sternickel, K., A. Effern, K. Lehnertz, T. Schreiber, et al., Nonlinear noise reduction using reference data. *Phys. Rev.*, 2001;**E63**: 036209.

24. Burghoff, M., J. Nenonen, L. Trahms, and T. Katila, Conversion of magnetocardiographic recordings between two

different multichannel SQUID devices. *IEEE Trans. Biomed. Eng.*, 2000;**47**: 869–875.

25. Numminen, J., S. Ahlfors, R. Ilmoniemi, J. Montonen, et al., Transformation of multichannel magnetocardiographic signals to standard grid form. *IEEE Trans. Biomed. Eng.*,1995;**42**: 72–78.

26. Cohen, D., Ferromagnetic contamination in the lungs and other organs of the human body. *Science*, 1973 May 18;**180**(87): 745–8.

27. Ribeiro, P.C., A.C. Bruno, P.L. Saboia e Silva, C.R. Barbosa, E.P. Ribeiro, E.C. Monteiro, and A.F. Costa, Detection of reentry currents in atrial flutter by magnetocardiography. *IEEE Trans. Biomed. Eng.*, 1999;**39**(8): 818–824.

28. Brazdeikis, A., C.W. Chu, P. Cherukuri, S. Litovsky, and M. Naghavi, Changes in magnetocardiogram patterns of infarcted-reperfused myocardium after injection of superparamagnetic contrast media. *Neurol. Clin. Neurophysiol.*, 2004;**30**: 16.

29. Brisinda, D., M.E. Caristo, and R. Fenici, Contactless magnetocardiographic mapping in anaesthetized Wistar rats: evidence of age-related changes of cardiac electrical activity. *Am. J. Physiol. Heart Circ. Physiol.*, 2005;Dec 22.

30. Mäkijärvi, M., J. Nenonen, L. Toivonen, J. Montonen, T. Katila, and P. Siltanen, Magnetocardiography: supraventricular arrhythmias and preexcitation syndromes. *Eur. Heart J.*, 1993;**14**(Suppl E): 46–52.

31. Moshage, W., S. Achenbach, K. Göhl, et al., Evaluation of the noninvasive localization accuracy of the cardiac arrhythmias attainable by multichannel magnetocardiography (MCG). *Int. J. Cardiac. Imag.*, 1996;**12**: 47–59.

32. Fenici, R., K. Pesola, P. Korhonen, M. Makijarvi, J. Nenonen, L. Toivonen, P. Fenici, and T. Katila, Magnetocardiographic pacemapping for nonfluoroscopic localization of intracardiac electrophysiology catheters. *PACE*, 1998,Nov;**21**(11 Pt 2): 2492–2499.

33. Fenici, R., D. Brisinda, J. Nenonen, and P. Fenici, Noninvasive study of ventricular preexcitation using multichannel magnetocardiography. *PACE*, 2003,Jan;**26**(1 Pt 2): 431–435.

34. Agren, P.L., H. Goranson, H. Jonsson, and L. Bergfeldt, Magnetocardiographic and magnetic resonance imaging for noninvasive localization of ventricular arrhythmia origin in a model of nonischemic cardiomyopathy. *PACE*, 2002,Feb;**25**(2): 161–166.

35. Leder, U., J. Haueisen, M. Pohl, R. Surber, J.P. Heyne, H. Nowak, H. R. Figulla, Localization of late potential sources in myocardial infarction. *Int. J. Cardiovasc. Imag.*, 2001,Aug;**17**(4): 315–325.

36. Grimm, B., J. Haueisen, M. Huotilainen, S. Lange, P. Van Leeuwen, T. Menendez, M. J. Peters, E. Schleussner, and U. Schneider, Recommended standards for fetal magnetocardiography. *PACE*, 2003 Nov;**26**(11): 2121–2126.

37. Stinstra, J., E. Golbach, P. van Leeuwen, S. Lange, T. Menendez, W. Moshage, E. Schleussner, C. Kaehler, H. Horigome, S. Shigemitsu, and M. J. Peters, Multicentre study of fetal cardiac time intervals using magnetocardiography. *BJOG*, 2002,Nov;**109**(11): 1235–1243.

38. Quinn, A., A. Weir, U. Shahani, et al., Antenatal fetal magnetocardiography: a new method for fetal surveillance? *Br. J. Obstet. Gynaecol.*, 1994;**101**: 866–870.

39. Menéndez, T., S. Achenbach, E. Beinder, et al., Usefulness of magnetocardiography for the investigation of fetal arrhythmias. *Am. J. Cardiol.*, 2001;**88**: 334–336.

40. Wakai, R. T., J. F. Strasburger, Z. Li, B. J. Deal, N. L. Gotteiner, Magnetocardiographic rhythm patterns at initiation and termination of fetal supraventricular tachycardia. *Circulation*, 2003 Jan 21;**107**(2): 307–12.

41. Cuneo, B.F., J.F. Strasburger, R.T. Wakai, and M. Ovadia, *Fetal Diagn. Ther.*, 2006;**21**(3): 307–313.

42. Menéndez, T., S. Achenbach, E. Beinder, et al., Prenatal diagnosis of QT prolongation by magnetocardiography. *PACE*, 2000;**23**: 1305–1307.

43. Van Leeuwen, P., B. Hailer, W. Bader, et al., Magnetocardiography in the diagnosis of fetal arrhythmia. *Br. J. Obstet. Gynaecol.*, 1999;**106**: 1200–1208.

44. Horigome, H., J. Shiono, S. Shigemitsu, et al., Detection of cardiac hypertrophy in the fetus by approximation of the current dipole using magnetocardiography. *Pediatr. Res.*, 2001;**50**: 242–245.

45. Van Leeuwen, P., S. Lange, A. Klein, D. Geue, and D.H. Gronemeyer, Dependency of magnetocardiographically determined fetal cardiac time intervals on gestational age, gender and postnatal biometrics in healthy pregnancies. *BMC Pregnancy Childbirth*, 2004,Apr 2;**4**(1): 6.

46. Van Leeuwen, P., Y. Beuvink, S. Lange, A. Klein, D. Geue, and D. Gronemeyer, Assessment of fetal growth on the basis of signal strength in fetal magnetocardiography. *Neurol. Clin. Neurophysiol.*, 2004, Nov 30;**47**(B).

47. Bolick, D.R., D.B. Hackel, K.A. Reimer, and R.E. Ideker, Quantitative analysis of myocardial infarct structure in patients with ventricular tachycardia. *Circulation*, 1986;**74**: 1266–1279.

48. Erne, S.N., R.R. Fenici, H.D. Hahlbom, W. Jaszczuk, H.P. Lehmann, and M. Masselli, High resolution magnetocardiographic recordings of the ST segment in patient with electrical late potentials. *Nuovo. Cimento.*, 1983;**2d**: 340–345.

49. Mäkijärvi, M., J. Montonen, L. Toivonen, P. Siltanen, M.S. Nieminen, M. Leiniö, and T. Katila, Identification of patients with ventricular tachycardia after myocardial infarction by high-resolution magnetocardography and electrocardiography. *J. Electrocardiol.*, 1993;**26**: 117–124.

50. Korhonen, P., J. Montonen, M. Mäkijärvi, T. Katila, M.S. Nieminen, and L. Toivonen, Late fields of the magnetocardiographic QRS complex as indicators of propensity to sustained ventricular tachycardia after myocardial infarction. *J. Cardiovasc. Electrophysiol.*, 2000;**11**: 413–420.

51. Müller, H.P., P. Gödde, K. Czerski, M. Oeff, R. Agrawal, P. Endt, W. Kruse, U. Steinhoff, and L. Trahms, Magnetocardiographic analysis of the two-dimensional distribution of intra-QRS fractionated activation. *Phys. Med. Biol.*, 1999;**44**: 105–120.

52. Korhonen, P., T. Husa, I. Tierala, H. Väänänen, M. Mäkijärvi, T. Katila, and L. Toivonen, Increased intra-QRS fragmentation in magnetocardiography as a predictor of arrhythmic events and mortality in patients with cardiac dysfunction after myocardial infarction. *J. Cardiovasc. Electrophysiol.*, 2006;**17**: 396–401.

53. Lant, J., G. Stroink, B. Ten Voorde, B. M. Horacek, and T. J. Montague, Complementary nature of electrocardiographic and magnetocardiographic data in patients with ischemic heart disease. *J. Electrocardiol.*, 1990;**23**: 315–322.

54. Nomura, M., K. Fujino, M. Katayama, A. Takeuchi, Y. Fukuda, M. Sumi, M. Murakami, Y. Nakaya, and H. Mori, Analysis of the T wave of the magnetocardiogram in patients with essential hypertensionby means of isomagnetic and vector array maps. *J. Electrocardiol.*, 1988;**21**: 174–182.

55. Oikarinen, L., M. Viitasalo, P. Korhonen, H. Väänänen, H. Hänninen, J. Montonen, M. Mäkijärvi, T. Katila, and L. Toivonen, Postmyocardial infarction patients susceptible to ventricular tachycardia show increased T wave dispersion independent

of delayed ventricular conduction. *J. Cardiovasc. Electrophysiol.*, 2001;**12**: 1115–1120.

56. Korhonen, P., H. Väänänen, M. Mäkijärvi, T. Katila, and L. Toivonen, Repolarization abnormalities detected by magnetocardiography in patients with dilated cardiomyopathy and ventricular arrhythmias. *J. Cardiovasc. Electrophysiol.*, 2001;**12**: 772–777.

57. Stroink, G., J. Lant, P. Elliot, P. Charlebois, and M.J. Gardner, Discrimination between myocardial infarct and ventricular tachycardia patients using magnetocardiographic trajectory plots and iso-integral maps. *J. Electrocardiol.*, 1992;**25**: 129–142.

58. Rovamo, L., M. Paavola, J. Montonen, M. Mäkijärvi, J. Nenonen, and T. Katila, Magnetocardioraphic repolarization maps in children with long QT syndrome, in *Biomagnetism: Fundamental Research and Clinical Applications*, C. Baumgartner, L. Deecke, G. Stroink, and S.J. Williamson, Editors. Amsterdam Oxford, Tokyo: IOS, 1995, pp. 615–618.

59. Haissaguerre, M., P. Jais, D. C. Shah, A. Takahashi, M. Hocini, G. Quiniou, S. Garrigue, A. Le Mouroux, P. Le Metayer, and J. Clementy, Spontaneous initiation of atrial fibrillation by ectopic beats originating in the pulmonary veins. *N. Engl. J. Med.*, 1998;**339**(10): 659–666.

60. Ausma, J., N. Litjens, M.H. Lenders, H. Duimel, F. Mast, L. Wouters, F. Ramaekers, M. Allessie, and M. Borgers, Time course of atrial fibrillation-induced cellular structural remodeling in atria of the goat. *J. Mol. Cell. Cardiol.*, 2001;**33**(12): 2083–2094.

61. Schotten, U., J. Ausma, C. Stellbrink, I. Sabatschus, M. Vogel, D. Frechen, F. Schoendube, P. Hanrath, and M.A. Allessie, Cellular mechanisms of depressed atrial contractility in patients with chronic atrial fibrillation. *Circulation*, 2001;**103**(5): 691–698.

62. Dilaveris, P.E., J.E. Gialafos, P-wave dispersion: a novel predictor of paroxysmal atrial fibrillation. *Ann. Noninvasive. Electrocardiol.*, 2001;**6**(2): 159–165.

63. Fukunami, M., T. Yamada, M. Ohmori, K. Kumagai, K. Umemoto, A. Sakai, N. Kondoh, T. Minamino, and N. Hoki, Detection of patients at risk for paroxysmal atrial fibrillation during sinus rhythm by P wave-triggered signal-averaged electrocardiogram. *Circulation*, 1991;**83**(1): 162–169.

64. Steinbigler, P. and R. Haberl B. Konig G. Steinbeck, P-wave signal averaging identifies patients prone to alcohol-induced paroxysmal atrial fibrillation. *Am J Cardiol*, 2003;**91**(4): 491–494.

65. Winklmaier, M., C. Pohle, S. Achenbach, M. Kaltenhauser, W. Moshage, and W.G. Daniel, P-wave analysis in MCG and ECG after conversion of atrial fibrillation. *Biomed. Tech. (Berl.)*, 1998;**43**(Suppl): 250–251.

66. Koskinen, R., M. Lehto, H. Vaananen, J. Rantonen, L.M. Voipio-Pulkki, M. Makijarvi, L. Lehtonen, J. Montonen, and L. Toivonen, Measurement and reproducibility of magnetocardiographic filtered atrial signal in patients with lone atrial fibrillation and in healthy subjects. *J. Electrocardiol.*, 2005;**38**(4): 330–336.

67. Hertervig, E., S. Yuan, S. Liu, O. Kongstad, J. Luo, S.B. Olsson, Electroanatomic mapping of transseptal conduction during coronary sinus pacing in patients with paroxysmal atrial fibrillation. *Scand. Cardiovasc. J.*, 2003;**37**(6): 340–343.

68. Markides, V. and R.J. Schilling, Atrial fibrillation: classification, pathophysiology, mechanisms and drug treatment. (Review) (5 refs) *Heart (British Cardiac. Soc.)*, 2003,Aug.; **89**(8): 939–943.

69. Verma, A., O.M. Wazni, N.F. Marrouche, D.O. Martin, F. Kilicaslan, S. Minor, R.A. Schweikert, W. Saliba, J. Cummings, J.D. Burkhardt, M. Bhargava, W.A. Belden, A. Abdul-Karim, and A. Natale, Pre-existent left atrial scarring in patients undergoing pulmonary vein antrum isolation: an independent predictor of procedural failure. *J. Am. Coll. Cardiol.*, 2005,Jan 18;**45**(2): 285–292.

70. Sumi, M., A. Takeuchi, M. Katayama, Y. Fukuda, M. Nomura, K. Fujino, M. Murakami, Y. Nakaya, H. Mori and P. Magnetocardiographic, Waves in normal subjects and patients with mitral stenosis. *Jpn. Heart J.*, 1986;**27**(5): 621–633.

71. Koskinen, R., H. Väänänen, V. Mäntynen, J. Montonen, J. Nenonen, L. Lehtonen, M. Mäkijärvi, and L. Toivonen, Field heterogeneity in magnetocardiographic atrial signals in patients with focally-triggered lone atrial fibrillation (abstract). *Heart Rhythm.*, 2004;**1**(1S): 226.

72. Kuusisto, J., R. Koskinen, V. Mäntynen, J. Nenonen, M. Mäkijärvi, J. Montonen, and L. Toivonen, Diversity in Activation of Healthy Atria by Magnetocardiographic Gradient Analysis (abstract), in *Proceedings of International Conference on Biomagnetism*, Boston, 2004: 407–408

73. Jurkko, R., V. Mäntynen, J. Tapanainen, J. Montonen, H. Väänänen, H. Parikka, L. Toivonen, Non-invasive detection of conduction pathways to left atrium using magnetocardiography: Validation by intracardiac electroanatomic mapping. *Europace* 2009;**11**: 169–177.

74. Jurkko, R., V. Mäntynen, M. Lehto, J.M. Tapanainen, J. Montonen, H. Parikka, L. Toivonen, Interatrial conduction in patients with paroxysmal atrial fibrillation and in healthy subjects. *Int. J. Cardiol.*, 2009, Jun 20.

75. Yamada, S., K. Tsukada, T. Miyashita, Y. Oyake, K. Kuga, I. Yamaguchi, Noninvasive diagnosis of partial atrial standstill using magnetocardiograms. *Circ. J.*, 2002;**66**(12): 1178–1180.

76. Kandori, A., T. Hosono, T. Kanagawa, S. Miyashita, Y. Chiba, M. Murakami, T. Miyashita, and K. Tsukada, Detection of atrial-flutter and atrial-fibrillation waveforms by fetal magnetocardiogram. *Med. Biol. Eng. Comput.*, 2002;**40**(2): 213–217.

77. Brockmeier, K., S. Comani, S. Erne, et al., Magnetocardiography and exercise testing. *J. Electrocardiol.*, 1994;**27**: 137–142.

78. Brockmeier, K., L. Schmitz, J.D. Bobadilla Chavez, et al., Magnetocardiography and 32-lead potential mapping: repolarization in normal subjects during pharmacologically induced stress. *J. Cardiovasc. Electrophysiol.*, 1997;**8**: 615–626.

79. Takala, P., H. Hänninen, J. Montonen, et al., Magnetocardiographic and electrocardiographic exercise mapping in healthy subjects. *Ann. Biomed. Eng.*, 2001;**46**: 975–982.

80. Van Leeuwen, P., B. Hailer, and M. Wehr, Changes in current dipole parameters in patients with coronary artery disease with and without myocardial infarction. *Biomed. Tech. (Berl.)*, 1997;**42**: 132–136.

81. Van Leeuwen, P., B. Hailer, S. Lange, et al., Spatial and temporal changes during the QT-interval in the magnetic field of patients with coronary artery disease. *Biomed. Tech. (Berl.)*, 1999;**44**: 139–142.

82. Hänninen, H., P. Takala, M. Mäkijärvi, et al., Detection of exercise induced myocardial ischemia by multichannel magnetocardiography in single vessel coronary artery disease. *Ann. Noninvas. Electrocardiol.*, 2000;**5**: 147–157.

83. Hänninen, H., P. Takala, P. Korhonen, et al., Features of ST segment and T-wave in exercise-induced myocardial ischemia evaluated with multichannel magnetocardiography. *Ann. Med.*, 2002;**34**: 1–10.

84. Takala, P., H. Hänninen, J. Montonen, et al., Heart rate adjustment of magnetic field map rotation in detection of myocardial

ischemia in exercise magnetocardiography. *Basic Res. Cardiol.*, 2002;**97**: 88–96.

85. Hänninen, H., P. Takala, M. Mäkijärvi, et al., Recording locations in multichannel magnetocardiography and body surface potential mapping sensitive for regional exercise-induced myocardial ischemia. *Basic Res. Cardiol.*, 2001;**96**: 405–414.

86. Tsukada, K., T. Miyashita, A. Kandori, et al., An iso-integral mapping technique using magnetocardiogram, and its possible use for diagnosis of ischemic heart disease. *Int. J. Card Imag.*, 2000;**16**: 55–66.

87. Seese, B., W. Moshage, S. Achenbach, et al., Magnetocardiographic (MCG) analysis of myocardial injury currents, in *Biomagnetism: Fundamental Research and Clinical Applications*, C. Baumgartner, et al., Editors. Amsterdam: Elsevier, 1995; 628–632.

88. Leder, U., H.P. Pohl, S. Michaelsen, et al., Non-invasive biomagnetic imaging in coronary artery disease based on individual current density. *Int. J. Cardiol.*, 1998;**64**: 83–92.

89. Pesola, K., H. Hänninen, K. Lauerma, J. Lötjönen, M. Mäkijärvi, J. Nenonen, P. Takala, L.M. Voipio-Pulkki, L. Toivonen, and T. Katila, Current densityestimation on the left ventricular epicardium: a potential method for ischemia localization. *Biomed. Tech. (Berl.)*, 1999b;**44**(suppl 2): 143–146.

90. Hailer, B., I. Chaikovsky, S. Auth-Eisernitz, H. Schafer, and P. Van Leeuwen, The value of magnetocardiography in patients with and without relevant stenoses of the coronary arteries using an unshielded system. *PACE*, 2005,Jan;**28**(1): 8–16.

91. Hailer, B., P. Van Leeuwen, I. Chaikovsky, S. Auth-Eisernitz, H. Schafer, and D. Gronemeyer, The value of magnetocardiography in the course of coronary intervention. *Ann. Noninvas. Electrocardiol.*, 2005,Apr;**10**(2): 188–196.

92. Tolstrup, K., B.E. Madsen, J.A. Ruiz, S.D. Greenwood, J. Camacho, R.J. Siegel, H.C. Gertzen, J.W. Park, and P.A. Smars, Non-invasive resting magnetocardiographic imaging for the rapid detection of ischemia in subjects presenting with chest pain. *Cardiology*, 2006;**106**(4): 270–276.

93. Park, J.W., P.M. Hill, N. Chung, P.G. Hugenholtz, and F. Jung, Magnetocardiography predicts coronary artery disease in patients with acute chest pain. *Ann. Noninvas. Electrocardiol.*, 2005,Jul;**10**(3): 312–323.

13 Polarcardiography

Gordon E. Dower

P. W. Macfarlane et al. (eds.), *Specialized Aspects of ECG*, DOI 10.1007/978-0-85729-880-5_13,
© Springer-Verlag London Limited 2012

13.1   Polarcardiography

Polarcardiography is a form of vectorcardiography. It provides a way of graphically representing the heart vector (❯ Chap. 7 of *Basic Electrocardiology: Cardiac Electrophysiology, ECG Systems and Mathematical Modeling*), but instead of doing so in the form of vectorcardiographic loops, which show only one beat and lack a time scale, the polarcardiograph separately plots the magnitude and direction of the heart vector against time. These are its polar coordinates, which are obtained from its rectangular, or *xyz*, coordinates by a simple mathematical transformation. Their use in electrocardiography goes back to Einthoven's manifest potential difference and electrical axis of the heart; that is, the magnitude and direction of the maximal heart vector in the frontal plane [1].

The choice of coordinate system can greatly affect the simplicity of certain mathematical problems. The rectangular coordinates of the heart vector are given directly by vectorcardiographic lead systems because of their simple relationship with potential differences on the body surface. The ideal vectorcardiographic lead system, however, would yield *xyz* signals as if they came from orthogonally placed surface electrodes on the body (assuming the body were a relatively large homogeneous sphere with the heart at its center). With this concept of the heart and body, it is natural to employ a spherical (polar) coordinate system. The most familiar application of such a system is to the terrestrial sphere. If altitude (radius) is ignored, only two coordinates, latitude and longitude, are required to fix a position on the earth's surface, whereas three rectangular coordinates would be needed.

It seemed intuitively obvious to Einthoven, and subsequently to several people [2], that polar coordinates, either in a plane or with respect to a sphere, should be helpful in studying the heart vector. For example, an increase in the peak magnitude of the heart vector, such as occurs in left ventricular hypertrophy (LVH), is an expected consequence of increase in the muscle mass of the left ventricle and is not affected by the orientation of the heart. In contrast, different orientations can produce various combinations of increased voltage in limb and precordial leads of the ECG, giving rise to a plethora of ECG voltage criteria.

Intriguing though the prospect was, the application of polarcardiography had to await the development of a device for continuously transforming rectangular into polar coordinates. The first clinically practical polarcardiograph was an analog computer completed in 1961 [3]. The polarcardiograms obtained from it provided the basis for developing diagnostic criteria covering a wide range of electrocardiographic conditions. It is important to appreciate that the transformation of coordinates does not increase information content, but it may display information in a manner that makes certain diagnostic features more obvious or discernible. Some polar criteria can be translated back into ECG or VCG criteria that had not previously been recognized, but others may be very difficult to discern in either of those displays.

The equipment now employed in computerized electrocardiography can execute the necessary transformations so that dedicated polarcardiographs are no longer needed; however, polar criteria and the polar approach play a useful role in the development of diagnostic programs. At the Woodward ECG computer system in the Vancouver General Hospital, polar coordinates form the basis of the measurement and analysis programs. These give the cardiologist information additional to that obtained from reading the ECG. However, the 12-lead ECG derived from the *xyz* signals (see ❯ Chap. 11 of *Basic Electrocardiology: Cardiac Electrophysiology, ECG Systems and Mathematical Modeling*) remains the primary graphic output of the system, with VCGs being generated when polar criteria for infarction are satisfied (see ❯ Fig. 13.18 and ❯ Table 13.3). Polarcardiograms can also be generated from any current or stored data, on request, although they are not used routinely for the following reasons:

(a) They are not really necessary, since the polar criteria have been satisfactorily programmed into the computer
(b) They are relatively voluminous, being written out at five times the paper speed of the conventional ECG and
(c) Most cardiologists are not familiar with them

However, polarcardiograms are used in problem cases, in research, and in the development of new criteria.

13.2   Spherical Coordinates Applied to the Body

❯ Figures 13.1 and ❯ 13.2 show how latitude and longitude are applied to the body to indicate the direction of the heart vector. The frontal plane of the body becomes the equatorial plane of the reference sphere. The angle in that plane α is the same as that used by Einthoven for the electrical axis of the heart. All points on a meridian of longitude have the same angle α. The angle of the heart vector with respect to the equatorial frontal plane (that is, anterior or posterior to it) is ψ. All points on a parallel of latitude have the same angle ψ.

Aitoff's equal-area projection (❷ Fig. 13.2) is a two-dimensional representation of the sphere that is useful in showing clustering of directions of corresponding heart vectors in groups of individuals (❷ Fig. 13.3). The orientation of the body in the Aitoff projection has been chosen so that the North–South axis corresponds to the posteroanterior (−z) axis of the transverse plane vector loop. Hence, anterior vectors are depicted downward in this form of Aitoff plot.

Elevation and azimuth are electrocardiographic synonyms for latitude and longitude, but they are less familiar terms to the general reader and have difficult dictionary definitions. Strictly, they are not appropriate because they define a direction with respect to an observer on the earth's surface. The celestial coordinates, declination, and right ascension would be conceptually more applicable, though not more so than latitude and longitude.

Although the position of a point on the surface of a sphere is defined by latitude and longitude, in order to fix that point in space, the radius of the sphere (R in ❷ Fig. 13.1) must also be specified. In polarcardiography, this third coordinate is known as magnitude, because it represents the magnitude of the heart vector.

13.3 Spatial Magnitude

For reasons of clarity, the magnitude coordinate will be discussed first. The spatial magnitude of the heart vector, when plotted against time, yields the M tracing. Magnitudes in the frontal, transverse, and sagittal planes (i.e., the distances from the origin in the corresponding VCG loops) are denoted by m_f, m_t, and m_s, respectively. The relationships between the magnitude tracings and their parent xyz signals are as follows:

$$M = \left(x^2 + y^2 + z^2\right)^{1/2}, M \geqslant 0$$

$$m_f = \left(x^2 + y^2\right)^{1/2}, m_f \geqslant 0$$

$$m_t = \left(x^2 + z^2\right)^{1/2}, m_t \geqslant 0$$

$$m_s = \left(y^2 + z^2\right)^{1/2}, m_s \geqslant 0$$

In the polarcardiographic examples in this chapter, the xyz signals have been derived from the Frank system (❷ Chap. 11 of *Basic Electrocardiology: Cardiac Electrophysiology, ECG Systems and Mathematical Modeling*).

At first sight, M tracings resemble ECGs and, so far as possible, they are similarly labeled. The P, QRS, and T events in the ECG have their counterparts in the M tracings (❷ Fig. 13.4). However, by definition, there cannot be Q or S waves because magnitudes are never negative. Although small initial peaks (e.g., ″r in ❷ Fig. 13.4) in the M tracing correspond approximately to the Q wave in the ECG, the degree of correspondence is variable and indefinite. It is useful, however, to retain the letters Q and S to denote the onset and offset points of the QRS complex. This is logical because it makes the time between the Q and S points equal to the QRS duration – a term desirable to retain, along with QRS complex and QT interval. Because of the multiplicity of peaks sometimes seen in QRS complexes in M tracings and the inapplicability of the terms Q wave and S wave, it is preferable not to refer to an R wave but rather to the individual R peaks in the manner shown in ❷ Fig. 13.4.

In left and right bundle branch block (LBBB and RBBB, respectively), the M tracing is very distinctive, the QRS complex being smooth in the former and notched in the latter (❷ Fig. 13.5). Nevertheless, angular data are included in the discrimination.

The M tracing is particularly valuable in determining QRS duration because of two useful properties. First, when the M tracing shows zero magnitude, all ECG leads must have zero signals, so problems relating to nonsimultaneity of the onset and offset of the QRS complex in various ECG leads (for example, an isoelectric Q wave) do not arise. Second, the M tracing returns, or almost returns, to the baseline to give a clear demarcation between QRS and ST events. (Exceptions to this are mentioned in ❷ Sect. 13.3.1.) The ECG does not give a good indication of this phenomenon and its QRS offset is often vague. The relative clarity of the Q and S points in the M tracing simplifies the programming of a computer to determine QRS duration [4]. This is a very important measurement in decision-tree logic leading to a diagnostic interpretation. Computer determinations of QRS durations based on the ECG show disappointing discrepancies from visual determinations. However, improving the agreement is difficult because visual determinations by different readers also

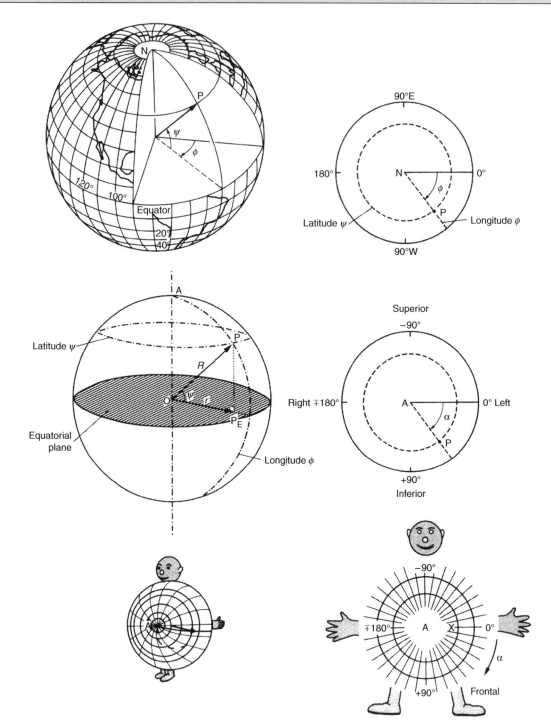

◘ Fig. 13.1

Definition of latitude and longitude. The vector from the center of the terrestrial sphere pierces the surface at P, the intersection of the meridian of longitude and the parallel of latitude. The angle Φ, between P meridian and reference (zero) meridian in the equatorial plane, is the longitude of P. The angle Ψ that the vector makes with respect to the equatorial plane is the latitude of P and is referred to as the posteroanterior (PA) latitude. Thus the latitude and longitude of P give spatial direction of the vector. The lower figures show spherical coordinates applied to the body: the North Pole becomes the anterior pole A, the equatorial plane becomes the frontal plane, and the angle Φ becomes α, following the tradition initiated by Einthoven

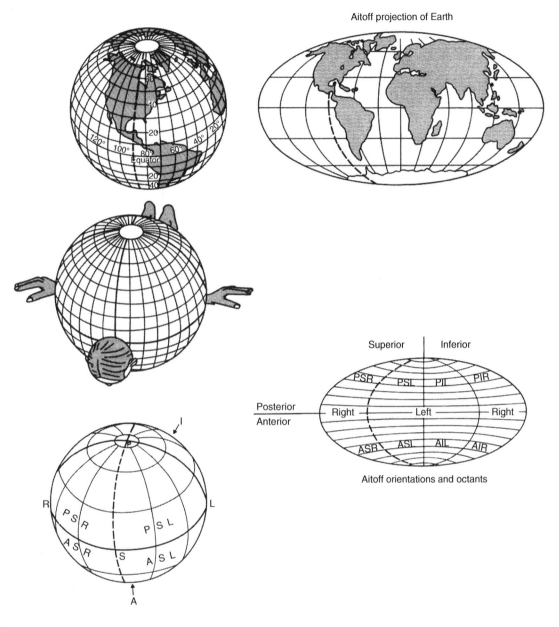

Aitoff projection of Earth

Aitoff orientations and octants

⬛ Fig. 13.2
The orientation of Aitoff equal-area projection for two-dimensional display of vector direction. The distribution of points on the sphere is uniform in this projection. *PSR* **posterior superior right,** *ASR* **anterior superior right,** *PSL* **posterior superior left,** *ASL* **anterior superior left,** *PIL* **posterior inferior left,** *AIL* **anterior inferior left,** *PIR* **posterior inferior right,** *AIR* **anterior inferior right**

vary a good deal. On the other hand, there is good agreement between computer and visual determinations of QRS duration using the spatial magnitude. The normal limits of QRS duration so determined are given in ❷ Tables 13.1 and ❷ 13.2 as diagnostic cut-off points used by the Woodward computers.

The ST segment is that part of the M tracing between S and T_i, the onset of the T wave. Sometimes, for example, in LBBB (❷ Fig. 13.5), the ST segment initially rises steeply for a short distance then abruptly changes its slope to a more gradual one, forming a knee. This knee is labeled J because of its resemblance to the J point in the ECG (❷ Fig. 13.4).

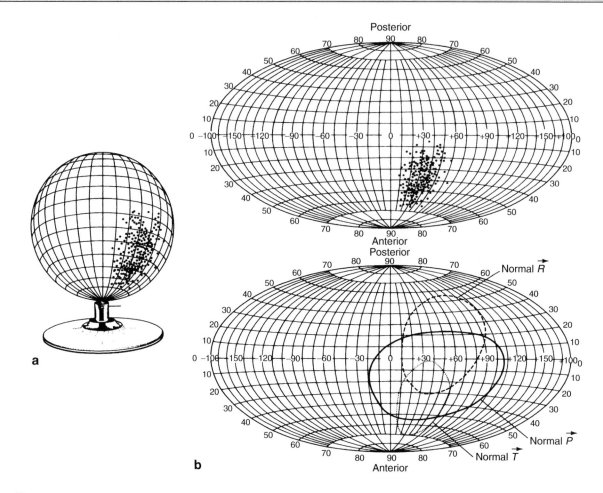

Fig. 13.3
Direction of *T* in 195 young adults. Clustering in the sphere (**a**) is equally well shown in the Aitoff projection (*top* part of **b**). Normal "continents" of $\vec{P}$, $\vec{R}$, and $\vec{T}$ directions are thus defined (*bottom* part of **b**)

Although, in the ECG, the J point is often used to mark the end of the QRS complex, the end of the QRS complex in the *M* tracing is defined as occurring at the S point because J is usually poorly defined.

M tracings reveal that there is not a clear-cut difference in identity between the ST segment and the T wave. However, it is useful to have some point in time that can be considered as representative of the ST segment so the ST point is taken as occurring midway between S and T, the peak of the T wave.

The points in the *M* tracing labeled P, R, ST, and T represent particular instants in time. A point U may often be identified also. These instants are not necessarily the same as those represented by similarly labeled points in the m_f, m_t, and m_s tracings. The vectors occurring at the points P, R, ST, and T in the *M* tracing are designated as $\vec{P}, \vec{R}, \vec{ST}$, and $\vec{T}$. The spatial magnitudes of these vectors are m_P, m_T, m_{ST}, and m_T: the heights of P, R, ST, and T above the baseline in the *M* tracing. By recording the *M*, m_f, m_t, and m_s tracings simultaneously, the magnitudes of these vectors in the frontal, transverse, and sagittal planes can be determined. These are designated as $m_f P$, $m_t P$, $m_s P$, and so on.

In vector loops, because of noise around the E point and lack of expansion on a time scale, the exact beginning of the QRS complex is difficult to determine, yet early QRS vectors, such as the 0.04 s vector, are often accorded considerable diagnostic importance. The timing of such vectors is clearly done more accurately from the *M* tracing. However, the greater detail afforded by the *M* tracing has disclosed that in many normal cases the development of early QRS vectors can be very gradual: a slight initial deflection, or foot (″r in ❷ Fig. 13.4) may be clearly discernible, conjectural, or absent from case to case (❷ Fig. 13.5) and sometimes from beat to beat. The presence or absence of this feature can make a

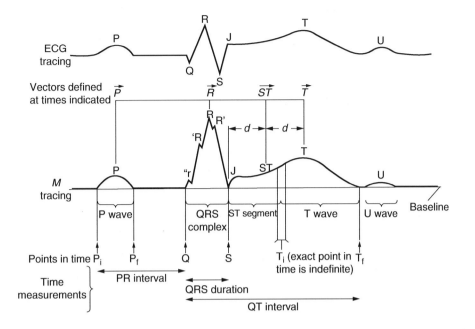

◻ Fig. 13.4
ECG and spatial vector magnitude (*M*) tracings are compared. All *M* deflections are above the baseline. The Q wave in the ECG corresponds to the so-called small foot ″r in the *M* tracing. Q and S points in the *M* tracing mark the beginning and end of the QRS complex to conform with terms PR and QT intervals, and QRS duration. The J point is not a useful time reference because it is often absent, whereas the nadir S is usually clear. P_i and P_f are P-wave onset and end, respectively; T_i and T_f are T-wave onset and end, respectively

difference of about 0.01 s to the QRS onset. This is something to be borne in mind when the QRS onset point is used as a time reference for defining QRS vectors. Its variability, however, still allows the *M* tracing to give a more consistent basis for determining QRS duration by computer than the QRS complex in the ECG [4].

The value of the *M* tracing in measuring QRS durations extends also to the determination of PR and QT intervals (❯ Table 13.3) for the same reason; namely, a zero value of the *M* tracing indicates that ECG signals are "zero," so that different ECG leads do not have to be compared.

13.3.1 Baseline Clamping

An interesting requirement of magnitude tracings, not obvious from the formulae for deriving them, is that the baselines preceding the QRS complex in the parent *xyz* signals should be clamped (that is, set to zero) before the transformation of coordinates is carried out. If this is not done, the apparent baseline of the magnitude tracing will ride above the zero level and there will appear to be negative deflections from that baseline, which may meet, but cannot cross that level. Negative magnitudes are of course impossible. The appearance of these pseudo negative deflections is obvious (❯ Fig. 13.6) and the consequent distortion is therefore avoidable. In fact, since the computer program clamps automatically and virtually without fail, this is no longer a problem, but the solution is not simple or obvious and, because of its crucial importance to polarcardiography, a brief account of it is merited.

The clamp point is located shortly before the Q point, at a time when signals are negligible in relation to an estimate of noise made in a 30 ms window in the region of the clamp point. The method used by the Woodward computers has not required alteration for several years and produces satisfactory *M* tracings in almost every case although rarely, P waves running into the QRS complex as is sometimes seen in the Wolff–Parkinson–White (WPW) syndrome, may give problems. The analysis program, however, bases its diagnosis of the WPW syndrome on the presence of delta waves in the ECG leads V_3–V_5, derived from the *xyz* signals. These signals are not distorted by clamping, since its effect is merely to

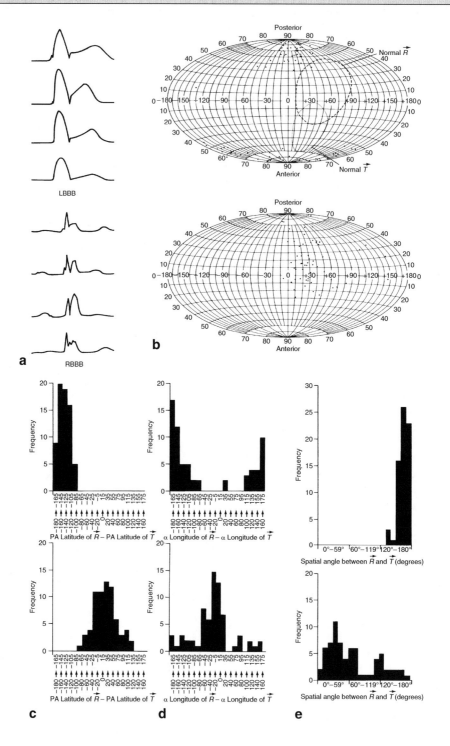

Fig. 13.5

Left bundle branch block (LBBB) as compared to right bundle branch block (RBBB). *M* tracings in eight typical examples of LBBB and RBBB (**a**) show marked differences in the smoothness of QRS contour. Note the variability of the initial small deflection, or foot, in LBBB. Aitoff plots (**b**) show directions of $\vec{R}$ and $\vec{T}$ in 69 cases each of LBBB (*top*) and RBBB (*bottom*). In LBBB, these are at opposite poles. This difference is also shown in histograms of latitude differences (**c**), but less so in longitude differences (**d**) and spatial angles between $\vec{R}$ and $\vec{T}$ (**e**)

◘ Table 13.1
Cutoff points for flagging interval measurements (ms): *I* interpolate according to age, *D* use default value

Interval	Flag	Default[a]	Age < 7	7 ⩽ age ⩽ 16	16 ⩽ age ⩽ 17
PR	>>	>210	> 180	I	>190 (rate > 100)
					>200 (rate ⩽ 100)
	<	<115	None	None	None
	<<	<106	<58	I	D
QRS	>>	>109	<88	I	D
	<<	<50	<46	I	D
QT$_c$	>>	>470	<473	I	D
	<<	<350	<300	I	D

[a]Age not otherwise specified

◘ Table 13.2
Cutoff points for flagging vector magnitudes (mV), ratios, and ischemic index $(M_s\theta)$: *I* interpolate, *D* use default value

Vector	Flag	Default	Age < 5	5 ⩽ age ⩽ 16	Age ⩾ 16 Female	16 ⩽ age ⩽ 28 Male
P	>>	>0.240	>0.290	I	D	D
	>	>0.200	>0.240	I	D	D
R	>>	>2.200	>3.320	I	>2.000	>2.400
	>	>2.100	>2.840	I	D	None
	<	None	<0.920	I	None	D
	<<	<0.850	<0.440	I	<0.750	D
m_t	>>	>2.150	>2.340	I	>1.850	>1.700
	>	>1.950	>2.030	I	>1.700	None
ST/R	>>	>0.25	D	D	D	>0.20[a]
T/R	>>	>0.75	>0.52	I	D	>0.60[a]
	<<	<0.10	<0.01	I	D	D
$M_s\theta$	*	⩾ 5	D	D	D	D
	*	⩾ 10	D	D	D	D

[a]For 16 ⩽ age ⩽ 30

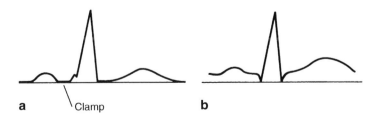

a ╲Clamp   b

◘ Fig. 13.6
M tracings from clamped *xyz* signals (**a**). If the baselines of *xyz* signals are not centered to zero (*clamped*) prior to transformation to polar coordinates, the magnitude tracing will show an upward displacement of the baseline and downward deflections (**b**)

● Table 13.3

Table of the information (with measurements made from polar coordinates) contained in computer outputs taken from a 99-year-old man with chest pain. Nine beats have been measured and analyzed. Measurements of time intervals are made from spatial magnitudes. Note the consistency of QRS durations, except for beat seven, which suggests aberrant conduction, probably owing to ectopy. P waves are not identified for every beat as they are rather small. R, ST, and T vectors all have abnormal longitudes (**); ($M_s\theta$) is increased (**). The extreme right-hand column gives baseline drift in 10 μV units. Under "computer comments," beats are ranked in order of increasing drift. Rows of asterisks indicate beats to which the comments apply, thus providing an indication of consistency. Criteria for anterior myocardial infarction (AMI) and inferior myocardial infarction (IMI) are present in each beat and are identified by letters in parentheses: B, a; T, b; d, i; y, g; G, c; where the upper case indicates a stronger positive criterion and the second lettered component refers to the lettered criterion in the text. For example, G, c indicates criterion c based on gamma downslope. "EQ vectors" refer to spherocardiographic criteria. The transverse QRS-vector loop indicates anterior infarction by having a notch in the efferent limb.

Beat	R-R	PR	QRS	QT	QT$_c$	M	Latitude	Longitude	M	Latitude	Longitude	M	Latitude	Longitude	M	Latitude	Longitude	m_rR	M_s	$M_s\theta$	Drift
1			82	382	409				1.80	29P	−5**	0.18	40A	−171**	0.32	40A	−171**	1.79	0.12	11**	12
2	874		82	385	412				1.83	27P	−5**	0.16	29A	−180**	0.31	31A	−171**	1.82	0.12	12**	3
3	863		82	383	410				1.83	27P	−5**	0.17	85A	−171**	0.31	31A	−171**	1.82	0.15	14**	8
4	868	160	83	368	394	0.10	36P	−14	1.81	29P	−5**	0.14	44A	−168*	0.32	34A	−167**	1.81	0.10	8*	8
5	845	161	84	398	426	0.06	45P	0	1.80	25P	−4**	0.22	33A	−180**	0.37	29A	−176**	1.80	0.12	11**	4
6	854		85	362	388				1.78	28P	−4**	0.13	38A	−143*	0.25	34A	−168**	1.78	0.06	5*	5
7	871	154	99	386	413	0.09	43P	−18	2.0	86A	−171**	0.20	36A	−180**	0.33	32A	−180**	2.10	0.14	13**	4
8	844		85	382	409				1.84	27P	−6**	0.13	38A	−168*	0.25	40A	−161**	1.83	0.10	9*	8
9	887	162	81	375	402	0.12	30P	−36**	1.78	29P	−7**	0.22	33A	−180**	0.38	31A	−176**	1.77	0.14	14**	

Computer comments

2 7 5 6 3 4 8 1 9   (valid for beats shown, in order or drift)

* Abnormally directed P vector

******** Unusual R-vector direction

\+ LVH by voltage: possible *(+)/probable(*)

+* QRS suggests (+)/indicates (*) AMI, (BT BT BT BT BT BT BT BT)

+** QRS suggests (+)/indicates (*) IMI (dy dy dy dy dy dyG dy)

|||||||| EQ vectors suggest apical (A), lateral (L) or inferior (I) MI.

******** Nonspecific T-wave abnormality

****** Nonspecific ST abnormality

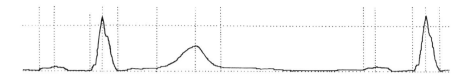

◻ Fig. 13.7
The normal spatial magnitude tracing in a computer-generated polarcardiogram. *Vertical dotted lines* show some computer-identified points in time. The time between dots horizontally is 10 ms. Note that the onset of each QRS in this *M* tracing is clamped to 0

straighten the baselines. Indeed, distortion resulting from drift tends to be reduced. The 12-lead ECGs derived from such clamped *xyz* signals (see ❯ Chap. 11 of *Basic Electrocardiology: Cardiac Electrophysiology, ECG Systems and Mathematical Modeling*) are free from baseline drift and are thereby much improved (❯ Fig. 13.18b). A record of the drift between beats is printed out by the computer in its table of measurements (❯ Table 13.3). The computer analyzes each beat separately and ranks its findings in order of increasing drift (❯ Table 13.3). If beats show excessive drift they can be rejected by the program. Distortion might be expected from the so-called atrial T wave, occurring just before and during the QRS complex. This turns out not to be a problem, however, because atrial T waves are small and of low frequency, so they do not disturb early QRS vectors important in the diagnosis of infarction.

The designation of part of the ECG as baseline is arbitrary because the actual DC level (see ❯ Chap. 12 of *Basic Electrocardiology: Cardiac Electrophysiology, ECG Systems and Mathematical Modeling*) is not measurable with conventional equipment. Two possible choices for the baseline are the PR and TP segments. Early analog polarcardiographs used the TP segment, clamping being triggered by the preceding R wave, followed by a time delay adjusted by the operator. Fast heart rates and U waves gave problems, however. When tape-recorded *xyz* signals became available, the PR segment became the baseline of choice. Two reproducing heads allowed the R wave, detected through circuitry linked to the first head, to trigger clamping before the same QRS complex arrived at the second head; a short time delay allowed the clamp point to be positioned just before QRS onset. When baseline drift occurred between beats, clamping resulted in a step resetting the *M* tracing to zero (❯ Fig. 13.8) prior to QRS onset. P vectors, preceding the clamp point, were thus affected by the total drift from the previous clamp. This problem was eliminated when digital signal-processing was adopted for polarcardiography, because baseline-drift removal could then be carried out forwards and backward between clamp points, so that drift corrections were linearly spread over the whole heart cycle. Digital processing, by allowing retrograde clamping, thus increased the accuracy of determinations of P-vector magnitudes and directions. It also permitted much refinement in the determination of the clamp points and eliminated operator adjustments.

It has been pointed out that no new information results from the transformation of rectangular to polar coordinates, although hidden features may be made obvious. It could be argued, however, that baseline clamping and straightening do add something to the tracings that is already known information but not contained in them, namely, that baseline wander or drift is non-cardiac in origin, and that the magnitude of the heart vector before the QRS complex may be taken as zero, to give a manifestly undistorted *M* tracing. The embodiment of this information in the polarcardiogram is, then, an addition. Clamping the *xyz* signals improves the quality and usefulness of the VCGs obtained from them because it provides accurate centering of the E point (❯ Fig. 13.11). This often cannot be achieved with VCG loops, because the E point is a blurred spot resulting from the telescoping of noise and small signals around it.

13.3.2 Some Characteristics of Magnitude Tracings

13.3.2.1 P Waves

Generally, in magnitude (M) tracings P waves appear much as in the ECG, except that they are always positive. Sometimes there are two P-wave peaks, suggesting interatrial block. The so-called atrial T wave, sometimes seen in the ECG, will not

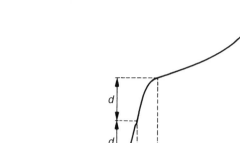
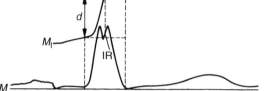

Fig. 13.8

The definition of a representative QRS vector IR when there are two equal peaks in the *M* tracing. In these tracings, produced by an analog polarcardiograph, the *M* tracing is recorded together with its integral, *MI*. The height midway between Q and S points in the integral tracing defines the half-area point, IR. Note the step after P wave, caused by baseline clamping

be observed directly in magnitude tracings because baselines are clamped during this period; however, its presence can be inferred because the baseline preceding the P wave will, in these cases, be displaced slightly upward. Atrial flutter and atrial fibrillation appear in magnitude tracings much as they do in the ECG. Large P waves in the M tracing, as in the ECG, suggest atrial hypertrophy. The cut-off point for the computer diagnosis of this condition is 0.22 mV.

13.3.2.2   QRS Complex

A typical normal QRS complex is shown in ◗ Fig. 13.7. It may begin with a decisive rise or show an initial foot. In myocardial infarction, the foot may be exaggerated and associated with diagnostic Q waves in the ECG. The foot may become diagnostic of infarction when it returns to the baseline before the main QRS deflection begins (◗ Fig. 13.11). When this happens in the transverse magnitude, the criterion $m_t \to 0$ (see ◗ Sect. 13.5.1.1) is positive for anterior or anteroseptal infarction. In the VCG, $m_t \to 0$ may be discernible (◗ Fig. 13.11 where the initial portion of the loop returns to the E point), but often it is lost in noise around the E point, in other parts of the QRS loop, or even in P and ST-T loops.

The peak of the QRS complex in the *M* tracing is usually distinct. The R vector whose magnitude is represented by this peak is then well defined. However, there may sometimes be two peaks of approximately equal magnitude and in this event the first or the second peak may alternately be the greater, from beat to beat. A useful definition of a characteristic QRS vector, in these cases, is the IR point, the point at which the area under the QRS complex is half its final value (◗ Fig. 13.8). This is a more reliable time reference than the Q point, which can be displaced by the initial foot as described above. Such a foot would have little effect on the timing of IR.

Deep notching of the QRS complex in the *M* tracing is a feature of RBBB (◗ Fig. 13.5); sometimes there appears to be a normal initial deflection followed by a delayed, slurred deflection, owing to the block. By contrast, in LBBB the QRS complex tends to be very smooth, but there is usually a small initial foot, corresponding to a small initial R wave in V_1 of the ECG. When magnitude and angle tracings are taken into account, the appearance of LBBB is so characteristic that myocardial infarction can sometimes be diagnosed in the presence of LBBB, which is much more difficult from the ECG (see also ◗ Chaps. 2 and ◗ 4 of *Electrocardiology: Comprehensive Clinical ECG*). Fine notching of the *M* tracing near the peak is not normal and is associated with patchy fibrosis.

Delta waves in the *M* tracing are present in WPW syndrome, but they are not diagnostic. The computer program obtains better results from searching for delta waves in leads V 3–V 5 in the derived ECG. As would be expected, ventricular ectopy produces QRS complexes strikingly different from normally conducted beats, and various types may be classified.

13.3.2.3 ST Segment

Normally, the S point has a magnitude that is zero, or close to it. It is characteristically elevated in stress-induced ischemia (❯ Fig. 13.9) and in injury currents from infarction or pericarditis. This provides a sensitive measure that is easy to quantify by computer. After the S point, the ST segment, normally, gradually slopes upward to become the T wave. In ischemia it may, however, be downsloping. In this case, the S point is at the junction between the steeply descending QRS and the gradually descending ST segment. Fortunately, this point is readily identified by the computer program. There is not, however, any readily identifiable point to be designated as a representative of the ST segment. Therefore, a point midway between the S and T points is used as mentioned in ❯ Sect. 13.3 (❯ Fig. 13.4). Sometimes, in gross recent infarction, the ST segment may join with the QRS complex to form a monophasic pattern reminiscent of transmembrane potentials.

13.3.2.4 T Wave

In normal and most abnormal *M* tracings, the T wave is simple and smooth. Rarely, in recent infarction, double T-wave humps occur. Evolving inferior infarction often produces a marked increase in the amplitude of the T wave (❯ Fig. 13.15). Myocardial ischemia usually reduces the relative amplitude of the T wave (❯ Fig. 13.9). U waves, when they appear at all, are often attached to the terminal downslope of the T wave. T waves that are diphasic, or inverted, in the ECG arise from changes in vector direction, more than vector magnitude, and the corresponding abnormalities in the *M* tracing are often minimal though they are revealed by angle tracings.

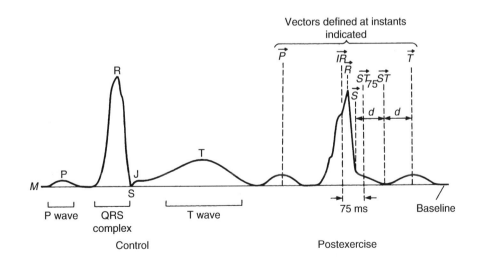

◘ Fig. 13.9

Spatial-magnitude changes in stress-induced ischemia, which causes the S-point to rise. The control *M* tracing is on the left and the post exercise *M* tracing on the right. The abnormal direction of ST_{75}, defined 75 ms after IR, is combined with the magnitude at S to give an ischemic index

13.4 Angle Tracings

Directions of the heart vector in the frontal, transverse, and (left) sagittal planes of the VCG are denoted by angles α, β, and γ which, when plotted against time, give three of the angle tracings of the polarcardiogram (❷ Fig. 13.10). The polarity chosen is such that positive angles appear in the lower half of the scale (❷ Fig. 13.11) in conformity with the vectorcardiographic tradition initiated by Einthoven for describing the electrical axis. Consequently, upslopes in any of these angle tracings indicate counterclockwise rotations of the VCG loops about the E point. Just as the transverse QRS VCG loop in normal subjects consistently shows a counterclockwise rotation, the tracing shows an even upslope (❷ Fig. 13.12). Downslopes in the tracing occur in anterior infarction (❷ Figs. 13.11 and ❷ 13.18) and LBBB. There may be a reversal of direction, in normal individuals; that is, a small β downslope near the maximal radius of the loop which corresponds to the peak of the m_t tracing. Downslopes in the β tracing often appear as kinks in the VCG loop (❷ Fig. 13.11). Though less consistent than the β tracing, the γ tracing is useful in revealing inferior infarction by downslopes occurring before the peak of the m_s tracing. However, there must be an initial Q wave in the y-signal tracing, while γ remains in the range $-175° < \gamma < -45°$. The α tracing, like the frontal loop, is much more variable in normal subjects and has not given rise to any polar criteria for infarction.

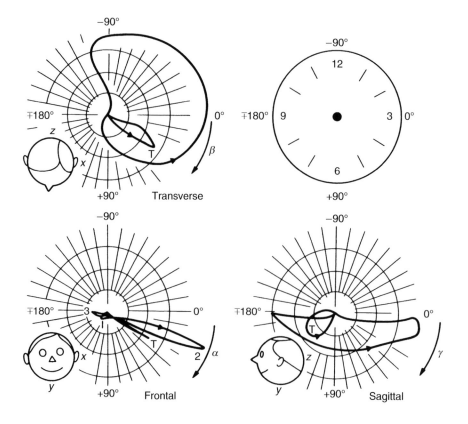

◼ Fig. 13.10

Using a clock face as reference for α, β, and γ angles in frontal, transverse, and left sagittal planes respectively, results in 0° at 3 o'clock, +90° at 6 o'clock, ±180° at 9 o'clock, and −90° at 12 o'clock

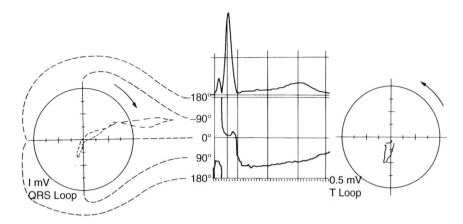

◘ Fig. 13.11

The relationship of the transverse QRS loop (*left*), T loop (*right*, amplification doubled), m_t magnitude, and angle tracings (*center*). Clockwise rotations of loops are associated with downsloping angle tracings. The example illustrates previous anterior infarction with $m_t \rightarrow 0$, indicated by the initial m_t deflection returning to the zero baseline and $\beta\downarrow$, indicated by the downsloping tracing, both of which criteria are present. That the initial lobe of the QRS loop returns exactly to the E point is indicated clearly by the m_t tracing; counterclockwise rotation of the T loop is indicated by the upsloping tracing opposite the T wave in the m_t tracing

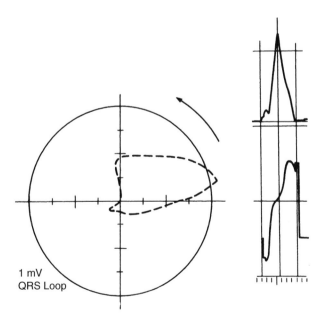

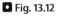 **Fig. 13.12**

A normal transverse plane QRS loop with m_t and β tracings. Note the counterclockwise rotation of the loop and upsloping β tracing

13.4.1 Latitudes and Longitudes

With the body conceptualized as a sphere, the frontal, transverse, and sagittal planes cut through the center to form equatorial planes of three different spherical polar coordinate systems. Each system has its respective polar axis: posteroanterior (PA), inferosuperior (IS), and right–left (RL). This polarity gives right-handed consistency of coordinates. The angles of the heart vector with respect to the planes give the PA-, IS- and RL-latitude tracings, respectively (❷ Fig. 13.13). Latitudes are expressed in degrees followed by one of the six letters to indicate the direction with respect to

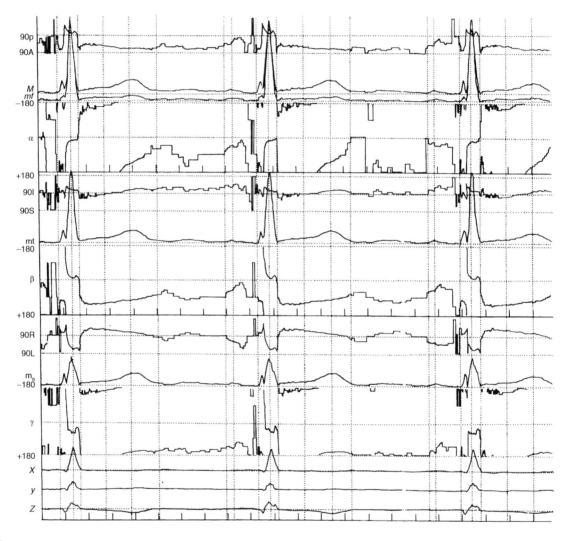

❑ Fig. 13.13

Polarcardiogram of the same patient as in ❷ Fig. 13.11 which shows the last of three beats displayed here. This beat had least baseline drift before clamping. Time marks occur every 10 ms. *XYZ* tracings (*bottom*) are of *xyz* signals which generate all other displays. *Vertical dotted lines* indicate computer-identified points (compare with ❷ Fig. 13.7) determined from the M tracing (second from *top*). Immediately below is the m_f tracing of frontal plane magnitude. Corresponding transverse and sagittal plane magnitudes appear lower down (m_t, m_s). Tracings of angles α, β, and γ appear below m_f, m_t, and m_s tracings, respectively. The remaining tracings are of angles anterior (*A*) and posterior (*P*) to the frontal plane, inferior (*I*) and superior (*S*) to the transverse plane, and right (*R*) and left (*L*) of the sagittal plane. Dots in vertical lines are 10° apart over angle ranges and 50 µV apart over magnitude ranges at standard recording sensitivity

one of the three equatorial planes. The difference between the latitude of the R and T vectors differs distinctly in RBBB and LBBB – more so than the corresponding differences in longitudes or the spatial angle between these vectors (❷ Fig. 13.5). Latitude tracings have been less productive of criteria than longitude tracings, although Bruce [5] has defined a criterion for apical infarction based on the RL-latitude tracing: a downslope from 45R or more within the initial 10 ms of QRS, crossing the zero-degree line after the first 10 ms, associated with a Q wave in the x-signal tracing and between $-45°$ and $-175°$. It is, of course, doubly redundant to use six angle coordinates to describe spatial directions and, in fact, this is not done. The directions of P, R, ST, and T, printed out by the measurement program, are given in terms of α longitude and PA latitude (of angle ψ in ❷ Fig. 13.1). Justification for displaying all six angle tracings in the polarcardiogram would be

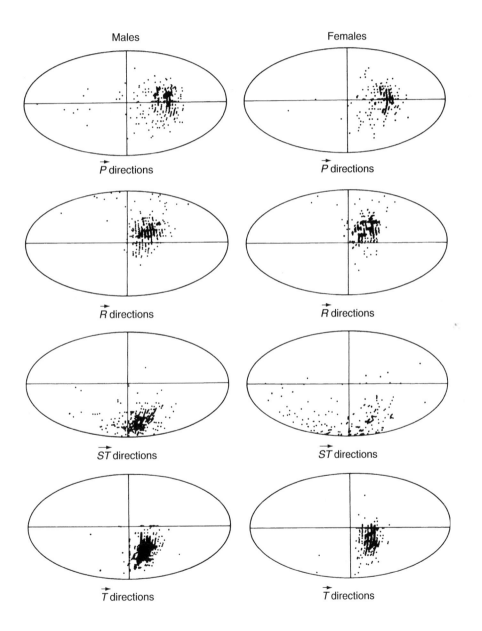

◘ Fig. 13.14

Directions of $\vec{P}$, $\vec{R}$, $\vec{ST}$ and $\vec{T}$ in 406 Cretan villagers. These findings should be compared with those of ❷ Fig. 13.3. Note that the T-vector distribution for women is slightly posterior to that for men

the same as that for displaying six limb leads in the ECG or three VCG views when only two are sufficient: abnormalities may show better in some than in others.

13.4.2   Normal Directions of Representative Heart Vectors

The normal directions of $\vec{P}, \vec{R},$ and $\vec{T}$ are shown in ❯ Fig. 13.3 for 195 young adults, and in ❯ Fig. 13.14 for 406 Cretan villagers. ❯ Figure 13.14 also shows the directions of the ST vectors. As vector magnitudes decrease toward zero, angular

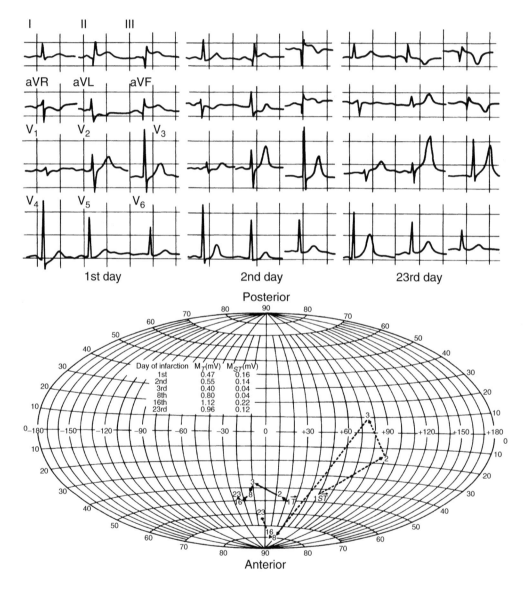

◻ Fig. 13.15

The typical migration of the T-wave vector in the Aitoff projection in evolving inferior infarction, with the movement toward "South America." The ST vector ultimately moves toward the same continent. ECGs (*above*) show evolving ST-T-wave changes. The spatial magnitudes of maximum $\vec{T}$ on first, second, third, eighth, 16th, and 23rd days are shown in the table (insert) together with the magnitudes of $\vec{ST}$. Note that on the 16th day, the magnitude of $\vec{T}$ is 2.4 times its initial value

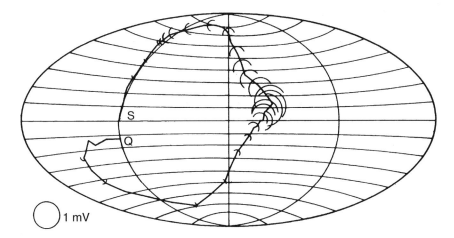

□ **Fig. 13.16**
A normal spherocardiogram of the same subject as in ❷ Fig. 13.12. The snakelike pattern starts in the anterior (*lower*) hemisphere and crosses the equator "east" of the vertical, zero-degree meridian. The beginning and end of the snake are marked Q and S, respectively. Semicircles are drawn every 2 ms. Their diameters indicate spatial magnitude; the reference *circle* represents 1 mV

directions have less resolution – at zero, directions are meaningless. This accounts for the wide scatter of $\vec{ST}$ directions among the women, whose $\vec{ST}$ magnitudes are often close to zero. In men, the $\vec{ST}$ tends to be larger and shows directions similar to those of the $\vec{T}$. The directions of $\vec{P}$ show considerable scatter, but it is the same in both sexes. $\vec{R}$ directions are well defined, but often change very quickly so that a few milliseconds difference in the timing of the R peak in the M tracing can result in a large difference in direction. This is responsible for some of the scatter seen for the $\vec{R}$ directions. $\vec{T}$, on the other hand, tends to change direction very gradually, if at all. It will be recalled that, in the VCG, the normal T loop is often a straight line. For this reason, and because magnitudes are large enough for accurate definition of direction, $\vec{T}$ directions show the least scatter. They form a well-defined "continent" that occupies only about 5% of the area of the globe (❷ Fig. 13.3).

Abnormal $\vec{P}$ directions are useful in detecting abnormalities that, in the ECG, might be interpreted as a result of a low atrial focus. They have not, however, proven of much value in detecting atrial hypertrophy, which is more reliably done from the magnitude of $\vec{P}$.

Unusual $\vec{R}$ directions are helpful but tend to occur too frequently to justify calling them abnormal, if that is the only finding. It will now be appreciated by the reader that the longitude of $\vec{R}$ is a measure of Einthoven's electrical axis, which is not to be confused with the mean electrical axis (see ❷ Sect. 13.5.4).

The most useful vector direction is that of $\vec{T}$. Directions of $\vec{T}$ that fail to lie within the normal continent (❷ Fig. 13.3) will give rise to abnormal T waves in the ECG. This efficient device for defining normality of T waves, presenting data in a way that immediately strikes the eye, should be compared with the prospect of defining T-wave normality on the basis of the 195 12-lead ECGs from the same subjects! It is an excellent example of the value of both the heart-vector concept and the use of spherical polar coordinates. It can also show subtle differences between populations. ❷ Figure 13.14 shows $\vec{T}$ distributions in male and female Cretan villagers: the center of the female distribution is slightly posterior to that of the male. A similar sex difference was observed in children aged 3–4 years [6] which is surprising in view of the similar body build at this age.

In evolving inferior infarction, there is a migration of $\vec{T}$ directions that is most characteristic (❷ Fig. 13.15). If the normal T continent is analogous to the continent of Africa, $\vec{T}$ migrates westward to lie in South America. The concomitant ECG change is the development of inverted T waves in inferior leads.

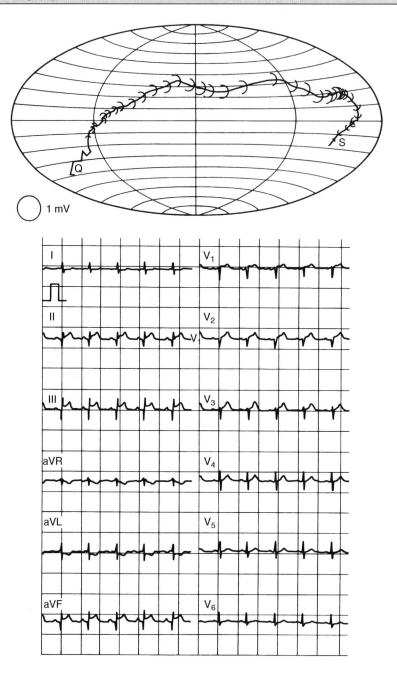

◘ Fig. 13.17

The spherocardiogram in inferior infarction. The "snake" begins in the anterior (*lower*) hemisphere and crosses the equator at longitude −80°. This should be compared with ❷ Fig. 13.16. The derived 12-lead ECG below shows recent inferior infarction

13.4.3 Spherocardiogram

Instead of plotting only a few vectors during the cardiac cycle, the Aitoff projection may be used to plot a full sequence of vectors, every 2 ms throughout the QRS complex (❷ Fig. 13.16). The spherocardiogram [7] is such a display: vector magnitudes are represented by the radii of semicircles whose centers indicate direction and whose convexities indicate the next plot in the sequence. The result resembles a snake which, for normal subjects, has the thickest part of its body in the region of the "continent" of the direction of the normal $\dot{R}$ (❯ Fig. 13.3). The head of the snake lies in the "southern" hemisphere and its body crosses the equator slightly to the "east" of the zero meridian. Absent initial anterior forces, as in anteroseptal infarction, result in the head lying on the equator or in the "northern" hemisphere. When the body of the snake crosses the equator to the west, inferior infarction is indicated (❯ Fig. 13.17). Although the spherocardiogram has been useful in developing computer criteria (see ❯ Sect. 13.5), like the polarcardiogram, it is not routinely generated. Despite being based on spherical polar coordinates, the spherocardiogram is more like a three-dimensional VCG: it suffers from the same shortcoming that phenomena are not displayed against a time coordinate.

13.5 Diagnostic Criteria

Rather than present the various criteria developed for visual interpretation of polarcardiograms, it is thought more useful to outline the criteria now used in the computer program for further analysis. These differ from the older analog criteria [8, 9] in several important ways: they are, of necessity, totally explicit; they are designed to give higher specificity, at the expense of some sensitivity; and they include some new criteria [10].

13.5.1 Criteria for Myocardial Infarction

13.5.1.1 Criteria Relating to the QRS Complex

(a) Polarcardiographic criteria
   (i) $\beta\downarrow$: a downslope in the tracing of the angle in the transverse plane (❯ Figs. 13.11 and ❯ 13.13), occurring 10 ms before the peak $m_t R$ of the transverse plane magnitude tracing (downslopes in the first 20 ms may be discounted). This is a criterion of anteroseptal or anterior infarction and corresponds to a region of clockwise rotation in the transverse plane vector loop (❯ Fig. 13.18a).

It must be noted that for the computer program, the definition of a downslope must be quite explicit. A downslope is an overall drop of $5°$ over a total downsloping time of at least 5 ms. A downslope begins at the onset of the first drop and ends at the beginning of the first rise following the fulfillment of its definition requirements of minimum time and overall drop. Small rises are allowed within a defined downslope provided that first, they are subtracted from the drop which has occurred up to that point and second, they do not thereby reduce the overall drop below $1°$. Horizontal segments are also allowed, but neither they nor the segments containing rises contribute to the total downsloping time. Downslopes terminating with a net drop $\geqslant 10°$ are rated very marked, otherwise they are rated as significant. An upslope is similarly defined except that drops become rises.

   (ii) $m_t \rightarrow 0$: a return to the baseline of the transverse magnitude tracing immediately following an initial deflection (❯ Fig. 13.11). This is a criterion for anterior infarction that is often not apparent in the vector loop because of ambiguity of the E point. It may not be present in every beat (❯ Fig. 13.13).

In the above criterion, "initial" means between 10 ms after the Q point and the time of the peak of the m_t tracing. Return to the baseline means falling to 0.01 mV or less, or to 0.02 mV if the estimate for baseline noise is at least 0.02 mY. Between Q and the return to the baseline there must be a deflection of the m_t tracing of more than 0.05 mV and this amount must be greater than twice the value of the noise estimate.

   (iii) $\gamma\downarrow$: a downslope in the tracing of the angle in the left sagittal plane occurring 10 ms after the Q point and 10 ms before the peak $m_s R$ of the sagittal plane magnitude tracing, provided that there is a Q wave in the Y tracing and longitude $< -45°$. This is a criterion of the inferior infarction; it corresponds to clockwise rotation in the initial anterosuperior segment of the left sagittal loop.

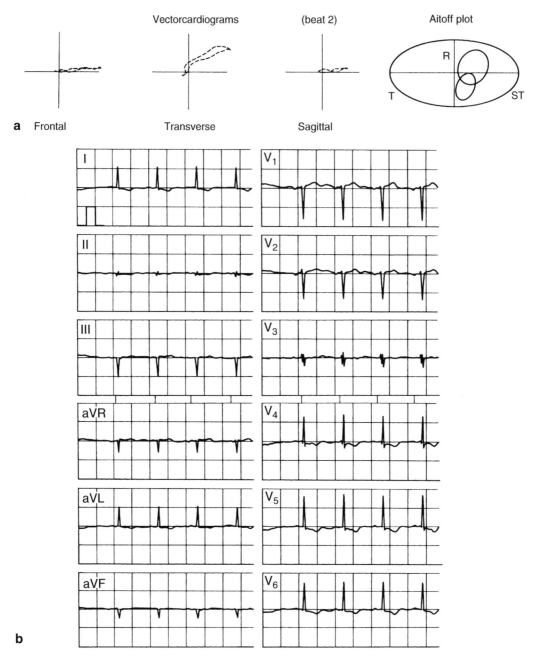

Vectorcardiograms (beat 2) Aitoff plot

a Frontal   Transverse   Sagittal

b

◘ **Fig. 13.18**
Part (a) shows VCGs and the Aitoff plot derived from the information for beat seven given in ❯ Table 13.3. The Aitoff plot illustrates that the directions of the R, ST, and T vectors are all outside the normal boundaries. Part (b) shows the ECG derived from three *xyz* signals of beats 1–4 (from ❯ Table 13.3); the ECG shows inferior infarction, but less-definite anterior infarction. Note the baseline drift prior to clamping of the first beat. Clamp points are indicated by short vertical lines between leads III and aVR, and V_3 and V_4

(b) Quasi-electrocardiographic criteria

(iv) Absence of initial anterior forces, indicating by an initial Q wave in the Z tracing. This is a criterion of anteroseptal infarction; it corresponds to Q waves in V_1 and V_2 of the ECG.

(v) Initial anterior forces do not exceed 6% of posterior forces, as indicated in the Z tracing. This is a weaker criterion of anteroseptal infraction than (iv).

(vi) Posterior forces in the Z tracing do not exceed 9% of M_R, the maximum spatial QRS vector. This is a criterion of true posterior infarction; it is invalidated by complete or partial RBBB. It has no ECG equivalent but corresponds approximately to the finding of a small S wave in V_2.

(vii) Initial superior forces exceed 35% of inferior forces, indicated in the Y tracing. M_R is substituted for the inferior forces if these become less than 20% of M_R. This is a criterion of inferior infarction and corresponds to a relatively large Q wave in aVF.

(viii) Initial rightward forces exceed 23% of leftward forces, indicated in the X tracing. This suggests apical or lateral infarction; it corresponds to a relatively large Q wave in leads I, aVL or V_6.

(ix) Duration of the Q wave in the Y tracing exceeds 40% of the QRS complex in the spatial magnitude tracing. This criterion of inferior infarction roughly corresponds to a wide Q wave in aVF.

(c) Spherocardiographic criteria

(x) The locus of QRS directions on the sphere crosses the equator outside the normal longitude range of $-15°$ to $+100°$. This suggests inferior, lateral, or apical infarction (I, L, or A) according to the following ranges: $-130° <$ longitude $< -15°$ for inferior infarction; $+100° <$ longitude $< +175°$ for lateral infarction; and $+175° <$ longitude $< -130°$ for apical infarction (range passes through $180°$). These criteria do not correspond to any ECG criteria.

Note that, near the crossing of the equator, the latitude must change from 5A to 5P within 10 ms. During this period, the vector magnitude must exceed 5% of M_R and the crossing must have occurred by 15 ms after the spatial magnitude tracing reaches its peak (M_R).

13.5.1.2 Non-QRS Criteria

(xi) $\vec{ST}$ suggests a current of injury if $M_S > 0.167 M_R$, where M_S is the magnitude of the spatial vector at the end of QRS, that is, the S point. This criterion has no ECG counterpart. There are refinements of this criterion which indicate the region of the injury such as anteroseptal, lateral apical, according to the direction of $\vec{ST}$.

(xii) $\vec{T}$ suggests an evolving or old inferior infarction at first, $M_T > 0.2 M_R$, where M_T is the spatial magnitude of the maximum $\vec{T}$; and second, this vector has a longitude between $-10°$ and $-60°$ and a latitude posterior to 70A and anterior to 20P.

(xiii) $\vec{T}$ suggests anterior injury if they have the following characteristics. First, $M_T > 0.2 M_R$; second, the longitude of the maximum $\vec{T}$ is between $-120°$ and $+165°$; third, M_T has a latitude posterior to 20P, but lies outside a region defined between longitudes $0°$ and $+45°$ and latitudes 19P and 45P; and finally, RBBB is not present. This corresponds to T-wave inversion in anterior precordial leads not of the type seen as a normal variant in women.

13.5.2 Evaluation of Performance of Infarction Criteria

The above criteria were evaluated with a test set of 369 subjects selected from a much larger population who were studied angiographically; 234 had 100% occlusion of a major coronary vessel and associated akinesia or dyskinesia (indicating infarction), and 135 had less than 50% occlusion, normal wall motion, normal hemodynamics, and no history of infarction [11]. The ECGs of the 369 subjects were separated into infarction and non-infarction groups by cardiologist ECG readers at two hospitals. A corresponding division was made by the computer using the above criteria. The computer's selection agreed slightly better with the angiographic evidence than the selections of the readers at the two hospitals: both its sensitivity and specificity were higher, though not significantly so. However, when the computer's selection of infarction cases was combined with the selections of either of the two groups of readers, the improvements in sensitivity were significant, while the corresponding reductions in specificity were not. This was satisfactory because the computer

◻ Table 13.4

Apparent (worst case) specificity of polar computer program with respect to myocardial infarction (MI) tested on 473 presumed healthy Cretan villagers in various age-groups

Age-group	Men Na	%	MI + veb	Specificity %
19–29	44	68	1	98
30–39	100	9	2	98
40–49	118	61	4	97
50–59	95	55	5	95
60–69	80	63	10	88
70–89	36	64	8	78
All	473	60	30	94

[a]Median ages for the men and women were both 46 years
[b]Positive diagnosis of previous infarction made by computer program

output was designed to be used as an aid to the cardiologist interpreting the ECG, rather than as an automated simulation of his interpretation. It is important to note, as an aside, that although the readers did not have VCGs for this evaluation, the computer generates these whenever it makes a diagnosis of infarction based on QRS evidence. This usually allows the reader to corroborate a positive diagnosis of infarction by the computer despite the lack of corroboration in the derived 12-lead ECG, that is, the ECGD (see ❷ Chap. 11 of *Basic Electrocardiology: Cardiac Electrophysiology, ECG Systems and Mathematical Modeling*). Sensitivity and specificity for the computer, alone, were 78% and 92%. However, the 92% specificity should be regarded as probably lower than it would be with a truly normal population because the 135 subjects who were negative angiographically could have had undetected lesions, since they all had sufficient chest pain to justify cardiac catheterization. When the computer criteria were applied to a test set of 118 Cretan villagers aged 40–49 years, the specificity was 97%. This is still probably lower than the true specificity because the Cretans were not examined – they were presumed healthy on the basis of the reported low prevalence of coronary artery disease among Cretan villagers [12]. ❷ Table 13.4 shows the specificity of the criteria in 473 Cretan villagers of various age-groups. Among the age-groups under 60 years, the specificity is 95% or better. There is a progressive decline in specificity with age, particularly after the age of 60 years. This decline is less than it appears, however, because 14 of the 30 positive cases had clear ECG evidence of previous myocardial infarction. Of course, it is possible to object that ECG evidence is inadmissible because it is not truly independent, but a cardiologist would find fault with failure of a computer program to detect "infarction" indicated by the ECG, so perhaps the program should not be faulted for those 14 cases. When this adjustment is made, the specificity for all subjects under 70% becomes 97%.

13.5.3 Criteria for Left Bundle Branch Block

This chapter would be unreasonably long if it contained every diagnostic criterion used by the polar analysis program. The myocardial infarction criteria have been given because of their importance and interest. The criteria for LBBB are also interesting and illustrate the polar approach when non-ECG evidence for a diagnosis is lacking.

Typical LBBB is recognized if:

(a) $\vec{R}$ is at least $70°$ posterior to $\vec{T}$
(b) The vector 30 ms before **IR** has transverse plane angle $< 30°$; that is, $\beta_{\text{IR}}-30\,\text{ms} < 30°$
(c) The spatial angle between R and $\vec{T}$ exceeds $120°$
(d) β increases by less than $20°$ from **IR** to **IR** + 20 ms
(e) $\beta_{IR+10\,\text{ms}} \leqslant \beta_{IR+10\,\text{ms}} + 22$ and
(f) QRS duration is flagged in the table of measurements ">>" (see ❷ Table 13.1)

If condition (a) is false and $90° \leqslant \vec{R} < -70°$, or if $\vec{R}$ is posterior to 30P, then the LBBB is considered atypical.

If LBBB is otherwise typical but M_S exceeds 5% of M_R, there is the probability of injury or aneurysm.

Left ventricular hypertrophy is probably present in addition to LBBB if M_R exceeds 4 mV; it is also possible if M_R exceeds 3 mV.

13.5.3.1 Developing Criteria for LBBB

The marked differences between the above criteria for LBBB and those employed in conventional electrocardiography exemplify the polar approach used by the computer program. A view concerning the development of diagnostic criteria for computer analysis of the ECG that has enjoyed recent currency is that, to be valid, such criteria must be based on independent, that is, non-ECG disease classification. Independent means for selecting suitable populations are available for myocardial infarction and LVH (so-called type A diagnosis) but not for LBBB, a condition identified, and therefore defined by the ECG (a type B diagnosis [13]). Because no independent "gold standard" is available for LBBB, it might appear most reasonable to employ ECG criteria in the computer program. Instead of this, the ECG was used to select cases of LBBB whose polarcardiograms were then studied for clearly identifiable characteristics. Several polarcardiograms appeared that could not be simply stated in terms of the ECG. For example, striking differences in the contours of the M tracings separated LBBB from RBBB (❯ Fig. 13.5). The $\vec{R}$ and $\vec{T}$ of these conditions show marked differences in latitudes (❯ Fig. 13.5).

The approach followed in developing LBBB criteria was as follows:

(a) Identify, from ECGs, a population (training set) with well-recognized LBBB
(b) Compare polarcardiograms and vector loops of this population with those of a non-LBBB population and observe any clear-cut characteristics that separate the populations
(c) Organize these into an effective tool for identifying LBBB, and
(d) Observe how well this tool performs, in a separate test set, when the ECG is ambiguous, and whether it misidentifies LBBB in those cases where the ECG is definite as a gold standard

This approach can produce a better indicator even when there is no independent standard. It has historical parallels. Wenckebach's phenomenon, although nowadays an ECG diagnosis, was originally identified in polygraph tracings. Its description predated that of the electrocardiograph by 4 years. The polygraph, however, did not give satisfactory recordings in every case and was supplanted by the ECG as a gold standard for this condition.

An approach similar to the above was undertaken for RBBB and IV conduction delay. Once the various subtleties for discriminating these conditions had been programmed, approximately 100 examples of each were selected by the computer from stored data which was not used in developing the criteria, and the derived 12-lead ECGs were studied to check the accuracy of the computer identifications. There were no discrepancies beyond what would be considered acceptable differences of opinion. Since the ECG criteria for diagnosing LBBB have served so well over the years, it might be asked what the benefit is from introducing others, even if they seem less ambiguous. An example of the value of this is that the distinction between LBBB and LVH with IV conduction delay is sometimes difficult from a single ECG, whereas the computer tends not to confuse them. The ability of the program to identify injury or aneurysm in LBBB is particularly interesting: in LBBB, the S point in the M tracing returns to the baseline as it does in the normal subject. Departures from this are unusual and appear to connote injury or perhaps aneurysm. This feature cannot be detected from the ECG.

13.5.4 Left Anterior Fascicular Block

Like LBBB, left anterior fascicular block is an entity defined by the ECG but it seems to be less clearly defined. Its diagnosis hinges on the mean QRS axis being less than $-45°$. The mean QRS axis is defined from leads I and III using the Einthoven triangle, except that, instead of taking simultaneous points in time in each lead, the sums of the positive and negative deflections are normally used. Unfortunately, because simultaneity is abandoned, the triangle scheme no longer applies, since the "deflections" in lead II no longer fit the "vector" constructed from the other two leads. The result is not a vector at all and lacks a physical basis. The mean QRS axis was introduced in order to determine some indication of axis *from* the nonsimultaneous data provided by the then-standard single-channel electrocardiograph. The α tracing is a continuous display of the electrical axis throughout the heart cycle with the improvement provided by a scientifically based lead system. With this available, there would seem to be little merit in persisting with a technically inferior and theoretically questionable measure, such as the mean QRS axis, as a diagnostic discriminator. However, with a continuous range of axes available, which should be selected as most representative of QRS events?

The polarcardiographic criteria for left anterior fascicular block are that the longitude of $I\vec{R}$ (❯ Fig. 13.8) is between $-110°$ and $-45°$ with QRS duration <110 ms. The diagnosis is excluded if LBBB, RBBB, LVH, low voltage, inferior infarction, injury, current, or recent infarction are diagnosed. The use of $I\vec{R}$ rather than $\vec{R}$ gives a little more consistency in cases where there are two peaks in the M tracing. The directions of $I\vec{R}$ are generally the same as those of $\vec{R}$ but show slightly less scatter.

Polarcardiographic study of left anterior fascicular block has not revealed any clear-cut set of discriminators, such as those described for LBBB. Perhaps this gives support to the doubts expressed by some concerning the validity of left anterior fascicular block as a clinical entity [14]. Clearly, in this case, some independent "gold standard" would be useful.

Although the computer comment suggesting left anterior fascicular block tends to agree with the visual reading of the derived 12-lead ECG, occasional examples of disagreement should not be a surprise in the light of the foregoing. Of course, these examples could be reduced to zero by the expedient of adopting the mean QRS axis, despite its faults, as the discriminator. This could easily be done but it seems like a backward step.

13.5.5 Left Ventricular Hypertrophy

In the course of developing polarcardiographic criteria for LVH, electrocardiographic and autopsy criteria were closely examined. Problems were encountered with both. Nevertheless, some correlation exists between the mass of cardiac muscle and the strength of the electric field generated by the heart. This is exploited in the voltage criteria of the ECG, but amplitudes in several leads must be measured and correlated because individual variations in the orientation of the maximum heart vector produce maximal projections on different leads. This problem is solved in polarcardiography in which the M tracing gives a direct indication of field strength. Thus, one measurement, M_R, the spatial magnitude of the maximum QRS vector, $\vec{R}$, can replace measurements of several limbs and chest leads of the ECG. Another measurement, m_tR, the magnitude of the projection of $\vec{R}$ in the transverse plane, is also useful because there is a tendency for LVH to be associated with a $20°$ change in longitude of $\vec{R}$ toward the transverse plane, so that m_tR is increased by these two effects. A study of 168 autopsied cases, comparing the ratio of heart weight to body length with M_R and m_tR yielded correlation coefficients of 0.48 and 0.50, respectively [15]. These are not impressive, but fibrosis and scarring was present in many of the cases, and these tend to reduce voltage. (Pure LVH, observed in children, yielded much higher correlations [16].) Performance of ECG voltage criteria, if measurements are carefully made, on tracings obtained with good equipment turns out to be about the same, but not all cases of LVH recognized electrocardiographically meet polarcardiographic criteria for LVH, and vice versa.

An exact definition of LVH is difficult. Heart weights in normal subjects show such a wide variation that a patient's heart weight may undergo 50% hypertrophy, yet still not exceed the upper bounds *for* normal [17]. Taking body length into consideration reduces the spread somewhat but the coefficients of correlation are very low [17]. Body-surface area is commonly employed as a correlate of LVH diagnosed by echocardiography (see also ❯ Chap. 3 of *Electrocardiology: Comprehensive Clinical ECG*). An echopolar study is overdue. Body build, athletic activity, and aging are normal factors that have a pronounced effect on body-surface voltages. If the effects of fibrosis, scarring, and myopathies are added to these, it is easy to appreciate that the diagnosis of LVH from body-surface potentials, whether these are studied as ECGs, VCGs, or vector magnitudes, is apt to be inexact. A further disquieting factor is that some patients show considerable day-to-day variations in voltage, beyond those attributable to differences in electrode placement or electrical activation.

The polarcardiographic criteria for LVH are indicated in ❯ Table 13.2. The appendix (Table A1.96) gives medians and upper 95 percentiles for 466 Cretan villagers for M_R and m_tR. Up to the age of 50 years, M_R is greater in males but gradually reduces with age in men, less clearly so in women. For the entire group, aged 19–82 years, for both sexes, the upper 95 percentiles for M_R and m_tR are 2.25 mV and 2.05 mV, respectively.

Of the ECG criteria of LVH – hypervoltage, left axis deviation, increased ventricular activation, and ST-T changes – only the first, and to some extent the second, have polarcardiographic equivalents (M_R and $m_t R$). The ST-T changes were considered secondary and nonspecific. When abnormal, ST-T-vector directions, as shown on the Aitoff plot, resemble those seen in ischemia. Ventricular activation time is based on the concept of intrinsicoid deflection, which is untenable vectorcardiographically since precordial-lead tracings can be simulated from derivations of the *xyz* signals.

13.5.6 Right Ventricular Hypertrophy

"Probable" right ventricular hypertrophy (RVH) is stated by the computer program if $\vec{R}$ is directed to the right, that is, if the longitude of $\vec{R}$ is not in the range $-90° <$ longitude of $R < +90°$, provided that:

(a) The ratio of maximum anterior forces to maximal posterior forces, during the QRS complex, exceeds 4
(b) $M_P > 0.22\,\text{mV}$
(c) T is not posterior to 50P, and
(d) RBBB is not diagnosed

It is also stated that if the direction of $\vec{R}$ is more than 10° outside the normal bounds, $I\vec{R}$ is not in the range $-I\,10° <$ longitude of $I\vec{R} < +120°$, and the angle between $\vec{R}$ and the direction of the lead I lead vector (59A, + 100) is less than 90°.

13.5.7 Ischemia

In myocardial ischemia, the **T** tend to be distributed around the 180° meridian (see **❯** Table 13.3), that is, approximately 180° from the normal direction of the $\vec{T}$. This corresponds to T-wave inversions in the ECG in ischemia. When ST segments of the ECG are depressed in ischemia, the directions of **ST** tend to parallel those of $\vec{T}$. During exercise testing, ischemia produces characteristic polarcardiographic changes which have been incorporated into an index of ischemia, $M_S\theta$. In the *M* tracing, the S point, instead of lying on or close to the zero baseline, becomes elevated (**❯** Fig. 13.9); M_S increases. The magnitude of the T wave, M_T in the *M* tracing tends to diminish, while that of the ST segment midway between the points S and T is variable. However, the directional change of *ST* is characteristic. The optimal time selected for sampling the directional *ST* changes is 75 ms after IR (**❯** Fig. 13.9) [18]. The directional change from normal is given by the spatial angle θ between the ST_{75} vector so defined and the normal direction of that vector, which is taken as (50A, +20) (latitude and longitude) after exercise, or (50A, +30) at rest. The product of M_S and θ gives the ischemic index $M_S\theta$. Because directions become meaningless as magnitudes reduce to zero, θ is considered to be zero if M_{ST75}, the spatial magnitude of the ST_{75} vector, is $\leqslant 0.04$ mV. For normal subjects, $M_S\theta < 7$ and the test is positive for ischemia if $M_S\theta$ exceeds 10.6; however, $M_S\theta$ may reach 60. Thus, ischemic changes seen in various leads of the ECG are reduced to a single number that has much more resolution than the microvolts of ST depression observed in various leads of the ECG. Furthermore, the ischemic index is easily programmed into the computer. It has shown statistically significant drug-induced changes that could not be demonstrated in the ECGs of the same patients [19].

13.6 Conclusion

The polar approach is but one of many means for studying and characterizing the electric field produced by the heart. Although it may strike the reader as strange, even alien, it often provides a relatively efficient means for categorizing abnormalities. In this regard, its very strangeness can be an asset since previously unrecognized features may be revealed. From a programming standpoint, the polar approach is attractive because it tends to be explicit.

References

1. Einthoven, W., G. Fahr, and A. De Waart, On the direction and manifest size of the variations of potential in the human heart and on the influence of the position of the heart on the form of the electrocardiogram. *Am. Heart J.*, 1950;**40**: 163–194.
2. Dower, G.E., *Polarcardiography*. Springfield, IL: Thomas, 1971, pp. 3–190.
3. Moore, A.D., P. Harding, and G.E. Dower, The polarcardiograph. An analogue computer that provides spherical coordinates of the heart vector. *Am. Heart J.*, 1962;**64**: 382–391.
4. Dower, G.E., D. Berghofer, and M. Kiely, Accuracy of computer measurements of QRS duration using spatial magnitude. Agreement with human readers. *Comput. Biomed. Res.*, 1983;**16**: 433–445.
5. Lerman, J., R.A. Bruce, and J.A. Murray, Correlation of polarcardiographic criteria for myocardial infarction with arteriographic and ventriculographic findings (substantiation of transmural and presentation of non-transmural criteria). *J. Electrocardiol.*, 1976;**9**: 219–226.
6. Niederberger, M., G.E. Dower, and H.B. Machado, Polarcardiographic and vectorcardiographic study of 70 normal children aged 3–4 years. *Clin. Cardiol.*, 1978;**1**: 142–151.
7. Niederberger, M. and G.A. Joskowicz, Global display of the heart vector (spherocardiogram). Applicability of vector and polarcardiographic infarct criteria. *J. Electrocardiol.*, 1977;**10**: 341–346.
8. Dower, G.E., H.E. Horn, and W.G. Ziegler, The polarcardiograph. Diagnosis of myocardial infarction. *Am. Heart J.*, 1965;**69**: 369–381.
9. Dower, G.E. and H.E. Horn, The polarcardiograph. Further studies of normal subjects, refinement of criteria for infarction, and a report on autopsied cases. *Am. Heart J.*, 1966;**72**: 451–462.
10. Dower, G.E., D. Berghofer, and M. Kiely, Polarcardiographic computer system vs cardiologists and derived ECG in diagnosis of infarction, in *Computers in Cardiology*, K.L. Ripley, Editor. New York: IEEE, 1982, pp. 75–80.
11. Dower, G.E., H. Bastos Machado, J.A. Osborne, D. Berghofer, and M. Kiely, Performance of computerized heart vector criteria in the diagnosis of myocardial infarction. *Rev. Port. Cardiol.*, 1984;**3**: 687–697.
12. Aravanis, C., A. Corcondilas, A.S. Dontas, D. Lekos, and A. Keys, IX The Greek islands of Crete and Corfu, in *Coronary Heart Disease in Seven Countries*, A. Keys, Editor. *Circulation*, 1910;**41**(Suppl I): 88–100.
13. Rautaharju, P.M., M. Ariet, T.A. Pryor, et al., Task Force III: computers in diagnostic electrocardiography. *Am. J. Cardiol.*, 1978;**41**: 158–170.
14. Rabkin, S.W., F.A.L. Mathewson, and R.B. Tate, Natural history of marked left axis deviation (left anterior hemiblock). *Am. J. Cardiol.*, 1979;**43**: 605–611.
15. Dower, G.E. and H.E. Horn, The polarcardiograph. Diagnosis of left ventricular hypertrophy. *Am. Heart J.*, 1967;**74**: 368–376.
16. Gamboa, R., P.G. Hugenholtz, and A.S. Nadas, Comparison of electrocardiograms and vectorcardiograms in congenital aortic stenosis. *Br. Heart J.*, 1965;**27**: 344–354.
17. Dower, G.E., H.E. Horn, and W.G. Ziegler, On electrocardiographic-autopsy correlations in left ventricular hypertrophy. A simple postmortem index of hypertrophy proposed. *Am. Heart J.*, 1967;**74**: 351–367.
18. Dower, G.E., R.A. Bruce, J. Pool, M.L. Simoons, M.W. Niederberger, and L.J. Meilink, Ischemic polarcardiographic changes induced by exercise: a new criterion. *Circulation*, 1973;**48**: 725–734.
19. Bruce, R.A., R. Alexander, Y.B. Li, et al., Electrocardiographic responses to maximal exercise in American and Chinese population samples, in *Measurement in Exercise Electrocardiography*, H. Blackburn, Editor. Springfield, IL: Thomas, 1969.

Appendix 1: Adult Normal Limits

P. W. Macfarlane et al. (eds.), *Specialized Aspects of ECG*, DOI 10.1007/978-0-85729-880-5,
© Springer-Verlag London Limited 2012

A1.1 Normal Limits of the 12-Lead ECG in White Caucasians

The data in the following tables have been derived from a study of over 1,450 apparently healthy Caucasians living in the west of Scotland. A few tables are based on smaller numbers. Further details can be found in ❯ Chap. 1 of *Electrocardiology: Comprehensive Clinical ECG*. The results are presented as mean ± standard deviation together with the 96% range; that is, 2% of measurements have been excluded from each extreme of the range. P-, Q, S, T- wave amplitudes are presented as negative measurements (❯ Tables A1.1–A1.31).

▣ Table A1.1
Interval and duration of measurements (in milliseconds) from Caucasian normals

Age-group	Sex	PR interval	QRS duration	QT interval	QTc interval Hodges[a]	QTc interval Bazett[b]	P-wave duration	Heart rate (bpm)
18→29	Male	152.5 ± 23.0	96.4 ± 8.6	385.5 ± 28.9	403.6 ± 19.0	413.9 ± 23.1	103.0 ± 14.2	70 ± 12
		112→208	80→114	336→442	368→444	370→463	72→128	48→98
		n = 265	n = 265	n = 265	n = 265	n = 265	n = 266	n = 266
	Female	145.9 ± 19.7	87.7 ± 7.8	380.0 ± 27.8	411.6 ± 18.0	429.7 ± 22.9	99.0 ± 12.7	76 ± 12
		114→194	72→104	322→440	378→451	386→477	70→122	55→108
		n = 317	n = 317	n = 317	n = 317	n = 317	n = 318	n = 318
30→39	Male	155.7 ± 21.4	95.4 ± 9.8	385.5 ± 29.5	404.8 ± 19.4	416.0 ± 22.9	105.0 ± 12.3	71 ± 12
		116→206	78→114	326→448	366→448	375→468	78→130	52→99
		n = 218	n = 218	n = 218	n = 218	n = 218	n = 221	n = 221
	Female	145.7 ± 18.6	88.6 ± 7.3	386.6 ± 27.7	415.2 ± 16.9	432.6 ± 20.9	99.0 ± 11.6	77 ± 13
		114→184	76→106	330→438	384→445	395→473	72→122	57→105
		n = 115	n = 115	n = 115	n = 115	n = 115	n = 118	n = 118
40→49	Male	157.2 ± 21.8	94.4 ± 9.9	390.8 ± 29.3	409.2 ± 17.9	420.0 ± 21.9	106.0 ± 11.2	70 ± 12
		116→210	78→114	340→450	377→450	377→464	84→128	49→96
		n = 119	n = 119	n = 119	n = 119	n = 119	n = 119	n = 119
	Female	154.9 ± 20.4	89.4 ± 7.9	386.1 ± 27.0	415.2 ± 22.5	433.7 ± 28.4	104.0 ± 12.9	77 ± 12
		108→200	74→108	328→434	347→457	350→483	78→128	59→106
		n = 72	n = 72	n = 72	n = 72	n = 72	n = 73	n = 73
50+	Male	161.5 ± 18.9	92.7 ± 9.3	385.5 ± 26.0	407.4 ± 17.5	420.9 ± 22.7	110.0 ± 10.5	73 ± 12
		120→196	74→112	320→434	374→444	380→475	86→134	54→100
		n = 123	n = 123	n = 123	n = 123	n = 123	n = 125	n = 125
	Female	155.6 ± 6.9	87.1 ± 8.7	390.7 ± 31.5	419.5 ± 22.7	438.2 ± 24.8	106.0 ± 9.5	77 ± 11
		122→196	68→104	336→488	376→486	392→506	88→126	59→104
		n = 79	n = 79	n = 79	n = 79	n = 79	n = 80	n = 80

[a]QTc = QT + 1.75 (rate – 60) – Ref. [107] in ❯ Chap. 1 of *Electrocardiology: Comprehensive Clinical ECG*
[b]QTc = QT (rate/60)$^{1/2}$ – Ref. [106] in ❯ Chap. 1. of *Electrocardiology: Comprehensive Clinical ECG*

▣ Table A1.2
Interval measurements (in milliseconds) from Caucasian normals versus heart rate

Heart rate (bpm)	PR interval	QT interval	QTc interval Hodges[a]	QTc interval Bazett[b]
<50	145.067 ± 18.19	443.6 ± 21.62	420.5 ± 20.49	391.537 ± 17.70
	116→176	396→482	376.75→459.25	357.864→426.6
	n = 15	n = 15	n = 15	n = 15
50→59	154.753 ± 25.81	417.425 ± 21.27	410.197 ± 21.08	402.633 ± 21.28
	110→220	378→468	370→458.5	358.078→454.235
	N = 146	N = 146	n = 146	n = 146

■ Table A1.2 (Continued)

Heart rate (bpm)	PR interval	QT interval	QT$_c$ interval Hodges[a]	QT$_c$ interval Bazett[b]
60→69	154.769 ± 22.62	399.339 ± 21.51	408.173 ± 20.54	415.549 ± 21.38
	116→208	354→444	368.75→450.25	372.64→462.2
	$n = 372$	$n = 372$	$n = 372$	$n = 372$
70→79	151.196 ± 20.28	382.44 ± 19.82	407.516 ± 19.18	425.481 ± 21.51
	114→196	344→426	372.25→452	388.32→477.234
	$n = 408$	$n = 408$	$n = 408$	$n = 408$
80→89	150.51 ± 20.19	367.522 ± 17.36	409.076 ± 16.93	434.074 ± 20.06
	114→194	332→406	376.5→444.5	395.044→474.053
	$n = 247$	$n = 247$	$n = 247$	$n = 247$
90→99	151.368 ± 17.52	356.842 ± 17.59	415.958 ± 17.34	446.019 ± 21.80
	114→182	320→388	383.5→449.25	405.54→488.23
	$n = 114$	$n = 114$	$n = 114$	$n = 114$
≥ 100	151.459 ± 14.14	328.108 ± 16.25	408.372 ± 18.63	435.705 ± 23.93
	130→180	298→352	377.25→439.5	395.685→476.246
	$n = 37$	$n = 37$	$n = 37$	$n = 37$

[a] $QT_c = QT + 1.75(\text{rate} - 60)$
[b] $QT_c = QT (\text{rate}/60)^{1/2}$

■ Table A1.3

Durations (in milliseconds) in Caucasian adults: lead I

Age-group	Sex	Q duration	R duration	S duration
18→29	Male	16 ± 5	45 ± 11	29 ± 11
		9 → 28	27 → 76	9 → 52
		$n = 126$	$n = 224$	$n = 168$
	Female	15 ± 4	46 ± 10	26 ± 9
		7 23	29 → 70	12 → 47
		$n = 127$	$n = 284$	$n = 155$
30→39	Male	17 ± 4	47 ± 12	28 ± 11
		8 → 26	29 → 80	12 → 53
		$n = 121$	$n = 212$	$n = 142$
	Female	16 ± 4	47 ± 11	25 ± 9
		8 → 26	29 → 68	11 → 46
		$n = 53$	$n = 125$	$n = 61$
40→49	Male	17 ± 4	48 ± 12	28 ± 11
		9 → 26	30 → 77	7 → 51
		$n = 115$	$n = 187$	$n = 110$
	Female	15 ± 4	49 ± 10	26 ± 8
		8 → 22	33 → 73	16 → 42
		$n = 52$	$n = 82$	$n = 31$
50+	Male	17 ± 4	50 ± 14	29 ± 10
		9 → 27	31 → 88	13 → 51
		$n = 122$	$n = 197$	$n = 99$
	Female	15 ± 4	50 ± 12	23 ± 7
		7 → 27	27 → 74	12 → 42
		$n = 74$	$n = 124$	$n = 43$

A1

◘ Table A1.4

Durations (in milliseconds) in Caucasian adults: lead II

Age-group	Sex	Q duration	R duration	S duration
18–29	Male	17 ± 5	52 ± 14	26 ± 11
		8 → 26	35 → 84	6 → 49
		n = 162	n = 230	n = 148
	Female	15 ± 4	47 ± 11	25 ± 9
		8 → 26	30 → 74	9 → 44
		n = 182	n = 287	n = 175
30–39	Male	17 ± 5	55 ± 15	27 ± 13
		9 → 28	31 → 88	6 → 56
		n = 118	n = 207	n = 115
	Female	16 ± 4	48 ± 10	24 ± 10
		10 → 23	33 → 72	6 → 46
		n = 95	n = 124	n = 65
40–49	Male	16 ± 4	54 ± 15	29 ± 14
		7 → 24	33 → 90	9 → 57
		n = 94	n = 182	n = 97
	Female	15 ± 4	51 ± 13	25 ± 10
		7 → 24	33 → 78	10 → 45
		n = 45	n = 80	n = 40
50+	Male	16 ± 4	53 ± 14	28 ± 13
		9 → 26	32 → 86	6 → 71
		n = 79	n = 195	n = 122
	Female	15 ± 4	52 ± 13	26 ± 11
		8 → 24	32 → 76	8 → 56
		n = 64	n = 129	n = 57

◘ Table A1.5

Durations (in milliseconds) in Caucasian adults: lead III

Age-group	Sex	Q duration	R duration	S duration
18–29	Male	23 ± 10	47 ± 20	30 ± 17
		10 → 50	11 → 87	6 → 84
		n = 128	n = 221	n = 116
	Female	22 ± 11	40 ± 16	29 ± 14
		9 → 80	10 → 74	7 → 68
		n = 166	n = 278	n = 160
30–39	Male	24 ± 12	42 ± 22	33 ± 20
		9 → 48	8 → 86	7 → 86
		n = 106	n = 205	n = 114
	Female	20 ± 7	41 ± 18	27 ± 16
		10 → 48	9 → 79	7 → 78
		n = 86	n = 123	n = 64

◘ Table A1.5 (Continued)

Age-group	Sex	Q duration	R duration	S duration
40–49	Male	23 ± 11	39 ± 21	37 ± 20
		8 → 58	11 → 86	6 → 79
		n = 72	n = 181	n = 114
	Female	22 ± 12	35 ± 18	36 ± 17
		12 → 78	12 → 74	9 → 70
		n = 33	n = 78	n = 48
50+	Male	26 ± 15	35 ± 20	41 ± 21
		9 → 100	10 → 83	10 → 90
		n = 68	n = 195	n = 137
	Female	22 ± 11	34 ± 18	35 ± 18
		9 → 62	8 → 76	6 → 70
		n = 49	n = 123	n = 82

◘ Table A1.6

Durations (in milliseconds) in Caucasian adults: lead aVR

Age-group	Sex	Q duration	R duration	S duration
18–29	Male	50 ± 13	19 ± 8	46 ± 11
		32 → 92	8 → 44	30 → 75
		n = 74	n = 208	n = 160
	Female	47 ± 9	18 ± 8	45 ± 9
		34 → 74	9 → 38	30 → 65
		n = 130	n = 248	n = 159
30–39	Male	51 ± 13	20 ± 10	50 ± 12
		34 → 84	9 → 50	32 → 78
		n = 91	n = 181	n = 125
	Female	46 ± 10	17 ± 6	45 ± 8
		36 → 78	8 → 39	34 → 65
		n = 41	n = 108	n = 85
40–49	Male	52 ± 12	20 ± 10	50 ± 12
		34 → 78	10 → 49	34 → 75
		n = 76	n = 157	n = 110
	Female	51 ± 13	17 ± 6	48 ± 9
		35 → 84	10 → 36	31 → 66
		n = 32	n = 67	n = 51
50+	Male	52 ± 13	20 ± 9	48 ± 13
		34 → 84	9 → 42	31 → 78
		n = 104	n = 159	n = 95
	Female	53 ± 13	18 ± 7	48 ± 12
		29 → 80	8 → 42	25 → 70
		n = 69	n = 92	n = 61

A1

◼ Table A1.7

Durations (in milliseconds) in Caucasian adults: lead aVL

Age-group	Sex	Q duration	R duration	S duration
18–29	Male	21 ± 13	35 ± 16	39 ± 18
		8 → 74	9 → 77	7 → 75
		n = 100	n = 219	n = 172
	Female	18 ± 6	38 ± 16	30 ± 14
		8 → 35	13 → 74	7 → 62
		n = 107	n = 284	n = 187
30–39	Male	20 ± 10	39 ± 17	37 ± 16
		9 → 68	11 → 79	7 → 71
		n = 114	n = 209	n = 158
	Female	18 ± 5	37 ± 16	33 ± 16
		9 → 29	10 → 76	8 → 66
		n = 40	n = 125	n = 82
40–49	Male	19 ± 7	41 ± 16	33 ± 15
		10 → 45	12 → 75	7 → 67
		n = 113	n = 186	n = 118
	Female	17 ± 4	45 ± 14	29 ± 13
		11 → 25	21 → 72	12 → 56
		n = 46	n = 82	n = 38
50+	Male	20 ± 10	46 ± 17	34 ± 16
		10 → 52	19 → 89	10 → 72
		n = 125	n = 196	n = 98
	Female	17 ± 6	45 ± 14	27 ± 13
		8 → 38	15 → 69	5 → 61
		n = 71	n = 124	n = 56

◼ Table A1.8

Durations (in milliseconds) in Caucasian adults: lead aVF

Age-group	Sex	Q duration	R duration	S duration
18–29	Male	19 ± 5	53 ± 17	28 ± 13
		9 → 27	15 → 90	8 → 69
		n = 143	n = 231	n = 129
	Female	17 ± 5	47 ± 12	27 ± 9
		8 → 28	25 → 74	12 → 49
		n = 174	n = 288	n = 162
30–39	Male	18 ± 5	55 ± 17	31 ± 16
		8 → 32	23 → 90	7 → 74
		n = 110	n = 208	n = 95
	Female	17 ± 4	47 ± 12	24 ± 10
		8 → 23	29 → 74	6 → 48
		n = 89	n = 124	n = 66

◘ Table A1.8 (Continued)

Age-group	Sex	Q duration	R duration	S duration
40–49	Male	17 ± 5	51 ± 19	32 ± 18
		9 → 28	13 → 92	6 → 80
		n = 76	n = 183	n = 102
	Female	16 ± 4	48 ± 14	27 ± 11
		9 → 24	20 → 76	11 → 53
		n = 36	n = 81	n = 43
50+	Male	18 ± 7	49 ± 18	33 ± 18
		9 → 52	15 → 88	8 → 79
		n = 73	n = 198	n = 125
	Female	16 ± 5	48 ± 15	31 ± 14
		8 → 28	18 → 78	9 → 69
		n = 55	n = 129	n = 62

◘ Table A1.9

Durations (in milliseconds) in Caucasian adults: lead V_1

Age-group	Sex	Q duration	R duration	S duration
18–29	Male	80	31 ± 6	55 ± 10
		80 → 80	20 → 46	30 → 76
		n = 1	n = 228	n = 229
	Female	57 ± 31	26 ± 5	54 ± 9
		3 → 78	14 → 37	32 → 71
		n = 5	n = 282	n = 282
30–39	Male	46 ± 31	28 ± 7	57 ± 9
		11 → 74	11 → 42	34 → 75
		n = 4	n = 210	n = 210
	Female		26 ± 5	55 ± 8
			16 → 36	37 → 68
			n = 126	n = 126
40–49	Male	68 ± 5	28 ± 7	57 ± 10
		58 → 72	15 → 45	29 → 75
		n = 6	n = 179	n = 179
	Female	60 ± 8	24 ± 5	57 ± 8
		54 → 66	12 → 32	45 → 78
		n = 2	n = 80	n = 80
50+	Male	38 ± 34	27 ± 6	56 ± 10
		14 → 62	15 → 45	34 → 79
		n = 2	n = 198	n = 198
	Female	9	24 ± 7	55 ± 9
		9 → 9	10 → 39	28 → 71
		n = 1	n = 125	n = 125

◘ Table A1.10

Durations (in milliseconds) in Caucasian adults: lead V_2

Age-group	Sex	Q duration	R duration	S duration
18–29	Male	74	33 ± 7	52 ± 9
		$74 \to 74$	$21 \to 48$	$36 \to 72$
		$n = 1$	$n = 228$	$n = 228$
	Female	9 ± 6	30 ± 7	52 ± 9
		$5 \to 13$	$17 \to 44$	$31 \to 70$
		$n = 2$	$n = 281$	$n = 280$
30–39	Male	41 ± 35	33 ± 9	54 ± 10
		$16 \to 66$	$20 \to 47$	$31 \to 73$
		$n = 2$	$n = 208$	$n = 207$
	Female		31 ± 6	52 ± 9
			$19 \to 45$	$29 \to 67$
			$n = 126$	$n = 126$
40–49	Male	72 ± 5	34 ± 8	51 ± 11
		$66 \to 76$	$19 \to 52$	$31 \to 75$
		$n = 3$	$n = 180$	$n = 180$
	Female	36 ± 40	30 ± 7	51 ± 10
		$8 \to 64$	$18 \to 47$	$29 \to 71$
		$n = 2$	$n = 82$	$n = 82$
50+	Male	30 ± 35	35 ± 8	49 ± 11
		$8 \to 82$	$20 \to 55$	$26 \to 73$
		$n = 4$	$n = 199$	$n = 199$
	Female	44 ± 42	30 ± 7	50 ± 9
		$14 \to 74$	$16 \to 45$	$27 \to 67$
		$n = 2$	$n = 126$	$n = 126$

◘ Table A1.11

Durations (in milliseconds) in Caucasian adults: lead V_3

Age-group	Sex	Q duration	R duration	S duration
18–29	Male	12 ± 5	43 ± 10	40 ± 13
		$8 \to 17$	$25 \to 62$	$16 \to 63$
		$n = 3$	$n = 229$	$n = 227$
	Female	23 ± 27	42 ± 9	37 ± 12
		$5 \to 62$	$23 \to 59$	$12 \to 60$
		$n = 4$	$n = 284$	$n = 275$
30–39	Male	14 ± 4	43 ± 10	42 ± 12
		$6 \to 18$	$26 \to 74$	$15 \to 62$
		$n = 8$	$n = 208$	$n = 204$
	Female		43 ± 10	38 ± 13
			$23 \to 74$	$15 \to 63$
			$n = 124$	$n = 118$

◘ Table A1.11   (Continued)

Age-group	Sex	Q duration	R duration	S duration
40–49	Male	14 ± 4	43 ± 9	41 ± 13
		9 → 18	26 → 62	14 → 65
		n = 5	n = 185	n = 182
	Female	13 ± 2	41 ± 8	39 ± 11
		11 → 14	22 → 60	18 → 58
		n = 2	n = 81	n = 79
50+	Male	12 ± 5	43 ± 10	41 ± 13
		5 → 21	27 → 66	18 → 68
		n = 13	n = 192	n = 190
	Female	12 ± 5	40 ± 8	39 ± 11
		8 → 20	22 → 58	18 → 60
		n = 5	n = 128	n = 125

◘ Table A1.12

Durations (in milliseconds) in Caucasian adults: lead V_4

Age-group	Sex	Q duration	R duration	S duration
18–29	Male	16 ± 6	46 ± 10	28 ± 11
		7 → 29	32 → 78	7 → 53
		n = 86	n = 227	n = 209
	Female	14 ± 4	44 ± 9	29 ± 9
		8 → 25	31 → 72	12 → 46
		n = 72	n = 284	n = 242
30–39	Male	14 ± 4	46 ± 10	32 ± 11
		8 → 27	33 → 86	11 → 57
		n = 62	n = 210	n = 193
	Female	16 ± 4	45 ± 9	32 ± 10
		8 → 24	33 → 73	15 → 53
		n = 35	n = 125	n = 97
40–49	Male	13 ± 4	46 ± 9	33 ± 12
		7 → 25	34 → 76	12 → 61
		n = 49	n = 184	n = 169
	Female	12 ± 4	44 ± 8	32 ± 11
		5 → 19	34 → 66	12 → 54
		n = 15	n = 80	n = 70
50+	Male	14 ± 4	44 ± 9	35 ± 13
		8 → 24	31 → 72	12 → 57
		n = 54	n = 199	n = 188
	Female	13 ± 4	42 ± 7	33 ± 10
		9 → 23	29 → 60	13 → 58
		n = 28	n = 128	n = 122

◘ Table A1.13

Durations (in milliseconds) in Caucasian adults: lead V_5

Age-group	Sex	Q duration	R duration	S duration
18–29	Male	17 ± 5	45 ± 12	27 ± 11
		9 → 27	30 → 80	6 → 49
		$n = 171$	$n = 230$	$n = 181$
	Female	14 ± 4	42 ± 9	27 ± 9
		8 → 24	29 → 69	10 → 46
		$n = 148$	$n = 288$	$n = 214$
30–39	Male	16 ± 5	46 ± 11	28 ± 12
		8 → 25	31 → 86	10 → 58
		$n = 127$	$n = 211$	$n = 179$
	Female	15 ± 5	43 ± 10	27 ± 9
		8 → 26	31 → 71	12 → 45
		$n = 79$	$n = 124$	$n = 88$
40–49	Male	15 ± 4	45 ± 10	29 ± 12
		7 → 24	33 → 79	8 → 55
		$n = 103$	$n = 186$	$n = 149$
	Female	13 ± 4	44 ± 9	29 ± 10
		8 → 20	33 → 67	12 → 51
		$n = 35$	$n = 81$	$n = 64$
50+	Male	15 ± 4	45 ± 11	33 ± 12
		8 → 26	31 → 78	11 → 68
		$n = 101$	$n = 198$	$n = 160$
	Female	14 ± 4	43 ± 9	28 ± 10
		8 → 25	28 → 66	13 → 49
		$n = 62$	$n = 128$	$n = 98$

■ Table A1.14

Durations (in milliseconds) in Caucasian adults: lead V_6

Age group	Sex	Q duration	R duration	S duration
18–29	Male	18 ± 5	47 ± 12	25 ± 11
		10 → 28	31 → 76	6 → 46
		n = 202	n = 228	n = 137
	Female	16 ± 4	44 ± 9	24 ± 8
		9 → 25	30 → 70	12 → 42
		n = 215	n = 289	n = 161
30–39	Male	17 ± 4	49 ± 13	26 ± 12
		8 → 26	31 → 82	8 → 58
		n = 159	n = 208	n = 129
	Female	17 ± 5	45 ± 9	25 ± 8
		10 → 28	34 → 71	11 → 45
		n = 104	n = 124	n = 59
40–49	Male	16 ± 4	50 ± 11	29 ± 11
		8 → 24	34 → 76	12 → 52
		n = 139	n = 186	n = 96
	Female	15 ± 4	47 ± 10	26 ± 8
		8 → 23	33 → 68	14 → 42
		n = 51	n = 82	n = 42
50+	Male	16 ± 4	48 ± 12	30 ± 11
		9 → 25	31 → 78	12 → 57
		n = 130	n = 195	n = 124
	Female	15 ± 4	48 ± 11	25 ± 9
		8 → 23	30 → 72	12 → 47
		n = 80	n = 128	n = 60

▢ Table A1.15

Amplitudes (in millivolts) in Caucasian adults: lead I

Age group	Sex	P+	P−	Q	R	S	STj	T+	T−
18–29	Male	0.099 ± 0.029 0.055–0.174 n = 224	−0.020 ± 0.000 −0.020–0.000 n = 1	−0.074 ± 0.051 −0.238–0.000 n = 126	0.756 ± 0.333 0.202–1.624 n = 224	−0.227 ± 0.139 −0.568–0.000 n = 168	0.031 ± 0.022 −0.006–0.077 n = 224	0.343 ± 0.116 0.116–0.641 n = 224	
	Female	0.101 ± 0.026 0.056–0.161 n = 283	−0.058 ± 0.011 −0.066–0.000 n = 2	−0.070 ± 0.046 −0.225–0.000 n = 127	0.699 ± 0.283 0.226–1.411 n = 284	−0.163 ± 0.096 −0.468–0.000 n = 155	0.011 ± 0.015 −0.022–0.038 n = 284	0.283 ± 0.093 0.112–0.506 n = 284	
30–39	Male	0.102 ± 0.027 0.056–0.163 n = 212	−0.019 ± 0.001 −0.019–0.000 n = 2	−0.070 ± 0.046 −0.223–0.000 n = 121	0.807 ± 0.353 0.251–1.685 n = 212	−0.189 ± 0.122 −0.536–0.000 n = 142	0.023 ± 0.019 −0.011–0.061 n = 212	0.300 ± 0.099 0.119–0.522 n = 212	
	Female	0.102 ± 0.032 0.051–0.202 n = 124	−0.023 ± 0.000 −0.023–0.000 n = 1	−0.070 ± 0.044 −0.208–0.000 n = 52	0.666 ± 0.290 0.198–1.557 n = 124	−0.145 ± 0.103 −0.622–0.000 n = 61	0.008 ± 0.017 −0.028–0.042 n = 124	0.257 ± 0.093 0.096–0.478 n = 124	
40–49	Male	0.098 ± 0.032 0.045–0.184 n = 207	−0.024 ± 0.016 −0.038–0.000 n = 4	−0.069 ± 0.041 −0.173–0.000 n = 125	0.791 ± 0.331 0.286–1.509 n = 207	−0.159 ± 0.100 −0.465–0.000 n = 121	0.019 ± 0.020 −0.017–0.074 n = 207	0.271 ± 0.105 0.105–0.547 n = 207	−0.087 ± 0.000 −0.087–0.000 n = 1
	Female	0.103 ± 0.026 0.055–0.184 n = 89	−0.038 ± 0.000 −0.038–0.000 n = 1	−0.068 ± 0.042 −0.191–0.000 n = 56	0.773 ± 0.256 0.374–1.414 n = 89	−0.129 ± 0.078 −0.351–0.000 n = 32	0.010 ± 0.018 −0.027–0.046 n = 89	0.245 ± 0.090 0.095–0.461 n = 89	−0.021 ± 0.000 −0.021–0.000 n = 1
50+	Male	0.097 ± 0.030 0.043–0.166 n = 200	−0.019 ± 0.008 −0.024–0.000 n = 2	−0.072 ± 0.045 −0.195–0.000 n = 125	0.800 ± 0.272 0.292–1.416 n = 200	−0.145 ± 0.087 −0.404–0.000 n = 99	0.015 ± 0.020 −0.028–0.060 n = 200	0.234 ± 0.097 0.079–0.502 n = 200	
	Female	0.102 ± 0.029 0.052–0.179 n = 125	−0.029 ± 0.000 −0.029–0.000 n = 1	−0.067 ± 0.043 −0.277–0.000 n = 54	0.807 ± 0.299 0.231–1.544 n = 125	−0.119 ± 0.081 −0.339–0.000 n = 44	0.004 ± 0.018 −0.039–0.032 n = 125	0.218 ± 0.098 0.060–0.452 n = 124	−0.036 ± 0.036 −0.087–0.000 n = 4

◼ Table A1.16
Amplitudes (in millivolts) in Caucasian adults: lead II

Age group	Sex	P+	P−	Q	R	S	STj	T+	T−
18–29	Male	0.148 ± 0.057 0.040–0.294 n = 229	−0.028–0.027 −0.124–0.000 n = 16	−0.089 ± 0.057 −0.251–0.000 n = 162	1.364 ± 0.428 0.566–2.357 n = 230	0.212 ± 0.126 −0.538–0.000 n = 148	0.041 ± 0.033 −0.015–0.117 n = 230	0.419 ± 0.141 0.150–0.780 n = 230	−0.022 ± 0.001 −0.023–0.000 n = 2
	Female	0.149 ± 0.055 0.052–0.305 n = 287	−0.029 ± 0.024 −0.086–0.000 n = 8	−0.075 ± 0.052 −0.202–0.000 n = 182	1.133 ± 0.340 0.523–1.828 n = 287	−0.169 ± 0.097 −0.437–0.000 n = 175	0.012 ± 0.024 −0.037–0.058 n = 287	0.334 ± 0.110 0.147–0.617 n = 287	
30–39	Male	0.150 ± 0.052 0.043–0.281 n = 207	−0.020 ± 0.004 −0.025–0.000 n = 7	−0.089 ± 0.061 −0.343–0.000 n = 118	1.118 ± 0.424 0.412–2.230 n = 207	−0.198 ± 0.143 −0.617–0.000 n = 115	0.033 ± 0.029 −0.025–0.101 n = 207	0.363 ± 0.131 0.142–0.710 n = 207	
	Female	0.158 ± 0.056 0.055–0.274 n = 123		−0.079 ± 0.044 −0.178–0.000 n = 95	1.080 ± 0.335 0.450–1.793 n = 123	−0.158 ± 0.110 −0.579–0.000 n = 65	0.007 ± 0.027 −0.069–0.074 n = 123	0.302 ± 0.106 0.118–0.554 n = 123	−0.064 ± 0.000 −0.064–0.000 n = 1
40–49	Male	0.145 ± 0.047 0.062–0.274 n = 200	−0.041 ± 0.013 −0.052–0.000 n = 4	−0.063 ± 0.039 −0.187–0.000 n = 103	0.911 ± 0.370 0.267–1.731 n = 201	−0.197 ± 0.147 −0.731–0.000 n = 108	0.026 ± 0.030 −0.042–0.088 n = 201	0.336 ± 0.125 0.136–0.656 n = 201	
	Female	0.144 ± 0.051 0.058–0.258 n = 87	−0.022 ± 0.008 −0.031–0.000 n = 3	−0.060 ± 0.037 −0.192–0.000 n = 48	0.886 ± 0.280 0.491–1.438 n = 87	−0.159 ± 0.111 −0.622–0.000 n = 43	0.014 ± 0.022 −0.029–0.053 n = 87	0.282 ± 0.095 0.100–0.523 n = 87	−0.027 ± 0.000 −0.027–0.000 n = 1
50+	Male	0.144 ± 0.047 0.047–0.242 n = 198	−0.018 ± 0.003 −0.023–0.000 n = 6	−0.072 ± 0.051 −0.200–0.000 n = 79	0.835 ± 0.368 0.258–1.980 n = 198	−0.188 ± 0.156 −0.719–0.000 n = 124	0.022 ± 0.026 −0.030–0.079 n = 198	0.304 ± 0.115 0.114–0.590 n = 198	−0.057 ± 0.000 −0.057–0.000 n = 1
	Female	0.153 ± 0.054 0.066–0.270 n = 130	−0.021 ± 0.013 −0.038–0.000 n = 5	−0.063 ± 0.037 −0.187–0.000 n = 64	0.865 ± 0.296 0.401–1.534 n = 130	−0.179 ± 0.106 −0.447–0.000 n = 57	0.005 ± 0.025 −0.066–0.053 n = 130	0.270 ± 0.101 0.079–0.498 n = 130	−0.067 ± 0.038 −0.131–0.000 n = 7

■ Table A1.17

Amplitudes (in millivolts) in Caucasian adults: lead III

Age group	Sex	P+	P-	Q	R	S	STJ	T+	T-
18–29	Male	0.086 ± 0.049 0.000–0.224 n = 197	−0.049 ± 0.030 −0.165–0.000 n = 104	−0.134 ± 0.111 −0.531–0.000 n = 128	0.777 ± 0.562 0.000–2.115 n = 221	−0.224 ± 0.230 −1.140–0.000 n = 116	0.009 ± 0.025 −0.053–0.062 n = 225	0.142 ± 0.095 0.000–0.381 n = 187	−0.101 ± 0.081 −0.304–0.000 n = 77
	Female	0.082 ± 0.048 0.000–0.220 n = 252	−0.038 ± 0.024 −0.104–0.000 n = 125	−0.110 ± 0.091 −0.562–0.000 n = 166	0.560 ± 0.391 0.000–1.475 n = 278	−0.209 ± 0.180 −0.912–0.000 n = 160	0.001 ± 0.019 −0.034–0.039 n = 282	0.093 ± 0.061 0.000–0.276 n = 245	−0.058 ± 0.044 −0.207–0.000 n = 109
30–39	Male	0.084 ± 0.045 0.000–0.206 n = 188	−0.044 ± 0.021 −0.105–0.000 n = 90	−0.130 ± 0.095 −0.429–0.000 n = 105	0.524 ± 0.477 0.000–1.813 n = 205	−0.328 ± 0.290 −1.261–0.000 n = 114	0.010 ± 0.021 −0.031–0.055 n = 206	0.123 ± 0.092 0.000–0.399 n = 172	−0.076 ± 0.052 −0.248–0.000 n = 78
	Female	0.088 ± 0.050 0.000–0.216 n = 113	−0.041 ± 0.022 −0.109–0.000 n = 51	−0.110 ± 0.085 −0.399–0.000 n = 86	0.542 ± 0.356 0.000–1.407 n = 122	−0.204 ± 0.198 −1.002–0.000 n = 63	−0.001 ± 0.021 −0.051–0.043 n = 124	0.089 ± 0.061 0.000–0.284 n = 106	−0.055 ± 0.043 −0.175–0.000 n = 59
40–49	Male	0.082 ± 0.042 0.000–0.190 n = 189	−0.044 ± 0.028 −0.134–0.000 n = 90	−0.116 ± 0.106 −0.478–0.000 n = 81	0.381 ± 0.307 0.000–1.483 n = 200	−0.348 ± 0.307 −1.120–0.000 n = 129	0.007 ± 0.025 −0.033–0.050 n = 204	0.123 ± 0.091 0.000–0.362 n = 164	−0.074 ± 0.057 −0.228–0.000 n = 80
	Female	0.072 ± 0.041 0.000–0.187 n = 80	−0.042 ± 0.024 −0.100–0.000 n = 38	−0.079 ± 0.058 −0.319–0.000 n = 35	0.295 ± 0.253 0.000–1.033 n = 85	−0.292 ± 0.245 0.000–1.269 n = 54	0.004 ± 0.016 −0.028–0.037 n = 86	0.080 ± 0.066 0.000–0.298 n = 73	−0.056 ± 0.040 −0.161–0.000 n = 35
50+	Male	0.081 ± 0.043 0.000–0.184 n = 190	−0.044 ± 0.023 −0.113–0.000 n = 90	−0.140 ± 0.143 −0.847–0.000 n = 68	0.322 ± 0.329 0.000–1.422 n = 198	−0.382 ± 0.315 −1.235–0.000 n = 140	0.007 ± 0.022 −0.038–0.064 n = 200	0.117 ± 0.094 0.000–0.423 n = 169	−0.068 ± 0.054 −0.236–0.000 n = 72
	Female	0.083 ± 0.045 0.000–0.209 n = 120	−0.039 ± 0.024 −0.126–0.000 n = 49	−0.103 ± 0.123 −0.849–0.000 n = 50	0.290 ± 0.249 0.000–0.944 n = 124	−0.336 ± 0.272 −1.080–0.000 n = 83	0.001 ± 0.019 −0.048–0.038 n = 126	0.091 ± 0.063 0.000–0.274 n = 109	−0.059 ± 0.050 −0.196–0.000 n = 47

Table A1.18

Amplitudes (in millivolts) in Caucasian adults: lead aVR

Age group	Sex	P+	P-	Q	R	S	STj	T+	T-
18–29	Male	0.024 ± 0.012 0.000–0.041 n = 4	-0.119 ± 0.034 -0.194 to -0.058 n = 231	-0.942 ± 0.237 -1.408–0.000 n = 74	0.093 ± 0.083 0.000–0.360 n = 208	-1.060 ± 0.261 -1.583–0.000 n = 160	-0.036 ± 0.025 -0.086–0.011 n = 231		-0.379 ± 0.109 -0.631 to -0.179 n = 231
	Female	0.023 ± 0.008 0.000–0.032 n = 3	-0.120 ± 0.033 -0.205 to -0.059 n = 289	-0.811 ± 0.226 -1.379–0.000 n = 130	0.085 ± 0.065 0.000–0.250 n = 248	-0.959 ± 0.230 -1.443–0.000 n = 160	0.012 ± 0.017 -0.051–0.020 n = 289		-0.307 ± 0.092 -0.504 to -0.153 n = 289
30–39	Male		-0.121 ± 0.031 -0.197 to -0.062 n = 215	-0.871 ± 0.248 -1.564–0.000 n = 91	0.104 ± 0.093 0.000–0.380 n = 181	-0.990 ± 0.275 -1.557–0.000 n = 125	-0.029 ± 0.022 -0.096–0.014 n = 215		-0.332 ± 0.098 -0.573 to -0.140 n = 215
	Female		-0.127 ± 0.035 -0.220 to -0.063 n = 124	-0.723 ± 0.212 -1.247–0.000 n = 41	0.071 ± 0.052 0.000–0.269 n = 107	-0.909 ± 0.242 -1.447–0.000 n = 84	-0.008 ± 0.020 -0.060–0.032 n = 124		-0.279 ± 0.090 -0.497 to -0.121 n = 124
40–49	Male	0.032 ± 0.007 0.000–0.026 n = 3	-0.115 ± 0.031 -0.196 to -0.060 n = 206	-0.764 ± 0.218 -1.210–0.000 n = 86	0.087 ± 0.084 0.000–0.310 n = 175	-0.893 ± 0.233 -1.403–0.000 n = 120	-0.022 ± 0.022 -0.080–0.019 n = 206		-0.302 ± 0.098 -0.539 to -0.146 n = 206
	Female	0.033 ± 0.000 0.000–0.033 n = 1	-0.121 ± 0.032 -0.194 to -0.062 n = 90	-0.719 ± 0.208 -1.357–0.000 n = 35	0.065 ± 0.043 0.000–0.239 n = 74	-0.872 ± 0.203 -1.310–0.000 n = 56	-0.011 ± 0.019 -0.049–0.024 n = 90	0.024 ± 0.000 0.000–0.024 n = 1	-0.263 ± 0.082 -0.413 to -0.096 n = 90
50+	Male	0.025 ± 0.000 0.000–0.025 n = 1	-0.115 ± 0.030 -0.176 to -0.057 n = 200	-0.748 ± 0.202 -1.352–0.000 n = 104	0.086 ± 0.074 0.000–0.372 n = 162	-0.840 ± 0.246 -1.404–0.000 n = 98	-0.018 ± 0.020 -0.063–0.024 n = 200		-0.268 ± 0.088 -0.468 to -0.115 n = 200
	Female	0.034 ± 0.000 0.000–0.034 n = 1	-0.122 ± 0.035 -0.195 to -0.061 n = 130	-0.766 ± 0.193 -1.238–0.000 n = 70	0.077 ± 0.056 0.000–0.215 n = 92	-0.877 ± 0.252 -1.407–0.000 n = 61	-0.005 ± 0.019 -0.037–0.040 n = 130	0.041 ± 0.023 0.000–0.072 n = 5	0.246 ± 0.086 -0.452 to -0.092 n = 128

Table A1.19

Amplitudes (in millivolts) in Caucasian adults: lead aVL

Age group	Sex	P+	P−	Q	R	S	STj	T+	T−
18–29	Male	0.055 ± 0.028 0.000–0.120 n = 197	−0.036 ± 0.021 −0.092–0.000 n = 106	−0.105 ± 0.113 −0.492–0.000 n = 100	0.311 ± 0.279 0.027–1.254 n = 219	−0.387 ± 0.261 −1.098–0.000 n = 172	0.011 ± 0.017 −0.019–0.045 n = 225	0.154 ± 0.096 0.020–0.412 n = 215	−0.043 ± 0.029 −0.124–0.000 n = 28
	Female	0.052 ± 0.023 0.000–0.111 n = 253	−0.032 ± 0.023 −0.100–0.000 n = 132	−0.082 ± 0.053 −0.254–0.000 n = 107	0.283 ± 0.223 0.040–0.980 n = 284	−0.253 ± 0.206 −0.871–0.000 n = 187	0.005 ± 0.012 −0.021–0.030 n = 285	0.124 ± 0.067 0.014–0.284 n = 280	−0.023 ± 0.018 −0.066–0.000 n = 22
30–39	Male	0.054 ± 0.024 0.000–0.114 n = 192	−0.033 ± 0.018 −0.097–0.000 n = 108	−0.086 ± 0.059 −0.287–0.000 n = 114	0.414 ± 0.310 0.040–1.199 n = 209	−0.288 ± 0.219 −0.845–0.000 n = 158	0.006 ± 0.013 −0.021–0.034 n = 212	0.136 ± 0.075 0.022–0.334 n = 197	−0.051 ± 0.034 −0.122–0.000 n = 24
	Female	0.053 ± 0.027 0.000–0.123 n = 103	−0.035 ± 0.022 −0.106–0.000 n = 66	−0.077 ± 0.047 −0.203–0.000 n = 39	0.256 ± 0.241 0.027–1.163 n = 124	−0.217 ± 0.147 −0.614–0.000 n = 82	0.005 ± 0.014 −0.030–0.030 n = 124	0.117 ± 0.068 0.010–0.307 n = 123	−0.030 ± 0.020 −0.071–0.000 n = 12
40–49	Male	0.055 ± 0.028 0.000–0.114 n = 176	−0.033 ± 0.017 −0.083–0.000 n = 107	−0.082 ± 0.048 −0.221–0.000 n = 123	0.430 ± 0.326 0.032–1.161 n = 206	−0.220 ± 0.166 −0.799–0.000 n = 130	0.006 ± 0.017 −0.023–0.039 n = 207	0.128 ± 0.081 0.015–0.348 n = 186	−0.051 ± 0.034 −0.155–0.000 n = 32
	Female	0.052 ± 0.024 0.000–0.113 n = 81	−0.029 ± 0.017 −0.088–0.000 n = 40	−0.081 ± 0.055 −0.298–0.000 n = 50	0.397 ± 0.255 0.040–1.070 n = 89	−0.173 ± 0.115 −0.456–0.000 n = 40	0.003 ± 0.013 −0.022–0.023 n = 89	0.114 ± 0.067 0.017–0.285 n = 85	−0.031 ± 0.015 −0.058–0.000 n = 9
50+	Male	0.055 ± 0.026 0.000–0.114 n = 171	−0.034 ± 0.017 −0.085–0.000 n = 117	−0.093 ± 0.054 −0.243–0.000 n = 128	0.478 ± 0.298 0.037–1.191 n = 199	−0.212 ± 0.156 −0.648–0.000 n = 98	0.004 ± 0.017 −0.032–0.050 n = 202	0.109 ± 0.077 0.010–0.324 n = 179	−0.050 ± 0.039 −0.181–0.000 n = 45
	Female	0.051 ± 0.024 0.000–0.121 n = 110	−0.033 ± 0.018 −0.097–0.000 n = 65	−0.081 ± 0.052 −0.302–0.000 n = 71	0.441 ± 0.293 0.028–1.209 n = 125	−0.159 ± 0.117 −0.468–0.000 n = 57	0.001 ± 0.013 −0.027–0.025 n = 126	0.096 ± 0.072 0.011–0.316 n = 119	−0.035 ± 0.029 −0.128–0.000 n = 26

Table A1.20

Amplitudes (in millivolts) in Caucasian adults: lead aVF

Age group	Sex	P+	P-	Q	R	S	STJ	T+	T-
18–29	Male	0.111 ± 0.054	−0.034 ± 0.025	−0.095 ± 0.058	1.038 ± 0.510	−0.186 ± 0.121	0.025 ± 0.027	0.258 ± 0.122	−0.056 ± 0.052
		0.000–0.257	−0.144–0.000	−0.257–0.000	0.038–2.117	−0.489–0.000	−0.037–0.085	0.034–0.576	−0.164–0.000
		n = 226	n = 39	n = 143	n = 231	n = 129	n = 231	n = 229	n = 10
	Female	0.109 ± 0.052	−0.026 ± 0.022	−0.079 ± 0.049	0.822 ± 0.363	−0.163 ± 0.106	0.007 ± 0.020	0.198 ± 0.085	−0.041 ± 0.012
		0.000–0.237	−0.119–0.000	−0.203–0.000	0.174–1.652	−0.500–0.000	−0.037–0.045	0.055–0.411	−0.062–0.000
		n = 283	n = 30	n = 174	n = 288	n = 162	n = 288	n = 287	n = 9
30–39	Male	0.112 ± 0.047	−0.028 ± 0.014	−0.085 ± 0.059	0.772 ± 0.458	−0.217 ± 0.167	0.022 ± 0.023	0.222 ± 0.114	−0.029 ± 0.010
		0.000–0.237	−0.062–0.000	−0.320–0.000	0.072–2.015	−0.770–0.000	−0.023–0.070	0.033–0.546	−0.036–0.000
		n = 202	n = 26	n = 110	n = 208	n = 95	n = 208	n = 208	n = 6
	Female	0.118 ± 0.053	−0.021 ± 0.013	−0.078 ± 0.048	0.781 ± 0.348	−0.143 ± 0.104	0.003 ± 0.023	0.180 ± 0.083	−0.038 ± 0.024
		0.000–0.243	−0.052–0.000	−0.182–0.000	0.085–1.533	−0.532–0.000	−0.056–0.058	0.031–0.366	−0.069–0.000
		n = 121	n = 11	n = 89	n = 123	n = 66	n = 123	n = 123	n = 6
40–49	Male	0.107 ± 0.045	−0.033 ± 0.021	−0.065 ± 0.040	0.575 ± 0.383	−0.194 ± 0.171	0.016 ± 0.026	0.207 ± 0.109	−0.031 ± 0.013
		0.000–0.224	−0.075–0.000	−0.179–0.000	0.047–1.466	−0.955–0.000	−0.032–0.067	0.040–0.501	−0.047–0.000
		n = 201	n = 20	n = 85	n = 203	n = 115	n = 203	n = 202	n = 9
	Female	0.013 ± 0.046	−0.027 ± 0.011	−0.059 ± 0.031	0.529 ± 0.284	−0.174 ± 0.145	0.009 ± 0.017	0.164 ± 0.078	−0.028 ± 0.013
		0.000–0.223	−0.049–0.000	−0.147–0.000	0.093–1.231	−0.910–0.000	−0.029–0.047	0.055–0.404	−0.046–0.000
		n = 87	n = 10	n = 38	n = 88	n = 46	n = 88	n = 88	n = 4
50+	Male	0.108 ± 0.044	−0.026 ± 0.015	−0.072 ± 0.050	0.499 ± 0.373	−0.222 ± 0.205	0.014 ± 0.022	0.191 ± 0.105	−0.031 ± 0.021
		0.000–0.211	−0.069–0.000	−0.233–0.000	0.032–1.778	−0.977–0.000	−0.037–0.065	0.033–0.486	−0.062–0.000
		n = 200	n = 27	n = 73	n = 202	n = 127	n = 202	n = 202	n = 7
	Female	0.113 ± 0.050	−0.028 ± 0.015	−0.057 ± 0.029	0.509 ± 0.297	−0.216 ± 0.149	0.003 ± 0.021	0.165 ± 0.078	−0.049 ± 0.041
		0.000–0.238	−0.067–0.000	−0.154–0.000	0.100–1.198	−0.709–0.000	−0.058–0.042	0.040–0.339	−0.156–0.000
		n = 129	n = 14	n = 55	n = 130	n = 62	n = 130	n = 130	n = 13

Table A1.21

Amplitudes (in millivolts) in Caucasian adults: lead V_1

Age group	Sex	P+	P-	Q	R	S	STJ	T+	T-
18–29	Male	0.073 ± 0.031 0.000–0.140 n = 229	−0.039 ± 0.017 −0.091–0.000 n = 151	−1.317 ± 0.000 −1.317–0.000 n = 1	0.392 ± 0.200 0.102–0.906 n = 229	−1.302 ± 0.455 −2.246 to −0.503 n = 229	0.055 ± 0.041 −0.029–0.135 n = 230	0.194 ± 0.147 0.000–0.593 n = 201	−0.115 ± 0.082 −0.290–0.000 n = 84
	Female	0.069 ± 0.030 0.000–0.135 n = 278	−0.033 ± 0.017 −0.079–0.000 n = 155	−1.059 ± 0.672 −1.544–0.000 n = 4	0.262 ± 0.148 0.050–0.648 n = 282	−1.075 ± 0.415 −1.995 to −0.369 n = 282	0.019 ± 0.028 −0.076–0.070 n = 285	0.086 ± 0.072 0.000–0.321 n = 192	−0.102 ± 0.063 −0.252–0.000 n = 193
30–39	Male	0.069 ± 0.028 0.000–0.143 n = 203	−0.046 ± 0.020 −0.101–0.000 n = 162	−0.860 ± 0.848 −1.594–0.000 n = 4	0.295 ± 0.207 0.040–1.030 n = 211	−1.158 ± 0.436 −2.328 to −0.265 n = 210	0.051 ± 0.033 −0.023–0.119 n = 213	0.179 ± 0.122 0.000–0.519 n = 194	−0.095 ± 0.075 −0.354–0.000 n = 54
	Female	0.064 ± 0.027 0.000–0.144 n = 121	−0.038 ± 0.020 −0.095–0.000 n = 80		0.251 ± 0.146 0.039–0.629 n = 125	−1.068 ± 0.384 −2.105 to −0.371 n = 125	0.020 ± 0.028 −0.076–0.056 n = 125	0.096 ± 0.073 0.000–0.316 n = 88	−0.101 ± 0.068 −0.272–0.000 n = 77
40–49	Male	0.061 ± 0.024 0.000–0.120 n = 194	−0.046 ± 0.023 −0.117–0.000 n = 165	−1.208 ± 0.318 −1.463–0.000 n = 6	0.258 ± 0.163 0.056–0.612 n = 199	−1.052 ± 0.408 −2.110 to −0.364 n = 199	0.045 ± 0.035 −0.019–0.119 n = 205	0.191 ± 0.123 0.000–0.495 n = 192	−0.087 ± 0.068 −0.305–0.000 n = 51
	Female	0.057 ± 0.022 0.000–0.104 n = 83	−0.040 ± 0.019 −0.097–0.000 n = 73	−1.007 ± 0.188 −1.140–0.000 n = 2	0.214 ± 0.131 0.029–0.634 n = 87	−0.951 ± 0.307 −1.518 to −0.505 n = 87	0.025 ± 0.018 −0.010–0.067 n = 89	0.079 ± 0.053 0.000–0.255 n = 73	−0.073 ± 0.059 −0.309–0.000 n = 50
50+	Male	0.057 ± 0.025 0.000–0.115 n = 193	−0.046 ± 0.021 −0.110–0.000 n = 190	−0.443 ± 0.576 −0.850–0.000 n = 2	0.229 ± 0.123 0.052–0.489 n = 201	−0.930 ± 0.365 −1.904 to −0.319 n = 201	0.047 ± 0.031 −0.005–0.113 n = 202	0.198 ± 0.117 0.000–0.513 n = 187	−0.097 ± 0.083 −0.337–0.000 n = 31
	Female	0.055 ± 0.024 0.000–0.114 n = 116	−0.047 ± 0.021 −0.105–0.000 n = 110	−0.029 −0.029–0.000 n = 1	0.201 ± 0.130 0.040–0.587 n = 126	−0.934 ± 0.340 −1.630 to −0.349 n = 126	0.030 ± 0.022 −0.006–0.083 n = 126	0.109 ± 0.065 0.000–0.291 n = 108	−0.077 ± 0.058 −0.319–0.000 n = 53

Table A1.22

Amplitudes (in millivolts) in Caucasian adults: lead V_2

Age group	Sex	P+	P-	Q	R	S	STJ	T+	T-
18–29	Male	0.094 ± 0.033 0.042–0.170 n = 228	-0.027 ± 0.011 -0.064–0.000 n = 39	-2.532 ± 0.000 -2.532–0.000 n = 1	0.833 ± 0.366 0.265–1.894 n = 228	-2.164 ± 0.711 -3.562 to -0.826 n = 228	0.164 ± 0.077 0.016–0.320 n = 229	0.887 ± 0.307 0.342–1.634 n = 229	
	Female	0.090 ± 0.030 0.040–0.157 n = 281	-0.021 ± 0.011 -0.050–0.000 n = 13	-0.026 ± 0.006 -0.030–0.000 n = 2	0.555 ± 0.259 0.145–1.206 n = 281	-1.458 ± 0.554 -2.889 to -0.550 n = 280	0.055 ± 0.046 -0.063–0.128 n = 281	0.483 ± 0.213 0.093–1.070 n = 281	-0.069 ± 0.041 -0.116–0.000 n = 3
30–39	Male	0.089 ± 0.032 0.033–0.176 n = 209	-0.030 ± 0.019 -0.118–0.000 n = 50	-0.969 ± 1.271 -1.868–0.000 n = 2	0.662 ± 0.355 0.139–1.640 n = 208	-1.863 ± 0.671 -3.518 to -0.664 n = 207	0.136 ± 0.069 -0.018–0.294 n = 209	0.784 ± 0.276 0.239–1.444 n = 208	-0.146 ± 0.110 -0.267–0.000 n = 3
	Female	0.085 ± 0.033 0.027–0.169 n = 125	-0.030 ± 0.019 -0.075–0.000 n = 16		0.505 ± 0.241 0.143–1.094 n = 125	-1.375 ± 0.610 -3.126 to -0.485 n = 125	0.050 ± 0.045 -0.030–0.154 n = 125	0.462 ± 0.182 0.095–0.874 n = 125	-0.146 ± 0.026 -0.174–0.000 n = 3
40–49	Male	0.084 ± 0.032 0.030–0.154 n = 201	-0.027 ± 0.014 -0.094–0.000 n = 64	-2.284 ± 0.215 -2.532–0.000 n = 3	0.604 ± 0.310 0.085–1.496 n = 199	-1.502 ± 0.559 -2.724 to -0.548 n = 199	0.114 ± 0.061 -0.021–0.265 n = 202	0.708 ± 0.243 0.240–1.256 n = 202	
	Female	0.078 ± 0.028 0.036–0.141 n = 90	-0.023 ± 0.008 -0.043–0.000 n = 15	-0.713 ± 0.969 -1.398–0.000 n = 2	0.430 ± 0.202 0.134–0.877 n = 89	-1.175 ± 0.456 -2.470 to -0.390 n = 89	0.053 ± 0.030 -0.003 ± 0.110 n = 90	0.418 ± 0.171 0.161–0.823 n = 90	
50+	Male	0.079 ± 0.031 0.028–0.155 n = 203	-0.025 ± 0.009 -0.047–0.000 n = 71	-0.428 ± 0.770 -1.583–0.000 n = 4	0.595 ± 0.331 0.148–1.497 n = 202	-1.285 ± 0.528 -2.425 to -0.271 n = 202	0.103 ± 0.061 -0.013–0.233 n = 203	0.659 ± 0.249 0.173–1.165 n = 202	-0.420 ± 0.000 -0.420–0.000 n = 1
	Female	0.074 ± 0.027 0.019–0.134 n = 128	-0.025 ± 0.012 -0.073–0.000 n = 48	-0.802 ± 1.076 -1.563–0.000 n = 2	0.453 ± 0.251 0.148–1.081 n = 127	-1.126 ± 0.397 -1.985 to -0.472 n = 127	0.053 ± 0.036 -0.033–0.132 n = 128	0.383 ± 0.154 0.073–0.672 n = 128	-0.066 ± 0.000 -0.066–0.000 n = 1

Table A1.23

Amplitudes (in millivolts) in Caucasian adults: lead V_3

Age group	Sex	P+	P−	Q	R	S	STj	T+	T−
18–29	Male	0.093 ± 0.030 0.038–0.160 n = 228	−0.024 ± 0.010 −0.049–0.000 n = 39	−0.061 ± 0.038 −0.103–0.000 n = 3	1.073 ± 0.506 0.326–2.344 n = 228	−1.294 ± 0.655 −2.840 to −0.213 n = 227	0.151 ± 0.069 0.033–0.305 n = 228	0.873 ± 0.280 0.380–1.474 n = 228	
	Female	0.085 ± 0.027 0.043–0.151 n = 283	−0.026 ± 0.036 −0.169–0.000 n = 18	−0.043 ± 0.037 −0.086–0.000 n = 3	0.761 ± 0.374 0.177–1.800 n = 284	−0.753 ± 0.374 −1.530 to −0.087 n = 275	0.041 ± 0.036 −0.019–0.108 n = 284	0.517 ± 0.204 0.160–1.012 n = 284	−0.130 ± 0.096 −0.198–0.000 n = 2
30–39	Male	0.092 ± 0.028 0.044–0.165 n = 208	−0.026 ± 0.011 −0.067–0.000 n = 29	−0.087 ± 0.068 −0.211–0.000 n = 8	0.983 ± 0.501 0.259–2.257 n = 208	−1.188 ± 0.515 −2.338 to −0.186 n = 204	0.119 ± 0.065 0.004–0.269 n = 208	0.779 ± 0.277 0.253–1.472 n = 208	
	Female	0.086 ± 0.028 0.031–0.174 n = 123	−0.028 ± 0.029 −0.116–0.000 n = 12		0.730 ± 0.367 0.180–2.174 n = 123	−0.765 ± 0.439 −1.870 to −0.134 n = 117	0.038 ± 0.037 −0.035–0.132 n = 123	0.499 ± 0.200 0.135–0.987 n = 122	−0.251 ± 0.208 −0.398–0.000 n = 2
40–49	Male	0.088 ± 0.028 0.039–0.152 n = 205	−0.022 ± 0.007 −0.044–0.000 n = 33	−0.066 ± 0.049 −0.150–0.000 n = 5	1.020 ± 0.506 0.250–2.221 n = 205	−1.015 ± 0.490 −2.037 to −0.217 n = 202	0.096 ± 0.059 −0.014–0.203 n = 205	0.731 ± 0.257 0.311–1.322 n = 205	
	Female	0.082 ± 0.025 0.038–0.139 n = 88	−0.022 ± 0.013 −0.047–0.000 n = 10	−0.062 ± 0.057 −0.128–0.000 n = 3	0.675 ± 0.329 0.187–1.633 n = 88	−0.719 ± 0.366 −1.657 to −0.193 n = 86	0.033 ± 0.032 −0.035–0.099 n = 88	0.457 ± 0.184 0.132–0.917 n = 88	
50+	Male	0.088 ± 0.027 0.040–0.167 n = 195	−0.023 ± 0.009 −0.052–0.000 n = 23	−0.066 ± 0.058 −0.219–0.000 n = 13	0.998 ± 0.506 0.200–2.235 n = 195	−0.994 ± 0.494 −2.080 to −0.178 n = 193	0.086 ± 0.060 −0.017–0.230 n = 195	0.687 ± 0.270 0.229–1.307 n = 194	
	Female	0.084 ± 0.026 0.037–0.148 n = 128	−0.021 ± 0.008 −0.039–0.000 n = 18	−0.051 ± 0.035 −0.108–0.000 n = 5	0.752 ± 0.409 0.183–1.811 n = 128	−0.768 ± 0.372 −1.696 to −0.214 n = 126	0.030 ± 0.035 −0.049–0.097 n = 128	0.436 ± 0.169 0.086–0.793 n = 128	−0.068 ± 0.059 −0.110–0.000 n = 2

◘ Table A1.24
Amplitudes (in millivolts) in Caucasian adults: lead V_4

Age group	Sex	P+	P-	Q	R	S	STj	T+	T-
18–29	Male	0.088 ± 0.028 0.033–0.158 n = 227	-0.018 ± 0.005 -0.025–0.000 n = 20	-0.090 ± 0.075 -0.307–0.000 n = 85	1.973 ± 0.702 0.792–3.558 n = 227	-0.584 ± 0.376 -1.660 to -0.074 n = 209	0.089 ± 0.054 -0.006–0.201 n = 227	0.705 ± 0.269 0.261–1.427 n = 227	
	Female	0.082 ± 0.027 0.038–0.150 n = 283	-0.022 ± 0.020 -0.089–0.000 n = 14	-0.064 ± 0.049 -0.271–0.000 n = 72	1.247 ± 0.453 0.452–2.264 n = 284	-0.372 ± 0.205 -0.832 to -0.075 n = 242	0.021 ± 0.027 -0.037–0.088 n = 284	0.413 ± 0.172 0.141–0.847 n = 284	-0.060 ± 0.000 -0.060–0.000 n = 1
30–39	Male	0.089 ± 0.027 0.042–0.152 n = 208	-0.021 ± 0.009 -0.041–0.000 n = 17	-0.076 ± 0.063 -0.335–0.000 n = 62	1.717 ± 0.601 0.658–3.257 n = 208	-0.627 ± 0.347 -1.571 to -0.113 n = 193	0.069 ± 0.050 -0.035–0.208 n = 208	0.625 ± 0.238 0.215–1.268 n = 208	
	Female	0.088 ± 0.028 0.032–0.155 n = 124	-0.020 ± 0.011 -0.032–0.000 n = 3	-0.073 ± 0.039 -0.197–0.000 n = 35	1.277 ± 0.509 0.285–2.705 n = 124	-0.433 ± 0.259 -1.050 to -0.097 n = 97	0.015 ± 0.031 -0.056–0.095 n = 124	0.418 ± 0.181 0.081–0.961 n = 124	-0.030 ± 0.000 -0.030–0.000 n = 1
40–49	Male	0.085 ± 0.024 0.044–0.142 n = 204	-0.022 ± 0.008 -0.041–0.000 n = 18	-0.060 ± 0.047 -0.306–0.000 n = 52	1.620 ± 0.629 0.516–3.222 n = 204	-0.571 ± 0.346 -1.425 to -0.074 n = 204	0.054 ± 0.046 -0.017–0.166 n = 204	0.593 ± 0.245 0.213–1.185 n = 204	-0.077 ± 0.000 -0.077–0.000 n = 1
	Female	0.085 ± 0.025 0.035–0.142 n = 87	-0.021 ± 0.012 -0.044–0.000 n = 6	-0.058 ± 0.048 -0.175–0.000 n = 87	1.110 ± 0.454 0.384–2.200 n = 87	-0.415 ± 0.257 -1.196 to -0.070 n = 76	0.010 ± 0.026 -0.046–0.075 n = 87	0.357 ± 0.159 0.094–0.787 n = 87	
50+	Male	0.086 ± 0.024 0.047–0.146 n = 202	-0.018 ± 0.004 -0.025–0.000 n = 10	-0.079 ± 0.055 -0.282–0.000 n = 54	1.592 ± 0.546 0.582–2.683 n = 202	-0.619 ± 0.377 -1.500 to -0.099 n = 191	0.045 ± 0.046 -0.044–0.159 n = 202	0.568 ± 0.248 0.166–1.249 n = 201	-0.135 ± 0.000 -0.135–0.000 n = 1
	Female	0.089 ± 0.027 0.041–0.151 n = 129	-0.019 ± 0.009 -0.036–0.000 n = 12	-0.048 ± 0.030 -0.148–0.000 n = 28	1.150 ± 0.454 0.435–2.326 n = 129	-0.444 ± 0.293 -1.473 to -0.072 n = 123	0.006 ± 0.030 -0.075–0.074 n = 129	0.352 ± 0.156 0.074–0.690 n = 129	-0.080 ± 0.045 -0.140–0.000 n = 4

◻ Table A1.25

Amplitudes (in millivolts) in Caucasian adults: lead V_5

Age group	Sex	P+	P-	Q	R	S	STJ	T+	T-
18–29	Male	0.082 ± 0.025	−0.020 ± 0.011	−0.101 ± 0.072	1.910 ± 0.598	−0.316 ± 0.228	0.051 ± 0.039	0.553 ± 0.226	
		0.028–0.136	−0.061–0.000	−0.324–0.000	0.958–3.530	−0.946 to −0.045	−0.010–0.155	0.194–1.152	
		n = 230	n = 20	n = 171	n = 230	n = 181	n = 230	n = 230	
	Female	0.079 ± 0.026	−0.016 ± 0.005	−0.070 ± 0.050	1.289 ± 0.383	−0.230 ± 0.131	0.013 ± 0.023	0.386 ± 0.141	
		0.037–0.143	−0.029–0.000	−0.233–0.000	0.574–2.112	−0.577 to −0.048	−0.032–0.061	0.149–0.720	
		n = 287	n = 14	n = 148	n = 288	n = 214	n = 287	n = 287	
30–39	Male	0.084 ± 0.023	−0.021 ± 0.008	−0.088 ± 0.069	1.761 ± 0.502	−0.330 ± 0.235	0.041 ± 0.039	0.497 ± 0.197	−0.370 ± 0.000
		0.035–0.135	−0.034–0.000	−0.283–0.000	0.756–3.012	−0.986 to −0.069	−0.029–0.154	0.181–1.028	−0.370–0.000
		n = 211	n = 11	n = 127	n = 211	n = 179	n = 211	n = 211	n = 1
	Female	0.084 ± 0.026	−0.011 ± 0.005	−0.074 ± 0.048	1.299 ± 0.411	−0.239 ± 0.162	0.010 ± 0.027	0.369 ± 0.151	
		0.030–0.146	−0.014–0.000	−0.197–0.000	0.502–2.372	−0.689 to −0.057	−0.040–0.087	0.126–0.827	
		n = 123	n = 2	n = 78	n = 123	n = 88	n = 123	n = 123	
40–49	Male	0.080 ± 0.022	−0.020 ± 0.010	−0.072 ± 0.049	1.576 ± 0.506	−0.306 ± 0.227	0.032 ± 0.034	0.458 ± 0.185	
		0.040–0.142	−0.044–0.000	−0.294–0.000	0.737–2.869	−0.952 to −0.049	−0.031–0.133	0.161–0.879	
		n = 206	n = 12	n = 111	n = 206	n = 165	n = 206	n = 206	
	Female	0.083 ± 0.026	−0.022 ± 0.012	−0.062 ± 0.046	1.190 ± 0.393	−0.247 ± 0.190	0.004 ± 0.024	0.323 ± 0.128	−0.077 ± 0.000
		0.044–0.138	−0.043–0.000	−0.202–0.000	0.625–2.092	−1.034 to −0.046	−0.056–0.052	0.085–0.616	−0.077–0.000
		n = 88	n = 8	n = 39	n = 88	n = 68	n = 88	n = 87	n = 1
50+	Male	0.081 ± 0.022	−0.020 ± 0.011	−0.080 ± 0.054	1.581 ± 0.470	−0.366 ± 0.237	0.023 ± 0.036	0.427 ± 0.190	−0.067 ± 0.000
		0.043–0.134	−0.047–0.000	−0.241–0.000	0.745–2.488	−0.967 to −0.053	−0.047–0.104	0.114–0.916	−0.067–0.000
		n = 201	n = 8	n = 102	n = 201	n = 162	n = 201	n = 201	n = 1
	Female	0.084 ± 0.026	−0.016 ± 0.012	−0.063 ± 0.037	1.241 ± 0.379	−0.261 ± 0.189	−0.001 ± 0.025	0.310 ± 0.139	−0.098 ± 0.044
		0.029–0.145	−0.033–0.000	−0.229–0.000	0.570–2.295	−0.837 to −0.049	−0.050–0.052	0.088–0.636	−0.158–0.000
		n = 129	n = 5	n = 62	n = 129	n = 99	n = 129	n = 128	n = 4

▣ Table A1.26
Amplitudes (in millivolts) in Caucasian adults: lead V_6

Age group	Sex	P+	P-	Q	R	S	STJ	T+	T-
18–29	Male	0.075 ± 0.023 0.032–0.125 n = 228	−0.011 ± 0.004 −0.020–0.000 n = 11	−0.106 ± 0.066 −0.262–0.000 n = 202	1.583 ± 0.463 0.766–2.806 n = 228	−0.197 ± 0.142 −0.572 to −0.039 n = 137	0.032 ± 0.028 −0.017–0.091 n = 228	0.424 ± 0.166 0.153–0.897 n = 228	
	Female	0.074 ± 0.025 0.031–0.137 n = 289	−0.020 ± 0.023 −0.075–0.000 n = 9	−0.076 ± 0.054 −0.257–0.000 n = 215	1.177 ± 0.319 0.611–1.966 n = 289	−0.143 ± 0.083 −0.359 to −0.046 n = 161	0.009 ± 0.023 −0.035–0.049 n = 289	0.327 ± 0.109 0.143–0.573 n = 289	−0.224 ± 0.168 −0.343–0.000 n = 2
30–39	Male	0.077 ± 0.022 0.040–0.131 n = 205	−0.019 ± 0.006 −0.026–0.000 n = 5	−0.090 ± 0.064 −0.271–0.000 n = 159	1.461 ± 0.456 0.623–2.540 n = 207	−0.187 ± 0.141 −0.564 to −0.025 n = 129	0.026 ± 0.028 −0.026–0.088 n = 207	0.390 ± 0.150 0.149–0.782 n = 207	
	Female	0.079 ± 0.024 0.032–0.140 n = 123	−0.013 ± 0.004 −0.018–0.000 n = 3	−0.083 ± 0.049 −0.229–0.000 n = 102	1.147 ± 0.323 0.605–1.978 n = 123	−0.153 ± 0.125 −0.724 to −0.032 n = 59	0.006 ± 0.023 −0.043–0.074 n = 123	0.302 ± 0.119 0.081–0.649 n = 123	
40–49	Male	0.075 ± 0.020 0.040–0.132 n = 206	−0.024 ± 0.012 −0.044–0.000 n = 8	−0.071 ± 0.043 −0.202–0.000 n = 152	1.291 ± 0.399 0.664–2.290 n = 206	−0.200 ± 0.137 −0.565 to −0.037 n = 109	0.021 ± 0.026 −0.031–0.094 n = 206	0.350 ± 0.140 0.137–0.680 n = 206	
	Female	0.079 ± 0.024 0.040–0.128 n = 89	−0.036 ± 0.000 −0.036–0.000 n = 1	−0.065 ± 0.042 −0.215–0.000 n = 55	1.068 ± 0.315 0.475–1.721 n = 89	−0.161 ± 0.127 −0.728 to −0.025 n = 45	0.004 ± 0.020 −0.037–0.049 n = 89	0.273 ± 0.104 0.091–0.500 n = 88	−0.057 ± 0.000 −0.057–0.000 n = 1
50+	Male	0.076 ± 0.020 0.038–0.117 n = 198	−0.014 ± 0.004 −0.016–0.000 n = 2	−0.078 ± 0.050 −0.233–0.000 n = 133	1.304 ± 0.409 0.649–2.287 n = 198	−0.200 ± 0.132 −0.591 to −0.046 n = 124	0.015 ± 0.029 −0.045–0.067 n = 198	0.318 ± 0.142 0.102–0.680 n = 198	−0.049 ± 0.028 −0.069–0.000 n = 2
	Female	0.080 ± 0.024 0.033–0.137 n = 129	−0.015 ± 0.008 −0.024–0.000 n = 6	−0.067 ± 0.040 −0.185–0.000 n = 80	1.100 ± 0.335 0.523–1.859 n = 129	−0.154 ± 0.084 −0.384 to −0.055 n = 61	−0.002 ± 0.021 −0.051–0.037 n = 129	0.259 ± 0.118 0.078–0.561 n = 128	−0.063 ± 0.042 −0.137–0.000 n = 6

◼ Table A1.27

R/S ratio in Caucasians: leads $V_1 - V_6$

Age group	Sex	V_1	V_2	V_3	V_4	V_5	V_6
18–29	Male	0.333 ± 0.21 0.053–0.913 n = 267	0.429 ± 0.25 0.089–1.191 n = 267	1.345 ± 2.03 0.180–6.82 n = 268	5.649 ± 7.15 0.699–36.66 n = 243	10.327 ± 10.11 1.188–44.53 n = 216	13.883 ± 12.47 2.211–62.125 n = 169
	Female	0.289 ± 0.19 0.042–0.803 n = 315	0.468 ± 0.31 0.104–1.55 n = 318	1.548 ± 1.84 0.211–8.31 n = 314	5.88 ± 8.07 0.831–36.74 n = 284	7.879 ± 7.42 1.30–27.13 n = 247	10.891 ± 8.81 2.417–40.64 n = 188
30–39	Male	0.30 ± 0.25 0.050–0.940 n = 214	0.420 ± 0.30 0.090–1.214 n = 215	1.218 ± 1.62 0.194–4.04 n = 214	4.623 ± 7.91 0.63–19.14 n = 202	8.298 ± 7.87 1.33–23.07 n = 181	13.093 ± 12.73 2.305–62.07 n = 137
	Female	0.272 ± 0.17 0.035–0.62 n = 116	0.480 ± 0.42 0.102–1.728 n = 114	2.188 ± 6.17 0.241–11.48 n = 113	4.482 ± 3.64 0.781–14.684 n = 96	8.197 ± 6.07 1.104–25.228 n = 88	13.757 ± 11.11 1.916–47.47 n = 63
40–49	Male	0.269 ± 0.17 0.031–0.711 n = 116	0.487 ± 0.48 0.087–1.40 n = 115	1.478 ± 2.73 0.184–5.265 n = 118	4.753 ± 6.47 0.481–34.40 n = 114	8.818 ± 9.93 1.097–47.43 n = 98	10.471 ± 9.22 1.877–31.14 n = 68
	Female	0.239 ± 0.14 0.034–0.519 n = 73	0.429 ± 0.26 0.092–1.311 n = 73	1.354 ± 1.39 0.125–4.044 n = 73	5.316 ± 7.79 0.572–43.119 n = 71	7.99 ± 5.85 1.554–26.21 n = 65	9.760 ± 6.18 1.993–22.516 n = 48
50+	Male	0.263 ± 0.17 0.046–0.75 n = 122	0.507 ± 0.35 0.133–1.428 n = 121	1.340 ± 1.42 0.313–5.767 n = 122	3.935 ± 3.71 0.789–13.33 n = 117	7.29 ± 7.48 1.371–28.674 n = 101	10.703 ± 10.62 1.575–45.51 n = 80
	Female	0.227 ± 0.14 0.044–0.626 n = 77	0.443 ± 0.28 0.049–1.082 n = 79	1.369 ± 1.41 0.203–6.578 n = 79	3.409 ± 3.07 0.564–14.904 n = 77	8.274 ± 7.90 1.568–34.44 n = 66	8.96 ± 6.93 2.37–17.65 n = 40

■ Table A1.28

Q/R ratios (%) in Caucasians: leads I, II, III, aVL, aVF, V_5, V_6

Age group	Sex	I	II	III	aVL	aVF	V_5	V_6
18–29	Male	9.0 ± 5.5	6.0 ± 3.6	18 ± 51.8	37 ± 78.5	8.0 ± 6.6	5.0 ± 3.7	7.0 ± 4.1
		0.0–23.4	0.0–14.8	0.0–81.5	0.0–188	0.0–19.3	0.0–14.9	0.0–17.8
		n = 143	n = 189	n = 154	n = 119	n = 166	n = 199	n = 230
	Female	8.0 ± 4.5	6.0 ± 3.6	23 ± 38.9	27 ± 41.9	8.0 ± 4.8	5.0 ± 3.1	6.0 ± 3.7
		0.0–22.3	0.0–14.9	0.0–139	0.0–75.0	0.0–19.5	0.0–12.6	0.0–16.0
		n = 132	n = 204	n = 192	n = 115	n = 202	n = 168	n = 236
30–39	Male	8.0 ± 4.9	7.0 ± 4.0	35 ± 83.6	25 ± 33.6	9.0 ± 5.0	5.0 ± 3.2	6.0 ± 3.8
		0.0–21.6	0.0–19.3	0.0–236	0.0–138	0.0–22.2	0.0–12.4	0.0–14.7
		n = 122	n = 129	n = 115	n = 110	n = 120	n = 137	n = 171
	Female	9.0 ± 4.5	7.0 ± 3.3	21 ± 33.6	29 ± 25.2	9.0 ± 4.3	5.0 ± 3.1	7.0 ± 3.8
		0.0–18.9	0.0–14.6	0.0–85.3	0.0–92.0	0.0–17.5	0.0–12.2	0.0–15.0
		n = 54	n = 90	n = 76	n = 40	n = 83	n = 78	n = 99
40–49	Male	8.0 ± 3.6	6.0 ± 2.4	56 ± 11.0	24 ± 43.1	13 ± 24.2	4.0 ± 1.9	6.0 ± 2.6
		0.0–15.7	0.0–11.0	0.0–154	0.0–160	0.0–86.0	0.0–8.2	0.0–10.8
		n = 72	n = 65	n = 47	n = 69	n = 51	n = 70	n = 91
	Female	7.0 ± 4.7	6.0 ± 3.2	24 ± 31.5	19 ± 16.9	10 ± 8.60	5.0 ± 2.8	6.0 ± 3.0
		0.0–18.8	0.0–13.4	0.0–92.8	0.0–38.2	0.0–29.7	0.0–11.7	0.0–13.2
		n = 47	n = 41	n = 31	n = 44	n = 38	n = 38	n = 50
50+	Male	8.0 ± 5.5	7.0 ± 4.7	80 ± 192.7	26 ± 42.2	17 ± 31.2	5.0 ± 4.1	6.0 ± 4.6
		0.0–31.3	0.0–20.5	0.0–740	0.0–238	0.0–64.0	0.0–21.5	0.0–19.8
		n = 79	n = 52	n = 45	n = 79	n = 43	n = 69	n = 84
	Female	8.0 ± 4.3	7.0 ± 4.7	52 ± 109.4	14 ± 7.70	11 ± 8.90	5.0 ± 3.9	6.0 ± 4.8
		0.0–16.7	0.0–14.6	0.0–335	0.0–27.4	0.0–36.7	0.0–13.0	0.0–13.9
		n = 46	n = 39	n = 38	n = 43	n = 35	n = 39	n = 51

Appendix 1: Adult Normal Limits

A1

663

■ Table A1.29
Miscellaneous measures

Age group	Sex	QRS axis (°)	T axis (°)	QRS–T angle (frontal plane) (°)	Lewis index[a] (mV)	SV_1+RV_5 (mV)	SV_1+RV_6 (mV)	SV_1+RV_6 (mV)
18–29	Male	57.5 ± 25.6 −10–91 n = 265	40.9 ± 16.7 2–69 n = 265	16.6 ± 23.9 −39–71 n = 265	−0.117 ± 0.956 −1.831–2.048 n = 266	3.331 ± 0.881 1.685–5.252 n = 264	3.905 ± 0.995 2.049–6.372 n = 265	2.99 ± 0.79 1.59–4.85 n = 265
	Female	51.2 ± 24.9 −9–91 n = 317	38.7 ± 15.0 6–65 n = 317	12.5 ± 25.1 −46–59 n = 317	0.110 ± 0.736 −1.288–1.574 n = 317	2.442 ± 0.690 1.112–3.816 n = 316	2.741 ± 0.727 1.430–4.635 n = 317	2.32 ± 0.64 1.20–3.68 n = 318
30–39	Male	46.5 ± 29.2 −22–92 n = 220	39.3 ± 17.2 −1–70 n = 220	7.2 ± 27.3 −61–59 n = 220	0.266 ± 0.899 −1.476–1.962 n = 221	3.007 ± 0.775 1.549–4.680 n = 220	3.430 ± 0.875 1.846–5.257 n = 219	2.69 ± 0.72 1.31–4.14 n = 220
	Female	49.6 ± 24.2 −14–81 n = 118	39.0 ± 15.4 1–66 n = 118	10.6 ± 21.7 −47–61 n = 118	0.129 ± 0.626 −1.011–1.293 n = 118	2.454 ± 0.644 0.483–4.287 n = 118	2.662 ± 0.834 1.565–4.803 n = 115	2.29 ± 0.60 1.43–3.59 n = 118
40–49	Male	37.7 ± 31.6 −37–85 n = 117	42.5 ± 17.3 5–71 n = 117	−4.8 ± 26.3 −67–37 n = 117	0.491 ± 0.892 −1.060–2.395 n = 118	2.702 ± 0.763 1.420–4.227 n = 118	2.842 ± 0.673 1.634–4.170 n = 117	2.39 ± 0.69 1.22–3.77 n = 118
	Female	36.2 ± 29.1 −53–85 n = 73	38.0 ± 15.7 5–67 n = 73	−1.8 ± 27.9 −86–40 n = 73	0.521 ± 0.698 0.762–1.818 n = 73	2.291 ± 0.634 1.087–3.411 n = 73	2.418 ± 0.566 1.429–3.433 n = 73	2.13 ± 0.57 1.07–3.16 n = 73
50+	Male	31.4 ± 30.6 −33–77 n = 125	44.4 ± 18.7 4–74 n = 125	−13.0 ± 27.1 −82–40 n = 125	0.627 ± 0.742 0.703–2.120 n = 125	2.709 ± 0.736 1.612–4.558 n = 125	2.746 ± 0.703 1.546–4.144 n = 124	2.35 ± 0.63 1.34–3.78 n = 125
	Female	26.9 ± 29.2 −36–73 n = 80	41.9 ± 15.9 4–72 n = 80	−15.0 ± 27.8 −89–26 n = 80	0.714 ± 0.691 0.578–2.165 n = 80	2.259 ± 0.567 1.086–3.635 n = 79	2.316 ± 0.574 1.298–3.419 n = 80	2.10 ± 0.55 0.94–3.14 n = 80

[a]Lewis index = (RI + SIII)–(SI + RIII).

◘ Table A1.30

ST slope (°) in selected leads in Caucasians

Age group	Sex	I	aVF	V₂	V₅	V₆
18–29	Male	19 ± 7 6–33 n = 265	12 ± 8 –2–31 n = 265	50 ± 12 21–69 n = 265	28 ± 10 11–51 n = 265	20 ± 8 6–38 n = 265
	Female	12 ± 6 3–24 n = 317	7 ± 5 –3–19 n = 318	31 ± 11 8–53 n = 317	15 ± 7 2–33 n = 318	11 ± 6 1–25 n = 318
30–39	Male	17 ± 8 3–36 n = 220	9 ± 7 –3–27 n = 220	46 ± 13 19–66 n = 220	26 ± 10 10–53 n = 220	18 ± 9 3–42 n = 220
	Female	10 ± 5 1–21 n = 118	6 ± 5 –4–16 n = 118	28 ± 10 10–50 n = 116	14 ± 7 0–33 n = 118	10 ± 6 0–25 n = 117
40–49	Male	13 ± 6 3–25 n = 118	9 ± 6 –1–22 n = 117	41 ± 13 13–63 n = 117	22 ± 9 7–43 n = 119	15 ± 7 2–31 n = 119
	Female	10 ± 5 2–20 n = 73	6 ± 6 –2–21 n = 73	25 ± 10 7–46 n = 73	13 ± 7 0–26 n = 73	10 ± 6 2–32 n = 73
50+	Male	12 ± 7 0–28 n = 125	9 ± 6 –1–24 n = 125	40 ± 12 15–61 n = 125	21 ± 13 2–43 n = 125	14 ± 8 0–31 n = 124
	Female	7 ± 4 0–14 n = 80	5 ± 5 –2–17 n = 80	24 ± 10 10–42 n = 80	12 ± 7 0–28 n = 80	7 ± 5 –1–19 n = 80

▪ Table A1.31

P terminal force in V_1, intrinsicoid deflection (ID) in V_5, V_6, and body-surface area (BSA) in the Caucasians studied as described in ❯ Chap. 1 of *Electrocardiology: Comprehensive Clinical ECG*.

Age group	Sex	P terminal force in V_1 (mV ms)	ID V_5 (ms)	ID V_6 (ms)	BSA (m²)
18–29	Male	1.09 ± 1.33	41 ± 13.4	41 ± 12.3	1.86 ± 0.15
		0.0–4.62	26–85	22–87	1.55–2.19
		n = 265	n = 265	n = 265	n = 257
	Female	0.75 ± 1.03	33 ± 8.40	35 ± 7.70	1.62 ± 0.14
		0.0–3.54	22–66	22–59	1.37–1.95
		n = 316	n = 318	n = 318	n = 315
30–39	Male	1.16 ± 1.21	37 ± 11.5	38 ± 10.7	1.89 ± 0.15
		0.0–3.94	22–79	22–84	1.60–2.26
		n = 219	n = 220	n = 220	n = 215
	Female	1.02 ± 1.25	35 ± 7.10	36 ± 6.90	1.62 ± 0.16
		0.0–4.29	22–48	24–47	1.38–2.07
		n = 118	n = 118	n = 117	n = 117
40–49	Male	1.49 ± 1.44	34 ± 9.40	35 ± 8.10	1.88 ± 0.17
		0.0–4.42	20–67	24–64	1.54–2.26
		n = 117	n = 119	n = 117	n = 115
	Female	1.57 ± 1.40	32 ± 6.70	33 ± 5.90	1.68 ± 0.16
		0.0–5.5	22–44	20–42	1.47–2.03
		n = 73	n = 73	n = 73	n = 69
50±	Male	1.47 ± 1.44	35 ± 10.7	33 ± 5.90	1.85 ± 0.14
		0.0–5.45	22–72	22–46	1.53–2.14
		n = 125	n = 175	n = 174	n = 121
	Female	1.42 ± 1.37	31 ± 6.30	32 ± 6.30	1.65 ± 0.11
		0.0–4.05	22–41	22–44	1.43–1.92
		n = 79	n = 80	n = 80	n = 79

A1.2   Normal Limits of the 12-Lead ECG in Chinese

The data in ❯ Tables A1.32–A1.38 were obtained from a study of 503 Chinese people with normal cardiovascular systems (see ❯ Chap. 1 of *Electrocardiology: Comprehensive Clinical ECG*). There were 255 males and 248 females. The most significant differences with the Caucasian data presented in ❯ Sect. A1.1 were in the QRS amplitudes, and for this reason, only some amplitude data are tabulated here. Fuller details are available in: Chen C Y, Chiang B N, Macfarlane P W. Normal limits of the electrocardiogram in a Chinese population. *J. Electrocardiol.* 1989;**22**(1): 1–15. Most of these tables are reproduced from that article with the permission of Churchill Livingstone, New York. Data are presented as mean ± standard deviation together with 96% ranges; that is, 2% of the measurements have been excluded from each extreme of the range. Where numbers of subjects studied in a subgroup is small, the full range is given. P-, Q, S, T- wave amplitudes are presented as positive measurements.

A1.3   Normal Limits of the 12-Lead ECG in Japanese

The data in ❯ Tables A1.39–A1.43 are taken from a study of 1,329 normal Japanese individuals. The ECGs were recorded on paper and measurements made by hand. For this reason, only selected amplitudes are presented. These data have been reproduced from: The normal value of electrocardiogram in the Japanese. *Jpn. Heart J.* 1963; **4**: 141–172 with the permission of the University of Tokyo Press, Tokyo. Note that the maximum and minimum values are presented and not the 96% range. Q, S wave amplitudes are treated as positive values.

◼ Table A1.32

Q-wave amplitude (millivolts) in normal Chinese in various age-groups: leads I-aVF

	18–29 Male (n = 56)	18–29 Female (n = 47)	30–39 Male (n = 50)	30–39 Female (n = 59)	40–49 Male (n = 50)	40–49 Female (n = 50)	50–59 Male (n = 50)	50–59 Female (n = 48)	60+ Male (n = 49)	60+ Female (n = 44)
I	0.07 ± 0.04	0.04 ± 0.02	0.05 ± 0.03	0.06 ± 0.03	0.07 ± 0.05	0.05 ± 0.02	0.07 ± 0.04	0.06 ± 0.03	0.07 ± 0.04	0.06 ± 0.02
	0.00–0.15	0.00–0.07	0.00–0.10	0.00–0.10	0.00–0.10	0.00–0.10	0.00–0.11	0.00–0.12	0.00–0.14	0.00–0.08
	n = 23	n = 14	n = 15	n = 15	n = 15	n = 15	n = 21	n = 17	n = 22	n = 16
II	0.10 ± 0.05	0.07 ± 0.06	0.07 ± 0.06	0.08 ± 0.05	0.07 ± 0.05	0.06 ± 0.03	0.07 ± 0.05	0.07 ± 0.05	0.07 ± 0.04	0.07 ± 0.06
	0.00–0.17	0.00–0.20	0.00–0.22	0.00–0.15	0.00–0.15	0.00–0.10	0.00–0.11	0.00–0.11	0.00–0.15	0.00–0.10
	n = 23	n = 25	n = 29	n = 25	n = 19	n = 17	n = 18	n = 15	n = 23	n = 10
III	0.11 ± 0.06	0.12 ± 0.08	0.13 ± 0.10	0.10 ± 0.08	0.15 ± 0.13	0.11 ± 0.12	0.11 ± 0.09	0.10 ± 0.08	0.14 ± 0.12	0.17 ± 0.13
	0.00–0.20	0.00–0.27	0.00–0.28	0.00–0.21	0.00–0.25	0.00–0.43	0.00–0.27	0.00–0.19	0.00–0.34	0.00–0.37
	n = 23	n = 28	n = 32	n = 34	n = 23	n = 24	n = 17	n = 19	n = 25	n = 18
aVR	0.79 ± 0.22	0.73 ± 0.14	0.79 ± 0.17	0.76 ± 0.18	0.71 ± 0.18	0.70 ± 0.20	0.70 ± 0.20	0.68 ± 0.18	0.69 ± 0.20	0.69 ± 0.21
	0.00–1.22	0.00–0.95	0.00–1.12	0.00–1.05	0.00–0.95	0.00–1.28	0.00–1.03	0.00–1.04	0.00–0.88	0.00–1.05
	n = 33	n = 33	n = 31	n = 35	n = 35	n = 36	n = 29	n = 38	n = 30	n = 36
aVL	0.10 ± 0.07	0.09 ± 0.08	0.11 ± 0.09	0.13 ± 0.15	0.12 ± 0.12	0.07 ± 0.04	0.10 ± 0.07	0.07 ± 0.05	0.09 ± 0.05	0.10 ± 0.08
	0.00–0.19	0.00–0.23	0.00–0.27	0.00–0.44	0.00–0.27	0.00–0.10	0.00–0.23	0.00–0.18	0.00–0.21	0.00–0.21
	n = 27	n = 16	n = 17	n = 22	n = 22	n = 20	n = 29	n = 24	n = 25	n = 23
aVF	0.10 ± 0.05	0.09 ± 0.06	0.08 ± 0.06	0.08 ± 0.05	0.08 ± 0.05	0.06 ± 0.02	0.07 ± 0.06	0.07 ± 0.04	0.08 ± 0.05	0.08 ± 0.07
	0.00–0.18	0.00–0.19	0.00–0.23	0.00–0.17	0.00–0.15	0.00–0.10	0.00–0.14	0.00–0.14	0.00–0.16	0.00–0.12
	n = 22	n = 26	n = 29	n = 30	n = 20	n = 18	n = 18	n = 12	n = 24	n = 13

Table A1.33

Q-wave amplitude (millivolts) in normal Chinese in various age-groups: leads $V_1 - V_6$

	18–29 Male n = 56	18–29 Female n = 47	30–39 Male n = 50	30–39 Female n = 59	40–49 Male n = 50	40–49 Female n = 50	50–59 Male n = 50	50–59 Female n = 48	60+ Male n = 49	60+ Female n = 44
V_1		1.08 ± 0.93			0.76 ± 0.81	0.98 ± 0.00	1.58 ± 0.00		0.33 ± 0.00	0.41 ± 0.01
		0.00–2.29			0.00–1.33	0.00–0.98	0.00–1.58		0.00–0.33	0.00–0.41
		n = 4			n = 2	n = 1	n = 1		n = 1	n = 3
V_2							0.04 ± 0.00		0.05 ± 0.00	0.04 ± 0.01
							0.00–0.04		0.00–0.05	0.00–0.04
							n = 1		n = 1	n = 3
V_3	0.07 ± 0.03	0.13 ± 0.06		0.03 ± 0.01			0.03 ± 0.00	0.23 ± 0.00	0.06 ± 0.01	0.06 ± 0.03
	0.00–0.09	0.00–0.18		0.00–0.04			0.00–0.03	0.00–0.23	0.00–0.07	0.00–0.10
	n = 2	n = 2		n = 3			n = 1	n = 1	n = 2	n = 4
V_4	0.11 ± 0.08	0.11 ± 0.10	0.07 ± 0.07	0.05 ± 0.02	0.09 ± 0.05	0.03 ± 0.01	0.07 ± 0.06	0.07 ± 0.07	0.09 ± 0.06	0.05 ± 0.04
	0.00–0.25	0.00–0.26	0.00–0.24	0.00–0.08	0.00–0.14	0.00–0.04	0.00–0.13	0.00–0.23	0.00–0.19	0.00–0.11
	n = 18	n = 7	n = 9	n = 14	n = 5	n = 5	n = 12	n = 8	n = 7	n = 13
V_5	0.11 ± 0.08	0.08 ± 0.07	0.09 ± 0.07	0.06 ± 0.03	0.08 ± 0.07	0.06 ± 0.02	0.08 ± 0.05	0.07 ± 0.05	0.07 ± 0.05	0.05 ± 0.03
	0.00–0.25	0.00–0.22	0.00–0.22	0.00–0.12	0.00–0.21	0.00–0.09	0.00–0.16	0.00–0.13	0.00–0.16	0.00–0.12
	n = 31	n = 14	n = 24	n = 22	n = 15	n = 13	n = 23	n = 14	n = 23	n = 19
V_6	0.11 ± 0.08	0.08 ± 0.06	0.09 ± 0.07	0.07 ± 0.03	0.08 ± 0.06	0.06 ± 0.03	0.08 ± 0.04	0.07 ± 0.04	0.07 ± 0.05	0.05 ± 0.03
	0.00–0.29	0.00–0.18	0.00–0.25	0.00–0.13	0.00–0.23	0.00–0.10	0.00–0.16	0.00–0.12	0.00–0.17	0.00–0.10
	n = 37	n = 21	n = 32	n = 36	n = 23	n = 20	n = 29	n = 20	n = 33	n = 21

◘ Table A1.34

R-wave amplitude (millivolts) in normal Chinese in various age-groups: leads I–aVF

	18–29 Male	18–29 Female	30–39 Male	30–39 Female	40–49 Male	40–49 Female	50–59 Male	50–59 Female	60+ Male	60+ Female
I	0.51 ± 0.23	0.41 ± 0.20	0.56 ± 0.25	0.50 ± 0.20	0.61 ± 0.30	0.60 ± 0.26	0.63 ± 0.30	0.61 ± 0.22	0.66 ± 0.29	0.66 ± 0.25
	0.13–1.00	0.08–0.86	0.22–1.14	0.17–0.87	0.17–1.27	0.25–1.21	0.17–1.27	0.30–1.07	0.23–1.37	0.19–1.11
	n = 56	n = 47	n = 50	n = 59	n = 50	n = 50	n = 50	n = 48	n = 49	n = 44
II	1.24 ± 0.42	1.19 ± 0.31	1.18 ± 0.40	1.09 ± 0.30	0.95 ± 0.41	0.93 ± 0.29	0.96 ± 0.41	0.81 ± 0.30	0.91 ± 0.45	0.78 ± 0.34
	0.49–2.17	0.68–1.65	0.58–2.21	0.53–1.70	0.21–1.60	0.51–1.47	0.25–1.97	0.39–1.37	0.30–1.90	0.35–1.49
	n = 56	n = 47	n = 50	n = 59	n = 50	n = 50	n = 50	n = 48	n = 49	n = 44
III	0.73 ± 0.49	0.90 ± 0.44	0.74 ± 0.51	0.72 ± 0.40	0.53 ± 0.42	0.46 ± 0.33	0.54 ± 0.50	0.39 ± 0.31	0.52 ± 0.48	0.35 ± 0.29
	0.02–1.71	0.21–1.85	0.04–2.08	0.06–1.46	0.04–1.38	0.04–1.10	0.05–1.94	0.05–1.36	0.05–1.63	0.04–1.16
	n = 56	n = 47	n = 50	n = 59	n = 49	n = 49	n = 50	n = 48	n = 49	n = 44
aVR	0.13 ± 0.12	0.11 ± 0.09	0.11 ± 0.09	0.08 ± 0.06	0.12 ± 0.09	0.09 ± 0.06	0.09 ± 0.08	0.11 ± 0.08	0.10 ± 0.06	0.11 ± 0.08
	0.00–0.43	0.00–0.32	0.00–0.37	0.00–0.23	0.00–0.31	0.00–0.24	0.00–0.23	0.00–0.24	0.00–0.26	0.00–0.28
	n = 51	n = 34	n = 43	n = 48	n = 41	n = 36	n = 39	n = 35	n = 40	n = 28
aVL	0.19 ± 0.16	0.16 ± 0.13	0.24 ± 0.19	0.18 ± 0.14	0.35 ± 0.27	0.27 ± 0.19	0.35 ± 0.31	0.32 ± 0.22	0.38 ± 0.32	0.38 ± 0.22
	0.04–0.59	0.04–0.52	0.04–0.59	0.00–0.54	0.00–0.98	0.04–0.69	0.05–1.07	0.07–0.83	0.04–1.07	0.06–0.83
	n = 56	n = 47	n = 49	n = 57	n = 48	n = 50	n = 49	n = 48	n = 49	n = 43
aVF	0.98 ± 0.48	1.04 ± 0.36	0.94 ± 0.46	0.90 ± 0.34	0.68 ± 0.44	0.68 ± 0.29	0.70 ± 0.48	0.55 ± 0.31	0.67 ± 0.49	0.49 ± 0.34
	0.09–2.07	0.48–1.81	0.13–2.13	0.28–1.56	0.07–1.50	0.13–1.34	0.04–1.92	0.03–1.27	0.09–1.73	0.03–1.24
	n = 56	n = 47	n = 50	n = 59	n = 50	n = 50	n = 50	n = 48	n = 49	n = 44

◻ Table A1.35
R-wave amplitude (millivolts) in normal Chinese in various age groups: leads $V_1 - V_6$

	18–29 Male n = 56	18–29 Female n = 47	30–39 Male n = 50	30–39 Female n = 59	40–49 Male n = 50	40–49 Female n = 50	50–59 Male n = 50	50–59 Female n = 48	60+ Male n = 49	60+ Female n = 44
V_1	0.43 ± 0.27	0.33 ± 0.28	0.33 ± 0.18	0.26 ± 0.12	0.27 ± 0.23	0.21 ± 0.13	0.27 ± 0.14	0.21 ± 0.15	0.27 ± 0.17	0.19 ± 0.12
	0.07–1.04	0.00–0.86	0.09–0.76	0.06–0.52	0.02–0.92	0.02–0.46	0.03–0.63	0.04–0.66	0.08–0.65	0.00–0.49
	n = 56	n = 44	n = 50	n = 59	n = 49	n = 49	n = 50	n = 48	n = 49	n = 41
V_2	0.92 ± 0.41	0.71 ± 0.41	0.85 ± 0.38	0.65 ± 0.25	0.72 ± 0.42	0.57 ± 0.28	0.73 ± 0.32	0.64 ± 0.30	0.76 ± 0.33	0.61 ± 0.35
	0.25–1.78	0.24–2.09	0.31–1.76	0.24–1.20	0.09–1.56	0.23–1.23	0.24–1.33	0.20–1.27	0.26–1.36	0.16–1.43
	n = 56	n = 47	n = 50	n = 59	n = 50	n = 50	n = 50	n = 48	n = 49	n = 44
V_3	1.21 ± 0.58	1.09 ± 0.47	1.21 ± 0.57	1.09 ± 0.48	0.99 ± 0.49	0.88 ± 0.39	1.19 ± 0.45	1.07 ± 0.50	1.30 ± 0.55	1.12 ± 0.46
	0.30–2.97	0.49–1.95	0.54–2.55	0.31–2.35	0.22–2.06	0.38–2.01	0.38–1.92	0.32–2.31	0.40–2.28	0.45–2.16
	n = 56	n = 47	n = 50	n = 59	n = 50	n = 50	n = 50	n = 48	n = 49	n = 44
V_4	2.06 ± 0.71	1.40 ± 0.45	1.83 ± 0.60	1.49 ± 0.48	1.76 ± 0.67	1.31 ± 0.40	1.85 ± 0.76	1.56 ± 0.48	1.97 ± 0.72	1.54 ± 0.48
	1.01–3.82	0.61–2.49	0.58–2.90	0.73–2.51	0.77–3.21	0.65–2.60	0.74–4.24	0.69–2.49	0.93–3.64	0.88–2.47
	n = 56	n = 47	n = 50	n = 59	n = 50	n = 50	n = 50	n = 48	n = 49	n = 44
V_5	1.84 ± 0.46	1.25 ± 0.38	1.83 ± 0.50	1.38 ± 0.35	1.83 ± 0.58	1.35 ± 0.39	1.82 ± 0.65	1.56 ± 0.45	1.89 ± 0.65	1.58 ± 0.47
	1.20–3.10	0.65–2.06	0.99–2.74	0.77–2.10	0.55–2.83	0.69–2.42	0.83–3.78	0.98–2.31	0.82–3.43	0.97–2.64
	n = 56	n = 47	n = 50	n = 59	n = 50	n = 50	n = 50	n = 48	n = 49	n = 44
V_6	1.43 ± 0.35	1.09 ± 0.32	1.50 ± 0.39	1.16 ± 0.26	1.47 ± 0.52	1.14 ± 0.34	1.48 ± 0.45	1.30 ± 0.41	1.47 ± 0.47	1.36 ± 0.43
	0.87–2.16	0.61–1.80	0.86–2.31	0.63–1.83	0.31–2.31	0.54–1.86	0.57–2.35	0.74–2.12	0.81–2.57	0.71–2.14
	n = 56	n = 47	n = 50	n = 59	n = 50	n = 50	n = 50	n = 48	n = 49	n = 44

◻ Table A1.36

S-wave amplitude (millivolts) in normal Chinese in various age-groups: leads I-aVF

	18–29 Male (n = 56)	18–29 Female (n = 47)	30–39 Male (n = 50)	30–39 Female (n = 59)	40–49 Male (n = 50)	40–49 Female (n = 50)	50–59 Male (n = 50)	50–59 Female (n = 48)	60+ Male (n = 49)	60+ Female (n = 44)
I	0.19 ± 0.13	0.18 ± 0.13	0.17 ± 0.09	0.14 ± 0.10	0.16 ± 0.11	0.13 ± 0.07	0.17 ± 0.11	0.16 ± 0.09	0.17 ± 0.09	0.14 ± 0.10
	0.00–0.49	0.00–0.44	0.00–0.33	0.00–0.40	0.00–0.44	0.00–0.29	0.00–0.41	0.00–0.36	0.00–0.30	0.00–0.34
	n = 47	n = 31	n = 42	n = 39	n = 40	n = 37	n = 30	n = 31	n = 39	n = 25
II	0.24 ± 0.16	0.17 ± 0.11	0.17 ± 0.13	0.17 ± 0.09	0.21 ± 0.12	0.15 ± 0.10	0.17 ± 0.13	0.20 ± 0.12	0.16 ± 0.07	0.18 ± 0.11
	0.00–0.63	0.00–0.43	0.00–0.48	0.00–0.48	0.00–0.48	0.00–0.33	0.00–0.35	0.00–0.44	0.00–0.26	0.00–0.37
	n = 39	n = 26	n = 28	n = 33	n = 34	n = 30	n = 30	n = 28	n = 31	n = 30
III	0.21 ± 0.16	0.17 ± 0.13	0.15 ± 0.14	0.15 ± 0.09	0.33 ± 0.28	0.17 ± 0.13	0.29 ± 0.36	0.27 ± 0.24	0.42 ± 0.31	0.32 ± 0.24
	0.00–0.55	0.00–0.42	0.00–0.48	0.00–0.33	0.00–0.90	0.00–0.41	0.00–1.36	0.00–0.79	0.00–0.91	0.00–0.81
	n = 43	n = 28	n = 27	n = 34	n = 33	n = 26	n = 36	n = 31	n = 26	n = 29
aVR	0.82 ± 0.36	0.80 ± 0.25	0.88 ± 0.30	0.76 ± 0.16	0.76 ± 0.40	0.85 ± 0.22	0.86 ± 0.18	0.62 ± 0.37	0.80 ± 0.29	0.70 ± 0.34
	0.00–1.43	0.00–1.33	0.00–1.39	0.00–1.16	0.00–1.72	0.00–1.19	0.00–1.22	0.00–1.07	0.00–1.30	0.00–1.15
	n = 26	n = 14	n = 20	n = 24	n = 17	n = 14	n = 21	n = 13	n = 21	n = 9
aVL	0.37 ± 0.21	0.41 ± 0.27	0.33 ± 0.24	0.32 ± 0.18	0.25 ± 0.16	0.20 ± 0.13	0.30 ± 0.28	0.22 ± 0.19	0.27 ± 0.24	0.17 ± 0.15
	0.00–0.89	0.00–0.98	0.00–0.92	0.00–0.72	0.00–0.55	0.00–0.45	0.00–0.99	0.00–0.75	0.00–0.71	0.00–0.52
	n = 50	n = 39	n = 45	n = 47	n = 38	n = 45	n = 34	n = 32	n = 41	n = 28
aVF	0.21 ± 0.14	0.15 ± 0.11	0.16 ± 0.10	0.16 ± 0.08	0.23 ± 0.16	0.14 ± 0.09	0.18 ± 0.23	0.19 ± 0.16	0.19 ± 0.14	0.18 ± 0.13
	0.00–0.51	0.00–0.34	0.00–0.32	0.00–0.31	0.00–0.54	0.00–0.33	0.00–0.98	0.00–0.44	0.00–0.49	0.00–0.39
	n = 40	n = 28	n = 22	n = 30	n = 34	n = 24	n = 31	n = 27	n = 30	n = 29

Table A1.37

S-wave amplitude (millivolts) in normal Chinese in various age-groups: leads V_1–V_6

	18–29 Male n = 56	18–29 Female n = 47	30–39 Male n = 50	30–39 Female n = 59	40–49 Male n = 50	40–49 Female n = 50	50–59 Male n = 50	50–59 Female n = 48	60+ Male n = 49	60+ Female n = 44
V_1	1.05 ± 0.43	0.86 ± 0.35	0.90 ± 0.34	0.83 ± 0.35	0.84 ± 0.36	0.84 ± 0.37	0.83 ± 0.43	0.77 ± 0.36	0.76 ± 0.43	0.64 ± 0.28
	0.25–1.97	0.00–1.54	0.36–1.57	0.28–1.78	0.00–1.49	0.14–1.54	0.21–2.06	0.24–1.42	0.12–1.73	0.00–1.21
	n = 56	n = 44	n = 50	n = 59	n = 48	n = 49	n = 49	n = 48	n = 49	n = 41
V_2	2.07 ± 0.67	1.29 ± 0.55	1.68 ± 0.57	1.22 ± 0.46	1.49 ± 0.61	1.26 ± 0.48	1.26 ± 0.62	1.16 ± 0.45	1.25 ± 0.58	0.97 ± 0.39
	0.84–3.43	0.46–2.67	0.63–2.76	0.31–2.17	0.32–2.69	0.50–2.35	0.11–2.75	0.42–2.14	0.18–2.60	0.19–1.84
	n = 56	n = 47	n = 49	n = 59	n = 50	n = 50	n = 50	n = 48	n = 49	n = 44
V_3	1.14 ± 0.46	0.68 ± 0.41	1.04 ± 0.50	0.66 ± 0.32	1.04 ± 0.42	0.77 ± 0.32	0.98 ± 0.47	0.79 ± 0.37	1.05 ± 0.46	0.79 ± 0.36
	0.40–2.15	0.00–1.56	0.00–2.20	0.00–1.25	0.27–1.86	0.24–1.32	0.00–1.98	0.24–1.77	0.37–1.89	0.10–1.47
	n = 56	n = 42	n = 48	n = 57	n = 50	n = 49	n = 47	n = 48	n = 49	n = 43
V_4	0.61 ± 0.33	0.41 ± 0.29	0.61 ± 0.38	0.38 ± 0.21	0.63 ± 0.32	0.44 ± 0.24	0.59 ± 0.35	0.52 ± 0.28	0.74 ± 0.36	0.56 ± 0.27
	0.00–1.25	0.00–1.20	0.00–1.43	0.00–0.82	0.00–1.18	0.00–0.94	0.00–1.57	0.09–1.02	0.00–1.46	0.00–1.20
	n = 50	n = 38	n = 41	n = 51	n = 48	n = 48	n = 45	n = 47	n = 46	n = 41
V_5	0.38 ± 0.23	0.29 ± 0.20	0.40 ± 0.25	0.25 ± 0.16	0.43 ± 0.26	0.33 ± 0.17	0.37 ± 0.25	0.35 ± 0.21	0.49 ± 0.29	0.39 ± 0.21
	0.00–0.94	0.00–0.81	0.00–1.01	0.00–0.65	0.00–0.87	0.00–0.64	0.00–1.07	0.00–0.76	0.00–1.01	0.00–0.88
	n = 45	n = 34	n = 38	n = 49	n = 46	n = 41	n = 44	n = 45	n = 46	n = 40
V_6	0.22 ± 0.14	0.20 ± 0.13	0.21 ± 0.15	0.15 ± 0.11	0.26 ± 0.17	0.18 ± 0.10	0.21 ± 0.16	0.21 ± 0.16	0.26 ± 0.15	0.23 ± 0.14
	0.00–0.57	0.00–0.38	0.00–0.50	0.00–0.44	0.00–0.56	0.00–0.43	0.00–0.61	0.00–0.50	0.00–0.57	0.00–0.49
	n = 45	n = 24	n = 36	n = 42	n = 42	n = 37	n = 39	n = 42	n = 42	n = 36

Table A1.38

Maximal T-wave amplitude (millivolts) in normal Chinese in various age-groups

	18–29		30–39		40–49		50–59		60+	
	Male $n = 56$	Female $n = 47$	Male $n = 50$	Female $n = 59$	Male $n = 50$	Female $n = 50$	Male $n = 50$	Female $n = 48$	Male $n = 49$	Female $n = 44$
I	0.28 ± 0.08 (0.12–0.44)	0.21 ± 0.06 (0.11–0.29)	0.25 ± 0.10 (0.10–0.47)	0.22 ± 0.06 (0.11–0.33)	0.22 ± 0.09 (0.08–0.41)	0.20 ± 0.07 (0.10–0.33)	0.22 ± 0.09 (0.08–0.41)	0.18 ± 0.07 (0.07–0.29)	0.18 ± 0.08 (0.08–0.35)	0.17 ± 0.07 (0.06–0.33)
II	0.37 ± 0.11 (0.17–0.58)	0.30 ± 0.12 (0.10–0.52)	0.35 ± 0.13 (0.11–0.58)	0.27 ± 0.10 (0.08–0.46)	0.28 ± 0.11 (0.12–0.52)	0.25 ± 0.08 (0.10–0.42)	0.29 ± 0.13 (0.07–0.58)	0.21 ± 0.09 (0.06–0.40)	0.27 ± 0.13 (0.12–0.62)	0.20 ± 0.10 (0.07–0.43)
III	0.11 ± 0.13 (−0.19–0.34)	0.11 ± 0.11 (−0.14–0.33)	0.10 ± 0.14 (−0.14–0.39)	0.06 ± 0.11 (−0.12–0.26)	0.07 ± 0.13 (−0.15–0.30)	0.06 ± 0.09 (−0.10–0.23)	0.09 ± 0.14 (−0.20–0.34)	0.03 ± 0.09 (−0.11–0.18)	0.09 ± 0.15 (−0.18–0.44)	0.04 ± 0.10 (−0.14–0.17)
aVR	−0.32 ± 0.08 (−0.50 to −0.20)	−0.26 ± 0.07 (−0.40 to −0.10)	−0.30 ± 0.09 (−0.46 to −0.10)	−0.26 ± 0.07 (−0.38 to −0.08)	−0.25 ± 0.08 (−0.42 to −0.12)	−0.22 ± 0.07 (−0.36 to −0.13)	−0.25 ± 0.09 (−0.42 to −0.07)	−0.19 ± 0.07 (−0.35 to −0.07)	−0.22 ± 0.08 (−0.44 to −0.10)	−0.18 ± 0.07 (−0.35 to −0.08)
aVL	0.09 ± 0.10 (−0.08–0.26)	0.06 ± 0.08 (−0.08–0.18)	0.08 ± 0.11 (−0.10–0.30)	0.09 ± 0.07 (−0.06–0.20)	0.08 ± 0.09 (−0.07–0.27)	0.09 ± 0.06 (−0.03–0.18)	0.07 ± 0.10 (−0.10–0.27)	0.08 ± 0.06 (−0.05–0.18)	0.05 ± 0.10 (−0.15–0.27)	0.08 ± 0.07 (−0.04–0.18)
aVF	0.24 ± 0.11 (0.04–0.45)	0.20 ± 0.11 (−0.09–0.42)	0.22 ± 0.12 (0.05–0.48)	0.17 ± 0.09 (−0.05–0.37)	0.18 ± 0.10 (0.03–0.41)	0.15 ± 0.07 (−0.03–0.29)	0.19 ± 0.12 (−0.10–0.50)	0.12 ± 0.08 (−0.06–0.26)	0.19 ± 0.12 (0.04–0.51)	0.12 ± 0.08 (−0.05–0.29)
V_1	0.17 ± 0.15 (−0.14–0.50)	−0.06 ± 0.14 (−0.24–0.23)	0.12 ± 0.16 (−0.25–0.35)	−0.05 ± 0.14 (−0.23–0.20)	0.09 ± 0.15 (−0.18–0.36)	−0.03 ± 0.09 (−0.22–0.17)	0.12 ± 0.16 (−0.21–0.39)	0.00 ± 0.11 (−0.19–0.19)	0.09 ± 0.15 (−0.15–0.33)	0.03 ± 0.09 (−0.18–0.10)
V_2	0.82 ± 0.25 (0.39–1.25)	0.32 ± 0.21 (0.08–0.84)	0.79 ± 0.27 (0.40–1.39)	0.33 ± 0.22 (−0.12–0.71)	0.62 ± 0.29 (0.09–1.18)	0.28 ± 0.19 (−0.10–0.65)	0.63 ± 0.22 (0.24–1.09)	0.30 ± 0.16 (0.10–0.54)	0.51 ± 0.22 (0.04–0.86)	0.25 ± 0.17 (−0.11–0.55)
V_3	0.90 ± 0.27 (0.37–1.40)	0.48 ± 0.20 (0.14–0.81)	0.81 ± 0.27 (0.36–1.34)	0.46 ± 0.25 (0.08–1.03)	0.68 ± 0.29 (0.11–1.48)	0.36 ± 0.23 (−0.13–0.83)	0.69 ± 0.24 (0.27–1.18)	0.37 ± 0.20 (0.10–0.83)	0.55 ± 0.25 (−0.07–1.07)	0.32 ± 0.13 (−0.04–0.80)
V_4	0.77 ± 0.28 (0.23–1.25)	0.45 ± 0.16 (0.16–0.71)	0.69 ± 0.27 (0.28–1.18)	0.41 ± 0.21 (0.07–0.91)	0.60 ± 0.30 (0.13–1.17)	0.34 ± 0.19 (0.05–0.86)	0.60 ± 0.28 (0.19–1.21)	0.33 ± 0.20 (0.08–0.90)	0.50 ± 0.26 (0.08–1.13)	0.29 ± 0.19 (0.03–0.71)
V_5	0.60 ± 0.20 (0.22–0.93)	0.41 ± 0.13 (0.20–0.65)	0.56 ± 0.23 (0.16–1.08)	0.38 ± 0.16 (0.09–0.73)	0.49 ± 0.20 (0.14–1.01)	0.33 ± 0.15 (0.06–0.59)	0.50 ± 0.26 (0.09–0.92)	0.31 ± 0.17 (0.07–0.71)	0.40 ± 0.21 (−0.09–0.84)	0.28 ± 0.15 (0.04–0.62)
V_6	0.44 ± 0.14 (0.18–0.72)	0.34 ± 0.10 (0.19–0.57)	0.43 ± 0.17 (0.13–0.80)	0.32 ± 0.11 (0.10–0.57)	0.38 ± 0.15 (0.14–0.74)	0.29 ± 0.10 (0.12–0.47)	0.39 ± 0.20 (0.08–0.75)	0.26 ± 0.14 (0.07–0.52)	0.32 ± 0.14 (0.08–0.59)	0.25 ± 0.12 (0.05–0.50)

Table A1.39

Amplitude of Q waves (in millimeters) in normal Japanese of various age-groups

Lead		Male 15–29 (n=61)	Female 15–29 (n=39)	Male 20–29 (n=165)	Female 20–29 (n=109)	Male 30–39 (n=119)	Female 30–39 (n=94)	Male 40–49 (n=153)	Female 40–49 (n=82)	Male 50–59 (n=135)	Female 50–59 (n=102)	Male 60–69 (n=101)	Female 60–69 (n=79)	Male 70+ (n=48)	Female 70+ (n=42)
I	Mn.	0.3	0.28	0.32	0.22	0.37	0.18	0.27	0.24	0.25	0.33	0.27	0.30	0.26	0.39
	Max.–Min.	1.9–0	1.5–0	1.4–0	1.5–0	2.47–0	1.8–0	2.1–0	2.0–0	1.7–0	2.0–0	2.3–0	2.3–0	2.0–0	1.7–0
II	Mn.	0.66	0.44	0.73	0.46	0.52	0.26	0.34	0.30	0.44	0.29	0.35	0.21	0.28	0.30
	Max.–Min.	3.2–0	2.5–0	9.2–0	2.7–0	3.2–0	1.9–0	2.4–0	2.1–0	5.6–0	1.1–0	2.0–0	1.7–0	1.1–0	1.7–0
III	Mn.	0.69	0.51	0.72	0.66	0.56	0.48	0.40	0.42	0.54	0.39	0.39	0.40	0.43	0.23
	Max.–Min.	3.0–0	3.2–0	8.8–0	3.2–0	2.9–0	2.11–0	2.9–0	5.6–0	11.0–0	4.4–0	2.0–0	2.3–0	2.6–0	2.9–0
aVR	Mn.	9.27	7.31	7.38	8.45	3.35	6.74	6.46	6.57	3.68	3.79	3.89	4.12	3.56	2.57
	Max.–Min.	2.0–0 (30)[a]	10.1–5.5	13.5–0	14.3–2.8 (47)[a]	12.9–0	11.5–0	18.2–0	14.5–0.8 (77)[a]	14.0–0 (96)[a]	10.9–0 (84)[a]	12.9–0 (74)[a]	9.9–0 (56)[a]	16.9–0 (23)[a]	1.39–0
aVL	Mn.	0.28	0.26	0.33	0.20	0.15	0.29	0.47	0.30	0.45	0.40	0.50	0.46	0.74	0.59
	Max.–Min.	2.0–0	2.1–0	4.0–0	3.0–0	3.2–0	4.4–0	5.2–0	1.8–0	3.8–0	2.6–0	4.1–0	4.1–0	5.3–0	3.2–0
aVF	Mn.	0.59	0.47	0.60	0.40	0.50	0.35	0.33	0.23	0.43	0.30	0.30	0.24	0.32	0.21
	Max.–Min.	3.8–0	2.4–0	5.8–0	2.5–0	3.0–0	3.4–0	3.1–0	2.2–0	5.3–0	2.6–0	2.0–0	1.7–0	1.1–0	1.4–0
V_4R	Mn.	0.3	0	0.15	0.03	0.11	0.01	0.15	0.18	0.23	0.09	0.07	0.18	0.01	0
	Max.–Min.	1.5–0 (31)[a]	0	1.4–0 (117)[a]	1.2–0 (95)[a]	4.6–0	0.2–0 (75)[a]	6.8–0	4.3–0	4.3–0	4.7–0	3.2–0	4.7–0	0.2–0	0
V_1	Mn.	0.03	0	0.01	0	0.01	0	0.11	0	0.09	0	0	0	0	0
	Max.–Min.	1.2–0	0	1.1–0	0	1.6–0	0	16.5–0	0	11.4–0	0	0	0.2–0	0	0.1–0
V_2	Mn.	0.04	0	0.01	0.01	0.01		0.10	0.01		0	0	0	0	0
	Max.–Min.	1.8–0	0	1.1–0	0.3–0	1.1–0	0.1–0	13.8–0	0.05–0	0	0.5–0	0	0	0.2–0	0
V_3	Mn.	0.03	0	0.01	0	0.01	0.01	0.04	0.02	0.02	0.01	0.03	0.01	0.04	0.04
	Max.–Min.	1.5–0	0	1.1–0	0	0.5–0	1.0–0	3.0–0	1.0–0	1.3–0	2.3–0	2.5–0	0.5–0	1.1–0	1.4–0
V_4	Mn.	0.35	0.16	0.31	0.13	0.4	0.01	0.27	0.70	0.24	0.25	0.26	0.23	0.35	0.50
	Max.–Min.	3.5–0	3.0–0	5.8–0	1.1–0	3.1–0	1.0–0	4.1–0	2.0–0	2.6–0	4.1–0	3.1–0	1.7–0	3.2–0	3.7–0
V_5	Mn.	1.01	0.39	0.87	0.33	0.70	0.04	0.52	0.39	0.51	0.34	0.53	0.34	0.36	0.59
	Max.–Min.	5.0–0	4.1–0	5.2–0	2.0–0	3.4–0	1.3–0	3.0–0	2.0–0	5.0–0	2.0–0	3.8–0	1.7–0	2.0–0	3.1–0
V_6	Mn.	0.95	0.56	0.92	0.45	0.58	0.39	0.59	0.48	0.31	0.49	0.52	0.36	0.45	0.52
	Max.–Min.	4.0–0	3.9–0	4.8–0	2.0–0	3.1–0	1.8–0	2.8–0	2.0–0	4.0–0	2.6–0	2.5–0	1.4–0	2.0–0	2.0–0

Mn., mean; Max., maximum; Min., minimum

[a] Number of cases in which measurement was made

◘ Table A1.40

Amplitude of R waves (in millimeters) in normal Japanese of various age-groups

Lead		15–29 Male (n = 61)	15–29 Female (n = 39)	20–29 Male (n = 165)	20–29 Female (n = 109)	30–39 Male (n = 119)	30–39 Female (n = 94)	40–49 Male (n = 153)	40–49 Female (n = 82)	50–59 Male (n = 135)	50–59 Female (n = 102)	60–69 Male (n = 101)	60–69 Female (n = 79)	70+ Male (n = 48)	70+ Female (n = 42)
I	Mn., SD	5.68, 2.34	5.41, 2.13	5.14, 2.67	5.56, 2.59	5.46, 2.38	5.38, 2.38	5.56, 2.70	5.71, 2.87	5.30, 2.36	6.46, 2.75	5.27, 2.98	6.34, 25.1	5.05, 2.62	6.55, 3.18
	Max.–Min.	13.0–2.0	10.0–2.2	15.3–0.26	15.3–0.43	12.9–1.0	14.2–1.0	14.6–0.3	14.3–0	15.9–0	14.9–0.0	16.9–0	12.9–0	16.9–1.0	15.9–1.0
II	Mn., SD	14.25, 4.65	11.67, 2.99	13.73, 4.69	11.64, 3.97	12.99, 3.82	15.35, 3.16	10.74, 4.20	9.91, 3.66	10.78, 4.11	9.17, 3.24	9.35, 3.98	7.44, 4.06	7.89, 3.23	7.28, 2.98
	Max.–Min.	22.1–6.0	17.5–6.5	23.8–4.2	22.7–2.0	23.9–3.0	19.1–3.33	21.0–0.2	17.0–0	25.9–3.0	17.9–0.0	18.9–1.0	33.4–0	15.9–2.0	16.9–2.0
III	Mn., SD	10.0, 2.97	7.39, 3.95	9.44, 4.86	7.44, 4.26	8.15, 4.19	5.36, 3.34	6.24, 6.20	5.16, 4.15	6.53, 4.36	4.42, 3.15	5.51, 3.16	3.34, 2.66	6.62, 3.39	3.18, 2.41
	Max.–Min.	23.1–25	15.7–0.2	22.1–0.1	21.5–0	19.9–0	15.3–0.4	17.5–0.3	17.0–0.5	21.9–0.0	14.9–0.0	14.9–0	12.4–0	12.4–0	11.9–0.0
aVR	Mn., SD	0.48, 0.24	0.32, 0.73	0.49, 0.56	0.63, 0.74	0.45, 0.72	0.50, 0.72	0.74, 0.00	0.19, 0.00	0.36, 0.17	0.35, 0.54	0.37, 0.24	0.32, 0.43	0.30, 0.48	0.43, 0.48
	Max.–Min.	3.69–0.02	1.5–0	3.2–0	3.2–0	4.9–0	2.4–0	11.9–0	1.4–0	2.4–0	1.9–0.0	2.4–0	1.9–0	1.4–0	1.9–0.0
aVL	Mn., SD	1.62, 1.17	3.06, 1.69	1.93, 2.21	1.71, 2.09	1.89, 1.48	2.21, 2.01	2.37, 2.52	2.29, 2.09	2.16, 2.42	3.15, 2.02	2.53, 2.24	3.29, 2.28	3.22, 2.28	3.86, 0.63
	Max.–Min.	6.44–0.1	6.9–0	16.2–0	13.2–0	11.9–0	9.1–0	14.9–0.1	10.5–0.1	12.9–0	9.9–0	8.9–0	11.9–0	14.9–0	13.9–0.0
aVF	Mn., SD	11.80, 3.53	9.55, 3.70	11.07, 4.76	10.00, 3.88	9.57, 3.93	7.45, 4.71	8.01, 4.25	7.47, 4.71	8.19, 4.34	6.52, 3.36	6.84, 4.81	4.76, 2.68	5.97, 3.32	4.74, 2.30
	Max.–Min.	21.8–1.2	17.5–3.0	25.9–0.5	20.9–0.4	19.9–0	15.4–0.2	17.2–0.4	16.5–0.49	22.9–0.0	16.9–0.0	15.9–0.0	13.9–0	13.0–0	15.9–0.0
V4R	Mn., SD	2.16, 3.26	1.43, 1.04	2.42, 1.65	1.51, 1.02	1.80, 1.05	0.98, 0.75	1.61, 0.00	5.50, 0.00	1.31, 0.74	1.04, 0.73	1.30, 0.96	1.09, 0.40	0.97	1.27, 0.85
	Max.–Min.	6.2–0.1	3.3–0	13.6–0	18.0–0	16.9–0	3.2–0.1	8.4–0.2	2.8–0.1	4.9–0	4.9–0.0	4.9–0	4.4–0	2.4–0	3.9–0.0
		(52)[a]	(34)[a]	(117)[a]	(97)[a]	(86)[a]	(76)[a]	(106)[a]	(76)[a]	(97)[a]	(80)[a]	(74)[a]			
V1	Mn., SD	5.54, 2.56	3.95, 2.44	5.05, 3.19	3.53, 2.55	3.67, 2.06	2.81, 1.66	3.17, 3.64	2.44, 1.62	3.40, 2.28	2.59, 1.67	3.22, 2.57	2.35, 1.89	2.14, 1.57	2.57, 1.47
	Max.–Min.	15.5–1.6	10.8–0	15.8–0.54	10.0–0.23	10.9–0	7.5–0.2	13.9–0.2	6.1–0.3	13.9–0.0	8.9–0.0	13.9–0	9.9–0	8.9–0	8.9–0
V2	Mn., SD	10.78, 4.16	7.32, 3.62	9.76, 4.69	7.10, 3.36	7.66, 3.95	6.48, 3.26	7.0, 4.12	5.52, 3.20	7.41, 4.27	5.95, 3.62	6.32, 3.38	6.38, 3.87	5.74, 3.87	6.28, 3.43
	Max.–Min.	15.7–3.5	18.0–0	22.4–0.8	23.7–1.0	17.9–0	12.5–1.2	18.6–1.0	17.2–0.7	21.9–0.0	15.9–0.0	17.9–0	23.9–0	14.4–0	13.9–0.0
V3	Mn., SD	13.66, 5.80	9.05, 3.22	11.56, 5.73	9.83, 4.50	10.10, 5.37	4.04, 5.34	9.74, 5.38	9.33, 5.66	11.13, 3.25	9.95, 5.77	10.75, 5.69	11.65, 4.98	11.58, 7.40	13.43, 6.10
	Max.–Min.	33.3–3.1	18.5–0.2	37.0–1.17	24.6–3.5	29.9–0	26.1–0.4	24.3–0.6	27.0–1.3	29.9–0.0	35.9–0.0	27.9–0	21.9–0	35.9–0	31.9–2.0
V4	Mn., SD	20.67, 7.05	13.49, 4.90	24.68, 7.53	14.60, 4.90	17.49, 7.35	14.65, 5.16	9.31, 6.51	15.86, 5.92	17.48, 6.04	15.99, 5.72	17.50, 8.41	17.29, 5.37	19.87, 7.94	21.09, 7.78
	Max.–Min.	35.8–2.3	24.8–6.8	53.2–5.0	30.6–2.87	41.9–2.0	34.0–7.1	33.8–3.4	26.8–5.5	35.9–0.0	37.9–0.0	49.9–2.0	37.4–2.0	37.9–0	39.9–6.0
V5	Mn., SD	18.87, 5.31	13.51, 3.44	17.45, 5.84	13.4, 4.46	15.85, 6.29	14.10, 4.48	16.45, 6.09	15.50, 5.0	16.2, 5.52	15.20, 5.29	16.87, 8.23	14.43, 4.88	16.74, 5.81	17.33, 6.05
	Max.–Min.	55.0–8.0	24.0–9.0	43.0–3.98	27.4–2.01	33.9–2.0	26.4–1.7	35.2–1.8	28.5–5.6	35.9–2.0	35.9–4.0	55.9–4.0	24.4–0	24.4–0	35.9–6.0
V6	Mn., SD	14.31, 4.31	11.56, 3.82	13.54, 5.11	11.07, 3.56	11.81, 4.54	11.65, 3.72	13.00, 5.06	11.88, 4.97	12.20, 4.27	11.85, 4.44	12.25, 5.99	10.30, 4.22	11.28, 4.05	10.0, 3.45
	Max.–Min.	28.2–7.0	21.8–7.0	29.0–2.4	23.7–1.2	23.9–2.0	24.9–1.1	24.7–0.9	26.1–1.7	25.9–2.0	23.9–0	37.9–2.0	23.9–0	23.9–20	17.9–4.0

Mn., mean; SD, standard deviation; Max., maximum; Min., minimum

[a] Number of cases in which measurement was made

Table A1.41

Amplitude of S wave (in millimeters) in normal Japanese of various age-groups

		15-19 Male n=61	15-19 Female n=39	20-29 Male n=165	20-29 Female n=109	30-39 Male n=119	30-39 Female n=94	40-49 Male n=153	40-49 Female n=82	50-59 Male n=135	50-59 Female n=102	60-69 Male n=101	60-69 Female n=79	70+ Male n=48	70+ Female n=42
I	Mn.	1.40	0.54	1.19	0.10	0.86	0.63	0.79	0.40	0.76	0.66	0.56	0.54	0.68	0.56
	Max.-Min.	5.7-0	3.4-0	5.35-0	4.0-0	3.9-0	2.7-0	5.0-0	3.1-0	3.9-0	3.4-0	3.4-0	3.4-0	3.4-0	2.4-0
II	Mn.	2.02	0.76	1.31	0.66	1.30	0.65	1.14	0.48	1.14	0.64	1.37	1.07	1.18	1.04
	Max.-Min.	5.8-0	2.9-0	6.2-0	6.2-0	6.9-0	4.6-0	9.1-0	3.7-0	7.9-0	4.9-0	8.4-0	8.9-0	5.9-0.0	4.9-0
III	Mn.	1.8	0.76	0.94	0.53	1.22	0.77	1.42	0.83	1.28	1.52	1.91	2.08	2.37	2.18
	Max.-Min.	4.9-0	4.8-0	8.9-0	6.2-0	11.9-0	4.1-0	14.0-0	5.5-0	11.9-0	8.9-0	9.9-0	12.9-0	11.9-0.0	10.9-0
aVR	Mn.	9.60	8.83	9.05	8.92	5.87	7.36	7.62	0.80	4.50	4.52	4.06	3.67	2.70	4.66
	Max.-Min.	14.4-0	11.2-5.6	21.7-0.17	21.0-4.0	15.9-0	11.6-3.6	14.0-0.7	13.8-0.1	17.9-0	15.9-0	19.9-0	13.9-0	11.9-0	15.9-0
aVL	Mn.	3.27	1.82	2.98	2.12	2.39	1.43	2.44	1.26	1.83	1.50	1.76	1.21	1.12	0.88
	Max.-Min.	9.5-0	7.1-0	14.2-0	12.0-0	15.9-0	7.2-0	8.8-0	8.2-0	8.9-0	5.9-0	7.9-0	5.9-0	5.9-0.0	3.4-0
aVF	Mn.	1.42	0.62	1.20	0.53	1.27	0.53	1.04	0.54	1.03	0.90	1.66	1.45	1.70	1.35
	Max.-Min.	5.84-0	2.2-0	12.0-0	3.2-0	12.9-0	2.0-0	7.1-0	3.8-0	8.9-0	4.9-0	22.9-0	10.9-0	6.9-0.0	5.9-0
V4R	Mn.	2.99	3.3	3.99	2.73	3.47	3.35	4.15	2.70	3.82	3.43	4.05	3.68	4.45	3.16
	Max.-Min.	8.05-0	8.4-0	11.0-0	14.0-0	8.9-0	10.2-0	18.6-0	9.4-0	13.9-0	10.9-0	10.9-0	20.9-0	9.9-0.0	6.9-0
		(49)[a]													
V1	Mn.	10.85	9.2	9.7	9.59	9.71	8.90	9.42	9.62	9.58	9.07	8.83	8.46	8.87	8.47
	Max.-Min.	22.7-0	22.0-0	27.4-0	24.5-2.3	1.9-0	15.5-0	24.2-0	23.3-1.1	21.9-0	21.9-0	19.9-0	21.9-0	17.9-0	17.9-0
V2	Mn.	18.04	15.8	20.05	14.06	15.37	13.38	13.97	12.26	14.14	13.25	12.55	13.08	13.03	12.38
	Max.-Min.	42.5-0	26.5-6.5	55.1-0	34.2-3.6	37.9-0	28.8-2.1	27.0-0	30.7-1.2	31.9-0	27.9-0	29.9-2.0	33.9-0	29.9-0.0	27.9-2.0
V3	Mn.	13.37	8.8	12.62	7.71	10.26	7.42	11.31	8.24	11.40	9.03	10.35	10.85	11.95	12.05
	Max.-Min.	25.0-0	17.0-0	34.0-0	16.0-0	27.9-0	16.9-0	29.5-0	19.4-0	27.9-2.0	27.9-0	27.9-0	37.9-0	27.9-0	29.9-0
V4	Mn.	7.22	4.5	6.46	6.42	5.54	4.00	6.43	3.91	6.82	5.85	7.01	6.36	7.66	7.38
	Max.-Min.	45.0-0	11.5-0	22.6-0	11.1-0	23.9-0	12.3-0	20.0-0	12.7-0	21.9-0	21.9-0	27.9-0	19.9-0	27.9-0	21.9-0
V5	Mn.	2.92	2.7	2.28	1.86	2.02	1.73	2.46	1.46	2.53	2.06	2.75	2.80	2.26	2.50
	Max.-Min.	40.0-0	5.1-0	10.0-0	6.4-0	14.9-0	5.55-0	11.5-0	6.3-0	18.9-0	10.9-0	16.9-0	23.9-0	7.9-0	10.9-0
V6	Mn.	1.32	0.62	0.99	0.54	0.85	0.51	0.64	0.39	0.91	0.72	0.99	0.94	0.80	0.84
	Max.-Min.	17.8-0	3.3-0	10.7-0	4.5-0	6.9-0	3.64-0	6.9-0	2.6-0.4	7.9-0	3.9-0	9.9-0	8.9-0	5.9-0	4.9-0

Mn., mean; Max., maximum; Min., minimum

[a]Number of cases in which measurement was made

◘ Table A1.42

ST segment "J" point (in millimeters) in normal Japanese of various age-groups

		15–29 Male (n=60)	15–29 Female (n=39)	20–29 Male (n=165)	20–29 Female (n=109)	30–39 Male (n=119)	30–39 Female (n=94)	40–49 Male (n=153)	40–49 Female (n=82)	50–59 Male (n=135)	50–59 Female (n=102)	60–69 Male (n=101)	60–69 Female (n=79)	70+ Male (n=48)	70+ Female (n=42)
I	Mn., SD	0.03, 0.21	0.1, 0.21	0.01, 0.25	−0.06, 0.23	0.08, 0.17	−0.01, 0.22	0.03, 0.17	0.08, 0.24	0.00, 0.22	−0.00, 0.18	0.06, 0.22	0.03, 0.10	0.00, 0.27	0.00, 0.09
	Max.–Min.	0.9 to −0.8	0.7 to −0.8	0.9 to −1.0	0.05 to −0.8	0.7 to −0.8	0.9 to −0.6	0.5 to −0.8	1.3 to −0.8	1.0 to −1.2	0.5 to −0.8	1.1 to −1.0	0.7 to −0.4	0.9 to −1.0	0.3 to −0.4
II	Mn., SD	0.02, 0.55	0.03, 0.45	0.13, 0.39	0.77, 0.42	0.16, 0.38	0.00, 0.23	0.03, 0.36	0.12, 0.46	0.07, 0.33	0.03, 0.26	0.05, 0.41	0.06, 0.08	0.00, 0.27	0.09, 0.41
	Max.–Min.	2.9 to −1.01	2.4 to −0.6	1.7 to −1.0	2.1 to −0.2	1.4 to −1.0	0.7 to −0.8	1.1 to −1.6	2.5 to −0.8	1.7 to −1.0	1.1 to −1.0	1.5 to −1.6	1.1 to −0.6	0.7 to −1.0	1.9 to −0.5
III	Mn., SD	0.05, 0.28	0.01, 0.30	0.07, 0.35	0.03, 0.40	0.15, 0.35	−0.01, 0.30	0.00, 0.41	0.07, 0.33	0.03, 0.28	0.06, 0.23	0.05, 0.38	0.09, 0.18	0.04, 0.17	0.03, 0.21
	Max.–Min.	1.1 to −1.2	1.5 to −0.6	1.9 to −0.8	1.3 to −0.8	1.9 to −0.8	1.3 to −1.0	1.1 to −1.2	1.1 to −1.0	1.0 to −1.1	0.9 to −1.0	1.1 to −2.0	1.1 to −0.6	0.5 to −0.4	1.9 to −0.5
aVR	Mn., SD	0.06, 0.41	−0.05, 0.20	0.00, 0.38	−0.05, 0.52	0.04, 0.34	0.01, 0.28	0.06, 0.29	0.04, 0.31	0.11, 0.28	0.04, 0.26	0.03, 0.29	0.04, 0.19	0.00, 0.23	−0.08, 0.19
	Max.–Min.	1.3 to −0.8	0.5 to −0.6	2.1 to −1.2	1.3 to −1.4	1.1 to −1.6	1.1 to −1.0	1.0 to −0.8	1.1 to −1.4	1.1 to −1.2	0.9 to −0.8	1.9 to −0.6	0.9 to −0.8	0.7 to −0.6	0.3 to −0.7
aVL	Mn., SD	−0.02, 0.23	0.03, 0.17	0.03, 0.31	0.20, 0.35	0.04, 0.19	−0.02, 0.27	0.06, 0.21	0.031, 0.22	−0.04, 0.21	0.05, 0.13	0.08, 0.17	0.02, 0.14	0.03, 0.13	0.02, 0.05
	Max.–Min.	0.9 to −0.8	0.5 to −0.6	1.3 to −1.2	1.5 to −0.6	0.9 to −2.0	1.0 to −1.8	1.1 to −1.0	0.7 to −1.2	0.7 to −1.0	0.7 to −0.6	1.3 to −0.6	0.3 to −0.6	0.3 to −0.6	0.2 to −1.0
aVF	Mn., SD	0.01, 0.35	0.3, 0.24	0.10, 0.41	0.53, 0.35	0.16, 0.35	0.00, 0.36	0.07, 0.37	0.09, 0.31	0.07, 0.33	0.04, 0.20	0.07, 0.37	0.09, 0.19	−0.03, 0.31	0.03, 0.30
	Max.–Min.	1.1 to −1.0	1.1 to −0.6	1.8 to −1.0	1.5 to −0.4	2.1 to −1.0	1.5 to −1.0	1.5 to −1.2	1.1 to −0.6	1.6 to −1.0	0.9 to −1.0	1.7 to −1.6	1.1 to −0.6	1.9 to −1.0	1.3 to −0.5
V4R	Mn., SD	0.23, 0.36	0.00, 0.23	0.02, 0.24	0.17, 0.26	0.11, 0.10	−0.02, 0.21	0.08, 0.24	−0.02, 0.21	0.02, 0.19	0.07, 0.21	0.13, 0.14	0.09, 0.18	0.16, 0.10	0.08, 0.10
	Max.–Min.	1.1 to −0.5	1.1 to −0.6	1.1 to −0.6	1.1 to −0.6	0.9 to −0.2	1.1 to −0.6	1.1 to −1.4	0.9 to −0.8	1.7 to −0.8	1.1 to −1.0	0.9 to −0.4	0.9 to −2.0	0.7 to −0.4	0.9 to −0.1
		(32)[a]	(36)[a]	(114)[a]	(94)[a]	(87)[a]	(68)[a]	(107)[a]	(74)[a]	(93)[a]	(78)[a]	(74)[a]	(56)[a]	(23)[a]	(17)[a]
V1	Mn., SD	0.28, 0.44	0.12, 0.35	0.44, 0.52	0.36, 0.29	0.38, 0.44	0.09, 0.25	0.39, 0.50	0.09, 0.38	0.39, 0.40	0.18, 0.25	0.08, 0.57	0.19, 0.30	0.46, 0.35	0.32, 0.39
	Max.–Min.	1.3 to −0.8	1.7 to −0.8	2.5 to −1.0	1.1 to −0.6	1.7 to −1.6	0.9 to −0.6	2.9 to −1.4	1.1 to −1.2	1.5 to −1.2	1.1 to −0.6	2.1 to −1.0	1.1 to −1.0	1.1 to −0.5	1.5 to −0.0
V2	Mn., SD	0.94, 0.87	0.26, 0.48	0.93, 0.89	0.47, 0.31	0.70, 0.30	0.28, 0.47	0.88, 0.86	0.32, 0.50	0.69, 0.79	0.40, 0.47	0.75, 0.48	0.51, 0.54	0.83, 0.63	0.62, 0.43
	Max.–Min.	3.3–0	1.1 to −1.4	4.1 to −1.0	1.3 to −0.4	4.1 to −1.4	2.7 to −0.8	6.1 to −0.6	2.1 to −1.2	2.8 to −2.6	1.9 to −1.0	3.3 to −0.5	2.7 to −1.0	2.5 to −0.5	1.5 to −0.7
V3	Mn., SD	1.00, 0.57	0.47, 0.57	0.87, 0.99	0.46, 0.29	0.67, 0.61	0.18, 0.44	0.76, 1.22	0.11, 0.93	0.56, 1.25	0.30, 0.62	0.60, 0.37	0.22, 0.40	0.59, 0.66	0.43, 0.57
	Max.–Min.	2.7 to −1.5	2.3 to −0.8	5.5 to −0.6	1.3 to −0.4	2.7 to −1.2	1.9 to −1.0	9.0 to −6.8	2.5 to −6.3	2.2 to −1.5	2.1 to −2.0	2.1 to −1.2	1.5 to −1.2	2.3 to −0.8	2.0 to −0.7
V4	Mn., SD	0.51, 0.72	0.10, 0.47	0.57, 0.90	0.37, 0.23	0.59, 0.79	0.04, 0.44	0.37, 0.59	0.01, 0.38	0.23, 0.50	0.04, 0.51	0.29, 0.55	0.03, 0.43	0.09, 0.57	0.06, 0.46
	Max.–Min.	2.9 to −1.0	2.3 to −0.8	6.4 to −1.0	1.1 to −0.4	5.1 to −1.6	1.7 to −0.8	3.3 to −2.4	2.1 to −1.0	1.8 to −1.4	2.5 to −1.2	1.9 to −2.0	1.5 to −1.6	1.7 to −1.6	1.0 to −1.0
V5	Mn., SD	0.35, 0.50	0.03, 0.31	0.26, 0.57	0.34, 0.22	0.25, 0.49	0.09, 0.33	0.19, 0.41	0.09, 0.54	0.05, 0.38	0.02, 0.35	0.09, 0.37	−0.02, 0.32	−0.02, 0.39	0.03, 0.25
	Max.–Min.	2.3 to −0.4	1.1 to −0.8	3.0 to −1.0	1.1 to −0.2	2.9 to −1.2	1.3 to −0.8	1.9 to −2.2	2.5 to −1.0	1.5 to −1.1	1.5 to −1.0	1.5 to −1.0	1.5 to −1.6	1.1 to −1.2	0.6 to −0.9
V6	Mn., SD	0.24, 0.50	0.0, 0.14	0.24, 0.50	0.34, 0.25	0.21, 0.41	0.13, 0.37	0.14, 0.26	0.20, 0.54	0.10, 0.32	0.06, 0.26	0.09, 0.33	0.09, 0.19	0.15, 0.30	0.05, 0.27
	Max.–Min.	2.2–0.4	0.7 to −0.4	5.1 to −0.6	1.3 to −0.2	2.5 to −2.1	1.5 to −1.0	1.1 to −1.2	2.5 to −0.6	1.5 to −1.0	1.9 to −0.6	1.5 to −1.0	1.1 to −0.6	0.7 to −1.0	1.0 to −0.7

Mn., SD, standard deviation; Max., maximum; Min., minimum

[a] Number of cases in which measurement was made

Table A1.43

Amplitude of T wave (in millimeters) in normal Japanese of various age-groups

		15–19 Male n=61	15–19 Female n=38	20–29 Male n=165	20–29 Female n=109	30–39 Male n=119	30–39 Female n=94	40–49 Male n=153	40–49 Female n=82	50–59 Male n=135	50–59 Female n=102	60–69 Male n=101	60–69 Female n=79	70+ Male n=48	70+ Female n=42
I	Mn., SD	3.21, 1.13	2.50, 0.88	2.80, 1.11	2.42, 0.98	2.42, 0.93	2.30, 0.79	2.42, 0.95	1.87, 0.89	2.23, 0.93	2.08, 0.81	2.07, 0.96	1.83, 0.96	1.54, 1.74	1.83, 0.78
	Max.-Min.	5.9–1.0	4.9–0.0	7.9–0.0	5.9–0.0	5.9–0.0	5.9 to –1.0	6.9–0.0	3.9–0.0	5.9–0.0	4.9–0.0	4.9–0.0	4.9–0.0	2.9 to –1.0	4.9 to –0.0
II	Mn., SD	4.65, 1.34	2.88, 1.04	4.26, 1.56	2.98, 1.40	3.79, 1.47	2.91, 1.15	3.63, 1.39	2.62, 1.02	3.40, 1.44	2.47, 1.22	3.18, 1.45	2.27, 1.02	2.56, 1.17	2.12, 0.87
	Max.-Min.	7.9–1.0	4.9–0.0	9.9–0.0	7.9 to –3.0	9.9–0.0	6.1–0.0	7.9–0.0	5.9–0.0	8.9 to –1.0	5.9 to –1.0	7.9–2.0	7.9–0.0	5.9–0.0	3.9–0.0
III	Mn., SD	1.93, 0.99	0.42, 0.95	1.78, 1.30	0.58, 1.10	1.65, 1.33	0.70, 0.76	1.45, 1.54	0.75, 0.99	1.40, 1.10	0.56, 0.90	1.46, 1.48	0.54, 1.07	1.33, 1.14	0.62, 0.78
	Max.-Min.	4.9 to –1.0	3.9 to –3.0	5.9 to –2.0	4.9 to –2.0	5.9 to –2.0	2.9 to –2.0	6.9 to –3.0	4.9 to –2.0	5.9 to –3.0	2.9 to –2.0	5.9 to –3.0	3.9 to –2.0	4.9 to –1.0	2.9 to –2.0
aVR	Mn., SD	–3.68, 1.58	2.42, 0.83	–2.37, 1.38	–0.3, 0.95	–2.74, 1.46	–2.50, 0.87	–2.00, 2.28	–1.55, 1.53	–2.31, 1.42	–1.88, 1.10	–2.16, 1.43	–1.58, 1.16	–0.16, 1.17	–1.12, 1.48
	Max.-Min.	–0.1 to –70	–0.1 to –5.0	–0.1 to –12.0	–0.1 to –5.0	3.9 to –7.6	–0.1 to –5.0	4.9 to –6	3.9 to –4.0	4.9 to –6.0	2.9 to –5.0	2.9 to –5.0	2.9 to –4.0	1.9 to –5.0	2.9 to –4.0
aVL	Mn., SD	1.05, 0.83	1.26, 0.83	0.89, 1.03	1.34, 1.02	0.70, 1.00	1.10, 0.72	0.87, 1.14	0.85, 0.66	0.73, 0.89	0.96, 0.72	0.52, 1.15	0.27, 0.84	0.52, 0.71	0.90, 0.85
	Max.-Min.	3.0 to –1.0	3.9 to –1.0	5.9 to –2.0	6.9 to –2.0	3.9 to –2.0	3.9 to –1.0	7.9 to –2.0	2.9 to –2.0	3.9 to –2.0	2.9 to –1.0	3.9 to –3.0	3.9 to –2.0	1.9 to –2.0	3.9 to –2.0
aVF	Mn., SD	3.18, 1.28	1.73, 0.95	2.98, 1.56	1.88, 1.20	2.62, 1.46	1.86, 0.93	2.45, 1.58	1.72, 0.90	2.21, 1.26	1.47, 0.86	2.43, 1.37	1.41, 0.75	1.75, 1.23	1.23, 1.06
	Max.-Min.	5.9–0.0	4.9 to –1.0	7.9 to –6.0	6.9 to –2.0	6.9 to –4.0	4.9 to –1.0	12.0 to –1.0	4.9 to –0.2	6.9 to –2.0	4.9 to –1.0	6.9 to –2.0	3.9 to –1.0	4.9 to –1.0	3.9 to –4.0
V4R	Mn., SD	–0.26, 1.10	–0.55, 0.78	0.17, 1.25	–0.68, 0.95	0.35, 1.02	0.67, 1.07	–0.01, 1.26	–0.49, 0.79	–0.02, 0.96	–0.42, 0.81	–0.26, 0.99	–0.55, 0.84	0.00, 1.16	–0.32, 0.57
	Max.-Min.	1.9 to –4.0	1.9 to –2.0	3.9 to –4.0	1.9 to –3.0	2.9 to –3.0	1.9 to –3.0	3.9 to –5.0	2.9 to –2.0	3.9 to –3.0	1.9 to –2.0	1.9 to –3.0	2.9 to –3.0	2.9 to –2.0	0.9 to –2.0
		(50)[a]	(37)[a]	(117)[a]	(96)[a]	(86)[a]	(67)[a]	(108)[a]	(74)[a]	(94)[a]	(78)[a]	(74)[a]	(56)[a]	(23)[a]	(17)[a]
V1	Mn., SD	1.42, 2.55	–0.15, 1.38	1.99, 1.81	–0.45, 1.65	1.77, 2.02	–0.19, 1.34	1.52, 4.21	0.53, 1.28	1.35, 2.10	–0.13, 1.45	1.20, 1.95	0.08, 1.45	1.63, 1.67	0.29, 1.86
	Max.-Min.	7.9 to –5.0	2.9 to –4.0	6.9 to –3.0	4.9 to –4.0	8.9 to –2.0	2.9 to –3.0	10.9 to –5.0	2.9 to –4.0	7.9 to –5.0	4.9 to –4.0	5.9 to –3.0	4.9 to –3.0	5.9 to –3.0	6.9 to –4.0
V2	Mn., SD	8.38, 3.67	3.20, 2.90	8.14, 3.65	2.96, 2.16	6.90, 3.57	3.17, 2.03	6.48, 3.04	2.78, 1.85	6.43, 3.01	3.35, 2.25	5.38, 2.90	3.08, 2.19	5.04, 2.80	3.24, 2.42
	Max.-Min.	19.9 to –1.0	10.9 to –3.0	23.9–0.0	8.9 to –4.0	18.9 to –2.0	8.9 to –2.0	13.9 to –1.0	7.9 to –2.0	13.9 to –3.0	9.9 to –3.0	11.9 to –5.0	10.9 to –2.0	11.9–0.0	9.9 to –3.0
V3	Mn., SD	9.92, 3.52	4.50, 2.24	8.86, 3.63	4.05, 2.16	7.58, 3.37	4.21, 2.17	7.92, 3.03	3.78, 2.14	7.95, 2.97	4.43, 2.52	7.27, 2.98	4.36, 2.37	7.08, 2.98	4.62, 2.41
	Max.-Min.	20.9–0.0	10.9–0.0	22.9–2.0	9.9 to –0.0	20.9–1.0	10.9–0.0	16.9–0.0	9.9 to –2.0	18.9–2.0	12.9 to –3.0	15.9 to –2.0	11.9 to –1.0	14.9–2.0	8.9 to –1.0
V4	Mn., SD	9.38, 3.75	5.15, 2.08	8.72, 3.93	4.80, 1.84	7.58, 3.89	4.87, 2.46	7.61, 3.35	4.36, 2.14	7.78, 2.93	4.32, 2.74	7.07, 3.27	4.22, 1.99	6.19, 2.63	4.33, 2.58
	Max.-Min.	16.9–1.0	10.9–0.0	24.9–1.0	10.9–0.0	40.9–1.0	13.0–0.0	26.9–1.0	11.9 to –1.0	18.9–2.0	13.9 to –2.0	17.4 to –5.0	12.9–0.0	13.9 to –4.0	11.9–0.0
V5	Mn., SD	8.53, 3.58	4.45, 1.70	5.30, 2.82	4.25, 1.65	5.44, 2.86	4.45, 2.01	5.54, 2.43	4.03, 1.95	5.50, 2.43	3.11, 1.66	5.48, 2.51	3.32, 1.77	4.42, 2.49	3.41, 1.66
	Max.-Min.	15.9–0.0	8.9–0.0	16.9–1.0	10.9 to –2.0	14.9–0.0	11.0–0.0	14.9–1.0	11.9–6	14.9 to –2.0	9.9–0.0	12.9–0.0	9.9–0.0	10.9 to –2.0	8.9–0.0
V6	Mn., SD	4.96, 2.21	3.69, 1.37	4.48, 2.15	3.43, 2.41	3.80, 1.85	3.55, 1.45	3.87, 1.75	3.12, 1.42	3.27, 1.60	2.98, 1.33	3.96, 2.06	2.45, 1.00	2.92, 1.54	2.34, 1.11
	Max.-Min.	11.9–0.0	6.9–0.0	14.9–0.0	8.9–0.0	8.9–0.0	7.9–1.0	9.9–0.0	7.9–0.0	8.9 to –1.0	7.9–0.0	13.9–0.0	4.9–0.0	6.9 to –1.0	4.9–0.0 (38)[a]

Mn., mean; SD, standard deviation; Max., maximum; Min., minimum

[a] Number of cases in which measurement was made

A1.4 Normal Limits of Right-Sided Chest Leads in Caucasians

The tables in this section were derived from 109 subjects with no evidence of heart disease (❯ Tables A1.44–A1.51b). The data is reproduced from: Andersen HR, Nielsen D, Hansen LG. The normal right chest electrocardiogram. *J. Electrocardiol.* 1987;**20**: 27–32 with the permission of Churchill Livingstone, New York.

◼ Table A1.44
R-wave amplitudes (millimeters)

	Median	95% fractile values	Mean $\bar{x}$	Range	Number n
V_3R	1.5	0.4–3.9	1.7	0.1–4.3	107
V_4R	1.0	0.3–3.3	1.2	0.2–4.2	101
V_5R	1.0	0.3–2.4	1.0	0.2–5.0	79
V_6R	0.7	0.2–2.6	0.9	0.2–5.1	59
V_7R	0.5	0.3–3.6	1.0	0.3–5.6	37

◼ Table A1.45
S-wave amplitudes (millimeters)

	Median	95% fractile values	Mean $\bar{x}$	Range	Number n
V_3R	5.1	1.7–11.4	5.7	0.9–13.5	108
V_4R	3.6	1.1–8.0	3.9	0.9–9.7	104
V_5R	3.6	1.0–7.7	3.5	0.5–8.8	89
V_6R	2.5	0.7–6.4	2.9	0.4–7.3	70
V_7R	2.7	0.8–5.4	2.8	0.7–6.8	45

◼ Table A1.46
Secondary r-wave (qr, rSr′) amplitudes (millimeters)

	Median	95% fractile values	Mean $\bar{x}$	Range	Number n
V_3R	0.8	0.5–1.5	0.9	0.4–1.5	6
V_4R	0.7	0.2–1.8	0.8	0.2–1.8	11
V_5R	0.8	0.3–2.5	1.0	0.2–2.5	36
V_6R	0.9	0.3–3.6	1.3	0.2–4.2	50
V_7R	0.0	0.3–3.6	1.2	0.1–4.8	71

◼ Table A1.47
Q-wave amplitudes (millimeters)

	Median	95% fractile values	Mean $\bar{x}$	Range	Number n
V_3R					2
V_4R	2.8	1.5–8.1	4.4	1.5–8.1	8
V_5R	2.5	0.8–5.3	2.7	0.7–5.9	30
V_6R	1.9	1.0–4.7	2.2	0.9–4.9	47
V_7R	1.8	0.9–3.9	2.0	0.6–4.1	71

◘ Table A1.48

r + r′ amplitudes (millimeters)

	Median	95% fractile values	Mean $\bar{x}$	Range	Number n
V_3R	1.5	0.3–3.9	1.7	0.0–4.3	109
$\sum_{V_3R}^{V_4R} r + r'$	2.5	0.5–6.8	2.8	0.3–8.1	109
$\sum_{V_3R}^{V_5R} r + r'$	3.5	0.5–9.1	3.8	0.3–13.3	109
$\sum_{V_3R}^{V_6R} r + r'$	4.0	0.8–11.3	4.9	0.4–15.7	109
$\sum_{V_3R}^{V_7R} r + r'$	4.9	1.4–14.8	6.0	0.4–20.5	109

◘ Table A1.49

J-point deviation (millimeters)

	Median	95% fractile values	Mean $\bar{x}$	Range	Number n
V_3R	−0.1	0.4 to −0.5	−0.1	−0.6 to +0.5	109
V_4R	−0.1	0.3 to −0.6	−0.1	−0.9 to +0.5	104
V_5R	0.0	0.3 to −0.7	−0.1	−0.8 to +0.5	107
V_6R	0.0	0.5 to −0.6	0.0	−0.8 to +0.5	108
V_7R	0.0	0.5 to −0.5	0.0	−0.9 to +0.6	103

◘ Table A1.50

ST-segment deviation (millimeters) 40 ms after last QRS deflection

	Median	95% fractile values	Mean $\bar{x}$	Range	Number n
V_3R	0.1	0.6 to −0.5	0.1	−1.2 to +0.8	109
V_4R	0.1	0.5 to −0.4	0.0	−1.4 to +0.6	109
V_5R	0.1	0.5 to −0.4	0.1	−0.8 to +0.6	109
V_6R	0.0	0.5 to −0.3	0.1	−0.5 to +1.0	109
V_7R	0.1	0.4 to −0.4	0.1	−0.5 to +0.9	109

◘ Table A1.51(a)

ST-segment deviation (millimeters) 80 ms after last QRS deflection

	Median	95% fractile values	Mean $\bar{x}$	Range	Number n
V_3R	0.3	0.9 to −0.3	0.3	−0.4 to +1.0	109
V_4R	0.2	0.6 to −0.3	0.2	−0.5 to +0.9	109
V_5R	0.1	0.5 to −0.3	0.1	−0.7 to +1.0	109
V_6R	0.0	0.5 to −0.3	0.0	−0.6 to +0.6	109
V_7R	0.0	0.4 to −0.3	0.0	−0.8 to +0.5	109

◘ Table A1.51(b)

Q-wave duration (ms)

	Median	95% fractile values	Mean $\bar{x}$	Range	Number n
V_3R					2
V_4R	53	20–80	50	20–81	8
V_5R	34	20–64	40	17–108	30
V_6R	34	17–74	36	17–81	47
V_7R	34	17–58	34	14–64	71

A1.5 Normal Limits of the Three-Orthogonal-Lead ECG

A1.5.1 Normal Limits in Males

Some of the earliest work on the three-orthogonal-lead ECG was undertaken in the laboratory of Pipberger. His group studied 510 men, including whites and blacks, and with the use of computer methods, analyzed the ECGs automatically. ❯ Tables A1.52–A1.61 are reproduced from Draper H W et al. The corrected orthogonal electrocardiogram and vectorcardiogram in 510 normal men (Frank-lead system). *Circulation* 1964;**30**: 853–864 with the permission of the American Heart Association, Dallas, Texas.

◻ Table A1.52

Measurements of P, QRS and T in scalar orthogonal leads *X*, *Y* and *Z*. The mean and standard deviation of each item is shown on the upper line. The second line indicates the limits of a 96 percentile range. A similar pattern is used for A1.52 to A1.61. Figures in parentheses in A1.52 show the actual number of measurements taken (e.g., Q waves in lead *X* were present in 306 cases only). Results not followed by a number in parentheses were obtained from the total series. All wave durations are based on the total QRS duration derived from the three leads. The earliest or last deflection in any one of the simultaneously recorded leads indicates onset or end of this complex

Item	X		Y		Z	
P amplitude (mV)	0.06 ± 0.03		0.11 ± 0.07		0.03 ± 0.0	
	0.03–0.12		0.05–0.23		−0.06–0.10	
Q amplitude (mV)	0.10 ± 0.05	(306)	0.10 ± 0.07	(333)	0.41 ± 0.21	
	0.03–0.25		0.01–0.29		0.09–0.93	
Q duration (s)	0.019 ± 0.004	(306)	0.021 ± 0.005	(333)	0.033 ± 0.007	
	0.012–0.028		0.008–0.032		0.020–0.048	
R amplitude (mV)	1.17 ± 0.37		1.03 ± 0.41		0.93 ± 0.35	
	0.51–1.97		0.35–1.95		0.36–1.79	
R duration (s)	0.051 ± 0.016		0.061 ± 0.019		0.059 ± 0.010	
	0.028–0.88		0.028–0.100		0.032–0.080	
S amplitude (mV)	0.27 ± 0.15	(407)	0.18 ± 0.12	(274)		
	0.06–0.68		0.03–0.49			
S duration (s)	0.039 ± 0.008	(407)	0.035 ± 0.010	(274)		
	0.024–0.056		0.020–0.056			
T amplitude (mV)	0.27 ± 0.13		0.22 ± 0.13		−0.28± 0.13	
	0.06–0.56		−0.11–0.48		−0.58 to −0.06	
Q/R amplitude ratio	0.08 ± 0.04	(306)	0.10 ± 0.05	(333)	0.49 ± 0.35	
	0.02–0.21		0.01–0.22		0.10–1.21	
R/S amplitude ratio	5.74 ± 4.62	(407)	9.07 ± 9.39	(274)		
	1.40–19.25		1.11–38.51			
R/T amplitude ratio	5.44 ± 4.01		5.18 ± 3.25		4.02 ± 2.66	
	1.63–20.16		1.67–13.79		1.12–12.42	
Time from beginning of QRS to largest R peak (s)	0.037 ± 0.005		0.039 ± 0.005		0.049 ± 0.006	
	0.028–0.048		0.028–0.052		0.036–0.064	

◻ Table A1.53

Time intervals obtained from three simultaneously recorded leads. The method of measurement is the same as indicated for Table A1.52

Item	Measurement (s)
P duration	0.102+0.016
	0.068–0.140
PR interval	0.153 ± 0.023
	0.112–0.204
PR segment	0.051 ± 0.019
	0.021–0.096
QRS duration	0.093 ± 0.009
	0.076–0.112
QT interval (uncorrected)	0.367 ± 0.034
	0.312–0.448

◻ Table A1.54

Maximal P, QRS and T vectors in the frontal, sagittal and horizontal planes together with spatial amplitude and orientation. The vectors in the plane projections were obtained from *XY*, *YZ* and *XZ* leads, respectively, and do not therefore represent projections of the spatial maximal vectors onto these planes

Item	Maximal P vector	Maximal QRS vector	Maximal T vector
Frontal plane			
Amplitude (mV)	0.18 ± 0.06	1.57 ± 0.42	0.36 ± 0.14
	0.08–0.31	0.81–2.53	0.12–0.69
Direction (°)	67 ± 18	41 ± 14	40 ± 20
	22–91	14–71	4–74
Sagittal plane			
Amplitude (mV)	0.17 ± 0.06	1.32 ± 0.45	0.36 ± 0.13
	0.06–0.31	0.60–2.42	0.13–0.67
Direction (°)	87 ± 23	48 ± 30	142 ± 23
	54–129	343–114	93–180
Horizontal plane			
Amplitude (mV)	0.09 ± 0.03	1.39 ± 0.36	0.40 ± 0.14
	0.04–0.14	0.74–2.19	0.15–0.72
Direction (°)	349 ± 41	327 ± 34	46 ± 19
	285–91	245–29	8–83
Spatial amplitude (m)V	0.18 ± 0.06	1.73 ± 0.44	0.46 ± 0.16
	0.09–0.32	0.92–2.75	0.18–0.82
Spatial orientation			
Azimuth (°)	342 ± 38	331 ± 27	44 ± 19
	277–75	263–23	4–79
Elevation (°)	63 ± 17	35 ± 13	29 ± 13
	20–86	7–60	2–58

■ Table A1.55

Quantitative analysis of early QRS vectors. The upper row provides mean ±SD and the lower row gives a 96% range

Instantaneous vectors[a]	Scalar amplitude (mV)			Planar direction (°)			Spatial magnitude and orientation		
	X	Y	Z	Frontal	Sagittal	Horizontal	Amplitude (mV)	Azimuth (°)	Elevation (°)
0.01 s after	−0.04± 0.04	−0.03± 0.06	−0.11± 0.06	210 ± 61	189 ± 36	110 ± 34	0.14 ± 0.06	110 ± 34	−10± 27
QRS onset	−0.14−0.07	−0.13−0.08	−0.25−0.01	59−330	79−242	17−168	0.05−0.29	17−168	−59−58
0.02 s after	0.05 ± 0.14	−0.01± 0.12	−0.31± 0.15	325 ± 87	180 ± 25	81 ± 26	0.37 ± 0.15	81 ± 26	−1± 20
QRS onset	−0.19−0.38	−0.25−0.29	0.68 to −0.06	162−136	117−220	23−124	0.12−0.75	23−124	−39−42
0.03 s after	0.56 ± 0.27	0.35 ± 0.25	−0.20± 0.32	29 ± 23	120 ± 40	21 ± 30	0.79 ± 0.30	21 ± 30	26 ± 15
QRS onset	0.06−1.19	−0.06−0.97	−0.89−0.48	350−59	41−186	319−79	0.29−1.52	319−79	−6−53
0.04 s after	1.05 ± 0.37	0.86 ± 0.37	0.34 ± 0.46	40 ± 16	72 ± 27	343 ± 25	1.51 ± 0.42	343 ± 25	35 ± 11
QRS onset	0.33−1.79	−0.24−1.79	−0.59−1.26	14−66	28−139	294−35	0.78−2.53	294 ± 35	13−59
0.05 s after	0.65 ± 0.51	0.74 ± 0.47	0.77 ± 0.40	52 ± 36	42 ± 24	307 ± 28	1.40 ± 0.50	307 ± 28	31 ± 16
QRS onset	−0.27−1.76	−0.09−1.74	−0.01−1.67	343−147	351−89	248−1	0.56−2.57	248−1	−5−59

[a]Scalar components, plane projections, spatial magnitude and orientation of five initial instantaneous QRS vectors taken 0.01 s intervals after the onset of QRS. As in all other tables the beginning of QRS is taken at the earliest deflection in any one of the simultaneously recorded scalar leads. In this as in all consecutive tables the ranges for azimuth are to be followed in clockwise direction

■ Table A1.56

Quantitative analysis of late QRS vectors. The upper row provides mean ±SD and the lower row gives a 96% range

Instantaneous vectors[a]	Scalar amplitude (mV)			Planar direction (°)			Spatial magnitude and orientation		
	X	y	Z	Frontal	Sagittal	Horizontal	Amplitude (mV)	Azimuth (°)	Elevation (°)
End of QRS or	0.01 ± 0.03	0.03 ± 0.04	−0.07 ± 0.04	79 ± 74	160 ± 30	83 ± 34	0.09 ± 0.04	83 ± 34	19 ± 27
J point	−0.06–0.08	−0.06–0.10	−0.17–0.00	279–241	95–227	9–153	0.03–0.19	9–153	−42–70
0.01 S before	−0.01 ± 0.06	0.01 ± 0.08	0.01 ± 0.08	156 ± 89	77 ± 97	197 ± 94	0.11 ± 0.05	197 ± 94	6 ± 45
End of QRS	−0.13–0.10	−0.13–0.15	−0.15–0.16	4–315	267–250	26–1	0.03–0.24	26–1	−72–79
0.02 S before	−0.09 ± 0.12	0.00 ± 0.16	0.24 ± 0.19	173 ± 72	358 ± 53	247 ± 52	0.34 ± 0.17	247 ± 52	−2 ± 34
End of QRS	−0.36–0.12	−0.30–0.33	−0.10–0.67	31–305	242–122	96–30	0.07–0.74	96–30	−74–63
0.03 S before	−0.03 ± 0.32	0.18 ± 0.33	0.60 ± 0.28	128 ± 74	12 ± 32	263 ± 32	0.76 ± 0.31	263 ± 32	10 ± 26
End of QRS	−0.51–0.95	−0.39–1.1	0.05–1.14	353–268	290–68	202–338	0.25–1.51	202–338	−54–55
0.04 S before	0.46 ± 0.59	0.61 ± 0.49	0.77 ± 0.37	69 ± 55	35 ± 29	295 ± 36	1.30 ± 0.48	295 ± 36	26 ± 20
End of QRS	−0.54–1.70	−0.31–1.66	−0.04–1.52	341–214	335–93	230–1	0.43–2.27	230–1	−26–58
0.05 S before	0.87 ± 0.48	0.81 ± 0.41	0.49 ± 0.50	46 ± 27	65 ± 32	331 ± 33	1.44 ± 0.48	331 ± 33	34 ± 13
End of QRS	−0.28–1.75	0.05–1.80	0.47–1.56	13–131	7–148	251–28	0.57–2.53	251–28	2–58

[a] Scalar components, planar projections, spatial magnitude and orientation of five terminal instantaneous QRS vectors taken in retrograde fashion from the end of QRS at 0.01 s intervals

■ Table A1.57

Quantitative analysis of ST segment. The upper row provides mean ±SD and the lower row gives a 96% range

Instantaneous vectors	Scalar amplitude (mV)			Spatial magnitude and orientation		
	X	Y	Z	Amplitude (mV)	Azimuth (°)	Elevation (°)
0.02 s after	0.01 ± 0.03	0.02 ± 0.04	−0.10 ± 0.04	0.11 ± 0.04	82 ± 22	12 ± 20
J point	−0.06–0.08	−0.06–0.10	−0.19 to −0.02	0.04–0.21	37–127	−35–55
0.04 s after	0.03 ± 0.03	0.03 ± 0.04	−0.11 ± 0.05	0.13 ± 0.05	77 ± 20	13 ± 19
J point	−0.04–0.10	−0.06–0.11	−0.22–0.03	0.05–0.24	35–117	−32–56
0.06 s after	0.04 ± 0.04	0.04 ± 0.04	−0.12 ± 0.05	0.15 ± 0.06	72 ± 19	16 ± 17
J point	−0.03–0.13	−0.05–0.14	−0.25 to −0.03	0.05–0.29	35–109	−22–54

☐ **Table A1.58**

Quantitative analysis of eight instantaneous QRS vectors

Instantaneous vectors [a]	Scalar amplitude (mV)			Spatial magnitude and orientation		
	X	Y	Z	Amplitude (mV)	Azimuth (°)	Elevation (°)
1/8 QRS	−0.04± 0.05	−0.03± 0.07	−0.14± 0.08	0.18 ± 0.07	108 ± 27	−10± 26
	−0.16–0.09	−0.18–0.10	−0.31–0.00	0.06–0.36	51–156	−59–58
2/8 QRS	0.17 ± 0.17	0.05 ± 0.13	−0.34± 0.19	0.44 ± 0.19	63 ± 27	7 ± 19
	−0.11–0.61	−0.21–0.34	−0.82–0.00	0.14–0.93	359–110	−30–50
3/8 QRS	0.87 ± 0.31	0.63 ± 0.30	0.03 ± 0.40	1.17 ± 0.37	359 ± 25	33 ± 11
	0.33–1.63	0.17–1.44	−0.74–0.90	0.59–2.19	308–47	12–55
4/8 QRS	0.89 ± 0.49	0.89 ± 0.44	0.70 ± 0.44	1.58 ± 0.48	320 ± 26	34 ± 14
	−0.15–1.84	0.02–1.85	−0.05–1.74	0.70–2.62	261–3	2–61
5/8 QRS	0.09 ± 0.40	0.34 ± 0.39	0.77 ± 0.29	1.00 ± 0.34	275 ± 30	18 ± 21
	−0.55–1.13	−0.36–1.28	0.10–1.38	0.39–1.73	224–341	−30–56
6/8 QRS	−0.13± 0.14	0.01 ± 0.19	0.34 ± 0.20	0.44 ± 0.18	248 ± 35	1 ± 29
	−0.41–0.17	−0.34–0.40	−0.04–0.76	0.12–0.89	153–328	−68–57
7/8 QRS	−0.02± 0.06	0.01 ± 0.09	0.02 ± 0.09	0.13 ± 0.05	288 ± 96	3 ± 45
	−0.15–0.11	−0.15–0.16	−0.15–0.20	0.04–0.27	116–101	−75–76
8/8 QRS (J point)	0.01 ± 0.03	0.03 ± 0.04	−0.07± 0.04	0.09 ± 0.04	83 ± 34	19 ± 27
	−0.06–0.08	−0.06–0.10	−0.17–0.00	0.03–0.19	9–153	−42–70

[a]Obtained after each eighth of the QRS duration

☐ **Table A1.59**

Quantitative analysis of ST and T vectors

Instantaneous vectors [a]	Scalar amplitude (mV)			Spatial magnitude and orientation		
	X	Y	Z	Amplitude (mV)	Azimuth (°)	Elevation (°)
1/8 (ST-T)	0.02 ± 0.02	0.00 ± 0.02	−0.04 ± 0.03	0.06 ± 0.02	67 ± 36	1 ± 29
	−0.02–0.06	−0.05–0.05	−0.10–0.02	0.02–0.10	317–133	−49–58
2/8 (ST-T)	0.04 ± 0.03	0.02 ± 0.03	−0.07 ± 0.04	0.10 ± 0.04	59 ± 23	11 ± 21
	−0.01–0.11	−0.04–0.08	−0.16–0.01	0.03–0.19	353–98	−33–52
3/8 (ST-T)	0.08 ± 0.05	0.05 ± 0.04	−0.12 ± 0.06	0.16 ± 0.07	55 ± 19	17 ± 15
	0.00–0.19	−0.03–0.15	−0.27 to −0.02	0.05–0.33	13–87	−16–48
4/8 (ST-T)	0.15 ± 0.08	0.10 ± 0.07	−0.19 ± 0.09	0.28 ± 0.11	52 ± 17	21 ± 12
	0.02–0.35	−0.01–0.29	−0.42 to −0.03	0.09–0.56	14–85	−3–47
5/8 (ST-T)	0.23 ± 0.11	0.18 ± 0.10	−0.25 ± 0.12	0.40 ± 0.15	46 ± 19	27 ± 12
	0.04–0.51	0.02–0.43	−0.51 to −0.02	0.14–0.73	6–81	5–55
6/8 (ST-T)	0.22 ± 0.12	0.20 ± 0.10	−0.17 ± 0.11	0.37 ± 0.14	37 ± 28	35 ± 15
	0.00–0.49	0.02–0.43	−0.38–0.02	0.06–0.68	352–81	8–68
7/8 (ST-T)	0.07 ± 0.05	0.08 ± 0.04	−0.04 ± 0.04	0.12 ± 0.06	28 ± 47	40 ± 22
	−0.02–0.17	−0.01–0.18	−0.11–0.03	0.02–0.24	244–163	−29–78

[a]Determined through time normalization of the ST-T segment

◻ Table A1.60

Time integrals of QRS and T derived from scalar leads X, Y and Z. Combinations of two scalar components lead to planar projections in the frontal, sagittal and horizontal planes. Spatial magnitude and orientation are obtained by vectorial addition of all three scalar components. Addition of the time integrals of QRS and T results in the ventricular gradient (VĜ). The P wave was included in the QRS time integral as described in the text. The QRS-T angle is derived from the two vectors of the respective time integrals

| Item | Planar direction (°) | | | Scalar amplitude (μVs) | | | Spatial magnitude, orientation and spatial angles | | |
	Frontal	Sagittal	Horizontal	X	Y	Z	Amplitude (μVs)	Azimuth (°)	Elevation (°)
SÂQRS	44 ± 23	53 ± 27	323 ± 25	22.20 ± 11.18	23.41 ± 13.36	17.11 ± 12.35	40.08 ± 13.51	323 ± 25	36 ± 17
	351–85	355–110	274–14	1.23–46.97	−2.83–51.87	−6.11–44.28	15.16–71.32	274–14	−5–71
SÂT	33 ± 24	152 ± 21	52 ± 18	29.09 ± 15.78	20.12 ± 14.73	−37.79 ± 17.50	54.97 ± 20.72	52 ± 18	21 ± 14
	338–78	106–197	13–86	2.33–64.86	−6.86–56.06	−76.45 to −6.65	20.29–106.33	13–86	−11–49
SVĜ	40 ± 14	114 ± 23	21 ± 19	51.29 ± 20.79	43.54 ± 21.28	−20.67 ± 19.99	74.35 ± 26.63	21 ± 19	36 ± 13
	9–67	71–159	340–58	15.30–102.55	5.51–94.79	−66.46–13.35	27.17–138.42	340–58	7–63
QRS-T angle	12 ± 33	97 ± 39	89 ± 31						78 ± 26
	0–88	24–163	23–148						26–134

◻ Table A1.61

Eigenvectors $\vec{A}$, $\vec{B}$ and $\vec{C}$ of the P, QRS, and T loops. The polar vector is identical with eigenvector $\vec{C}$. The ratios between eigenvectors give an estimate of the planarity of the loop and its configuration. The magnitude of the polar vector is based on the area of the loop in its 'broadside' projection. A multiplication constant was used for P and T because of their small magnitude

Item	P loop	QRS loop	T loop
Eigenvector $\vec{C}$ (polar vector)			
Azimuth (°)	35 ± 34	339 ± 30	337 ± 24
	304–95	285–46	292–36
Elevation (°)	−14 ± 15	−50 ± 12	−31 ± 17
	−50–11	−73 to −25	−63–8
Eigenvector $\vec{B}$			
Azimuth (°)	122 ± 31	65 ± 37	97 ± 33
	64–183	329–143	27–170
Elevation (°)	11 ± 15	3 ± 23	−37 ± 18
	−26–43	−45–49	−69–6
Eigenvector $\vec{A}$			
Azimuth (°)	352 ± 35	332 ± 42	39 ± 21
	293–79	244–56	354–79
Elevation (°)	62 ± 20	30 ± 15	31 ± 15
	0–84	−6–57	1–61
Eigenvector ratios			
C/B	0.20 ± 0.16	0.02 ± 0.04	0.05 ± 0.09
	0.00–0.65	0.00–0.10	0.00–0.38
B/A	0.21 ± 0.17	0.41 ± 0.20	0.17 ± 0.13
	0.00–0.67	0.06–0.85	0.01–0.51
C/A	0.03 ± 0.03	0.01 ± 0.01	0.01 ± 0.01
	0.00–0.14	0.00–0.03	0.00–0.03
Spatial amplitude of the Polar vector (area of "broadside" projection of the spatial loop) (mV^2)	$6.16 ± 3.43 \times 10^{-3}$	1.62 ± 0.85	$5.03 ± 3.48 \times 10^{-2}$
	$1.69–15.76 \times 10^{-3}$	0.45–3.89	$0.66–14.76 \times 10^{-2}$

A1.5.2 Normal Limits in Females

The group of Pipberger, in a later paper, published data on the normal limits of the Frank orthogonal-lead ECG in 450 women, including both whites and blacks. ❷ Tables A1.62–A1.68 are reproduced from Nemati M et al. The orthogonal electrocardiogram in normal women. Implications of sex differences in diagnostic electrocardiography. *Am. Heart J.* 1978;**95**: 12–21, with the permission of Mosby, St. Louis, Missouri.

■ Table A1.62

Measurements of P, QRS and T in orthogonal *X*, *Y* and *Z* leads

Item	X		Y		Z	
P amplitude[a]	0.05 ± 0.02[c]		0.09 ± 0.04		Positive component	
	0.02–0.09[d]		0.02–0.17		0.03 ± 0.02	
					0–0.08	
					Negative	
					component	
					−0.03 ± 0.02	
					−0.07–0	
Q amplitude	−0.08 ± 0.05	(237)[e]	−0.08 ± 0.05	(238)	−0.31 ± 0.17	(446)
	−0.22 to −0.01		−0.23 to −0.01		−0.77 to −0.07	
R amplitude	0.94 ± 0.35		0.81 ± 0.33		0.68 ± 0.25	
	0.35–1.75		0.27–1.55		0.22–1.25	
S amplitude	−0.17 ± 0.11	(319)	−0.17 ± 0.12	(252)	−0.19 ± 0.17	(9)
	−0.47 to −0.01		−0.52 to −0.01		−0.60 to −0.04	
T amplitude	0.22 ± 0.10		0.16 ± 0.09		−0.08 ± 0.10	
	0.05–0.44		−0.03–0.39		−0.31–0.10	
Q/R amplitude ratio	0.07 ± 0.04	(237)	0.09 ± 0.06	(238)	0.54 ± 0.42	(446)
	0.01–0.18		0.01–0.22		0.10–1.73	
R/S amplitude ratio	11.36 ± 18.00	(319)	9.20 ± 13.00	(252)	4.00 ± 3.30	(9)
	1.12–71.70		0.64–56.00		0.70–12.00	
Q duration[b]	0.016 ± 0.003	(237)	0.017 ± 0.004	(238)	0.030 ± 0.008	(446)
	0.010–0.024		0.009–0.028		0.014–0.047	
R duration	0.045 ± 0.012		0.050 ± 0.014		0.048 ± 0.010	
	0.028–0.071		0.028–0.081		0.028–0.069	
S duration	0.029 ± 0.009	(319)	0.028 ± 0.090	(252)	0.028 ± 0.009	(9)
	0.012–0.048		0.012–0.049		0.018–0.044	
R peak time	0.037 ± 0.005		0.039 ± 0.005		0.048 ± 0.006	
(instrinsicoid deflection)	0.028–0.048		0.027–0.050		0.036–0.062	
RX + RZ	1.60 ± 0.42					
	0.87–2.50					

[a]Amplitudes are in millivolts [b]Durations are in seconds [c]Mean ± standard deviation of each item [d]Limits of a 96 percentile range [e]Figures in parentheses show the actual number of observation: results not followed by a number in parentheses were obtained from total series

A1.5.3 Effect of Age, Build and Race on the Orthogonal-Lead ECG

The correlation of various ECG parameters with age and race (black and white) was investigated by Pipberger *et al.* In general terms, voltages were higher in black men than in white men. ❷ Tables A1.69–A1.73 are reproduced from Pipberger HV et al. Correlations of the orthogonal electrocardiogram and vectorcardiogram with constitutional variables in 518 normal men. *Circulation* 1967;**35**: 536–551 with the permission of the American Heart Association, Dallas, Texas. ❷ Table A1.69 sets out the distribution of ages of subjects in ❷ Tables A1.70–A1.73.

◻ Table A1.63

Measurements of initial, terminal and instantaneous vectors in orthogonal X, Y and Z leads

	X	Y	Z
Initial vectors from the onset of QRS			
0.01 s	−0.01 ± 0.05	−0.00 ± 0.06	−0.11 ± 0.06
	−0.11−0.10	−0.13−0.12	−0.23−0.01
0.02 s	0.16 ± 0.16	0.10 ± 0.14	−0.22 ± 0.16
	−0.13−0.56	−0.13−0.45	−0.51−0.14
0.03 s	0.62 ± 0.27	0.44 ± 0.26	−0.13 ± 0.31
	0.10−1.25	−0.01−1.07	−0.66−0.65
0.04 s	0.77 ± 0.41	0.63 ± 0.38	0.39 ± 0.36
	0.00−1.70	−0.08−1.46	−0.53−1.10
Terminal vectors from the end of QRS			
J point	0.00 ± 0.03	0.00 ± 0.03	0.01 ± 0.03
	−0.06−0.05	−0.06−0.06	−0.07−0.04
0.01 s	−0.01 ± 0.05	0.00 ± 0.08	0.09 ± 0.07
	−0.12−0.11	−0.15−0.14	−0.07−0.22
0.02 s	−0.03 ± 0.15	0.00 ± 0.17	0.31 ± 0.17
	−0.27−0.36	−0.28−0.38	−0.04−0.62
0.03 s	0.19 ± 0.38	0.21 ± 0.32	0.52 ± 0.26
	−0.29−1.18	−0.35−0.97	−0.05−1.04
0.04 s	0.61 ± 0.48	0.53 ± 0.40	0.44 ± 0.36
	−0.25−1.61	−0.29−1.32	−0.31−1.16
Instantaneous ST vectors			
0.02 s after J point	−0.02 ± 0.07	−0.03 ± 0.04	−0.01 ± 0.05
	−0.10−0.06	−0.12−0.07	−0.09−0.07
0.04 s after J point	−0.01 ± 0.07	−0.03 ± 0.05	−0.02 ± 0.04
	−0.09−0.07	−0.12−0.07	−0.09−0.05
0.06 s after J point	0.00 ± 0.08	−0.02 ± 0.07	−0.02 ± 0.04
	−0.08−0.07	−0.11−0.07	−0.10−0.05

◻ Table A1.64

Measurements of P, PR, QRS and QT

Item	Measurement (s)
P duration	0.106 ± 0.019
	0.064−0.142
PR interval	0.154 ± 0.022
	0.112−0.208
PR segment	0.048 ± 0.018
	0.020−0.096
QRS duration	0.084 ± 0.008
	0.068−0.104
QT interval (uncorrected)	0.372 ± 0.026
	0.319−0.428

■ Table A1.65

Measurement of P, QRS and T vectors in frontal, left sagittal and horizontal plane

Item	Frontal Amplitude	Angle	Left sagittal Amplitude	Angle	Horizontal Amplitude	Angle
Maximal P vector	0.01 ± 0.04^a	61^b	0.10 ± 0.04	96	0.06 ± 0.02	14
	0.04–0.19	$0–93^b$	0.03–0.18	178–44	0.03–0.12	115 to −98
Maximal QRS vector	1.24 ± 0.38	41	1.00 ± 0.31	125	1.10 ± 0.32	29
	0.63–2.19	10–88	0.49–1.70	−156–48	0.55–1.84	114 to −35
Maximal T vector	0.28 ± 0.11	32	0.20 ± 0.08	62	0.25 ± 0.10	−17
	0.10–0.57	2–68	0.07–0.42	170 to −88	0.09–0.49	42 to −70
Half-area QRS vector	1.12 ± 0.45	42	0.93 ± 0.36	120	0.97 ± 0.33	29
	0.22–2.20	−1–82	0.24–1.71	−174–52	0.36–1.70	78 to −22
Initial QRS vectors						
0.01 s	0.07 ± 0.04	-137^c	0.13 ± 0.05	−4	0.13 ± 0.05	−95
	0.01–0.18	20 to −10	0.03–0.24	80 to −58	0.03–0.24	−5 to −146
0.02 s	0.23 ± 0.17	28	0.29 ± 0.14	24	0.32 ± 0.14	−54
	0.02–0.69	−129–174	0.04–0.62	144 to −30	0.06–0.69	38 to −115
0.03 s	0.78 ± 0.32	34	0.53 ± 0.27	88	0.69 ± 0.27	−2
	0.17–1.51	1–64	0.04–1.16	156–10	0.12–1.32	54 to −57
0.04 s	1.06 ± 0.45	39	0.84 ± 0.35	124	0.96 ± 0.36	30
	0.10–2.00	−4–84	0.10–1.59	−168–42	0.20–1.75	88 to −26
Terminal QRS vectors						
0.01 s	0.08 ± 0.05	-150^c	0.12 ± 0.06	−172	0.11 ± 0.06	96^c
	0.01–0.20	16 to −18	0.01–0.24	−32–82	0.01–0.23	−98 to −36
0.02 s	0.18 ± 0.14	-169^c	0.36 ± 0.16	−177	0.35 ± 0.17	99
	0.03–0.55	15 to −30	0.05–0.69	−82–108	0.03–0.72	−150–16
0.03 s	0.45 ± 0.35	63^c	0.64 ± 0.27	163	0.66 ± 0.29	78
	0.04–1.44	−20 to −80	0.12–1.24	−124–84	0.13–1.34	150 to −5
0.04 s	0.90 ± 0.49	43	0.81 ± 0.34	132	0.89 ± 0.36	41
	0.06–2.00	−25 to −160	0.19–1.56	−140–54	0.18–1.75	122 to −26

[a]Amplitudes are in millivolts [b]Angles are in °. All angular ranges should be read in a clockwise sequence [c]Angles show no significant clustering as evidenced by wide 96 percentile ranges

■ Table A1.66

Spatial magnitude and orientation of maximal P, QRS and T vectors

Item	Magnitude (mV)	Azimuth (°)	Elevation (°)
Maximal P*XYZ* vector	0.11 ± 0.04	14	48
	0.05–0.20	115 to −98[a]	−22–80
Maximal QRS*XYZ* vector	1.35 ± 0.36	29	34
	0.75–2.25	114 to −35	−5–61
Maximal T*XYZ* vector	0.33 ± 0.13	−17	31
	0.12–0.64	42 to −70	−50–64

[a]Angular ranges should be read in a clockwise sequence

◻ Table A1.67

Direction of inscription of QRS loops in the frontal, left sagittal and horizontal planes in 450 normal women: CW, clockwise; CW/CCW, figure-of-eight, clockwise then counterclockwise; CCW/CW, figure-of-eight, counterclockwise then clockwise; CCW, counterclockwise

	Frontal	Left sagittal	Horizontal
CW	230 (51%)	8 (2%)	0 (0%)
CW/CCW	37 (8%)	12 (3%)	0 (0%)
CCW/CW	61 (14%)	27 (6%)	8 (2%)
CCW	122 (27%)	403 (89%)	442 (98%)

◻ Table A1.68

Sex-specific limits. Data are derived from records of 510 normal men and 450 normal women, unless indicated otherwise in parentheses ($p < 0.001$ for all measurements)

Item	Men		Women	
Scalar measurements				
QRS duration[a]	0.093 ± 0.009		0.084 ± 0.008	
	0.076–0.112		0.068–0.104	
QZ amplitude[b]	−0.41 ± 0.21		−0.31 ± 0.17	(446)
	−0.93 to −0.09		−0.77 to −0.07	
RX amplitude	1.17 ± 0.37		0.94 ± 0.35	
	0.51–1.97		0.35–1.75	
RY amplitude	1.03 ± 0.41		0.81 ± 0.33	
	0.35–1.95		0.27–1.55	
RZ amplitude	0.93 ± 0.35		0.68 ± 0.25	
	0.36–1.79		0.22–1.25	
SX amplitude	−0.27 ± 0.15	(407)	−0.17 ± 0.11	(319)
	−0.68 to −0.06		−0.47 to −0.01	
TZ amplitude	−0.28 ± 0.13		−0.08 ± 0.10	
	−0.58 to −06		−0.31–0.10	
Q/RZ amplitude ratio	0.50 ± 0.35		0.54 ± 0.42	(446)
	0.10–1.20		0.10–1.73	
RX + RZ amplitude	2.00 ± 0.52		1.60 ± 0.42	
	1.06–3.10		0.87–2.50	
J point in lead Z	−0.07 ± 0.04		−0.01 ± 0.03	
	−0.17–0.00		−0.07–0.04	

A1.6 Normal Limits of Polarcardiographic Data

The technique of polarcardiography is explained in ❷ Chap. 13 of *Specialized Aspects of ECG*. As an adjunct, some tables of normal limits derived from the work of Dower are presented in ❷ Tables A1.74 to ❷ A1.77. The terminology is also discussed in the chapter. In addition, data from exercise testing of normals is included.

⬛ Table A1.68   (Continued)

Item	Men		Women	
Planar measurements				
Max. QRSXY amplitude	1.57 ± 0.42		1.24 ± 0.38	
	0.81–2.53		0.63–2.19	
Max. QRSZY amplitude	1.32 ± 0.45		1.00 ± 0.31	
	0.60–2.42		0.49–1.71	
Max. QRSXZ amplitude	1.39 ± 0.36		1.10 ± 0.31	
	0.74–2.19		0.55–1.83	
Max. TZY amplitude	0.36 ± 0.13		0.20 ± 0.08	
	0.13–0.67		0.07–0.42	
Max. TXZ amplitude	0.40 ± 0.14		0.25 ± 0.10	
	0.15–0.72		0.09–0.49	
Max. TZY angle[c]	38		62	
	87–0		170 to −88	
Max. TXZ angle	−46		−17	
	−8 to −83		42 to −70	
Spatial measurements				
Max. QRSXYZ magnitude	1,073 ± 0.44		1.35 ± 0.36	
	0.92–2,075		0.75–2.25	
Max. TXYZ magnitude	0.46 ± 0.16		0.30 ± 0.12	
	0.18–0.82		0.09–0.59	

[a] Duration are in seconds [b] Amplitudes are in millivolts [c] Angles are in degrees

⬛ Table A1.69
Age distribution of subjects included in the study

Age-group	20–29	30–39	40–49	50–59	60–78	total
Number of cases	78	179	151	56	54	518

Note that in ❷ Table A1.74, the median values were obtained from grouped data. Prominent sex differences can be seen by comparing adjacent columns marked*. Progressive change with age can be seen by comparing corresponding columns at the same level; for example, systolic blood pressure (BP) increases from 120 to 145 mmHg for male and female (M + F) with increasing age.

With increasing age, the R vector decreases in magnitude and tends toward the transverse and frontal planes (longitude and latitude of R); the ST vector tends to be greater in the men than in the women; the longitude difference between the T and R vectors (long. T–long. R) also tends to decrease. Offered for comparative purposes the systolic blood pressure shows an increase with age, especially in the women.

With respect to sex differences the T vector is more anterior (latitude of T) in the men, and its magnitude is greater, especially in the 20–29 age-group. Relative to the R vector, the T vector is more strongly anterior (lat. T–lat. R) in the men, and of greater magnitude (M_T/M_R) (❷ Tables A1.75–A1.79).

Table A1.70

Correlations between age-groups and ECG measurements. The means and standard deviations in this and the following tables are shown in the upper line of each measurement. The lower line indicates the limits of 96 percentile ranges. In the last column results of t-tests are given, comparing the youngest and oldest age-groups. Vector magnitude is denoted vc

	Correlation coefficient	Age-group (years)					p (youngest vs. oldest group)
		20–29	30–39	40–49	50–59	60–78	
Wave durations							
P duration (s)	0.223	0.096 ± 0.012	0.098 ± 0.012	0.099 ± 0.011	0.104 ± 0.011	0.104 ± 0.013	<0.01
		0.072–0.116	0.072–0.116	0.076–0.124	0.088–0.124	0.080–0.128	
Scalar QRS measurements							
RY (mV)	−0.338	1.25 ± 0.42	1.06 ± 0.39	1.02 ± 0.42	0.88 ± 0.38	0.72 ± 0.37	<0.001
		0.53–2.08	0.47–1.95	0.34–1.99	0.26–1.69	0.24–1.63	
RZ (mV)	−0.277	1.03 ± 0.37	0.98 ± 0.35	0.89 ± 0.31	0.78 ± 0.26	0.74 ± 0.33	<0.001
		(78)	(179)	(151)	(56)	(54)	
		0.51–1.71	0.42–1.76	0.38–1.54	0.33–1.24	0.28–1.74	
SX (mV)	−0.214	−0.27 ± 0.21	−0.26 ± 0.16	−0.25 ± 0.15	−0.24 ± 0.16	−0.15 ± 0.10	<0.01
		(37)	(100)	(86)	(42)	(41)	
		−0.04 to −0.79	−0.01 to −0.64	−0.03 to −0.57	−0.01 to −0.55	−0.01 to −0.34	
Initial 0.02 s lead Z (mV)	0.268	−0.30 ± 0.19	−0.26 ± 0.16	−0.24 ± 0.13	−0.18 ± 0.10	−0.17 ± 0.12	<0.001
		(78)	(179)	(151)	(56)	(54)	
		−0.63 to −0.13	−0.62 to −0.05	−0.63 to −0.03	−0.47 to −0.02	−0.45 to −0.03	
Initial 0.02 s lead Z (mV)	0.192	0.29 ± 0.47	0.34 ± 0.49	0.21 ± 0.41	0.15 ± 0.38	0.07 ± 0.42	<0.01
		−0.50–1.22	−0.51–1.23	−0.54–1.11	−0.61–0.77	−0.81–0.91	
Initial 0.05 s lead Z (mV)	−0.257	0.83 ± 0.44	0.76 ± 0.42	0.65 ± 0.39	0.53 ± 0.37	0.50 ± 0.40	<0.001
		0.10–1.56	−0.07–1.67	−0.12–1.38	−0.12–1.16	−0.26–1.43	
Planar QRS measurements							
Maximal vc. sagittal plane (mV)	−0.371	1.56 ± 0.46	1.37 ± 0.45	1.27 ± 0.41	1.12 ± 0.36	0.97 ± 0.42	<0.001
		0.73–2.46	0.72–2.39	0.59–2.25	0.43–2.00	0.48–2.03	
Maximal vc. direction, frontal plane (°)	−0.288	50 ± 15	41 ± 13	42 ± 15	38 ± 18	32 ± 16	<0.001
		17–77	17–66	13–73	6–74	3–56	
Maximal vc. direction, horizontal plane (°)	−0.217	312 ± 30	325 ± 32	326 ± 36	331 ± 36	340 ± 36	<0.001
		254–354	250–26	243–19	241–20	264–46	

◻ Table A1.70   (Continued)

	Correlation coefficient	Age-group (years)					p (youngest vs. oldest group)
		20–29	30–39	40–49	50–59	60–78	
Spatial QRS measurements							
Maximal vc.	−0.367	1.88 ± 0.42	1.80 ± 0.43	1.65 ± 0.45	1.45 ± 0.33	1.36 ± 0.48	<0.001
(mV)		1.13–2.82	0.96–2.76	0.94–2.74	0.91–2.19	0.77–2.47	
Initial 0.02 s vc.	−0.269	0.36 ± 0.16	0.31 ± 0.17	0.27 ± 0.14	0.24 ± 0.11	0.22 ± 0.11	<0.001
(mV)		0.15–0.69	0.11–0.68	0.10–0.68	0.08–0.51	0.05–0.48	
Initial 0.05 s vc.	−0.359	1.65 ± 0.44	1.49 ± 0.47	1.36 ± 0.45	1.19 ± 0.41	1.07 ± 0.46	<0.001
(mV)		0.91–2.54	0.77–2.48	0.55–2.42	0.49–1.91	0.40–2.00	
Spatial ST-T measurements							
Maximal T vc.	−0.312	0.50 ± 0.17	0.45 ± 0.15	0.42 ± 0.14	0.40 ± 0.13	0.31 ± 0.12	<0.001
(mV)		0.26–0.82	0.20–0.80	0.16–0.75	0.20–0.71	0.10–0.61	
0.04 s ST-T vc.	−0.213	0.12 ± 0.05	0.11 ± 0.05	0.11 ± 0.04	0.09 ± 0.04	0.09 ± 0.04	<0.01
(mV)		0.02–0.22	0.04–0.23	0.03–0.20	0.02–0.17	0.03–0.20	
3/8 ST-T vc.	−0.361	0.19 ± 0.08	0.17 ± 0.07	0.15 ± 0.06	0.13 ± 0.06	0.10 ± 0.05	<0.001
(mV)		0.08–0.36	0.05–0.32	0.04–0.32	0.04–0.25	0.03–0.24	
4/8 ST-T vc.	−0.376	0.30 ± 0.11	0.26 ± 0.10	0.24 ± 0.10	0.21 ± 0.09	0.15 ± 0.07	<0.001
(mV)		0.11–0.54	0.10–0.48	0.06–0.46	0.09–0.42	0.05–0.32	
Time integrals							
SÂQRS	−0.243	42.0 ± 13.0	42.0 ± 14.5	39.5 ± 13.0	34.5 ± 11.4	32.4 ± 13.4	<0.001
(μVs)		18.7–65.6	15.0–72.1	18.9–74.0	16.9–56.2	12.3–62.7	
SÂT	−0.352	57.8 ± 22.8	52.8 ± 20.0	47.0 ± 17.7	44.0 ± 17.3	31.9 ± 14.9	<0.001
(μVs)		26.5–100.0	17.1–95.9	13.4–90.4	19.3–92.5	6.3–58.7	
SVĜ	−0.343	78.9 ± 27.5	73.3 ± 25.7	66.3 ± 24.4	59.4 ± 24.4	46.2 ± 20.8	<0.001
(μVs)		36.2–140.0	31.7–133.0	20.8–120.0	15.9–115.0	16.1–92.2	

◻ **Table A1.71**

Correlations between subjects of the white and black race

	Correlation coefficient	Race White		Black		p (W versus B)
Scalar QRS measurements						
QRS duration (s)	−0.320	0.098 ± 0.009		0.091 ± 0.009		<0.001
		0.080–0.116		0.076–0.108		
QX duration (s)	−0.160	0.019 ± 0.006	(173)	0.017 ± 0.004	(96)	<0.02
		0.008–0.028		0.008–0.024		
QY duration (s)	−0.377	0.021 ± 0.007	(133)	0.015 ± 0.006	(72)	<0.001
		0.008–0.032		0.008–0.028		
QY (mV)	−0.267	0.09 ± 0.07	(133)	0.06 ± 0.05	(72)	<0.001
		0.01–0.27		0.01–0.23		
RX (mV)	0.264	1.06 ± 0.35		1.25 ± 0.36		<0.001
		0.49–1.84		0.63–1.94		
RY (mV)	0.197	1.96 ± 0.42		1.13 ± 0.41		<0.001
		0.28–1.99		0.41–1.99		
RZ (mV)	0.275	1.84 ± 0.30		1.04 ± 0.37		<0.001
		0.33–1.53		0.44–1.98		
Q/RX ratio	−0.128	0.06 ± 0.05	(173)	0.05 ± 0.03	(96)	<0.05
		0.00–0.20		0.00–0.11		
Q/RY ratio	−0.392	0.09 ± 0.06	(133)	0.05 ± 0.03	(72)	<0.001
		0.01–0.23		0.00–0.14		
Initial 0.04 s, lead X (mV)	0.280	1.88 ± 0.32		1.08 ± 0.38		<0.001
		0.31–1.59		0.44–1.79		
Initial 0.02 s, lead Y (mV)	0.279	−0.02 ± 0.09		0.04 ± 0.13		<0.001
		−0.22–0.15		−0.20–0.31		
Initial 0.03 s, lead Y (mV)	0.315	0.19 ± 0.20		0.33 ± 0.23		<0.001
		−0.09–0.73		−0.02–0.90		
Initial 0.04 s, lead Y (mV)	0.297	0.67 ± 0.36		0.91 ± 0.41		<0.001
		0.10–1.62		0.23–1.76		
Terminal 0.03 s, lead Z (mV)	0.284	0.51 ± 0.27		0.69 ± 0.30		<0.001
		0.06–1.12		0.13–1.37		
Planar QRS measurements						
Maximal vc. frontal (mV)	0.299	1.44 ± 0.41		1.70 ± 0.42		<0.001
		0.73–2.38		0.96–2.65		
Maximal vc. sagittal plane (mV)	0.238	1.22 ± 0.44		1.45 ± 0.46		<0.001
		0.52–2.12		0.73–2.46		
Maximal vc. horizontal plane (mV)	0.312	1.26 ± 0.34		1.49 ± 0.36		<0.001
		0.65–2.05		0.89–2.24		
Spatial QRS measurements						
Maximal vc. (mV)	0.305	1.58 ± 0.43		1.87 ± 0.45		<0.001
		0.83–2.52		1.06–2.94		
Initial 0.02 s vc., elevation angle (°)	0.256	−3 ± 22		9 ± 22		<0.001
		−44–47		−25–60		
Initial 0.03 s vc. (mV)	0.348	0.56 ± 0.25		0.77 ± 0.31		<0.001
		0.18–1.16		0.28–1.50		
Initial 0.04 s vc. (mV)	0.386	1.21 ± 0.40		1.58 ± 0.46		<0.001
		0.52–2.17		0.74–2.58		
Terminal 0.05 s vc., azimuth angle (°)	0.243	324 ± 37		342 ± 34		<0.001
		240–28		266–42		

◼ Table A1.72

Correlations between chest configuration and ECG measurements. The ratio SD/TD was derived from sagittal and transverse chest diameters. Note the small increases of the mean Q/RY ratio accompanied by a marked increase of 136% of the upper limit of the 96 percentile range. Mean results failed frequently to reflect the magnitude of changes in range limits

	Correlation coefficient	Chest configuration				p (first versus fourth subgroup)
		0.69 (SD/TD)	0.70–0.74 (SD/TD)	0.75–0.79 (SD/TD)	0.80 (SD/TD)	
Scalar QRS measurements						
RY (mV)	−0.227	1.16 ± 0.45	1.09 ± 0.40	0.96 ± 0.42	0.91 ± 0.39	<0.001
		0.40–2.1	0.34–2.02	0.28–1.86	0.27–1.72	
RZ (mV)	−0.237	1.02 ± 0.33	0.94 ± 0.32	0.93 ± 0.36	0.80 ± 0.33	<0.001
		0.46–1.67	0.42–1.74	0.33–1.98	0.33–1.41	
Initial 0.04 s, lead Y (mV)	−0.220	0.85 ± 0.43	0.81 ± 0.39	0.72 ± 0.39	0.65 ± 0.36	<0.001
		0.23–1.85	0.20–1.71	0.08–1.75	0.03–1.40	
Initial 0.04 s, lead Z (mV)	−0.235	0.37 ± 0.49	0.29 ± 0.45	0.26 ± 0.47	0.10 ± 0.38	<0.001
		−0.50–1.23	−0.51–1.14	−0.55–1.27	−0.58–0.96	
Q/RY ratio	0.147	0.06 ± 0.04	0.07 ± 0.05	0.08 ± 0.06	0.09 ± 0.07	<0.05
		(38)	(67)	(41)	(59)	
		0.01–0.14	0.00–0.18	0.01–0.21	0.01–0.33	
Planar QRS measurements						
Maximal vc. direction, frontal plane (°)	−0.218	46 ± 16	44 ± 14	40 ± 14	37 ± 17	<0.001
		16–79	16–71	10–72	5–66	
Maximal vc. direction, horizontal plane (°)	0.195	320 ± 32	320 ± 34	326 ± 34	335 ± 36	<0.001
		252–13	239–19	247–24	248–36	
Spatial QRS measurements						
Maximal vc. (mV)	−0.200	1.81 ± 0.42	1.74 ± 0.44	1.64 ± 0.48	1.57 ± 0.46	<0.001
		1.01–2.69	0.94–2.76	0.84–2.81	0.81–2.64	
Initial 0.04 s vc., azimuth angle (°)	0.206	341 ± 28	345 ± 28	347 ± 25	355 ± 22	<0.001
		296–40	298–38	302–34	312–40	
Initial 0.04 s vc, elevation angle (°)	−0.190	37 ± 12	35 ± 12	33 ± 12	31 ± 14	<0.01
		15–60	14–58	5–55	2–54	
Spatial ST-T measurements						
0.04 s ST-T vc. (mV)	−0.196	0.12 ± 0.05	0.11 ± 0.04	0.10 ± 0.05	0.09 ± 0.04	<0.001
		0.05–0.23	0.03–0.19	0.03–0.26	0.03–0.19	

Table A1.73

Correlation between body weight and ECG measurements. When relative body weight or deviations from ideal weight were used instead of absolute weight, ECG items exhibiting significant relationships were almost identical but most correlation coefficients decreased noticeably

	Correlation coefficient	Weight				p (first versus fourth subgroup)
		≤134 (lb)	135–159 (lb)	160–184 (lb)	≥185 (lb)	
Scalar QRS measurements						
RZ (mV)	−0.171	0.99 ± 0.39 / 0.41–1.94	0.94 ± 0.35 / 0.36–1.74	0.89 ± 0.32 / 0.41–1.65	0.82 ± 0.29 / 0.38–1.44	<0.01
Initial 0.05 s, lead X (mV)	0.233	0.51 ± 0.49 / −0.35–1.49	0.70 ± 0.49 / −0.18–1.56	0.80 ± 0.50 / −0.28–1.77	0.86 ± 0.48 / −0.06–1.72	<0.001
Initial 0.04 s, lead Z (mV)	−0.316	0.43 ± 0.43 / −0.34–1.23	0.33 ± 0.45 / −0.44–1.22	0.16 ± 0.43 / −0.58–0.106	0.04 ± 0.41 / −0.61–0.95	<0.001
Initial 0.05 s, lead Z (mV)	−0.270	0.82 ± 0.41 / 0.13–1.64	0.75 ± 0.41 / −0.10–1.67	0.62 ± 0.40 / −0.30–1.38	0.52 ± 0.42 / −0.34–1.29	
Planar QRS measurements						
Maximal vc. direction, frontal plane (°)	−0.262	47 ± 15 / 19–74	43 ± 15 / 13–69	40 ± 14 / 11–70	35 ± 17 / 6–73	<0.001
Maximal vc. Direction, horizontal plane (°)	0.261	310 ± 35 / 243–4	352 ± 34 / 248–32	326 ± 33 / 248–19	339 ± 32 / 263–38	<0.001
Spatial QRS measurements						
Maximal vc., azimuth angle (°)	0.232	318 ± 27 / 265–5	329 ± 24 / 271–15	330 ± 28 / 252–18	339 ± 30 / 274–24	<0.001
Initial 0.04 s vc., azimuth angle (°)	0.313	336 ± 26 / 296–27	344 ± 27 / 298–36	353 ± 25 / 302–42	358 ± 22 / 308–35	<0.001
Initial 0.04 s vc., elevation angle (°)	−0.263	38 ± 11 / 17–52	36 ± 12 / 13–58	32 ± 13 / 9–53	29 ± 12 / 6–56	<0.001
Initial 0.05 s vc., azimuth angle (°)	0.295	301 ± 29 / 250–352	310 ± 27 / 259–5	320 ± 29 / 249–19	325 ± 29 / 265–15	<0.001
Spatial ST-T measurements						
7/8 ST-T vc., elevation angle (°)	−0.190	42 ± 14 / 13–68	41 ± 14 / 16–71	37 ± 13 / 9–66	35 ± 14 / 6–58	<0.01
Polar vectors						
P, elevation angle (°)	−0.260	−5 ± 19 / −41–29	−9 ± 20 / −54–32	−13 ± 19 / −62–20	−21 ± 21 / −63–17	<0.001
QRS, elevation angle (°)	−0.229	−46 ± 12 / −67 to −24	−48 ± 12 / −75 to −25	−51 ± 12 / −76 to −32	−55 ± 13 / −81 to −28	<0.001
T, elevation angle (°)	−0.176	−27 ± 19 / −58–5	−29 ± 20 / −64–8	−35 ± 17 / −70–5	−36 ± 19 / −63–11	<0.01

◻ Table A1.74

Polarcardiographic median normal values of Cretan villagers. See Chapter 45 for definitions.

Age-groups	20–82			20–29			30–39			40–49			50–59			60–82		
	M	F	M+F	M	F	M+F	M	F	M+F	M	F	M+F	M	F	M+F	M	F	M+F
Number of cases	275	191	466	30	16	46	53	42	95	70	46	116	51	43	94	71	44	115
Median age (years)	46	48	48	26	26	26	36	36	36	44	46	44	54	54	54	68	68	68
Intervals (ms): PR	135	135	135	130	125	130	135	135	135	140	135	135	130	135	135	145	135	140
QRS	85	80	80	80	80	80	85	80	80	85	80	80	85	85	85	85	75	80
QT$_c$	370	360	370	350	360	360	370	360	360	360	370	360	370	360	360	390	370	380
Latitudes: P	10A	10A	10A	10A	10A	10A	10A	10A	10A	10A	10A	10A	10A	0	10P	0	0	0
R	10P	20P	20P	20P	20P	20P	10P	20P	20P	10P	20P	20P	20P	10P	10P	10P	10P	10P
ST	60A	50A	60A	60A	60A	60A	60A	60A	60A	60A	60A	60A	60A	40A	60A	60A	50A	60A
T	40A*	20A	30A	40A	20A	30A	30A	30A	30A	40A	20A	30A	40A	10A	30A	30A	30A	30A
Lat. T–Lat. R	50	40	40	50	40	50	50	40	50	50	40	40	50	20	40	40	40	40
Longitudes: P	+60	+70	+70	+70	+70	+70	+70	+70	+70	+70	+70	+70	+70	+60	+70	+70	+60	+70
R	+30	+40	+30	+40	+50	+50	+40	+40	+30	+30	+30	+30	+30	+30	+30	+20	+30	+30
ST	+30	+50	+40	+50	–90	+40	+30	+50	+30	+30	+20	+30	+20	+70	+40	+50	+65	+50
T	+30	+40	+30	+30	+40	+40	+30	+40	+30	+30	+30	+30	+30	+40	+40	+30	+40	+30
Long. T–Long. R	–10	0	0	–10	–10	–10	0	–10	–10	0	–10	0	0	0	0	10	10	10
Magnitudes (mV): P	0.14	0.14	0.14	0.17	0.13	0.16	0.14	0.15	0.15	0.15	0.14	0.14	0.14	0.15	0.15	0.13	0.14	0.13
R	1.55	1.50	1.50	1.75	1.65	1.75	1.60	1.55	1.55	1.60	1.45	1.50	1.45	1.45	1.45	1.45	1.45	1.45
ST	0.14*	0.08	0.11	0.21	0.08	0.17	0.17	0.07	0.12	0.15	0.07	0.10	0.14	0.06	0.10	0.12	0.08	0.10
T	0.500*	0.350	0.450	0.625	0.400	0.575	0.525	0.400	0.475	0.500	0.325	0.450	0.500	0.325	0.400	0.475	0.350	0.425
m_1R	1.30	1.25	1.30	1.55	1.25	1.35	1.25	1.20	1.25	1.35	1.15	1.30	1.20	1.25	1.25	1.30	1.25	1.25
S	0.045	0.040	0.045	0.045	0.045	0.045	0.060	0.040	0.050	0.045	0.030	0.040	0.045	0.030	0.040	0.040	0.040	0.040
M$_S,\theta$	1	1	1	1	1	1	1	1	1	1	1	1	1	1	1	1	1	1
M$_T$/M$_R$	0.32*	0.24	0.30	0.36	0.24	0.30	0.34	0.28	0.30	0.30	0.26	0.28	0.34	0.22	0.30	0.32	0.22	0.30
M$_P$/M$_R$	0.08	0.10	0.08	0.08	0.08	0.08	0.10	0.10	0.10	0.08	0.10	0.10	0.10	0.12	0.10	0.08	0.10	0.08
Systolic BP (mmHg)	130	130	130	125	120	120	125	125	125	130	130	130	130	135	135	140	150	145

◻ Table A1.75

Magnitudes in space (M_R) and transverse plane (m_tR) in Cretan villagers. Up to age 50, M_R is greater in males, but not m_tR. In males, M_R reduces with age, also in FEMALEs but only up to age 50. In females m_tR tends to increase with age, but not in males. No overall sex difference for M_R and m_tR, but younger males show greater M_R. Medians of M_R are always greater than m_tR, also 95 percentiles. 95 percentiles for R or T in either sex do not show change with age, but numbers are too small to draw a reliable conclusion

Age-group	Sex	n	M_R(mV) median	M_R (mV) upper 95%	m_t R (mV) median	m_t R (mV) upper 95%
20–82	M+F	466	1.50	2.25	1.30	2.05
	M	275	1.55	2.30	1.30	2.10
	F	191	1.50	2.10	1.25	1.85
20–29	M+F	46	1.75	2.50	1.35	2.15
	M	30	1.75	2.40	1.55	2.15
	F	16	1.65	2.20	1.25	1.50
30–39	M+F	95	1.55	2.15	1.25	1.75
	M	53	1.65	2.15	1.25	1.80
	F	42	1.50	2.10	1.20	1.75
40–49	M+F	116	1.50	2.30	1.30	1.95
	M	70	1.60	2.25	1.35	2.00
	F	46	1.45	1.95	1.15	1.65
50–59	M+F	94	1.45	2.10	1.25	1.95
	M	51	1.45	2.10	1.20	1.95
	F	43	1.45	2.05	1.25	1.90
60–82	M+F	115	1.40	2.35	1.25	2.10
	M	71	1.45	2.35	1.30	2.00
	F	44	1.40	2.10	1.25	2.05

◻ Table A1.76

Normal lower and upper 2½ percentiles (After Dower G. Polarcardiography. 1961. © Thomas: Springfield, Illinois. Reproduced with permission)

	74 young women on university campus		121 young men on university campus		192 elderly men with normal ECGs	
	Lower	Upper	Lower	Upper	Lower	Upper
PR interval (s)	0.111	0.202	0.113	0.207	0.111	0.200
QRS duration (ms)	62.0	105.0	70.0	109.0	61.0	106.0
QT_C interval (s)	0.369	0.451	0.357	0.442		
QT interval (ms)					0.302	0.426
M_P (mV)	0.028	0.182	0.042	0.198		
M_R (Mv)	0.751	2.172	0.951	2.111	0.695	2.028
M_{ST} (mV)	0.042	0.193	0.088	0.332	0.000	0.222
M_T (mV)	0.209	0.654	0.300	0.875	0.193	0.742
M_{ST}/M_R	0.035	0.133	0.064	0.240	0.000	0.151
M_T/M_R	0.147	0.536	0.207	0.700	0.141	0.604
Latitude difference (°)	−78.0	−9.50	−105.0	−11.7		
Longitude difference (°)	−7.88	43.8	−18.7	73.3		
Angle between $\hat{R}$ and $\hat{T}$ (°)	14.7	80.9	14.9	114.5	18.2	149.6

◻ Table A1.77

Lower 2½ percentiles, medians, and upper 2½ percentiles for various polarcardiographic quantities (measured by computer in apparently healthy hospital staff). M_P, spatial magnitude of maximum P vector, $\vec{P}$; M_R, spatial magnitude of maximum QRS vector, $\vec{R}$; M_T spatial magnitude of maximum T vector, $\vec{T}$; m_tR, magnitude of maximum transverse plane QRS vector; M_{ST}, spatial magnitude of vector $\vec{ST}$ occurring midway in time between end of QRS complex and $\vec{T}$; lat., latitude posterior or anterior to frontal plane; long., longitude, or angle α in the frontal plane (After Dower G E, Osborne JA. Polarcardiographic study of hospital staff-abnormalities found in smokers. *J. Electrocardiol*. 1972; **5**: 273–80. © Churchill Livingstone, New York. Reproduced with permission)

	137 women, median age 47			117 men, median age 51		
	Lower 2½ percentile	Median	Upper 2½ percentile	Lower 2½ percentile	Median	Upper 2½ percentile
PR interval (s)	0.10 (0.11)[a]	0.14	0.19 (0.20)[a]	0.11 (0.11)	0.16	0.19 (0.21)[a]
QRS duration (ms)	60 (62)	80	100 (105)	70 (70)	80	100 (109)
QT$_C$ interval (s)	0.36 (0.37)	0.41	0.45 (0.45)	0.35 (0.36)	0.40	0.44 (0.44)
M_P (mV)	0.06 (0.03)	0.14	0.26 (0.18)	0.06 (0.04)	0.14	0.24 (0.20)
			0.22 (0.17)[b]			0.22 (0.19)[b]
M_R (mV)	0.82 (0.75)	1.41	2.24 (2.17)	1.02 (0.95)	1.50	2.20 (2.11)
			1.98 (1.82)[b]			2.14 (1.90)[b]
m_tR (mV)	0.72 (0.56)	1.16	1.84 (1.40)	0.77 (0.77)	1.31	2.13 (1.68)
			1.71 (1.28)[b]			1.95 (1.59)[b]
M_{ST} (mV)	0.04 (0.04)	0.12	0.22 (0.19)	0.09 (0.09)	0.21	0.35 (0.33)
M_T (mV)	0.21 (0.21)	0.44	0.82 (0.65)	0.28 (0.30)	0.60	0.92 (0.88)
M_{ST}/M_R	0.02 (0.04)	0.08	0.20 (0.13)	0.06 (0.06)	0.13	0.27 (0.24)
M_T/M_R	0.13 (0.15)	0.31	0.68 (0.54)	0.19 (0.21)	0.39	0.68 (0.70)
Lat. difference between $\vec{R}$ and $\vec{T}$ (°)	−115 (−80)	−44	+3 (−10)	−109 (−105)	−47	−2 (−10)
Long. difference between $\vec{R}$ and $\vec{T}$ (°)	−41 (−10)	+5	+139 (+45)	−45 (−20)	0	157 (+75)
Angle between $\vec{R}$ and $\vec{T}$ (°)	9 (15)	46	134 (81)	11 (15)	50	125 (115)

[a]Corresponding values from 74 young women and 121 young men
[b]Upper 5 percentiles

A1.7 Linear and Directional Statistics

A1.7.1 Acknowledgment

The work in this section has been compiled by Dr. Jerome Liebman of the Rainbow Babies and Children's Hospital, Cleveland, Ohio.

A1.7.2 Linear Statistics

Linear statistics are utilized for all linear measurements such as durations and magnitudes. Standard statistical methods are readily available, although there are many issues which must be understood in order to ensure appropriate use.

First, most standard ECGs are recorded with a maximal frequency response of 100–125 Hz, as are some orthogonal ECGs. However, for most orthogonal ECGs, the frequency response has been at least 250 Hz, often 500 Hz. In the author's laboratory, for recording the standard ECG, an upper frequency response limit above 250 Hz is preferred while

■ Table A1.78

PCG variables, at rest and after maximal exercise, in 30 healthy middle-aged men and 32 healthy young men compared. (After Bruce R A, Li Y B, Dower G E, Nilson K. Polarcardiographic responses to maximal exercise and to changes in posture in healthy middle aged men. J. Electrocardiol. 1973; 6: 91–6. Γ Churchill Livingstone, New York. Reproduced with permission)

| Variables | At rest | | | | | After exercise | | | | | Middle-aged rest versus exercise |
| | Middle-aged | | Young | | | Middle-aged | | Young | | | |
	X	σ	X	σ	p	X	Σ	X	σ	p	p
Heart rate (bmp)	67	11	72	13	NS	155	8	197	8	<0.001	<0.0001
PR interval (ms)	158	24	128	28	<0.001	121	15	110	15	<0.01	<0.0001
QRS duration (ms)	68	2	80	8	<0.05	75	6	79	8	<0.05	NS
RT interval (ms)	237	40				145	15				<0.0001
QT interval (ms)	360	30	341	30	<0.05	228	22	214	15	<0.01	<0.0001
$\hat{P}$: M (mV)	0.14	0.05	0.14	0.05	NS	0.20	0.05	0.27	0.08	<0.001	<0.0001
α long. (°)	+45	28	+57	49	NS	+57	42	+63	41	NS	NS
PA lat. (°)	6P	23	2P	22	NS	7A	21	13A	23	NS	0.03
$\hat{R}$: M (mV)	1.48	0.36	1.76	0.46	NS	1.30	0.38	1.42	0.55	NS	NS
α long. (°)	+27	35	+42	15	<0.05	+38	57	+34	81	NS	NS
PA lat. (°)	26P	16	19P	22	NS	31P	28	43	20	NS	NS
$\hat{ST}$: M (mV)	0.15	0.05	0.20	0.06	<0.002	0.11	0.05	0.22	0.08	<0.001	<0.01
α long. (°)	+28	19	+33	18	NS	−8	94	+20	48	NS	NS
PA lat. (°)	41A	25	39A	24	NS	49A	26	43A	27	NS	NS
$\hat{T}$: M (mV)	0.56	0.17	0.59	0.18	<0.01	0.60	0.15	0.67	0.17	NS	NS
α long. (°)	+24	11	+33	12	<0.01	+26	20	+30	21	NS	NS
PA lat. (°)	29A	19	29A	16	NS	39A	20	35A	21	NS	NS

◘ Table A1.79

Polarcardiographic responses in 72 apparently healthy middle-aged women and 40 young women before and after maximal exercise. M, spatial magnitude (After Bruce RA, Dower GE, Whitkanack S, Voigt AE. Polar-cardiographic responses to maximal exercise in middle-aged women. *J. Electrocardiol.* 1974; **7**: J15–22. © Churchill Livingstone, New York. Reproduced with permission)

Variables	Before maximal exercise			After maximal exercise			Before versus after exercise middle aged p
	Young	(Mean ± SD) Middle-aged	p	Young	(Mean ± SD) Middle-aged	p	
Heart-rate (bpm)	81.0 ± 15.0	74.7 ± 10.6	0.01	192.2 ± 9.0	151.6 ± 17.1	0.00001	0.00001
PR interval (ms)	138 ± 26	141 ± 17	NS	108 ± 14	129 ± 16	0.00001	0.001
QRS duration (ms)	73 ± 6	77 ± 8	0.01	72 ± 10	76 ± 7	0.05	NS
QT interval (ms)	339 ± 43	351 ± 25	NS	215 ± 15	248 ± 23	0.00001	0.00001
$\hat{P}$: M (mV)	0.15 ± 0.07	0.14 ± 0.06	NS	0.22 ± 0.06	0.23 ± 0.09	NS	0.00001
α longitude (°)	62.0 ± 44.0	30.5 ± 38.4	0.001	69.0 ± 37.0	32.8 ± 48.0	0.0001	NS
PA latitude (°)	A4.6 ± 29.0	A1.5 ± 27.3	NS	A10.0 ± 31.0	A11.1 ± 31.1	NS	0.05
$\hat{R}$: M (mV)	1.40 ± 0.34	1.49 ± 0.37	NS	1.23 ± 34.0	1.32 ± 32.3	NS	NS
α longitude (°)	46.0 ± 20.0	32.7 ± 22.6	0.01	41.0 ± 50.0	39.2 ± 30.6	NS	NS
PA latitude (°)	P27.0 ± 18.0	P26.2 ± 22.7	NS	P40.0 ± 21.0	P32.9 ± 22.6	NS	NS
ST: M (mV)	0.10 ± 0.05	0.10 ± 0.04	NS	0.16 ± 0.07	0.10 ± 0.04	0.00001	NS
α longitude (°)	29.0 ± 34.0	8.7 ± 48.5	0.05	16.0 ± 60.0	−9.5 ± 72.4	NS	NS
PA latitude (°)	A36.0 ± 23.0	A57.7 ± 212	0.00001	A41.0 ± 30.0	A53.7 ± 29.2	0.05	NS
$\hat{T}$: M (mV)	0.37 ± 0.15	0.42 ± 0.14	NS	0.53 ± 0.16	0.45 ± 0.12	0.01	NS
α longitude (°)	33.0 ± 13.0	21.4 ± 13.7	0.0001	33.0 ± 20.0	17.9 ± 33.3	0.05	NS
PA latitude (°)	A15.0 ± 20.0	A27.0 ± 13.2	0.001	A35.0 ± 18.0	A40.0 ± 17.2	NS	0.00001

the machine which is regularly used has an upper limit listed at 700 Hz. Although it is not well known by most electro-cardiographers, the higher-frequency response electrocardiograph allows detection of higher-frequency content in the ECG. It has been shown that in order to detect a frequency *content* of at least 100 Hz, it is necessary that the instrument have a frequency *response* of at least 200 Hz [1]. It should be appreciated that, in the *same patient*, with the electrodes attached and an appropriate electrocardiograph running, merely switching from the normal high-frequency response to the low-frequency response usually to avoid ac interference produces a significant decrease in QRS voltage. Therefore, separate tables of normal ranges should be available [2, 3] for both low-frequency response machines and high-frequency response machines. This is particularly true for the pediatric ECG. Manufacturers have a responsibility to produce equipment that meets the required standards. Nowadays, equipment has to meet strict standards but technical staff often opt for a low frequency setting to reduce noise, thereby running the risk of distorting the ECG.

A second issue is that from puberty, different age/sex groups have different normal voltage ranges. Pediatric cardiologists are aware that the voltages in pubescent females are lower than those of males. The same is true in virtually all age-groups through adulthood. In addition, for each decade throughout adulthood, total voltage decreases in both males and females, so that standards should be available for each, throughout the decades [4].

Prior to puberty, there is no difference in normal ECG ranges between males and females.

However, of great interest is the fact that the newborn baby has lower voltages than older infants and children, and these increase dramatically from the newborn period till about the age of 3 months. It is also striking that the prematurely-born infant has even lower voltages than does the full-term baby [5, 6]. Catch-up occurs at varying ages for each individual baby, and usually at about 3 months.

Racial differences are also important, but, again, probably not until puberty. Blacks may have much higher voltages than whites, and, occasionally, individual normal black teenagers may have extremely high voltages, with no available explanation. Unfortunately, separate large tables for normal blacks are not available.

A fourth major issue is that electrocardiographic amplitude data is skewed. The mean and the median are rarely the same, the distribution in the various age ranges not being Gaussian [2, 3]. Almost always the 50th percentile is below the mean, in addition to which the mean plus twice standard deviation may be higher than the maximal value recorded. Therefore, the use of means and standard deviations for magnitude is not appropriate, which is why the use of percentiles to describe the distribution is necessary (see ❷ Chap. 1 of *Electrocardiology: Comprehensive Clinical ECG*). In describing the complete distribution, as is frequently done, a series of percentiles is optimal. In using the percentiles to describe low and high limits of the normal range, the $2\frac{1}{2}$ and $97\frac{1}{2}$ percentiles are recommended. However, because of known inaccuracies of measurement, the 5th and 95th percentiles denoted p_5 and p_{95} are considered as being satisfactory by the author.

A1.7.3 Directional Statistics

For directional (circular and spherical) data, linear statistics are not appropriate. The fallacies in employing linear methods for directional statistics are easily understood, although, because of the lack of available methodology, such incorrect measurements were almost invariably used [7]. For example, if two vectors, 1° and 359° are grouped, the mean of 360°/2 = 180° is obviously incorrect, since it is 180° away from the true average direction of 0°. Why not, therefore, change the terminology to +1° and −1°? The mean of 0°/2 = 0° would be correct. However, suppose two vectors at 179° and 181° were then averaged. According to the new terminology, the electrocardiographer would then have to average +179° and −179° in order to be consistent. The average of +179° and −179° = 0°/2 = 0°, which is again 180° away from the true average direction of 180°. Some of these rotational adjustments have been reported [8], but in using linear statistics, the adjustments have a minimal error only when there is an intense clustering of the data. Every linear treatment of directional data has inherent error. Whether the angles are, measured from −180° to +180°, or from 0° to 360°, and so on, some of the observations (actually close together) *must inevitably be treated as being far apart*. Therefore, appropriate statistical analyses of planar data as well as spherical data were developed by Downs et al. [9, 10], based upon the Von Mises distribution [11–13]. This new set of statistics was termed the "center of gravity method." In linear analysis, there is an arithmetic mean. In circular analysis, there is a prevalent direction.

◻ Table A1.80

Segment of a table from 50 premature infants where the ECG was recorded with the Frank-lead system. n_f, n_s, n_h are the number of angles under study; d_f, d_s, d_h are the distances to the center of gravity; $\widehat{a}_f$, $\widehat{a}_s$, $\widehat{a}_h$ are the prevalent directions of the vector. All parameters represent measurements taken in the frontal, sagittal and horizontal planes, respectively (denoted by the subscripts f, s, h)

Age (h)	Times vector (ms)	n_f	d_f	$\widehat{a}_f$	X_f^2	n_s	d_s	$\widehat{a}_s$	X_s^2	n_h	d_h	$\widehat{a}_h$	X_h^2
24	10	50	0.41	7	16.4	50	0.95	178	90.6	50	0.96	83	91.6

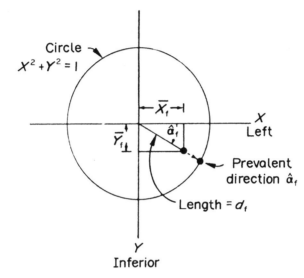

◻ Fig. A1.1

The center of gravity (X_f, Y_f) or, in polar coordinates (d_f, α_f) of points (x_f, y_f) on the circle $X^2 + Y^2 = 1$ in the frontal plane

For details of the methods, the reader is referred to pertinent literature, including utilization with tabular data. However, some explanations and descriptions will be given here. ❯ Table A1.80 is a segment of a table from 50 premature infants where the ECG was recorded with the Frank system.

Imagine the data for the 10 ms vector of the 50 premature infants to be on a circular disk, balanced on a fulcrum at its center. If all the observations were in approximately the same direction, then they would all cluster together and the disk would tilt maximally. The direction of tilt would be toward the center of gravity of the points: this is termed the prevalent direction. If the points were scattered equally around the disk, there would be no tilt and there would be no prevalent direction.

In calculating the prevalent direction $\widehat{a}_f$ the "average" of the 50 10 ms angles (each α_f) in the frontal plane, reference is made to ❯ Fig. A1.1.

For each angle α_f, X_f and Y_f are computed as follows.

$$X_f = \cos \alpha_f, \qquad Y_f = \sin \alpha_f \tag{A1.1}$$

The means are then computed from:

$$\overline{X}_f = \sum X_f / n_f \qquad \overline{Y}_f = \sum Y_f / n_f \tag{A1.2}$$

where n_f is number of angles under study in the frontal plane.

The center of gravity corresponds to the point $(\overline{X}_f, \overline{Y}_f)$ and the distance d_f to the center of gravity is then

$$d_f = \left(\overline{X}_f + \overline{Y}_f\right) \tag{A1.3}$$

The direction α_f toward the center of gravity is calculated from

$$\cos \hat{\alpha}_f = \overline{X}_f / d_f \quad \text{or} \quad \sin \hat{\alpha}_f = \overline{Y}_f / d_f \tag{A1.4}$$

where d_f is termed the precision. If it is zero, then there is no prevalent direction. If it is 1.0, then *all* the individual measurements are the same. The higher the precision d, the more the clustering; the lower the precision d, the more the scatter.

In order to determine whether a calculated prevalent direction can be trusted, that is, whether a true prevalent direction actually exists, a χ^2 value can be calculated where:

$$\chi_f^2 = 2n_f d_f^2 \tag{A1.5}$$

Values of χ^2 greater than 5.99 are significant at the 5% level, and values of χ^2 greater than 9.21 are significant at the 1% level.

For ❯ Table A1.80, d_f is not high (0.41), so that there is little cluster of the $\hat{\alpha}_f$. However, the prevalent direction of $7°$ can be trusted, since the $\chi_f^2 = 16.4$. For the sagittal and horizontal planes, the values of χ^2 are extremely high at 90.6 and 91.6 so that the high precisions $d_s = 0.95$ and $d_b = 0.96$ (and thus high cluster) can be very reliably trusted. (To determine whether a particular measured angle α is likely to be within the accepted normal range, it is only necessary to determine whether the angle is between the p_5 and p_{95} for the normal population.)

For spatial data, a methodology has been developed similar to that of the above planar data. In this case, consider that there exists a sample of spatial vectors with coordinates (X, Y, Z) and that it is desired to determine an "average" spatial direction for n measurements. Imagine a sphere placed in the surface of a liquid. If the n measurements cluster about some direction, then the sphere will rotate in the liquid until the center of gravity of the n measurements points downward. This is the spatial prevalent direction (❯ Fig. A1.2).

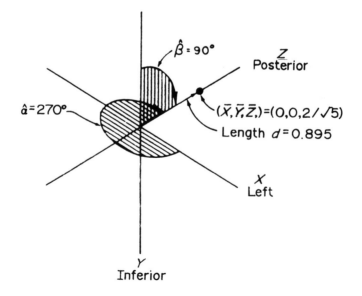

◻ Fig. A1.2
An example of the spatial prevalent direction expressed in spherical and Cartesian coordinates

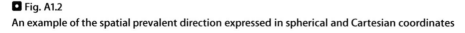

■ Table A1.81

Segment of spatial data for the same 50 premature babies tabulated in ❯ Table A1.80

Age (h)	Timed vector (ms)	X	Y	Z	d	$\hat{\alpha}$ (°)	β (°)	χ^2	n
24	10	0.122	0.045	-0.910	0.920	82	93	127.1	50

As before, the distance from the center of the sphere to the center of gravity $(\overline{X}, \overline{Y}, \overline{Z})$ is a measure of how much the observations cluster, and is called the *spatial precision*. The center of gravity $(\overline{X}, \overline{Y}, \overline{Z})$ can also be expressed in spherical coordinates $(d, \hat{\alpha}, \widehat{\beta})$ where $\hat{\alpha}$ is the longitude or angular deviation from the left in the horizontal plane (0–360°) and $\widehat{\beta}$ is the colatitude or angular deviation from the superior (0–180°). (The spherical α is identical to the planar α_h.) The spatial prevalent direction is $(\hat{\alpha}, \widehat{\beta})$ and can be determined uniquely.

A χ^2 can be calculated to test whether the clustering about the spatial prevalent direction can be trusted. Values of χ^2 greater than 7.81 are significant at the 5% level and values of χ^2 larger than 11.34 are significant at the 1% level. For further details and the methodology (with equations) for calculation of the above, the reader is referred to an original paper and a recent summary [14].

❯ Table A1.81 is a segment of spatial data for the same 50 premature babies given in ❯ Table A1.80.

The d and χ^2 are both very high, consistent with the high d for the horizontal and sagittal planes, despite the low d for the frontal plane. The α of 82° is actually the $\hat{\alpha}_h$. The $\widehat{\beta}$ of 93° has no corollary in the planar directions. However, from these spatial data, all the planar data can be calculated.

For detailed research (as well as descriptive) purposes, this methodology has been very satisfactory. As with linear statistics, for example, it is frequently necessary to determine whether two different samples of directional measurements are from the same or different populations. The necessary methodology is detailed in the appendix to [9].

References

1. Thomas, C., Electrocardiographic measurement system response, in *Pediatric Electrocardiography*, J. Liebman, R. Plonsey, and P. Gillette, Editors. Baltimore: Williams and Wilkins, 1982, Chap. 5, pp. 40–59.

2. Liebman, J. and R. Plonsey, Electrocardiography, in *Moss' Heart Disease in Infants, Children and Adolescents*, H. Adams and G.C. Emmanouillides, Editors. Baltimore: Williams and Wilkins, 1983, Chap. 3.

3. Liebman, J., Tables of normal standards, in *Pediatric Cardiology*, J. Liebman, R. Plonsey, and P. Gillette, Editors. Baltimore: Williams and Wilkins, 1982, Chap. 8, pp. 82–133.

4. Pipberger, H.V., M.J. Goldman, D. Littman, F.P. Murphy, J. Cosma, and J.R. Snyder, Correlations of the orthogonal electrocardiogram and vectorcardiogram with constitutional variables in 518 normal men. *Circulation*, 1967; **35**: 536.

5. Sreenivasan, V.V, B.J. Fisher, J. Liebman, and T.D. Downs, A longitudinal study of the standard electrocardiogram in the healthy premature infant during the first year of life. *Am. J. Cardiol.*, 1973; **31**: 57.

6. Liebman, J., H.C. Romberg, T.D. Downs, and R. Agusti, The Frank QRS vectorcardiogram in the premature infant, in *Vectorcardiography, 1965*, I. Hoffman and R.C. Taymore, Editors. Amsterdam: North-Holland, 1966.

7. Hugenholtz, P.C. and J. Liebman, The orthogonal electrocardiogram in 100 normal children (Frank system), with some comparative data recorded by the cube system. *Circulation*, 1962; **26**: 891.

8. Liebman, J., C. Doershuk, C. Rapp, and L. Matthews, The vectorcardiogram in cycstic fibrosis: diagnostic significance and correlation with pulmonary function tests. *Circulation*, 1967; **32**: 552.

9. Downs, T.D., J. Liebman, R. Agusti, and H.C. Romberg, The statistical treatment of angular data in vectocardiography, in *Vectorcardiography, 1965*, I. Hoffman and R.C. Traymore, Editors. Amsterdam: North-Holland, 1966, p. 272.

10. Downs, T.D. and J. Liebman, Statistical methods for vectorcardiographic directions. *IEEE Trans. Biomed. Eng.*, 1969; **16**: 87.

11. Stephens, M.A., *The Statistics of Directions. The Von Mises and Fisher Distributions*, PhD thesis. Tornto: University of Toronto, 1962.

12. Downs, T.D., *The Von Mises Distribution: Derived Distributions Regression Theory, and Some Applications to Meterological Problems*, PhD thesis. Ann Arbor: University of Michigan, 1965.

13. Downs, T.D., Some relationships amont the von Mises distributions of different dimensions. *Biometrika*, 1966; **53**: 269.

14. Liebman, J., Statistics related to electrocardiographic interpretation, in *Pediatric Electrocardiography*, J. Liebman, R. Plonsey, and P. Gillete, Editors. Baltimore: Williams and Wilkins, 1982, Chap. 7, pp. 76–81.

Appendix 2: Paediatric Normal Limits

A2.1   Normal Limits of the Paediatric 12-Lead ECG

This appendix is based on a series of 1,784 ECGs collected from neonates, infants and children in Glasgow, Scotland in the late 1980s. Some outline information was previously published [1, 2] but the detailed normal limits as presented in this chapter have never previously been published. Lead V_{4R} has been recorded to the exclusion of lead V_3. Precordial leads are therefore presented in the sequence V_1, V_2, V_{4R}, V_4, V_5, V_6.

One of the significant aspects of this data is the availability of ECGs from over 500 neonates from birth to 7 days of life. Nowadays, new mothers tend to be discharged from hospital within 24–48 h and so the difficulty of collecting such a database is significantly increased.

The standard presentation of mean together with standard deviation and 96 percentile range has been used throughout. (❷ Tables A2.1–A2.24) With small numbers in some groups this leads to an irregular upper limit of normal for some measures but in practice, continuous equations for normal limits can be developed (see ❷ Chap. 1 of *Electrocardiology: Comprehensive Clinical ECG*).

❑ Table A2.1

Durations (in milliseconds) in Caucasian children: lead I

Age-group	Q duration	S duration	R duration	R′ duration
<24 h	36 ± 17	16 ± 4	29 ± 4	
	6 → 62	10 → 23	22 → 40	
	n = 10	n = 35	n = 35	
<1 day	33 ± 15	17 ± 7	29 ± 4	
	9 → 52	6 → 25	22 → 40	
	n = 36	n = 112	n = 110	
<2 days	29 ± 17	17 ± 5	28 ± 5	24
	8 → 56	6 → 26	19 → 38	24 → 24
	n = 34	n = 99	n = 99	n = 1
<3 days	30 ± 16	17 ± 5	28 ± 5	30
	8 → 56	7 → 28	17 → 38	30 → 30
	n = 41	n = 80	n = 79	n = 1
<1 week	23 ± 17	16 ± 5	29 ± 6	17
	8 → 56	5 → 27	20 → 43	17 → 17
	n = 38	n = 104	n = 104	n = 1
<1 month	16 ± 15	18 ± 5	26 ± 6	
	5 → 52	11 → 32	17 → 43	
	n = 14	n = 43	n = 43	
<3 months	11 ± 5	22 ± 6	24 ± 6	24
	6 → 30	10 → 34	13 → 34	24 → 24
	n = 34	n = 66	n = 65	n = 1
<6 months	12 ± 4	24 ± 5	25 ± 6	
	5 → 18	17 → 41	14 → 35	
	n = 21	n = 50	n = 46	
<1 year	12 ± 3	24 ± 5	24 ± 7	33
	8 → 19	14 → 38	14 → 42	33 → 33
	n = 40	n = 73	n = 70	n = 1
1–2 years	13 ± 4	27 ± 7	24 ± 7	24 ± 2
	5 → 25	16 → 46	10 → 39	22 → 25
	n = 69	n = 111	n = 95	n = 2

◻ Table A2.1   (Continued)

Age-group	Q duration	S duration	R duration	R′ duration
3–4 years	14 ± 4	30 ± 7	28 ± 8	
	7 → 21	20 → 51	14 → 45	
	n = 77	n = 141	n = 109	
5–6 years	14 ± 5	31 ± 6	27 ± 8	
	6 → 40	21 → 46	13 → 44	
	n = 71	n = 155	n = 136	
7–8 years	13 ± 5	32 ± 8	27 ± 8	10
	7 → 21	21 → 54	14 → 45	10 → 10
	n = 80	n = 141	n = 114	n = 1
9–10 years	13 ± 4	36 ± 9	27 ± 9	17 ± 5
	7 → 21	24 → 64	6 → 45	13 → 22
	n = 49	n = 115	n = 92	n = 3
11–12 years	14 ± 4	37 ± 7	29 ± 9	
	8 → 29	24 → 55	14 → 50	
	n = 62	n = 119	n = 90	
13–14 years	15 ± 4	39 ± 8	28 ± 10	23 ± 6
	7 → 27	27 → 63	12 → 55	19 → 27
	n = 62	n = 141	n = 113	n = 2
15–16 years	15 ± 5	39 ± 9	30 ± 11	
	8 → 29	27 → 63	11 → 61	
	n = 46	n = 92	n = 71	
17–18 years	32			
	32 → 32			
	n = 1			

◻ Table A2.2

Durations (in milliseconds) in Caucasian children: lead II

Age-group	Q duration	S duration	R duration	R′ duration
<24 h	18 ± 11	21 ± 8	18 ± 5	
	9 → 68	9 → 39	12 → 35	
	n = 41	n = 41	n = 22	
<1 day	16 ± 5	21 ± 9	19 ± 6	19 ± 13
	7 → 24	7 → 41	10 → 39	5 → 38
	n = 132	n = 136	n = 71	n = 5
<2 days	16 ± 5	21 ± 9	19 ± 7	18 ± 9
	9 → 38	7 → 44	10 → 45	12 → 28
	n = 106	n = 116	n = 69	n = 3
<3 days	16 ± 6	22 ± 12	19 ± 6	23 ± 12
	10 → 38	7 → 43	7 → 32	12 → 36
	n = 102	n = 105	n = 56	n = 3
<1 week	17 ± 6	19 ± 6	20 ± 7	15 ± 0
	9 → 44	7 → 35	6 → 37	15 → 15
	n = 115	n = 114	n = 75	n = 2

◨ Table A2.2   (Continued)

Age-group	Q duration	S duration	R duration	R′ duration
<1 month	16 ± 3	21 ± 6	19 ± 6	24
	11 → 23	9 → 39	12 → 32	24 → 24
	n = 41	n = 45	n = 28	n = 1
<3 months	16 ± 3	25 ± 7	17 ± 4	26 ± 0
	12 → 24	11 → 45	12 → 26	26 → 26
	n = 58	n = 67	n = 46	n = 2
<6 months	16 ± 5	27 ± 6	19 ± 6	19 ± 6
	6 → 24	19 → 38	13 → 34	15 → 23
	n = 40	n = 49	n = 32	n = 2
<1 year	14 ± 5	29 ± 7	21 ± 6	36
	6 → 26	18 → 54	12 → 34	36 → 36
	n = 54	n = 73	n = 52	n = 1
1–2 years	16 ± 4	32 ± 9	23 ± 7	21 ± 7
	8 → 26	21 → 56	12 → 37	13 → 26
	n = 79	n = 111	n = 74	n = 3
3–4 years	16 ± 4	34 ± 10	24 ± 9	17 ± 4
	7 → 23	23 → 57	8 → 41	14 → 21
	n = 106	n = 141	n = 98	n = 3
5–6 years	15 ± 4	36 ± 9	23 ± 8	24
	7 → 22	24 → 60	12 → 43	24 → 24
	n = 118	n = 155	n = 114	n = 1
7–8 years	15 ± 6	37 ± 8	25 ± 9	18
	7 → 24	26 → 61	13 → 46	18 → 18
	n = 94	n = 141	n = 115	n = 1
9–10 years	15 ± 4	40 ± 9	23 ± 10	17 ± 5
	7 → 21	26 → 64	7 → 47	14 → 23
	n = 86	n = 115	n = 84	n = 3
11–12 years	14 ± 5	43 ± 11	25 ± 9	17 ± 1
	7 → 26	29 → 78	7 → 45	16 → 18
	n = 83	n = 119	n = 87	n = 3
13–14 years	14 ± 4	43 ± 11	26 ± 10	13 ± 4
	7 → 25	30 → 75	9 → 50	7 → 17
	n = 100	n = 141	n = 111	n = 5
15–16 years	16 ± 6	45 ± 12	28 ± 11	16
	7 → 37	29 → 76	11 → 53	16 → 16
	n = 60	n = 92	n = 67	n = 1
17–18 years	15	22		
	15 → 15	22 → 22		
	n = 1	n = 1		

● Table A2.3

Durations (in milliseconds) in Caucasian children: lead III

Age-group	Q duration	S duration	R duration	R' duration
<24 h	17 ± 3	28 ± 7	18 ± 4	12
	12 → 23	15 → 41	12 → 21	12 → 12
	n = 41	n = 43	n = 4	n = 1
<1 day	18 ± 3	28 ± 8	15 ± 3	32 ± 6
	13 → 23	12 → 44	11 → 21	27 → 39
	n = 131	n = 138	n = 32	n = 3
<2 days	17 ± 3	27 ± 8	15 ± 5	16 ± 7
	9 → 24	7 → 44	7 → 32	9 → 25
	n = 110	n = 119	n = 32	n = 5
<3 days	17 ± 3	28 ± 12	15 ± 3	20 ± 3
	10 → 25	8 → 56	8 → 22	15 → 23
	n = 101	n = 106	n = 22	n = 6
<1 week	17 ± 3	27 ± 8	16 ± 4	14 ± 6
	10 → 24	8 → 43	12 → 31	9 → 20
	n = 115	n = 117	n = 32	n = 3
<1 month	19 ± 4	28 ± 9	15 ± 4	26 ± 7
	13 → 28	9 → 54	8 → 22	21 → 31
	n = 41	n = 45	n = 11	n = 2
<3 months	20 ± 3	27 ± 8	17 ± 5	24 ± 5
	13 → 28	8 → 43	10 → 32	18 → 30
	n = 59	n = 67	n = 17	n = 7
<6 months	22 ± 4	25 ± 9	17 ± 7	23 ± 5
	14 → 30	6 → 42	8 → 41	14 → 31
	n = 38	n = 50	n = 20	n = 9
<1 year	21 ± 4	23 ± 9	16 ± 6	22 ± 10
	14 → 30	5 → 38	8 → 39	5 → 53
	n = 47	n = 73	n = 35	n = 23
1–2 years	21 ± 6	25 ± 11	20 ± 11	20 ± 8
	9 → 54	7 → 54	8 → 63	8 → 39
	n = 68	n = 110	n = 63	n = 33
3–4 years	21 ± 6	31 ± 13	22 ± 12	24 ± 9
	6 → 32	6 → 64	6 → 58	9 → 44
	n = 94	n = 140	n = 79	n = 23
5–6 years	18 ± 5	33 ± 13	19 ± 10	26 ± 7
	5 → 27	6 → 60	6 → 49	13 → 43
	n = 106	n = 155	n = 84	n = 22
7–8 years	19 ± 6	35 ± 13	24 ± 11	28 ± 14
	8 → 28	7 → 62	7 → 53	8 → 48
	n = 82	n = 141	n = 94	n = 19
9–10 years	19 ± 4	39 ± 14	21 ± 11	23 ± 12
	9 → 28	13 → 72	5 → 60	5 → 47
	n = 78	n = 115	n = 70	n = 15

◨ Table A2.3   (Continued)

Age-group	Q duration	S duration	R duration	R′ duration
11–12 years	18 ± 6	40 ± 16	24 ± 12	23 ± 12
	7 → 32	7 → 80	5 → 51	5 → 45
	n = 75	n = 119	n = 74	n = 14
13–14 years	19 ± 6	41 ± 17	26 ± 13	26 ± 17
	8 → 31	9 → 79	6 → 57	5 → 71
	n = 88	n = 141	n = 93	n = 21
15–16 years	19 ± 6	44 ± 17	28 ± 14	28 ± 14
	9 → 37	8 → 82	6 → 67	11 → 48
	n = 55	n = 92	n = 55	n = 8
17–18 years	14	17		
	14 → 14	17 → 17		
	n = 1	n = 1		

◨ Table A2.4

Durations (in milliseconds) in Caucasian children: lead aVR

Age-group	Q duration	S duration	R duration	R′ duration
<24 h	17 ± 7	22 ± 13	16 ± 6	21 ± 7
	8 → 30	8 → 68	6 → 31	11 → 31
	n = 15	n = 42	n = 24	n = 15
<1 day	20 ± 6	22 ± 12	15 ± 7	19 ± 6
	8 → 35	8 → 50	6 → 40	0 → 33
	n = 46	n = 135	n = 73	n = 57
<2 days	21 ± 6	19 ± 10	14 ± 5	22 ± 6
	13 → 38	7 → 46	5 → 30	11 → 42
	n = 35	n = 117	n = 72	n = 62
<3 days	20 ± 6	20 ± 11	15 ± 6	20 ± 7
	8 → 33	7 → 48	6 → 35	11 → 32
	n = 26	n = 105	n = 67	n = 51
<1 week	18 ± 7	19 ± 11	14 ± 4	21 ± 5
	10 → 34	8 → 56	5 → 22	12 → 33
	n = 20	n = 116	n = 86	n = 80
<1 month	22 ± 3	15 ± 7	16 ± 4	21 ± 6
	17 → 27	8 → 42	8 → 26	13 → 37
	n = 8	n = 45	n = 36	n = 33
<3 months	26 ± 7	14 ± 5	21 ± 4	20 ± 5
	11 → 41	5 → 29	14 → 34	12 → 28
	n = 13	n = 67	n = 55	n = 48
<6 months	26 ± 4	16 ± 6	24 ± 3	21 ± 5
	18 → 31	6 → 33	20 → 34	13 → 32
	n = 16	n = 50	n = 34	n = 27
<1 year	28 ± 5	16 ± 8	26 ± 6	21 ± 6
	11 → 37	6 → 36	17 → 46	12 → 38
	n = 25	n = 72	n = 49	n = 37

■ Table A2.4 (Continued)

Age-group	Q duration	S duration	R duration	R′ duration
1–2 years	29 ± 7	17 ± 7	28 ± 6	22 ± 8
	11 → 46	7 → 35	19 → 45	8 → 38
	n = 33	n = 107	n = 80	n = 56
3–4 years	35 ± 8	17 ± 7	31 ± 6	24 ± 8
	24 → 72	8 → 38	21 → 51	12 → 43
	n = 39	n = 133	n = 102	n = 78
5–6 years	35 ± 7	17 ± 7	32 ± 5	23 ± 8
	27 → 68	7 → 36	24 → 48	12 → 44
	n = 52	n = 148	n = 103	n = 79
7–8 years	35 ± 4	18 ± 8	34 ± 7	25 ± 8
	29 → 46	8 → 44	24 → 51	12 → 40
	n = 45	n = 140	n = 96	n = 75
9–10 years	37 ± 5	17 ± 8	36 ± 7	23 ± 9
	29 → 48	7 → 41	27 → 62	7 → 49
	n = 43	n = 108	n = 72	n = 55
11–12 years	39 ± 7	19 ± 9	39 ± 8	25 ± 8
	28 → 60	8 → 46	28 → 67	13 → 44
	n = 48	n = 112	n = 71	n = 50
13–14 years	41 ± 8	19 ± 9	39 ± 7	25 ± 9
	33 → 74	8 → 43	29 → 62	12 → 52
	n = 59	n = 135	n = 83	n = 69
15–16 years	44 ± 9	22 ± 10	39 ± 6	27 ± 9
	33 → 68	9 → 48	30 → 60	15 → 50
	n = 41	n = 82	n = 50	n = 37
17–18 years		18	7	
		18 → 18	7 → 7	
		n = 1	n = 1	

■ Table A2.5

Durations (in milliseconds) in Caucasian children: lead aVL

Age-group	Q duration	S duration	R duration	R′ duration
<24 h	24 ± 17	16 ± 4	31 ± 4	
	9 → 40	10 → 22	23 → 42	
	n = 4	n = 41	n = 41	
<1 day	25 ± 18	17 ± 4	30 ± 5	13 ± 1
	7 → 54	11 → 23	21 → 41	0 → 13
	n = 8	n = 136	n = 134	n = 2
<2 days	23 ± 16	17 ± 4	30 ± 5	15 ± 4
	7 → 46	9 → 25	19 → 39	12 → 17
	n = 11	n = 116	n = 114	n = 2

■ Table A2.5   (Continued)

Age-group	Q duration	S duration	R duration	R′ duration
<3 days	20 ± 15	16 ± 4	30 ± 5	21 ± 7
	7 → 52	8 → 25	20 → 44	15 → 28
	n = 12	n =102	n = 102	n = 3
<1 week	16 ± 17	17 ± 4	30 ± 6	13 ± 5
	6 → 56	8 → 26	18 → 42	8 → 22
	n = 9	n = 115	n = 115	n = 6
<1 month	39 ± 27	19 ± 4	28 ± 6	12 ± 0
	9 → 62	11 → 29	16 → 47	12 → 12
	n = 5	n = 42	n = 42	n = 2
<3 months	12 ± 7	21 ± 4	27 ± 6	11 ± 2
	6 → 32	12 → 32	13 → 37	9 → 12
	n = 13	n = 66	n = 66	n = 2
<6 months	11 ± 4	24 ± 6	26 ± 6	20
	6 → 19	13 → 50	17 → 35	20 → 20
	n = 13	n = 50	n = 48	n = 1
<1 year	12 ± 5	22 ± 5	26 ± 7	25 ± 18
	6 → 26	12 → 37	13 → 41	12 → 37
	n = 30	n = 73	n = 71	n = 2
1–2 years	13 ± 5	24 ± 7	25 ± 8	17 ± 5
	6 → 28	14 → 52	8 → 43	13 → 26
	n = 54	n = 111	n = 98	n = 6
3–4 years	15 ± 8	25 ± 9	30 ± 10	19 ± 6
	6 → 40	10 → 49	6 → 48	6 → 33
	n = 60	n = 140	n = 118	n = 15
5–6 years	15 ± 10	23 ± 8	31 ± 11	18 ± 5
	5 → 62	8 → 44	9 → 51	12 → 28
	n = 58	n = 154	n = 140	n = 26
7–8 years	18 ± 10	25 ± 12	30 ± 12	21 ± 6
	6 → 54	10 → 60	6 → 53	12 → 35
	n = 71	n = 140	n = 115	n = 33
9–10 years	21 ± 17	25 ± 10	34 ± 12	21 ± 8
	7 → 76	10 → 57	10 → 60	9 → 44
	n = 37	n = 112	n = 99	n = 24
11–12 years	20 ± 10	27 ± 13	32 ± 14	23 ± 8
	10 → 57	6 → 66	7 → 59	7 → 39
	n = 49	n = 117	n = 100	n = 23
13–14 years	19 ± 11	29 ± 14	34 ± 16	22 ± 9
	6 → 74	9 → 69	6 → 72	7 → 42
	n = 55	n = 139	n = 118	n = 37
15–16 years	24 ± 17	30 ± 14	34 ± 14	22 ± 10
	8 → 78	10 → 63	6 → 65	7 → 45
	n = 41	n = 88	n = 70	n = 19
17–18 years		13	22	
		13 → 13	22 → 22	
		n = 1	n = 1	

◯ Table A2.6

Durations (in milliseconds) in Caucasian children: lead aVF

Age-group	Q duration	S duration	R duration	R' duration
<24 h	16 ± 4	24 ± 8	17 ± 8	
	11 → 24	10 → 41	6 → 37	
	n = 42	n = 43	n = 14	
<1 day	17 ± 4	25 ± 9	17 ± 5	21 ± 14
	10 → 24	11 → 45	11 → 36	9 → 37
	n = 133	n = 137	n = 44	n = 3
<2 days	17 ± 3	24 ± 8	17 ± 7	15 ± 3
	8 → 23	7 → 39	7 → 46	13 → 19
	n = 110	n = 119	n = 50	n = 3
<3 days	17 ± 4	25 ± 12	18 ± 5	22 ± 10
	10 → 27	5 → 51	10 → 31	15 → 29
	n = 101	n = 106	n = 36	n = 2
<1 week	17 ± 3	22 ± 7	18 ± 7	
	11 → 26	8 → 37	10 → 54	
	n = 116	n = 117	n = 56	
<1 month	17 ± 3	25 ± 7	17 ± 4	
	8 → 25	13 → 43	12 → 24	
	n = 43	n = 45	n = 19	
<3 months	17 ± 3	27 ± 8	15 ± 5	25 ± 8
	12 → 23	11 → 50	8 → 26	16 → 36
	n = 57	n = 67	n = 28	n = 6
<6 months	19 ± 4	26 ± 7	17 ± 7	20 ± 3
	11 → 27	8 → 42	8 → 38	16 → 24
	n = 40	n = 50	n = 26	n = 5
< 1 year	18 ± 4	28 ± 9	19 ± 7	26 ± 11
	11 → 28	5 → 58	7 → 36	5 → 36
	n = 50	n = 73	n = 40	n = 7
1–2 years	18 ± 5	30 ± 9	21 ± 9	23 ± 11
	8 → 27	9 → 52	5 → 46	5 → 38
	n = 73	n = 111	n = 66	n = 9
3–4 years	18 ± 4	35 ± 12	22 ± 10	23 ± 6
	11 → 26	8 → 62	6 → 41	10 → 31
	n = 95	n = 141	n = 85	n = 9
5–6 years	16 ± 4	36 ± 10	22 ± 8	29 ± 2
	7 → 24	13 → 62	12 → 43	27 → 31
	n = 114	n = 155	n = 99	n = 3
7–8 years	17 ± 6	38 ± 10	25 ± 10	18 ± 10
	7 → 24	24 → 68	7 → 47	6 → 33
	n = 87	n = 141	n = 97	n = 6
9–10 years	16 ± 4	42 ± 11	24 ± 10	16 ± 3
	7 → 22	25 → 72	9 → 53	13 → 19
	n = 79	n = 115	n = 74	n = 4
11–12 years	16 ± 5	44 ± 12	26 ± 10	10
	6 → 27	28 → 80	12 → 46	10 → 10
	n = 76	n = 119	n = 77	n = 1

◘ Table A2.6   (Continued)

Age-group	Q duration	S duration	R duration	R′ duration
13–14 years	16 ± 5	44 ± 13	28 ± 10	19 ± 6
	8 → 26	29 → 80	9 → 48	13 → 27
	n = 94	n = 141	n = 96	n = 4
15–16 years	17 ± 6	45 ± 13	27 ± 12	44 ± 18
	6 → 38	24 → 76	6 → 53	24 → 57
	n = 57	n = 92	n = 63	n = 3
17–18 years	14	17		
	14 → 14	17 → 17		
	n = 1	n = 1		

◘ Table A2.7

Durations (in milliseconds) in Caucasian children: lead V_1

Age-group	Q duration	S duration	R duration	R′ duration
<24 h		30 ± 7	23 ± 6	30
		19 → 44	14 → 36	30 → 30
		n = 43	n = 40	n = 1
<1 day	9 ± 1	32 ± 7	23 ± 6	
	8 → 10	21 → 52	12 → 35	
	n = 2	n = 137	n = 124	
<2 days	11 ± 8	33 ± 8	21 ± 6	
	5 → 17	20 → 54	13 → 37	
	n = 2	n = 117	n = 100	
<3 days	12 ± 6	32 ± 7	22 ± 10	11 ± 5
	8 → 16	20 → 48	12 → 42	7 → 17
	n = 2	n = 102	n = 93	n = 3
<1 week		35 ± 9	20 ± 5	
		23 → 60	12 → 34	
		n = 114	n = 99	
<1 month	10	35 ± 8	21 ± 6	
	10 → 10	24 → 62	13 → 36	
	n = 1	n = 41	n = 37	
<3 months	10 ± 3	33 ± 9	24 ± 8	7 ± 2
	8 → 12	20 → 56	7 → 55	6 → 10
	n = 2	n = 62	n = 56	n = 4
<6 months		31 ± 8	28 ± 9	12 ± 5
		20 → 60	9 → 43	9 → 19
		n = 49	n = 48	n = 4
<1 year		29 ± 8	29 ± 10	23 ± 11
		15 → 55	8 → 50	9 → 44
		n = 70	n = 69	n = 10
1–2 years	12 ± 6	28 ± 8	37 ± 9	14 ± 8
	8 → 16	14 → 58	12 → 51	6 → 32
	n = 2	n = 107	n = 103	n = 10
3–4 years	86	25 ± 5	39 ± 12	21 ± 9
	86 → 86	16 → 39	13 → 59	6 → 36
	n = 1	n = 135	n = 135	n = 27

Table A2.7 (Continued)

Age-group	Q duration	S duration	R duration	R' duration
5–6 years	28 ± 28	25 ± 5	42 ± 11	18 ± 10
	8 → 48	13 → 40	15 → 55	4 → 43
	n = 2	n = 146	n = 146	n = 23
7–8 years		25 ± 4	43 ± 11	22 ± 9
		18 → 34	16 → 59	12 → 49
		n = 135	n = 135	n = 28
9–10 years		25 ± 4	42 ± 11	23 ± 11
		17 → 38	15 → 61	5 → 45
		n = 108	n = 108	n = 25
11–12 years		25 ± 5	44 ± 12	24 ± 9
		16 → 37	22 → 65	9 → 46
		n = 104	n = 104	n = 27
13–14 years	48 ± 36	25 ± 5	47 ± 13	23 ± 14
	8 → 76	13 → 36	18 → 82	6 → 59
	n = 3	n = 107	n = 107	n = 27
15–16 years	39 ± 38	26 ± 5	45 ± 13	28 ± 11
	12 → 66	15 → 37	11 → 67	11 → 49
	n = 2	n = 70	n = 70	n = 17
17–18 years		27	20	
		27 → 27	20 → 20	
		n = 1	n = 1	

Table A2.8

Durations (in milliseconds) in Caucasian children: lead V_2

Age-group	Q duration	S duration	R duration	R' duration
<24 h		26 ± 5	29 ± 6	8!
		19 → 46	19 → 42	8 → 8
		n = 43	n = 42	n = 1
<1 day	13	26 ± 4	29 ± 5	10
	13 → 13	19 → 32	18 → 41	10 → 10
	n = 1	n = 137	n = 136	n = 1
<2 days	6	27 ± 5	28 ± 5	13
	6 → 6	19 → 45	19 → 48	13 → 13
	n = 1	n = 116	n = 114	n = 1
<3 days	10 ± 5	27 ± 5	27 ± 10	10 ± 4
	4 → 15	18 → 42	16 → 43	7 → 13
	n = 4	n = 104	n = 104	n = 2

◻ Table A2.8   (Continued)

Age-group	Q duration	S duration	R duration	R′ duration
<1 week	10	29 ± 8	26 ± 5	10
	10 → 10	20 → 64	17 → 38	10 → 10
	n = 1	n = 114	n = 111	n = 1
<1 month	9	28 ± 6	26 ± 5	
	9 → 9	23 → 62	18 → 38	
	n = 1	n = 42	n = 41	
<3 months	8	30 ± 5	28 ± 5	
	8 → 8	22 → 46	19 → 50	
	n = 1	n = 63	n = 62	
<6 months	7 ± 1	29 ± 4	32 ± 5	
	6 → 8	22 → 42	23 → 40	
	n = 2	n = 48	n = 48	
<1 year	6	29 ± 6	35 ± 7	21 ± 8
	6 → 6	22 → 66	14 → 51	15 → 26
	n = 1	n = 73	n = 72	n = 2
1–2 years	11 ± 2	28 ± 6	39 ± 7	21 ± 16
	9 → 13	14 → 46	21 → 52	9 → 32
	n = 3	n = 106	n = 106	n = 2
3–4 years	21	27 ± 4	42 ± 8	21 ± 5
	21 → 21	19 → 39	19 → 59	14 → 30
	n = 1	n = 140	n = 140	n = 11
5–6 years	6 ± 3	26 ± 4	44 ± 7	17 ± 8
	4 → 8	18 → 36	26 → 57	5 → 29
	n = 2	n = 155	n = 155	n = 8
7–8 years		27 ± 4	45 ± 8	16 ± 6
		18 → 39	25 → 59	6 → 25
		n = 140	n = 140	n = 10
9–10 years		27 ± 4	46 ± 9	24 ± 9
		20 → 36	21 → 62	11 → 44
		n = 114	n = 114	n = 11
11–12 years	6	28 ± 6	47 ± 10	20 ± 10
	6 → 6	18 → 43	22 → 66	4 → 34
	n = 1	n = 119	n = 119	n = 10
13–14 years	43 ± 49	28 ± 6	46 ± 12	22 ± 9
	8 → 78	16 → 40	23 → 71	9 → 38
	n = 2	n = 138	n = 138	n = 29
15–16 years	9	29 ± 6	47 ± 11	23 ± 6
	9 → 9	17 → 40	28 → 69	12 → 34
	n = 1	n = 89	n = 89	n = 13
17–18 years		24	25	
		24 → 24	25 → 25	
		n = 1	n = 1	

■ Table A2.9

Durations (in milliseconds) in Caucasian children: lead V_{4R}

Age-group	Q duration	S duration	R duration	R' duration
<24 h	11 ± 5	34 ± 6	17 ± 3	
	6 → 18	22 → 50	12 → 28	
	n = 7	n = 43	n = 29	
<1 day	13 ± 3	34 ± 7	18 ± 4	30
	9 → 18	21 → 50	12 → 29	0 → 30
	n = 14	n = 136	n = 93	n = 1
<2 days	10 ± 4	35 ± 7	17 ± 4	27
	6 → 20	23 → 52	12 → 30	27 → 27
	n = 19	n = 116	n = 72	n = 1
<3 days	10 ± 3	37 ± 8	16 ± 4	34
	6 → 15	24 → 56	12 → 28	34 → 34
	n = 15	n = 102	n = 52	n = 1
<1 week	10 ± 3	38 ± 8	16 ± 4	31
	6 → 16	23 → 56	12 → 35	31 → 31
	n = 15	n = 113	n = 62	n = 1
<1 month	12 ± 3	38 ± 8	17 ± 10	21 ± 3
	8 → 16	15 → 56	6 → 59	18 → 24
	n = 5	n = 44	n = 24	n = 3
<3 months	12 ± 8	36 ± 11	19 ± 7	19 ± 6
	5 → 25	14 → 66	5 → 52	9 → 27
	n = 5	n = 65	n = 47	n = 8
<6 months	18 ± 9	34 ± 11	19 ± 8	15 ± 6
	12 → 28	18 → 53	5 → 37	7 → 26
	n = 3	n = 49	n = 44	n = 9
<1 year	11 ± 3	30 ± 10	23 ± 11	18 ± 8
	6 → 14	16 → 70	6 → 44	7 → 45
	n = 4	n = 70	n = 66	n = 20
1–2 years	14 ± 9	27 ± 9	28 ± 13	15 ± 8
	8 → 33	13 → 54	5 → 53	6 → 34
	n = 7	n = 110	n = 106	n = 26
3–4 years	15 ± 12	25 ± 7	36 ± 13	17 ± 8
	8 → 40	14 → 44	9 → 54	4 → 35
	n = 6	n = 137	n = 136	n = 24
5–6 years	24 ± 28	25 ± 7	40 ± 12	14 ± 7
	5 → 56	15 → 48	11 → 54	5 → 28
	n = 3	n = 146	n = 145	n = 18
7–8 years	11	26 ± 6	43 ± 12	17 ± 10
	11 → 11	16 → 47	10 → 58	5 → 38
	n = 1	n = 136	n = 134	n = 13
9–10 years	12 ± 9	26 ± 8	43 ± 12	16 ± 10
	5 → 25	13 → 52	14 → 63	7 → 35
	n = 4	n = 109	n = 107	n = 10

■ Table A2.9   (Continued)

Age-group	Q duration	S duration	R duration	R′ duration
11–12 years	33 ± 27	25 ± 7	46 ± 11	21 ± 11
	7 → 64	13 → 43	20 → 64	7 → 40
	n = 5	n = 102	n = 102	n = 10
13–14 years	38 ± 31	26 ± 8	45 ± 14	21 ± 12
	10 → 72	13 → 59	8 → 66	4 → 44
	n = 4	n = 109	n = 107	n = 17
15–16 years	31 ± 33	27 ± 9	45 ± 14	19 ± 9
	7 → 54	12 → 64	9 → 68	5 → 32
	n = 2	n = 73	n = 71	n = 12
17–18 years		28	17	
		28 → 28	17 → 17	
		n = 1	n = 1	

■ Table A2.10

Durations (in milliseconds) in Caucasian children: lead V_4

Age-group	Q duration	S duration	R duration	R′ duration
<24 h	9 ± 2	26 ± 4	26 ± 5	
	6 → 11	18 → 34	18 → 43	
	n = 8	n = 43	n = 42	
<1 day	9 ± 3	25 ± 5	26 ± 5	
	4 → 13	16 → 35	16 → 38	
	n = 23	n = 138	n = 137	
<2 days	9 ± 3	26 ± 5	25 ± 6	
	4 → 15	14 → 36	13 → 38	
	n = 20	n = 119	n = 119	
<3 days	9 ± 3	25 ± 6	23 ± 6	22 ± 8
	5 → 15	13 → 37	8 → 34	17 → 32
	n = 25	n = 106	n = 104	n = 3
<1 week	10 ± 4	24 ± 6	23 ± 7	19
	4 → 33	13 → 39	12 → 40	19 → 19
	n = 57	n = 116	n = 115	n = 1
<1 month	10 ± 3	23 ± 5	24 ± 8	
	4 → 16	16 → 37	15 → 67	
	n = 20	n = 45	n = 45	
<3 months	11 ± 4	25 ± 7	24 ± 5	
	6 → 21	15 → 52	15 → 38	
	n = 35	n = 67	n = 65	
<6 months	12 ± 4	27 ± 6	26 ± 6	
	5 → 16	19 → 45	16 → 40	
	n = 20	n = 50	n = 50	

◼ **Table A2.10** (Continued)

Age-group	Q duration	S duration	R duration	R′ duration
<1 year	12 ± 4	27 ± 6	27 ± 8	22
	6 → 20	15 → 43	12 → 49	22 → 22
	n = 27	n = 72	n = 71	n = 1
1–2 years	13 ± 4	28 ± 7	27 ± 8	24 ± 6
	6 → 25	11 → 41	12 → 44	19 → 32
	n = 47	n = 110	n = 108	n = 4
3–4 years	13 ± 4	33 ± 7	28 ± 9	17 ± 5
	7 → 22	21 → 47	10 → 45	14 → 25
	n = 50	n = 141	n = 134	n = 4
5–6 years	12 ± 5	35 ± 7	28 ± 9	16 ± 7
	6 → 32	24 → 49	12 → 47	8 → 27
	n = 56	n = 155	n = 152	n = 5
7–8 years	13 ± 6	36 ± 7	30 ± 9	17 ± 7
	6 → 40	23 → 49	9 → 48	12 → 30
	n = 39	n = 141	n = 140	n = 5
9–10 years	11 ± 5	38 ± 6	29 ± 10	18 ± 7
	4 → 21	27 → 51	10 → 48	10 → 34
	n = 25	n = 115	n = 111	n = 7
11–12 years	13 ± 5	40 ± 8	31 ± 10	15 ± 2
	7 → 26	28 → 63	12 → 51	13 → 16
	n = 26	n = 119	n = 115	n = 2
13–14 years	12 ± 4	42 ± 7	32 ± 9	14
	6 → 18	31 → 52	14 → 54	14 → 14
	n = 26	n = 141	n = 138	n = 1
15–16 years	13 ± 6	42 ± 6	32 ± 11	
	6 → 25	30 → 57	10 → 56	
	n = 17	n = 91	n = 90	
17–18 years		25	22	
		25 → 25	22 → 22	
		n = 1	n = 1	
<24 h	11 ± 3	20 ± 5	24 ± 6	
	4 → 16	29 → 12	16 → 42	
	n = 22	n = 43	n = 41	
<1 day	11 ± 3	20 ± 6	23 ± 5	
	5 → 17	12 → 37	14 → 37	
	n = 77	n = 137	n = 134	
<2 days	12 ± 3	21 ± 6	24 ± 6	
	7 → 20	12 → 34	13 → 36	
	n = 59	n = 118	n = 116	

■ Table A2.11

Durations (in milliseconds) in Caucasian children: lead V₅

Age-group	Q duration	S duration	R duration	R′ duration
<3 days	11 ± 3	20 ± 6	22 ± 5	57 ± 24
	5 → 15	12 → 31	13 → 32	40 → 74
	n = 59	n = 106	n = 104	n = 2
<1 week	12 ± 4	18 ± 4	23 ± 7	
	6 → 18	11 → 35	12 → 39	
	n = 96	n = 116	n = 109	
<1 month	13 ± 3	19 ± 5	22 ± 6	30 ± 23
	8 → 23	14 → 38	13 → 40	14 → 46
	n = 36	n = 44	n = 42	n = 2
<3 months	13 ± 3	21 ± 5	22 ± 6	20
	5 → 23	14 → 36	12 → 33	20 → 20
	n = 56	n = 66	n = 65	n = 1
<6 months	14 ± 4	22 ± 4	23 ± 6	23
	8 → 24	15 → 31	12 → 38	23 → 23
	n = 38	n = 48	n = 46	n = 1
<1 year	14 ± 4	23 ± 6	24 ± 7	36 ± 18
	7 → 26	13 → 44	12 → 42	23 → 48
	n = 58	n = 73	n = 67	n = 2
1–2 years	15 ± 5	25 ± 7	24 ± 8	28 ± 15
	8 → 26	9 → 46	10 → 38	9 → 50
	n = 83	n = 111	n = 100	n = 5
3–4 years	15 ± 4	29 ± 7	25 ± 9	16 ± 2
	8 → 24	21 → 53	5 → 45	13 → 17
	n = 121	n = 140	n = 120	n = 4
5–6 years	14 ± 4	30 ± 6	25 ± 8	16 ± 9
	7 → 23	23 → 54	11 → 43	9 → 35
	n = 125	n = 155	n = 142	n = 7
7–8 years	15 ± 5	31 ± 6	27 ± 8	14 ± 3
	6 → 26	23 → 45	12 → 44	12 → 18
	n = 118	n = 141	n = 134	n = 3
9–10 years	15 ± 4	33 ± 8	25 ± 10	17 ± 5
	6 → 24	22 → 64	7 → 44	13 → 32
	n = 97	n = 115	n = 106	n = 10
11–12 years	15 ± 5	36 ± 8	26 ± 10	16 ± 2
	6 → 27	25 → 63	10 → 50	14 → 18
	n = 91	n = 118	n = 106	n = 4
13–14 years	16 ± 5	37 ± 7	28 ± 9	17 ± 6
	8 → 26	27 → 52	10 → 47	12 → 29
	n = 87	n = 140	n = 135	n = 6
15–16 years	16 ± 6	39 ± 8	29 ± 12	19 ± 4
	8 → 34	28 → 64	6 → 59	15 → 22
	n = 50	n = 92	n = 86	n = 3
17–18 years	12	15	17	
	12 → 12	15 → 15	17 → 17	
	n = 1	n = 1	n = 1	

◼ Table A2.12

Durations (in milliseconds) in Caucasian children: lead V_6

Age-group	Q duration	S duration	R duration	R′ duration
<24 h	16 ± 10	18 ± 5	22 ± 8	
	8 → 60	12 → 31	12 → 45	
	n = 36	n = 40	n = 32	
<1 day	15 ± 8	18 ± 7	22 ± 6	18 ± 2
	6 → 50	7 → 39	9 → 40	0 → 19
	n = 100	n = 127	n = 104	n = 3
<2 days	14 ± 8	17 ± 6	22 ± 6	16 ± 4
	6 → 48	8 → 42	12 → 37	13 → 20
	n = 85	n = 111	n = 100	n = 3
<3 days	14 ± 8	18 ± 6	21 ± 6	21 ± 7
	6 → 48	9 → 34	10 → 32	14 → 27
	n = 81	n = 99	n = 79	n = 3
<1 week	15 ± 6	17 ± 5	21 ± 7	21 ± 4
	7 → 46	10 → 35	12 → 38	18 → 24
	n = 99	n = 110	n = 87	n = 2
<1 month	14 ± 3	18 ± 4	20 ± 6	22 ± 1
	9 → 23	10 → 27	12 → 37	21 → 22
	n = 38	n = 45	n = 40	n = 2
<3 months	14 ± 3	22 ± 5	20 ± 5	
	8 → 26	16 → 35	12 → 31	
	n = 61	n = 65	n = 53	
<6 months	15 ± 4	22 ± 4	20 ± 7	30 ± 1
	8 → 25	13 → 36	12 → 38	29 → 31
	n = 42	n = 49	n = 41	n = 2
<1 year	15 ± 4	24 ± 9	21 ± 7	24 ± 6
	7 → 23	8 → 64	10 → 38	18 → 33
	n = 59	n = 73	n = 60	n = 5
1–2 years	17 ± 5	27 ± 7	21 ± 7	30 ± 10
	7 → 27	11 → 50	11 → 34	18 → 43
	n = 91	n = 110	n = 76	n = 5
3–4 years	16 ± 4	29 ± 7	24 ± 8	29 ± 16
	8 → 25	19 → 52	12 → 44	16 → 48
	n = 131	n = 140	n = 99	n = 4
5–6 years	16 ± 4	31 ± 6	23 ± 7	13
	8 → 22	23 → 48	12 → 42	13 → 13
	n = 139	n = 154	n = 119	n = 1
7–8 years	16 ± 4	31 ± 6	24 ± 8	26 ± 16
	8 → 24	23 → 47	12 → 43	15 → 37
	n = 129	n = 140	n = 119	n = 2
9–10 years	16 ± 4	34 ± 8	23 ± 9	17 ± 1
	8 → 24	25 → 64	6 → 42	15 → 18
	n = 107	n = 115	n = 88	n = 4
11–12 years	16 ± 4	37 ± 8	25 ± 9	9 ± 2
	8 → 29	27 → 64	13 → 47	7 → 10
	n = 104	n = 117	n = 86	n = 2

☐ Table A2.12   (Continued)

Age-group	Q duration	S duration	R duration	R′ duration
13–14 years	16 ± 5	37 ± 6	25 ± 9	15 ± 5
	8 → 29	29 → 58	5 → 44	12 → 21
	n = 124	n = 140	n = 122	n = 3
15–16 years	17 ± 5	40 ± 10	28 ± 10	38
	9 → 34	27 → 76	13 → 59	38 → 38
	n = 58	n = 88	n = 72	n = 1
17–18 years	15	16		
	15 → 15	16 → 16		
	n = 1	n = 1		

☐ Table A2.13

Amplitudes (in μV) in Caucasian children: lead I

Age-group	P+	P−	Q	R	S	STj	T+	T−
<24 h	80 ± 27	−59 ± 0	−428 ± 311	208 ± 181	−742 ± 312	10 ± 18	84 ± 51	−70 ± 95
	37 → 136	−59 → −59	−903 → −36	30 → 906	−1,586 → −296	37 → −42	23 → 231	−378 → −12
	n = 43	n = 1	n = 10	n = 35	n = 35	n = 43	n = 41	n = 14
<1 day	81 ± 27	−42 ± 49	−427 ± 315	206 ± 161	−711 ± 227	18 ± 21	93 ± 50	−57 ± 38
	23 → 142	−137 → −11	−1,199 → −27	25 → 595	−1,392 → −347	−15 → 62	18 → 219	−158 → −12
	n = 138	n = 6	n = 36	n = 112	n = 110	n = 138	n = 133	n = 34
<2 days	79 ± 25	−26 ± 10	−333 ± 251	214 ± 145	−687 ± 202	22 ± 26	116 ± 57	−39 ± 25
	43 → 146	−37 → −17	−752 → −29	30 → 599	−1,171 → −335	−34 → 76	31 → 261	−95 → −12
	n = 119	n = 3	n = 34	n = 99	n = 99	n = 119	n = 119	n = 12
<3 days	82 ± 33	−22 ± 12	−303 ± 207	210 ± 141	−658 ± 239	28 ± 28	125 ± 54	−49 ± 30
	39 → 147	−41 → −8	−674 → −34	54 → 631	−1,193 → −240	−10 → 125	38 → 291	−101 → −7
	n = 106	n = 8	n = 41	n = 80	n = 79	n = 106	n = 106	n = 9
<1 week	83 ± 28	−25 ± 12	−244 ± 275	191 ± 138	−643 ± 198	37 ± 31	151 ± 58	−69 ± 49
	27 → 141	−43 → −10	−952 → −29	32 → 615	−1,185 → −351	−4 → 139	35 → 276	−138 → −22
	n = 116	n = 7	n = 38	n = 104	n = 104	n = 117	n = 117	n = 5
<1 month	89 ± 30	−37 ± 18	−141 ± 206	282 ± 199	−556 ± 197	37 ± 25	209 ± 76	−28 ± 3
	33 → 176	−48 → −16	−743 → −24	49 → 759	−1,043 → −215	−7 → 93	68 → 400	−30 → −26
	n = 45	n = 3	n = 14	n = 43	n = 43	n = 45	n = 45	n = 2
<3 months	96 ± 27		−78 ± 62	626 ± 291	−474 ± 185	28 ± 35	257 ± 89	−64 ± 47
	44 → 168		−350 → −23	56 → 1,270	−870 → −55	−98 → 101	64 → 457	−117 → −28
	n = 67		n = 34	n = 66	n = 65	n = 69	n = 66	n = 3
<6 months	102 ± 27	−23 ± 0	−107 ± 74	807 ± 230	−467 ± 206	34 ± 23	288 ± 85	
	48 → 197	−23 → −23	−336 → −22	321 → 1,307	−1,019 → −147	−12 → 85	159 → 539	
	n = 50	n = 1	n = 21	n = 50	n = 46	n = 50	n = 50	

⬛ Table A2.13   (Continued)

Age-group	P+	P–	Q	R	S	STj	T+	T–
<1 year	112 ± 31	−53 ± 24	−107 ± 71	870 ± 330	−374 ± 206	35 ± 31	310 ± 92	−47 ± 23
	41 → 188	−95 → −31	−334 → −33	339 → 1,714	−1,054 → −94	−36 → 139	89→524	−63 → −31
	n = 73	n = 5	n = 40	n = 73	n = 70	n = 74	n = 73	n = 2
1–2 years	112 ± 28	−75 ± 49	−130 ± 96	821 ± 364	−311 ± 161	25 ± 33	330 ± 120	−50 ± 0
	61 → 197	−128 → −23	−501 → −22	238 → 1,838	−695 → −71	−25 → 146	112 → 680	−50 → −50
	n = 110	n = 5	n = 69	n = 111	n = 95	n = 116	n = 111	n = 1
3–4 years	99 ± 21	−28 ± 8	−103 ± 62	684 ± 261	−278 ± 141	14 ± 19	281 ± 87	−89 ± 50
	59 → 145	−34 → −19	−280 → −28	252 → 1,248	−614 → −67	−22 → 68	130 → 463	−136→−37
	n = 141	n = 3	n = 77	n = 141	n = 109	n = 141	n = 141	n = 3
5–6 years	97 ± 20	−59 ± 26	−89 ± 55	624 ± 238	−244 ± 127	11 ± 24	276 ± 86	−62 ± 40
	58 → 141	−77 → −40	−263 → −22	185 → 1,259	−581→−64	−60 →71	123 → 433	−94→−17
	n = 154	n = 2	n = 71	n = 155	n = 136	n = 155	n = 154	n = 3
7–8 years	95 ± 21	−45 ± 42	−80 ± 61	592 ± 278	−220 ± 140	11 ± 22	279 ± 88	−86 ± 64
	60 → 140	−74 → −15	−203 → −21	187 → 1,354	−781 → −62	−36 → 74	132 → 481	−131 → −40
	n = 140	n = 2	n = 80	n = 141	n = 114	n = 141	n = 141	n = 2
9–10 years	97 ± 26	−38 ± 0	−72 ± 53	541 ± 219	−202 ± 130	14 ± 24	285 ± 98	−57 ± 9
	50 → 162	−38 → −38	−259 → −21	190 → 1,042	−668 → −41	−19 → 73	103 → 519	−66 → −48
	n = 115	n = 1	n = 49	n = 115	n = 92	n = 115	n = 115	n = 3
11–12 years	101 ± 24	−102 ± 0	−80 ± 48	649 ± 245	−233 ± 121	10 ± 28	281 ± 86	−75 ± 42
	64 → 153	−102 → −102	−241 → −23	230 → 1,250	−563 → −70	−43 → 106	135 → 518	−135 → −41
	n = 118	n = 1	n = 62	n = 119	n = 90	n = 119	n = 119	n = 4
13–14 years	99 ± 25		−78 ± 57	630 ± 274	−221 ± 121	17 ± 32	297 ± 102	−146 ± 0
	58 → 153		−378 → −23	232 → 1,390	−491 → −46	−17 → 128	106 → 557	−146 → −146
	n = 141		n = 62	n = 141	n = 113	n = 141	n = 140	n = 1
15–16 years	92 ± 22	−37 ± 0	−71 ± 54	625 ± 308	−243 ± 153	13 ± 28	275 ± 107	−124 ± 40
	48 → 149	−37 → −37	−226 → −23	169 → 1,469	−761 → −46	−47 → 81	129 → 576	−152 → −95
	n = 92	n = 1	n = 46	n = 92	n = 71	n = 92	n = 91	n = 2
17–18 years	132 ± 0		−606 ± 0			24 ± 0	158 ± 0	
	132 → 132		−606 → −606			24 → 24	158 → 158	
	n = 1		n = 1			n = 1	n = 1	

⬛ Table A2.14

Amplitudes (in μV) in Caucasian children: lead II

Age-group	P+	P–	Q	R	S	STj	T+	T–
<24 h	146 ± 50		−208 ± 143	597 ± 303	−393 ± 197	46 ± 30	149 ± 65	−117 ± 81
	65 → 276		−722 → −47	111 → 1,398	−961 → −178	−3 → 131	55 → 314	−174 → −59
	n = 43		n = 41	n = 41	n = 22	n = 43	n = 42	n = 2
<1 day	157 ± 48	−16 ± 0	−208 ± 127	618 ± 365	−433 ± 193	48 ± 32	157 ± 65	−147 ± 204
	56 → 258	−16 → −16	−526 → −34	53 → 1,389	−966 → −55	1 → 115	51 → 299	−597 → −20
	n = 138	n = 1	n = 132	n = 136	n = 71	n = 138	n = 137	n = 7
<2 days	164 ± 53	−35 ± 19	−204 ± 107	579 ± 300	−460 ± 204	51 ± 31	182 ± 70	−99 ± 66
	68 → 298	−54 → −17	−510 → −44	116 → 1,348	−905 → −165	−9 → 121	47 → 404	−175 → −60
	n = 118	n = 3	n = 106	n = 116	n = 69	n = 119	n = 118	n = 3

A2

◨ **Table A2.14   (Continued)**

Age-group	P+	P−	Q	R	S	STj	T+	T−
<3 days	163 ± 61	−36 ± 24	−210 ± 126	542 ± 303	−425 ± 229	58 ± 35	199 ± 69	−32 ± 13
	60 → 322	−77 → −19	−609 → −42	86 → 1,399	−976 → −94	−9 → 169	70 → 394	−41 → −22
	n = 105	n = 5	n = 102	n = 105	n = 56	n = 106	n = 106	n = 2
<1 week	168 ± 53	−25 ± 0	−239 ± 107	662 ± 345	−453 ± 220	65 ± 37	222 ± 72	−58 ± 0
	73 → 305	−25 → −25	−542 → −27	104 → 1,485	−975 → −89	−14 → 173	100 → 398	−58 → −58
	n = 117	n = 1	n = 115	n = 114	n = 75	n = 117	n = 117	n = 1
<1 month	159 ± 46	−23 ± 8	−199 ± 103	695 ± 312	−308 ± 160	47 ± 43	260 ± 84	−29 ± 0
	88 → 250	−29 → −17	−567 → −70	86 → 1,392	−662 → −94	−1 → 274	135 → 607	−29 → −29
	n = 45	n = 2	n = 41	n = 45	n = 28	n = 45	n = 45	n = 1
<3 months	150 ± 32		−218 ± 108	1,029 ± 407	−226 ± 76	44 ± 35	287 ± 91	
	87 → 231		−470 → −43	99 → 2,177	−405 → −111	−23 → 162	123 → 568	
	n = 67		n = 58	n = 67	n = 46	n = 69	n = 67	
<6 months	150 ± 39		−209 ± 132	1,067 ± 360	−247 ± 129	47 ± 32	293 ± 84	
	72 → 274		−492 → −34	404 → 1,830	−732 → −108	−22 → 127	126 → 560	
	n = 50		n = 40	n = 49	n = 32	n = 50	n = 50	
<1 year	159 ± 35	−96 ± 23	−178 ± 137	1,112 ± 445	−260 ± 116	55 ± 35	327 ± 102	
	81 → 241	−113 → −70	−676 → −22	468 → 2,666	−510 → −87	−19 → 164	84 → 597	
	n = 73	n = 3	n = 54	n = 73	n = 52	n = 74	n = 73	
1–2 years	146 ± 43	−39 ± 44	−169 ± 123	1,068 ± 379	−257 ± 121	28 ± 35	299 ± 112	
	50 → 240	−100 → 0	−480 → −29	349 → 1,928	−561 → −43	−20 → 161	93 → 579	
	n = 111	n = 4	n = 79	n = 111	n = 74	n = 116	n = 111	
3–4 years	149 ± 42	−29 ± 16	−140 ± 87	1,252 ± 381	−233 ± 125	13 ± 27	361 ± 127	
	73 → 241	−40 → −18	−332 → −23	475 → 2,119	−507 → −52	−41 → 66	129 → 653	
	n = 140	n = 2	n = 106	n = 141	n = 98	n = 141	n = 141	
5–6 years	136 ± 53	−27 ± 11	−126 ± 87	1,342 ± 420	−236 ± 113	16 ± 30	370 ± 108	
	36 → 277	−47 → −12	−357 → −22	637 → 2,394	−531 → −58	−35 → 92	171 → 594	
	n = 155	n = 12	n = 118	n = 155	n = 114	n = 155	n = 155	
7–8 years	137 ± 49	−35 ± 26	−119 ± 96	1,317 ± 380	−249 ± 137	15 ± 30	398 ± 118	−57 ± 0
	45 → 242	−105 → −18	−329 → −22	708 → 2,205	−620 → −54	−29 → 93	196 → 685	−57 → −57
	n = 140	n = 10	n = 94	n = 141	n = 115	n = 141	n = 141	n = 1
9–10 years	129 ± 53	−22 ± 8	−109 ± 62	1,423 ± 378	−218 ± 120	21 ± 38	401 ± 134	
	38 → 253	−38 → −13	−260 → −24	619 → 2,180	−497 → −55	−39 → 200	173 → 705	
	n = 115	n = 8	n = 86	n = 115	n = 84	n = 115	n = 115	
11–12 years	137 ± 49	−23 ± 13	−89 ± 55	1,413 ± 379	−245 ± 137	16 ± 31	391 ± 125	−62 ± 9
	37 → 232	−45 → −10	−217 → −23	759 → 2,342	−617 → −54	−60 → 122	148 → 672	−68 → −55
	n = 119	n = 6	n = 83	n = 119	n = 87	n = 119	n = 119	n = 2
13–14 years	125 ± 61	−27 ± 12	−90 ± 64	1,368 ± 408	−271 ± 152	23 ± 45	393 ± 137	−231 ± 0
	21 → 250	−60 → −14	−303 → −23	584 → 2,387	−740 → −47	−33 → 139	172 → 736	−231 → −231
	n = 139	n = 16	n = 100	n = 141	n = 111	n = 141	n = 140	n = 1
15–16 years	141 ± 59	−36 ± 23	−94 ± 65	1,290 ± 407	−278 ± 183	16 ± 41	366 ± 123	−77 ± 9
	35 → 297	−82 → −18	−394 → −27	593 → 2,089	−732 → −54	−77 → 98	144 → 631	−87 → −67
	N = 91	n = 6	n = 60	n = 92	n = 67	n = 92	n = 92	n = 4
17–18 years	270 ± 0		−284 ± 0	792 ± 0		85 ± 0	246 ± 0	
	270 → 270		−284 → −284	792 → 792		85 → 85	246 → 246	
	n = 1		n = 1	n = 1		n = 1	n = 1	

◾ Table A2.15

Amplitudes (in µV) in Caucasian children: lead III

Age-group	P+	P−	Q	R	S	STj	T+	T−
<24 h	83 ± 46	−26 ± 10	−289 ± 157	1,072 ± 443	−377 ± 244	35 ± 30	103 ± 72	−30 ± 15
	18 → 198	−41 → −6	−731 → −78	209 → 2,028	−725 → −162	−15 → 114	14 → 110	−55 → −16
	n = 41	n = 15	n = 41	n = 43	n = 4	n = 43	n = 43	n = 7
<1 day	89 ± 45	−26 ± 15	−311 ± 145	1,048 ± 419	−228 ± 95	30 ± 22	97 ± 56	−67 ± 131
	14 → 195	−64 → −12	−651 → −101	49 → 1,954	−428 → −108	−10 → 85	15 → 272	−612 → −7
	n = 135	n = 29	n = 131	n = 138	n = 32	n = 138	n = 135	n = 20
<2 days	101 ± 43	−42 ± 27	−290 ± 143	950 ± 413	−212 ± 121	28 ± 32	98 ± 51	−61 ± 43
	27 → 213	−104 → −15	−655 → −72	32 → 2,017	−497 → −74	−30 → 96	22 → 240	−174 → −14
	n = 112	n = 23	n = 110	n = 119	n = 32	n = 119	n = 109	n = 20
<3 days	98 ± 50	−39 ± 18	−271 ± 128	882 ± 374	−197 ± 107	30 ± 29	105 ± 57	−51 ± 27
	26 → 225	−86 → −16	−621 → −59	54 → 1,859	−445 → −52	−38 → 100	15-277	−108 → −13
	n = 99	n = 23	n = 101	n = 106	n = 22	n = 106	n = 97	n = 17
<1 week	102 ± 47	−28 ± 14	−304 ± 126	972 ± 412	−209 ± 105	27 ± 26	104 ± 57	−37 ± 23
	17 → 223	−69 → −5	−626 → −92	97 → 2,095	−506 → −91	−34 → 82	19-241	−102 → −10
	n = 113	n = 22	n = 115	n = 117	n = 32	n = 117	n = 112	n = 26
<1 month	86 ± 51	−29 ± 12	−263 ± 126	913 ± 375	−158 ± 69	9 ± 40	86 ± 55	−42 ± 26
	10 → 208	−44 → −13	−575 → −77	23 → 1,571	−277 → −57	−29 → 208	13 → 228	−88 → −11
	n = 44	n = 13	n = 41	n = 45	n = 11	n = 45	n = 37	n = 16
<3 months	73 ± 31	−30 ± 18	−348 ± 166	909 ± 456	−220 ± 163	15 ± 31	88 ± 64	−78 ± 51
	16 → 168	−78 → −12	−726 → −76	54 → 2,038	−704 → −77	−24 → 141	16 → 317	−210 → −16
	n = 65	n = 18	n = 59	n = 67	n = 17	n = 69	n = 57	n = 22
<6 months	64 ± 25	−24 ± 14	−372 ± 139	765 ± 450	−256 ± 203	11 ± 29	79 ± 52	−79 ± 67
	25 → 130	−67 → −10	−682 → −104	24 → 1,816	−876 → −72	−36 → 63	20 → 218	−315 → −21
	n = 50	n = 16	n = 38	n = 50	n = 20	n = 50	n = 36	n = 30
<1 year	66 ± 28	−38 ± 28	−373 ± 170	651 ± 482	−291 ± 206	19 ± 24	88 ± 58	−85 ± 45
	17 → 123	−162 → −16	−807 → −122	25 → 1,575	−824 → −60	−28 → 76	18 → 314	−230 → −29
	n = 70	n = 34	n = 47	n = 73	n = 35	n = 74	n = 57	n = 35
1–2 years	64 ± 36	−36 ± 22	−280 ± 140	563 ± 432	−289 ± 243	2 ± 19	69 ± 53	−98 ± 56
	12 → 158	−109 → −10	−751 → −61	25 → 1,739	−967 → −47	−35 → 39	13 → 262	−248 → −28
	n = 101	n = 56	n = 68	n = 110	n = 64	n = 116	n = 66	n = 77
3–4 years	76 ± 39	−34 ± 16	−232 ± 138	817 ± 524	−204 ± 147	−2 ± 22	131 ± 86	−73 ± 51
	15 → 177	−99 → −13	−648 → −27	35 → 1,893	−604 → −40	−37 → 43	14 → 352	−232 → −15
	n = 127	n = 57	n = 94	n = 140	n = 79	n = 141	n = 121	n = 46
5–6 years	74 ± 38	−41 ± 20	−191 ± 126	903 ± 550	−156 ± 112	4 ± 21	125 ± 78	−51 ± 30
	14 → 174	−91 → −13	−456 → −24	34 → 2,102	−335 → −41	−44 → 62	17 → 361	−153 → −14
	n = 126	n = 76	n = 106	n = 155	n = 84	n = 155	n = 146	n = 43
7–8 years	71 ± 37	−40 ± 23	−177 ± 118	882 ± 527	−217 ± 159	3 ± 23	140 ± 90	−45 ± 25
	16 → 169	−113 → −13	−528 → −25	28 → 1,972	−722 → −47	−33 → 96	26 → 366	−129 → −16
	n = 120	n = 72	n = 82	n = 141	n = 94	n = 141	n = 139	n = 31
9–10 years	67 ± 41	−44 ± 26	−162 ± 98	1,035 ± 518	−163 ± 110	6 ± 27	150 ± 96	−71 ± 58
	13 → 183	−132 → −9	−416 → −27	45 → 1,973	−589 → −36	−37 → 79	23 → 402	−265 → −16
	n = 92	n = 70	n = 78	n = 115	n = 70	n = 115	n = 107	n = 28
11–12 years	71 ± 35	−42 ± 20	−126 ± 78	908 ± 527	−193 ± 151	6 ± 22	142 ± 84	−62 ± 40
	14 → 149	−108 → −14	−2, 901 → −21	38 → 2,271	−808 → −28	−43 → 53	21 → 346	−163 → −13
	n = 100	n = 65	n = 75	n = 119	n = 74	n = 119	n = 111	n = 30

◧ Table A2.15 (Continued)

Age-group	P+	P−	Q	R	S	STj	T+	T−
13–14 years	71 ± 44	−51 ± 25	−111 ± 66	878 ± 511	−227 ± 158	5 ± 26	133 ± 78	−63 ± 37
	13 → 220	−114 → −18	−303 → −24	34 → 1,985	−736 → −31	−46 → 71	21 → 341	−140 → −13
	n = 105	n = 90	n = 88	n = 141	n = 93	n = 141	n = 126	n = 35
15–16 years	82 ± 53	−38 ± 21	−123 ± 81	797 ± 482	−225 ± 158	3 ± 26	121 ± 78	−56 ± 28
	14 → 219	−137 → −14	−402 → −27	31 → 1,805	−751 → −41	−55 → 54	20 → 125	−156 → −23
	n = 77	n = 53	n = 55	n = 92	n = 55	n = 92	n = 89	n = 30
17–18 years	138 ± 0		−241 ± 0	1,399 ± 0		61 ± 0	95 ± 0	
	138 → 138		−241 → −241	1,399 → 1,399		61 → 61	95 → 95	
	n = 1		n = 1	n = 1		n = 1	n = 1	

◧ Table A2.16

Amplitudes (in μV) in Caucasian children: lead aVR

Age-group	P+	P−	Q	R	S	STj	T+	T−
<24 h		−110 ± 32	−188 ± 180	273 ± 245	−228 ± 132	−28 ± 19	84 ± 87	−113 ± 49
		−181 → −60	−671 → −31	22 → 974	−533 → −64	−64 → 14	23 → 229	−231 → −46
		n = 43	n = 15	n = 42	n = 24	n = 43	n = 5	n = 42
<1 day	15 ± 2	−116 ± 32	−269 ± 155	283 ± 227	−263 ± 170	−32 ± 25	65 ± 72	−121 ± 50
	13 → 16	−181 → −46	−662 → −42	30 → 786	−778 → −46	−88 → 11	12 → 300	−237 → −42
	n = 2	n = 138	n = 46	n = 135	n = 73	n = 138	n = 18	n = 137
<2 days	9 ± 0	−118 ± 34	−286 ± 130	217 ± 197	−237 ± 141	−36 ± 24	51 ± 34	−147 ± 55
	9 → 9	−209 → −60	−571 → −42	22 → 809	−625 → −35	−96 → 11	14 → 114	−289 → −39
	n = 1	n = 119	n = 35	n = 117	n = 72	n = 119	n = 6	n = 117
<3 days	34 ± 33	−119 ± 42	−264 ± 124	218 ± 181	−248 ± 152	−43 ± 28	47 ± 22	−160 ± 51
	11 → 57	−203 → −42	−484 → −36	27 → 659	−723 → −42	−105 → 29	31 → 62	−289 → −68
	n = 2	n = 106	n = 26	n = 105	n = 67	n = 106	n = 2	n = 106
<1 week	22 ± 4	−122 ± 34	−240 ± 145	202 ± 183	−305 ± 173	−51 ± 31	59 ± 33	−183 ± 57
	19 → 24	−217 → −54	−638 → −77	29 → 892	−696 → −74	−130 → 0	36 → 97	−332 → −83
	n = 2	n = 117	n = 20	n = 116	n = 86	n = 117	n = 3	n = 117
<1 month	23 ± 10	−121 ± 29	−384 ± 121	151 ± 134	−389 ± 221	−42 ± 29	33 ± 8	−233 ± 69
	14 → 33	−193 → −62	−533 → −235	25 → 680	−1,050 → −114	−84 → 11	27 → 39	−430 → −112
	n = 3	n = 45	n = 8	n = 45	n = 36	n = 45	n = 2	n = 45
<3 months		−119 ± 24	−609 ± 260	138 ± 105	−786 ± 272	−37 ± 32		−269 ± 79
		−190 → −78	−1,017 → −74	24 → 465	−1,262 to −309	−114 → 80		−511 → −92
		n = 67	n = 13	n = 67	n = 55	n = 69		n = 67
<6 months		−122 ± 32	−792 ± 259	188 ± 152	−906 ± 190	−41 ± 24		−288 ± 70
		−233 → −56	−1,246 to −79	26 → 730	−1,264 to −615	−92 → 11		−523 → −154
		n = 50	n = 16	n = 50	n = 34	n = 50		n = 50
<1 year	62 ± 36	−132 ± 29	−852 ± 299	179 ± 153	−980 ± 303	−45 ± 31		−316 ± 86
	27 → 99	−208 → −72	−1,478 → −81	20 → 729	−2,188 to −616	−94 → 51		−454 → −117
	n = 3	n = 73	n = 25	n = 72	n = 49	n = 74		n = 73
1–2 years	89 ± 34	−125 ± 29	−711 ± 231	174 ± 119	−983 ± 270	−26 ± 32		−313 ± 106
	65 → 113	−187 → −74	−1,118 → −97	22 → 501	−1,426 to −499	−87 → 24		−646 → −126
	n = 2	n = 110	n = 33	n = 107	n = 80	n = 116		n = 111
3–4 years		−120 ± 26	−797 ± 185	122 ± 89	−948 ± 221	−13 ± 20		−319 ± 93
		−177 → −69	−1,362 → −457	23 → 392	−1,405 to −466	−55 → 28		−552 → −149
		n = 141	n = 39	n = 133	n = 102	n = 141		n = 141

Table A2.16 (Continued)

Age-group	P+	P−	Q	R	S	STj	T+	T−
5–6 years	27 ± 18	−112 ± 31	−824 ± 166	125 ± 91	−975 ± 259	−13 ± 25	38 ± 0	−321 ± 87
	15 → 58	−184 → −54	−1,288 → −553	23 → 363	−1,568 → −607	−67 → 67	38 → 38	−495 → −148
	n = 5	n = 155	n = 52	n = 148	n = 103	n = 155	n = 1	n = 155
7–8 years	86 ± 0	−113 ± 28	−842 ± 251	114 ± 96	−924 ± 241	−13 ± 23	127 ± 0	−337 ± 91
	86 → 86	−184 → −65	−1,451 → −463	21 → 384	−1,459 → −535	−70 → 27	127 → 127	−562 → −183
	n = 1	n = 140	n = 45	n = 140	n = 96	n = 141	n = 1	n = 141
9–10 years	21 ± 0	−110 ± 30	−837 ± 194	103 ± 83	−977 ± 218	−17 ± 28	35 ± 0	−341 ± 102
	21 → 21	−182 → −57	−1,240 → −521	22 → 364	−1,578 → −585	−73 → 27	35 → 35	−560 → −166
	n = 1	n = 115	n = 43	n = 108	n = 72	n = 115	n = 1	n = 115
11–12 years	67 ± 0	−115 ± 30	−908 ± 177	122 ± 107	−1,041 ± 223	−12 ± 27	58 ± 0	−334 ± 92
	67 → 67	−181 → −59	−1,290 → −610	23 → 479	−1,662 → −650	−77 → 81	58 → 58	−570 → −179
	n = 1	n = 118	n = 48	n = 112	n = 71	n = 119	n = 1	n = 119
13–14 years	14 ± 3	−107 ± 37	−826 ± 214	126 ± 107	−1,036 ± 265	−20 ± 36	182 ± 0	−343 ± 110
	11 → 18	−176 → −41	−1,414 → −465	21 → 401	−1,573 → −522	−113 → 29	182 → 182	−600 → −145
	n = 4	n = 141	n = 59	n = 135	n = 83	n = 141	n = 1	n = 140
15–16 years	17 ± 10	−111 ± 33	−805 ± 277	139 ± 129	−1,035 ± 241	−13 ± 32	84 ± 10	−317 ± 107
	9 → 31	−196 → −40	−1,675 → −352	23 → 521	−1,737 → −582	−63 → 75	77 → 91	−584 → −125
	n = 4	n = 92	n = 41	n = 82	n = 50	n = 92	n = 2	n = 92
17–18 years		−200 ± 0		166 ± 0	−108 ± 0	−54 ± 0		−199 ± 0
		−200 → −200		166 → 166	−108 → −108	−54 → −54		−199 → −199
		n = 1		n = 1	n = 1	n = 1		n = 1

Table A2.17

Amplitudes (in μV) in Caucasian children: lead aVL

Age-group	P+	P−	Q	R	S	STj	T+	T−
<24 h	34 ± 17	−29 ± 20	−295 ± 283	224 ± 160	−865 ± 322	−12 ± 19	47 ± 28	−62 ± 62
	9 → 65	−90 → −9	−681 → −47	34 → 731	−1,654 → −394	−49 → 27	11 → 119	−369 → −15
	n = 31	n = 28	n = 4	n = 41	n = 41	n = 43	n = 22	n = 34
<1 day	31 ± 18	−30 ± 26	−291 ± 286	223 ± 140	−832 ± 251	−5 ± 15	51 ± 45	−57 ± 37
	7 → 76	−96 → −7	−759 → −36	46 → 546	−1,518 → −465	−33 → 31	11 → 147	−165 → −12
	n = 104	n = 90	n = 8	n = 136	n = 134	n = 138	n = 79	n = 88
<2 days	24 ± 22	−32 ± 18	−264 ± 261	211 ± 131	−780 ± 250	−3 ± 25	57 ± 42	−40 ± 24
	0 → 92	−78 → −9	−609 → −24	42 → 582	−1,563 → −354	−49 → 112	13 → 164	−113 → −9
	n = 119	n = 81	n = 11	n = 116	n = 114	n = 119	n = 82	n = 67
<3 days	33 ± 25	−31 ± 26	−177 ± 210	191 ± 118	−718 ± 230	−1 ± 22	53 ± 42	−45 ± 31
	6 → 86	−182 → −6	−548 → −24	32 → 535	−1,318 → −308	−44 → 59	10 → 182	−159 → −6
	n = 75	n = 69	n = 12	n = 102	n = 102	n = 106	n = 78	n = 52
<1 week	29 ± 20	−31 ± 21	−158 ± 240	206 ± 111	−750 ± 248	5 ± 21	64 ± 38	−51 ± 31
	6 → 81	−101 → −5	−659 → −22	36 → 488	−1,490 → −373	−41 → 47	11 → 139	−161 → −11
	n = 82	n = 90	n = 9	n = 115	n = 115	n = 117	n = 94	n = 44

◘ Table A2.17 (Continued)

Age-group	P+	P−	Q	R	S	STj	T+	T−
<1 month	40 ± 22	−33 ± 24	−353 ± 396	225 ± 123	−703 ± 232	14 ± 25	98 ± 52	−56 ± 26
	9 → 93	−88 → −9	−912 → −26	65 → 625	−1,147 → −243	−69 → 55	12 → 233	−93 → −17
	n = 34	n = 26	n = 5	n = 42	n = 42	n = 45	n = 40	n = 8
<3 months	40 ± 22	−22 ± 14	−76 ± 65	397 ± 199	−647 ± 246	7 ± 28	125 ± 69	−54 ± 59
	10 → 123	−76 → −6	−236 → −20	58 → 988	−1,205 → −174	−110 → 59	25 → 322	−216 → −14
	n = 61	n = 38	n = 13	n = 66	n = 66	n = 69	n = 64	n = 11
<6 months	40 ± 19	−18 ± 10	−88 ± 46	480 ± 188	−598 ± 232	11 ± 19	154 ± 77	−30 ± 33
	14 → 83	−41 → −4	−163 → −25	110 → 1,092	−1,159 → −208	−21 → 61	15 → 427	−78 → −4
	n = 50	n = 24	n = 13	n = 50	n = 48	n = 50	n = 49	n = 4
<1 year	52 ± 24	−23 ± 14	−103 ± 63	522 ± 238	−474 ± 224	8 ± 21	160 ± 70	−42 ± 24
	9 → 108	−73 → −9	−245 → −28	136 → 1,199	−1,089 → −112	−32 → 57	32 → 331	−71 → −5
	n = 69	n = 33	n = 30	n = 73	n = 71	n = 74	n = 71	n = 8
1–2 years	56 ± 25	−30 ± 26	−117 ± 89	475 ± 275	−386 ± 207	11 ± 20	188 ± 90	−48 ± 17
	12 → 133	−132 → −9	−460 → −26	93 → 1,287	−1,035 → −50	−22 → 68	27 → 410	−72 → −26
	n = 106	n = 38	n = 54	n = 111	n = 98	n = 116	n = 110	n = 5
3–4 years	48 ± 20	−27 ± 17	−106 ± 84	336 ± 185	−447 ± 272	8 ± 16	121 ± 65	−53 ± 38
	13 → 84	−88 → −9	−407 → −23	66 → 756	−10−74 → −48	−21 → 41	19 → 269	−159 → −7
	n = 127	n = 64	n = 60	n = 140	n = 118	n = 141	n = 132	n = 21
5–6 years	49 ± 22	−25 ± 13	−86 ± 69	255 ± 156	−454 ± 259	3 ± 17	109 ± 60	−46 ± 31
	10 → 94	−70 → −6	−410 → −22	38 → 719	−1,114 → −59	−41 → 40	15 → 245	−136 → −10
	n = 146	n = 58	n = 58	n = 154	n = 140	n = 155	n = 145	n = 28
7–8 years	48 ± 23	−24 ± 13	−104 ± 77	248 ± 183	−440 ± 279	4 ± 17	102 ± 61	−43 ± 26
	11 → 98	−63 → −7	−483 → −23	43 → 768	−1,176 → −46	−32 → 38	14 → 240	−107 → −8
	n = 129	n = 58	n = 71	n = 140	n = 115	n = 141	n = 130	n = 34
9–10 years	53 ± 28	−26 ± 15	−130 ± 129	197 ± 131	−484 ± 260	4 ± 16	110 ± 72	−51 ± 38
	11 → 127	−72 → −8	−473 → −23	41 → 558	−1,104 → −63	−31 → 33	14 → 347	−169 → −13
	n = 105	n = 42	n = 37	n = 112	n = 99	n = 115	n = 107	n = 23
11–12 years	53 ± 23	−26 ± 17	−116 ± 97	232 ± 190	−415 ± 260	2 ± 19	109 ± 62	−52 ± 33
	13 → 104	−88 → −8	−595 → −28	38 → 867	−976 → −38	−44 → 51	20 → 262	−145 → −15
	n = 112	n = 47	n = 49	n = 117	n = 100	n = 119	n = 107	n = 18
13–14 years	60 ± 24	−29 ± 20	−110 ± 111	228 ± 196	−389 ± 235	7 ± 18	114 ± 67	−32 ± 20
	17 → 117	−96 → −9	−699 → −25	27 → 790	−945 → −43	−26 → 56	18 → 261	−81 → −7
	n = 134	n = 43	n = 55	n = 139	n = 118	n = 141	n = 136	n = 20
15–16 years	48 ± 23	−36 ± 18	−125 ± 124	231 ± 191	−373 ± 261	6 ± 19	111 ± 69	−55 ± 42
	11 → 103	−81 → −11	−537 → −21	46 → 884	−1,050 → −56	−24 → 49	8 → 281	−169 → −16
	n = 85	n = 40	n = 41	n = 88	n = 70	n = 92	n = 85	n = 18
17–18 years		−16 ± 0		113 ± 0	−1,002 ± 0	−18 ± 0	39 ± 0	
		−16 → −16		113 → 113	−1,002 → −1,002	−18 → −18	39 → 39	
			n = 1	n = 1	n = 1	n = 1	n = 1	

Table A2.18

Amplitudes (in μV) in Caucasian children: lead aVF

Age-group	P+	P−	Q	R	S	STj	T+	T−
<24 h	111 ± 48	−16 ± 9	−226 ± 114	798 ± 360	−260 ± 184	40 ± 28	120 ± 58	−34 ± 38
	221 → 21	−25 → −7	−541 → −47	82 → 1,492	−703 → −70	−1 → 117	34 → 296	−78 → −11
	n = 43	n = 4	n = 42	n = 43	n = 14	n = 43	n = 43	n = 3
<1 day	121 ± 45	−22 ± 14	−251 ± 113	811 ± 380	−309 ± 131	39 ± 26	121 ± 55	−150 ± 253
	36 → 227	−40 → −8	−428 → −74	73 → 1,725	−691 → −106	0 → 98	29 → 260	−601 → −20
	n = 138	n = 5	n = 133	n = 137	n = 44	n = 138	n = 137	n = 5
<2 days	129 ± 50	−39 ± 23	−233 ± 112	723 ± 353	−316 ± 156	40 ± 28	135 ± 58	−42 ± 53
	21 → 247	−79 → −12	−555 → −36	38 → 1,462	−657 → −90	95 → −19	31 → 293	−150 → −13
	n = 118	n = 9	n = 110	n = 119	n = 50	n = 119	n = 117	n = 6
<3 days	128 ± 54	−29 ± 17	−232 ± 106	675 ± 337	−314 ± 141	44 ± 29	142 ± 63	−14 ± 0
	37 → 268	−58 → −11	−541 → −58	27 → 1,571	−622 → −141	−15 → 134	28 → 322	−14 → −14
	n = 104	n = 9	n = 101	n = 106	n = 36	n = 106	n = 106	n = 1
<1 week	132 ± 50	−15 ± 8	−264 ± 104	783 ± 373	−316 ± 149	46 ± 28	155 ± 61	−15 ± 0
	34 → 241	−22 → −6	−517 → −71	139 → 1,801	−785 → −65	−7 → 110	53 → 312	−15 → −15
	n = 117	n = 4	n = 116	n = 117	n = 56	n = 117	n = 117	n = 1
<1 month	120 ± 47	−21 ± 2	−212 ± 104	780 ± 300	−221 ± 101	27 ± 40	160 ± 72	
	44 → 225	−22 → −19	−571 → −62	276 → 1,377	−454 → −85	−14 → 241	72 → 480	
	n = 45	n = 2	n = 43	n = 45	n = 19	n = 45	n = 45	
<3 months	109 ± 30		−255 ± 126	880 ± 427	−154 ± 74	30 ± 28	172 ± 72	−42 ± 1
	55 → 176		−579 → −52	34 → 2,049	−351 → −66	−22 → 111	67 → 358	−43 → −41
	n = 67		n = 58	n = 67	n = 28	n = 69	n = 65	n = 2
<6 months	105 ± 30	−31 ± 0	−254 ± 114	831 ± 380	−158 ± 86	29 ± 28	158 ± 74	−60 ± 2
	53 → 185	−31 → −31	−459 → −62	46 → 1,671	−421 → −59	−26 → 92	30 → 316	−61 → −58
	n = 50	n = 1	n = 40	n = 50	n = 26	n = 50	n = 50	n = 2
<1 year	108 ± 30	−45 ± 43	−235 ± 136	788 ± 474	−160 ± 76	37 ± 26	185 ± 78	−69 ± 66
	35 → 171	−136 → −16	−628 → −53	26 → 1,819	−384 → −53	−6 → 94	72 → 454	−116 → −22
	n = 73	n = 7	n = 50	n = 73	n = 40	n = 74	n = 72	n = 2
1–2 years	100 ± 38	−28 ± 15	−183 ± 122	746 ± 405	−178 ± 87	15 ± 23	146 ± 78	−33 ± 20
	32 → 177	−52 → −12	−553 → −27	24 → 1,769	−353 → −49	69 → −24	17 → 329	−77 → −16
	n = 109	n = 10	n = 73	n = 111	n = 66	n = 116	n = 110	n = 10
3–4 years	107 ± 42	−24 ± 12	−165 ± 92	998 ± 469	−182 ± 106	6 ± 23	230 ± 107	−68 ± 33
	24 → 191	−57 → −11	−413 → −30	42 → 1,955	−512 → −45	44 → −42	25 → 466	−116 → −46
	n =140	n = 11	n = 95	n = 141	n = 85	n = 141	n = 139	n = 4
5–6 years	96 ± 49	−25 ± 13	−135 ± 100	1,113 ± 466	−183 ± 89	10 ± 23	237 ± 90	−35 ± 0
	14 → 228	−56 → −8	−366 → −21	111 → 2,245	−405 → −59	−34 → 73	87 → 452	−35 → −35
	n = 152	n = 34	n = 114	n = 155	n = 99	n = 155	n = 155	n = 1
7–8 years	99 ± 44	−31 ± 21	−133 ± 96	1,093 ± 426	−219 ± 133	9 ± 25	262 ± 100	−64 ± 20
	25 → 206	−74 → −11	−409 → −23	329 → 2,033	−551 → −48	−29 → 70	104 → 509	−78 → −50
	n = 136	n = 24	n = 87	n = 141	n = 97	n = 141	n = 141	n = 2
9–10 years	92 ± 48	−26 ± 15	−128 ± 76	1,237 ± 410	−189 ± 99	13 ± 30	263 ± 114	−52 ± 32
	15 → 216	−63 → −8	−304 → −29	414 → 2,072	−516 → −42	−41 → 137	43 → 539	−83 → −20
	n = 109	n = 25	n = 79	n = 115	n = 74	n = 115	n = 115	n = 3

Table A2.18 (Continued)

Age-group	P+	P–	Q	R	S	STj	T+	T–
11–12 years	98 ± 42	–24 ± 15	–97 ± 58	1,161 ± 428	–202 ± 111	11 ± 23	254 ± 107	–47 ± 28
	20 → 185	–68 → –5	–233 → –273	404 → 2,170	–477 → –52	–39 → 66	45 → 494	–91 → –17
	n = 115	*n* = 22	*n* = 76	*n* = 119	*n* = 77	*n* = 119	*n* = 119	*n* = 5
13–14 years	94 ± 51	–32 ± 18	–93 ± 62	1,117 ± 433	–249 ± 137	14 ± 33	250 ± 106	–54 ± 48
	13 → 211	–94 → –12	–287 → –24	309 → 2,144	–683 → –57	–35 → 89	77 → 484	–138 → –23
	n = 125	*n* = 47	*n* = 94	*n* = 141	*n* = 96	*n* = 141	*n* = 140	*n* = 5
15–16 years	104 ± 57	–26 ± 22	–98 ± 67	1,020 ± 434	–228 ± 157	9 ± 32	237 ± 90	–53 ± 21
	21 → 259	–105 → –10	–295 → –21	201 → 1,861	–605 → –275	–69 → 74	96 → 417	–80 → –15
	n = 89	*n* = 20	*n* = 57	*n* = 92	*n* = 63	*n* = 92	*n* = 91	*n* = 7
17–18 years	204 ± 0		–263 ± 0	1,095 ± 0		73 ± 0	171 ± 0	
	204 → 204		–263 → –263	1,095 → 1,095		73 → 73	171 → 171	
	n = 1		*n* = 1	*n* = 1		*n* = 1	*n* = 1	

Table A2.19
Amplitudes (in μV) in Caucasian children: lead V_1

Age-group	P+	P–	Q	R	S	STj	T+	T–
<24 h	93 ± 44	–40 ± 14		1,248 ± 547	–764 ± 458	–18 ± 31	175 ± 120	–121 ± 68
	28 → 186	–74 → –19		481 → 2,291	–1, 780 → –141	–75 → 47	15 → 590	–254 → –39
	n = 40	*n* = 25		*n* = 43	*n* = 40	*n* = 43	*n* = 33	*n* = 22
<1 day	90 ± 52	–39 ± 16	–36 ± 7	1,169 ± 487	–786 ± 503	–24 ± 37	148 ± 102	–111 ± 57
	13 → 201	–83 → –13	–41 → –31	329 → 2,370	–2, 176 → –74	–112 → 53	31 → 432	–281 → –24
	n = 132	*n* = 65	*n* = 2	*n* = 137	*n* = 124	*n* = 137	*n* = 12	*n* = 99
<2 days	83 ± 50	–49 ± 24	–69 ± 59	1,102 ± 524	–603 ± 379	–28 ± 40	124 ± 83	–145 ± 78
	25 → 244	–133 → –15	–110 → –27	404 → 2,592	–1, 530 → –137	–110 → 64	18 → 320	–355 → –34
	n = 106	*n* = 58	*n* = 2	*n* = 117	*n* = 100	*n* = 117	*n* = 76	*n* = 102
<3 days	85 ± 43	–44 ± 26	–87 ± 70	1,102 ± 536	–615 ± 385	–37 ± 69	98 ± 52	–182 ± 104
	18 → 199	–121 → –15	–136 → –37	363 → 2,832	–1, 718 → –145	–136 → 62	35 → 261	–621 → –47
	n = 97	*n* = 40	*n* = 2	*n* = 102	*n* = 93	*n* = 102	*n* = 57	*n* = 97
<1 week	86 ± 49	–44 ± 31		1,085 ± 445	–494 ± 326	–47 ± 42	102 ± 67	–211 ± 79
	17 → 249	–229 → –18		2,078 → 354	–1, 530 → –103	–137 → 15	25 → 332	–428 → –70
	n = 109	*n* = 51		*n* = 114	*n* = 99	*n* = 114	*n* = 28	*n* = 110
<1 month	83 ± 49	–40 ± 20	–28 ± 0	873 ± 391	–463 ± 346	–32 ± 42	102 ± 68	–192 ± 102
	29 → 237	–81 → –10	–28 → –28	425 → 2,303	–1, 529 → –102	–105 → 53	30 → 224	–467 → –58
	n = 38	*n* = 16	*n* = 1	*n* = 41	*n* = 37	*n* = 41	*n* = 16	*n* = 38
<3 months	65 ± 34	–45 ± 21	–134 ± 117	772 ± 345	–496 ± 337	–20 ± 60	102 ± 75	–251 ± 143
	17 → 144	–98 → –14	–217 → –51	194 → 1,656	–1, 735 → –120	–137 → 336	38 → 314	–465 → 0
	n = 52	*n* = 40	*n* = 2	*n* = 63	*n* = 56	*n* = 65	*n* = 12	*n* = 65
<6 months	59 ± 28	–45 ± 28		829 ± 413	–511 ± 358	–19 ± 45	80 ± 46	–319 ± 99
	16 → 131	–127 → –18		298 → 2,222	–1, 660 → –96	–92 → 192	40 → 156	–493 → –139
	n = 41	*n* = 32		*n* = 49	*n* = 48	*n* = 49	*n* = 5	*n* = 48
<1 year	68 ± 29	–53 ± 35		779 ± 420	–538 ± 330	–22 ± 27	160 ± 83	–343 ± 97
	21 → 142	–194 → –15		47 → 2,037	–1, 562 → –95	–74 → 106	77 → 243	–577 → –204
	n = 59	*n* = 43		*n* = 70	*n* = 69	*n* = 71	*n* = 3	*n* = 69

⬤ Table A2.19   (Continued)

Age-group	P+	P−	Q	R	S	STj	T+	T−
1–2 years	91 ± 33	−57 ± 36	−114 ± 59	807 ± 382	−771 ± 385	−3 ± 31	126 ± 64	−317 ± 105
	26 → 152	−204 → −21	−155 → −72	99 → 1,804	−1,701 → −183	−86 → 65	46 → 224	−578 → −139
	n = 100	n = 46	n = 2	n = 107	n = 103	n = 112	n = 7	n = 105
3–4 years	95 ± 36	−56 ± 32	−526 ± 0	610 ± 244	−895 ± 394	13 ± 30	85 ± 37	−270 ± 92
	30 → 168	−153 → −16	−526 → −526	106 → 1,112	−1,893 → −205	−45 → 91	43 → 163	−467 → −88
	n = 129	n = 57	n = 1	n = 135	n = 135	n = 136	n = 25	n = 136
5–6 years	98 ± 35	−55 ± 25	−342 ± 409	509 ± 232	−1,008 ± 398	22 ± 28	77 ± 31	−249 ± 96
	33 → 182	−132 → −24	−631 → −53	84 → 1,020	−2,011 → −395	−28 → 88	40 → 155	−448 → −51
	n = 141	n = 62	n = 2	n = 146	n = 146	n = 147	n = 37	n = 145
7–8 years	88 ± 35	−54 ± 30		483 ± 283	−969 ± 426	25 ± 26	78 ± 37	−251 ± 98
	28 → 166	−180 → −17		142 → 1,388	−1,921 → −264	−37 → 78	38 → 185	−431 → −76
	n = 133	n = 69		n = 135	n = 135	n = 135	n = 34	n = 129
9–10 years	76 ± 32	−49 ± 25		403 ± 191	−1,090 ± 462	31 ± 31	111 ± 98	−218 ± 99
	21 → 150	−115 → −15		131-919	−2,213 → −214	−25 → 145	32 → 468	−436 → −43
	n = 104	n = 73		n = 108	n = 108	n = 108	n = 35	n = 102
11–12 years	75 ± 31	−57 ± 37		383 ± 225	−1,130 ± 451	30 ± 33	129 ± 121	−206 ± 99
	22 → 148	−228 → −16		66 → 1,090	−2,366 → −363	−33 → 109	34 → 573	−488 → −35
	n = 97	n = 70		n = 104	n = 104	n = 104	n = 39	n = 87
13–14 years	70 ± 30	−58 ± 32	−788 ± 692	329 ± 196	−1,097 ± 418	33 ± 36	91 ± 65	−176 ± 92
	25 → 136	−151 → −18	−1,364 → −20	52 → 912	−2,265 → −366	−26 → 164	31 → 342	−450 → −32
	n = 99	n = 81	n = 3	n = 107	n = 107	n = 109	n = 44	n = 96
15–16 years	72 ± 34	−54 ± 25	−115 ± 99	348 ± 211	−1,194 ± 529	38 ± 36	79 ± 114	−156 ± 93
	22 → 232	−110 → −19	−185 → −45	71 → 1,186	−2,303 → −98	−43 → 140	492 → 0	−420 → −37
	n = 65	n = 50	n = 2	n = 70	n = 70	n = 71	n = 71	n = 48
17–18 years	56 ± 0	−26 ± 0		1,028 ± 0	−466 ± 0	−17 ± 0		−139 ± 0
	56 → 56	−26 → −26		1,028 → 1,028	−466 → −466	−17 → −17		−139 → −139
	n = 1	n = 1		n = 1	n = 1	n = 1		n = 1

⬤ Table A2.20
Amplitudes (in μV) in Caucasian children: lead V_2

Age-group	P+	P−	Q	R	S	STj	T+	T−
<24 h	123 ± 55	−19 ± 8		1,642 ± 621	−1,758 ± 690	−17 ± 38	198 ± 151	−113 ± 57
	15 → 238	−33 → −13		709 → 3,673	−2,967 → −618	−77 → 77	21 → 487	−226 → −35
	n = 43	n = 5		n = 43	n = 42	n = 43	n = 35	n = 19
<1 day	114 ± 52	−51 ± 71	−36 ± 0	1,402 ± 500	−1,534 ± 674	−35 ± 48	169 ± 98	−133 ± 88
	36 → 229	−342 → −12	−36 → −36	494 → 2,393	−2,927 → −405	−119 → 70	25 → 417	−352 → −25
	n = 133	n = 21	n = 1	n = 137	n = 136	n = 137	n = 103	n = 91
<2 days	103 ± 47	−33 ± 17	−60 ± 0	1,402 ± 536	−1,346 ± 609	−27 ± 44	133 ± 91	−138 ± 75
	28 → 230	−65 → −8	−60 → −60	484 → 2,536	−2,887 → −414	−111 → 77	21 → 407	−313 → −28
	n = 116	n = 22	n = 1	n = 116	n = 114	n = 116	n = 84	n = 93
<3 days	111 ± 39	−33 ± 25	−83 ± 65	1,343 ± 504	−1,278 ± 556	−29 ± 72	125 ± 79	−179 ± 114
	32 → 192	−77 → −9	−166 → −21	501 → 2,689	−2,895 → −300	−161 → 76	26 → 376	−595 → −34
	n = 102	n = 9	n = 4	n = 104	n = 104	n = 104	n = 56	n = 89

■ **Table A2.20** (Continued)

Age-group	P+	P−	Q	R	S	STj	T+	T−
<1 week	110 ± 53	-57 ± 55	-60 ± 0	$1,332 \pm 480$	$-1,130 \pm 499$	-35 ± 63	116 ± 75	-210 ± 128
	$17 \rightarrow 248$	$-219 \rightarrow -21$	$-60 \rightarrow -60$	$583 \rightarrow 2,542$	$-2,070 \rightarrow -238$	$-172 \rightarrow 86$	$16 \rightarrow 326$	$-574 \rightarrow -37$
	$n = 112$	$n = 16$	$n = 1$	$n = 114$	$n = 111$	$n = 114$	$n = 43$	$n = 102$
<1 month	108 ± 54	-36 ± 31	-52 ± 0	$1,159 \pm 519$	$-1,000 \pm 494$	0 ± 63	118 ± 78	-145 ± 110
	$22 \rightarrow 235$	$-87 \rightarrow -10$	$-52 \rightarrow -52$	$380 \rightarrow 3,156$	$-2,431 \rightarrow -276$	$-99 \rightarrow 92$	$33 \rightarrow 302$	$-500 \rightarrow -20$
	$n = 42$	$n = 6$	$n = 1$	$n = 42$	$n = 41$	$n = 42$	$n = 32$	$n = 24$
<3 months	102 ± 40	-49 ± 27	-56 ± 0	$1,406 \pm 411$	-972 ± 433	11 ± 61	144 ± 94	-209 ± 134
	$33 \rightarrow 224$	$-96 \rightarrow -20$	$-56 \rightarrow -56$	$566 \rightarrow 2,292$	$-2,306 \rightarrow -307$	$-87 \rightarrow 343$	$42 \rightarrow 474$	$-554 \rightarrow -50$
	$n = 63$	$n = 6$	$n = 1$	$n = 63$	$n = 62$	$n = 65$	$n = 35$	$n = 47$
<6 months	96 ± 43	-32 ± 14	-33 ± 11	$1,449 \pm 464$	$-1,015 \pm 489$	0 ± 44	121 ± 91	-269 ± 142
	$19 \rightarrow 184$	$-56 \rightarrow -5$	$-41 \rightarrow -25$	$750 \rightarrow 2,829$	$-2,142 \rightarrow -344$	$-86 \rightarrow 101$	$24 \rightarrow 397$	$-638 \rightarrow -48$
	$n = 48$	$n = 10$	$n = 2$	$n = 48$	$n = 48$	$n = 48$	$n = 18$	$n = 42$
<1 year	104 ± 42	-44 ± 25	-134 ± 0	$1,520 \pm 463$	$-1,083 \pm 466$	1 ± 38	99 ± 40	-271 ± 132
	$23 \rightarrow 251$	$-82 \rightarrow -15$	$-134 \rightarrow -134$	$736 \rightarrow 3,269$	$-2,650 \rightarrow -378$	$-74 \rightarrow 155$	$28 \rightarrow 187$	$-671 \rightarrow -58$
	$n = 73$	$n = 12$	$n = 1$	$n = 73$	$n = 72$	$n = 74$	$n = 24$	$n = 71$
1–2 years	114 ± 37	-77 ± 63	-70 ± 24	$1,473 \pm 593$	$-1,478 \pm 688$	11 ± 46	134 ± 70	-307 ± 160
	$31 \rightarrow 193$	$-200 \rightarrow -14$	$-84 \rightarrow -43$	$275 \rightarrow 2,720$	$-2,722 \rightarrow -185$	$-108 \rightarrow 124$	$51 \rightarrow 380$	$-695 \rightarrow -36$
	$n = 101$	$n = 13$	$n = 3$	$n = 106$	$n = 106$	$n = 111$	$n = 46$	$n = 89$
3–4 years	110 ± 36	-48 ± 20	-362 ± 0	$1,285 \pm 442$	$-1,703 \pm 613$	38 ± 39	156 ± 83	-222 ± 112
	$187 \rightarrow 44$	$-95 \rightarrow -21$	$-362 \rightarrow -362$	$434 \rightarrow 2,200$	$-3,188 \rightarrow -572$	$-50 \rightarrow 142$	$43 \rightarrow 396$	$-486 \rightarrow -50$
	$n = 140$	$n = 11$	$n = 1$	$n = 140$	$n = 140$	$n = 140$	$n = 107$	$n = 96$
5–6 years	110 ± 32	-34 ± 9	-28 ± 10	$1,090 \pm 385$	$-1,819 \pm 639$	54 ± 46	184 ± 119	-154 ± 85
	$60 \rightarrow 214$	$-48 \rightarrow -25$	$-35 \rightarrow -21$	$399 \rightarrow 2,004$	$-3,161 \rightarrow -647$	$-28 \rightarrow 175$	$46 \rightarrow 478$	$-339 \rightarrow -38$
	$n = 155$	$n = 8$	$n = 2$	$n = 155$	$n = 155$	$n = 155$	$n = 133$	$n = 85$
7–8 years	106 ± 36	-29 ± 16		$1,030 \pm 444$	$-1,822 \pm 638$	58 ± 41	198 ± 128	-141 ± 93
	$45 \rightarrow 208$	$-57 \rightarrow -15$		$353 \rightarrow 2,050$	$-3,224 \rightarrow -713$	$-23 \rightarrow 184$	$47 \rightarrow 547$	$-540 \rightarrow -34$
	$n = 140$	$n = 13$		$n = 140$	$n = 140$	$n = 140$	$n = 131$	$n = 58$
9–10 years	102 ± 34	-25 ± 13		870 ± 344	$-1,891 \pm 624$	67 ± 46	280 ± 179	-129 ± 72
	$41 \rightarrow 211$	$-45 \rightarrow -13$		$314 \rightarrow 1,707$	$-3,635 \rightarrow -744$	$-18 \rightarrow 198$	$52 \rightarrow 865$	$-259 \rightarrow -27$
	$n = 113$	$n = 9$		$n = 114$	$n = 114$	$n = 114$	$n = 105$	$n = 32$
11–12 years	94 ± 33	-44 ± 26	-21 ± 0	718 ± 295	$-1,704 \pm 590$	69 ± 51	285 ± 184	-108 ± 61
	$36 \rightarrow 177$	$-109 \rightarrow -18$	$-21 \rightarrow -21$	$208 \rightarrow 1,465$	$-3,335 \rightarrow -644$	$-19 \rightarrow 212$	$50 \rightarrow 809$	$-237 \rightarrow -32$
	$n = 118$	$n = 18$	$n = 1$	$n = 119$	$n = 119$	$n = 119$	$n = 117$	$n = 23$
13–14 years	83 ± 34	-42 ± 27	$-1,079 \pm 1,484$	650 ± 336	$-1,562 \pm 611$	66 ± 47	281 ± 186	-84 ± 54
	$26 \rightarrow 160$	$-125 \rightarrow -12$	$-2,128 \rightarrow -30$	$170 \rightarrow 1,493$	$-2,910 \rightarrow -387$	$-10 \rightarrow 194$	$43 \rightarrow 781$	$-244 \rightarrow -21$
	$n = 134$	$n = 32$	$n = 2$	$n = 138$	$n = 138$	$n = 139$	$n = 134$	$n = 20$
15–16 years	84 ± 29	-38 ± 17	-26 ± 0	632 ± 356	$-1,603 \pm 584$	78 ± 59	367 ± 238	-117 ± 68
	$34 \rightarrow 152$	$-69 \rightarrow -10$	$-26 \rightarrow -26$	$183 \rightarrow 2,034$	$-2,888 \rightarrow -645$	6-242	$69 \rightarrow 1,125$	$-228 \rightarrow -49$
	$n = 86$	$n = 21$	$n = 1$	$n = 89$	$n = 89$	$n = 89$	$n = 87$	$n = 5$
17–18 years	113 ± 0			$1,481 \pm 0$	$-1,599 \pm 0$	-43 ± 0	75 ± 0	-131 ± 0
	$113 \rightarrow 113$			$1,481 \rightarrow 1,481$	$-1,599 \rightarrow -1,599$	$-43 \rightarrow -43$	75-7-5	$-131 \rightarrow -131$
	$n = 1$			$n = 1$	$n = 1$	$n = 1$	$n = 1$	$n = 1$

◘ Table A2.21

Amplitudes (in μV) in Caucasian children: lead V$_{4R}$

Age-group	P+	P−	Q	R	S	STj	T+	T−
<24 h	75 ± 42	−40 ± 14	−64 ± 76	989 ± 365	−344 ± 169	−6 ± 27	116 ± 87	−82 ± 53
	17 → 178	−69 → −20	−225 → −22	307 → 1,747	−749 → −156	−55 → 74	17 → 440	−244 → −7
	n = 39	n = 24	n = 7	n = 43	n = 29	n = 43	n = 34	n = 23
<1 day	86 ± 43	−36 ± 20	−72 ± 31	992 ± 339	−359 ± 263	−13 ± 24	107 ± 71	−85 ± 49
	11 → 200	−142 → −13	−121 → −22	373 → 1,653	−1, 273 → −93	−66 → 36	22 → 292	−228 → −17
	n = 123	n = 69	n = 14	n = 136	n = 93	n = 136	n = 99	n = 103
<2 days	80 ± 39	−37 ± 22	−55 ± 34	980 ± 338	−298 ± 181	−15 ± 28	81 ± 52	−109 ± 65
	19 → 189	−149 → −12	−143 → −20	288 → 1,993	−804 → −36	−65 → 61	17 → 291	−285 → −24
	n = 110	n = 57	n = 19	n = 116	n = 72	n = 116	n = 70	n = 98
<3 days	74 ± 39	−35 ± 17	−39 ± 18	924 ± 321	−262 ± 161	−23 ± 48	67 ± 36	−129 ± 69
	16 → 166	−102 → −13	−73 → −20	405 → 1,713	−658 → −67	−84 → 30	25 → 199	−322 → −32
	n = 97	n = 47	n = 15	n = 102	n = 52	n = 102	n = 43	n = 99
<1 week	88 ± 44	−40 ± 30	−47 ± 22	962 ± 345	−299 ± 214	−34 ± 40	80 ± 59	−165 ± 62
	19 → 235	−169 → −12	−113 → −23	415 → 1,747	−1, 508 → −68	−170 → 29	26 → 328	−295 → −57
	n = 107	n = 34	n = 15	n = 113	n = 62	n = 113	n = 34	n = 109
<1 month	77 ± 44	−38 ± 22	−56 ± 57	758 ± 335	−242 ± 232	−28 ± 32	86 ± 43	−152 ± 71
	12 → 161	−110 → −9	−155 → −20	95 → 1,629	−1, 106 → −52	−91 → 82	13 → 167	−342 → −51
	n = 41	n = 20	n = 5	n = 44	n = 24	n = 44	n = 14	n = 42
<3 months	60 ± 26	−37 ± 25	−89 ± 91	551 ± 243	−241 ± 126	−26 ± 31	60 ± 46	−225 ± 88
	16 → 121	−105 → −11	−238 → −23	102 → 1,257	−553 → −65	−80 → 34	13 → 128	−464 → −51
	n = 60	n = 40	n = 5	n = 65	n = 47	n = 67	n = 7	n = 62
<6 months	53 ± 26	−35 ± 21	−232 ± 255	514 ± 237	−257 ± 210	−18 ± 26	56 ± 0	−236 ± 77
	15 → 144	−104 → −8	−526 → −76	110 → 1,189	−1, 088 → −54	−57 → 31	56 → 56	−466 → −110
	n = 46	n = 25	n = 3	n = 49	n = 44	n = 49	n = 1	n = 49
<1 year	58 ± 21	−35 ± 19	−38 ± 8	426 ± 221	−247 ± 148	−14 ± 28	61 ± 24	−234 ± 75
	22 → 123	−104 → −13	−47 → −29	95 → 1,248	−896 → −44	−79 → 116	48 → 97	−474 → −99
	n = 65	n = 38	n = 4	n = 70	n = 66	n = 71	n = 4	n = 69
1–2 years	63 ± 25	−36 ± 35	−92 ± 110	348 ± 173	−302 ± 201	−4 ± 37	83 ± 79	−192 ± 78
	16 → 131	−220 → −12	−341 → −35	89 → 835	−1, 026 → −42	−84 → 104	14 → 285	−407 → −52
	n = 102	n = 46	n = 7	n = 110	n = 106	n = 115	n = 10	n = 108
3–4 years	73 ± 31	−27 ± 12	−82 ± 68	349 ± 171	−419 ± 229	3 ± 24	46 ± 20	−175 ± 81
	22 → 135	−59 → −12	−202 → −29	77 → 745	−991 → −95	−40 → 62	18 → 100	−352 → −37
	n = 135	n = 41	n = 6	n = 137	n = 136	n = 137	n = 43	n = 136
5–6 years	68 ± 30	−28 ± 14	−117 ± 131	295 ± 140	−477 ± 236	10 ± 18	57 ± 60	−166 ± 75
	15 → 131	−75 → −10	−267 → −27	81 → 624	−1, 046 → −104	−24 → 45	26 → 419	−332 → 0
	n = 142	n = 65	n = 3	n = 146	n = 145	n = 147	n = 41	n = 147
7–8 years	66 ± 29	−28 ± 13	−70 ± 0	287 ± 151	−488 ± 249	11 ± 18	51 ± 29	−171 ± 74
	12 → 123	−63 → −10	−70 → −70	75 → 648	−1, 109 → −100	−36 → 49	20 → 164	−318 → −35
	n = 129	n = 63	n = 1	n = 136	n = 134	n = 136	n = 42	n = 128

◘ **Table A2.21   (Continued)**

Age-group	P+	P–	Q	R	S	STj	T+	T–
9–10 years	59 ± 29	−31 ± 16	−27 ± 7	245 ± 122	−536 ± 304	13 ± 21	59 ± 39	−160 ± 75
	16 → 142	−115 → −12	−37 → −21	46 → 579	−1,679 → −109	−42 → 63	26 → 204	−348 → −26
	n = 101	n = 67	n = 4	n = 109	n = 107	n = 109	n = 35	n = 104
11–12 years	59 ± 24	−32 ± 15	−270 ± 387	222 ± 131	−539 ± 287	9 ± 24	50 ± 26	−146 ± 80
	17 → 110	−93 → −11	−934 → −20	40 → 631	−1,277 → −144	−57 → 47	21 → 172	−362 → −33
	n = 95	n = 71	n = 5	n = 102	n = 102	n = 104	n = 44	n = 95
13–14 years	46 ± 27	−34 ± 15	−282 ± 278	190 ± 115	−486 ± 274	13 ± 17	41 ± 22	−113 ± 63
	10 → 102	−76 → −12	−569 → −20	43 → 575	−1,460 → −36	−26 → 51	13 → 94	−318 → −18
	n = 95	n = 90	n = 4	n = 109	n = 107	n = 111	n = 45	n = 103
15–16 years	51 ± 25	−29 ± 14	−166 ± 206	184 ± 135	−482 ± 320	13 ± 24	59 ± 49	−104 ± 66
	13 → 109	−76 → −11	−311 → −20	25 → 914	−1,209 → −31	−36 → 83	15 → 219	−298 → −16
	n = 66	n = 46	n = 2	n = 73	n = 71	n = 74	n = 38	n = 55
17–18 years	24 ± 0	−48 ± 0		655 ± 0	−249 ± 0	−16 ± 0		−132 ± 0
	24 → 24	−48 → −48		655 → 655	−249 → −249	−16 → −16		−132 → −132
	n = 1	n = 1		n = 1	n = 1	n = 1		n = 1

◘ **Table A2.22**

Amplitudes (in μV) in Caucasian children: lead V$_4$

Age-group	P+	P–	Q	R	S	STj	T+	T–
<24 h	139 ± 43	−78 ± 86	−83 ± 39	1,554 ± 484	−1,573 ± 562	10 ± 51	187 ± 128	−92 ± 40
	66 → 250	−177 → −24	−156 → −32	700 → 2,427	−3,213 → −592	−65 → 141	42 → 177	−175 → −51
	n = 42	n = 3	n = 8	n = 43	n = 42	n = 43	n = 38	n = 11
<1 day	141 ± 58	−104 ± 108	−72 ± 50	1,578 ± 483	−1,565 ± 560	7 ± 53	178 ± 135	−134 ± 93
	57 → 279	−313 → −24	−233 → −20	2,513 → 536	−2,834 → −530	−110 → 125	24 → 776	−446 → −24
	n = 138	n = 6	n = 23	n = 138	n = 137	n = 138	n = 113	n = 56
<2 days	134 ± 40	−62 ± 66	−107 ± 83	1,567 ± 510	−1,439 ± 524	14 ± 52	144 ± 111	−115 ± 78
	62 → 236	−160 → −18	−367 → −30	540 → 3,072	−2,608 → −424	−132 → 117	15 → 429	−350 → −250
	n = 119	n = 4	n = 20	n = 119	n = 119	n = 119	n = 89	n = 57
<3 days	144 ± 39	−39 ± 11	−91 ± 67	1,545 ± 534	−1,254 ± 539	25 ± 69	139 ± 99	−166 ± 113
	69 → 229	−47 → −31	−218 → −20	67 → 2,847	−2,502 → −132	−110 → 152	15 → 440	−580 → −43
	n = 106	n = 2	n = 25	n = 106	n = 104	n = 106	n = 75	n = 57
<1 week	143 ± 44	−71 ± 75	−116 ± 98	1,645 ± 542	−1,173 ± 489	36 ± 63	178 ± 97	−187 ± 121
	56 → 251	−157 → −19	−481 → −20	695 → 3,126	−2,392 → −261	−98 → 180	39 → 402	−644 → −54
	n = 116	n = 3	n = 57	n = 116	n = 115	n = 116	n = 79	n = 56
<1 month	142 ± 43	−72 ± 0	−140 ± 97	1,497 ± 463	−954 ± 369	32 ± 57	259 ± 127	−193 ± 129
	55 → 239	−72 → −72	−373 → −23	732 → 2,757	−2,350 → −317	−76 → 157	41 → 561	−442 → −25
	n = 45	n = 1	n = 20	n = 45	n = 45	n = 45	n = 38	n = 11
<3 months	113 ± 37	−26 ± 8	−156 ± 123	1,983 ± 489	−863 ± 355	44 ± 61	273 ± 155	−162 ± 187
	48 → 208	−35 → −16	−540 → −26	1,094 → 3,084	−1,649 → −150	−36 → 373	21 → 735	−647 → −40
	n = 67	n = 4	n = 35	n = 67	n = 65	n = 69	n = 63	n = 9
<6 months	104 ± 43	−29 ± 10	−185 ± 152	1,741 ± 549	−795 ± 331	48 ± 37	257 ± 180	−132 ± 65
	49 → 276	−38 → −18	−428 → −20	877 → 3,202	−1,659 → −307	−11 → 162	58 → 910	−233 → −39
	n = 50	n = 3	n = 20	n = 50	n = 50	n = 50	n = 46	n = 11

⬛ Table A2.22 (Continued)

Age-group	P+	P−	Q	R	S	STj	T+	T−
<1 year	109 ± 40	−31 ± 19	−190 ± 184	1,792 ± 675	−794 ± 410	44 ± 48	270 ± 148	−223 ± 162
	49 → 257	−52 → −16	−777 → −25	541 → 3,768	−2,462 → −222	−42 → 263	52 → 663	−713 → −63
	n = 72	n = 3	n = 27	n = 72	n = 71	n = 73	n = 63	n = 16
1–2 years	86 ± 27	−37 ± 28	−179 ± 129	1,668 ± 668	−741 ± 414	36 ± 33	282 ± 187	−147 ± 94
	25 → 155	−89 → −15	−549 → −25	50 → 3,095	−1,995 → −165	−23 → 114	24 → 719	−348 → −27
	n = 109	n = 10	n = 47	n = 110	n = 108	n = 115	n = 98	n = 32
3–4 years	87 ± 27	−17 ± 5	−143 ± 113	2,125 ± 724	−861 ± 482	34 ± 33	433 ± 259	−113 ± 122
	41 → 150	−26 → −11	−523 → −22	886 → 3,760	−2,083 → −145	−39 → 105	49 → 993	−443 → −31
	n = 141	n = 12	n = 50	n = 141	n = 134	n = 141	n = 140	n = 10
5–6 years	86 ± 25	−23 ± 12	−134 ± 118	2,263 ± 828	−963 ± 532	44 ± 41	523 ± 223	−206 ± 52
	43 → 154	−49 → −12	−613 → −21	929 → 4,305	−2,694 → −200	−20 → 153	138 → 987	−261 → −158
	n = 155	n = 17	n = 56	n = 155	n = 152	n = 155	n = 153	n =3
7–8 years	84 ± 28	−25 ± 12	−110 ± 93	2,063 ± 793	−1,037 ± 566	44 ± 42	571 ± 246	−129 ± 0
	47 → 159	−51 → −14	−459 → −24	911 → 3,804	−2,307 → −114	−36 → 122	150 → 1,232	−129 → −129
	n = 141	n = 13	n = 39	n = 141	n = 140	n = 141	n = 141	n = 1
9–10 years	82 ± 24	−22 ± 6	−100 ± 80	1,955 ± 771	−972 ± 510	56 ± 51	652 ± 264	
	44 → 151	−37 → −14	−312 → −22	878 → 4,040	−2,359 → −136	−19 → 198	168 → 1,328	
	n = 115	n = 12	n = 25	n = 115	n = 111	n = 115	n = 115	
11–12 years	87 ± 25	−25 ± 22	−102 ± 82	1,864 ± 686	−891 ± 495	45 ± 51	589 ± 251	
	43 → 145	−86 → −10	−292 → −22	713 → 3,400	−2,475 → −149	−47 → 200	203 → 1,292	
	n = 118	n = 10	n = 26	n = 119	n = 115	n = 119	n = 119	
13–14 years	79 ± 28	−23 ± 12	−55 ± 32	1,632 ± 624	−1,045 ± 547	68 ± 64	602 ± 251	−48 ± 0
	27 → 137	−47 → −7	−174 → −24	607 → 3,010	−2,342 → −206	−21 → 253	168 → 1,176	−48 → −48
	n = 140	n = 22	n = 26	n = 141	n = 138	n = 141	n = 141	n = 1
15–16 years	83 ± 27	−19 ± 7	−85 ± 97	1,638 ± 735	−898 ± 554	60 ± 67	587 ± 289	−109 ± 58
	31 → 144	−38 → −10	−381 → −20	582 → 3,787	−2,332 → −168	−38 → 229	188 → 1,314	−150 → −68
	n = 91	n = 11	n = 17	n = 91	n = 90	n = 91	n = 91	n = 2
17–18 years	199 ± 0			1,687 ± 0	−2,201 ± 0	72 ± 0	143 ± 0	
	199 → 199			1,687 → 1,687	−2,201 → −2,201	72 → 72	143 → 143	
	n = 1			n = 1	n = 1	n = 1	n = 1	

⬛ Table A2.23

Amplitudes (in µV) in Caucasian children: lead V₅

Age-group	P+	P−	Q	R	S	STj	T+	T−
<24 h	110 ± 40	−99 ± 109	−132 ± 102	924 ± 419	−893 ± 427	29 ± 41	161 ± 104	−55 ± 32
	45 → 218	−176 → −22	−381 → −22	292 → 1,890	−1,848 → −148	−53 → 157	18 → 440	−98 → −11
	n = 42	n = 2	n = 22	n = 43	n = 41	n = 43	n = 43	n = 8
<1 day	112 ± 51	−60 ± 32	−104 ± 64	999 ± 434	−964 ± 470	29 ± 34	154 ± 88	−66 ± 39
	55 → 213	−102 → −13	−278 → −23	296 → 1,886	−1,958 → −206	−37 → 106	29 → 385	−151 → −20
	n = 135	n = 7	n = 77	n = 137	n = 134	n = 137	n = 131	n = 33
<2 days	105 ± 33	−24 ± 10	−127 ± 100	941 ± 419	−924 ± 451	33 ± 38	173 ± 90	−64 ± 49
	43 → 205	−40 → −10	−543 → −27	221 → 1,840	−2,171 → −210	−65 → 117	27 → 458	−204 → −11
	n = 116	n = 6	n = 59	n = 118	n = 116	n = 118	n = 110	n = 20

◻ **Table A2.23** (Continued)

Age-group	P+	P–	Q	R	S	STj	T+	T–
<3 days	115 ± 35	−34 ± 24	−124 ± 69	1,002 ± 427	−876 ± 477	52 ± 40	192 ± 91	−106 ± 65
	55 → 186	−51 → −17	−256 → −24	291 → 2,255	−2,343 → −225	−30 → 138	51 → 436	−278 → −22
	n = 106	n = 2	n = 59	n = 106	n = 104	n = 106	n = 97	n = 18
<1 week	114 ± 36	−26 ± 15	−172 ± 101	1,090 ± 473	−794 ± 385	59 ± 50	243 ± 114	−170 ± 167
	38 → 191	−40 → −11	−466 → −28	273 → 2,412	−1,685 → −154	−60 → 205	42 → 519	−510 → −18
	n = 116	n = 3	n = 96	n = 116	n = 109	n = 117	n = 109	n = 13
<1 month	119 ± 44	−45 ± 2	−184 ± 114	1,163 ± 538	−647 ± 375	42 ± 46	310 ± 150	−34 ± 16
	58 → 298	−46 → −43	−478 → −43	324 → 2,690	−1,767 → −112	−32 → 172	90 → 696	−45 → −22
	n = 43	n = 2	n = 36	n = 44	n = 42	n = 44	n = 43	n = 2
<3 months	101 ± 33	−24 ± 10	−228 ± 159	1,849 ± 630	−578 ± 272	47 ± 43	358 ± 130	−93 ± 0
	39 → 220	−38 → −17	−959 → −32	913 → 3,271	−1,367 → −177	−25 → 202	86 → 648	−93 → −93
	n = 66	n = 4	n = 56	n = 66	n = 65	n = 68	n = 66	n = 1
<6 months	96 ± 51	−31 ± 30	−195 ± 117	1,569 ± 563	−536 ± 329	60 ± 51	357 ± 202	−130 ± 0
	31 → 277	−75 → −9	−496 → −35	572 → 3,111	−1,368 → −157	−11 → 203	107 → 928	−130 → −130
	n = 48	n = 4	n = 38	n = 48	n = 46	n = 48	n = 47	n = 1
<1 year	94 ± 36	−29 ± 13	−218 ± 159	1,758 ± 667	−481 ± 272	53 ± 42	364 ± 148	−72 ± 18
	34 → 293	−52 → −18	−891 → −38	59 → 3,238	−1,277 → −95	−5 → 317	35 → 748	−88 → −45
	n = 73	n = 5	n = 58	n = 73	n = 67	n = 74	n = 73	n = 4
1–2 years	84 ± 48	−34 ± 27	−224 ± 155	1,569 ± 690	−379 ± 234	30 ± 48	333 ± 160	−109 ± 47
	29 → 391	−103 → −13	−626 → −35	35 → 3,080	−999 → −65	−25 → 120	63 → 724	−172 → −35
	n = 109	n = 13	n = 83	n = 111	n = 100	n = 116	n = 107	n = 6
3–4 years	78 ± 21	−18 ± 11	−189 ± 126	2,003 ± 661	−388 ± 234	15 ± 26	465 ± 204	−37 ± 26
	35 → 116	−45 → −6	−596 → −26	803 → 3,381	−1,047 → −56	−38 → 71	62 → 877	−76 → −21
	n = 140	n = 10	n = 121	n = 140	n = 120	n = 140	n = 140	n = 4
5–6 years	78 ± 22	−22 ± 16	−185 ± 130	2,443 ± 684	−493 ± 294	20 ± 33	578 ± 196	
	36 → 120	−85 → −12	−534 → −20	1,227 → 3,889	−1,475 → −105	−60 → 98	235 → 1,065	
	n = 155	n = 18	n = 125	n = 155	n = 142	n = 155	n = 155	
7–8 years	76 ± 21	−39 ± 62	−160 ± 114	2,392 ± 640	−488 ± 276	14 ± 32	627 ± 196	
	41 → 134	−267 → −11	−481 → −21	1,302 → 4,029	−1,159 → −109	−48 → 87	262 → 1,131	
	n = 139	n = 16	n = 118	n = 141	n = 134	n = 141	n = 141	
9–10 years	74 ± 21	−17 ± 4	−154 ± 108	2,373 ± 606	−424 ± 278	22 ± 34	676 ± 226	
	39 → 136	−23 → −12	−411 → −23	1,209 → 3,918	−1,200 → −86	−34 → 110	219 → 1,146	
	n = 115	n = 11	n = 97	n = 115	n = 106	n = 115	n = 115	
11–12 years	81 ± 23	−26 ± 29	−123 ± 91	2,317 ± 686	−430 ± 264	16 ± 41	604 ± 255	−110 ± 0
	43 → 153	−90 → −10	−346 → −20	933 → 3,796	−1,169 → −77	−58 → 152	200 → 1,286	−110 → −110
	n = 117	n = 7	n = 91	n = 118	n = 106	n = 118	n = 118	n = 1
13–14 years	74 ± 27	−19 ± 9	−123 ± 108	2,272 ± 795	−519 ± 309	29 ± 46	598 ± 240	−51 ± 0
	18 → 130	−43 → −5	−441 → −25	973 → 4,521	−1,213 → −126	−46 → 153	208 → 1,192	−51 → −51
	n = 138	n = 24	n = 87	n = 140	n = 135	n = 140	n = 139	n = 1
15–16 years	79 ± 24	−16 ± 4	−117 ± 94	1,901 ± 738	−508 ± 394	25 ± 39	515 ± 237	−101 ± 25
	35 → 150	−21 → −10	−383 → −23	665 → 3,687	−1,691 → −70	−23 → 105	186 → 1,089	−129 → −81
	n = 92	n = 8	n = 50	n = 92	n = 86	n = 92	n = 92	n = 3
17–18 years	146 ± 0		−125 ± 0	969 ± 0	−426 ± 0	69 ± 0	241 ± 0	
	146 → 146		−125 → −125	969 → 969	−426 → −426	69 → 69	241 → 241	
	n = 1		n = 1	n = 1	n = 1	n = 1	n = 1	

◻ Table A2.24

Amplitudes (in μV) in Caucasian children: lead V_6

Age-group	P+	P–	Q	R	S	STj	T+	T–
<24 h	83 ± 30	−97 ± 91	−140 ± 92	521 ± 258	−372 ± 198	26 ± 37	162 ± 124	−40 ± 23
	42 → 166	−199 → −24	−412 → −26	83 → 1,118	−867 → −139	−29 → 200	36 → 604	−88 → −21
	n = 41	n = 3	n = 36	n = 40	n = 32	n = 42	n = 42	n = 8
<1 day	83 ± 31	−41 ± 28	−133 ± 84	563 ± 389	−467 ± 353	22 ± 28	131 ± 69	−54 ± 36
	29 → 136	−76 → −10	−328 → −22	67 → 1,705	−1,708 → −55	−32 → 81	28 → 323	−137 → −10
	n = 127	n = 11	n = 100	n = 127	n = 104	n = 132	n = 128	n = 16
<2 days	82 ± 30	−39 ± 29	−116 ± 83	488 ± 314	−438 ± 324	32 ± 42	159 ± 81	−75 ± 38
	38 → 161	−85 → −2	−380 → −22	38 → 1,328	−1,326 → −100	−24 → 130	37 → 464	−134 → −21
	n = 110	n = 7	n = 85	n = 111	n = 100	n = 115	n = 107	n = 10
<3 days	92 ± 34	−13 ± 4	−122 ± 82	545 ± 345	−493 ± 361	44 ± 38	173 ± 76	−83 ± 37
	30 → 177	−17 → −8	−377 → −24	68 → 1,562	−1,558 → −60	−21 → 171	51 → 391	−129 → −20
	n = 101	n = 4	n = 81	n = 99	n = 79	n = 103	n = 100	n = 9
<1 week	86 ± 33	−30 ± 22	−163 ± 99	574 ± 368	−407 ± 244	53 ± 65	203 ± 105	−55 ± 44
	29 → 177	−73 → −3	−388 → −27	69 → 1,814	−998 → −66	−38 → 301	25 → 493	−148 → −6
	n = 109	n = 8	n = 99	n = 110	n = 87	n = 112	n = 109	n = 9
<1 month	100 ± 39	−42 ± 33	−183 ± 93	743 ± 456	−339 ± 230	41 ± 50	267 ± 122	−7 ± 0
	40 → 225	−93 → −23	−346 → −49	43 → 1,867	−1,023 → −68	−12 → 237	90 → 666	−7 → −7
	n = 45	n = 4	n = 38	n = 45	n = 40	n = 45	n = 45	n = 1
<3 months	96 ± 30	−30 ± 21	−223 ± 127	1,359 ± 581	−361 ± 223	39 ± 36	330 ± 106	
	52 → 219	−55 → −17	−738 → −31	538 → 2,976	−1,087 → −60	−25 → 133	126 → 603	
	n = 64	n = 3	n = 61	n = 65	n = 53	n = 67	n = 65	
<6 months	88 ± 37	−33 ± 26	−200 ± 110	1,193 ± 472	−326 ± 212	52 ± 35	326 ± 143	−167 ± 0
	39 → 277	−73 → −11	−479 → −35	142 → 2,321	−820 → −64	−7 → 178	140 → 843	−167 → −167
	n = 48	n = 5	n = 42	n = 49	n = 41	n = 49	n = 48	n = 1
<1 year	91 ± 53	−31 ± 21	−223 ± 135	1,230 ± 561	−274 ± 223	51 ± 54	349 ± 113	−183 ± 0
	34 → 411	−57 → −6	−740 → −26	30 → 2,539	−1,600 → −42	−20 → 334	159 → 651	−183 → −183
	n = 72	n = 8	n = 59	n = 73	n = 60	n = 74	n = 72	n = 1
1–2 years	75 ± 29	−30 ± 22	−216 ± 134	1,196 ± 547	−227 ± 151	23 ± 30	282 ± 119	−55 ± 24
	28 → 146	−65 → −6	−539 → −23	54 → 2,324	−701 → −56	−25 → 120	54 → 550	−83 → −24
	n = 109	n = 9	n = 91	n = 110	n = 76	n = 115	n = 109	n = 4
3–4 years	74 ± 20	−28 ± 36	−179 ± 109	1,428 ± 511	−211 ± 109	7 ± 22	367 ± 135	−99 ± 104
	36 → 113	−135 → −6	−530 → −28	435 → 2,320	−442 → −66	−41 → 45	100 → 642	−255 → −37
	n = 138	n = 12	n = 131	n = 140	n = 99	n = 140	n = 137	n = 4
5–6 years	72 ± 21	−19 ± 8	−181 ± 112	1,747 ± 477	−240 ± 149	11 ± 29	434 ± 148	−63 ± 13
	26 → 115	−37 → −11	−511 → −25	803 → 2,974	−650 → −56	−51 → 85	168 → 801	−72 → −54
	n = 154	n = 10	n = 139	n = 154	n = 119	n = 154	n = 154	n = 2
7–8 years	72 ± 20	−27 ± 15	−162 ± 98	1,797 ± 538	−239 ± 153	9 ± 31	487 ± 150	
	40 → 120	−60 → −11	−417 → −35	968 → 3,137	−799 → −51	−51 → 110	234 → 908	
	n = 139	n = 13	n = 129	n = 140	n = 119	n = 140	n = 140	
9–10 years	70 ± 20	−14 ± 4	−153 ± 92	1,851 ± 453	−221 ± 140	13 ± 30	519 ± 173	
	30 → 125	−21 → −9	−404 → −28	1,030 → 3,135	−642 → −53	−37 → 136	193 → 946	
	n = 115	n = 12	n = 107	n = 115	n = 88	n = 115	n = 115	
11–12 years	76 ± 21	−22 ± 18	−130 ± 79	1,836 ± 478	−239 ± 134	7 ± 29	463 ± 173	
	42 → 121	−65 → −8	−306 → −23	907 → 3,022	−573 → −76	−55 → 121	892 → 163	
	n = 116	n = 9	n = 104	n = 117	n = 86	n = 117	n = 117	

Table A2.24   (Continued)

Age-group	P+	P–	Q	R	S	STj	T+	T–
13–14 years	70 ± 26	–21 ± 12	–117 ± 92	1,762 ± 515	–244 ± 139	15 ± 40	450 ± 177	–89 ± 49
	20 → 127	–45 → –6	–391 → –23	874 → 3,107	–384 → –36	–65 → 151	204 → 983	–124 → –54
	n = 136	n = 17	n = 124	n = 140	n = 122	n = 140	n = 139	n = 2
15–16 years	75 ± 23	–14 ± 6	–118 ± 74	1,574 ± 498	–267 ± 206	11 ± 29	395 ± 170	–127 ± 66
	28 → 144	–96 → –11	–377 → –26	656 → 2,691	–1,075 → –62	–34 → 64	135 → 806	–226 → –89
	n = 87	n = 6	n = 58	n = 88	n = 72	n = 88	n = 87	n = 4
17–18 years	136 ± 0		–177 ± 0	595 ± 0		44 ± 0	153 ± 0	
	136 → 136		–177 → → 177	595 → 595		44 → 44	153 → 153	
	n = 1		n = 1	n = 1		n = 1	n = 1	

A2.2   Percentile Charts

The following percentile charts showing normal 12-lead ECG limits were obtained from a study of 2,141 white children between birth and 16 years. Data were derived from computer-assisted methods where the sampling rate was 333 samples per second so that there may be some underestimation of upper limits of normal. The charts are reproduced from: Davignon A *et al*. Normal ECG standards for infants and children. *Pediatr. Cardiol.* 1979/1980; **1**: 133–52 with the permission of Springer, New York. Note that V$_3$R was included while V$_3$ was omitted in this study (❷ Figs. A2.1–A2.39).

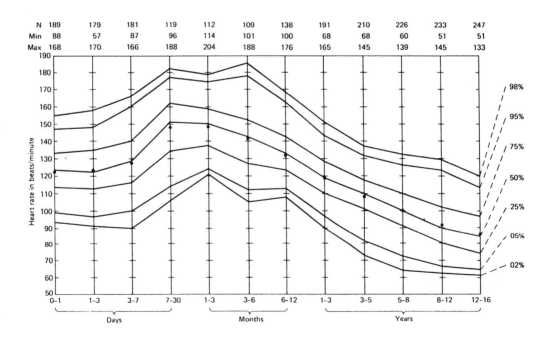

Fig. A2.1
Heart rate versus age (•, mean)

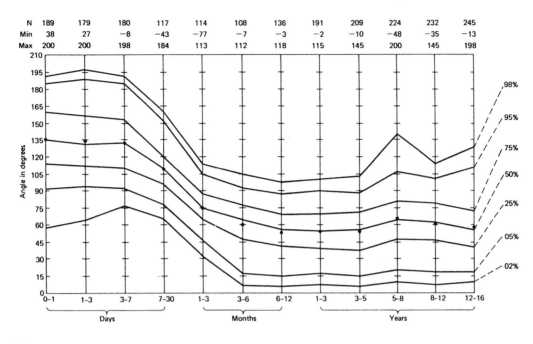

□ Fig. A2.2
Frontal plane QRS angle versus age (•, mean)

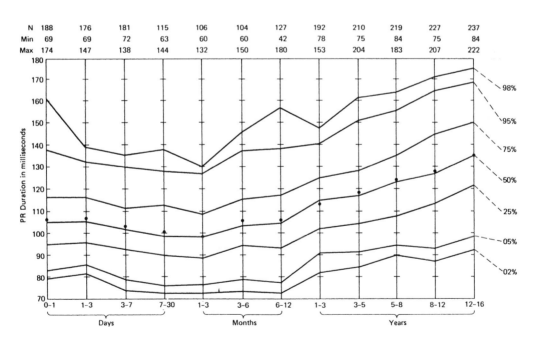

□ Fig. A2.3
PR duration in lead II versus age (•, mean)

N	179	179	112	130	145	158	126	145	129	181	102	107	161	222
Min	81	69	75	72	80	72	81	69	45	51	51	60	54	57
Max	207	201	171	183	222	180	183	192	183	171	153	144	144	138

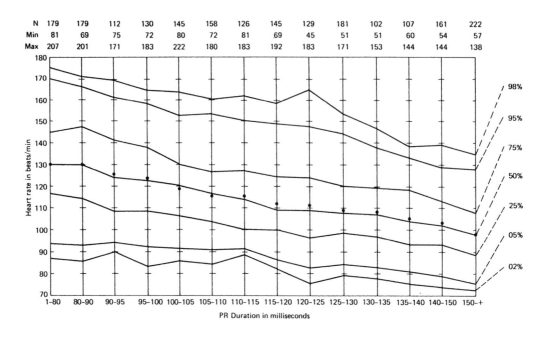

Fig. A2.4

Heart rate versus PR duration in lead II (•, mean)

N	187	176	180	117	115	108	135	192	210	223	229	244
Min	18	30	27	36	33	27	30	33	39	42	39	27
Max	78	69	72	84	84	81	81	78	78	90	87	99

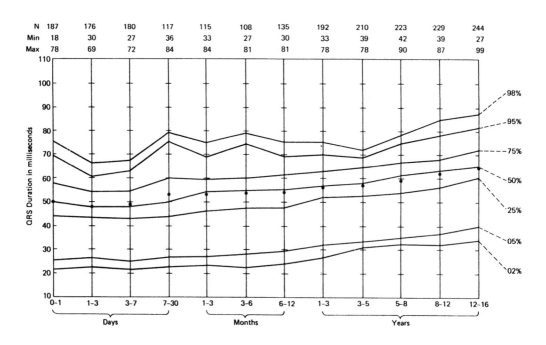

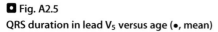

Fig. A2.5

QRS duration in lead V_5 versus age (•, mean)

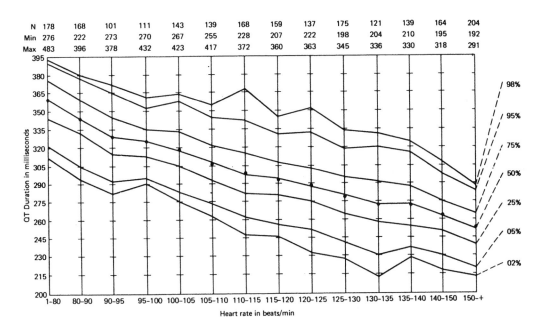

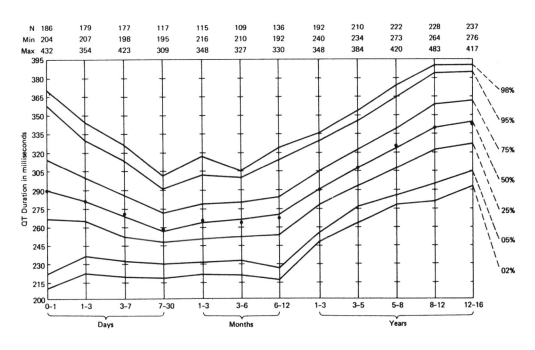

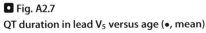

Fig. A2.6

QT duration in lead V₅ versus heart rate (•, mean)

Fig. A2.7

QT duration in lead V₅ versus age (•, mean)

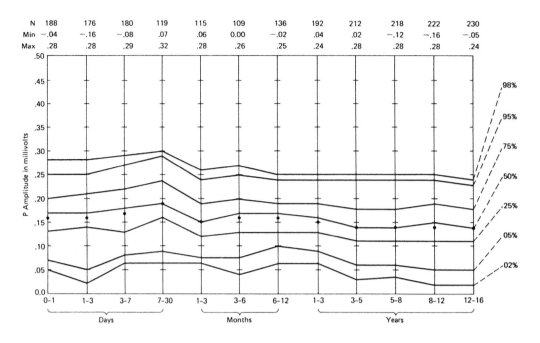

■ Fig. A2.8
P amplitude in lead II versus age (•, mean)

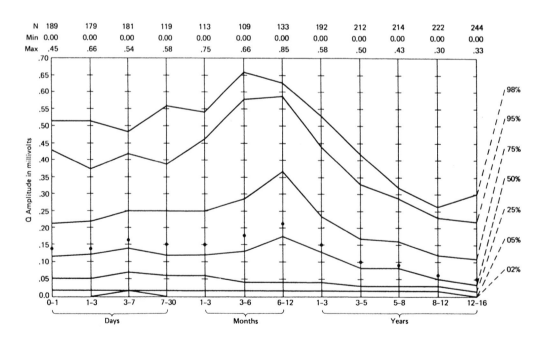

■ Fig. A2.9
Q amplitude in lead III versus age (•, mean)

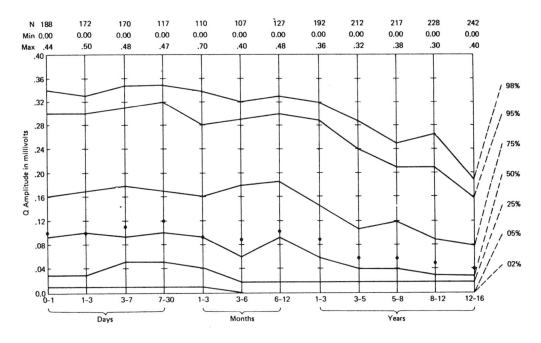

Fig. A2.10
Q amplitude in lead a VF versus age (•, mean)

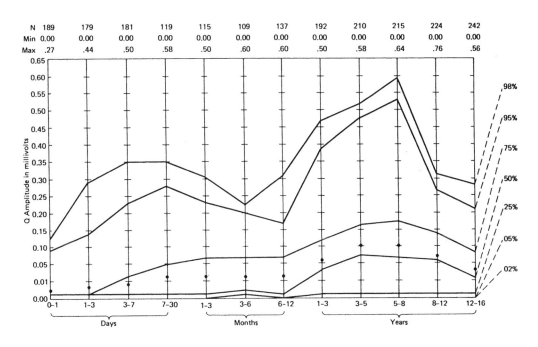

Fig. A2.11
Q amplitude in lead V₅ versus age (•, mean)

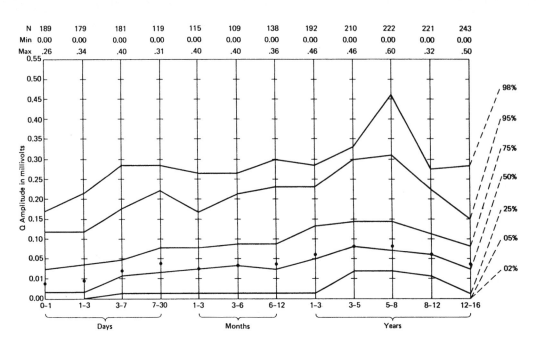

Fig. A2.12

Q amplitude in lead V$_6$ versus age (•, mean)

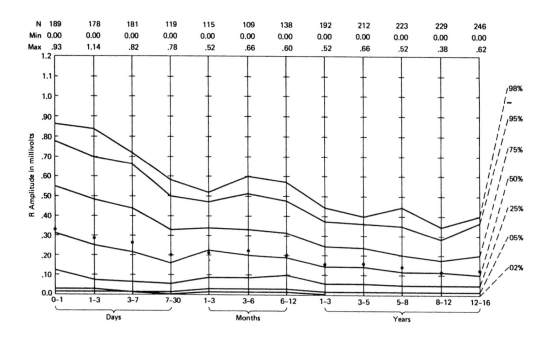

Fig. A2.13

R amplitude in lead aVR versus age (•, mean)

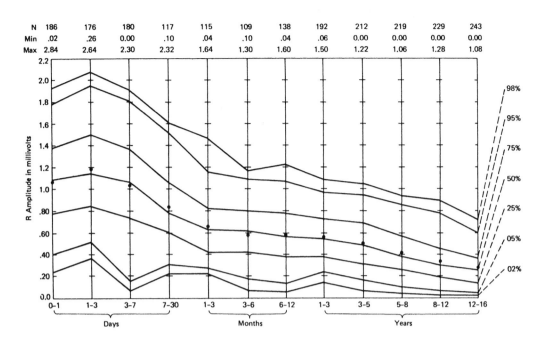

N	186	176	180	117	115	109	138	192	212	219	229	243
Min	.02	.26	0.00	.10	.04	.10	.04	.06	0.00	0.00	0.00	0.00
Max	2.84	2.64	2.30	2.32	1.64	1.30	1.60	1.50	1.22	1.06	1.28	1.08

Fig. A2.14

R amplitude in lead V_3R versus age (•, mean)

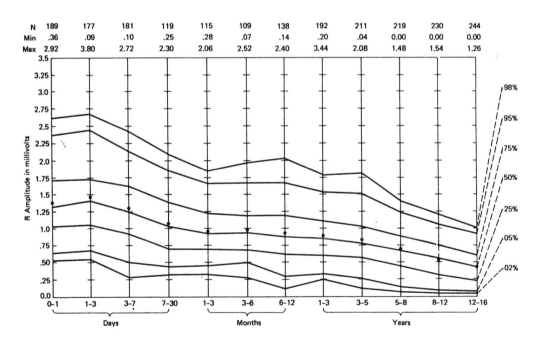

N	189	177	181	119	115	109	138	192	211	219	230	244
Min	.36	.09	.10	.25	.28	.07	.14	.20	.04	0.00	0.00	0.00
Max	2.92	3.80	2.72	2.30	2.06	2.52	2.40	3.44	2.08	1.48	1.54	1.26

Fig. A2.15

R amplitude in lead V_1 versus age (•, mean)

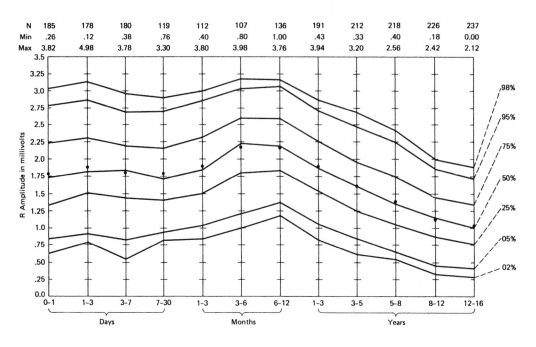

Fig. A2.16

R amplitude in lead V₂ versus age (•, mean)

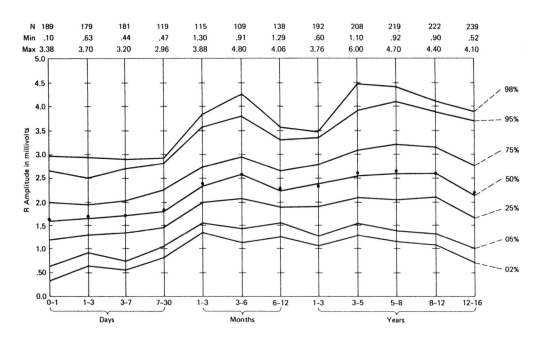

Fig. A2.17

R amplitude in lead V₄ versus age (•, mean)

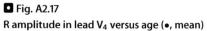

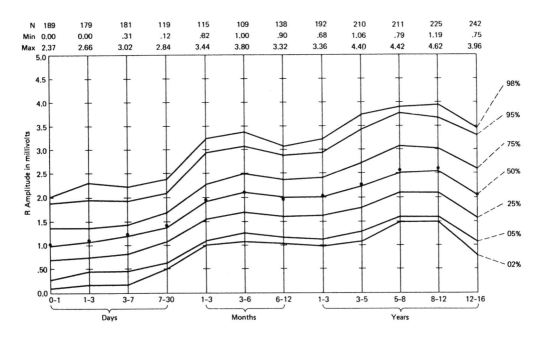

N	189	179	181	119	115	109	138	192	210	211	225	242
Min	0.00	0.00	.31	.12	.82	1.00	.90	.68	1.06	.79	1.19	.75
Max	2.37	2.66	3.02	2.84	3.44	3.80	3.32	3.36	4.40	4.42	4.62	3.96

◨ Fig. A2.18
R amplitude in lead V$_5$ versus age (•, mean)

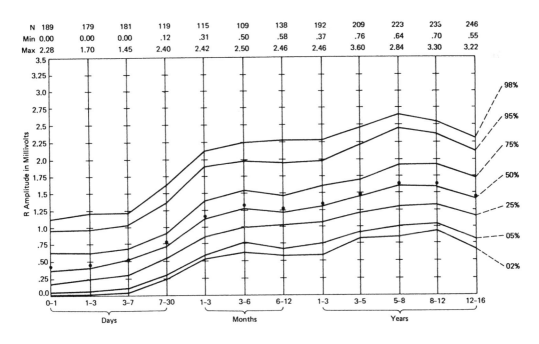

N	189	179	181	119	115	109	138	192	209	223	235	246
Min	0.00	0.00	0.00	.12	.31	.50	.58	.37	.76	.64	.70	.55
Max	2.28	1.70	1.45	2.40	2.42	2.50	2.46	2.46	3.60	2.84	3.30	3.22

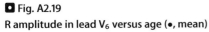

◨ Fig. A2.19
R amplitude in lead V$_6$ versus age (•, mean)

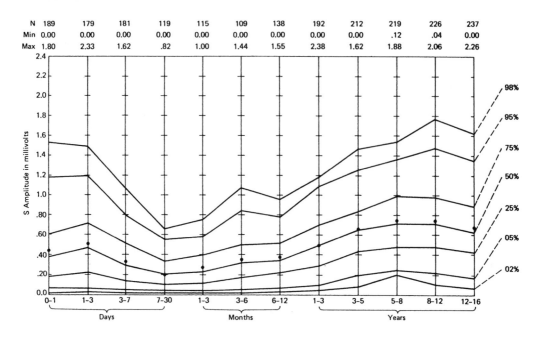

Fig. A2.20

S amplitude in lead V₃R versus age (•, mean)

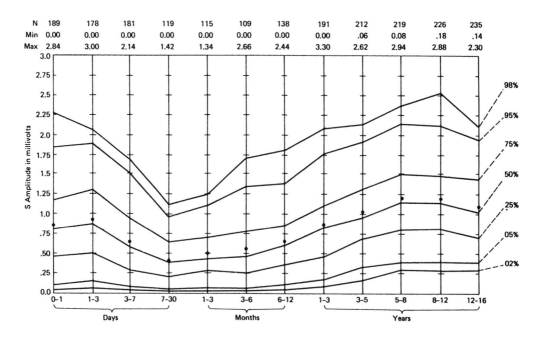

Fig. A2.21

S amplitude in lead V₁ versus age (•, mean)

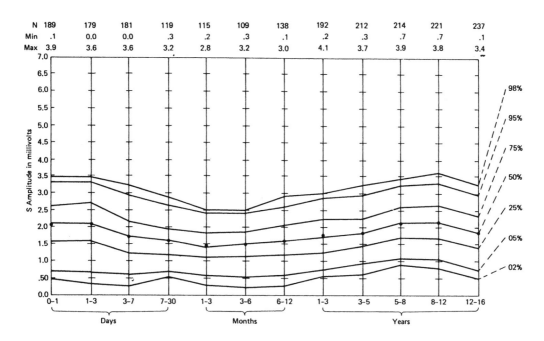

Fig. A2.22
S amplitude in lead V_2 versus age (•, mean)

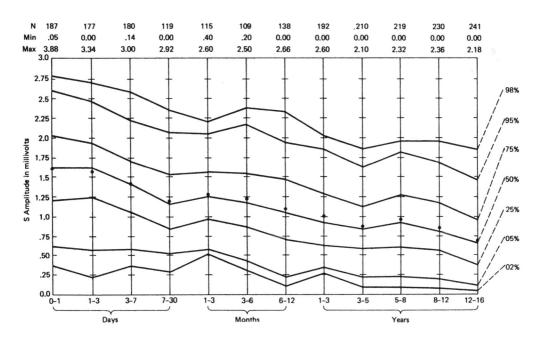

Fig. A2.23
S amplitude in lead V_4 versus age (•, mean)

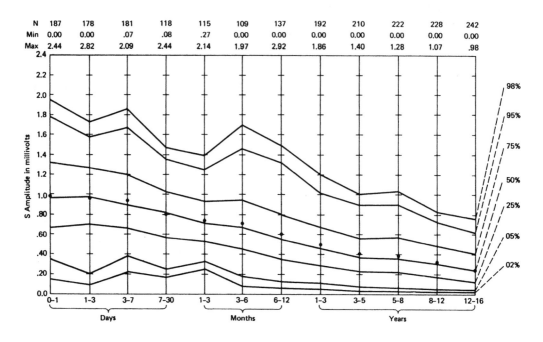

N	187	178	181	118	115	109	137	192	210	222	228	242
Min	0.00	0.00	.07	.08	.27	0.00	0.00	0.00	0.00	0.00	0.00	0.00
Max	2.44	2.82	2.09	2.44	2.14	1.97	2.92	1.86	1.40	1.28	1.07	.98

Fig. A2.24

S amplitude in lead V₅ versus age (•, mean)

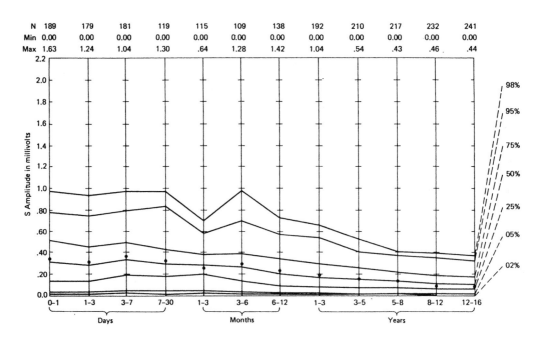

N	189	179	181	119	115	109	138	192	210	217	232	241
Min	0.00	0.00	0.00	0.00	0.00	0.00	0.00	0.00	0.00	0.00	0.00	0.00
Max	1.63	1.24	1.04	1.30	.64	1.28	1.42	1.04	.54	.43	.46	.44

Fig. A2.25

S amplitude in lead V₆ versus age (•, mean)

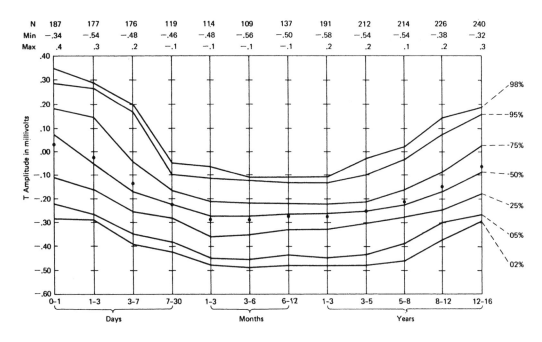

Fig. A2.26

T amplitude in lead V₃R versus age (•, mean)

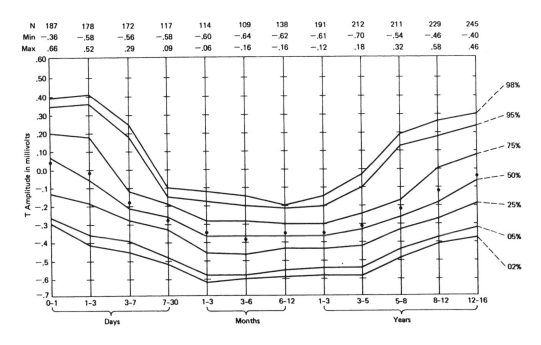

Fig. A2.27

T amplitude in lead V₁ versus age (•, mean)

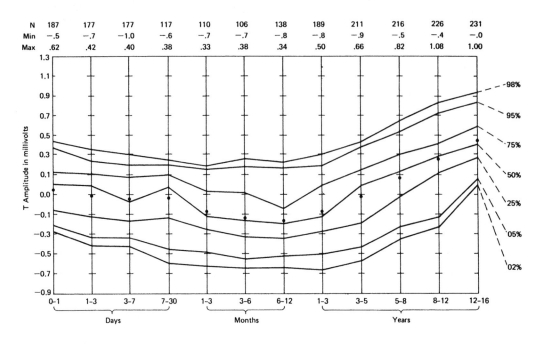

N	187	177	177	117	110	106	138	189	211	216	226	231
Min	−.5	−.7	−1.0	−.6	−.7	−.7	−.8	−.8	−.9	−.5	−.4	−.0
Max	.62	.42	.40	.38	.33	.38	.34	.50	.66	.82	1.08	1.00

● Fig. A2.28

T amplitude in lead V_2 versus age (●, mean)

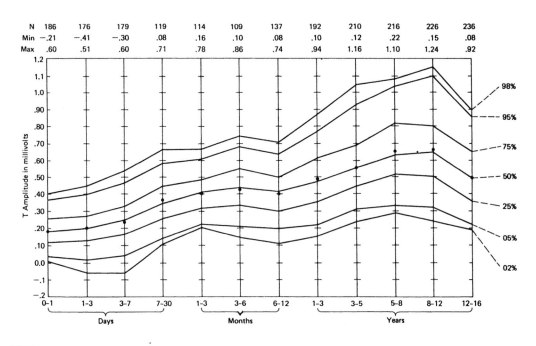

N	186	176	179	119	114	109	137	192	210	216	226	236
Min	−.21	−.41	−.30	.08	.16	.10	.08	.10	.12	.22	.15	.08
Max	.60	.51	.60	.71	.78	.86	.74	.94	1.16	1.10	1.24	.92

● Fig. A2.29

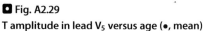

T amplitude in lead V_5 versus age (●, mean)

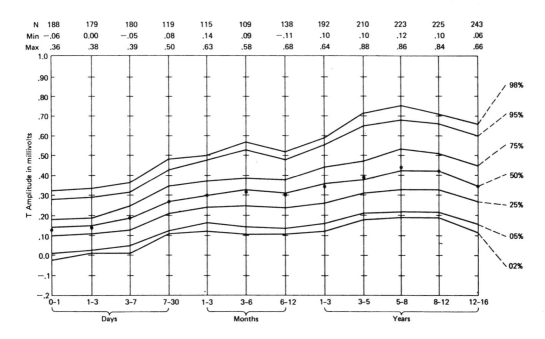

Fig. A2.30

T amplitude in lead V_6 versus age (•, mean)

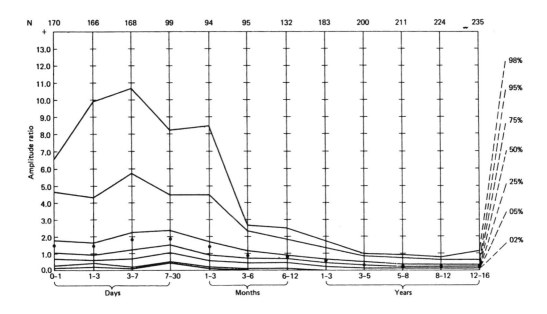

Fig. A2.31

R/S amplitude ratio in lead V_3R versus age (•, mean)

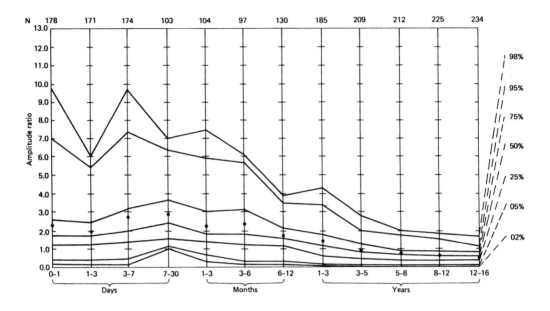

◘ Fig. A2.32

R/S amplitude ratio in lead V₁ versus age (●, mean)

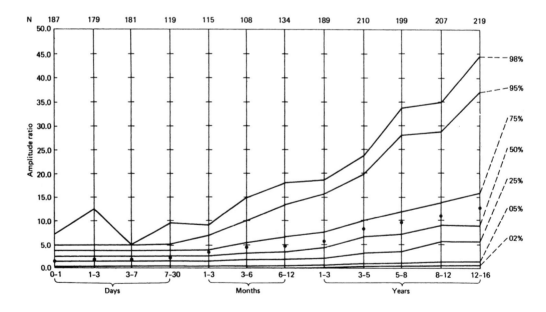

◘ Fig. A2.33

R/S amplitude ratio in lead V₅ versus age (●, mean)

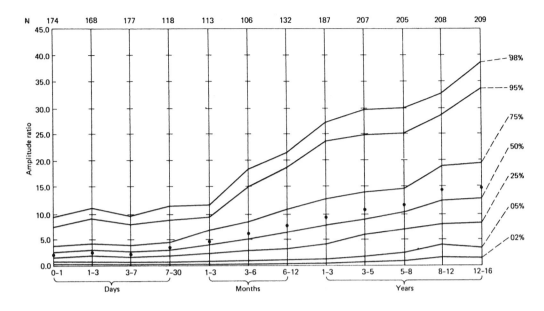

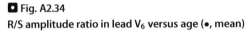

Fig. A2.34

R/S amplitude ratio in lead V_6 versus age (•, mean)

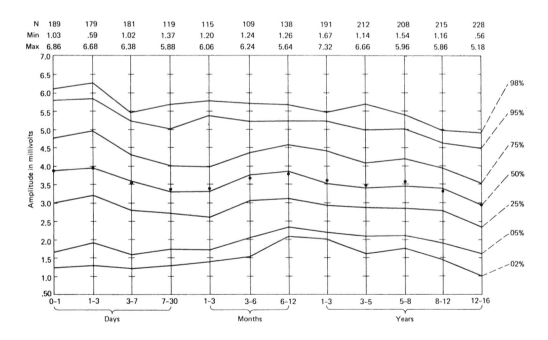

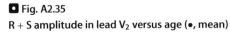

Fig. A2.35

R + S amplitude in lead V_2 versus age (•, mean)

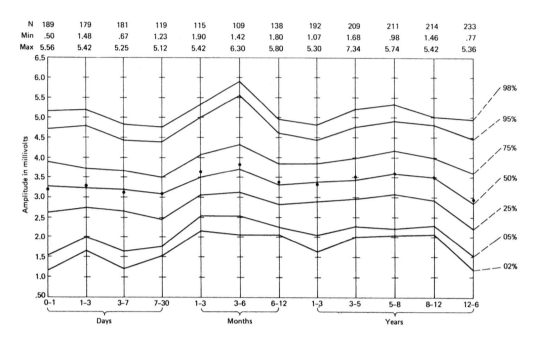

N	189	179	181	119	115	109	138	192	209	211	214	233
Min	.50	1.48	.67	1.23	1.90	1.42	1.80	1.07	1.68	.98	1.46	.77
Max	5.56	5.42	5.25	5.12	5.42	6.30	5.80	5.30	7.34	5.74	5.42	5.36

Fig. A2.36

R + S amplitude in lead V_4 versus age (•, mean)

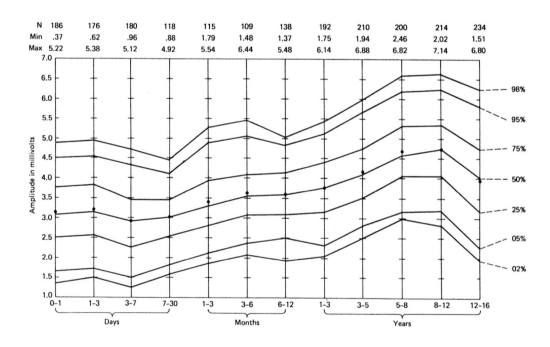

N	186	176	180	118	115	109	138	192	210	200	214	234
Min	.37	.62	.96	.88	1.79	1.48	1.37	1.75	1.94	2.46	2.02	1.51
Max	5.22	5.38	5.12	4.92	5.54	6.44	5.48	6.14	6.88	6.82	7.14	6.80

Fig. A2.37

R amplitude in lead V_5 + S amplitude in lead V_2 versus age (•, mean)

N	189	179	181	119	115	109	138	192	210	217	225	235
Min	.14	.16	.28	.27	.68	.66	.61	.58	1.04	1.24	1.41	.69
Max	4.08	3.28	2.72	2.40	3.02	4.22	3.44	5.18	4.54	5.24	5.74	4.36

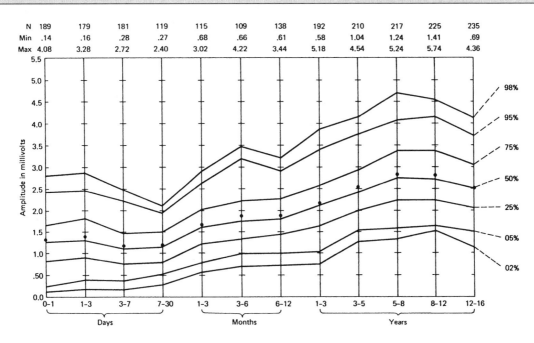

Fig. A2.38

R amplitude in lead V_6 + S amplitude in lead V_1 versus age (•, mean)

N	189	179	181	118	115	109	138	192	210	225	231	246
Min	9	9	10	9	12	15	10	15	15	15	18	15
Max	33	27	30	30	30	36	42	36	39	39	45	45

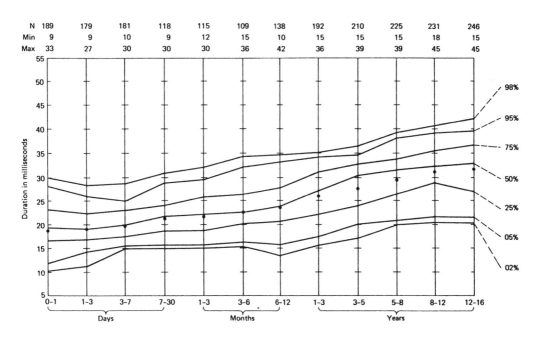

Fig. A2.39

Ventricular activation time in lead V_5 versus age (•, mean)

A2

A2.3   Additional 12-Lead Pediatric ECG Normal Limits

Liebman, who has contributed ❯ Chap. 9 of *Electrocardiology: Comprehensive Clinical ECG* as well as a short technical note on linear and directional statistics (see ❯ Appendix 1, Sect. A1.7), has published extensively on normal limits of the pediatric and adolescent ECG. He has stressed the difference between using equipment with high (adequate) and low (poor) frequency response. Some tables which are mostly complementary to ❯ Sect. A2.2 are reproduced from: Liebman J, Plonsey R, Gillette PC, eds. *Pediatric Cardiology.* 1982, with the permission of Williams and Wilkins, Baltimore, Maryland. These include a mixture of "high-" and "low-frequency data." The former are more correct for use with modern recording equipment (❯ Tables A2.25–A2.30).

◘ Table A2.25
High-frequency data

Age	Heart rate (bpm)						PR interval (s)					
	Min	5%	Mean	95%	Max.	SD	Min	5%	Mean	95%	Max.	SD
0–24 h	85	94	119	145	145	16.1	0.07	0.07	0.10	0.12	0.13	0.012
1–7 days	100	100	133	175	175	22.3	0.5	0.07	0.09	0.12	0.13	0.014
8–30 days	115	115	163	190	190	19.9	0.07	0.07	0.09	0.11	0.13	0.010
1–3 months	115	124	154	190	205	18.6	0.07	0.07	0.10	0.13	0.17	0.017
3–6 months	115	111	140	179	205	21.0	0.07	0.07	0.10	0.13	0.13	0.014
6–12 months	115	112	140	177	175	18.7	0.07	0.08	0.10	0.13	0.15	0.013
1–3 years	100	98	126	163	190	19.8	0.07	0.08	0.11	0.15	0.17	0.019
3–5 years	55	65	98	132	145	18.0	0.09	0.09	0.12	0.15	0.17	0.015
5–8 years	70	70	98	115	145	16.1	0.09	0.10	0.13	0.16	0.19	0.017
8–12 years	55	55	79	107	115	15.0	0.09	0.10	0.14	0.17	0.27	0.022
12–16 years	55	55	75	102	115	13.5	0.09	0.11	0.14	0.16	0.21	0.018
	P-wave duration (s)						QRS duration (s)					
0–24 h	0.040	0.040	0.051	0.065	0.075	0.066	0.05	0.05	0.065	0.084	0.09	0.010
1–7 days	0.035	0.038	0.046	0.061	0.065	0.066	0.04	0.04	0.056	0.079	0.08	0.010
8–30 days	0.040	0.040	0.048	0.057	0.065	0.064	0.04	0.04	0.057	0.073	0.08	0.009
1–3 months	0.040	0.040	0.046	0.058	0.065	0.063	0.05	0.05	0.062	0.080	0.08	0.007
3–6 months	0.040	0.040	0.049	0.065	0.065	0.072	0.06	0.06	0.068	0.080	0.08	0.008
6–12 months	0.040	0.046	0.058	0.068	0.075	0.058	0.05	0.05	0.065	0.080	0.08	0.008
1–3 years	0.045	0.053	0.065	0.082	0.085	0.090	0.05	0.05	0.064	0.080	0.08	0.008
3–5 years	0.040	0.051	0.069	0.087	0.095	0.108	0.06	0.06	0.072	0.084	0.09	0.009
5–8 years	0.050	0.059	0.070	0.084	0.095	0.095	0.05	0.05	0.067	0.080	0.08	0.017
8–12 years	0.050	0.061	0.075	0.092	0.105	0.098	0.05	0.05	0.073	0.084	0.09	0.008
12–16 years	0.060	0.064	0.081	0.095	0.105	0.095	0.04	0.04	0.068	0.080	0.10	0.010

◼ Table A2.26

Heart rate and durations: adolescents

	Sex	Mean	SD	5%	50%	95%
Heart rate	Male	69	11	52	70	90
	Female	73	12	57	70	92
	Total	71	12	55	70	90
P-wave duration	Male	0.09	0.02	0.06	0.08	0.11
	Female	0.09	0.02	0.06	0.09	0.12
	Total	0.09	0.02	0.06	0.09	0.11
PR interval	Male	0.15	0.03	0.10	0.15	0.20
	Female	0.15	0.02	0.12	0.15	0.19
	Total	0.15	0.02	0.11	0.15	0.20
QRS duration	Male	0.08	0.01	0.06	0.08	0.10
	Female	0.08	0.01	0.05	0.08	0.09
	Total	0.08	0.01	0.06	0.08	0.10
QT interval	Male	0.38	0.04	0.32	0.38	0.42
	Female	0.37	0.03	0.32	0.38	0.42
	Total	0.37	0.04	0.32	0.38	0.43
T-wave duration	Male	0.21	0.06	0.16	0.20	0.35
	Female	0.19	0.04	0.15	0.18	0.28
	Total	0.20	0.05	0.15	0.20	0.31

◼ Table A2.27

Heart rate (bpm): prematures

Infants		Mean	Percentile	
Age	Number	Heart rate	5th	95th
24 h	66	141	109	173
72 h	69	150	127	182
1 week	62	164	134	200
1 month	42	170	133	200
2 months	30	171	128	203
3 months	24	159	130	202
6 months	16	145		
1 year	18	142		

◼ Table A2.28

P amplitude in lead II ×10 (mV): prematures

Infants		Mean	Percentile	
Age	Number	P amplitude	5th	95th
24 h	65	1.1	0.5	2.0
72 h	69	1.3	0.5	2.0
1 week	62	1.3	0.5	2.6
1 month	40	0.8	0.3	1.5
2 months	30	0.9	0.4	1.5
3 months	24	1.0	0.5	1.9
6 months	16	1.1		
1 year	18	1.2		

◘ Table A2.29

Amplitudes in V$_3$(high-frequency data) ×10 (mV)

Age	R wave						S wave					
	Min.	5%	Mean	95%	Max.	SD	Min.	5%	Mean	95%	Max.	SD
0–24 h	12.0	12.7	18.8	26.7	28.0	4.12	10.0	12.0	25.0	32.0	38.0	6.05
1–7 days	4.0	8.8	18.1	30.0	40.0	6.55	0.0	2.	17.1	33.0	38.0	8.37
8–30 days	0.0	8.3	18.8	33.8	36.0	7.50	2.0	4.2	12.4	20.0	26.0	5.47
1–3 months	12.0	13.5	21.8	29.1	32.0	4.50	2.0	4.9	14.0	21.3	22.0	4.95
3–6 months	12.0	14.5	20.1	30.0	32.0	4.56	2.0	4.5	14.7	23.5	26.0	6.14
6–12 months	8.0	9.7	17.8	23.5	24.0	4.32	0.0	4.9	14.2	22.6	26.0	5.94
1–3 years	8.0	8.8	15.4	27.0	32.0	4.92	2.0	4.5	13.4	23.5	26.0	5.24
3–5 years	4.0	6.0	15.0	22.7	24.0	4.49	2.0	3.3	12.2	20.0	26.0	6.00
5–8 years	0.0	4.5	13.1	23.2	32.0	5.81	0.0	3.7	15.0	24.8	30.0	6.10
8–12 years	0.0	4.4	10.8	21.0	32.0	5.22	0.0	2.4	13.2	24.0	30.0	6.80
12–16 years	0.0	3.8	10.0	19.6	28.0	5.34	0.0	2.2	10.8	25.4	34.0	6.82

◘ Table A2.30

Amplitude in lead V$_4$R (low-frequency data) ×10 (mV)

Age	R wave					S wave				
	Min.	5%	Mean	95%	Max.	Min.	5%	Mean	95%	Max.
30 h	3.5	4.0	8.6	14.2	15.0	0.0	0.2	3.8	13.0	12.0
1 month	3.0	3.3	6.3	8.5	12.0	0.0	0.8	1.8	4.6	9.0
2–3 months	0.5	1.1	5.1	10.1	15.0	0.0	0.0	3.4	9.3	15.0
4–5 months	2.0	2.4	5.2	7.5	9.0	1.0	0.3	3.5	6.7	9.0
6–8 months	2.0	1.3	4.4	7.1	7.0	0.0	0.2	3.9	11.7	10.0
9 months–2 years	1.0	0.2	4.0	6.6	8.0	0.0	0.8	4.9	8.1	10.5
2–5 years	1.0	1.6	3.4	7.4	8.0	1.0	1.2	4.8	9.5	12.0
6–13 years	0.2	0.6	2.5	5.7	7.0	0.5	0.9	5.8	12.5	20.0

A2.4 Normal Limits of the Pediatric Orthogonal-Lead ECG

A number of tables are included to provide an indication of the normal limits of the orthogonal-lead ECG in infants and children. The terminology is discussed in ❷ Chap. 9 of *Electrocardiology: Comprehensive Clinical ECG* and in addition, the concept of prevalent direction is described in Appendix 1, ❷ Sect. A1.7 by Liebman. Tables have been reproduced from Liebman J, Plonsey R, Gillette PC. *Pediatric Electrocardiography*. 1982, with the permission of Williams and Wilkins, Baltimore, Maryland. However, some of these tables are from earlier publications and the list at the end of the section relates to the identifying superscript in the legend to each table (❷ Tables A2.31–A2.51). ❷ Figures A2.40 and ❷ A2.41 are reproduced from the work of Davignon and Rautaharju with the permission of Springer (❷ See A2.2).

■ Table A2.31

Direction of inscription of the QRS complex: adolescents[a]

	Sex	Number	Clockwise		Figure-of-eight		Counterclockwise	
			No.	%	No.	%	No.	%
Frontal plane	male	67	42	62.6	2	2.9	23	34.3
	female	47	29	61.7	3	6.3	15	31.9
	total	114	71	62.2	5	4.3	38	33.3
Horizontal plane	male	67	0	0	1	1.4	66	98.5
	female	47	0	0	2	4.2	45	95.7
	total	114	0	0	3	2.6	111	97.3

■ Table A2.32

Direction of inscription of the QRS complex: prematures C, clockwise; CC, counterclockwise[b]

	Frontal plane		Horizontal plane			
Age of infants	C (%)	CC (%)	C (%)	CC (%)	Figure-of-eight initially CC (%)	Narrow[a] loop (%)
24 h	97	3	1.5	11	34	54
72 h	98.5	1.5	1.5	16.5	43.5	39
1 week	97	3		21.5	54	24.5
1 month	97.5	2.5	2.5	17	51	29.5
2 months	93.5	6.5	3.5	30	53.5	13.5
3 months	100		4.5	29	62.5	4
6 months	100		6	37.5	50	6
1 year	100		5.5	61	28	5.5

[a]Presence of a QRS loop so narrow that the specific direction of inscription has no significance

■ Table A2.33

Evolution of the Frank vectorcardiogam in normal infants. In frontal plane, initial QRS to left 66.6% from birth to 30 days; initial QRS to left 55.5% from 1 to 2 months; initial QRS to left 10.5% from to 2 to 3 months; initial QRS to left 6.2% by 6–8 months[c]

	Frontal			Horizontal		
Groups	CW	Figure-of-eight	CCW	CW	Figure-of-eight	CCW
I (birth–30 h)	91.3	7.0	1.7	61.5	19.2	19.3
II (1 month)	88.9	11.1	0	18.5	40.7	40.8
III (2–3 months)	97.4	0	2.6	2.6	39.5	57.9
IV (4–5 months)	87.0	6.5	6.5	0	35.5	64.5
V (6–8 months)	87.6	6.2	6.2	0	21.9	78.1
VI (12–18 months)	83.3	10.0	6.7	0	6.6	93.4

■ Table A2.34
Prevalent direction of the QRS in the frontal plane: adolescents[a]

Prevalent direction							
Sex	Age	d	χ^2	$\hat{\alpha}_f$	5%	50%	95%
Male	11 → 15	0.94	51.2	65	10	70	90
Male	16 → 19	0.92	63.9	63	9	70	91
Female	11 → 15	0.97	48.5	62	38	60	87
Female	16 → 19	0.93	36.0	56	11	65	80
Male	11 → 19	0.93	115.0	64	10	70	90
Female	11 → 19	0.95	84.2	59	15	60	80
Total	11 → 19	0.93	198.9	62	14	65	90

■ Table A2.35
Prevalent direction of the QRS in the horizontal plane: adolescents[a]

Prevalent direction							
Sex	Age	d	χ^2	$\hat{\alpha}_h$	5%	50%	95%
Male	11 → 15	0.94	51.6	330	292	335	8
Male	16 → 19	0.92	64.4	333	289	340	8
Female	11 → 15	0.96	48.0	334	290	340	354
Female	16 → 19	0.95	38.2	332	300	340	0
Male	11 → 19	0.93	116.0	332	292	340	5
Female	11 → 19	0.96	86.2	333	292	340	0
Total	11 → 19	0.94	202.1	332	293	340	0

■ Table A2.36
Prevalent direction of the T in the frontal plane: adolescents[a]

Prevalent direction							
Sex	Age	d	χ^2	$\hat{\alpha}_f$	5%	50%	95%
Male	11 → 15	0.96	53.8	42	15	45	60
Male	16 → 19	0.94	67.7	48	5	55	70
Female	11 → 15	0.98	49.6	42	17	45	60
Female	16 → 19	0.96	39.0	42	3	45	74
Male	11 → 19	0.95	121.2	45	7	45	70
Female	11 → 19	0.97	88.6	42	17	45	60
Total	11 → 19	0.96	209.6	44	10	45	63

■ Table A2.37

Prevalent direction of the T in the horizontal plane: adolescents[a]

Prevalent direction							
Sex	Age	d	χ^2	$\hat{\alpha}_h$	5%	50%	95%
Male	11 → 15	0.90	47.5	15	310	15	60
Male	16 → 19	0.88	58.3	24	338	15	74
Female	11 → 15	0.96	48.4	12	335	15	38
Female	16 → 19	0.97	39.2	12	310	15	25
Male	11 → 19	0.89	105.1	20	334	15	60
Female	11 → 19	0.97	87.6	12	335	15	33
Total	11 → 19	0.92	191.4	17	335	15	60

■ Table A2.38

Frontal angular deviation of T from QRS: adolescents[a]

Prevalent direction							
Sex	Age	d	χ^2	$\hat{\alpha}_f$	5%	50%	95%
Male	11 → 15	0.90	46.9	337	285	335	40
Male	16 → 19	0.94	66.6	345	305	345	17
Female	11 → 15	0.97	48.8	340	302	340	0
Female	16 → 19	0.93	36.0	346	316	340	42
Male	11 → 19	0.92	113.0	342	299	340	34
Female	11 → 19	0.95	84.5	343	309	340	15
Total	11 → 19	0.93	197.5	342	305	340	18

■ Table A2.39

Horizontal angular deviation of T from QRS: adolescents[a]

Prevalent direction							
Sex	Age	d	χ^2	$\hat{\alpha}_h$	5%	50%	95%
Male	11 → 15	0.85	41.8	45	330	35	98
Male	16 → 19	0.83	52.8	52	334	45	108
Female	11 → 15	0.95	46.4	39	4	35	80
Female	16 → 19	0.92	35.2	39	330	35	75
Male	11 → 19	0.84	94.3	49	339	45	103
Female	11 → 19	0.93	81.7	39	4	35	78
Total	11 → 19	0.87	174.3	45	356	40	93

◻ Table A2.40
Prevalent direction of QRS: prematures[b]

| Age of infants | Frontal plane | | | | First horizontal vector | | | | Second horizontal vector | | | |
	No. of infants	Prevalent direction	5%	95%	No. of infants	Prevalent Direction	5%	95%	No. of Infants	Prevalent direction	5%	95%
24 h	60	127	75	194	58	74	338	340	16	239		
72 h	68	121	75	195	59	84	295	220	15	233		
1 week	61	117	75	165	54	69	332	216	21	231	9	332
1 month	42	80	17	171	35	58	340	115	13	232		
2 months	30	63	345	105	30	46	340	60	8	231		
3 months	24	59	352	105	23	51	346	108	2	223		
6 months	15	58			16	30			1	240		
1 year	18	46			18	12			2	253		

◻ Table A2.41
Prevalent direction of T: prematures[b]

| Age of infants | Frontal plane | | | | Horizontal plane | | | |
	No. of infants	Prevalent direction	5%	95%	No. of infants	Prevalent direction	5%	95%
24 h	52	41	319	84	56	314	240	111
72 h	65	28	315	60	61	318	241	101
1 week	60	31	345	75	59	335	290	15
1 month	42	53	30	75	36	346	281	52
2 months	30	43	353	67	30	334	259	15
3 months	24	47	19	74	24	335	295	14
6 months	14	41			15	333		
1 year	18	46			18	343		

◻ Table A2.42
QRS magnitudes ×10 (mV): prematures[b]

Age of infants	No. of infants	R wave	5%	95%	No. of infants	S wave	5%	95%
			Lead V_5 (X axis)					
24 h	64	6.5	2.0	12.6	61	6.8	0.06	17.6
72 h	65	7.4	2.6	14.9	64	6.5	1.00	16.0
1 week	61	8.7	3.8	16.8	56	6.8	0.00	15.0
1 month	38	13.0	6.2	21.6	38	6.2	1.20	14.0
2 months	30	18.3	12.1	31.5	29	7.0	0.96	15.0
3 months	24	21.0	14.6	31.5	24	6.7	1.30	21.4
6 months	16	20.3			16	6.8		
1 year	18	17.5			17	3.0		

■ Table A2.42 (Continued)

Age of infants	No. of infants	R wave	5%	95%	No. of infants	S wave	5%	95%
Lead aVF (Y axis)								
24 h	63	6.7	0.85	16.6	28	0.96	0.00	4.5
72 h	68	7.1	0.86	13.9	33	1.20	0.00	5.5
1 week	61	7.6	1.3	14.1	30	0.98	0.00	3.3
1 month	42	9.0	1.8	18.8	20	0.86	0.00	4.0
2 months	30	10.0	1.2	21.7	13	0.90	0.00	5.3
3 months	24	11.1	1.9	23.0	14	0.77	0.00	3.8
6 months	16	12.0			9	0.53		
1 year	18	9.1			9	0.56		
Lead V_2 (Z axis)								
24 h	65	11.4	3.5	21.3	65	15.0	2.5	26.5
72 h	66	11.9	5.0	20.8	66	13.5	2.6	26.0
1 week	60	12.3	4.0	20.5	60	14.0	3.0	25.0
1 month	41	15.0	8.3	21.0	41	14.0	5.1	26.3
2 months	30	19.0	8.6	32.0	30	17.1	8.0	34.5
3 months	23	20.1	13.3	30.0	23	16.1	6.0	37.6
6 months	16	20.6			16	18.5		
1 year	18	16.3			18	16.0		

■ Table A2.43

Spatial magnitude and orientation (MSVR in mV). M, male; F, female; T, total[d]

	n	$\hat{\alpha}$	β	D	χ^2	MSVR mean mag.	SD	$P_{2.5}$	P_5	P_{10}	P_{50}	P_{90}	P_{95}	$P_{97.5}$
Frank-lead system														
M 2-5	23	246	108	0.58	22.8	1.11	0.46		0.33	0.44	1.10	1.80	1.86	
M 6-10	60	254	107	0.73	96.6	1.11	0.41	0.45	0.49	0.59	1.02	1.78	1.99	214.
M 2-10	83	252	107	0.69	117.8	1.11	0.42	0.36	0.47	0.58	1.04	1.79	1.92	2.08
F 2-5	29	257	113	0.74	47.4	1.06	0.35		0.44	0.60	1.09	1.56	1.65	
F 6-10	63	253	109	0.69	90.3	1.01	0.39	0.20	0.34	0.51	0.95	1.46	1.80	2.05
F 2-10	92	254	111	0.71	137.5	1.02	0.38	0.25	0.39	0.56	0.95	1.52	1.67	1.97
T 2-5	52	252	111	0.66	68.6	1.08	0.40	0.33	0.34	0.58	1.10	1.69	1.80	1.85
T 6-10	123	254	108	0.71	186.7	1.06	0.40	0.33	0.47	0.56	0.99	1.62	1.91	2.08
T 2-10	175	253	109	0.70	254.9	1.07	0.40	0.33	0.46	0.58	1.02	1.65	1.81	2.02
T 2-19	341	252	112	0.63	406.5	0.94	0.43	0.22	0.30	0.40	0.92	1.51	1.71	1.94

□ Table A2.44

Spatial magnitude and orientation (MSVL). M, male; F, female; T, total[d]

	n		β	D	χ	MSVR mean mag.	SD	P2.5	P5	P10	P50	P90	P95	P97.5
Frank-lead system														
M 2-5	23		347	129	0.85	50.2	1.73	0.60		0.83	0.87	1.80	2.59	2.74	
M 6-10	60		329	133	0.87	135.9	1.82	0.53	1.00	1.10	1.13	1.77	2.67	2.93	3.15
M 2-10	83		334	133	0.86	183.9	1.80	0.55	0.85	0.96	1.10	1.80	2.59	2.81	3.05
F 2-5	29		341	133	0.83	60.0	1.71	0.44		1.02	1.10	1.69	2.13	2.66	
F 6-10	63		340	138	0.93	162.5	1.77	0.44	1.03	1.10	1.13	1.76	2.36	2.60	2.80
F 2-10	92		340	136	0.90	221.7	1.75	0.44	1.02	1.09	1.13	1.75	2.31	2.58	2.81
T 2-5	52		344	131	0.84	109.9	1.72	0.51	0.93	0.88	1.01	1.76	2.40	2.70	2.97
T 6-10	123		334	136	0.90	296.5	1.80	0.49	1.05	1.10	1.13	1.76	2.43	2.77	2.93
T 2-10	175		337	135	0.88	404.5	1.77	0.49	0.95	1.05	1.12	1.76	2.42	2.75	2.89
T 2-19	341		336	136	0.88	801.1	1.71	0.48	0.88	1.00	1.11	1.69	2.31	2.59	2.82

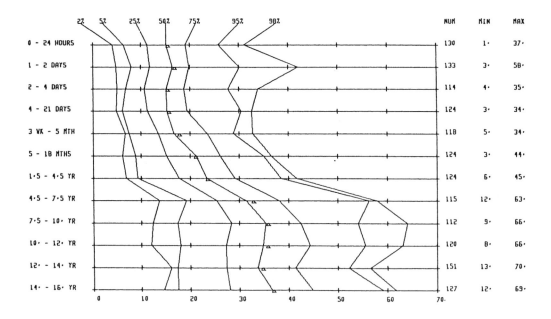

□ Fig. A2.40

Percentile distributions for the spatial magnitude of the QRS integral sector in normal children from birth to aged 16 years[g]

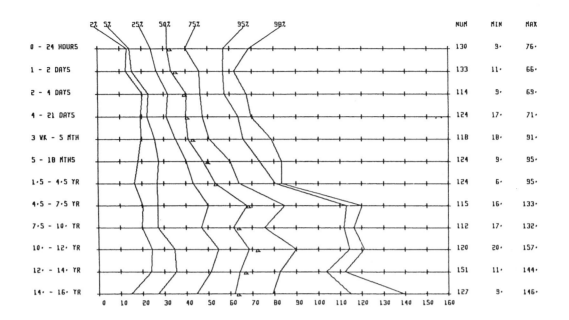

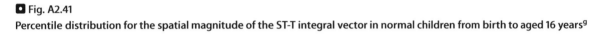

Fig. A2.41
Percentile distribution for the spatial magnitude of the ST-T integral vector in normal children from birth to aged 16 years[g]

Table A2.45
Maximal projections. M, male; F, female; T, total[d]: Magnitude is in mV

| | n | Frank system | | | | | | | | |
		Mean mag.	SD	$p_{2.5}$	p_5	p_{10}	p_{50}	p_{90}	p_{95}	$p_{97.5}$
X initial right										
M 2-5	23	0.18	0.16		0.00	0.00	0.15	0.41	0.51	
M 6-10	60	0.12	0.12	0.00	0.00	0.00	0.09	0.28	0.36	0.48
M 2-10	83	0.14	0.14	0.00	0.00	0.00	0.11	0.33	0.36	0.55
F 2-5	29	0.11	0.09		0.00	0.00	0.11	0.24	0.26	
F 6-10	63	0.10	0.09	0.00	0.00	0.00	0.09	0.21	0.25	0.39
F 2-10	92	0.10	0.08	0.00	0.00	0.00	0.09	0.22	0.25	0.35
T 2-5	52	0.14	0.13	0.00	0.00	0.00	0.11	0.32	0.38	0.50
T 6-10	123	0.11	0.11	0.00	0.00	0.00	0.09	0.25	0.35	0.38
T 2-10	175	0.12	0.11	0.00	0.00	0.00	0.09	0.25	0.35	0.40
T 2-19	341	0.10	0.10	0.00	0.00	0.00	0.08	0.23	0.30	0.36

■ Table A2.45   (Continued)

	n	Frank system Mean mag.	SD	$p_{2.5}$	p_5	p_{10}	p_{50}	p_{90}	p_{95}	$p_{97.5}$
X left										
M 2-5	23	1.23	0.52		0.49	0.55	1.22	2.02	2.22	
M 6-10	60	1.17	0.47	0.37	0.41	0.68	1.09	1.80	2.23	2.47
M 2-10	83	1.19	0.48	0.40	0.49	0.60	1.14	1.81	2.22	2.34
F 2-5	29	1.15	0.47		0.55	0.60	1.16	1.60	2.21	
F 6-10	63	1.08	0.36	0.18	0.46	0.65	1.08	1.55	1.66	1.89
F 2-10	92	1.10	0.40	0.28	0.52	0.60	1.10	1.55	1.64	2.03
T 2-5	52	1.19	0.49	0.49	0.53	0.59	1.18	1.79	2.15	2.62
T 6-10	123	1.13	0.42	0.34	0.46	0.68	1.08	1.66	1.82	2.25
T 2-10	175	1.14	0.44	0.40	0.52	0.61	1.10	1.68	1.90	2.25
T 2-19	341	1.06	0.44	0.35	0.46	0.56	1.04	1.60	1.80	1.99
X terminal right										
M 2-5	23	0.32	0.23		0.00	0.01	0.28	0.66	0.69	
M 6-10	60	0.29	0.20	0.00	0.00	0.03	0.30	0.52	0.58	0.84
M 2-10	83	0.30	0.21	0.00	0.00	0.02	0.30	0.55	0.65	0.70
F 2-5	29	0.30	0.21		0.00	0.06	0.25	0.62	0.75	
F 6-10	63	0.23	0.17	0.00	0.00	0.02	0.24	0.48	0.52	0.78
F 2-10	92	0.25	0.19	0.00	0.00	0.02	0.24	0.50	0.63	0.79
T 2-5	52	0.31	0.22	0.00	0.00	0.03	0.26	0.64	0.68	0.80
T 6-10	123	0.26	0.19	0.00	0.00	0.02	0.26	0.50	0.55	0.75
T 2-10	175	0.27	0.20	0.00	0.00	0.02	0.26	0.52	0.63	0.74
T 2-19	341	0.23	0.19	0.00	0.00	0.00	0.20	0.50	0.55	0.65

■ Table A2.46

Maximal projections. M, male; F, female; T total[d]: Magnitude is in mV

	n	Frank-lead system Mean Mag.	SD	$p_{2.5}$	p_5	p_{10}	p_{50}	p_{90}	p_{95}	$p_{97.5}$
X initial superior										
M 2-5	23	0.12	0.12		0.00	0.00	0.10	0.28	0.46	
M 6-10	60	0.11	0.09	0.00	0.00	0.00	0.08	0.26	0.30	0.32
M 2-10	83	0.11	0.10	0.00	0.00	0.00	0.10	0.26	0.30	0.35
F 2-5	29	0.10	0.10		0.00	0.00	0.08	0.24	0.37	
F 6-10	63	0.10	0.09	0.00	0.00	0.00	0.08	0.21	0.30	0.37
F 2-10	92	0.10	0.09	0.00	0.00	0.00	0.08	0.22	0.31	0.38
T 2-5	52	0.11	0.11	0.00	0.00	0.00	0.10	0.25	0.36	0.47
T 6-10	123	0.10	0.09	0.00	0.00	0.00	0.08	0.22	0.30	0.35
T 2-10	175	0.10	0.10	0.00	0.00	0.00	0.08	0.24	0.30	0.35
T 2-19	341	0.10	0.08	0.00	0.00	0.00	0.08	0.20	0.25	0.30

◘ Table A2.46 (Continued)

	n	Frank-lead system								
		Mean Mag.	SD	$p_{2.5}$	p_5	p_{10}	p_{50}	p_{90}	p_{95}	$p_{97.5}$
Y inferior										
M 2-5	23	1.02	0.45		0.39	0.45	1.00	1.78	1.98	
M 6-10	60	1.17	0.41	0.51	0.56	0.64	1.09	1.76	1.97	2.15
M 2-10	83	1.13	0.43	0.45	0.47	0.58	1.04	1.76	1.96	2.05
F 2-5	29	1.09	0.32		0.46	0.71	1.12	1.50	1.54	
F 6-10	63	1.27	0.40	0.64	0.68	0.72	1.30	1.82	2.00	2.24
F 2-10	92	1.22	0.39	0.58	0.67	0.72	1.21	1.64	1.97	2.07
T 2-5	52	1.06	0.38	0.36	0.42	0.50	1.06	1.51	1.71	1.97
T 6-10	123	1.22	0.41	0.56	0.63	0.70	1.20	1.77	2.00	2.10
T 2-10	175	1.17	0.41	0.46	0.56	0.66	1.16	1.69	1.96	2.03
T 2-19	341		0.40	0.47	0.58	0.65	1.12	1.70	1.88	2.02
Y terminal superior										
M 2-5	23	0.11	0.11		0.00	0.00	0.07	0.24	0.40	
M 6-10	60	0.13	0.11	0.00	0.00	0.00	0.15	0.28	0.32	0.38
M 2-10	83	0.12	0.11	0.00	0.00	0.00	0.10	0.27	0.32	0.43
F 2-5	29	0.08	0.10		0.00	0.00	0.06	0.23	0.35	
F 6-10	63	0.11	0.15	0.00	0.00	0.00	0.04	0.28	0.40	0.61
F 2-10	92	0.10	0.14	0.00	0.00	0.00	0.04	0.26	0.39	0.47
T 2-5	52	0.09	0.10	0.00	0.00	0.00	0.07	0.23	0.32	0.45
T 6-10	123	0.12	0.13	0.00	0.00	0.00	0.08	0.28	0.32	0.44
T 2-10	175	0.11	0.12	0.00	0.00	0.00	0.08	0.26	0.32	0.44
T 2-19	341	0.10	0.12	0.00	0.00	0.00	0.07	0.26	0.32	0.38

◘ Table A2.47

Maximal projections. M, male; F, female; T total[d]: Magnitude is in mV

	n	Frank-lead system								
		Mean mag.	SD	$p_{2.5}$	p_5	p_{10}	p_{50}	p_{90}	p_{95}	$p_{97.5}$
Z anterior										
M 2-5	23	0.86	0.41		0.36	0.42	0.78	1.52	2.02	
M 6-10	60	0.64	0.27	0.23	0.28	0.31	0.60	1.00	1.18	1.37
M 2-10	83	0.70	0.32	0.25	0.30	0.36	0.62	1.09	1.25	1.68
F 2-5	29	0.72	0.30		0.26	0.34	0.70	1.10	1.35	
F 6-10	63	0.62	0.21	0.17	0.22	0.36	0.62	0.90	1.01	1.15
F 2-10	92	0.65	0.24	0.19	0.24	0.36	0.65	0.95	1.09	1.24
T 2-5	52	0.78	0.35	0.25	0.31	0.37	0.74	1.10	1.64	1.97
T 6-10	123	0.63	0.24	0.20	0.26	0.33	0.62	0.95	1.05	1.24
T 2-10	175	0.67	0.29	0.22	0.28	0.36	0.64	1.01	1.16	1.42
T 2-19	341	0.57	0.29	0.12	0.16	0.23	0.55	0.94	1.08	1.25

◻ Table A2.47 (Continued)

	n	Frank-lead system								
		Mean mag.	SD	$p_{2.5}$	p_5	p_{10}	p_{50}	p_{90}	p_{95}	$p_{97.5}$
Z posterior										
M 2-5	23	1.02	0.44		0.29	0.45	1.04	1.70	1.72	
M 6-10	60	1.15	0.37	0.64	0.68	0.70	1.12	1.72	1.86	2.10
M 2-10	83	1.11	0.39	0.41	0.62	0.65	1.08	1.70	1.79	2.03
F 2-5	29	1.09	0.26		0.65	0.75	1.10	1.44	1.53	
F 6-10	63	0.97	0.39	0.18	0.23	0.56	0.94	1.41	1.87	2.01
F 2-10	92	1.01	0.35	0.22	0.42	0.61	0.99	1.42	1.63	1.93
T 2-5	52	1.06	0.35	0.31	0.48	0.63	1.08	1.54	1.70	1.71
T 6-10	123	1.06	0.39	0.23	0.56	0.66	1.00	1.65	1.85	2.04
T 2-10	175	1.06	0.38	0.26	0.55	0.65	1.02	1.58	1.75	1.93
T 2-19	341	0.97	0.40	0.22	0.32	0.48	0.94	1.45	1.70	1.90

◻ Table A2.48

Ratios of maximal projections. M, male; F, female; T, total[d]: Magnitude is in mV

	X terminal right/X left						Y terminal superior/Y interior					Z anterior/Z posterior							
	n	Mean mag.	SD	P_{50}	P_{90}	P_{95}	Mean mag.	SD	P_{50}	P_{90}	P_{95}	n	Mean mag.	SD	P_5	P_{10}	P_{50}	P_{90}	P_{95}
Frank-lead system																			
M 11-15	62	0.23	0.21	0.18	0.63	0.75	0.10	0.12	0.06	0.28	0.42	62	0.57	0.28	0.21	0.24	0.52	0.94	1.11
M 16-19	30	0.29	0.46	0.15	0.53	1.55	0.14	0.13	0.11	0.30	0.43	29	0.54	0.24	0.21	0.25	0.50	0.92	0.97
M 11-19	92	0.25	0.31	0.17	0.55	0.75	0.11	0.12	0.08	0.28	0.28	91	0.56	0.27	0.21	0.26	0.50	0.94	1.04
F 11-15	42	0.26	0.40	0.13	0.71	0.83	0.08	0.13	0.02	0.21	0.46	42	0.85	1.44	0.15	0.17	0.56	1.35	1.98
F 16-19	32	0.23	0.25	0.12	0.65	0.88	0.12	0.13	0.09	0.29	0.28	32	0.63	0.50	0.13	0.16	0.49	1.47	1.95
F 11-19	74	0.25	0.34	0.13	0.69	0.84	0.10	0.13	0.03	0.26	0.43	74	0.76	1.13	0.14	0.17	0.50	1.33	1.94
F 11-15	104	0.24	0.30	0.15	0.67	0.75	0.09	0.12	0.04	0.26	0.43	104	0.68	0.94	0.18	0.22	0.53	1.10	1.36
T 16-19	62	0.26	0.37	0.13	0.55	0.85	0.13	0.13	0.11	0.29	0.32	61	0.59	0.40	0.15	0.21	0.50	1.11	1.53
Total	166	0.25	0.32	0.15	0.59	0.75	0.10	0.12	0.06	0.27	0.40	165	0.65	0.79	0.18	0.22	0.50	1.10	1.36

◻ Table A2.49

Maximal spatial angles and magnitudes- QRS + T. M, male; F, female; T, total[d]: Magnitude is in mV

	n		β	D	χ	Mean Mag.	SD	$P_{2.5}$	P_5	P_{10}	P_{50}	P_{90}	P_{96}	$P_{97.5}$
Frank-lead system														
QRS														
M 2-5	23	347	129	0.85	49.5	1.73	0.60		0.83	1.87	1.81	2.59	2.74	
M 6-10	60	327	133	0.85	130.7	1.83	0.53	1.00	1.11	1.14	1.77	2.67	2.93	3.15
M 2-10	83	332	133	0.84	177.6	1.80	0.55	0.85	0.96	1.11	1.80	2.59	2.81	3.05
F 2-5	29	341	133	0.83	59.4	1.72	0.44		1.02	1.15	1.69	2.13	2.66	
F 6-10	63	336	138	0.90	152.1	1.79	0.43	1.08	1.12	1.15	1.76	2.36	2.60	2.80
F 2-10	92	338	136	0.87	210.9	1.76	0.43	1.07	1.11	1.15	1.76	2.31	2.58	2.81
T 2-5	52	344	131	0.83	108.6	1.72	0.51	0.83	0.88	1.01	1.76	2.40	2.70	2.97
T 6-10	123	331	136	0.87	281.3	1.81	0.48	1.07	1.11	1.15	1.76	2.43	2.77	2.93
T 2-10	175	335	135	0.86	387.5	1.78	0.49	0.95	1.06	1.13	1.76	2.42	2.75	2.89
T 2-19	341	334	136	0.87	772.9	1.71	0.48	0.91	1.02	1.12	1.69	2.31	2.59	2.82

◻ Table A2.49   (Continued)

	n		β	D	χ	Mean Mag.	SD	$P_{2.5}$	P_5	P_{10}	P_{50}	P_{90}	P_{96}	$P_{97.5}$
T wave														
M 2-5	22	33	123	0.89	51.7	0.48	0.15		0.18	0.25	0.53	0.68	0.72	
M 6-10	58	360	128	0.93	149.2	0.54	0.18	0.22	0.27	0.32	0.49	0.79	0.83	1.00
M 2-10	80	352	127	0.90	195.3	0.52	0.17	0.20	0.25	0.31	0.51	0.76	0.79	0.92
F 2-5	29	341	121	0.91	72.3	0.51	0.18		0.25	0.28	0.51	0.81	0.90	
F 6-10	62	0	132	0.91	153.4	0.51	0.20	0.18	0.23	0.28	0.51	0.77	0.93	1.11
F 2-10	91	354	129	0.90	220.6	0.51	0.19	0.21	0.23	0.28	0.51	0.78	0.89	1.03
T 2-5	51	338	122	0.90	123.6	0.50	0.17	0.18	0.23	0.28	0.53	0.68	0.82	0.93
T 6-10	120	360	130	0.92	302.2	0.52	0.19	0.21	0.25	0.29	0.51	0.78	0.83	1.05
T 2-10	171	353	128	0.90	415.9	0.52	0.18	0.21	0.24	0.29	0.51	0.77	0.82	0.96
T 2-19	335	5	130	0.88	781.6	0.48	0.18	0.18	0.21	0.28	0.48	0.72	0.79	0.94

◻ Table A2.50

Normal values – magnitudes – Frank scalars (atrial)[f]

Age	Median	n	Mean	SD	p_5	p_{10}	p_{50}	p_{90}	p_{96}
X left (μV)									
Birth–6 months	1.8 months	27	102	37	44	61	100	167	188
6 months–5 years	2.5 years	22	78	26	38	43	76	127	139
5–12 years	8.1 years	42	76	17	47	54	76	95	117
12–19 years	15.6 years	24	69	17	42	46	66	93	97
Entire group	6.6 years	115	81	27	45	51	76	117	134
Y interior (μV)									
Birth–6 months	1.8 months	27	114	43	45	62	112	175	189
6 months–5 years	2.5 years	22	134	41	25	64	135	175	191
5–12 years	8.1 years	42	118	47	43	55	114	187	202
12–19 years	15.6 years	24	137	45	55	69	150	171	189
Entire group	6.6 years	115	124	45	48	68	124	179	193
Z interior (μV)									
Birth–6 months	1.8 months	27	41	24	6	11	40	72	92
6 months–5 years	2.5 years	22	45	15	18	22	44	65	76
5–12 years	8.1 years	42	44	16	20	24	43	62	80
12–19 years	15.6 years	24	40	17	18	20	36	67	76
Entire group	6.6 years	115	43	18	18	20	41	65	77
Z posterior (μV)									
birth–6 months	1.8 months	27	40	24	0	18	42	76	85
6 months–5 years	2.5 years	22	32	19	1	14	30	64	67
5–12 years	8.1 years	42	30	16	1	18	27	54	57
12–19 years	15.6 years	24	26	18	1	9	20	57	61
Entire group	6.6 years	115	32	18	0	15	29	58	65

◻ Table A2.50 (Continued)

Age	Median	n	Mean	SD	p_5	p_{10}	p_{50}	P_{90}	p_{96}
Spatial voltage anterior (μV)									
Birth–6 months	1.8 months	27	117	42	52	65	113	182	201
6 months–5 years	2.5 years	22	94	31	50	57	91	145	150
5–12 years	8.1 years	42	93	30	41	53	93	134	150
12–19 years	15.6 years	24	109	37	42	65	104	168	173
Entire group	6.6 years	115	102	36	50	60	99	151	167
Spatial voltage posterior (μV)									
Birth–6 months	1.8 months	27	109	58	0	0	110	189	196
6 months–5 years	2.5 years	22	113	58	3	23	115	195	213
5–12 years	8.1 years	42	85	38	2	35	82	126	157
12–19 years	15.6 years	24	84	44	7	39	68	160	179
Entire group	6.6 years	115	36	50	0	30	92	166	185

◻ Table A2.51

Normal values (timing) – Frank scalars (atrial)[f]

Age	Median	n	Mean	SD	p_5	p_{10}	p_{50}	p_{90}	p_{96}
P duration (ms)									
Birth–6 months	1.8 months	27	63	12	44	48	65	85	89
6 months–5 years	2.5 years	22	77	9	58	64	78	90	92
5–12 years	8.1 years	42	85	8	67	77	84	95	102
12–19 years	15.6 years	24	91	10	75	77	91	103	114
Entire group	6.6 years	115	80	14	55	60	82	95	100
PR interval (ms)									
Birth–6 months	1.8 months	27	107	13	84	87	108	124	126
6 months–5 years	2.5 years	22	125	15	97	108	125	146	146
5–12 years	8.1 years	42	137	20	107	112	133	161	161
12–19 years	15.6 years	24	144	17	108	126	140	165	165
Entire group	6.6 years	115	120	21	91	101	130	160	160
Macruz index									
birth–6 months	1.8 months	27	1.58	0.61	0.82	0.91	1.41	2.72	3.23
6 months–5 years	2.5 years	22	1.80	0.80	1.10	1.13	1.56	3.46	3.99
5–12 years	8.1 years	42	1.81	0.58	0.89	1.08	1.75	2.76	2.89
12–19 years	15.6 years	24	1.93	0.77	0.92	1.19	1.85	2.68	4.18
Entire group	6.6 years	115	1.78	0.68	0.91	1.13	1.61	2.67	3.05

⬛ Table A2.51 (Continued)

Age	Median	n	Mean	SD	p_5	p_{10}	p_{50}	p_{90}	p_{96}
Time maximal anterior (%)									
Birth–6 months	1.8 months	27	39	11	19	23	40	52	64
6 months–5 years	2.5 years	22	34	17	20	25	35	43	45
5–12 years	8.1 years	42	38	9	27	28	37	51	56
12–19 years	15.6 years	24	37	7	26	27	37	48	51
Entire group	6.6 years	115	37	9	24	27	37	48	53
Time ant.-post. shift (%)									
Birth–6 months	1.8 months	27	59	14	32	42	54	76	96
6 months–5 years	2.5 years	22	57	13	40	42	57	83	87
5–12 years	8.1 years	42	61	10	44	48	59	85	91
12–19 years	15.6 years	24	62	14	44	48	59	85	91
Entire group	6.6 years	115	60	12	43	47	58	78	84

(a) Strong, W.B., T.F. Downs, J. Liebman, and R. Liebowitz, The normal adolescent electrocardiogram. *Am. Heart J.*, 1972;**83**: 115. The tables are reproduced with the permission of Mosby, St Louis, Missouri.

(b) Sreenivasan, V.V., B.J. Fisher, J. Liebman, and T.D. Downs, A longitudinal study of the standard electrocardiogram in the healthy premature infant during the first year of life. *Am. J. Cardiol.*, 1973;**31**: 57. The tables are reproduced with the permission of Yorke Medical Group, New York.

(c) Namin, E.P., R.A. Arcilla, I.A. D'Cruz, and B.M. Gasul, Evolution of the Frank vectorcardiogram in normal infants. *Am. J. Cardiol.*, 1964;**13**: 757. The tables are reproduced with the permission of Yorke Medical Group, New York.

(d) Kan, J.S., J. Liebman, M.H. Lee, and A. Whitney, Quantification of the normal Frank and McFee-Parungao orthogonal electrocardiogram at ages two to ten years. *Circulation*, 1977;**55**: 31. The tables are reproduced with the permission of the American Heart Association, Dallas, Texas.

(e) Liebman, J., M.H. Lee, P.S. Rao, and W. McKay, Quantification of the normal and Frank-McFee-Parungao orthogonal electrocardiogram in the adolescent. *Circulation*, 1973;**48**: 735. The tables are reproduced with the permission of the American Heart Association, Dallas, Texas.

(f) Ferrer, P.L. and R.C. Ellison, The Frank scalar atrial vectorcardiogram in normal children. *Am. Heart J.*, 1974;**88**: 467. The tables are reproduced with the permission of Mosby, St Louis, Missouri.

(g) Rautaharju, P.M., A. Davignon, F. Soumis, E. Boiselle, and C. Hoquette, Evolution of QRS- T relationship from birth to adolescence in Frank-lead orthogonal electrocardiograms of 1492 normal children. *Circulation*, 1979;**60**: 196–204. The tables are reproduced with the permission of the American Heart Association, Dallas, Texas.

References

1. Macfarlane, P.W., E.N. Coleman, E.O. Pomphrey, S. McLaughlin, A. Houston, and T. Aitchison, Normal limits of the high-fidelity pediatric ECG. *J. Electrocardiol.*, 1989;**22**(Suppl): 162–168.

2. Macfarlane, P.W., S.C. McLaughlin, and J.C. Rodger, Influence of lead selection and population on automated measurement of QT dispersion. *Circulation*, 1998;**98**: 2160–2167.

Appendix 3: Instrumentation Standards and Recommendations

A3.1   Introduction

All ECG instruments such as direct writing electrocardiographs, cardiac monitors, ambulatory monitoring electrocardiographic devices, stress ECG machines, fetal monitors and other ECG devices that process signals from galvanic biopotential sensors share the same design principles. Modern ECG equipment utilizes integrated digital signal processors (DSP) to perform signal amplification, analog-to-digital conversion, digital filtering, formatting and communication.

This section lists several of the available standards and recommendations related to the design of such instruments. The concepts discussed and their terminology are introduced in ❷ Sect. 12.4 (Vol. 1).

A3.2   General Design Considerations

Electrocardiographs have been optimized to best suit their particular application. The function of the analog processor is to form an ECG lead signal, amplify it, eliminate the common mode noise, and minimize the external interference.

The front-end, which is responsible for processing of the body surface potentials must be able to work with low voltage alternating current (AC) signals ranging from 0.01 to 5.0 mV, combined with a direct current (DC) common-mode component of up to ±300 mV resulting from the electrode–skin interface and a common-mode noise of up to 1.5 V AC.

The bandwidth of the electrocardiograph depends on the application and can range from 50 Hz for monitoring applications to 1 kHz for late-potential measurements. The bandwidth is of great importance in ECG diagnosis since many interpretation criteria are based on exact measurements of small notches and slurs. The faithful reproduction of the lower frequency regions, such as the ST segment, is essential since these have a critical diagnostic value. Many studies have been carried out for determining the frequency content of the adult and pediatric ECGs. The American Heart Association (AHA) recommends 150 Hz as minimum bandwidth and 500 Hz as minimum sampling rate for recording adult and pediatric ECGs. The report also states that it is unknown how far the bandwidth of systems may need to be extended, due to limitations of previous studies [1].

The analog ECG signal is then sampled and converted into digital data (❷ Sect. 12.A). In modern electrocardiographs, the sampling rate is usually much higher than is required by the Nyquist criterion and may be as high as 50 kHz in some cases (❷ Sect. 12.A.1.2). The advantage of sampling at such a high rate is the elimination of the need for using anti-aliasing filters at the front-end and to facilitate the reduction of noise in the input signal by computing running averages.

Rijnbeek et al. [2] reported on normal ECG features observed when using the higher sampling rate of 1,200 sps. On the basis of this study, a minimum bandwidth of 250 Hz for recording pediatric ECGs was recommended. He showed that with a bandwidth of 150 Hz, 38% of the cases in the study had an error >25 μV in the maximum positive deflection in lead V4. For leads V2 and V6, these percentages were 25% and 23%, respectively. Furthermore, 15% of the positive deflections and 7% of the negative deflections in V4 have amplitude errors >50 μV when a 150 Hz filter is used. The effect of age on the frequency content of the ECG signals was also addressed. It was found that the frequency content gradually decreases from infancy to adulthood. The data for children aged 12 to 16 years indicate that the system bandwidth should be 150 Hz to yield amplitude errors less than 25μV in 95% of the cases in this age group. This is close to the 125 Hz recommendation of the AHA for the adult ECG [3]. In vectorcardiographic leads, Berson et al. [4] found amplitude errors >50 μV in 8% of the R-wave amplitudes and 5% of the S-wave amplitudes when using a 150 Hz filter.

The differences between the results of the two studies may, in part, be explained by the difference in the sampling rates used (500 versus 1,200 sps) and by the use of different lead systems. Furthermore, the analyses by Berson et al. [4] were not performed on separate leads but on leads X, Y, and Z combined, which is likely to underestimate the effect of filtering on individual lead signals. More importantly, it was concluded that a threshold of 25 μV instead of 50 μV is preferable for measuring the effect of a reduced bandwidth on signal amplitudes.

Rijnbeek recommended using the minimum bandwidth of 250 Hz for the entire pediatric population. The higher bandwidth demands the sampling rate to be at least twice the bandwidth of the signal (❷ Sect. 12.A.2). In order to facilitate a high quality data representation, the AHA recommends a sampling rate of at least two or three times this theoretical minimum. As a rule of thumb, the pediatric ECG should be sampled at least at 1,000 samples per second.

A3.2.1 FDA Performance Standards

All diagnostic pieces of ECG equipment are classified by the Federal Drug Administration as Class II devices. Hence their design is subject both to safety and performance standards. These standards have been developed by the American Association of Medical Instrumentation and adopted by the American National Standards Institute as ANSI/AAMI EC11:1991/(R)2001. The standards establish minimum safety and performance requirements for ECG systems with direct-writing devices that are intended for use under the operating conditions specified. Also included are standards for the analysis of rhythm and of detailed morphology of complex cardiac complexes. Subject to this standard are all parts of the ECG system necessary to (a) obtain the signal from the surface of the patient's body, (b) amplify this signal, and (c) display it in a form suitable for diagnosing the heart's electrical activity. Hence, this standard includes requirements for the entire electrocardiographic recording system, ranging from the input electrodes right up to the displayed output.

Included within the scope of this standard are:

1. Direct-writing electrocardiographs.
2. Electrocardiographs used in other medical devices (e.g., patient monitors, defibrillators, stress testing devices), when such devices are intended for use in obtaining diagnostic ECG signatures.
3. Electrocardiographs having a display that is remote from the patient (via cable, telephone, telemetry, or storage media), when such devices are intended for use in obtaining ECG signatures. These devices are subject to the functional performance requirements at the system output-input levels.

Excluded from the scope of this standard are:

1. Devices that collect ECG data from locations other than the external surface of the body
2. Devices for interpretation and pattern recognition (e.g., QRS detectors, alarm circuits, rate meters, diagnostic algorithms)
3. Fetal ECG monitors
4. Ambulatory monitoring electrocardiographic devices, including ECG recorders and associated scanning and read-out devices
5. Diagnostic electrocardiographic devices utilizing non-permanent displays
6. Vectorcardiographs, that is, a device for displaying loops derived from X,Y,Z leads (see ❯ Chap. 11 of *Basic Electrocardiology: Cardiac Electrophysiology, ECG Systems and Mathematical Modeling*)
7. Electrocardiographic devices intended for use under extreme or uncontrolled environmental conditions outside of a hospital environment or physician's office
8. Cardiac monitorsl

See FDA: http://www.fda.gov/cdrh/ode/ecgs.pdf for further details

A3.2.2 Guidance for Diagnostic ECG

The Industry Diagnostic ECG Guidance (including Non-Alarming ST Segment Measurement) was issued on November 5, 1998. This guidance applies to most of the diagnostic electrocardiographs covered by the ANSI/AAMI EC11-1991 standard for Electrocardiographs (EC-11 standard). Included in the EC-11 standard are ECG devices intended for diagnostic purposes.

The Guidance for Industry, Cardiac Monitors (including Cardiotachometer and Rate Alarm) was issued on: November 5, 1998. See

http://www.fda.gov/cdrh/ode/cmonitor.pdf

This guidance applies to most of the cardiac monitors covered by the ANSI/AAMI EC13-1992 standard for Cardiac Monitors, Heart Rate Meters, and Alarms (EC13 standard). Included in the EC13 standard are ECG devices intended for monitoring purposes.

A3.2.3 Typical Design Specifications for an Electrocardiograph

Sampling rate:

- Digital sampling rate: 4,000 sps/channel
- 10,000 samples/s/channel used for pacemaker spike detection
- ECG analysis frequency: 500 sps

Dynamic range:

- AC differential: ±10 mV DC offset: ±320 mV
- Resolution: 4.88 µV/LSB @ 500 sps
- Frequency response: −3 dB @ 0.01–150 Hz
- Common mode rejection: >140 dB (123 dB with AC filter disabled)
- Input impedance: >10 MΩ @ 10 Hz, defibrillator protected
- Patient leakage: <10 µA
- Pace detect: Orthogonal LA, LL and V6; 750 µV @ 50 µs

Communication:

- Modem and Fax transmission, WI-FI wireless 802.11X

Writers:

- Writer technology: Thermal dot array
- Writer speeds: 5, 12.5, 25 and 50 mm/s (same as displayed)
- Number of traces: 3, 6, 12 or 15, user selectable (same as displayed)
- Writer sensitivity/gain: 2.5, 5, 10, 20, 10/5 (split calibration) mm/mV (same as displayed)
- Writer speed accuracy: ±2%
- Writer amplitude accuracy: ±5%
- Writer resolution: Horizontal: 1,000 dpi @ 25 mm/s, Vertical: 200 dpi

Electrical power:

- Power supply: AC or battery operation
- Voltage: 100–240 VAC +10, −15%
- Current: 0.5A @ 115 VAC, 0.3 A @ 240 VAC, typical
- Mains Frequency: 50–60 Hz ± 10%
- Battery type: User replaceable, 18 V @ 3.5 AH ± 15%, rechargeable NiMH

A3.2.4 Typical Performance Requirements for Cardiac Monitors

Cardiac monitors, with or without heart rate meters and alarms, are intended primarily for detecting cardiac rhythm and are covered by the ANSI/AAMI standard for cardiac monitors, heart rate meters and alarms – ANSI/AAMI EC 13-2002. A separate AAMI standard EC 38-1998 covers the Ambulatory Electrocardiographs. The objective of these standards was to provide minimum labeling, performance, and safety requirements and to help ensure a reasonable level of clinical efficacy and patient safety in the use of cardiac monitors. With the few exceptions noted below, performance and disclosure requirements in that standard remain appropriate.

  In one section, the standard defines performance requirements, specifying a minimum, a maximum or a range of values, as applicable, that must be met. A separate section lists several performance parameters without specifying values; the requirement is for disclosure of the achieved value to the consumer in a standardized manner. For example, a minimum heart rate meter accuracy for irregular rhythms is not specified, but the accuracy of detecting several types of defined ECG complexes must be disclosed. Designation of specifications as either performance requirements or disclosures is appropriate. The reader is referred to standard-10 for further details, including test procedures and rationale. Below is a partial listing of some important parameters in each category:

1. Protection from overload: Protection should be adequate (no damage) for 1 V (peak to peak), 60 Hz, applied for 10 s to any electrode connection. The device should recover within 8 s after defibrillation shocks of up to at least 5,000 V, delivered with energies up to 360 J.
2. Isolated patient connection: The system should include isolated patient connections to meet standards defined in the publication: American National Standard for Safe Current Limits for Electromedical Apparatus: 11.

The American Heart Association has also published its own set of instrumentation and practice standards for electrocardiographic monitoring in coronary care units, intensive care units, telemetry units, surgical suites, emergency rooms, and all other areas in which ECG monitoring functions are performed. These were directed primarily at the cardiac monitors that detect and diagnose arrhythmias and also at those that detect ST segment changes that suggest myocardial ischemia. The AHA felt that specific guidelines for ECG monitors are required, even though much of the technology is similar to other forms of ECG measurement. The clinical environment, including severity and acuteness of illness and immediacy of treatment, combined with limited time for over-reading and editing, and initiation of urgent therapy by non-physicians mandate more critical evaluation of automated arrhythmia detection and diagnostic systems.

A3.2.5 Typical Specifications for the ECG Monitoring Devices

Frequency response	−3 dB @ 0.01–150 Hz
Sampling Frequency	500 samples per second (sps)
Dynamic range	AC differential: ±10 mV
	DC offset: ±320 mV
Resolution	4.88 µV/LSB @ 500 sps
Common mode rejection	>140 dB
Input impedance	>10MΩ@10 Hz, defibrillator protected
Patient leakage current	<10 µA
Pace detect	750 µV @ 50 µs
Front-end circuits	See below

To ensure correct operation with typical electrode-skin impedances and typical interference sources, the front-end of an electrocardiograph should meet the following demands:

- Very high common mode input impedance (>100 MΩ at 50/60 Hz)
- High differential mode input impedance (>10 MΩ at 50/60 Hz)
- Equal common mode input impedances for all inputs
- High common mode rejection ratio (>80 dB at 50/60 Hz)

A3.3 Patient Safety Standards

Power-line–operated electromedical equipment, connected to patients for monitoring, may permit accidental flow (leakage) of weak alternating current (AC) through a patient's body to ground. An intracardiac catheter may provide a low-resistance path to ground through the patient's heart and thereby place the patient at risk for electrically induced ventricular tachycardia (VT) or ventricular fibrillation (VF).

In addition to the performance standards, the Safe Current Limits for Electromedical Apparatus (ANSI/AAMI ES1-1993) standards apply to all electrocardiograph designs. It states that: "The electrocardiographic (ECG) or vectorcardiographic apparatus shall be designed so that no more than 50 µA root mean square, from direct current component to the tenth harmonic of the power line frequency shall flow through any patient-connected lead under either normal or single-fault conditions." This raised the limit from 10 to 50 µA [5], the value of the European standard since 1988 [6]. Both the 10-µA standard [7, 8] and the 50-µA standard were based on estimates of the risk of AC-induced VF. However, AC may cause cardiovascular collapse at levels that are below the VF threshold [9–13]. This adverse response to AC was not considered in the selection of either safety standard. Furthermore, safe levels of AC have not been determined in closed-chest humans.

The 10-µA standard was adopted in 1967 to ensure patient safety during cardiac catheterization [14] and pacemaker [15] procedures. The annual number of invasive cardiac procedures in the United States has increased from less than 60,000 when the 10-µA standard was adopted to more than 3 million today. The potential number of adverse outcomes from leakage current increased correspondingly.

Electromedical devices contain electrical isolation circuits and insulation to limit leakage current. Manufacturers continue to comply with the original 10-µA standard, but they may realize substantial cost savings by equipment designs that comply only with the newer 50-µA standard [16]. However, the American Heart Association continues to recommend the 10-µA standard [17–19].

A3.4   Recommendations for the Standardization and Interpretation of the Electrocardiogram

Around 2005, the American Heart Association, the American College of Cardiology Foundation and the Heart Rhythm Society agreed to collaborate on the establishment of a series of recommendations for the standardization and interpretation of the ECG. A number of working groups were set up and over the next few years, various publications emerged on the topic. These were all endorsed by the International Society for Computerized Electrocardiology. The six papers form an important contribution to the field and are recommended as essential reading for anyone interested in the development of diagnostic criteria, particularly for computer assisted interpretation of the ECG.

The titles of the different papers are self explanatory and there is no need to expand on the content. However, it is worth mentioning that the first paper [20] is wide ranging and includes many aspects of ECG recording through electrode positioning to requirements for digital filters. The other papers deal with terminology [21], intraventricular conduction disturbances [22], the ST Segment, T and U Waves, and the QT Interval [23], cardiac chamber hypertrophy [24] and acute ischemia/infarction [25].

It is also relevant to highlight again the guidelines published over 30 years ago in a paper [8] entitled "Recommendations for standardization of leads and their specifications for instruments in electrocardiography and vectorcardiography," which still contains many points that are of relevance in this area.

A3.5   Guidelines

A3.5.1   Heart Rate Variability

A Task Force of the European Society of Cardiology and the North American Society of Pacing and Electrophysiology produced a guideline paper relating to heart rate variability [26]. The paper dealt with standards of measurement, physiological interpretation and clinical use.

A3.5.2 Electrocardiographic Monitoring in Hospital Settings

A scientific statement for the American Heart Association Councils on Cardiovascular Nursing, Clinical Cardiology and Cardiovascular disease in the young, dealing with electrocardiographic monitoring in hospital settings was published in 2004 [27]. This sets out recommendations for the different types of monitoring that are necessary in the hospital environment, ranging from arrhythmia analysis through to ischemia monitoring and QT interval assessment. Different types of ECG lead systems for monitoring are described and recommendations relating to staffing, training and quality improvement are given.

A3.5.3 Recommendations for Ambulatory Electrocardiography

A paper on instrumentation and ambulatory electrocardiography published as a set of recommendations was published in 1985 [28]. Much of the information there is still of relevance although equipment is now predominantly based around digital recording techniques. A follow up paper was published in 1999 [29]. These more recent guidelines review equipment and also deal with assessment of symptoms that may be related to disturbances of rhythm and assessment of risk in patients without symptoms of arrhythmias.

A3.5.4 Exercise Testing

Guidelines for clinical exercise testing laboratories were published in 1995 [30]. These outlined the environment in which exercise testing should be undertaken and discussed equipment requirements, etc. Clinical guidelines were published in 1997 [31] and updated in 2002 [32]. These papers essentially deal with the conditions under which exercise testing is deemed to be appropriate.

A3.5.5 Clinical Competence

The ACC and AHA issued a statement on competence for reporting ECGs and ambulatory ECGs [33]. This publication outlines the diagnostic areas where physicians are expected to have a high degree of competence in reporting resting and ambulatory ECGs.

A3.5.6 Pacemakers/Electrophysiology Testing

One of the earliest guidelines on electrophysiology testing and pacemakers was published in 1984 [34]. This outlined the three position and the five position coding scheme for pacemakers. This was updated in 2002 [35]. A paper on guidelines for implantation of pacemakers, which was published in 2002 [36], contained earlier 1998 guidelines together with updated guidelines.

References

1. Kligfield, P., L.S. Gettes, J.J. Bailey, et al., Recommendations for the standardization and interpretation of the electrocardiogram: Part I: the electrocardiogram and its technology. A scientific statement from the American Heart Association Electrocardiography and Arrhythmias Committee, Council on Clinical Cardiology; the American College of Cardiology Foundation; and the Heart Rhythm Society Endorsed by the International Society for Computerized Electrocardiology. *Circulation*, 2007;**115**(10).

2. Rijnbeek, P.R., J.A. Kors, and M. Witsenburg, Minimum bandwidth requirements for recording of pediatric electrocardiograms. *Circulation*, 2001;**104**(25): 3087–3090.

3. Bailey, J.J., A.S. Berson, A. Garson, Jr., L.G. Horan, P.W. Macfarlane, D.W. Mortara, and C. Zywietz, Recommendations for standardization and specifications in automated electrocardiography: bandwidth and digital signal processing. *Circulation*, 1990;**81**: 730–739.

4. Berson, A.S., Y.K. Francis, B.A. Lau, J.M. Wojick, and H.V. Pipberger, Distortions in infant electrocardiograms caused by inadequate high-frequency response. *Am. Heart J.*, 1977;**93**: 730–734.

5. *Safe Current Limits for Electromedical Apparatus.* 1993, Association for the Advancement of Medical Instrumentation.

6. Medical Electrical Equipment- Part 1: General Requirements for Safety in Collateral Standard: Electromagnetic Compatibility – Requirements and Test. 1993.

7. Pipberger, H.V., R.C. Arzbaecher, A.S. Berson, et al., Amendment of recommendations for standardization of specifications for instruments in electrocardiography and vectorcardiography concerning safety and electrical shock hazards. 1972; Committee of Electrocardiography, American Heart Association. *Circulation*, 1972;**46**: 1–2.

8. Pipberger, H.V., R.C. Arzbaecher, A.S. Berson, et al., Recommendations for standardization of leads and of specifications for instruments in electrocardiography and vectorcardiography. 1975. Committee on Electrocardiography, American Heart Association. *Circulation*, 1975;**52**: 11–31.

9. Green, H., E.B. Raftery, and I.C. Gregory, Ventricular fibrillation threshold of healthy dogs to 50 Hz current in relation to earth leakage currents of electromedical equipment. *Biomed. Eng.*, 1972;**7**: 408–414.

10. Raftery, E., H. Green, and I. Gregory, Disturbances of heart rhythm produced by 50 Hz leakage currents in dogs. *Cardiovasc. Res.*, 1975;**9**: 256–262.

11. Raftery, E.B., H.L. Green, and M.H. Yacoub, Disturbances of heart rhythm produced by 50 Hz leakage currents in human subjects. *Cardiovasc. Res.*, 1975;**9**: 263–265.

12. Roy, O.Z., J.R. Scott, and G.C. Park, 60 Hz ventricular fibrillations and pump failure thresholds versus electrode area. *IEEE Eng. Med. Biol.*, 1976;**BME-23**: 45–48.

13. Graystone, P. and J. Ledsome, Microshock hazards in hospital: fibrillation thresholds: the wrong parameter, in *Digest of the 10th International Conference on Medical and Biologic Engineering*, Dresden, Germany, 1973.

14. Weinberg, D.I., J.L.D. Artley, R.E. Whalen, and H.D. Mcintosh, Electric shock hazards in cardiac catheterization. *Circ. Res.*, 1962;**11**: 1004–1009.

15. Whalen, R.E., C.F. Starmer, and H.D. McIntosh, Electrical hazards associated with cardiac pacemaking. *Ann. NY Acad. Sci.*, 1964;**111**: 922–931.

16. Bruner, J.M.R. and P.F. Leonard, Codes and standards: who makes the rules?, in *Electricity, Safety and the Patient*. Chicago: Year Book Medical Publishers, 1989, pp. 240–279.

17. Laks, M.M., R. Arzbaecher, D. Geselowitz, et al., Will relaxing safe current limits for electromedical equipment increase hazards to patients? *Circulation*, 2000;**102**: 823.

18. Laks, M.M., R. Arzbaecher, J.J. Bailey, et al., Recommendations for safe current limits for electrocardiographs: a statement for healthcare professionals from the Committee of Electrocardiography; American Heart Association. *Circulation*, 1996;**93**: 837–839.

19. Laks, M.M., R. Arzbaecher, J.J. Bailey, et al., Comments on "Special report: recommendations for safe current limits for electrocardiographs". *Circulation*, 1997;**95**: 277–278.

20. Kligfield, P., L.S. Gettes, J.J. Bailey, et al., AHA/ACC/HRS recommendations for the standardization and interpretation of the electrocardiogram. Part I: The electrocardiogram and its technology. A scientific statement From the American Heart Association Electrocardiography and Arrhythmias Committee, Council on Clinical Cardiology; the American College of Cardiology Foundation; and the Heart Rhythm Society (Endorsed by the International Society for Computerized Electrocardiology). *J. Am. Coll. Cardiol.*, 2007;**49**: 1109–1127, doi:10.1016/j.jacc.2007.01.024.

21. Mason, J.W., E.W. Hancock, and L.S. Gettes, AHA/ACC/HRS recommendations for the standardization and interpretation of the electrocardiogram. Part II: Electrocardiography diagnostic statement list. A scientific statement from the American Heart Association Electrocardiography and Arrhythmias Committee, Council on Clinical Cardiology; the American College of Cardiology Foundation; and the Heart Rhythm Society. (Endorsed by the International Society for Computerized Electrocardiology). *J. Am. Coll. Cardiol.*, 2007;**49**: 1128–1135, doi:10.1016/j.jacc.2007.01.025.

22. Surawicz, B., R. Childers, B.J. Deal, and L.S. Gettes, AHA/ACC/HRS recommendations for the standardization and interpretation of the electrocardiogram. Part III: Intraventricular conduction disturbances. A scientific statement from the American Heart Association Electrocardiography and Arrhythmias Committee, Council on Clinical Cardiology; the American College of Cardiology Foundation; and the Heart Rhythm Society. (Endorsed by the International Society for Computerized Electrocardiology). *J. Am. Coll. Cardiol.*, 2009;**53**: 976–981, doi:10.1016/j.jacc.2008.12.013.

23. Rautaharju, P.M., B. Surawicz, and L.S. Gettes, AHA/ACCF/HRS recommendations for the standardization and interpretation of the electrocardiogram. Part IV: The ST segment, T and U waves, and the QT interval. A scientific statement from the American Heart Association Electrocardiography and Arrhythmias Committee, Council on Clinical Cardiology; the American College of Cardiology Foundation; and the Heart Rhythm Society. (Endorsed by the International Society for Computerized Electrocardiology). *J. Am. Coll. Cardiol.*, 2009;**53**: 982–991, doi:10.1016/j.jacc.2008.12.014.

24. Hancock, E.W., B.J. Deal, D.M. Mirvis, et al., AHA/ACCF/HRS recommendations for the standardization and interpretation of the electrocardiogram. Part V: Electrocardiogram changes associated with cardiac chamber hypertrophy. A scientific statement from the American Heart Association Electrocardiography and Arrhythmias Committee, Council on Clinical Cardiology; the American College of Cardiology Foundation; and the Heart Rhythm Society. (Endorsed by the International Society for Computerized Electrocardiology). *J. Am. Coll. Cardiol.*, 2009;**53**: 992–1002, doi:10.1016/j.jacc.2008.12.015.

25. Wagner, G.S., P.W. Macfarlane, H. Wellens, et al., AHA/ACCF/HRS recommendations for the standardization and interpretation of the electrocardiogram. Part VI: Acute ischemia/infarction. A scientific statement from the American Heart Association Electrocardiography and Arrhythmias Committee, Council on Clinical Cardiology; the American College of Cardiology Foundation; and the Heart Rhythm Society Endorsed by the International Society for Computerized Electrocardiology. *J. Am. Coll. Cardiol.*, 2009;**53**: 1003–1011, doi:10.1016/j.jacc.2008.12.016.

26. Task Force of the European Society of Cardiology and the North American Society of Pacing Electrophysiology, Heart rate variability. Standards of measurement, physiological interpretation, and clinical use. *Circulation*, 1996;**93**: 1043–1065.

27. Drew, B., R.M. Califf, M. Funk, et al., AHA scientific statement. Practice standards for electrocardiographic monitoring in hospital settings. *Circulation*, 2004;**110**: 2721–2746.

28. Sheffield, L.T., A. Berson, and D. Bragg-Remschel, Recommendations for standards and instrumentation and practice in the use of ambulatory electrocardiography. The Task force of the Committee on Electrocardiography and Cardiac Electrophysiology of the Council on Clinical Cardiology. *Circulation*, 1985;**71**: 626A–636A.

29. Crawford, M.H., S.J. Bernstein, P.C. Deedwania, et al., ACC/AHA guidelines for ambulatory electrocardiography. Executive summary and recommendations: A report of the American College of Cardiology/American Heart Association Task Force on Practice Guidelines (Committee to Revise the Guidelines for Ambulatory Electrocardiography). *Circulation*, 1999;**100**: 886–893.

30. Pina, I.L., G.J. Balady, P. Hanson, A.J. Labovitz, D.W. Madonna, and J. Myers, Guidelines for clinical exercise testing laboratories. A statement for healthcare professionals from the Committee on Exercise and Cardiac Rehabilitation, American Heart Association. *Circulation*, 1995;**91**: 912–921.

31. Gibbons, R., G.J. Balady, J.W. Beasley, et al., ACC/AHA guidelines for exercise testing. A report of the American College of Cardiology/American Heart Association Task Force on Practice Guidelines (Committee on Exercise Testing). *J. Am. Coll. Cardiol.*, 1997;**30**: 260–311.

32. Gibbons, R., G.J. Balady, J.T. Bricker, et al., ACC/AHA 2002 guideline update for exercise testing: summary article. A report of the American College of Cardiology/American Heart Association Task Force on Practice Guidelines (Committee to Update the 1997 Exercise testing Guidelines). *Circulation*, 2002;**106**: 1883–1892.

33. Kadish, A.H., A.E. Buxton, H.L. Kennedy, B.P. Knight, C.D. Schuger, and C.M. Tracy, A report of the ACC/AHA/ACP-ASIM task force on clinical competence (ACC/AHA Committee to develop a clinical competence statement on electrocardiography and ambulatory electrocardiography). *Circulation*, 2001;**104**: 3169–3178.

34. Gettes, L.S., D.P. Zipes, P.C. Gillette, et al., Personnel and equipment required for electrophysiologic testing. Report of the committee on electrocardiography and cardiac electrophysiology, Council on Clinical Cardiology, the American Heart Association. *Circulation*, 1984;**69**: 1219A–1221A.

35. Bernstein, A.D., J.-C. Daubert, R.D. Fletcher, et al., The revised NASPE/BPEG generic code for antibradycardia, adaptive-rate, and multisite pacing. *PACE*, 2002;**25**: 260–264.

36. Gregoratis, G., J. Abrams, A.E. Epstein, et al., ACC/AHA/NASPE 2002 guideline update for implantation of cardiac pacemakers and antiarrhythmia devices: Summary article. A report of the American College of Cardiology/American Heart Association Task Force on Practice Guidelines (ACC/AHA/NASPE Committee to Update the 1998 Pacemaker Guidelines). *Circulation*, 2002;**106**: 2145–2161.

Appendix 4: Coding Schemes

A4.1   The Minnesota Code

The Minnesota code was initially developed and published in 1960 (see Ref. [20] in (❯ Chap. 1 of *Electrocardiology: Comprehensive Clinical ECG*). It remains the most widely used ECG coding scheme in epidemiological practice and has recently been revised and extended. The following section has been reprinted from: Prineas RJ, Crow RS, Zhang Z-M. The Minnesota Code Manual of Electrocardiographic Findings. 2009, with the permission of Springer, New York.

A4.1.1   Minnesota Code 2009

A4.1.1.1   Q and QS Patterns

(Do not code in the presence of Wolff-Parkinson-White (WPW) code 6-4-1), or artificial pacemaker code 6-8 or code 6-1, 8-2-1, 8-2-2, or 8-4-1 with a heart rate $\geq$ 140. To qualify as a Q wave, the deflection should be at least 0.1 mV (1 mm in amplitude).

Anterolateral site (leads I, aVL, V_6)

- 1-1-1   Q/R amplitude ratio $\geq$1/3, plus Q duration $\geq$0.03 s in lead I or V_6.
- 1-1-2   Q duration $\geq$0.04 s in lead I or V_6.
- 1-1-3   Q duration $\geq$0.04 s, plus R amplitude $\geq$3 mm in lead aVL.
- 1-2-1   Q/R amplitude ratio $\geq$1/3, plus Q duration $\geq$0.02 s and <0.03 s in lead I or V_6.
- 1-2-2   Q duration $\geq$0.03 s and <0.04 s in lead I or V_6.
- 1-2-3   QS pattern in lead I. Do not code in the presence of 7-1-1.
- 1-2-8   Initial R amplitude decreasing to 2 mm or less in every beat (and absence of codes 3-2, 7-1-1, 7-2-1 or 7-3) between V_5 and V_6. (All beats in lead V_5 must have an initial R >2 mm.)
- 1-3-1   Q/R amplitude ratio $\geq$1/5 and <1/3, plus Q duration $\geq$0.02 s and <0.03 s in lead I or V_6.
- 1-3-3   Q duration $\geq$0.03 s and <0.04 s, plus R amplitude $\geq$3 mm in lead aVL.
- 1-3-8[1]   Initial R amplitude decreasing to 2 mm or less in every beat (and absence of codes 3-2, 7-1-1, 7-2-1, or 7-3) between V_5 and V_6 (All beats in lead V_5 must have an initial R > 2 mm.)

Posterior (inferior) site (leads II, III, aVF).

- 1-1-1   Q/R amplitude ratio $\geq$1/3, plus Q duration $\geq$0.03 s in lead II.
- 1-1-2   Q duration $\geq$0.04 s in lead II.
- 1-1-4   Q duration $\geq$0.05 s in lead III, plus a Q-wave amplitude $\geq$1.0 mm in the majority of beats in lead aVF.
- 1-1-5   Q duration $\geq$0.05 s in lead aVF.
- 1-2-1   Q/R amplitude ratio $\geq$1/3, plus Q duration $\geq$0.02 s and<0.03 s in lead II.
- 1-2-2   Q duration $\geq$0.03 s and <0.04 s in lead II.
- 1-2-3   QS pattern in lead II. Do not code in the presence of 7-1-1.
- 1-2-4   Q duration $\geq$0.04 s and <0.05 s in lead III, plus a Q wave $\geq$1.0 mm amplitude in the majority of beats in aVF.
- 1-2-5   Q duration $\geq$0.04 s and <0.05 s in lead aVF.
- 1-3-1   Q/R amplitude ratio $\geq$1/5 and <1/3, plus Q duration $\geq$0.02 s and <0.03 s in lead II.
- 1-3-4   Q duration $\geq$0.03 s and <0.04 s in lead III, plus a Q wave $\geq$1.0 mm amplitude in the majority of beats in lead aVF.
- 1-3-5   Q duration $\geq$0.03 s and <0.04 s in lead aVF.
- 1-3-6   QS pattern in each of leads III and aVF. (Do not code in the presence of 7-1-1.)
- 1-3-7[2]   QS pattern in lead a aVF only. (Do not code in the presence of 7-1-1)

Anterior site (leads V_1, V_2, V_3, V_4, V_5)

- 1-1-1   Q/R amplitude ratio ≥1/3 plus Q duration ≥0.03 s in any of leads V_2, V_3,V_4,V_5.
- 1-1-2   Q duration ≥0.04 s in any of leads V_1, V_2, V_3, V_4, V_5.
- 1-1-6   QS pattern when initial R wave is present in adjacent lead to the right on the chest, in any of leads V_2, V_3, V_4, V_5, V_6.
- 1-1-7   QS pattern in all of leads V_1–V_4 or V_1–V_5.
- 1-2-1   Q/R amplitude ratio ≥1/3, plus Q duration ≥0.02 s and <0.03 s, in any leads V_2, V_3, V_4, V_5.
- 1-2-2   Q duration ≥0.03 s and <0.04 s in any leads V_2, V_3, V_4, V_5.
- 1-2-7   QS pattern in all of lead V_1, V_2, and V_3. (Do not code in the presence of 7-1-1.)
- 1-3-1   Q/R amplitude ratio ≥1/5 and <1/3 plus Q duration ≥0.02 s and <0.03 s in any of leads V_2, V_3, V_4, V_5.
- 1-3-2   QS pattern in lead V_1 and V_2. (Do not code in the presence of 3-1 or 7-1-1.)
- 1-3-8[1]   Initial R amplitude decreasing to 2.0 mm or less in every beat (and absence of codes 3-2, 7-1-1, 7-2-1, or 7-3) between any of leads V_2 and V_3, V_3, and V_4, or V_4 and V_5. (All beats in the lead immediately to the right on the chest must have an initial R > 2 mm.)

A4.1.1.2   QRS Axis Deviation

(Do not code in presence of low-voltage QRS code 9-1, WPW 6-4-1, artificial pacemaker code 6-8, ventricular conduction defects 7-1-1, 7-2-1, 7-4 or 7-8.)

- 2-1   Left. QRS axis from −30° through −90° in leads I, II, III. (The algebraic sum of major positive and major negative QRS waves must be 0 or positive in I, negative in III, and 0 or negative in II).
- 2-2   Right. QRS axis from +120° through −150° in leads I, II, III. (The algebraic sum of major positive and major negative QRS waves must be negative in I, and zero or positive in III, and in I must be one half or more of that in III.)
- 2-3   Right (optional code when 2-2 is not present). QRS axis from +90° through +119° in leads I, II, III. (The algebraic sum of major positive and major negative QRS waves must be zero or negative in I and positive in II and III.)
- 2-4   Extreme axis deviation (usually S1, S2, S3 pattern). QRS axis from −90° through −149° in leads I, II and III. (The algebraic sum of major positive and major negative QRS waves must be negative in each of leads I, II and III.)
- 2-5   Indeterminate axis. QRS axis approximately 90° from the frontal plane. (The algebraic sum of major positive and major negative QRS waves is zero in each of leads I, II and III, or the information from these three leads is incongruous.)

A4.1.1.3   High-Amplitude R Waves

Do not code in the presence of codes 6-4-1, 6-8, 7-1-1, 7-2-1, 7-4, or 7-8.

- 3-1   Left: R amplitude >26 mm in either V_5 or V_6, or R amplitude >20.0 mm in any of leads I, II, III, aVF, or R amplitude >12.0 mm in lead aVL measured only on second to last complete normal beat.

- 3-2 Right: R amplitude ≥5.0 mm and R amplitude ≥S amplitude in the majority of beats in lead V_1, when S amplitude is >R amplitude somewhere to the left on the chest of V_1 (codes 7-3 and 3-2, if criteria for both are present).
- 3-3 Left (optional code when 3-1 is not present): R amplitude >15.0 mm but ≤20.0 mm in lead I, or R amplitude in V_5 or V_6, plus S amplitude in V_1 > 35.0 mm.
- 3-4 Criteria for 3-1 and 3-2 both present.

A4.1.1.4   ST Junction (J) and Segment Depression

(Do not code in the presence of codes 6-4-1, 6-8, 7-1-1, 7-2-1, 7-4, or 7-8. When 4-1, 4-2, or 4-3 is coded, then a 5-code most often must also be assigned except in lead V_1.)

Anterolateral site (leads I, aVL, V_6)

- 4-1-1 STJ depression ≥2.0 mm and ST segment horizontal or downward sloping in any of leads I, aVL, or V_6
- 4-1-2 STJ depression ≥1.0 mm but <2.0 mm, and ST segment horizontal or downward sloping in any of leads I, aVL, or V_6
- 4-2 STJ depression ≥0.5 mm and <1.0 mm and ST segment horizontal or downward sloping in any of leads I, aVL, or V_6
- 4-3 No STJ depression as much as 0.5 mm but ST segment downward sloping and segment or T-wave nadir ≥0.5 mm below P-R baseline, in any of leads I, aVL, or V_6
- 4-4 STJ depression ≥1.0 mm and ST segment upward sloping or U-shaped, in any of leads I, aVL, or V_6

Posterior (inferior) site (leads II, III, aVF)

- 4-1-1 STJ depression ≥2.0 mm and ST segment horizontal or downward sloping in lead II or aVF
- 4-1-2 STJ depression ≥1.0 mm but <2.0 mm and ST segment horizontal or downward sloping in lead II or aVF
- 4-2 STJ depression ≥0.5 mm and <1.0 mm and ST segment horizontal or downward sloping in lead II or aVF
- 4-3 No STJ depression as much as 0.5 mm, but ST segment downward sloping and segment or T-wave nadir ≥0.5 mm below P-R baseline in lead II
- 4-4 STJ depression ≥1.0 mm and ST segment upward sloping, or U shaped, in lead II

Anterior site (leads V_1, V_2, V_3, V_4, V_5)

- 4-1-1 STJ depression ≥2.0 mm and ST segment horizontal or downward sloping in any of leads V_1, V_2, V_3, V_4, V_5
- 4-1-2 STJ depression ≥1.0 mm but <2.0 mm and ST segment horizontal or downward sloping in any of leads V_1, V_2, V_3, V_4, V_5
- 4-2 STJ depression ≥0.5 mm and <1.0 mm and ST segment horizontal or downward sloping in any of leads V_1, V_2, V_3, V_4, V_5
- 4-3 No STJ depression as much as 0.5 mm, but ST segment downward sloping and segment or T-wave nadir ≥0.5 mm below P-R baseline in any of leads V_2, V_3, V_4, V_5
- 4-4 STJ depression ≥1.0 mm and ST segment upward sloping or U-shaped in any of leads V_1, V_2, V_3, V_4, V_5

A4.1.1.5   T-Wave Items

(Do not code in the presence of codes 6–4–1, 6-8, 7–1–1, 7–2–1, 7-4, or 7–8.)

Anterolateral site (leads I, aVL, V_6)

- 5-1   T amplitude negative 5.0 mm or more in either of leads I, V_6, or in lead aVL when R amplitude is $\geq$5.0 mm
- 5-2   T amplitude negative or diphasic (positive–negative or negative–positive type) with negative phase at least 1.0 mm but not as deep as 5.0 mm in lead I or V_6, or in lead aVL when R amplitude is $\geq$5.0 mm
- 5-3   T amplitude zero (flat), or negative, or diphasic (negative-positive type only) with less than 1.0 mm negative phase in lead I or V_6, or in lead aVL when R amplitude is $\geq$5.0 mm
- 5-4   T amplitude positive and T/R amplitude ratio <1/20 in any of leads I, aVL, V_6; R-wave amplitude must be $\geq$10.0 mm

Posterior (inferior) site (leads II, III, aVF)

- 5-1   T amplitude negative 5.0 mm or more in lead II, or in lead aVF when QRS is mainly upright
- 5-2   T amplitude negative or diphasic with negative phase (negative–positive or positive–negative type) at least 1.0 mm but not as deep as 5.0 mm in lead II, or in lead aVF when QRS is mainly upright
- 5-3   T amplitude zero (flat), or negative, or diphasic (negative-positive type only) with less than 1.0 mm negative phase in lead II; not coded in lead aVF
- 5-4   T amplitude positive and T/R amplitude ratio <1/20 in lead II; R-wave amplitude must be $\geq$10.0 mm

Anterior site (leads V_2, V_3, V_4, V_5)

- 5-1   T amplitude negative 5.0 mm or more in any of leads V_2, V_3, V_4, V_5
- 5-2   T amplitude negative (flat) n any codes, or diphasic (negative–positive or positive–negative type) with negative phase at least 1.0 mm but not as deep as 5.0 mm, in any of leads V_2, V_3, V_4, V_5
- 5-3   T amplitude zero (flat), or negative, or diphasic (negative–positive type only) with less than 1.0 mm negative phase, in any of leads V_3, V_4, V_5
- 5-4   T amplitude positive and T/R amplitude ratio <1/20 in any of leads V_3, V_4, V_5; R-wave amplitude must be $\geq$10.0 mm

A4.1.1.6   AV Conduction Defect in Codes

- 6-1   Complete (third degree) AV block (permanent or intermittent) in any lead. Atrial and ventricular complexes independent, and atrial rate faster than ventricular rate, with ventricular rate <60.
- 6-2-1   Mobitz type II (occurrence of P wave on time with dropped QRS and T).
- 6-2-2   Partial (second degree) AV block in any lead (2:1 or 3:1 block).
- 6-2-3   Wenckebach's phenomenon (PR interval increasing from beat to beat until QRS and T dropped).
- 6-3   PR(PQ) interval $\geq$0.22 s in the majority of beats in any of leads I, II, III, aVL, aVF.
- 6-4-1   Wolff-Parkinson-White pattern (WPW), persistent. Sinus P wave. PR interval <0.12 s, plus QRS duration $\geq$0.12 s, plus R peak duration $\geq$0.06 s, coexisting in the same beat and present in the majority of beats in any of leads I, II, aVL, V_4, V_5, V_6. (6-4-1 suppresses 1-2-3, 1-2-7, 1-3-2, 1-3-6, 1-3-8, all 3, 4, 5, 7, 9-2, 9-4, 9-5 codes.)

- 6-4-2   WPW pattern, intermittent. WPW pattern in ≤50% of beats in appropriate leads.
- 6-5   Short PR interval. PR interval <0.12 s in all beats of any two of leads I, II, III, aVL, aVF.
- 6-6   Intermittent aberrant atrioventricular conductions. PR > 0.12 s (except in presence of 6-5 or heart rate greater than 100); wide QRS complex >0.12 s; normal P wave when most beats are sinus rhythm. (Do not code in the presence of 6-4-2.)
- 6-8   Artificial pacemaker.

A4.1.1.7   Ventricular Conduction Defect in Codes

- 7-1-1   Complete left bundle branch block (LBBB). (Do not code in presence of 6-1, 6-4-1, 6-8, 8-2-1 or 8-2-2,) QRS duration ≥0.12 s in a majority of beats (of the same QRS pattern) in any of leads I, II, III, aVL, aVF, *plus* R peak duration ≥0.06 s in a majority of beats (of the same QRS pattern) in any of leads I, II aVL, V_5, V_6 (7-1-1 suppresses 1-2-3, 1-2-7, 1-2-8, 1-3-2, 1-3-6, all 2, 3, 4, 5, 9-2, 9-4, 9-5 codes. If any other codable Q wave coexists with the LBBB pattern, code the Q and diminish the 7-1-1 code to a 7-4 code.)
- 7-1-2   Intermittent LBBB. Same as 7-1-1 but with presence of normally conducted QRS complexes of different shape than the LBBB pattern.
- 7-2-1   Complete right bundle branch block (RBBB). (Do not code in the presence of 6-1, 6-4-1, 6-8, 8-2-1 or 8-2-2.) QRS duration ≥0.12 s in a majority of beats (of the same QRS pattern) in any of leads I, II, III, aVL, aVF, *plus*: R' > R in V_1 or QRS mainly upright, *plus* R peak duration ≥0.06 s in V_1 or V_2; or S duration > R duration in all beats in lead I or II. (Suppresses 1-2-8 + 1-3-8, all 2-, 3-, 4- and 5- codes, 9-2, 9-4, 9-5.)
- 7-2-2   Intermittent RBBB. Same as 7-2-1 but with presence of normally conducted QRS complexes of different shape than the RBBB pattern.
- 7-3   Incomplete right bundle branch block. QRS duration <0.12 s in each of leads I, II, III, aVL, aVF, and R' > R in either of leads V_1, V_2. (Code as 3-2 in addition if those criteria are met. 7-3 suppresses code 1-2-8.)
- 7-4   Intraventricular block. QRS duration ≥0.12 s in a majority of beats in any of leads I, II, III, aVL. (7-4 suppresses all 2, 3, 4, 5, 9-2, 9-4, 9-5 codes.)
- 7-5   R-R' pattern in either of leads V_1, V_2 with R' amplitude ≤ R.
- 7-6   Incomplete LBBB. (Do not code in the presence of any codable Q or QS wave.) QRS duration ≥0.10 and <0.12 s in the majority of beats of each of leads I, aVL, and V_5 or V_6.
- 7-7   Left anterior hemiblock (LAH). QRS duration <0.12 s in the majority of beats in leads I, II, III, aVL, aVF, *plus* Q-wave amplitude ≥0.25 mm and <0.03 s duration in lead I, *plus* left axis deviation of −45° or more negative. (In presence of 7-2, code 7-8 if axis is <−45° and the Q wave in lead I meets the above criteria).
- 7-8   Combination of 7-7 and 7-2.
- 7-9-1[2]   Type 1 Brugada pattern convex (coved) ST segment elevation ≥ 2 mm *plus* T-wave negative with little or no isoelectric (baseline) separation in at least 2 leads of $V_1 - V_3$.
- 7-9-2[2]   Type 2 Brugada pattern ST segment elevation ≥ 2 mm *plus* T-wave positive or diphasic that results in a "saddle-back" shape in at least 2 leads of $V_1 - V_3$.
- 7-9-3[2]   Type 3 Brugada pattern. 7-2-1 *plus* ST segment elevation ≥ 1 mm *plus* a "saddle-back" configuration in at least 2 leads of $V_1 - V_3$.
- 7-10[2]   Fragmented QRS.

A4.1.1.8   Arrhythmias

- 8-1-1   Presence of frequent atrial or junctional premature beats (10% or more of recorded complexes).
- 8-1-2   Presence of frequent ventricular premature beats (10% or more of recorded complexes).

- 8-1-3 Presence of both atrial and/or junctional premature beats and ventricular premature beats (so that individual frequencies are <10% but *combined* premature beats are ≥10% of complexes).
- 8-1-4 Wandering atrial pacemaker.
- 8-1-5 Presence of 8-1-2 and 8-1-4.
- 8-2-1 Ventricular fibrillation or ventricular asystole.
- 8-2-2 Persistent ventricular (idioventricular) rhythm.
- 8-2-3 Intermittent ventricular tachycardia. Three or more consecutive ventricular premature beats occurring at a rate ≥100. This includes more persistent ventricular tachycardia.
- 8-2-4 Ventricular parasystole (should not be coded in presence of 8-3-1).
- 8-3-1 Atrial fibrillation (persistent).
- 8-3-2 Atrial flutter (persistent).
- 8-3-3 Intermittent atrial fibrillation (code if 3 or more clear-cut, consecutive sinus beats are present in any lead).
- 8-3-4 Intermittent atrial flutter (code if 3 or more clear-cut, consecutive sinus beats are present in any lead).
- 8-4-1 Supraventricular rhythm persistent. QRS duration <0.12 s; and absent P waves or presence of abnormal P waves (inverted or flat in aVF); and regular rhythm.
- 8-4-2 Supraventricular tachycardia intermittent. Three consecutive atrial or junctional premature beats occurring at a rate ≥100 min^{-1}.
- 8-5-1 Sinoatrial arrest. Unexpected absence of P, QRS and T, plus a R-R interval at a fixed multiple of the normal interval, ±10%.
- 8-5-2 Sinoatrial block. Unexpected absence of P, QRS and T, preceded by progressive shortening of P-P intervals, (R-R interval at a fixed multiple of the normal interval, ±10%).
- 8-6-1 AV dissociation with ventricular pacemaker (without capture). Requires: P-P and R-R to occur at variable rates with ventricular rate as fast as or faster than the atrial rate plus variable PR intervals, plus no capture beats.
- 8-6-2 AV dissociation with ventricular pacemaker (with capture).
- 8-6-3 AV dissociation with atrial pacemaker (without capture).
- 8-6-4 AV dissociation with atrial pacemaker (with capture).
- 8-7 Sinus tachycardia (≥ 100 min^{-1}).
- 8-8 Sinus bradycardia (≤ 50 min^{-1}).
- 8-9 Other arrhythmias. Heart rate may be recorded as a continuous variable.

A4.1.1.9 ST-Segment Elevation

Do not code in the presence of codes 6-4-1, 6-8, 7-1-1, 7-2-1, 7-4, or 7-8.

Anterolateral site (leads I, aVL, V_6)

- 9-2 ST-segment elevation ≥1.0 mm in any of leads I, aVL, V_6.

Posterior (inferior) site (leads II, III, aVF)

- 9-2 ST-segment elevation ≥1.0 mm in any of leads II, III, aVF.

Anterior site (leads V_1, V_2, V_3, V_4, V_5)

- 9-2 ST-segment elevation ≥1.0 mm in lead V_5 or ST-segment elevation ≥2.0 mm in any of leads V_1, V_2, V_3, V_4.

A4.1.1.10   Miscellaneous Items

- 9-1   Low QRS amplitude. QRS peak-to-peak amplitude <5 mm in all beats in each of leads I, II, III, or <10 mm in all beats in each of leads V_1, V_2, V_3, V_4, V_5, V_6. (Check calibration before coding).
- 9-3   P-wave amplitude ≥2.5 mm in any of leads II, III, aVF, in a majority of beats.
- 9-4-1   QRS transition zone at V_3 or to the right of V_3 on the chest. (Do not code in the presence of 6-4-1, 6-8, 7-1-1, 7-2-1, 7-4, or 7-8.)
- 9-4-2   QRS transition zone at V_4 or to the left of V_4 on the chest. (Do not code in the presence of 6-4-1, 6-8, 7-1-1, 7-2-1, 7-4, or 7-8.)
- 9-5   T-Wave amplitude >12 mm in any of leads I, II, III, aVL, aVF, V_1, V_2, V_3, V_4, V_5, V_6. (Do not code in the presence of 6-4-1, 6-8, 7-1-1, 7-2-1, 7-4, or 7-8.
- 9-6[2]   Notched and widened P wave (duration ≥ 0.12 s) in frontal plane (usually lead II), and/or deep negative component to the P wave in lead V_1 duration ≥ 0.04 s and depth ≥ 1 mm.
- 9-7-1[2] Definite Early Repolarization. STJ elevation ≥ 1 mm in the majority of beats, T wave amplitude ≥ 5 mm prominent J point, upward concavity of the ST segment, and a distinct notch or slur on the down-stroke of the R wave in any of V_3 – V_6, OR STJ elevation ≥ 2 mm in the majority of beats and T wave amplitude ≥ 5 mm prominent J point, and upward concavity of the ST segment in any of V_3 – V_6.
- 9-7-2[2] Probable Early Repolarization. STJ elevation ≥ 1 mm in the majority of beats, prominent J point, and upward concavity of the ST segment in any of V_3 – V_6 and T wave amplitude ≥ 8 mm in any of the leads V_3 – V_6.
- 9-8-1[2] Uncorrectable lead reversal.
- 9-8-2[3] Poor Quality/Technical problems which interfere with coding.
- 9-8-3[2] Correctable lead reversal.
  - i.   Correctable limb lead connection error.
  - ii. Correctable chest lead connection error in V_1 – V_3.
  - iii. Correctable chest lead connection error in V_4 – V_6.
  - iv. Correctable other chest lead connection error.
- 9-8-4[3] Technical problems that do not interfere with coding.

A4.1.1.11   Incompatible Codes

❯ Table A4.1 gives a list of incompatible codes. The codes in the left-hand column suppress the codes in the right-hand column.

A4.1.1.12   ECG Criteria for Significant Serial ECG Change

A detailed explanation of criteria for serial change can be found in Chapter 15 of the recently published Minnesota Code Manual of Electrocardiographic Findings (RJ Prineas, RS Crow, Z-M Zhang, Springer, 2009). An extract is given here.

Evolving Q-wave

Q1.   No Q-code in reference ECG followed by a record with a diagnostic Q-code (MC 1-1-1 through 1-2-7) **OR** an Equivocal Q-code (1-3-x) in reference ECG followed by record with any code 1-1-x Q-code.

---

[1]1-3-8 was previously 1-2-8

[2]New code from first edition

[3]9-8-2 in the first edition was 9-8-1, and 9-8-4 was 9-8-2 in the first edition.

◘ Table A4.1

Incompatible codes

Code	Suppresses this code(s)
All Q, QS codes	7-6
Q ≥ 0.03 in Lead I	7-7
3-1	1-3-2
3-2	1-3-8, 7-3
6-1	All other codes except 8-2
6-4-1	All other codes
6-8	All other codes
7-1-1	1-2-3, 1-2-7, 1-3-2, 1-3-6, 1-3-7, 1-3-8, all 2-, 3-, 4-, and 5-codes, 7-7, 7-8, 7-9, 7-10, 9-2, 9-4, 9-5, 9-7-1, 9-7-2
7-2-1	1-3-8, all 2-, 3-, 4-, and 5-codes, 9-2, 9-4, 9-5, 9-7-1, 9-7-2
7-3	1-3-8
7-4	All 2-, 3-, 4-, and 5-codes, 9-2, 9-4, 9-5
7-8	1-3-8, all 2-, 3-, 4-, and 5-codes, 9-2, 9-4, 9-5, 9-7-1, 9-7-2
8-1-2	8-2-4
8-1-4	8-1-1, 9-3
8-2-1	All other codes
8-2-2	All other codes
8-2-3	8-1-2
8-3-1	8-1-1, 8-1-2
8-3-2	6-2-2, 8-1-1, 8-1-2
8-3-3	8-1-1, 8-1-2
8-3-4	6-2-2
8-4-1	6-5
8-4-1 + heart rate ≥140 bpm	All other codes except 7-4 or 6-2
Heart rate >100 bpm	6-5
8-4-2	8-1-1
9-1	All 2-codes

Q2.   An Equivocal Q-code (any MC 1-3 x code) and no major ST-segment depression (MC 4-0, 4-4, 4-3) in reference ECG followed by a record with a diagnostic Q-code (MC 1-2-1 – 1-2-7) *Plus* a major ST-segment depression (MC 4-1-x or 4-2).

Q3.   An Equivocal Q-code (any MC 1-3-x) and no major T-wave inversion (MC 5–4, 5-3 or 5-0) in reference ECG followed by a record with a diagnostic Q-code (MC1-2-1 through 1-2-7) *Plus* a major T-wave inversion (MC 5-1 or 5-2).

Q4.   An Equivocal Q-code (any MC 1-3-x) and Q-code (MC 1-2-1 through 1-2-7) *Plus* and ST-segment elevation (MC 9-2).

Q5.   No Q-code and no MC 4-1-x or 4-2 in reference ECG followed by a record with an Equivocal Q-code (any MC 1-3-x) *Plus* MC 4-1-x or 4-2.

Q6.   No Q-code and no MC 5-1 or 5-2 in reference ECG followed by a record with an Equivocal Q-code (any MC 1-3-x) *Plus* a MC 5-1 or 5-2.

Q7.   No Q-code and no MC 9-2 in reference ECG followed by a record with an Equivocal Q-code (any MC 1-3-x) *Plus* a MC 9-2.

Evolving ST-Elevation

STE-1   MC 9-0 in reference ECG followed by a record with MC 9-2 in at least 2 leads and > 100% increase ST elevation in both leads.

STE-2   MC 9-2 in reference ECG followed by a record with MC 9-2 in at least 2 leads and > 100% increase in ST elevation in both leads.

STE-3   MC 9-2 and no MC 5-1 or 5-2 in reference ECG followed by a record appearance of MC 5-1 or 5-2 with 100% increase in T wave inversion in at least 2 leads.

STE-4   Reversal of evolving STE-1 (within the hospital ECG only).

STE-5   Reversal of evolving STE-2 (within the hospital ECG only).

Evolving ST-Depression/T Wave Inversion

ST-T1   Either MC 4-0 (no 4-code), 4–4 or 4–3 in reference ECG followed by a record with MC 4–2 or 4-1-2 or 4-1-1 and > 100% increase in ST segment depression.

ST-T2   Either MC 4-2 4–1–2 in reference ECG followed by a record with MC 4–1–1 and > 100% increase in ST segment depression.

ST-T3   Either MC 5-0, 5-4 or 5-3 in reference ECG followed by a record with MC 5-2 or 5-1 and > 100% increase in T-wave inversion.

ST-T4   MC 5-2 in reference ECG followed by a record with MC 5-1 and > 100% in T-wave inversion.

ST-T5   MC 4–1-1 in reference ECG followed by a record with MC 4–1–1 and > 100% increase in ST depression.

ST-T6   MC 5-1 in reference ECG followed by a record with MC 5-1 and > 100% increase in T-wave inversion

ST-T7   MC 5-2 in reference ECG followed by a record with MC 5-2 and > 100% increase in T-wave inversion.

ST-T1R   Reverse of ST-T1[4]

ST-T2R   Reverse of ST-T2[4]

ST-T3R   Reverse of ST-T3[4]

ST-T4R   Reverse of ST-T4[4]

ST-T5R   Reverse of ST-T5[4]

ST-T6R   Reverse of ST-T6[4]

ST-T7R   Reverse of ST-T7[4]

Evolving Bundle Branch Block

E-BBB1   No MC 7-1 in the reference ECG followed by an ECG with MC 7-1-1 in follow-up ECG **and** QRS duration increase by > 0.02 s.

E-BBB2   No MC 7-2 in the reference ECG followed by an ECG with MC 7-2-1 in follow-up ECG **and** QRS duration increase by > 0.02 s.

E-BBB3   No MC 7-4 in the reference ECG followed by an ECG with MC 7–4 in follow-up ECG **and** QRS duration increase by > 0.02 s.

Evolving ECG – LVH

E-LVH 1   MC 3-0 in reference ECG flowed by an ECG with a MC 3-1 in the follow-up ECG, confirmed as a significant increase.

---

[4] Requires > 100% decrease in ST depression or T-wave inversion of follow-up record compared to reference ECG, and code changes must occur in the same lead groups.

E-LVH 2   MC 3-0 in reference ECG flowed by an ECG with a MC 3-3 in the follow-up ECG, confirmed as a significant increase.

E-LVH 3   MC 3-1 in reference ECG flowed by an ECG with a MC 3-0 in the follow-up ECG, confirmed as a significant decrease.

E-LVH 4   MC 3-3 in reference ECG flowed by an ECG with a MC 3-0 in the follow-up ECG, confirmed as a significant decrease.

E-LVH 5   MC 3-1 in reference ECG flowed by an ECG with a MC 3-1 in the follow-up ECG, confirmed by a significant increase or a significant decrease.

E-LVH 6   MC 3-3 in reference ECG flowed by an ECG with a MC 3-3 in the follow-up ECG, confirmed by a significant increase or a significant decrease.

A4.2   The Punsar Code

One of the authors of the original publication of the Minnesota code, Punsar, developed an alternative scheme, in collaboration with others, for classifying the ST-T segment. The code is described simply in ❷ Table A4.2 and ❷ Fig. A4.1 which is reproduced from: Punsar S, Pyorala K, Siltanen P. Classification of electrocardiographic ST segment changes in epidemiological studies of coronary heart disease. Ann. Med. Intern. Fenn. 1968; **57**:53–63, with the permission of Annales Medicinae Internae Fenniae, Helsinki.

The authors tested their code in a 5-year follow-up of 1,534 men aged 40–59. The incidence of events including death or myocardial infarction was highest in the ischemic group and decreased in the remaining groups in a progressive fashion. It was also noted that with each group, the prognosis varied according to the amount of ST depression present.

◻ Table A4.2

Correspondence of the items in the new, modified code to those in the Minnesota code

Modified code		Minnesota code				
		At rest		Postexercise[a]		
I	1	IV	1	XI	1
	2		1		1
	3		2		2
	4		3		3
	5				
S	1	IV	4	XI	4
	2		4		4
	3				
	4				
R	1	IV	4		4
	2		4	XI	4
	3				

[a]The original 1960 Minnesota code had postexercise classifications, coded X to XVI

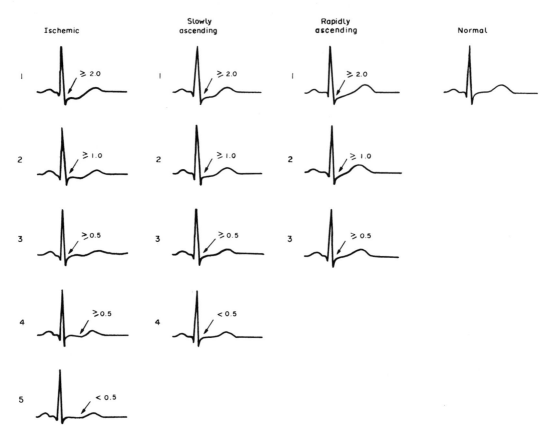

◾ **Fig. A4.1**
Categories of ST-segment changes in the new, modified classification (the Punsar code). Note that the figures beside each arrow indicate the amount of ST depression in millimeters

Appendix 5: Normal Limits of the 12 Lead Vectorcardiogram

Appendix 5A   Normal Limits of Adult 12-Lead Vectorcardiogram

The tables of amplitudes and durations in this Appendix have been obtained from the X, Y, Z leads derived from the 12-lead ECG according to the methods described in ➋ Chap. 11, ➋ Sect. 11.6 and using the coefficients presented in Table 11.6. Data have been derived from 1,555 adult ECGs whose age distribution is shown in the lower part of ➋ Table 11.1. The 215 males over 50 have been subdivided, with 38 men being aged 60 and over, while similarly 139 females include 19 aged 60 and over.

Data are expressed as mean ± standard deviation below which is given the 96 percentile ranges, i.e., 2% of values are excluded at either end of the distribution except in the case of the groups aged 60 and over where the 100% range is presented. Angular data are presented with respect to the reference frames illustrated in ➋ Fig. 11.9 of *Specialized Aspects of ECG*.

A5.1   Scalar Measurements from the Leads X, Y, and Z

A5.1.1   P Wave Amplitude and Duration

◼ Table A5.1

P wave amplitudes (mV) in males

Age (years)	X	Y	Z
18–29	0.07 ± 0.02	0.11 ± 0.05	0.05 ± 0.02
	0.03 → 0.12	0.02 → 0.25	0.02 → 0.10
30–39	0.07 ± 0.02	0.11 ± 0.04	0.04 ± 0.02
	0.03 → 0.12	0.01 → 0.22	0.01 → 0.11
40–49	0.07 ± 0.02	0.11 ± 0.04	0.04 ± 0.02
	0.03 → 0.14	0.03 → 0.22	0.00 → 0.09
50–59	0.07 ± 0.02	0.11 ± 0.04	0.04 ± 0.02
	0.04 → 0.13	0.04 → 0.20	0.01 → 0.08
60–	0.07 ± 0.03	0.11 ± 0.04	0.04 ± 0.03
	0.03 → 0.11	0.04 → 0.18	0.00 → 0.08

◼ Table A5.2

P wave amplitudes (mV) in females

Age (years)	X	Y	Z
18–29	0.07 ± 0.02	0.11 ± 0.05	0.04 ± 0.02
	0.03 → 0.13	0.02 → 0.26	0.01 → 0.08
30–39	0.08 ± 0.02	0.12 ± 0.05	0.04 ± 0.02
	0.04 → 0.13	0.03 → 0.24	0.01 → 0.09
40–49	0.08 ± 0.02	0.11 ± 0.04	0.04 ± 0.02
	0.04 → 0.12	0.03 → 0.24	0.01 → 0.08
50–59	0.08 ± 0.02	0.11 ± 0.04	0.04 ± 0.02
	0.04 → 0.13	0.03 → 0.22	0.00 → 0.07
60–	0.08 ± 0.03	0.12 ± 0.06	0.04 ± 0.01
	0.03 → 0.14	0.03 → 0.23	0.01 → 0.06

◘ Table A5.3

P wave durations (ms) in males

Age (years)	X	Y	Z
18–29	93 ± 14	98 ± 14	98 ± 14
	66 → 122	66 → 122	66 → 122
30–39	103 ± 11	103 ± 11	103 ± 11
	78 → 124	78 → 124	78 → 124
40–49	107 ± 11	107 ± 11	107 ± 11
	86 → 128	86 → 128	86 → 128
50–59	108 ± 11	108 ± 11	108 ± 11
	80 → 128	80 → 128	80 → 128
60–	110 ± 12	110 ± 12	110 ± 12
	90 → 130	90 → 130	90 → 130

◘ Table A5.4

P wave durations (ms) in females

Age (years)	X	Y	Z
18–29	97 ± 11	97 ± 11	97 ± 11
	72 → 116	72 → 116	72 → 116
30–39	100 ± 10	100 ± 10	100 ± 10
	78 → 116	78 → 116	78 → 116
40–49	104 ± 10	104 ± 10	104 ± 10
	82 → 124	82 → 124	82 → 124
50–59	104 ± 13	104 ± 13	104 ± 13
	64 → 128	64 → 128	64 → 128
60–	104 ± 12	104 ± 12	104 ± 12
	88 → 130	88 → 130	88 → 130

A5.1.2 Q Wave Amplitude and Duration

◘ Table A5.5

Q wave amplitude (mV) in males

Age (years)	X	Y
18–29	−0.11 ± 0.09	−0.10 ± 0.06
	−0.37 → −0.02	−0.29 → −0.02
30–39	−0.09 ± 0.08	−0.10 ± 0.06
	−0.33 → −0.02	−0.30 → −0.02
40–49	−0.08 ± 0.05	−0.07 ± 0.04
	−0.21 → −0.02	−0.17 → −0.02
50–59	−0.09 ± 0.06	−0.07 ± 0.05
	−0.26 → −0.02	−0.21 → −0.02
60–	−0.07 ± 0.04	−0.08 ± 0.05
	−0.14 → −0.02	−0.21 → −0.02

◻ **Table A5.6**

Q wave amplitude (mV) in females

Age (years)	X	Y
18–29	−0.08 ± 0.06	−0.10 ± 0.06
	−0.25 → −0.02	−0.29 → −0.02
30–39	−0.09 ± 0.06	−0.08 ± 0.05
	−0.26 → −0.02	−0.20 → −0.02
40–49	−0.07 ± 0.05	−0.06 ± 0.03
	−0.22 → −0.02	−0.13 → −0.02
50–59	−0.06 ± 0.04	−0.06 ± 0.03
	−0.17 → −0.02	−0.16 → −0.02
60–	−0.07 ± 0.04	−0.05 ± 0.03
	−0.14 → −0.02	−0.10 → −0.03

◻ **Table A5.7**

Q wave durations (ms) in males

Age (years)	X	Y
18–29	17 ± 5	19 ± 7
	8 → 28	8 → 27
30–39	16 ± 6	19 ± 5
	8 → 27	7 → 31
40–49	16 ± 4	17 ± 5
	7 → 23	6 → 25
50–59	16 ± 4	18 ± 5
	10 → 24	6 → 27
60–	15 ± 3	19 ± 5
	10 → 23	5 → 29

◻ **Table A5.8**

Q wave durations (ms) in females

Age (years)	X	Y
18–29	15 ± 4	17 ± 5
	7 → 25	7 → 26
30–39	16 ± 4	16 ± 4
	7 → 24	6 → 24
40–49	15 ± 3	14 ± 4
	9 → 21	8 → 24
50–59	14 ± 4	16 ± 4
	7 → 22	8 → 24
60–	15 ± 4	13 ± 6
	9 → 24	5 → 21

A5.1.3 R Wave Amplitude and Duration

◼ Table A5.9

R wave amplitudes (mV) in males

Age (years)	X	Y	Z
18–29	1.66 ± 0.46	1.16 ± 0.46	0.52 ± 0.23
	0.08 → 2.86	0.31 → 2.23	0.13 → 1.02
30–39	1.53 ± 0.43	0.91 ± 0.46	0.42 ± 0.24
	0.69 → 2.44	0.14 → 2.13	0.09 → 1.07
40–49	1.40 ± 43	0.69 ± 0.39	0.37 ± 0.19
	0.66 → 2.41	0.04 → 1.51	0.04 → 0.87
50–59	1.38 ± 0.38	0.58 ± 0.34	0.36 ± 0.17
	0.72 → 2.01	0.11 → 1.46	0.10 → 0.76
60–	1.20 ± 0.36	0.65 ± 0.39	0.30 ± 0.19
	0.75 → 1.93	0.08 → 1.50	0.05 → 0.67

◼ Table A5.10

R wave amplitudes (mV) in females

Age (years)	X	Y	Z
18–29	1.23 ± 0.34	0.91 ± 0.34	0.33 ± 0.15
	0.56 → 1.96	0.32 → 1.75	0.07 → 0.70
30–39	1.23 ± 0.37	0.87 ± 0.32	0.32 ± 0.15
	0.58 → 1.97	0.29 → 1.48	0.10 → 0.67
40–49	1.11 ± 0.32	0.66 ± 0.26	0.25 ± 0.12
	0.62 → 1.75	0.24 → 1.16	0.04 → 0.49
50–59	1.11 ± 0.29	0.61 ± 0.31	0.26 ± 0.14
	0.60 → 1.76	0.14 → 1.31	0.04 → 0.73
60–	1.28 ± 0.46	0.55 ± 0.21	0.32 ± 0.14
	0.54 → 2.23	0.25 → 1.16	0.04 → 0.56

◼ Table A5.11

R wave durations (ms) in males

Age (years)	X	Y	Z
18–29	45 ± 15	55 ± 17	32 ± 9
	27 → 79	28 → 86	20 → 45
30–39	46 ± 14	57 ± 16	31 ± 9
	28 → 84	26 → 86	17 → 44
40–49	47 ± 14	55 ± 18	32 ± 8
	31 → 82	15 → 90	15 → 48
50–59	46 ± 14	55 ± 17	33 ± 8
	30 → 79	22 → 90	21 → 52
60–	43 ± 11	54 ± 15	29 ± 8
	29 → 62	34 → 86	14 → 40

■ Table A5.12

R wave durations (ms) in females

Age (years)	X	Y	Z
18–29	44 ± 12	47 ± 13	28 ± 6
	27 → 76	24 → 78	15 → 41
30–39	44 ± 12	48 ± 12	28 ± 5
	31 → 67	31 → 72	17 → 38
40–49	45 ± 11	52 ± 14	27 ± 7
	31 → 71	28 → 86	10 → 41
50–59	44 ± 11	52 ± 15	27 ± 7
	26 → 86	20 → 77	11 → 43
60–	44 ± 11	51 ± 13	32 ± 5
	28 → 64	33 → 72	24 → 46

A5.1.4 S Wave Amplitude and Duration

■ Table A5.13

S wave amplitudes (mV) in males

Age (years)	X	Y	Z
18–29	−0.27 ± 0.18	−0.16 ± 0.09	−1.38 ± 0.47
	−0.68 → −0.05	−0.41 → −0.03	−2.50 → −0.59
30–39	−0.26 ± 0.20	−0.18 ± 0.16	−1.05 ± 0.37
	−0.71 → −0.05	−0.44 → −0.04	−1.70 → −0.49
40–49	−0.29 ± 0.18	−0.17 ± 0.13	0.37 ± 0.19
	−0.73 → −0.06	−0.44 → −0.03	0.04 → 0.87
50–59	−0.25 ± 0.17	−0.17 ± 0.16	0.36 ± 0.17
	−0.68 → 0.04	−0.60 → −0.05	0.10 → 0.76
60–	−0.35 ± 0.18	−0.18 ± 0.14	−0.81 ± 0.31
	−0.54 → −0.17	−0.28 → −0.06	−1.04 → −0.48

■ Table A5.14

S wave amplitudes (mV) in females

Age (years)	X	Y	Z
18–29	−0.17 ± 0.10	−0.15 ± 0.09	−0.92 ± 0.34
	−0.52 → −0.05	0.42 → 0.04	−1.65 → −0.35
30–39	−0.20 ± 0.11	−0.14 ± 0.12	−0.92 ± 0.33
	−0.39 → −0.06	−0.36 → −0.05	−1.65 → −0.35
40–49	−0.18 ± 0.14	−0.14 ± 0.11	−0.99 ± 0.39
	−0.34 → −0.04	−0.25 → −0.04	−1.54 → −0.46
50–59	−0.20 ± 0.14	−0.16 ± 0.09	−0.74 ± 0.30
	−0.42 → −0.06	−0.29 → −0.06	−1.32 → 0.34
60–	−0.16 ± 0.10	0.18 ± 0.10	−0.66 ± 0.25
	−0.19 → −0.11	−0.17 → −0.12	−0.79 → −0.50

◘ Table A5.15

S wave durations (ms) in males

Age (years)	X	Y	Z
18–29	26 ± 12	26 ± 10	53 ± 8
	6 → 48	7 → 48	35 → 71
30–39	28 ± 13	29 ± 14	54 ± 10
	7 → 57	8 → 60	31 → 71
40–49	31 ± 12	32 ± 15	52 ± 11
	10 → 55	7 → 68	25 → 70
50–59	32 ± 12	30 ± 15	50 ± 11
	11 → 53	8 → 67	27 → 73
60–	33 ± 12	28 ± 11	53 ± 9
	12 → 56	11 → 50	31 → 67

◘ Table A5.16

S wave durations (ms) in females

Age (years)	X	Y	Z
18–29	24 ± 9	25 ± 9	51 ±9
	7 → 41	10 → 45	30 → 67
30–39	28 ± 9	23 ± 10	52 ± 8
	8 → 43	8 → 43	35 → 64
40–49	26 ± 10	26 ± 10	52 ± 8
	12 → 41	12 → 50	27 → 75
50–59	27 ± 10	27 ± 11	51 ± 9
	12 → 47	11 → 58	30 → 64
60–	29 ± 11	33 ± 15	47 ± 10
	13 → 53	12 → 50	20 → 59

A5.1.5 T Wave Amplitude

◘ Table A5.17

T wave amplitudes (mV) in males

Age (years)	X	Y	Z
18–29	0.46 ± 0.19	0.25 ± 0.11	0.47 ± 0.18
	0.10 → 0.95	0.02 → 0.55	0.14 → 0.86
30–39	0.42 ± 0.16	0.21 ± 0.10	0.42 ± 0.16
	0.12 → 0.80	0.03 → 0.48	0.08 → 0.80
40–49	0.38 ± 0.17	0.19 ± 0.10	0.39 ± 0.15
	0.08 → 0.82	0.03 → 0.43	0.12 → 0.72
50–59	0.35 ± 0.16	0.17 ± 0.08	0.38 ± 0.16
	0.09 → 0.72	0.04 → 0.38	0.07 → 0.74
60–	0.36 ± 0.18	0.21 ± 0.12	0.33 ± 0.17
	0.06 → 0.66	0.08 → 0.38	0.12 → 0.73

■ Table A5.18
T wave amplitudes (mV) in females

Age (years)	X	Y	Z
18–29	0.34 ± 0.12	0.20 ± 0.08	0.23 ± 0.11
	0.14 → 0.60	0.04 → 0.46	0.04 → 0.56
30–39	0.33 ± 0.13	0.18 ± 0.08	0.22 ± 0.11
	0.12 → 0.64	0.05 → 0.37	0.02 → 0.43
40–49	0.28 ± 0.11	0.16 ± 0.07	0.20 ± 0.09
	0.05 → 0.51	0.05 → 0.33	0.06 → 0.43
50–59	0.27 ± 0.11	0.17 ± 0.07	0.20 ± 0.09
	0.07 → 0.56	0.03 → 0.32	0.03 → 0.36
60–	0.26 ± 0.14	0.17 ± 0.08	0.21 ± 0.08
	0.03 → 0.62	0.10 → 0.30	0.04 → 0.37

A5.2 Planar and Spatial Measurements

A5.2.1 Direction of Inscription in the QRS Vector Loop

■ Table A5.19
Direction of inscription of the QRS vector loop in males (%)

	Frontal	Left sagittal	Transverse
Counterclockwise	22.9	88.0	98.1
Figure of 8	19.1	8.4	0.9
Clockwise	58.0	3.6	1.0

■ Table A5.20
Direction of inscription of the QRS vector loop in females (%)

	Frontal	Left sagittal	Transverse
Counterclockwise	21.8	94.5	97.9
Figure of 8	25.3	3.9	1.2
Clockwise	52.9	1.6	0.9

A5.2.2 Magnitude of Maximal Spatial QRS Vector

■ Table A5.21
Magnitude of maximal spatial QRS vector (mV)

Age (years)	Males	Females
18–29	2.39 ± 0.62	1.76 ± 0.47
	1.07 → 3.97	0.75 → 3.06
30–39	2.07 ± 0.58	1.74 ± 0.46
	1.00 → 3.61	0.92 → 2.77

◉ Table A5.21 (Continued)

Age (years)	Males	Females
40–49	1.79 ± 0.49	1.46 ± 0.41
	0.85 → 2.94	0.79 → 2.26
50–59	1.65 ± 0.45	1.46 ± 0.37
	0.86 → 2.91	0.78 → 2.22
60–	1.57 ± 0.42	1.37 ± 0.51
	0.99 → 2.20	1.00 → 1.90

A5.2.3 Magnitude of Maximal Planar QRS Vector

◉ Table A5.22
Magnitude of the maximal QRS vector in frontal, sagittal, and transverse planes (mV) in males

Age (years)	Frontal	Sagittal	Transverse
18–29	2.04 ± 0.52	1.75 ± 0.60	2.09 ± 0.52
	0.99 → 3.26	0.70 → 3.41	1.02 → 3.39
30–39	1.80 ± 0.49	1.48 ± 0.58	1.85 ± 0.48
	0.82 → 3.03	0.52 → 3.11	0.92 → 2.95
40–49	1.59 ± 0.46	1.23 ± 0.45	1.64 ± 0.43
	0.69 → 2.82	0.45 → 2.26	0.83 → 2.78
50–59	1.50 ± 0.42	1.07 ± 0.40	1.54 ± 0.39
	0.77 → 2.70	0.44 → 2.05	0.84 → 2.76
60–	1.40 ± 0.37	1.12 ± 0.41	1.42 ± 0.36
	0.92 → 2.03	0.64 → 1.91	0.89 → 2.08

◉ Table A5.23
Magnitude of the maximal QRS vector in frontal, sagittal, and transverse planes (mV) in females

Age (years)	Frontal	Sagittal	Transverse
18–29	1.54 ± 0.40	1.28 ± 0.44	1.51 ± 0.39
	0.67 → 2.56	0.49 → 2.48	0.67 → 2.58
30–39	1.51 ± 0.42	1.25 ± 0.43	1.50 ± 0.40
	0.62 → 2.42	0.60 → 2.25	0.88 → 2.51
40–49	1.29 ± 0.33	1.02 ± 0.35	1.31 ± 0.36
	0.68 → 1.96	0.40 → 1.78	0.84 → 2.76
50–59	1.29 ± 0.33	1.02 ± 0.36	1.31 ± 0.31
	0.68 → 1.96	0.42 → 1.86	0.69 → 2.01
60–	1.27 ± 0.52	0.82 ± 0.30	1.27 ± 0.48
	0.99 → 1.88	0.60 → 1.18	0.93 → 1.77

A5.2.4 Maximal Planar QRS Vector Angle

◘ Table A5.24

96-Percentile ranges of maximal QRS vector angle (degrees) in males

Age (years)	Frontal	Sagittal	Transverse
18–29	34 ± 14	40 ± 24	−37 ± 26
	12 → 62	0 → 96	−105 → 14
30–39	28 ± 14	38 ± 36	−32 ± 28
	3 → 54	−12 → 144	−99 → 19
40–49	23 ± 19	33 ± 34	−28 ± 31
	−2 → 53	−13 → 140	−103 → 27
50–59	20 ± 13	31 ± 41	−25 ± 36
	−5 → 43	−23 → 150	−117 → 25
60–	22 ± 35	32 ± 33	−32 ± 0.35
	0 → 58	0 → 84	−103 → 25

◘ Table A5.25

96-Percentile ranges of maximal QRS vector angle (degrees) in females

Age (years)	Frontal	Sagittal	Transverse
18–29	34 ± 15	40 ± 22	−35 ± 19
	13 → 59	−9 → 89	−85 → 3
30–39	35 ± 11	44 ± 20	−36 ± 22
	14 → 55	−13 → 79	−97 → −2
40–49	27 ± 19	37 ± 31	−33 ± 25
	6 → 48	−20 → 99	−109 → 9
50–59	27 ± 12	34 ± 28	−31 ± 27
	6 → 23	−15 → 142	−108 → 16
60–	21 ± 10	42 ± 54	−16 ± 31
	0 → 47	−41 → 180	−107 → 27

A5.2.5 Maximal T Vector Angle

◘ Table A5.26

96-Percentile ranges of maximal T vector angle (degrees) in males

Age (years)	Frontal	Sagittal	Transverse
18–29	28 ± 15	154 ± 18	45 ± 17
	−6 → 60	110 → 184	13 → 81
30–39	25 ± 17	154 ± 21	44 ± 17
	6 → 48	96 → 180	5 → 78
40–49	27 ± 16	155 ± 18	46 ± 17
	5 → 56	113 → 180	9 → 76
50–59	25 ± 14	156 ± 21	46 ± 20
	3 → 51	98 → 181	2 → 78
60–	32 ± 18	147 ± 26	38 ± 25
	10 → 81	95 → 176	2 → 65

◘ Table A5.27
96-Percentile ranges of maximal T vector angle (degrees) in females

Age (years)	Frontal	Sagittal	Transverse
18–29	30 ± 19	134 ± 26	28 ± 18
	8 → 50	61 → 178	−15 → 62
30–39	29 ± 10	137 ± 26	−30 ± 19
	9 → 48	80 → 183	−15 → 68
40–49	30 ± 16	140 ± 21	34 ± 17
	9 → 56	98 → 185	10 → 77
50–59	29 ± 26	140 ± 26	33 ± 29
	8 → 53	82 → 187	−13 → 76
60–	38 ± 30	144 ± 22	40 ± 24
	0 → 153	78 → 180	−6 → 105

Appendix 5B   Normal Limits of Paediatric 12-Lead Vectorcardiogram

The vector data presented in this Appendix have been obtained from X, Y, Z leads derived from the 12-lead ECG according to the methods described in 11.6 and using the coefficients presented in ❷ Table 11.9 *Basic Electrocardiology: Cardiac Electrophysiology, ECG Systems and Mathematical Modeling*. Data have been derived from 1,782 neonates, infants, and children, whose age distribution is shown in the upper part of ❷ Table 11.1 of *Specialized Aspects of ECG*.

Data are expressed as mean ± standard deviation below which is given the 96 percentile ranges, i.e., 2% of values are excluded at either end of the distribution except when the total number in the age group is small, in which case the 100% range is presented. Angular data are presented with respect to the reference frames illustrated in ❷ Fig. 11.9 of *Specialized Aspects of ECG*.

B5.1   Scalar Measurements from the Leads X, Y and Z

◘ Table B5.1
Maximal spatial P, QRS, and T magnitudes (mV)

Age	Max P	Max QRS	Max T
< 24 h	0.16 ± 0.05	1.83 ± 0.48	0.25 ± 0.08
	0.09 → 0.25	0.95 → 2.76	0.08 → 0.41
1 day	0.17 ± 0.05	1.71 ± 0.43	0.23 ± 0.07
	0.09 → 0.25	1.03 → 2.48	0.11 → 0.38
2 days	0.17 ± 0.05	1.62 ± 0.41	0.25 ± 0.08
	0.10 → 0.27	0.93 → 2.51	0.12 → 0.43
3 days	0.17 ± 0.04	1.60 ± 0.41	0.28 ± 0.08
	0.10 → 0.25	1.00 → 2.48	0.14 → 0.43
≤ 1 week	0.18 ± 0.05	1.53 ± 0.35	0.34 ± 0.10
	0.10 → 0.31	0.99 → 2.36	0.16 → 0.55
≤ 1 month	0.18 ± 0.06	1.38 ± 0.40	0.37 ± 0.10
	0.08 → 0.26	0.76 → 2.04	0.19 → 0.60
≤ 3 months	0.16 ± 0.04	1.87 ± 0.45	0.43 ± 0.09
	0.07 → 0.24	1.17 → 2.95	0.28 → 0.60
≤ 6 months	0.15 ± 0.04	1.70 ± 0.38	0.44 ± 0.12
	0.09 → 0.27	1.02 → 2.35	0.27 → 0.67

◻ Table B5.1   (Continued)

Age	Max P	Max QRS	Max T
≤ 1 year	0.17 ± 0.05	1.81 ± 0.48	0.49 ± 0.11
	0.11 → 0.25	1.09 → 2.80	0.30 → 0.69
1–2 years	0.15 ± 0.04	1.86 ± 0.49	0.47 ± 0.14
	0.09 → 0.24	1.03 → 2.82	0.22 → 0.70
3–4 years	0.15 ± 0.04	2.20 ± 0.53	0.53 ± 0.15
	0.09 → 0.24	1.25 → 3.21	0.21 → 0.84
5–6 years	0.14 ± 0.04	2.46 ± 0.55	0.58 ± 0.15
	0.08 → 0.24	1.56 → 3.61	0.31 → 0.87
7–8 years	0.14 ± 0.04	2.43 ± 0.48	0.61 ± 0.15
	0.08 → 0.23	1.56 → 3.38	0.36 → 0.90
9–10 years	0.14 ± 0.04	2.51 ± 0.53	0.65 ± 0.18
	0.07 → 0.23	1.55 → 3.33	0.34 → 1.00
11–12 years	0.14 ± 0.05	2.43 ± 0.52	0.60 ± 0.19
	0.07 → 0.24	1.45 → 3.51	0.30 → 0.92
13–14 years	0.14 ± 0.05	2.29 ± 0.59	0.58 ± 0.20
	0.06 → 0.25	1.25 → 3.60	0.26 → 1.00
15–16 years	0.14 ± 0.05	2.17 ± 0.61	0.55 ± 0.20
	0.07 → 0.27	1.20 → 3.23	0.24 → 0.95

◻ Table B5.2

Maximal P, QRS, and T vector angles in transverse plane (degrees)

Age	Max P	Max QRS	Max T
< 24 h	22 ± 38	−6 ± 108	23 ± 69
	−42 → 70	−131 → 181	−76 → 136
1 day	28 ± 35	−10 ± 113	−4 ± 68
	−47 → 78	−139 → 216	−105 → 132
2 days	25 ± 35	26 ± 111	−32 ± 49
	−49 → 83	−135 → 217	−92 → 92
3 days	26 ± 31	10 ± 99	−43 ± 42
	−45 → 73	−138 → 206	−100 → 66
≤ 1 week	24 ± 33	34 ± 88	−44 ± 31
	−46 → 73	−130 → 210	−92 → 20
≤ 1 month	15 ± 36	29 ± 89	−25 ± 33
	−63 → 66	−126 → 185	−80 → 10
≤ 3 months	8 ± 37	14 ± 37	−31 ± 26
	−67 → 62	−111 → 62	−93 → 31
≤ 6 months	6 ± 33	10 ± 44	−38 ± 22
	−41 → 59	−107 → 74	−72 → 14
≤ 1 year	11 ± 34	13 ± 38	−45 ± 19
	−62 → 67	−45 → 83	−87 → −13
1–2 years	23 ± 36	−19 ± 50	−38 ± 25
	−50 → 69	−110 → 89	−83 → 5
3–4 years	20 ± 36	−28 ± 28	−22 ± 21
	−48 → 76	−109 → 27	−64 → 16
5–6 years	28 ± 37	−29 ± 21	−10 ± 17
	−43 → 87	−96 → 7	−45 → −23

■ Table B5.2   (Continued)

Age	Max P	Max QRS	Max T
7–8 years	19 ± 39	−30 ± 21	−4 ± 17
	−46 → 82	−63 → 16	−40 → 35
9–10 years	17 ± 37	−31 ± 30	3 ± 18
	−50 → 87	62 → 10	−31 → 43
11–12 years	14 ± 39	−33 ± 19	9 ± 17
	−53 → 82	−78 → 4	−21 → 51
13–14 years	10 ± 44	−32 ± 27	9 ± 17
	−62 → 90	−71 → 9	−20 → 41
15–16 years	4 ± 43	−29 ± 50	20 ± 20
	−57 → 81	−93 → 204	−19 → 56

■ Table B5.3

Maximal P, QRS, and T vector angles in frontal plane (degrees)

Age	Max P	Max QRS	Max T
< 24 h	54 ± 14	79 ± 87	76 ± 69
	27 → 74	−90 → 208	25 → 151
1 day	58 ± 16	88 ± 80	67 ± 39
	18 → 78	−106 → 190	18 → 135
2 days	58 ± 21	77 ± 81	62 ± 43
	12 → 83	−71 → 191	23 → 102
3 days	52 ± 23	67 ± 79	54 ± 22
	−41 → 72	−68 → 194	16 → 106
≤ 1 week	57 ± 14	62 ± 65	51 ± 22
	22 → 77	−46 → 186	19 → 94
≤ 1 month	54 ± 14	61 ± 68	42 ± 19
	30 → 81	−19 → 190	18 → 82
≤ 3 months	56 ± 12	36 ± 25	38 ± 22
	25 → 79	4 → 135	18 → 94
≤ 6 months	56 ± 13	35 ± 27	36 ± 13
	26 → 77	−7 → 105	13 → 56
≤ 1 year	56 ± 14	31 ± 35	41 ± 16
	18 → 76	−18 → 97	21 → 75
1–2 years	57 ± 14	41 ± 38	38 ± 17
	5 → 73	−73 → 151	16 → 72
3–4 years	58 ± 16	39 ± 23	34 ± 10
	23 → 82	12 → 127	18 → 55
5–6 years	52 ± 28	37 ± 20	29 ± 9
	−36 → 82	13 → 101	11 → 46
7–8 years	54 ± 22	38 ± 18	29 ± 8
	3 → 75	13 → 63	12 → 46
9–10 years	50 ± 25	41 ± 19	26 ± 8
	−21 → 80	15 → 65	12 → 45
11–12 years	53 ± 22	39 ± 17	28 ± 8
	−26 → 85	15 → 72	9 → 42
13–14 years	44 ± 41	41 ± 17	28 ± 8
	−91 → 81	13 → 74	12 → 46
15–16 years	50 ± 34	47 ± 32	28 ± 9
	−90 → 82	11 → 181	11 → 47

Index

Note: The page numbers that appear in bold type indicates a substantive discussion of the topic.